Practical Paediatric Problems

A Textbook for MRCPCH

Edited by

Dr Jim Beattie
Consultant Paediatrician and Nephrologist,
Royal Hospital for Sick Children, Yorkhill,
Glasgow, UK

Professor Robert Carachi
Head of Section of Surgical Paediatrics,
Division of Paediatric Surgery,
University of Glasgow,
Honorary Consultant Paediatric Surgeon,
Royal Hospital for Sick Children,
Yorkhill, Glasgow, UK

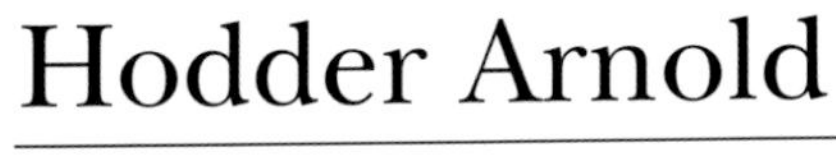

A MEMBER OF THE HODDER HEADLINE GROUP

First published in Great Britain in 2005 by
Hodder Education, a member of the Hodder Headline Group
338 Euston Road, London NW1 3BH

http://www.hoddereducation.co.uk

Distributed in the United States of America by
Oxford University Press Inc.
198 Madison Avenue, New York, NY10016
Oxford is a registered trademark of Oxford University Press

British Library Cataloguing in Publication Data
A catalogue record for this book is available from the British Library

Library of Congress Cataloging-in-Publication Data
A catalog record for this book is available from the Library of Congress

ISBN 0 340 80932 9
ISBN 0 340 80933 7 (International Students' Edition, restricted territorial availability)

1 2 3 4 5 6 7 8 9 10

Commissioning Editor: Sarah Burrows
Project Editor: Naomi Wilkinson
Production Controller: Joanna Walker
Cover Design: Georgina Hewitt
Indexers: Indexing Specialists (UK) Ltd

Typeset in 10/13 Rotis Serif by Charon Tec Pvt. Ltd, Chennai, India
www.charontec.com
Printed and bound in India by Replika Press Pvt. Ltd.

To Wilma and Annette, for their patience while this book was being written.

Contents

Contributors

Jack Beattie
Consultant in Emergency Medicine
Acute Ambulatory Assessment Unit
Royal Hospital for Sick Children
Yorkhill
Glasgow

Jim Beattie
Consultant Paediatrician and Nephrologist
Royal Hospital for Sick Children
Yorkhill
Glasgow

Amir F Azmy
Consultant Paediatric Urologist
Royal Hospital for Sick Children
Yorkhill
Glasgow

A David Burden
Consultant Dermatologist
Western Infirmary
Glasgow

Robert Carachi
Professor, Division of Paediatric Surgery
Royal Hospital for Sick Children
Yorkhill
Glasgow

J Brian S Coulter
Senior Lecturer in Tropical Child Health
Liverpool School of Tropical Medicine
Liverpool

Jonathan Coutts
Consultant Neonatalogist
Queen Mother's Hospital
Yorkhill
Glasgow

Malcolm DC Donaldson
Senior Lecturer in Child Health
University Department of Child Health
Royal Hospital for Sick Children
Yorkhill
Glasgow

Roderick Duncan
Consultant Paediatric Orthopaedic Surgeon and
Honorary Clinical Senior Lecturer
Royal Hospital for Sick Children
Glasgow

Paul Galea
Consultant Paediatrician
Royal Hospital for Sick Children
Yorkhill
Glasgow

Janet Gardner-Medwin
Senior Lecturer in Paediatric Rheumatology and
Honorary Consultant
University Department of Child Health
Royal Hospital for Sick Children
Yorkhill
Glasgow

Neil Gibson
Consultant in Paediatric Respiratory Medicine
Royal Hospital for Sick Children
Yorkhill
Glasgow

Brenda Gibson
Consultant Haematologist
Royal Hospital for Sick Children
Yorkhill
Glasgow

Peter Gillett
Consultant Paediatric Gastroenterologist
Royal Hospital for Sick Children
Sciennes Road
Edinburgh

Rosie Hague
Consultant in Paediatric Infectious Disease and Immunology
Royal Hospital for Sick Children
Yorkhill
Glasgow

David Hallworth
Consultant in Anaesthesia and Intensive Care
Royal Hospital for Sick Children
Yorkhill
Glasgow

Anne Marie Heuchen
Consultant Neonatologist
Queen Mother's Hospital
Yorkhill
Glasgow

Alan Houston
Consultant Cardiologist
Royal Hospital for Sick Children
Yorkhill
Glasgow

Iain J Horrocks
Specialist Registrar in Paediatric Neurology
Royal Hospital for Sick Children
Yorkhill
Glasgow

Alison M Kelly
Specialist Registrar in Paediatric Gastroenterology, Hepatology and Nutrition
Royal Hospital for Sick Children
Yorkhill
Glasgow

Rosemary Lever
Consultant Dermatologist
Royal Hospital for Sick Children
Yorkhill
Glasgow

Elaine Lockhart
Consultant Child and Adolescent Psychiatrist
Royal Hospital for Sick Children
Yorkhill
Glasgow

Robert McWilliam
Consultant Paediatric Neurologist
Royal Hospital for Sick Children
Yorkhill
Glasgow

Michael Morton
Consultant Child and Adolescent Psychiatrist
Department of Child and Family Psychiatry
Royal Hospital for Sick Children
Yorkhill
Glasgow

William Newman
Consultant Paediatric Ophthalmologist
Royal Liverpool Children Hospital
Alder Hey
Liverpool

Wendy Paterson
Auxologist
Department of Child Health
Royal Hospital for Sick Children
Yorkhill
Glasgow

Trevor Richens
Consultant Cardiologist
Royal Hospital for Sick Children
Yorkhill
Glasgow

Kenneth J Robertson
Consultant Paediatrician
Royal Hospital for Sick Children
Yorkhill
Glasgow

Peter Robinson
Consultant in Paediatric Metabolic Disease
Royal Hospital for Sick Children
Yorkhill
Glasgow

Judith H Simpson
Consultant Neonatologist
Queen Mother's Hospital
Yorkhill
Glasgow

Diane M Snowdon
Specialist Registrar in Paediatric Gastroenterology, Hepatology and Nutrition
Royal Hospital for Sick Children
Yorkhill
Glasgow

David Tappin
Senior Lecturer in Community Child Health
PEACH Unit
Royal Hospital for Sick Children
Yorkhill
Glasgow

John Tolmie
Consultant in Medical Genetics
Duncan Guthrie Institute
Yorkhill
Glasgow

Lawrence T Weaver
Professor of Child Health
University Department of Child Health
Royal Hospital for Sick Children
Yorkhill
Glasgow

Foreword

When Professor James Holmes Hutchison wrote his preface to the first edition of *Practical Paediatric Problems*, published in 1964, he acknowledged 'that a textbook by a single author on a subject as vast as paediatrics must to some extent be selective; for the author must write only of what he knows.' There was at that time no MRCPCH but there was a requirement to pass a membership examination of one of the three UK Royal Colleges in general medicine before entry to training for a hospital consultant post could even be contemplated.

Forty years on and we, thankfully, find that there has been an exponential increase in our knowledge and understanding of childhood health problems and how best to deal with and to prevent many of them.

Specialist training for a career in paediatric medicine has also changed considerably and the answer to the question 'what is a paediatrician?' has been well expressed in the Royal College of Paediatrics and Child Health document *A Framework of Competences for Basic Specialist Training in Paediatrics*. This document is for doctors in basic specialist training in paediatrics and their tutors and educational supervisors.

The authors and editors of this edition of *Practical Paediatric Problems* have, like Professor Hutchison, been selective and each has written only of what they know. The result is a comprehensive distillate of their knowledge and practical experience which will not only clearly guide their readers to achieve success in Basic Specialist Training and the MRCPCH examinations, but will also give them an excellent basis for higher specialist training. It will also enable them to deal with practical paediatric problems throughout their subsequent careers as paediatricians.

Forrester Cockburn
Emeritus Professor of Child Health
University of Glasgow
May 2005

Preface

In the 40 years since the publication of the first edition of *Practical Paediatric Problems*, paediatrics has become a large, highly developed, sophisticated and technically demanding area of health care. Advances in the understanding of paediatric clinical physiology and pathophysiology have enabled a better understanding of disease processes resulting in radically improved outcome.

Doctors undergoing General Professional or Basic Specialist Training (GPT/BST) in paediatrics have to master a considerable breadth and depth of core scientific and clinical knowledge along with important clinical, technical and practical skills. In addition they must acquire appropriate attitudes in order to deal with the challenges of their chosen specialty.

Although restructuring of postgraduate medical training in the UK is planned, including the introduction of newer methods of assessment, examinations are likely to remain a necessary hurdle in professional development. For trainees in paediatrics, achievement of the MRCPCH is a vital step in the progress from GPT/BST to Higher Specialist Training. The aims of the MRCPCH examination are to assess the candidate's knowledge, clinical judgement and ability to organize a management plan. We hope this book will help those preparing for both parts of the MRCPCH examination worldwide, but particularly for Part 2.

We elected not to replicate the MRCPCH examination format, examples of which are available on the Royal College of Paediatrics and Child Health (RCPCH) website (www.rcpch.ac.uk) and in a number of other texts but have attempted to present a structured, contemporary and comprehensive approach modelled closely on the 'core knowledge' and 'particular problems' identified in the RCPCH publication, *A Syllabus and Training Record for General Professional Training in Paediatrics and Child Health* (1999). We believe the content will also help trainees achieve the required standards in the more recent RCPCH publication, *A Framework of Competences for Basic Specialist Training in Paediatrics* (2004).

Major reference textbooks in paediatrics are either system or disease based; however, as in other areas of clinical medicine, patients frequently present with ill structured problems and there is therefore a need for a symptom-based text to assist in clinical problem solving. In this regard we hope that the book will be of value to practising paediatricians, paediatric surgeons, accident and emergency staff, general practitioners and indeed any clinician whose practice includes children and young people.

By necessity, this book is multi-author and all the authors in this book are experts from a broad range of disciplines within paediatrics, but we acknowledge and apologize in advance for any gaps that are inevitable in a book of this size. We hope the provision of reference sources with each chapter will go some way in addressing any deficiencies and we would welcome readers' suggestions and criticisms. In addition, while every effort has been made to ensure accuracy of information, especially with regard to drug selection and dosage, appropriate information sources should be accessed, particularly *Medicines for Children* (2003).

We are indebted to all the contributors for their hard work, to Joanna Koster, Sarah Burrows and Naomi Wilkinson of Hodder Arnold for their immense patience and support, to Dr Peter Galloway, Consultant in Medical Biochemistry, RHSC, Yorkhill, to our respective secretaries Lynda Lawson and Kay Byrne for their expert and willing help in a project that inevitably took a lot longer than planned and finally to our wives and families for their forbearance.

Jim Beattie and Robert Carachi
RHSC, Yorkhill, Glasgow
May 2005

Royal College of Paediatrics and Child Health (1999) *A Syllabus and Training Record for General Professional Training in Paediatrics and Child Health*. London: RCPCH Publications Ltd.

Royal College of Paediatrics and Child Health and the Neonatal Paediatric Pharmacists Group (2003) *Medicines for Children*, 2nd edn. London: RCPCH Publications Ltd.

Royal College of Paediatrics and Child Health (2004) *A Framework of Competences for Basic Specialist Training in Paediatrics*. London: RCPCH Publications Ltd.

Chapter 1

Community child health, child development and learning difficulties

David Tappin

HISTORY OF COMMUNITY CHILD HEALTH

Before 1974, the care of children outside hospital in the UK was undertaken either by general practitioners (GPs) or by community health services, which were part of the local authority as opposed to the health authority. Reforms in 1973 (the National Health Service Reorganisation Act 1973) brought together most of the child health services under a 'health' umbrella. The government commissioned a review chaired by Donald Court, which reported in 1976 and set out a blueprint for the care of children. This integrated vision of child health care moved much of the routine work provided by community child health services – vaccination, child health surveillance, school health – to general practice under the care of a general practitioner. The more specialist paediatric aspects of the community health services – adoption and fostering, child protection, developmental paediatrics particularly in relation to special schools – were to be undertaken by consultant community paediatricians. Although it has taken time, many of Court's recommendations have come about. Consultant paediatricians, working mainly outside hospital, have gradually replaced retiring senior clinical medical officers and most have a primary general paediatric qualification (MRCP[UK] or MRCPCH). General practice paediatricians have not emerged in the UK, and vaccination and child health surveillance are now performed by health visitors and GPs.

The following sections are taken from *Health for All Children: Guidance on Implementation in Scotland.* This document has been produced by the Scottish Executive (2004) as a consultation document, but is likely to provide the framework in Scotland for preventive childcare services.

KEY LEARNING POINT

The Court Report (1976) produced a framework for the integration of hospital, community and general practice care of children, which has slowly come about.

HEALTH FOR ALL CHILDREN

Parts of this section in quotes, quotation marks and boxes, are taken directly from *Health for All Children: Guidance on Implementation in Scotland* (Scottish Executive, 2004, © Crown copyright). Readers are referred directly to the document for further information.

In 1988, the Royal College of Paediatrics and Child Health established a multi-disciplinary working group to review routine health checks for young children. It's [*sic*] report, first published in 1989, was entitled *Health for All Children*. In later years, the remit of the review was extended beyond routine checks to detect abnormalities or disease, to include activity designed to prevent illness and efforts by health professionals to promote good health. Sir David Hall, Professor of Paediatrics and past-President of the RCPCH, chairs the working group. The report of the most recent RCPCH review of child health screening and surveillance programmes in the UK was published in February 2003 as the fourth edition of the report *Health for All Children*, and is commonly referred to as *Hall 4*. (Scottish Executive, 2004)

There will always be a need to ensure universal provision of a health promotion and surveillance programme for all children and young people to enable families to take well informed decisions about their child's health and development; to identify children with particular health or developmental problems; and to recognise and respond when a child may be in need. However, each family's circumstances and needs are different. Some parents need only information and ready access to professional advice when their child is injured or unwell or when they are worried about their child's development or welfare. Other parents may need considerable support, guidance and help at specific times, or over a continuous period, perhaps because of their child's serious ill health or disability, or because of their own personal circumstances. (Scottish Executive, 2004)

KEY LEARNING POINT

Over 15 years, Hall reports 1, 2, 3 and 4 have sought evidence for routine child health surveillance. They have driven a rationalization and standardization of child health contacts in the community.

CORE PROGRAMME FOR CHILD HEALTH SCREENING AND SURVEILLANCE

'**Child health surveillance** – used to describe routine child health checks and monitoring.

Child health screening – the use of formal tests or examination procedures on a population basis to identify those who are apparently well, but who may have a disease or defect, so that they can be referred for a definitive diagnostic test.

Health promotion – used to describe planned and informed interventions that are designed to improve physical or mental health or prevent disease, disability and premature death. Health in this sense is a positive holistic state.' (Scottish Executive, 2004)

The Core Child Health Programme begins at birth. On the labour ward, a card is completed for the Notification of Birth Acts 1907, 1915 and 1965, and sent to the local health board (health authority). All contacts are scheduled and organized centrally at health board level.

KEY LEARNING POINTS

- All families with children receive the core programme of child health contacts (Figure 1.1).
- The core programme includes health promotion, screening and detecting problems vaccination and child health surveillance during infancy and pre-school years (Table 1.1) as well as for school-aged children and young people (Table 1.2).
- The reduction from the previous routine contacts schedule allows giving additional support to certain groups and intensive support to vulnerable families who need it.

This programme adheres to the recommendations of the fourth UK report (*Hall 4*) from the Royal College of Paediatrics and Child Health (RCPCH), *Health for All Children* (Hall and Elliman, 2003).

'TARGETING SUPPORT FOR VULNERABLE CHILDREN' (SCOTTISH EXECUTIVE, 2004)

Vulnerable groups include:

- 'Children at vulnerable points of transition (e.g. moving from one location to another, changing schools, moving from children's to adult services)
- Children not registered with a General Practitioner
- Children living away from home
- Children excluded by language barriers
- Traveller families
- Families living in temporary or bed and breakfast accommodation
- Children of troubled, violent or disabled parents
- Children who care for disabled parents
- Children who are involved with, or whose families are involved with, substance misuse, crime or prostitution
- Runaways and street children
- Asylum seekers and refugees, particularly if unaccompanied
- Children in secure settings
- Children of parents in prison'

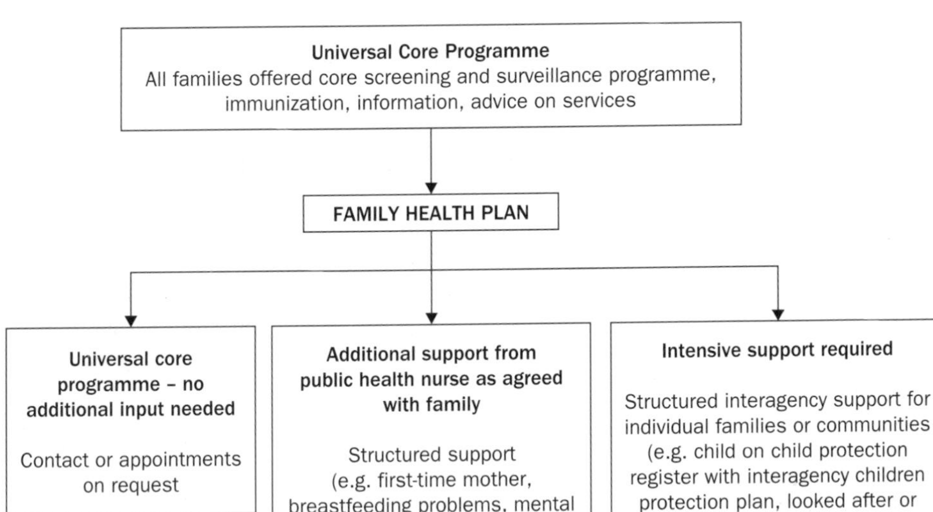

Figure 1.1 Plan to target support for those who need it most (redrawn with permission from Scottish Executive (2004) *Health for All Children: Guidance on Implementation in Scotland*. A draft for consultation. Edinburgh: Scottish Executive)

Table 1.1 The Universal Core Child Health Screening and Surveillance Programme – pre-school years

Neonate first 24 hours

Action: Child health professional – GP, midwife, junior doctor, consultant paediatrician

Record birth weight
Record head circumference
Record length (only if abnormality suspected)
Record length of pregnancy in weeks
Record problems during pregnancy/birth
Vitamin K administration
Hip test for dislocation (Ortolani and Barlow manoeuvres)
Inspection of eyes and examination of red reflex
Thorough check of cardiovascular system for congenital heart disease
Check genitalia (undescended testes, hypospadias, other anomalies)
Check femoral pulses
Neonatal hearing screening – to be phased in by April 2005
Record feeding method at discharge
Review any problems arising or suspected from antenatal screening, family history or labour
Health promotion – discuss:

- Baby care
- Feeding
- Jaundice
- Vitamin K
- Reducing SIDS risks
- Hepatitis B and bCG vaccines
- Smoking
- Oral health
- Any parental concerns

Provide information about local support networks and contacts for additional advice or support when needed
Identify parents who might have major problems with their infant (e.g. depression, domestic violence, substance abuse, learning difficulties, mental health problems)

Neonatal hearing screen
HDL (2001) 51, which issued in June 2001, advised the service about the introduction of universal neonatal hearing screening. The introduction of hearing tests for all neonates is also a Partnership Agreement commitment. Implementation is underway with the establishment of two pathfinder sites in Tayside and Lothian, where screening began in January 2003 and March 2003, respectively. NHS Boards are expected to implement the screening programme by April 2005

Vitamin K
Each NHS Board area should have a single protocol for the administration of Vitamin K, with which every member of staff involved with maternity and neonates is familiar

Screening
Advise that no screening test is perfect. Details of signs and potential emerging problems in PCHR and who to contact if concerned

(*Continued*)

Table 1.1 *(Continued)*

Within first 10 days of life	
Action: Lead health professional is normally the community midwife, but may be hospital midwife, GP or public health nurse in unusual circumstances	
Weight (where appropriate on clinical suspicion) Blood spot test for – phenylketonuria (PKU), hypothyroidism and cystic fibrosis Record feeding method Smokers in household Record diagnoses or concerns (coded): • Feeding • Weight • Illness • Sleeping • Crying • Child protection issues • Appearance • Other Impairment/abnormalities in infant Mother's health and wellbeing Discussion of birth registration Health promotion – discuss: • Reducing SIDS risks • Parenting skills • Immunisation schedule • Support networks and services • Safety • Smoking • Feeding • Any parental concerns • Oral health	Cystic fibrosis screening HDL (2001) 73, which issued in October 2001, advised about the introduction of a neonatal screening programme for cystic fibrosis using the existing blood spot test. The programme was introduced across Scotland in February 2003 PKU and congenital hypothyroidism HDL (2001) 34, which issued in April 2001, provided guidance on the organisation of neonatal screening for PKU and congenital hypothyroidism Haemoglobinopathies Assessment work in relation to screening for haemoglobinopathies is currently underway. No decision has yet been taken in relation to a screening programme in Scotland Screening advice Advise that no screening test is perfect. Details of signs and potential emerging problems in PCHR and who to contact if concerned Frequency of visits Visits to the family home are usual on several occasions within the first 10 days of life. Some new parents may need to be seen more frequently than others. In particular, additional support should be provided for babies who have special needs or who needed treatment in the neonatal intensive care unit Weight Whoever is responsible for weight measurement must be able to deal with questions about the interpretation of the weight chart
6–8 Weeks – must be completed by 8 weeks	
Action: Lead professional is Public Health Nurse and/or GP and may be others in unusual circumstances	
Immunisation – DTP-Hib, PV + MenC Repeat hip test for dislocation (Ortolani and Barlow manoeuvres) Repeat inspection of eyes and examination of red reflex Repeat thorough check of cardiovascular system for congenital heart disease Repeat check of genitalia (undescended testes, hypospadias, other anomalies) Check femoral pulses Check blood spot result Weight BCG considered/been done? (for targeted population) Record smokers in household (pre-school) Feeding method Diagnoses/concerns (coded): • Feeding • Hearing • Illness • Eyes	Immunisation Whoever is responsible for immunisation must be able to deal with questions about vaccines Can be combined with the postnatal examination at which physical health, contraception, social support, depression, etc. can be discussed as appropriate Weight Whoever is responsible for weight measurement must be able to deal with questions about the interpretation of the weight chart Head circumference If no concern at this stage, no further routine measurement required

(Continued)

Table 1.1 *(Continued)*

- Crying
- Appearance
- Behaviour
- Weight gain
- Growth
- Movement
- Sleeping
- Child protection issues
- Other

Gross motor:
- Pull to sit
- Ventral suspension
- Handling

Hearing and communication
- Response to sudden sound
- Response to unseen mothers voice

Vision and social awareness
- Intent regard mothers face
- Follow angling object past midline
- Social smile

Length (only in infant who had a low birth weight, where disorder is suspected or present, or where health, growth or feeding pattern causing concern).
Head circumference
Parents' health and wellbeing
Enter national special needs system when clinical diagnosis recorded
Health promotion – discuss:
- Nutrition
- Development
- Safety
- Smoking
- Oral health
- Immunisation schedule
- Parenting skills
- Support networks and services
- Any parental concerns
- Sleeping position

Review family's circumstances and needs to make an initial plan with them for support and contact over the short to medium term. Identify high-risk situations and carry out a risk assessment

3 Months

Action: Lead professional, GP, practice nurse or public health nurse

Immunisation – DTP-Hib + PV + Men C
Weight
Health promotion – discuss:
- Nutrition
- Development
- Safety
- Smoking
- Oral health
- Immunisation schedule
- Parenting skills
- Support networks and services
- Any parental concerns

Immunisation
Whoever is responsible for immunisation must be able to deal with questions about vaccines

Weight
Whoever is responsible for weight measurement must be able to deal with questions about the interpretation of the weight chart

4 Months

Action: Lead professional, GP, public health nurse

Immunisation – DTP-Hib + PV + Men C
Weight
Health promotion – discuss:
- Weaning
- Nutrition
- Oral health
- Immunisation schedule

Immunisation
Whoever is responsible for immunisation must be able to deal with questions about vaccines

(Continued)

Table 1.1 (*Continued*)

• Development • Safety • Smoking • Parenting skills • Support networks and services • Any parental concerns	Weight Whoever is responsible for weight measurement must be able to deal with questions about the interpretation of the weight chart
12–15 months	
Action: Primarily GP, practice nurse or public health nurse	
Immunisation – MMR Weight measurement Health promotion – discuss: • Nutrition • Development • Safety • Smoking • Oral health • Immunisation schedule • Parenting skills • Support networks and services • Any parental concerns	Immunisation Whoever is responsible for immunisation must be able to deal with questions about vaccines Weight Whoever is responsible for weight measurement must be able to deal with questions about the interpretation of the weight chart
3–4 years	
Action: Lead professionals could be public health nurse, GP, practice nurse or community paediatrician	
Immunisation – PV + MMR + DTP Weight measurement Health promotion – discuss: • Development • Safety • Nutrition • Smoking • Oral health • Registration with dentist • Parenting skills • Support networks and services • Any parental concerns	Immunisation Whoever is responsible for immunisation must be able to deal with questions about vaccines Weight Whoever is responsible for weight measurement must be able to deal with questions about the interpretation of the weight chart
4–5 years	
Action: Orthoptist	
Vision screen	Where pre-school orthoptist vision screening cannot be implemented immediately, children should instead be screened on school entry. As a minimum, training and monitoring should be provided by an orthoptist

Source: With permission from the Scottish Executive (2004) *Health for All Children: Guidance on Implementation in Scotland.* Edinburgh: Scottish Executive.

GP, general practitioner; NHS, National Health Service; PCHR, personal child health record; SIDS, sudden infant death syndrome.

Table 1.2 The Universal Core Child Health Screening and Surveillance Programme – school years

Entry to primary school	
Action: School health service and community dental service	
Height Weight Record body mass index (BMI) *for public health monitoring purposes only*	Height The 1990 nine-centile charts have been agreed as the standard measurement of height by the Royal College of Paediatrics and Child Health

(*Continued*)

Table 1.2 *(Continued)*

Sweep test of hearing (continue pending further review) Identify children who may not have received pre-school health care programme for any reason Identify any physical, developmental or emotional problems that have been missed and initiate intervention Check that pre-school vision screening undertaken and make appropriate arrangements where not Ensure all children have access to primary health and dental care Dental check at P1 through the National Dental Inspection Programme Oral health promotion: • Dentist registration and attendance • Twice daily supervised brushing • Reducing sugary food and drink consumption	Physical examination There is no evidence to justify a full physical examination or health review based on questionnaires or interviews on school entry Vision testing Vision testing on school entry should only be undertaken where a universal pre-school orthoptic vision screening programme is not in place Dental checks National Dental Inspection Programme identifies children at greatest risk of oral disease and is used to inform the school health plan
Primary 7 **Action: School health service and community dental service**	
Dental check through the National Dental Inspection Programme Oral health promotion: • Dentist registration and attendance • Twice daily supervised brushing • Reducing sugary food and drink consumption Other health promotion activity should include: • Smoking • Nutrition • Physical activity • Substance use • Sexual health • Personal safety • Mental health and wellbeing	Dental checks National Dental Inspection Programme identifies children at greatest risk of oral disease and is used to inform the school health plan Health promotion Development of an effective core programme of health promotion in schools is premised on the roll out of Health Promoting Schools
Secondary school **Action: School health service and community dental service**	
Age 10–14 years – BCG immunisation In areas where vision is checked at 11 years old, this should continue pending further review by the National Screening Committee. If not being undertaken, it should not be introduced Age 13–18 years – PV + Td immunisation Dental check at S3 through the National Dental Inspection Programme Oral health promotion: • Dentist registration and attendance • Twice daily supervised brushing • Reducing sugary food and drink consumption Other health promotion activity should include: • Smoking • Nutrition • Physical activity • Substance use • Sexual health • Personal safety • Mental health and wellbeing	Dental checks National Dental Inspection Programme identifies children at greatest risk of oral disease and is used to inform the school health plan Health promotion Development of an effective core programme of health promotion in schools is premised on the roll out of Health Promoting Schools
Source: with permission from the Scottish Executive (2004) *Health for All Children: Guidance for Implementation in Scotland.* Edinburgh: Scottish Executive.	

'Assessing vulnerability' (Scottish Executive, 2004)

'Assessment of children and their needs should include consideration of:

- **The child's developmental needs**, including health and education, identity and family and social relationships, emotional and behavioural development, presentation and self-care.
- **Parenting capacity**, including ability to provide good basic care, stimulation and emotional warmth, guidance and boundaries, ensuring safety and stability.
- **Wider family and environmental factors**, including family history and functioning, support from extended family and others, financial and housing circumstances, employment, social integration and community resources.'

No one agency can undertake a comprehensive assessment within and across all these domains without support from colleagues in other services and sectors. But where a single agency is in touch with a child or family and identifies problems or stresses in any one of these areas, this should signal the need to involve others to accurately assess whether the child and family may be in need of additional or intensive support, and agree how this should best be provided. The universal core programme should provide information to enable health professionals to identify vulnerable children and their needs, and to ensure appropriate planning and referral for additional or intensive support when necessary. The national child health demonstration project in Scotland, Starting Well, has utilised a simple 3 point scale for community workers.

'Starting Well Demonstration Project – Family Need Score'

'The Family Need Score (FNS) is a three point scale used by Starting Well public health nurses to indicate the vulnerability of each Starting Well family. Based on professional judgement, public health nurses give families a Family Need Score of 1, 2 or 3:

- FNS 1 – Indicates that the family requires less than routine visiting outlined in core visiting schedule.
- FNS 2 – Indicates that the family requires routine visiting outlined in core visiting schedule.
- FNS 3 – Indicates that the family requires more than routine visiting outlined in core visiting schedule.

The family's score is reviewed approximately every three months and is recorded in the Family Health Plan. The data are also entered on the Starting Well database to enable on-going population needs assessment. Whilst recording a FNS for the family, public health nurses also indicate whether there are any special issues evident for that family in relation to drugs and/or alcohol.' (Scottish Executive, 2004)

'As well as assessing and targeting individual vulnerable children and families, NHS Boards should assess the level of vulnerability of communities. This will mean targeting resources such as Public Health Nurses to the most deprived communities in their population' (Scottish Executive, 2004).

KEY LEARNING POINTS

- Targeting support for vulnerable families often requires multi-agency assessment of vulnerability, which should include consideration of the child's developmental needs, parenting capacity, and wider family and environmental factors.
- Support required is likely to be from more than one agency and needs coordination to avoid duplication or omission.

'Child protection' (Scottish Executive, 2004)

All agencies and professionals in contact with children and families have an individual and shared responsibility to contribute to the welfare and protection of vulnerable children and young people. This applies to services for adults working with parents to tackle problems which may have a negative impact on their care of children. Preventing child abuse and neglect must be one of the key aims of the universal core programme to support child health. Where abuse and neglect has occurred, children are entitled to support and therapy to address the consequences, help them recover from the effects of abuse and neglect, and keep them safe from future harm. This is a key objective of multi-agency support programmes for children at risk of significant harm. Every professional in contact with children or their families must be aware of their duty to recognise and act on concerns about child abuse.

'Induction for staff working with children in all agencies should include:

- Training to raise awareness of child abuse and neglect and agency responsibilities for child protection.
- Familiarity with child protection procedures.
- The name and contact details of a designated person in their agency with lead responsibility for advising on child protection matters and local referral arrangements in the event of concern about a particular child' (Scottish Executive, 2004).

'Domestic abuse is a serious social problem in its own right. It is now also recognised that exposure to family violence is profoundly damaging to children's emotional and social development' (Scottish Executive, 2004).

KEY LEARNING POINT

Child protection requires 'All agencies and professionals in contact with children and families to have an individual and shared responsibility to contribute to the welfare and protection of vulnerable children and young people' (Scottish Executive, 2004).

'INFORMATION COLLECTION AND SHARING' (SCOTTISH EXECUTIVE, 2004)

All agencies gather information from children and families to enable them to decide how best to help, and to keep records of their contact with children and families including details of their assessments, plans for intervention, treatment and support.

'Systems for recording, storing and retrieving information gathered from children and families or generated in the course of professionals work provide:

- A record for the clinician or practitioner of the work undertaken and the outcomes to assist their ongoing work with the family and to ensure they are accountable to their patient or client, to their profession and to their employing organisation or equivalent.
- Aggregate information about presenting conditions and problems, what was done and the outcome to assist managers and planners to assess needs and plan services.
- Information for families about their child's health status and treatment or care' (Scottish Executive, 2004).

'National guidance sets out the requirements for effective working in partnership with parents. This depends on good information for parents from professionals' (Scottish Executive, 2004).

'Achieving partnerships with parents and children in the planning and delivery of services to children requires that:

- They have sufficient information at an early stage both verbally and in writing to make informed choices.
- They are aware of the various consequences of the decisions they may take.
- They are actively involved wherever appropriate in assessments, decision-making, care reviews and conferences.
- They are given help to express their views and wishes and to prepare written reports and statements for meetings where necessary.
- Professionals and other workers listen to and take account of parents' and carers' views.
- Families are able to challenge decisions taken by professionals and make a complaint if necessary.
- Families have access to independent advocacy when appropriate' (Scottish Executive, 2004).

'Health professionals should inform and advise parents and, where appropriate, children, that to provide proper care, information is recorded in written records and on computer. Sharing information between professionals and agencies should be based on parental consent unless there are concerns about a child's welfare or safety which would override patient confidentiality' (Scottish Executive, 2004).

KEY LEARNING POINT

'Sharing information between professionals and agencies should be based on parental consent unless there are concerns about a child's welfare or safety, which would override patient confidentiality' (Scottish Executive, 2004).

'The Scottish Executive is working with local authority and health partners in Aberdeen, Glasgow, Dumfries and Galloway and Lanarkshire to pilot the following:

- **An Integrated Children's Service Record** to define and develop the structures and standards for an integrated care record for children, integrating health, social work and education.
- **A Single Assessment Framework** that will allow the sharing of assessment information between the partner agencies.
- **A Personal Care Record** to provide a secure store for the records of a child from health, education, and social services and the Scottish Children's Reporters Administration.
- **An Integrated Child Protection Framework** to extend the technologies and processes currently used to share information on older people in Lanarkshire, to children with child protection issues' (Scottish Executive, 2004).

'Child health information' (Scottish Executive, 2004)

The current child health systems are well established, though with the exception of the Scottish Immunisation and Recall System (SIRS), they are not used in all NHS Board areas. They are primarily clinical systems (as opposed to being merely data collection systems) and provide useful support to clinicians dealing with children.

'Effective monitoring' (Scottish Executive, 2004)

Current child health information systems provide invaluable information about the uptake of screening programmes, referrals of children with development problems or disabilities, time lapses between referral and diagnosis and between diagnosis and treatment. It is important to keep under review age at diagnosis, false positive rates, waiting times at each point in the network of services and differences between age of diagnosis for high risk and low risk cases. Standardisation of records would facilitate comparisons between areas. This will be considered in the child health information strategy.

'The Parent Held Child Health Record' (Scottish Executive, 2004)

Hall 4 reviewed the use and content of the Parent Held Child Health Record (PHCHR), introduced a decade ago to facilitate partnership with parents and empower them in overseeing their child's development and health care. Parents and primary care professionals value the record but other health professionals make more limited use of the PHCHR. Whether professionals make entries in the book or ask for it at health appointments or at contact with services such as attendance at Accident and Emergency Departments is important to parents and influences how they view the book. There is the potential to integrate the information in the PHCHR into the Family Health Plan once it comes on line. In the meantime, NHS Boards should adopt the PHCHR as a basis for recording information on child health.

SECONDARY AND TERTIARY CARE FOR CHILDREN

Secondary care for children takes place in both a hospital and a community setting. Paediatricians based in hospital have traditionally seen all acutely ill children referred from primary care, have looked after premature or ill babies after birth and have been referred 'medical' and 'surgical' paediatric problems to be seen as outpatients. Paediatricians based outside hospital have often dealt with 'educational' medicine, have looked after children 'in care' for fostering and adoption, have dealt with 'developmental' problems and have increasingly been passed the responsibility for 'child protection'. Over the past 10 years, secondary care paediatrics has become more *combined* as consultant paediatricians have been appointed to replace senior clinical medical officers in the community. Future plans are based around the community health partnerships (CHPs), where seven or eight consultant paediatricians (some mostly working in a hospital setting and some in the community) will look after the child health needs of a CHP area to provide an *integrated* service for a total population of around 150 000. Two such CHP areas would feed into one district general hospital. The eight paediatricians will be trained in complementary special interests so that all common paediatric problems can be dealt with effectively. These special interests would be augmented by attachment to tertiary care specialist centres to provide an *integrated* clinical network and a *seamless* service for children.

TERTIARY CARE FOR CHILDREN

'Hospital' paediatrics has become as specialized as adult medicine at a tertiary level. Paediatric tertiary specialties include respiratory disease, rheumatology, nephrology, child and family psychiatry, neurology, neonatology, emergency medicine, intensive care, infectious diseases, endocrinology, diabetes, metabolic disease, dermatology, cardiology, leukaemia and cancer care, and a number of paediatric surgical specialties. It is likely that tertiary specialties will develop within community based paediatrics and may include disability, social paediatrics – child protection, adoption and fostering, and looked after/vulnerable children, child mental health – which may include educational medicine and public health paediatrics.

OUTREACH: HOSPITAL AT HOME/DIRECT ACCESS

Secondary and tertiary care paediatric problems lend themselves to outreach work. The aim is to keep children in their own environment away from hospital care when this is possible. 'Outreach' nurses provide specialist care, e.g. for children with cystic fibrosis. Most antibiotic therapy can now be given at home by parents. Intravenous access can be replaced by nurses in the child's home. Diabetic liaison nurses provide ongoing advice and training at home so that admission at diagnosis is often not necessary for the 'walking-wounded'. Specialist nurses are a resource for schools so that teachers can learn to cope with common problems and the child is more secure in the school environment. Paediatric nephrology has been at the forefront of 'Hospital at Home' initiatives. Now children with chronic renal failure are treated by parents at home using overnight peritoneal dialysis. Children with asthma that is difficult to control may be granted 'direct access' to paediatric units so that delay in treatment is minimized. Initiatives will increase as technology improves so that long-term admission for chronic problems such as overnight ventilation will become a thing of the past.

SOCIAL PAEDIATRICS

The following section has been largely taken from the website of the Children's Hearings (www.childrens-hearings.co.uk).

The Children's Hearings system and the reporter

Successive UK governments have highlighted the difficulty of dealing with children who offend. The need for a system different from juvenile courts is well recognized. In Scotland such a system has been in place for over 30 years. The system is not concerned with guilt or innocence but the welfare or best interests of the child. This principle is applied whether the child has offended or has been offended against or abused. One system deals with juvenile criminal justice and children's welfare.

KEY LEARNING POINT

The Children's Hearings system is not concerned with guilt or innocence but with the welfare and best interests of the child.

How the system came about

In the late 1950s and early 1960s it had become increasingly evident that change was required in how society dealt with children and young people. To this end a committee was set up under Lord Kilbrandon to investigate possible solutions. The principles underlying the Children's Hearings system were recommended by the Committee on Children and Young Persons (the Kilbrandon Committee) which reported in 1964. The Committee found that children and young people appearing before the courts whether they had committed offences or were in need of care or protection had common needs for social and personal care. The Committee considered that juvenile courts were unsuited for dealing with these problems because they had to combine the characteristics of a criminal court of law with those of a treatment agency. Separation of those functions was therefore recommended; the establishment of the facts where disputed was to remain with the courts, but decisions on treatment were to be the responsibility of a new and unique kind of hearing. The Hearings system represents one of the radical changes initiated by the Social Work (Scotland) Act 1968. On 15 April 1971 the Hearings took over from the courts most of the responsibility for dealing with children and young people under the age of 16 years who commit offences or who are in need of care or protection.

Why are children brought to the attention of a hearing?

The grounds on which a child or young person may be brought before a hearing are set down in the Children (Scotland) Act 1995. These grounds include the child who is:

- beyond the control of parents or other relevant person
- exposed to moral danger
- likely to suffer unnecessarily or suffer serious impairment to health or development through lack of parental care
- the victim of an offence including physical injury or sexual abuse
- failing to attend school
- indulging in solvent abuse
- misusing alcohol or drugs or has committed an offence.

The reporter

The reporter is an official employed by the Scottish Children's Reporters Administration. All referrals regarding children and young people who may be deemed to need compulsory measures of supervision must be made to the reporter. The main source of referrals is the police, but referrals can be made by other agencies such as social work, education or health – in fact any member of the public may make a referral to the Reporter. The Reporter then has a duty to make an initial investigation before deciding what action, if any is necessary in the child's interests. First, the Reporter must consider the sufficiency of evidence with regard to the grounds for referral and thereafter decide whether there is a case for seeking compulsory measures of supervision.

KEY LEARNING POINTS

- All children and young people who may be deemed to need compulsory measures of supervision must be referred to the Reporter.
- Social workers provide most referrals, health-care workers also do so, but anybody can make a referral.
- The Reporter looks at the evidence and decides if there is a case for seeking compulsory supervision.

The Reporter is given a statutory discretion in deciding the next step in the procedure.

- The Reporter may decide that no further action is required, and the child or young person and parent or other relevant person is then informed of the decision. It is not unusual for the Reporter to convey this decision in person in offence cases when the child may be warned about their future behaviour
- The Reporter may refer the child or young person to the local authority with the request that social workers arrange for such advice, guidance and assistance, on an informal basis, as may be appropriate for the child
- The Reporter may arrange to bring the child to a hearing because in his or her view the child is in need of compulsory measures of supervision.

KEY LEARNING POINT

The Reporter may decide on no further action; refer for social work help for the child/family; arrange to bring the child to a hearing of a children's panel because the Reporter is of the opinion that compulsory supervision is required.

Children under 16 years are only considered for prosecution in court where serious offences such as murder or assault to the danger of life are in question or where they are involved in offences where disqualification from driving is possible. However, in cases of this kind it is by no means automatic that prosecution will occur, and where the public interest allows, children in these categories are referred to the Reporter by the Procurator Fiscal for decision on referral to a hearing. Where the child or young person is prosecuted in court, the court may refer the case to a hearing for advice on the best method of dealing with them. The court on receipt of that advice or in certain cases without seeking advice first, may remit the case for disposal by a hearing.

Children's panels

Members of a children's panel volunteer to serve and come from a wide range of occupations, neighbourhood and income groups. All have experience of and interest in children and the ability to communicate with them and their families. There is an approximate balance between men and women and individuals aged between 18 and 60 years can apply to become panel members. The panel members are carefully prepared for their task through initial training programmes and have continuing opportunities during their period of service to develop their knowledge and skills and attend in-service training courses.

KEY LEARNING POINT

Children's panels are made up of trained volunteers – local men and women.

SELECTION AND APPOINTMENT OF PANEL MEMBERS

People are appointed or reappointed to panels by Scottish ministers. The task of selection is the responsibility of the Children's Panel Advisory Committee (CPAC) for the local authority area. The selection procedure adopted by the CPAC involves application forms, interviews and group discussions. The initial period of appointment for a panel member is up to five years and is renewable on the recommendation of the CPAC. Over Scotland as a whole, there are over 2000 panel members.

The hearings

The Hearing is a lay tribunal comprising three members including male and female members charged with making decisions on the needs of children and young people. The Hearing can consider cases only where the child or young person, parents or other relevant person accept the grounds for referral stated by the Reporter, or where they accept them in part and the Hearing considers it proper to proceed. Where the grounds for referral are not accepted or the child does not understand them, the Hearing must (unless it decides to discharge the referral) direct the Reporter to apply to the Sheriff to decide whether the grounds are established.

The Sheriff decides if there is 'proof' of grounds for referral to the Children's Hearing. The level of proof is *on the balance of probabilities*, which allows the children's panel to act where a criminal court, which requires proof *beyond reasonable doubt*, could not. If the Sheriff is satisfied that any of these grounds are established, they remit the case to the Reporter to make arrangements for a Hearing. In certain specified circumstances a child or young person may be detained in a place of safety as defined in the Children (Scotland) Act 1995 by warrant pending a decision of a hearing for a period not exceeding 22 days in the first instance.

The Hearing, or the Sheriff in certain court proceedings, may appoint a person known as a Safeguarder. The role of the Safeguarder is to prepare a report that assists the panel in reaching a decision in the child's best interests.

KEY LEARNING POINTS

- A hearing is presided over by three children's panel members and can only consider cases if the parents or child accept the grounds for referral stated by the Reporter. Otherwise, the Sheriff must first decide if there is 'proof' of grounds, in which case they are likely to pass the case back to the children's panel hearing.
- The level of proof is *on the balance of probabilities*, which allows the children's panel to act where a criminal court, which requires proof *beyond reasonable doubt*, could not. This allows 'child protection' to proceed more easily.

ATTENDANCE AT A HEARING

A hearing is usually held at a place in the child or young person's home area. The layout of the room where the Hearing takes place is informal with the participants generally sitting round a table. Normally, the child or young person must attend. They have the right to attend all stages of their own Hearing. The Hearing may, however, suggest that they need not attend certain parts of the hearing or even the whole proceedings – for example, if matters might arise that could cause distress.

It is important that both the child's parents or other relevant person are present when the Hearing considers his or her problem so that they can take part in the discussion and help the Hearing to reach a decision. Their attendance is compulsory by law, and failure to appear may result in prosecution and a fine. The parents or other relevant person may take a representative to help them at the Hearing or each may choose a separate representative.

Other persons may also be present, with the approval of the Chairman of the Hearing. No one is admitted unless they have a legitimate concern in the case or with the panel system. The Hearing is, therefore, a small gathering able to proceed in an informal way and to give the child and his or her parents the confidence to take a full part in the discussion.

The Hearing's task is to decide on the measures of supervision that are in the best interest of the child or young person. It receives a report on the child and his or her social background from the social work department of the local authority and, where appropriates, a report from the child's school. Medical, psychological or psychiatric reports may also be requested. Parents are provided with copies of these reports.

The Hearing discusses the situation fully with the parents, child or young person and any representatives, the social worker and the teacher, if present. As the Hearing is concerned with the wider picture and the long-term wellbeing of the child, the measures that it decides on will be based on the best interests of the child. They may not appear to relate directly to the reasons that were the immediate cause of the child's appearance. For example, the Hearing may decide that a child or young person who has committed a relatively serious offence should not be removed from home, because their difficulties may be adequately dealt with and their need for supervision adequately met within the treatment resources available in their home area. In contrast, a child or young person who has come to the Hearing's attention because of a relatively minor offence may be placed away from home for a time if it appears that their home background is a major cause of their difficulties and the Hearing considers that removal from home would be in their best interest.

KEY LEARNING POINT

The Hearing's task is to decide on the measures of supervision that are in the best interest of the child or young person.

SUPERVISION

If the Hearing thinks compulsory measures of supervision are appropriate it will impose a supervision requirement, which may be renewed until the child is 18 years old. Most children will continue to live at home but will be under the supervision of a social worker. Sometimes, the Hearing will decide that a child should live away from their home with relatives or foster parents, or in one of several establishments managed by local authority or voluntary organizations, such as children's homes or other residential schools. No power has been given to a hearing to fine the child or young person or their parents. All decisions made by hearings are legally binding on that child or young person.

APPEALS

The child or young person or their parents may appeal to the Sheriff against the decision of a hearing, but must do so within 21 days. Once an appeal is lodged it must be heard within 28 days. Any Safeguarder who has been appointed also has the right of appeal against the decision of a hearing. Thereafter on a point of law only, the Sheriff's decision may be appealed to the Sheriff Principal or the Court of Session.

LEGAL ADVICE AND AID

Legal advice is available free or at reduced cost under the Legal Advice and Assistance Scheme to inform a child or their parents about their rights at the Hearing and to advise about acceptance of the ground for referral. Legal aid is not available for representation at the Hearing, but may be obtained for appearances in the Sheriff Court either when the case has been referred for establishment of the facts or in appeal cases.

REVIEW HEARING

The Hearing may suggest a review date. A supervision requirement lapses after a year unless it is reviewed earlier. At the Review Hearing, which is attended by the parents or other relevant person and normally the child, the supervision requirement may be discharged, continued or altered. A child, parent or other relevant person can request the review after three months, but the social work department may recommend a review at any time. The reporter arranges review hearings.

RESOURCES

In addition to funding the Scottish Children's Reporters Administration, which costs around £14 million, the Scottish Executive contributes over £500 000 annually to the training of panel members. This funding provides for training organizers, who prepare and deliver training based at Aberdeen, Edinburgh, Glasgow and St Andrews universities. Responsibility for meeting the costs of this training rests with local authorities who are also responsible for providing appropriate facilities for the assessment and supervision of children and for carrying out the supervision requirements made by hearings.

RESEARCH AND STATISTICS

Much research has been conducted on the Hearings system; most of it has been carried out by researchers based at Scottish universities, sometimes with the support of funds from other countries. A review of the research and a number of other significant studies have been published. Detailed references to recent or significant publications are available from the Children's Hearings website (www.childrens-hearings.co.uk).

Child protection

England and Wales

Children Act 1989

- Social workers have a statutory duty to investigate reports and take appropriate action to safeguard a child's welfare.

- Case conference to decide if measures of supervision are required and if child should be put on child protection register.
- Proceedings for protection of children under the Children Act take place in civil courts and are focused on the interests of the child which need proof *on the balance of probabilities.*

(From Department of Health (1991) *Working Together Under the Children Act.* London: HMSO.)

Scotland

Children (Scotland) Act 1995

- Social workers have a statutory duty to investigate reports and take appropriate action to safeguard a child's welfare.
- Case conference to decide if measures of supervision are required and if child should be put on child protection register.
- If compulsory supervision is likely to be required the case goes to the Reporter to the Children's panel. If after investigation he/she decides it is, the case is referred to the Children's Hearings system for a decision on compulsory supervision required to safeguard the child. If parents contest the grounds then the Reporter takes it to a 'proof' hearing with the Sheriff, who examines the grounds and decides *on the balance of probabilities* if they are valid. If they are, he passes the case back to the Children's Hearings to decide compulsory supervision required.

(From Scottish Office (2000) *Protecting Children – A Shared Responsibility: Guidance for Health Professionals.* London: HMSO.)

KEY LEARNING POINTS

- The Victoria Climbié report and recommendations make it clear that every professional in contact with children or their families must be aware of their duty to recognize and act on concerns about child abuse.
- A definition of child abuse is circumstances where a child's basic needs are not being met in a manner which is appropriate to his or her individual needs and stages of development and the child is, or will be, at risk through avoidable acts of commission or omission on the part of their custodian.
- Child protection is when a child needs protection from child abuse.

Signs of abuse

A child who has been abused or neglected may show obvious physical signs; however, many children without such signs signal possible abuse through their behaviour. When professionals listen to and take seriously what children say they are far more likely to detect abuse. Children with special needs are particularly vulnerable. Categories of abuse are often mixed but have been labelled physical abuse, physical neglect, non-organic failure to thrive, sexual abuse and emotional abuse. A rare form of abuse is simulated or induced illness (factitious illness syndrome, Munchausen syndrome by proxy).

PHYSICAL INJURY POSSIBLY CAUSED BY ABUSE

Bruising

- Black eyes as most accidents only cause one.
- Bruising in or around the mouth, a torn frenulum.
- Grasp marks on the arms or chest.
- Finger marks, e.g. on each side of the face.
- Symmetrical bruising, often on the ears.
- Outline bruising caused by belts or a hand print.
- Linear bruising particularly on the buttocks and back.
- Bruising on soft tissue with no good explanation.
- Bruising of different ages.
- Tiny red marks on face, in or around eyes indicating constriction or shaking.
- Petechial bruising around the mouth or neck.
- It is rare to have accidental bruising on the back, back of legs, buttocks, neck, mouth, cheeks, behind the ear, stomach, chest, under the arm, in the genital or rectal area.
- Mongolian blue spots are patches of blue-black pigmentation classically found on the lumbar and sacral regions of Afro-Caribbean children at birth but also on children of other skin colours including white.

Bites

- Bites leave clear impressions of the teeth.

Burns, scalds

- Burns and scalds with clear outlines are suspicious.
- A child is unlikely to sit down voluntarily in a hot bath and will have scalding of the feet if they have

got in themselves. They will have splash marks where they struggled to get out.
- Small round burns may be cigarette burns.

Scars

- Many children have scars but many of different ages, large scars from burns that did not receive medical attention and small round scars possibly from cigarette burns should be sought.

Fractures

- These should be suspected if there is pain, swelling and discoloration over a bone or joint.
- The commonest non-accidental fractures are to the long bones.
- Due to lack of mobility and stage of development it is rare for a child under the age of 12 months to sustain a fracture accidentally.
- Fractures cause pain.
- It is difficult for a parent to be unaware that a child has been hurt.

Genital, anal bruises

- It is unusual for a child to have bruising or bleeding in this area.

Shaken baby

- Subdural haemorrhages, retinal haemorrhages, fractures of ribs or long bones.

Poisoning

- May occur in factitious illness syndrome (Munchausen by proxy).

Definition for registration

Actual or attempted physical injury to a child under the age of 16 years where there is definite knowledge or reasonable suspicion that the injury was inflicted or knowingly not prevented.

CASE STUDY: Bruising

A 3-year-old child was admitted with marks on the leg and small bruises to both sides of the face. Grandmother explained that this was how she had held her own children by the face when telling them off. The leg bruises were linear smack marks. Photographs were taken. Social workers gained a place of safety order and after review it was deemed the child remained at risk and was fostered.

CASE STUDY: Fractures

A 4-month-old infant was admitted with a cough and difficulty breathing with persistent crying. Routine chest radiograph showed multiple rib fractures confirmed by a paediatric radiologist.

CASE STUDY: Fractures

An 18-month-old was admitted after a two-month history of a limp after a fall. A healed tibial fracture was seen on radiograph. A significant gap between the event and presentation was present and therefore non-accidental injury (NAI) suspected. Expert opinion from a paediatric orthopaedic surgeon described this as a 'typical' toddler's fracture and as social workers and health visitor had no worries about the family, NAI was ruled out.

CASE STUDY: Shaken baby

An infant presented after being looked after by stepfather with a history of stopping breathing and requiring mouth-to-mouth resuscitation. The infant was brought in by blue light ambulance not breathing. On examination there was a full fontanelle and tonic decerebrate movements. The infant was ventilated in the intensive care unit and had retinal haemorrhages – **make sure that the most senior ophthalmologist is brought in to document the retinal haemorrhages.** Post-mortem showed large subdural haematomas – **make sure that early neurological assessment is made so that intervention can be performed.**

Rib fracture in infancy should be taken as very suspicious of non-accidental injury (NAI) until proved otherwise. It is always important to be sure of evidence so opinion from an expert radiologist should be sought.

PHYSICAL NEGLECT

The following indicators, singly or in combination should alert workers:

- lack of appropriate food
- inappropriate or erratic feeding

- hair loss
- lack of adequate clothing
- circulation disorders
- unhygienic home conditions
- lack of protection from exposure to dangers
- failure or delay in seeking appropriate medical attention
- failure to reach developmental milestones.

CASE STUDY: Neglect

A 6-year-old child had attended with his mother for soiling for a number of years. His mother said that she gave him his medication. The child and his brothers ran wild to the extent that when the child and mother were brought in to hospital for enemas and toilet training over a weekend, the mother was called a number of times by neighbours to inform her that the other children were running riot around the neighbourhood. The child was discharged with little improvement. Eventually he was taken into care along with his brothers for lack of parental supervision and being out of control. The child was seen three months later at clinic in the care of a foster parent. She had stopped his medication but had instituted a programme of 50 pence for sitting each evening and passing a stool and £1 if he did it without moaning. His soiling had resolved.

CASE STUDY: Neglect

A mother who was a registered drug addict on a methadone programme was admitted with her 6-week-old infant who was reported by her health visitor not to be gaining weight and to be a poor feeder but very irritable. The child was irritable but fed reasonably well with the ward nurses. Mum was an infrequent visitor to the ward, and when she did come, there were two episodes where Mum was drowsy and nearly dropped the child onto the floor. A further episode took place where Mum fell asleep in a chair, lying over the child, and the child had to be removed from Mum's arms. A case conference was convened by the social work department. Nursing evidence and other concerns were enough for the social work department to obtain a place of safety order. The child was taken into foster placement and thrived.

Definition for registration

This occurs when a child's essential needs are not met and this is likely to cause impairment to physical health and development. Such needs include food, clothes, cleanliness, shelter and warmth. A lack of appropriate care results in persistent or severe exposure, through negligence, to circumstances that endanger the child.

SEXUAL ABUSE

Children can make statements spontaneously or in a planned way and this is often dependent on their age. The following indicators should alert workers to the possibility of the child being a victim of sexual abuse.

Physical indicators

These include injuries in the genital area, infections or abnormal discharge in the genital area, complaints of genital itching or pain, depression or withdrawal, wetting or soiling, day or night, sleep disturbances or nightmares, chronic illnesses, especially throat infections, venereal disease *which may be diagnostic*, anorexia or bulimia, unexplained pregnancy, phobias or panic attacks.

CASE STUDY: Rectal bleeding

A 2-year-old girl was presented by grandfather with a history of bright red rectal bleeding after eating a sausage roll which grandfather said had glass in it. The child had iron-deficiency anaemia. No blood was ever seen and no sausage roll with glass. Mother was very quiet and lived with grandfather and grandmother. Grandmother was said to be bedridden, mother was 17 years old and the child's father was not 'in contact'. The child presented again 10 years later with abdominal pain and vomiting. Mother had eventually moved out and was living with her boyfriend. Mother and boyfriend wanted counselling about 'issues' before mother would agree to marry her boyfriend.

General indicators

These include self-harm, excessive sexual awareness or knowledge of sexual matters inappropriate for the child's age, acting in a sexually explicit manner, displays of affection in a sexual way inappropriate to age, sudden changes in behaviour or school performance or school avoidance, tendency to cling or need constant reassurance, tendency to cry easily, regression to younger behaviour such as thumb sucking, playing with discarded toys, acting like a baby, distrust of a familiar or anxiety about being left with a relative, a babysitter or a lodger, unexplained gifts or money, secretive behaviour, eating disorders, fear of undressing for gym, phobias or panic attacks.

CASE STUDY: Overt sexualized behaviour

A 13-year-old presented with abnormal behaviour. She did not recognize her parents or others around her. She proceeded to move into a fugue-like state where she alternated between being very active and sitting silently on her bed. The active phases included episodes where she would take all her clothes off and imitate sexual acts.

Definition for registration

Any child below the age of 16 years may be deemed to have been sexually abused when person(s), by design or neglect exploits the child, directly or indirectly, with any activity intended to lead to sexual arousal or other forms of gratification of that person or any other person(s) including organized networks.

NON-ORGANIC FAILURE TO THRIVE

The following indicators should alert workers to the possibility of abuse:

- diarrhoea
- child having little interest in food
- child thriving away from home
- unresponsive child
- staying frozen in one position for an unnaturally long time
- poor skin or muscle tone
- circulatory disorders
- lethargic child
- height and weight centile falling away
- abnormal relationships particularly at mealtimes, e.g. persistent withholding of food as a punishment.

CASE STUDY: Non-organic failure to thrive

A 2-year-old was seen in clinic with failure to thrive below the 2nd centile having started out on the 50th. No weight had been gained for a year. Parents said that she would not eat. Family were well known to social services as Mum was on a methadone programme. Food diary showed that the child was largely given fizzy juice and ate crisps. The family had no real mealtimes and just ate in front of the television. The child was allowed to run around and started each meal with a large drink of juice. Father seemed controlling and the family were very difficult to engage.

Definition for registration

Children who significantly fail to reach normal growth and developmental milestones (i.e. physical growth, weight, motor skills). Organic reasons must have been medically eliminated and a diagnosis of non-organic failure to thrive established.

FACTITIOUS ILLNESS SYNDROME (MUNCHAUSEN SYNDROME BY PROXY)

Parents (often mothers) report fraudulent signs and may even simulate symptoms such as bleeding and fever. Children are exposed to needless investigation and hospital admission.

CASE STUDY: Vomiting blood

A 3-year-old was admitted with a history of vomiting bright red blood. No further vomiting of blood took place on the ward. The parents were very worried and father was upper middle class and quite aggressive. Investigation including bloods and barium meal failed to show a cause. The child was sent home but one month later presented again, this time with a pillow case covered in blood. Endoscopy was performed but nothing found. Six months later, the child was seen at a tertiary referral centre for paediatric gastroenterology. Eventually, a further hospital pillowcase appeared with blood on it. It was shown that the blood group of the child did not match the blood group on the pillow.

Roles of agencies in child protection

All children have the right to protection and all adults have responsibilities to ensure that children receive such protection. *The welfare of children is the responsibility of the whole local authority including social work, health, police and education services.* Social work services assess the needs of children and provide appropriate services.

They make enquiries into the circumstances of children who may require compulsory measures of supervision. The role of the police is to prevent child abuse, protect the victim(s) and detect the offender. Health professionals may be the first to see symptoms of abuse and should share information about concerns with social workers, police or the Reporter to the Children's Hearing system at an early stage. General practitioners, general paediatricians and specialist paediatricians in child protection may take referrals from social work, police, education and legal departments to assess the needs and management of a child's health in the context of interagency concerns about abuse.

The role of health professionals in child protection:

- recognizing children in need of protection
- contributing to enquiries including examination of children
- participating in child protection conferences
- providing therapeutic help to abused children and their parents
- playing a part through the child protection plan in safeguarding children.

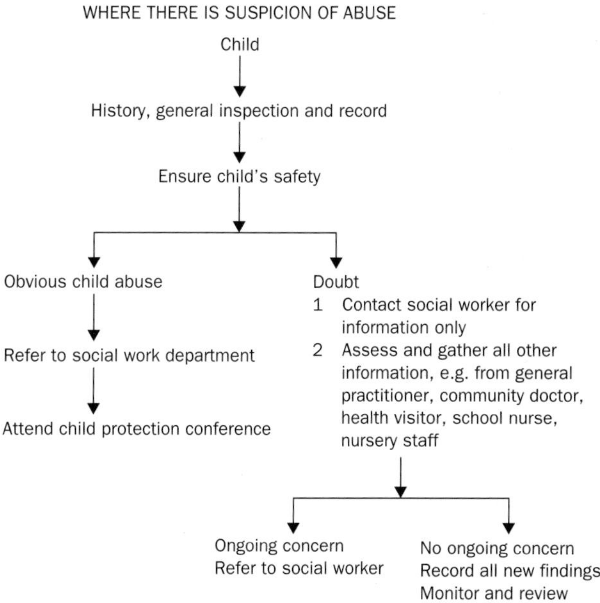

Figure 1.2 The steps to follow when there is suspicion of abuse

Teachers are likely to have the greatest level of routine contact with children. Educational professionals have a major responsibility in identifying cases of child abuse. Any person may refer a child to the Reporter if they have reasonable cause to believe that the child may be in need of compulsory measures of supervision, that is measures of protection, guidance, treatment or control. The Procurator Fiscal is the local representative of the Lord Advocate in Scotland who is responsible for the prosecution of crime. To prosecute a perpetrator in the criminal courts proof must be *beyond reasonable doubt*, but lack of this does not stop the Children's Hearings system providing a supervision order to protect a child when proof is at the level of *balance of probabilities*.

Deciding on how to respond

Referrals about concerns over a child's welfare will not always require a response under child protection procedures. In every referral professional judgement will need to be exercised to decide upon the most appropriate response (Figure 1.2). The local authority social work service has the statutory duty to protect children, in partnership with other agencies. It should be stressed, however, that no one agency can or should work in isolation from the others. Therefore when deciding how best to respond to a referral, agencies should consult and discuss the information available with each other. When doing so the paramount consideration should be the welfare of the child. It is important that a distinction be made between agency checks and referrals.

KEY LEARNING POINTS

In all cases of suspected abuse:

- inform senior colleague who is ultimately responsible for the case
- inform social work department and discuss management
- inform parent (unless it puts child at risk of harm)
- record accurate details of history and clinical findings with diagrams
- send report to relevant trust health professional with responsibility for child protection
- send report to manager of social work department for child protection conference purposes
- attend child protection case conference.

The medical examination

Where abuse is suspected, a full health assessment should be carried out including a detailed medical history and general physical examination including health and emotional needs. A two doctor examination should be conducted in cases of suspected child sexual abuse by doctors experienced in forensic examination at a time and in a place appropriate to the case to avoid duplication of examination. Examinations should be sensitive, child-centred and conducive to the best outcome for the child. A medical examination may not provide evidence that child abuse has occurred, and absence of medical evidence does not automatically mean absence of abuse. Information from medical examinations should be considered alongside information from social workers, police and any other relevant agency.

The purpose of the medical examination is:

- to provide a full health assessment of the child's needs
- to establish what immediate treatment the child may require
- to provide an opinion on whether or not child abuse has occurred
- to provide evidence where appropriate to support a referral to the Children's Hearings system (via the Reporter) or for criminal proceedings
- to secure any further medical assistance for the child if required
- where appropriate to reassure the child and family that no long-term physical damage has occurred.

WHERE TO ARRANGE A MEDICAL EXAMINATION AND/OR ASSESSMENT

An appropriately equipped paediatric facility with experienced paediatric nursing staff is required. For physical injury, access to a good X-ray facility and high-quality medical photography are essential. For sexual abuse specialist video-colposcopy facilities are required.

WHEN TO ARRANGE A MEDICAL EXAMINATION FOR SUSPECTED CHILD ABUSE

There should be a three-way discussion between social workers, the police and a medical practitioner (consultant paediatrician in child protection, general paediatric consultant, community paediatrician or a GP) to decide whether and when a medical examination is required.

Some circumstances which require a medical examination

- A child has physical injuries which he or she states were inflicted.
- A child has injuries and the explanation is not consistent with the injuries.
- A child appears to be suffering from physical neglect.
- Any allegation of child sexual abuse including touching over clothes, fondling, attempted or actual digital penetration, a penetrative episode.
- Concern about non-organic failure to thrive.

WHO DECIDES TO ARRANGE A MEDICAL EXAMINATION?

The senior social worker should discuss with police and relevant medical personnel (as above) and agreement should be reached on whether a medical examination is required and what it will achieve, type of medical required, who should conduct it, where and when it should be conducted. Whether face to face or on the telephone, discussions and decisions on how to proceed should be clearly documented. If it is agreed to arrange a medical examination or assessment it is important that the examining doctors have clear information about the causes of concern, the social background including previous instances of known or suspected abuse.

TIMING

With physical injury, it is important to arrange a medical examination as soon as possible so that signs of injury such as bruising do not fade. With sexual abuse, if there has been any form of recent sexual assault it is imperative to arrange a medical examination within 72 hours of the last incident in order to obtain forensic evidence. If more than 72 hours has passed since sexual assault allegedly occurred then time could be spent planning the medical. In situations where the GP is unsure whether the clinical presentation is due to abuse or illness, for example a child with unexplained severe bruising which could be due to a haematological condition, referral to the hospital for a paediatric opinion prior to initiating interagency discussions may be indicated. It is important to provide the hospital paediatricians with available social background that may suggest abuse.

RECORD KEEPING

Records should be detailed and legible as original records may be required later for criminal proceedings. Special sheets, which include diagrams of body parts and detailed diagrams of the genitalia, should be available to aid description of injuries. Detailed measurements should be included. Details of the full names, addresses and contact telephone numbers of family members and friends and other professionals involved are invaluable and should be clearly documented in the notes. It is important for clinicians to note carefully any explanations given for injuries. Records should note the date and time of any incident and the date and time the record was made. Written reports of findings should be provided at an early stage to the police and local authority (social work) if the child's case is the subject of court proceeding or a children's hearing. Professional records may need to be made available to the police, the Reporter and the courts.

Records should include:

- details of any concerns about the child and family
- details of contact with the family or other agencies
- the findings of any assessment
- decisions made about the case within each agency or in discussions with other agencies
- a note of information shared with other agencies, with whom and when.

KEY LEARNING POINT

Good record keeping is essential both for protecting the child and for evidential purposes. Take the full name, address and telephone number of everybody involved including police, social worker, the Reporter, parents, grandparents, etc. Make sure your notes are legible and detailed. Make sure if you are a junior, whoever is supervising you also writes in the notes.

CONSENT

The Age of Legal Capacity (Scotland) Act 1991 provides that a person under the age of 16 years shall have the legal capacity to consent on his or her own behalf to any surgical, medical or dental procedure or treatment, including psychological or psychiatric examination, where, in the opinion of an attending qualified medical practitioner, he or she is capable of understanding the nature and possible consequences of the procedure or treatment. If the local authority believes that a medical examination is required to find out whether concerns about a child's safety or welfare are justified, and parents refuse consent, the local authority may apply to a sheriff for a Child Assessment Order. The child, if deemed to have legal capacity, can still refuse the examination as a whole or any part of it, e.g. photography.

KEY LEARNING POINT

Child can decline examination if deemed to have legal capacity.

PHOTOGRAPHY

For both physical abuse and sexual abuse, high-quality photography is an essential part of recording of injuries. This is aided by colposcopy in cases of sexual abuse.

KEY LEARNING POINT

A doctor above senior house officer (SHO) level must be present and witness medical photographs to be used in court.

Referral to the Reporter of the Children's Hearings system

This guidance reflects the 1998 Scottish Office guidelines *Protecting Children – A Shared Responsibility.* Ensuring the swift and well-informed referral of vulnerable children who require compulsory support, guidance, protection and control is the overriding consideration. The decision to refer a child to the children's Reporter is a significant step with potentially far-reaching consequences for the child and his/her family/carers. A number of general principles should be applied when decisions are being taken.

- The child's welfare shall be the paramount consideration when deciding whether or not to refer a child to the Reporter.
- Agencies are required to take into account the views of children and families and to work in partnership with them.
- Local authorities (e.g. social work department) have a statutory duty to safeguard and promote the welfare of children.

There are different statutory provisions relating to referral of a child to the Reporter. The law recognizes three distinct providers of such information.

- The local authority (e.g. social work department) should refer to the Reporter all cases of suspected child abuse.
- The police inform the Reporter of abuse cases with criminal proceeding.

- Any other person (e.g. health professionals) should refer a case to the Reporter if compulsory measures of care, protection or control may be, in their opinion, in the best interests of the child.

Grounds for referral of children to the Reporter and to the Children's Hearings system

A child may be in need of compulsory measures of supervision if any of the following conditions is satisfied with respect to her or him (section 52(2) of the Children (Scotland) Act 1995).

a is beyond control of any relevant person
b is falling into bad associations or is exposed to moral danger
c is likely:
  i to suffer unnecessarily or
  ii to be impaired seriously in his health or development, due to a lack of parental care
d is a child in respect of whom any of the offences mentioned in Schedule 1 to the Criminal Procedure (Scotland) Act 1995 has been committed (Note: These are offences against children to which special provisions apply. Among the most common of these are sexual offences against children, assault, neglect and abandonment)
e is, or is likely to become, a member of the same household as a child in respect of whom any offences referred to in paragraph d above has been committed
f is, or is likely to become a member of the same household as a person who has committed any of the offences referred to in paragraph d
g is, or is likely to become, a member of the same household as a person in respect of whom an offence under sections 1 to 3 of the Criminal Law (Consolidation) (Scotland) Act 1995 (incest and intercourse with a child by a step-parent or person in position of trust) has been committed by a member of that household;
h has failed to attend school regularly without reasonable excuse
i has committed an offence
j has misused alcohol or any drug, whether or not a controlled drug within the meaning of the Misuse of Drugs Act 1971
k has misused a volatile substance by deliberately inhaling its vapour, other than for medical purpose
l is being provided with accommodation by a local authority under section 25, or is the subject of a parental responsibilities order obtained under section 86 of the Act and, in either case, his behaviour is such that special measures are necessary for his adequate supervision in his interest or the interest of others.

Most referrals by health professionals are likely to arise from concerns relating to childcare and protection. They should also consider referral of children on other grounds, e.g. school-related issues or misuse of drugs, alcohol or volatile substances.

CASE STUDY: Child with speech delay

A 4-year-old girl had been referred to the child development centre (CDC) with speech delay at age 2 years. The child attended the CDC once but did not attend for follow-up or for a hearing test with the educational audiologist or for blood tests or for assessment by a speech and language therapist. Every time the educational psychologist tried to see the child in the nursery placement Mum failed to arrive. The speech and language therapist made appointments with the mother to meet her at home but she was never there. The child was due to go to school, the nursery thought the child needed further help perhaps from the language unit, but nobody had managed to make a complete assessment of the child due to parental non-cooperation/neglect. After discussions at a language panel meeting this child was referred to the Reporter by the community paediatrician. Suddenly, all appointments were kept and the assessment proceeded quickly.

When making a referral to the Children's Reporter, agencies or individuals must *not* take into consideration whether they believe there is sufficient evidence for grounds for referral to be established. Considerations relating to sufficiency of evidence and standard of proof are exclusively a matter for the Reporter. Referral should be made where a health professional has reasonable cause to believe that a child may be in need of compulsory measures of supervision. In terms of the Children (Scotland) Act 1995, 'supervision' in this context may include measures taken for the protection, guidance, treatment, or control of the child. It is essential that sufficient and speedy referral be made. Consultation by telephone is encouraged before making a referral. Each referral should be dated and signed by the author.

All referrals to the Reporter should contain the following information (if known):

- full name, address (present and normal address), and date of birth of child/children being referred
- any special requirements of the child or family, e.g. religion, disability, ethnic origin, language, etc.
- details of all other children in the household with a clear indication of whether the agency also intends to refer them
- full names and address of parents/carers
- name of child's GP and health visitor
- a clear indication of whether the child is subject to any orders or legal requirements including details of any restrictions on contact
- whether or not the referral has been discussed with the family
- whether or not the child is attending child and adolescent mental health services
- a summary of the reason(s) for referral to the Reporter
- a factual account of the circumstances relating to the referral and names and addresses of all parties involved, e.g. how, when and by whom the incident was discovered.

Referrals to the police

Although the police have a clear role in investigating offences against children, it is the responsibility of social work services to assess the needs and possible risks to a child about whom concerns have been expressed. A referral to the police should be made when there is reason to believe child protection measures are required. In order to determine whether such measures are required, there is an onus on social work services to assess the situation and circumstances of the child.

Child protection conference

Child protection conferences are an important stage in the child protection process and provide a forum for professionals to share information and make plans to protect children. A key function is to consider the need for registration but equal emphasis should be placed on identifying a child protection plan to safeguard the child. There are four types of conference: initial, review, pre-birth and transfer (to another geographic area). Social work services are responsible for convening, chairing and minuting a child protection conference, but any agency can request a child protection conference by contacting the team leader for social work in the area the child resides. Parental involvement at child protection conferences should be the rule rather than the exception. It is vital that health professionals in the primary care team and any other medical or health staff involved attend to describe and interpret medical findings and relevant background information. Health professionals should normally provide written reports of their involvement and any assessment and findings.

Tasks undertaken by a child protection conference

- Ensure that all relevant information is shared and collated.
- Assess the degree of existing and likely future risk to the child.
- Identify the child's needs and any services required to help him or her.
- Formulate or review a child protection plan which includes a decision whether to place a child on the Child Protection Register.

CASE STUDY

A 6-year-old child arrived at school with a black eye. When asked by a teacher how he had bruised his eye, he said that his stepfather punched him. At the case conference the community police officer, social worker, school teacher, probation officer for stepfather, hospital doctor and mother were present. Mother said that the stepfather was no longer living in the house. However, it became clear that she did not believe the boy's story and she was therefore deemed unable to protect him. He was put on the 'at-risk register' and the mother was told that if evidence came to light from community police or elsewhere that the stepfather was still in the house, a Child Protection Order would be sought and the boy would be taken into the care of the local authority.

KEY LEARNING POINT

The child protection conference has an important role to formulate a child protection plan to protect a child from further abuse. It is important for all professionals and parents to be there as together they are likely to have all the information to achieve a competent plan. If part of the picture is missing then a competent plan may not be achieved and the child may remain at risk.

Communication

In some cases of child abuse, problems have arisen when professionals fail to communicate effectively and share information both vertically within a professional structure and between professional agencies involved with the child and family. It is crucial for the benefit of the child that key people communicate effectively across professional boundaries in an atmosphere of trust.

Child Protection Register

The purpose of the Register is to provide a record of children who are in need of protection by means of an interagency child protection plan. The Register can provide a central point for enquiry for professional staff who are concerned about a child. The management and upkeep of the Child Protection Register is the responsibility of social work services. The Child Protection Register is not a legal order but rather an interagency internal 'highlighter' to flag up children who are felt to be at risk of abuse or in need of protection. Enquiries are made via the social work area team or standby out of hours. The decision to place a child's name on or take it off the Child Protection Register is taken at the child protection conference. There are five categories of registration corresponding to the different forms of child abuse: physical injury, sexual abuse, non-organic failure to thrive, emotional abuse and physical neglect.

The Children's Hearings system in child protection in Scotland

Important measures are available to protect children who have been the victims of offences whether or not there is a prosecution or conviction maintained *beyond reasonable doubt* in a criminal court. Such offences can be established within the Children's Hearings system by proof (deemed sufficient at a sheriff's proof hearing) *on the balance of probabilities*. Children, who are not themselves victims, but are at risk of abuse through their contact with the person responsible, can also be protected.

KEY LEARNING POINT

The Children's Hearings system can protect children even if criminal proceedings do not succeed. By working on proof at the *level of the balance of probabilities*, compulsory supervision, which may include care outside the home, can still be invoked.

Orders

An application for a Child Protection Order can be made by any person to a sheriff who must be satisfied that there are reasonable grounds to believe that the child is being treated in a manner to cause significant harm or will suffer such harm if not removed to a place of safety. A 24-hour Emergency Order can be made to a Justice of the Peace or a police constable can remove a child for 24 hours if a sheriff is not available. A Child Assessment Order from a sheriff is intended to enable an assessment of a child's health or development to be made. A local authority may apply to a sheriff for an Exclusion Order to exclude a 'named person' from the house of a particular child or children.

CASE STUDY: An infant hit by a parent

A mother was at a bus stop at 10 pm on a Saturday night with her 9-month-old infant in a pram. A bus stopped and passengers witnessed the mother hitting the child who was crying. The bus driver separated the mother from the child with the help of some passengers and a passing police car stopped. An Emergency Child Protection Order was taken out by the police officer who brought the child to the hospital as a place of safety. The sheriff granted a Child Protection Order to the social work department the next day.

THE LOCAL CHILD PROTECTION COMMITTEE

The committee is an interagency forum for developing, monitoring and reviewing child protection policies. The membership includes representatives of social work, education and health services (managerial and professional including the designated doctor and nurse, a GP for primary care), the police, the National Society for the Prevention of Cruelty for Children (NSPCC), the probation service, and may include a lawyer, the Procurator Fiscal and other voluntary agencies. Members are accountable to their own agencies and have authority to speak on their agency's behalf. Committees produce written guidelines for the management of child abuse in their area to foster close interagency cooperation.

Fostering and adoption: the role of the community paediatrician

There is obviously a close link between child protection and fostering and adoption, as many children who are fostered and adopted have been the subject of some kind of abuse. In Glasgow, community paediatricians have taken on the task of tracking children who are looked after by the local authority, fostered and eventually adopted. Over 1000 children are in the care of the local authority at any one time in Glasgow with 300 new 'receipts into care' each year. A database of children received into care has been established over the past 10 years. The aim is to improve the healthcare provision for this transient group of children. Each child requires a medical examination by a doctor before or soon after being received into care. This contact allows a health appraisal to be undertaken and appropriate management to be implemented.

Adoption panels decide on the placement of a child who either voluntarily or by the order of the court has been 'freed' from parental responsibility and requires and is willing to be permanently placed with new permanent carers who will assume parental responsibility. Each adoption panel has at least one medical adviser. The role of the medical adviser is to provide the panel and the prospective adopters with a full detailed account of the child's medical background and what may be required in the future including operations and outpatient attendance. This may require full assessment of the child by the panel adviser with the help of other specialists. A separate medical adviser may be employed for the health of prospective adopters. The panel needs to be sure that adopters will be able and healthy until the child is able to achieve an independent life. The medical adviser has to attend adoption panel meetings and is an important person to advocate for the best interests of the child.

CHILD DEVELOPMENT AND LEARNING DIFFICULTIES

Child disability services are a core part of community child health. All children deserve access to a range of high-quality services that will help them attain optimal health and wellbeing and to become healthy and well-adjusted adults. Children with physical or mental illness or disability with often economic and social disadvantage require additional help and support to reach their potential. Although many chronic illnesses cause children to have disability and consequent special needs, 90 per cent are caused by impaired function of the nervous system.

These children require a different service to simple hospital inpatient and outpatient care. A child with multiple disabilities including complex neurological problems compounded by psychological and behavioural difficulties needs a dedicated *multidisciplinary interagency* approach. Child development teams may include a specialist health visitor, a clinical psychologist, a speech therapist, a physiotherapist, an occupational therapist, a social work resource worker and a community paediatrician. The social work resource worker is especially important for families of disabled children who often are in need of extra benefits, particularly Disability Living Allowance, which is not means tested.

KEY LEARNING POINT

Children with developmental problems require assessment and help from a multidisciplinary group of experts usually working in a number of different agencies including health, education and social services.

Educational input will be coordinated by an educational psychologist and may include assessments by an educational audiologist, a home visiting teacher and teachers and nurses within the nursery and school system. Parent support groups can help 'new' parents to come to terms with their child's disability by seeing how other families have coped. Disabled children often require input from other specialties particularly neurology, ophthalmology, genetics, ENT, orthopaedics and child and family psychiatry. The primary care team needs to be closely involved. There is a changing population of disabled children with increasing numbers who have more complex difficulties. Children with cerebral palsy experience greater impairment than previously.

Over recent years there have been increasing referrals to disability services, with public awareness and knowledge particularly with regard to conditions such as autism and attention deficit hyperactivity disorder.

Multidisciplinary team requirements

- Child and family
- Community paediatrician
- Nursing staff
- Specialist health visitor
- School nurses
- Physiotherapist
- Speech and language therapist
- Occupational therapist
- Social work resource worker
- Clinical psychologist
- Administrative support
- Equipment
- Accommodation which allows effective team work to take place

Interagency groups

- Health
- Education
- Social work
- Housing
- Voluntary organizations and charities
- Parental support groups

In Scotland the links between health, education and social work are often formalized for an individual child through **PRESCAT** (pre-school community assessment team) for planning prior to school entry. For school-age children interagency working is often brought together through the **Record of Special Educational Needs** process.

KEY LEARNING POINT

Early referral to education of children who may require assessment to decide appropriate school placement is essential.

CHILD DEVELOPMENT TEAMS

The child development team should be a full multidisciplinary specialist team as recommended by the Court Report in 1976, and subsequently by the British Association for Community Child Health (2001). Ideally, the team should be based within a purpose-built child development centre that should be based in a community setting but with good links to both hospital and primary care services. The aim is to provide assessment and care and to work closely with education so that a child is placed correctly in primary education to achieve the best possible outcome. The child development team works primarily with pre-school children who have or who may have significant developmental problems. Older children may continue to be managed by the child development team, or their care may be passed to other services such as school health or learning disability teams.

The primary aims of the child development team are:

- to assess the child's development and healthcare needs
- to plan and review the paediatric care of the child
- to implement the care of the child in respect to the team's specialist resources
- to make appropriate referrals to, and to carry out liaison with, other child health services, for example audiology and ophthalmology
- to make appropriate referral to, and to work with external agencies, particularly education and social work services
- to work with the family to promote the best interests of the child
- to work closely with the primary care team and hospital-based colleagues.

Links with neonatal care

Lower gestational age infants are now more likely to survive but major handicap is often present in very preterm babies. In Glasgow, close links have been formed between the child development teams and neonatal follow-up through a combined clinic system usually sited at the neonatal unit. This allows early planning and assessment as well as intervention. Neonatal survivors, however, make up only about 10 per cent of the workload of the child development teams.

KEY LEARNING POINT

Graduates of neonatal intensive care units only make up a small proportion of infants referred to a child development centre.

INVESTIGATION OF DEVELOPMENTAL DELAY

Developmental delay or learning difficulties are probably among the commonest problems encountered in community paediatric practice. The latter term should be used when it is obvious that the child will not 'catch up' with his peer group as the persistent use of the term 'delay' may give parents an unrealistic expectation that the problem is a temporary one.

KEY LEARNING POINT

As with other paediatric problems, a comprehensive history, examination and a few special investigations are required to work up a child with developmental delay. In only about 50 per cent is a specific reason or diagnosis made for their delay.

Developmental delay can be assessed with a variety of scales. Many developmental paediatricians use the Griffiths Developmental Assessment tool. In Glasgow's community child development centres the practice is to use a simple practical tool called the Schedule of Growing Skills (version II). It comes complete in a box with understandable instructions and uses a combination of measures based on history and examination. It is useful for pre-school children and generates a simple multicopy report, which can be sent to other therapists and agencies such as education or to inform PRESCAT.

It is important to investigate children with developmental delay, primarily to try to identify causation and also to assist with management and to give some information about prognosis, recurrence risks and future prevention strategies. Developmental delay can be defined as significant delay in two or more developmental domains – gross/fine motor; speech/language; cognition; personal/social and activities of daily living. A comprehensive history is essential and should include pre-, peri- and postnatal history including threatened miscarriage and drug exposure, and a detailed family history. It should be ascertained whether the child is simply delayed or is showing signs of regression. A complete physical examination should include measurement of occipitofrontal circumference (OFC) (and comparison with parents if abnormal), observation of gait, a search for neurocutaneous stigmata, abdominal examination for visceromegaly, check of the spine and reflexes and ophthalmological examination. Genetics referral is particularly useful for the evaluation of dysmorphic features and abnormal growth including head size, if there is associated visual or hearing impairment or an unusual behaviour pattern and if there is a positive family history.

It is important to undertake routine investigation of all children with developmental delay if the diagnosis is not apparent after history and examination as above. A suggested first-line screen should include chromosomes (including specific fragile X examination), urea and electrolytes, creatine kinase and thyroid function. Full blood count and ferritin will detect cases of iron-deficiency anaemia, which may contribute to developmental delay. There are a number of conditions that are rare, but treatable, and as such deserve specific consideration. These include lead poisoning and biotinidase deficiency.

Second-line investigations should be selective and guided by clues in the history and examination. These consist of neuroimaging, metabolic investigation and electroencephalography. Neuroimaging should be considered in cases of abnormal head size, focal neurology (spasticity, dystonia, ataxia, increase or loss of reflexes or seizures), and any unexpected change in the child's condition. Magnetic resonance imaging (MRI) is the investigation of choice, although computed tomography (CT) is better for bony structures or calcification.

Metabolic investigations have the disadvantage of a high frequency of non-specific, non-diagnostic abnormalities but should be considered in the following situations:

- Positive family history
- Parental consanguinity
- Developmental regression
- Recurrent unexplained illness
- Hypotonia
- Eye abnormalities, e.g. cataract
- Hepatosplenomegaly
- Structural hair abnormalities
- Unexplained deafness.

CASE STUDY

An 18-month-old infant with slow speech was seen. She had significant upper airway obstruction. The Schedule of Growing Skills showed her to have normal development apart from hearing and speech. Hearing was assessed and an ENT referral made which showed conductive deafness associated with significant upper airway obstruction. Blood tests for fragile X carrier, thyroid function and creatine kinase were normal. Grommets were inserted and it was noted that she was very difficult to intubate and her neck was quite 'stiff'. At nursery she remained very quiet but did well with non-verbal tasks. At an appointment with another community paediatrician, the child was noted to be 'funny looking' with coarse facies and hair. At a further hearing assessment the audiologist had seen a child like this before. Urine examination confirmed type 1 mucopolysaccharidosis.

KEY LEARNING POINT

Rare diseases do occur.

Check that the neonatal Guthrie screen has been done. Other suggested investigations are urine amino and organic acids, mucopolysaccharides, blood lactate and ammonia, serum lactate, plasma biotinidase and amino acids, and very long chain fatty acids. Electroencephalography should only be done if there is a history suggestive of seizures or regression in speech suggestive of Landau-Kleffner syndrome. It can also be done if there is a recognized associated phenotype, e.g. Angelman syndrome. It is important to remember that investigations are not a substitute for detailed history and examination, but that they can be a useful adjunct in determining the aetiology of developmental delay.

Referral to other therapists in the child development team is often required for therapeutic assessment but is also required for diagnosis particularly to educational audiology and speech and language therapy for diagnosis in children with speech delay. Educational audiologists have the necessary skills to test the hearing of difficult to test children including those who have multiple developmental problems.

HEARING SCREENING

All areas should be planning to introduce Universal Newborn Hearing Screening (UNHS) in line with national guidance from the UK National Screening Committee and HDL(2001)51, which was issued in June 2001 to advise NHS Scotland about the introduction of UNHS. Implementation is underway, with the establishment of two pathfinder sites in Tayside and Lothian, where screening began in January and March 2003, respectively. NHS boards are expected to implement the UNHS programme by April 2005. Once UNHS is in place, universal distraction testing at 7–9 months should be abandoned. The National Hearing Screening Implementation Group for UNHS is currently considering the period for which UNHS must be in place before universal distraction testing should be abandoned and is expected to issue advice. The Group has already recommended increased vigilance among professionals in relation to risk groups such as children who have suffered from meningitis, received ototoxic drugs (i.e. those which may damage the hearing mechanism), children with middle ear disease and children with developmental disorders which may mimic hearing loss or be associated with hearing loss. The school entry hearing sweep test should continue while further evidence about its effectiveness is collected and evaluated. No further routine hearing testing should be undertaken beyond this test on entry to primary school. Audiology services must be able to respond to the concerns of referrers and parents promptly. NHS boards should therefore review the local arrangements regarding access to paediatric audiology services and training of staff to ensure children with suspected hearing loss can be fast tracked for hearing testing. Audiological assessment and follow-up should be arranged automatically for any child who has had bacterial meningitis, prolonged treatment with ototoxic drugs or severe head injury before or soon after discharge.

AUDIOLOGICAL ASSESSMENT

Many health authorities are now using auditory brainstem response (ABR) to examine the hearing integrity of at-risk infants from neonatal units. These techniques require the infant to be asleep or anaesthetized and are therefore most appropriate for young infants while asleep. Stimulus clicks are entered using earphones. Electroencephalographic recording is made to assess response. Problems include difficulty in distinguishing between purely high-tone hearing loss and overall hearing loss. When retested later, children with a threshold greater than 60 dBA of hearing loss by ABR usually have some degree of sensorineural hearing loss. The ABR is often mistakenly viewed as the 'gold standard' audiological assessment, but interpretation must always be made in conjunction with ongoing behavioural assessment.

Infants between the ages of 6 and 18 months are tested using the Distraction Test. This screening test, employed by health visitors at the eight-month child health surveillance examination, is to be discontinued. The test is based on the principle that the normal response when the sound is presented is for the baby to turn his or her head to locate the source of the sound. The sound presentation level should be 30 dBA. Minimal voice, high-frequency rattle, and sibilant 's' should all be presented at 1 m from the child's ear and at an angle of 45° which should be outside the child's field of vision. Warble tones are presented at 50 cm from the child's ear on the same plane and at an angle of 45°.

> Requirements for a distraction hearing test
>
> - A quiet room of minimum floor area of 16 m^2 with ambient noise level not exceeding 25–30 dBA.
> - A low table.
> - A selection of frequency-specific sounds: warble tones, 1 and 4 kHz high-frequency rattle.
> - A sound meter.

The test is undertaken with the baby seated on the parent's knee facing forward and sitting erect (Figure 1.3). The parent should be instructed not to react in any way when stimulus sounds are presented. The role of another person at the front is to attract the baby's attention by using a small spinning toy on the low table, and then cover the object, with fingers or remove it from the table. The person presenting the stimuli should be in position at the back of the baby. As soon as the person at the front has removed the object, the sound stimulus should be introduced on the same plane as the baby's ear. To be credited with a response the baby must hear the signal, turn and locate its position. This response should be recorded by the person presenting the stimulus. The person at the front is the judge of what is or is not a response. The person at the front then attracts the baby's attention as before and the person presenting the stimuli moves to the other side

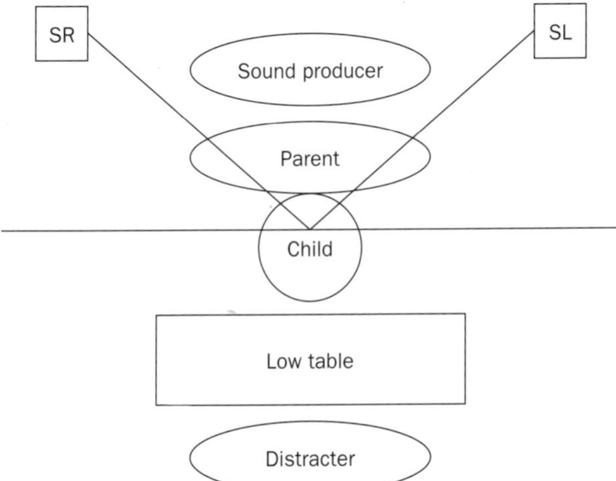

Figure 1.3 Test arrangements for a distraction test. SL, stimulus left; SR, stimulus right

and presents a different stimulus again at an angle of 45° and in the same plane. Great care has to be taken not to work in a regular pattern and not to stop the sound too quickly as some babies take time to respond. This method is used until all stimuli have been presented and results recorded. Some babies 'hunt' for stimuli, and this should be assessed and recorded using a 'no sound test'.

Some common pitfalls with the distraction hearing test are visual cueing where the rear tester or his or her shadow moves into the peripheral vision of the baby; tactile cueing by the breath of the tester when delivering the stimulus or the mother squeezing the child to encourage a response; auditory cueing such as wearing creaking shoes; and olfactory cueing wearing strong perfume may then turn the baby to the olfactory stimulus.

Hearing assessment of children with disability can be difficult and should be undertaken by a person with experience and training such as an educational audiologist. Children who have a significant hearing loss are referred to and managed by the hearing impairment assessment team (HIAT). This group has representatives from health, education and social services to maximize the child's opportunities.

> **KEY LEARNING POINT**
>
> Hearing and vision assessment on children with developmental delay can be difficult and should be undertaken by an expert. These children will benefit greatly from correction of hearing or vision abnormalities.

VISION SCREENING

All children should be screened by an orthoptist in their pre-school year, between the ages of 4 and 5 years, removing the need for vision testing on school entry. This reflects recommendations by the UK National Screening Committee and Hall 4, and is already being implemented in some areas using a database to manage orthoptist screening in pre-school centres, health centres and primary schools to achieve maximum coverage. Until an orthoptist pre-school vision screening programme is in place, children's visual acuity should be tested on school entry by an orthoptist, or through a programme supervised by an orthoptist or an optometrist. The evidence for screening in secondary school remains inconclusive. On that basis, if screening on a single occasion is already in place, it should continue, but more frequent screening should cease, and no new vision screening should be introduced in secondary school. There is little evidence of the benefits of screening for colour vision defects and no attempt should be made to screen for colour vision defects in primary school. If screening is already in place for adolescents, it should continue, but no new colour vision screening should be introduced. Adolescents whose career planning might be affected by an impaired colour vision should be advised to visit an optometrist for expert advice and assessment. Arrangements should be made for any child undergoing assessment for educational underachievement or other school problems to have a visual acuity check. Vision screening should also be undertaken in schools for children with hearing impairment. One person in each NHS board area should take overall responsibility for monitoring vision screening.

Visual acuity assessment can be difficult in children with developmental problems. Specially trained orthoptists are likely to provide the best measure of visual acuity in tandem with an experienced optometrist to test for refractive errors. It is vital that visual acuity and hearing are optimized as soon as possible using hearing aids and glasses if required. This will allow children the best chance to learn at home and in future educational settings. Children with significant visual impairment are referred to and managed by the visual impairment assessment team (VIAT). Like the HIAT (see above) this group includes representatives from health, education and social services and aims to maximize the child's potential.

Tests of vision for developmental screening

Vision should be tested at each developmental assessment. The nature of the test varies according to age. Postnatal examination should involve simple inspection and confirmation of the presence of the red reflex. At 6 weeks fixation and horizontal following should be confirmed in addition to the red reflex. By 8 months, test the full range of eye movements, symmetry of corneal reflections, and cover test if required, in addition to the red reflex. If screening is performed at 21 months vision testing should follow the same pattern as at 8 months. The first screening test of acuity can be performed at 3.5 years but this may be deferred if a universal orthoptic screening programme is in place for 4 year olds. Visual acuity is tested using a single-letter matching test (Sheridan–Gardiner or Stycar), should be uniocular with adequate occlusion and be performed at 3 or 6 m. A picture matching test (Kay pictures) may be used in the developmentally less able. No test of near acuity is required. If orthoptic testing is carried out, log Mar tests may be used (Glasgow cards). Eye movements, corneal reflections, red reflex or fundal examination should be repeated and a cover test performed with the child fixed on a far and then a near target. Distance visual acuity should be checked at school entry and, although crowded tests are preferable, a single-letter test is often required. Later tests of acuity should be using a Snellen chart at 6 m. If the acuity is reduced, the test should be repeated with a pinhole to indicate simple refractive errors. If colour vision is being tested, Ishihara plates should be used.

Learning difficulties with visual impairment

The true incidence of visual impairment in children with learning difficulties (or indeed the true incidence in the general population) is not known but is becoming increasingly recognized, particularly those with cerebral visual impairment. As the severity of the learning difficulties increases so does the likelihood of visual impairment. At least 20 per cent of children with severe learning difficulties have a significant visual impairment and refractive error is four times more common than in the general population. Sixty per cent of children who have a visual impairment have additional difficulties. There should be a high index of suspicion with certain other impairments: cerebral palsy, particularly diplegia or athetosis, and hydrocephalus. Visual impairment compounds the effects of learning difficulty affecting all areas of development: early bonding, language (verbal and non-verbal), gross and fine motor skills, spatial concepts, self-help, feeding, dressing, washing, toileting and sleep. Early recognition of visual difficulty is vital as some conditions, e.g. cataract, may be treatable and in non-treatable conditions in order that early intervention from home visiting teachers and therapists can be introduced to promote development and support parents.

Dual sensory impairment

Classically, the 'deaf-blind' child is affected by rubella or other congenital infections. In the UK, but not worldwide however, immunization has altered this and now the vast majority of children who have both a hearing and a visual impairment also have learning and other difficulties. These children are now more likely to have prematurity, cerebral malformation, postnatal meningitis/ encephalitis or a primary syndrome as a cause. The term multidisabled visually impaired (MDVI) is generally used in education and the voluntary agencies to describe these children's difficulties. Much of that which applies to the visually impaired child with learning difficulties also applies to these children. All children with developmental delay or learning difficulty need their vision and hearing assessed. Early diagnosis of these impairments is vital to avoid the risks of children 'shutting off' and rejection of, e.g. hearing aids, if prescribed later. Promoting the use of residual hearing or vision is important and experience through touch, smell, taste, etc. is required. A structured approach is required to aid children's understanding and the early introduction of objects of reference is useful. Parental support is necessary to promote bonding, etc., and this is usually provided by the preschool home visiting teacher service or education sensory support service.

Tests of vision at different ages

The commonest test of vision is visual acuity and this can be measured from birth using electrophysiological techniques. Other tests of vision, visual fields, contrast sensitivity, colour discrimination and light/dark adaptation, require more cooperation and therefore are used later. A gross measure of vision in the very young can also be achieved by inducing nystagmus using an optokinetic drum or spinning the child, indicating that some vision is present. From the age of 6 months, a measure of acuity can be made by preferential looking techniques – Keller cards. These can be used until around 18 months when interest is lost, and from 1 year, other preferential looking cards – Cardiff cards, can be used which may hold interest until 2.5 years. Picture (Kay) or letter (Stycar or Sheridan–Gardiner) matching tests can be used as soon as children can match. From 3 years, the standard test is a single-letter matching test. Crowded tests are superior to single-letter tests and should be used as soon as children are able – this may not be until the age of 6 or 7 years depending on experience and developmental level. In the past, the Snellen chart was seen as the 'gold standard' but this has been superseded by log Mar charts, particularly Glasgow cards.

Links with ENT and ophthalmology

Children may present with purely hearing or visual impairment, although many have other disabilities. Specialist visual impairment (VIAT) and hearing impairment teams (HIAT) include representatives from health often a community paediatrician, education and social services. These teams aim to maximize a child's potential and work closely with schools for the blind and deaf.

KEY LEARNING POINT

Close liaison between hearing assessment and ENT and vision assessment and ophthalmology is essential if defects are to be treated promptly and effectively.

COMMUNICATION: SPEECH AND LANGUAGE DEVELOPMENT

Normal developing children move through the stages of communication development at more or less the same time (Tables 1.3 and 1.4). By the age of 5 years, most children will have learned to use language to express their emotions, interact with others and manipulate their immediate environment. Children progress from using non-verbal communication, for example sending messages through sounds, actions, eye gaze and facial expression, to using spoken language. Although most children say their first

Table 1.3 The stages and variations that normally developing children go through as they develop communication

Age	Level of communication
Birth to 3 months	The infant communicates effectively using cries, comfort sounds and body movements
3–8 months	The infant shows an interest in people but does not yet communicate intentionally
8–13 months	The infant communicates with intention using sounds as if they were words and imitates adult sounds
12–18 months	The infant uses first words and communicates primarily for social reasons
18–24 months	Although using many single words the infant will now combine single words into two-word sentences. Vocabulary may increase to about 200 words
14–26 months	The child uses three-, four- and five-word sentences and good functional communication
3–5 years	The child uses long and complex sentences

Table 1.4 Speech sound development

Age	Speech sounds
3 years	m, b, p, h, w
4 years	k, g, t, d, n, ng, f
5 years	s, z, l, v, y, th, sh, cl
6 years	r, j

spoken words around 14 months they start learning about communication right from birth and continue to develop throughout childhood and early adulthood. Infants learn that their behaviour has an effect on others, and from that realization evolves intentional non-verbal communication, which forms the foundation for future communication.

There are several components in the development of communication. These include comprehension, expressive language, speech and language use. They must develop together in order that the result is effective communication. Certain prerequisites are necessary for the development of communication:

- Motivation
- Cognitive skills
- Short- and long-term memory
- Attention and listening skills
- Ability to symbolize.

Referral to education PRESCAT

Referral to an educational psychologist is made early often at the first child development clinic visit. This is often through the PRESCAT structure (see above), where health, education and social work professionals meet on a formal basis to discuss individual children.

ROLE OF EDUCATIONAL SPECIALISTS

Pre-school

Frequently, the educational psychologist will be given overall responsibility for coordinating the process of assessing and recording a child's special educational needs. Various education professionals, including psychologists, class teachers and learning support specialists, undertake educational psychological assessment and intervention. In the case of pre-school children, an educational home visitor may also contribute. The pre-school nursery is often the best place to judge the communication and concentration skills of young children. Certainly, autistic children will have difficulty and exhibit diagnostic traits in this 'normal' environment. Special nursery placement will also be able to assess how well an autistic child is likely to integrate into mainstream education and what level of learning support is likely to be needed. Nursery is also a sensible place to judge how difficult it will be to teach a child with attention deficit hyperactivity disorder in a mainstream school, the support that is likely to be needed and the effect of medication on ability to concentrate. Nursery teachers are in an ideal position to make assessment over time of whether a child has difficulties which will interfere with normal learning at school and judge progress over a prolonged period often as long as 24 months from 3 to 5 years of age.

School

Once at school, where the support normally provided in the class does not meet the child's needs, the member of teaching staff with responsibility for special educational needs (special needs coordinator) will decide whether to involve learning support staff. This specialist teacher will be able to advise on a suitable intervention and assist in the formulation of an individualized educational programme. Educational authorities should discover, at the earliest opportunity, those children with special educational needs to ensure that any necessary provision is made and to allow for planning of appropriate interventions. Again, a multidisciplinary approach to assessment is recommended and the team should include parents as well as professionals. Sharing of information and regular review are essential and parents and children should be empowered to feel they are partners in the process. Case conferences provide helpful means of enabling the team to achieve a more precise identification of the child's needs.

In the case of children with long-term and significant needs, the education authority may decide to open a Record of Needs. This statutory document summarizes the assessments undertaken, and outlines the services to be put in place to meet the special educational needs that have been identified.

Consequences of learning difficulties for a child may vary depending on the degree and nature of the difficulties. The severity of the learning difficulties can limit access to learning situations and restrict the variety of experience available to the child and there may be social, behavioural, medical and educational implications. Reflecting the philosophy of the European Convention on Human Rights, the Standard in Scotland's Schools (Scotland) Act 2000 introduced a statutory requirement of a presumption of mainstream schooling for all children, and states that only in exceptional circumstances should a child be educated in specialist provision. It is acknowledged that children with learning difficulties can show increased vulnerability and may need additional support or protection. However, it is essential to offer them the least restrictive environment possible and provide the opportunities for practising those skills learned in class.

The commonest referral to the child development team

The commonest reason by far for referral to child development teams in Glasgow is for speech delay. Children not speaking at their 22-month routine child health surveillance examination in primary care are often reviewed and commonly are referred to child development teams at about 2 years of age. We will have to wait and see if removing routine surveillance at 22 months (recommended in Hall 4) is detrimental. Parents are often worried about autism and feel that lack of progress or even regression took place at 12–15 months of age at the time of the measles, mumps, rubella (MMR) vaccination.

The first contact after a GP or health visitor referral will be with the specialist health visitor from the child development team, often in the patient's home. This important contact will allow background problems such as housing and other social circumstances to be assessed. Appointment at the child development centre will be with a community paediatrician, preferably in conjunction with a speech and language therapist. Full history and examination including an overall assessment of development (Schedule of Growing Skills version II) will be undertaken, with an examination of communication skills. From this early assessment, a plan will be constructed for further assessment for diagnosis and treatment.

A child with obvious significant problems in the area of communication will be referred to the community autism team for diagnosis, for hearing assessment by an educational audiologist and to PRESCAT who will allocate the case to an educational psychologist. Blood samples will be taken which will include fragile X as this condition has been associated with autism. Once a diagnosis of autistic spectrum disorder has been made, the family will meet and discuss the diagnosis with the community paediatrician and speech and language therapist attached to the community autism team. The educational psychologist will meet the family and discuss special nursery placement for assessment and therapy. The family will be referred to the social work resource worker to help the family successfully claim Disability Living Allowance. Six months or so prior to school entry a special educational needs assessment, initiated by the child's educational psychologist, will formalize all the assessments made by each professional group. This will involve the child's parents as pivotal members of a multidisciplinary team to try to find the most appropriate school placement for the child. The parents always have the last say as to which school their child attends be it mainstream or special.

A child whose communication skills are not in question at first assessment may undergo blood tests and will have a hearing assessment by an educational audiologist. Follow-up with results will be made after perhaps six months to assess progress. Speech and language follow-up may be made at home or in a nursery setting where the nursery staff will provide information on progress and the child can be assessed in a 'normal' environment.

CASE STUDY

A 3-year-old child was referred with speech delay and a lack of concentration. He was so difficult to control that the nursery initially refused to take him as he disrupted the class. He was a big boy and he was noted to be quite clumsy. He was impossible to engage in the Schedule of Growing Skills developmental assessment. Blood tests including fragile X were normal. Hearing test though difficult was normal. He was assessed in a special nursery for children with speech and language/communication disorders by an educational psychologist and speech and language therapist. He was diagnosed as being on the autistic spectrum.

CASE STUDY

A pair of 15-month-old twins who were much wanted *in vitro* fertilization (IVF) infants were seen after referral because one twin would not engage in play. Mother had experienced postnatal depression. The 'normal' twin was said to play well with his cousins and had a number of words. The 'abnormal' twin sat in a corner and would not engage in play associated with the Schedule of Growing Skills. He did not approach his parents and had poor eye contact. He said little and repeated 'dada' for all adults. Blood tests and hearing test were normal. He was assessed by the 'community autism team', which included a community paediatrician and a specialist speech and language therapist. After a number of visits to a group for children with speech and language disorders the 'abnormal' boy started to engage more and after a few months became as sociable as his twin.

KEY LEARNING POINT

The diagnosis of autism is often made by a team of speech and language therapists with help from community paediatricians (community autism team) who liaise for training with the Department of Child and Family Psychiatry. Educational assessment is made at special nurseries where teachers, speech therapists and an educational psychologist work with parents to decide appropriate school placement.

Many children with disability enter school with a diagnosis, having been through the process of multidisciplinary interagency evaluation that may lead to the opening of a Record of Special Needs. Some with learning difficulties will not present until after starting school. Some children will become newly disabled, e.g. after a severe head injury. School-age services for children with disability may be organized in different ways from pre-school services, however, the same professions need to be represented. Once a child starts in school, there must remain a forum so that health professionals can influence school-based therapies even to the extent of change of placement. Such advice and follow-up should be part of a child's 'individual educational programme'.

CASE STUDY

A child had a severe head injury in a road traffic accident. His cognitive function was mildly impaired, he had difficulty with concentration but he had a dense hemiparesis that had improved with daily physiotherapy in hospital. He started at a school for mild learning impairment and had once weekly physiotherapy by a non-resident physiotherapist who covered a large number of schools in the area. He managed in class but his hemiparesis was not improving. A multidisciplinary meeting decided after strong advice from the physiotherapist and the community paediatrician that this child required placement in a specialist school for physically handicapped children for assessment and treatment of his evolving hemiparesis.

This approach to the management of health issues in schools is supported by legislation, e.g. the Education (Scotland) Act 1980: 'An education authority can only lawfully establish that a child has pronounced specific or complex needs such as require continuing review and record him if he has undergone a process of observation and assessment including educational, psychological and medical assessment.' 'An education authority must ensure that the provision made by them for a recorded child or young person includes provision for his special educational needs that require assistance from health.' More recent legislation focuses on the disabled child: 'Every child has the right to receive school education and it is the duty of the education authority to secure education directed at the development of the child or young person to their fullest potential' (Standards in Scotland's Schools Act 2000).

Transition to adult care

A challenge for professionals working with disabled children is ensuring appropriate effective transition to adult services. This is often of great concern to families who perceive a loss of support. The Education Scotland Act 1980 supplies some supportive legislation for young people with a record of needs: 'Formal assessment is required to identify a child's "future" needs, which will include a medical assessment for children with health problems.' This process should start well before school leaving to allow appropriate planning. In practice, paediatric services often remain involved into early adulthood.

PAEDIATRIC PUBLIC HEALTH

Paediatric public health has both academic and service components. Academic paediatric public health focuses on obtaining grant funding for discrete pieces of research and publishing the findings in peer-reviewed journals. Paediatric public health physicians are also active in service planning and funding both nationally and locally. They work closely with health promotion departments as well as with primary, secondary and tertiary sick children's services, attempting to marry needs with limited resources.

Community paediatricians are involved in both academic and other aspects of paediatric public health and need to understand broader public health issues. This will allow them to access child health data, to look at population statistics and to use both parametric and non-parametric statistical analysis. Large child health surveillance datasets are established and added to on a routine basis. Little of this is collated and used for any purpose. This goldmine of information needs urgent attention and is ideal for small trainee projects.

An example

The Newborn Screening Laboratory performs tests for phenylketonuria, congenital hypothyroidism and cystic fibrosis on all neonates in Scotland using heel prick blood collected onto a Guthrie card from 7-day-old neonates by community midwives at home (see Table 1.1, page 3). Information is collected about type of feeding (breast/bottle) and hospital of birth. This information has been collated and is sent to all maternity units on an annual basis. Significant publications have emanated from this routinely collected data.

Child health promotion is a likely term to supersede child health surveillance. Examples of preventive activity include advice about immunization, reducing the risks of cot death, encouraging breastfeeding, dental prophylaxis, avoiding passive smoking, avoiding behaviour problems and accident prevention. Examples of a child health issue that touches all levels of paediatric care is childhood accidents and poisonings. Establishing an injury surveillance system is the first step towards preventing future accidents. Documenting *who, when, where, why* and *how* will pinpoint reasons for common accidents and assess the effect of intervention.

KEY LEARNING POINT

Like most health specialties, there are two components to paediatric public health: academic and NHS.

School nurses

School nurses have an important role as they are often the only healthcare workers in mainstream schools. As well as providing part of the immunization programme in school, they are increasingly involved in health promotion. School nurses have traditionally provided teaching within the curriculum on the subject of puberty. Other areas are now being targeted, including healthy eating. In special schools the school nurse is the primary healthcare worker backed up by a community paediatrician.

The problems of so-called elimination disorders, wetting and soiling, are common and distressing to both the child, family and to teaching staff. School nurses are now becoming experts in managing both night-time and day-time wetting and will perhaps in the future be experts at treating soiling. Clinics are emerging for these problems where school nurses work alongside community paediatricians. The Enuresis Resource and Information Centre (ERIC) has led the way in how to provide services for children who wet and soil (34 Old School House, Britannia Road, Kingswood, Bristol BS15 8DB, UK; tel: +44(0)117 9603060; email: info@eric.org.uk; website: www.eric.org.uk).

KEY LEARNING POINT

School nursing is moving towards a more population based public health role from a role that included more individual service provision.

CHILD MENTAL HEALTH

Over the past 10 years clinical psychology has emerged from its Cinderella status to be a part of mainstream community child health. Many children have behavioural difficulties which cause significant problems both within and outwith the family. Clinical psychologists are now members of the child development team and run behaviour clinics often in conjunction with a community paediatrician.

Autism has now come under the umbrella of the child development team with a diagnosis made on the International Classification of Diseases (ICD) 10 criteria after assessment by a speech and language therapy team that includes a developmental paediatrician.

It is likely in the future that follow-up of children with attention deficit hyperactivity disorder will fall under the umbrella of the child development team. At present, diagnosis and treatment is often established by child and family psychiatric services. This initial assessment may remain, but transfer to community paediatric care would allow close liaison with nursery and school. Adjustment to medication and liaison with clinical psychology to provide a behavioural programme would fit well with follow-up at nursery and school.

KEY LEARNING POINTS

- Community-based services are ideally placed to expand provision for problems with a significant behavioural aspect.
- Children with autism have specific educational requirements as do children with attention deficit hyperactivity disorder.
- Attention deficit hyperactivity disorder will become a disorder managed by a community child health multidisciplinary team.

REFERENCES

British Association for Community Child Health (2001). *Standards for Child Development Services*. London: Royal College of Paediatrics and Child Health.

Court SDM (1976) *Fit for the Future. Report of the Committee on Child Health Services*. London: HMSO.

Department of Health (1991) *Working Together Under the Children Act*. London: HMSO.

Hall DMB, Elliman D (eds) (2003) *Health for All Children*. Oxford: Oxford University Press.

Royal College of Paediatrics and Child Health (2002) *Strengthening the Care of Children in the Community. A Review of Community Child Health in 2001*. London: Royal College of Paediatrics and Child Health.

Scottish Executive (2004) *Health for All Children: Guidance on Implementation in Scotland*. A draft for consultation. Edinburgh: Scottish Executive.

Scottish Office (1997) *Scotland's Children: The Children (Scotland) Act 1995, Regulations and Guidance*. Vol. 1: Support and protection for children and their families; Vol. 2: Children looked after by the local authority; and Vol. 3: Adoption and Parental Responsibilities Orders, Edinburgh: Scottish Office.

Scottish Office (2000) *Protecting Children – A Shared Responsibility: Guidance for Health Professionals*. Edinburgh: Scottish Office.

Chapter 2

Behavioural and emotional problems

Michael Morton and Elaine Lockhart

APPROACHES TO CHILD AND ADOLESCENT MENTAL HEALTH

CLINICAL SKILLS FOR MANAGING BEHAVIOURAL AND EMOTIONAL PROBLEMS

The 'general goals' for general professional training in paediatrics and child health provide a good foundation for working with children with behavioural and emotional problems. The physical setting is important and should be welcoming, child friendly and low on distractions. Staff attitudes and values are also important and roles need to be clear. Clarity about responsibility helps to ensure that powerful emotional issues are well managed. An understanding of the management of anxiety in social systems is helpful. In working with emotional issues, practitioners need to ensure that they are not being driven by irrational anxieties generated within themselves or from the powerful feelings of others. Knowledge of mental mechanisms is essential and is discussed later. Discussion within a multidisciplinary team or with colleagues supports safe practice.

Assessment and communication

Assessment of individual and family functioning forms a basis for good communication. Thought needs to be given to the impact on families of the style of communication from the clinic, e.g. appointment letters and information leaflets. The appearance, dress and behaviour of staff may facilitate or inhibit communication. To facilitate communication with children, play and drawing materials should be available. Decisions need to be made about seeing children and young people separately from parents and parents away from children and about the time that can be given. Important issues of capacity and consent need time. Communication is supported by written information, e.g. writing to families after clinic attendance (Graham *et al.*, 1999).

It is essential to recognize non-verbal communications and physiological signs of arousal. The elements of the mental state assessment are shown in the box below. This approach may be needed with children or parents. Recognition of parental mental disorder may clarify children's needs. Maternal depression is a common harmful complication of the puerperium.

> Headings in a mental state examination
>
> General appearance (includes age appropriateness and dysmorphism)
>
> Level of awareness
>
> Motor activity
>
> Language and verbal communication
>
> Emotional presentation and reported mood
>
> Disturbance of thought (includes attentional difficulties, problems with memory and orientation)
>
> Perception (including signs of hallucination and other perceptual disturbance)
>
> Insight (capacity to reflect on psychological basis for difficulties)

Physical assessment will be directed by the presentation. Specific systematic examination will be more or less important according to presentation (e.g. abdominal examination in encopresis) and an understanding of the possible organic basis of symptoms. It may be necessary to look for signs of congenital disorder, including neurocutaneous syndromes. Neurological examination may be required. Physical investigation should be undertaken with attention to the possibility that unnecessary investigation may heighten anxiety or increase concerns about possible somatic disorder in an unhelpful fashion.

Family assessment requires training. Practitioners should note gross family dysfunction, such as parental mental illness or explicit emotional or physical abuse taking place in the consulting room. It is important to be aware of norms of behaviour and to identify children who are excessively clingy or dependent, as well as those who are unusually self reliant. In discussion of presenting symptoms and family understanding of difficulties and strategies to manage them, it may be possible to identify both strengths and deficits within the family. Family functioning can be thought about in terms of defined variables, e.g. quality of communication, allocation of roles within the family, behavioural controls, etc.

To understand family functioning it is important to consider input from grandparents or young children who may highlight difficulties that will not otherwise be apparent.

Relationship skills

Every contact between child and family and the health service is part of that family's relationship to the service. Negative experiences in the past may impact on current difficulties. It has been recognized that in chronic conditions a continuous relationship with one or more key professionals is valuable but often difficult to achieve. In behavioural and emotional disorders, the importance of the relationship between child and family and practitioner is crucial and factors within this relationship can determine the outcome of therapeutic interventions. Systems need to recognize the importance of relationships between families and clinicians and care needs to be taken with inevitable changeovers, such as junior doctor rotations. The longer the relationship, the more thought must be given to its termination, and planning for discharge or handover to adult services is recommended.

Therapeutic skills

An understanding of basic behavioural management, recognition of covert rewards for disruptive behaviour and acknowledgement of the value of rewarding good behaviour may be all that is required in simpler behaviour disorders. Rewards can be meaningfully linked to behaviour by the use of diaries or behaviour charts. Measuring difficult behaviours puts them in context and shows progress.

An understanding of cognitive difficulties that may entrench disorder and discussion with children and families about dysfunctional cognitions can be valuable. For example in psychological seizure, simple explanation of the disorder and the possible underlying mechanisms can lead to a resolution of difficulties. Emotional difficulties may need to be ventilated and the practitioner should be able to listen sympathetically to distress and support simple problem-solving approaches. More complex emotional difficulties may need more detailed assessment approaches, referral or specific treatment within the paediatric service. Many forms of psychological treatment require specialist training and it is helpful for a potential referrer to understand the principles of therapeutic modalities that may be available, including cognitive behavioural therapy, individual psychotherapy, play therapy, expressive therapies (art, music and drama) and family therapy. Group interventions may be particularly valuable in adolescents. Support groups for children with chronic illness require considerable commitment but can lead to positive outcomes. Group activities in residential settings such as camps for young patients with diabetes provide an opportunity to support healthy mental development and address problems in treatment adherence and adjustment to illness.

Drug treatments for child and adolescent emotional and behavioural disorders are generally the preserve of specialist practitioners and require careful assessment and monitoring (Kutcher, 1997). Many psychiatric indications for psychotropic treatment are not covered by drug licences and require discussion of the implications of their unlicensed status with children and families. (The Royal College of Paediatrics and Child Health (RCPCH) (2000) information sheet on this topic is most helpful).

Sedation needs to take account of physical risks and also the possible impact on learning and development of chronic use of sedative medications. Melatonin may be useful in some children with sleep disorders but should only be initiated after assessment of sleep hygiene (Ross *et al.*, 2002). Drug treatments may be valuable in enuresis and constipation related to encopresis. Methylphenidate may be prescribed in attentional disorders and should be initiated by a specialist (National Institute for Clinical Excellence (NICE), 2000). Long-term monitoring arrangements must be in place if the prescription is to be continued and consideration needs to be given to reviewing the use of this drug as it is to be hoped that children will not need to remain on medication throughout their development. Other drug treatments for attentional disorders require more specialist assessment (Scottish Intercollegiate Guidelines Network (SIGN), 2001).

It is now recognized that antidepressants have a place in the treatment of obsessional-compulsive disorders and possibly also in childhood depression. Specific serotonin reuptake inhibitors have little cardiotoxicity and reduced risk in overdose although like the older tricyclic antidepressants they can have other side effects that may interfere with adherence and outweigh the therapeutic benefit. Carbamazepine and sodium valproate have recognized functions in stabilizing mood disorders in adults and may be beneficial in mood and behavioural disorders in some children. Psychotic disorders require antipsychotic medication as in adult psychiatry.

Although there is limited anecdotal literature of the use of drugs to help conduct symptoms and aggression, in general this is not justified. Specific circumstances such as developmental disorder or learning disability may mean that drug treatments have more of a place if alternative treatment approaches fail. It is sometimes necessary for specialist clinics to consider whether the risks associated with prescribing are outweighed by the harm that may come to children as a result of family or school placement breakdown where behavioural disturbance has not been manageable in other ways. In an acute situation the use of drugs that help to control impulsivity may contain a crisis but it is generally preferable to use human supports for children rather than drug treatment. Benzodiazepines may be helpful in crisis but a proportion of children will become disinhibited.

Capacity for reflection

Although specific clinical skills are valuable in the management of emotional and behavioural disorders the importance of reflection on the process of decision making cannot be underestimated. Psychiatric training emphasizes the importance of supervision and consultation with colleagues.

KEY LEARNING POINTS

- Tackling behavioural and emotional disorders requires careful attention to communication and to the setting in which families are seen.
- Important information can be gathered by assessing the mental state of both children and parents.
- Assessment of a family's strengths and weaknesses is helpful for understanding and addressing problems.
- Paediatricians should develop basic skills and be aware of the range of therapies available.

ORGANIZATION OF SERVICES FOR CHILD AND ADOLESCENT MENTAL HEALTH AND MULTIDISCIPLINARY WORKING

All professionals working with children have a role to play in the promotion of psychological wellbeing, prevention of emotional and behavioural disorders and their early detection. The further management of these problems will depend upon the complexity of the difficulties and the local availability of specialized mental health practitioners.

The promotion of mental health and wellbeing and prevention of disorder

Opportunities for promotion of children's mental health arise in all encounters with them regardless of the setting, e.g. Health, Education, etc. Healthy development is promoted by good antenatal care, support for new mothers, parenting programmes, availability of good quality childcare and pre-school facilities, supportive educational environments, etc. There is a clear link between adverse socioeconomic factors, e.g. unemployed parents, poor housing and low income and an increased rate of mental health disorders and mild learning disability. Health services need to work with other agencies and at a higher political level to devise social policies that will have a beneficial effect on the mental health of a community as a whole.

The above could be described as primary prevention. Professionals working with children will be involved in a range of preventive strategies.

Pre-school services

Most services set up for children in the community focus primarily on health surveillance and early interventions. At this stage, it is almost impossible and unwise to separate detection of physical disorders from those of an emotional and behavioural nature and a trained practitioner will evaluate the global developmental progress of children. In addition to planned checks, health visitors, general practitioners and practice nurses will have other contacts with families which allow for further assessment and discussion of problems. Most children attend nursery placement for at least a year prior to school entry. This is the setting for many behavioural and developmental problems to be uncovered and assessed. Some children will need to be referred to specialist child and adolescent mental health services but most will be treated by parents and nursery staff, sometimes with the help of a psychologist.

CASE STUDY

A 4-year-old boy at nursery was referred by staff to the child development clinic with delayed speech, solitary play and aggression. Assessment involved the community paediatrician, speech therapist and clinical psychologist. A diagnosis of autism was made. These professionals liaised with educational staff regarding school placement and he was referred to a pre-school programme run by his local department of child psychiatry.

School services

Once children start school they will have contact with health services in this setting. In the UK, educational psychologists work in schools assessing children with suspected psychological or learning difficulties and providing short treatment programmes.

Throughout childhood, social services play a major role in care and protection issues and in supporting families with difficulties. Frequently different agencies – health services, education and social services – work separately, even with the same families, but there is a move towards more joint planning and delivery of services, e.g. joint assessment teams in schools.

Multidisciplinary teams in hospitals

In the hospital setting many different professionals work with children, whether in a multidisciplinary team or by contributing their expertise on a case by case basis.

Within paediatric teams, doctors, nurses and other professionals contribute to assessments and treatment plans which include psychosocial aspects of care. Emotional and behavioural problems are often picked up by those working most closely with children, e.g. nurses, play therapists, physiotherapists, etc. How this is managed will depend upon local availability of mental health professionals, e.g. a clinical psychologist may be attached to the team, there may be a psychiatric liaison service or cases may be referred on to community-based clinics. In complex cases, a range of disciplines may have a role, e.g. speech and language therapy, occupational therapy, teachers and hospital-based social workers.

Child and adolescent mental health services

Well resourced child and adolescent mental health services (CAMHS) will have a variety of professionals working together in a multidisciplinary team. Usually teams will have psychiatrists, nurses, psychologists and social workers. Other professionals may also be present, e.g. art therapists, family therapists, psychotherapists, speech and language therapists and teachers. Effective team functioning requires attention to be paid to communication between team members, clarity about roles and responsiveness to changing need.

Child and adolescent mental health services are generally organized on a tiered basis ranging from tier one primary care workers to tier four inpatient and regional services (NHS Health Advisory Service, 1995). Integrated services aim to provide seamless care according to the severity and complexity of children's difficulties. There is much scope for joint training, service planning and working between paediatrics and CAMHS given that many of the children are seen by both or have similar problems.

KEY LEARNING POINTS

- All professionals working with children can promote mental health as well as implementing preventive and treatment work.
- Health professionals need to work with other agencies in planning and providing services for children's health, both physical and emotional.
- Well functioning multidisciplinary teams allow professionals to contribute their expertise to the assessment and treatment of children.

NORMAL EMOTIONAL AND BEHAVIOURAL DEVELOPMENT AND THE DEVELOPMENT OF PERSONALITY

Genetic and environmental factors play a complex interactive role in how the child develops physically, cognitively and emotionally from their prenatal state onwards (Goodman and Scott, 1997). Brain development is largely under genetic control, with usually multiple genes being involved but requires a nurturing environment which meets the infant's biological and emotional needs.

The fetal brain needs a healthy environment free of illness or toxins to develop normally. A traumatic or prolonged delivery may result not only in physical disability, e.g. cerebral palsy, epilepsy or learning disabilities, but also in an associated non-specific increase in risk of developing emotional or behavioural problems.

Temperament and personality

Historically, it was believed that babies were born in a helpless state and their development was totally dependent upon their environment. Chess and Thomas (1995) established that babies are temperamentally different, categorizing them as being 'easy', 'difficult' or 'slow to warm up' in terms of how they establish feeding routines, respond to people, etc. These categories demonstrate consistency throughout childhood. A baby's temperament can have either a positive or adverse effect on the quality of care he or she receives.

Feeding

Establishing successful feeding in the early days is essential for providing adequate nutrition to the developing, growing baby. It also facilitates the development of a mutually rewarding relationship with the main caregiver. Problems may arise due to illness in the baby or the mother, abnormalities of the baby's mouth and gastrointestinal system or maternal anxiety, especially if breastfeeding.

Attachment theory and personality

Bowlby (1988) developed a theory (attachment theory) which describes how from birth babies will, in a genetically predetermined manner, establish an intense two-way relationship with their caregivers. He described attachment as an adaptive, biological process by which babies maintains close contact with their mothers to meet their needs for care and protection.

Ainsworth and colleagues (1978) developed attachment styles further. They described children as having the following attachment styles:

- Secure
- Anxious/resistant
- Anxious/avoidant
- Disorganized/disorientated.

There is evidence that children who establish a secure attachment with their mothers and other family members later have an enhanced capacity to develop social relationships. Conversely, those with poor attachment patterns struggle with developing relationships, both socially and in the quality of their relationships with their own children.

Progress through childhood

Children need not only adequate care, nutrition, housing and security but also an appropriate environment that encourages their development through play and exploration of their surroundings. Their development needs to be viewed in the context of their family's life cycle (Carr, 1999), e.g. their arrival creates a significant shift in how their parents view themselves and their changed circumstances. As children grow older their parents are confronted by their own parents' increasing age and frailty. How children manage their developmental tasks will be significantly influenced by how their parents are managing their own challenges and by the support they receive.

In adolescence, the task is to negotiate increased autonomy and peer relations while maintaining supportive family bonds. At different ages, young people acquire legal rights to engage in activities such as buying cigarettes, sexual intercourse, driving cars and voting. Most young people maintain reasonable relationships with significant adults but views may differ and rebellion is seen as normal.

KEY LEARNING POINTS

- Genetic and environmental factors play an interactive role in emotional and behavioural development.
- Temperamental styles and patterns of attachment in early life predict later emotional well-being and quality of relationships.
- Children require a nurturing environment which fosters growth and development.

Effects of stress on children at different ages

Stress may be physical or psychological in nature. It arises as a result of life events and is maintained by chronic adversities. The effects of stress in childhood are to varying degrees mediated by adults. The fetal response is almost inseparable from the mother's. The response to stress is physiological in the fetus and neonate and has an increasingly psychological component as cognitive and emotional maturation proceeds. The hypothalamic–pituitary–adrenal axis and the autonomic nervous system mediate physiological stress responses. Although the acute effects of stress are well known, the chronic physical effects of stress are less well described. Some children may be physically or psychologically more resilient and an interaction with environmental supports and family vulnerabilities determines individual responses.

Psychological reactions to stress may be divided between principally conscious behavioural strategies, described as coping behaviours, and predominantly unconscious reactions known as defence mechanisms.

Coping behaviours depend on cognitive capacity. They include the strategy of seeking a rational understanding for the causes of stress, particularly valuable to the school-age child. Anticipated difficulties may be helped by rehearsal in play. Development of problem solving skills may be encouraged to support the process of adjustment to stress.

Psychological defence mechanisms are not as reliably adaptive as coping behaviours. Defence mechanisms may provide an individual with a way of managing unbearable stress and should not be regarded as maladaptive unless there is evidence that the nature or persistence of the mechanism is interfering with the process of adjustment. Common defence mechanisms include **denial**, which can be useful. **Displacement** of feelings is also common, for example a child who has not grieved for the death of a parent might become severely angry as a result of the loss of a favourite toy. This should be distinguished from **projection** of feelings where an individual who is not able to deal with their own emotional state identifies and responds to these feelings as if they were located in someone else. **Rationalization** is the mechanism whereby an individual discounts the importance of emotion by attribution of false meaning. Regression is seen when a child in need of additional support adopts a more infantile pattern of behaviour with which such support is more normally associated.

> Some examples of mental mechanisms
>
> **Denial:** An adolescent with a terminal cancer persists in a false hope of recovery, without conscious awareness of the falseness of their position. By not facing facts the young person is able to avoid unbearable feelings and pass time constructively.
>
> **Projection:** A child is very angry with his teacher but is frightened to express that anger. The child wrongly believes that the teacher is angry with him.
>
> **Rationalization:** A boy with behaviour problems arising from distress at family conflict which is impairing his education may be described by parents as having normal problems in the classroom 'like any boy'.

Doctors working with children and young people under stress will find many examples of psychological defence mechanisms. Regression is common and adaptive as long as the child and family are able to move on as part of the progress towards health. If unrecognized, projection is one of the most damaging defence mechanisms in clinical practice and can lead to intense but misplaced emotions around the ill child. Clinicians should seek to support effective coping strategies, which minimize the need for defence mechanisms. Defence mechanisms should be recognized and respected, being challenged only when they are impeding recovery.

When stress is overwhelming

Extreme stress, or trauma, may overwhelm an individual's capacity for coping and overcome defence mechanisms. Psychological reactions to overwhelming stress may be acute and transient but the effects may persist in the form of post-traumatic stress disorder (page 50). Less extreme maladaptive responses to stress in childhood may be categorized as externalizing or internalizing mechanisms. Externalization is a process by which stressed children cause distress in others. This may be adaptive if the child's behaviour leads to adult help being mobilized.

> ### CASE STUDY: Successful externalization
>
> A 7-year-old boy suddenly develops oppositional behaviour, which alerts his teacher to his mother's treatable depression.

Internalization describes an emotional process that is easier to understand but often overlooked. Depression, fearfulness and social withdrawal are common signs of internalized distress. Somatic symptoms may occur in internalizing disorders but in some children somatic symptoms are found as a result of stress without any associated emotional state. Somatization (the expression of distress through bodily complaints) is more likely to occur in individuals who lack the capacity to express feelings more directly. Developmental factors are important in understanding this process, found at its simplest in the recurrence of bed-wetting in a child under stress.

KEY LEARNING POINTS

- The hypothalamic–pituitary–adrenal axis and autonomic nervous system mediate physiological stress responses accompanied by a psychological component.
- It is helpful for paediatricians to understand conscious coping behaviours and unconscious defence mechanisms.
- Overwhelming stress may lead to externalizing and internalizing reactions.

PSYCHOLOGICAL ASPECTS OF PHYSICAL ILLNESS

Stress and support associated with illness and treatment

Illness and treatment may be significant stressors, but advantages may come from illness as well as difficulties. Stress can be modified by factors relating to the disease, the child, the family and wider social systems.

Education support may make a significant difference to long-term adjustment. School health services and educational psychologists can ensure access to the curriculum and modify the school environment to minimize disadvantages in relation to illness and treatment.

Some children benefit from considerable social supports, as well as financial support, whereas others receive few benefits. Provision of expenses to allow hospital visiting and respite support may allow families to organize themselves around the needs of the sick child and siblings. Family assessment highlights family strengths and areas where support may be required. A good marriage, realistic attitudes, satisfactory adaptation, stability, warmth, cohesion and satisfactory parental communication predict a better outcome (Lask and Fosson, 1989). Psychosocial assessment may be particularly important where demanding treatment depends upon family support. Such assessments have been used to support decisions about prioritization, for example in the early days of renal transplantation. A sick child depends on communication amongst adults involved. Difficulties are magnified where the impact of illness on the child is not well understood and even more so where there are conflicting views about the illness, treatment and supports required.

Hospitalization affects the whole family. The pre-school child is particularly vulnerable and 'rooming in' practices of children's wards reflect this. Home-based treatments are preferable, but hospitalization can provide respite. The provision of resources for play and education, as well as family support, may reduce the stress of hospitalization. Good quality information reduces fear and pretreatment visits and play interventions can be helpful. Intensive care settings are particularly stressful.

The death of a child carries particular resonance. There are different views within society about postmortem care. Consideration needs to be given to information available to children and their families. Perceived risks of death should be acknowledged even where professionals do not see the same level of risk as the family. Some experiences carry fear of death, which may be compounded by a lack of understanding.

CASE STUDY

A parent's experience of their 4-year-old's first seizure was dominated by a fear that the child was dying. Until this was identified and discussed the parent continued to have excessive anxiety in relation to seizure events and was not reassured by the diagnosis of epilepsy.

Illness-specific stresses

It is important to define specific stresses associated with illness, which specific interventions may alleviate. For example, disfiguring conditions may affect self-perception, which develops in the context of the reaction of others. Early cosmetic correction may improve outcome. In cleft lip and palate, external appearance may be corrected but it is also important to address the disruption of communication arising from disorder. There is more uncertainty about the benefits of early surgery to correct facial stigmata of Down syndrome. There is debate about the extent to which defects should be addressed within the child as opposed to tackling societal attitudes to disfigurement and disability.

In some circumstances, illness-specific factors lead to behavioural disturbance. For example, parathyroid disorder may be associated with specific behavioural disturbance, alleviated by better control of calcium levels. Behavioural disturbance also may arise as a result of treatment, e.g. the behavioural side effects of steroids. An organically based deterioration in behaviour may be better tolerated if the cause is understood. On the other hand, undue allowances for the effects of organic illness may entrench difficulties. Thoughtful discussion of these issues with parents and teachers is required.

Psychophysiological cycles

The interaction between anxiety and autonomic arousal is central to the interaction between stress and physical illness. Symptoms are modified by emotional state and the meaning attributed to it. High anxiety may lead to magnified perception of minor symptoms. Children in distress require adult understanding. Some adults may be excessively anxious that the extreme nature of the child's distress may indicate extreme physical pathology. Other adults may respond that the child is 'putting it on'. Children who are generally distressed find inappropriate adult responses unhelpful and may become even more distressed and insistent upon their symptoms. Differences between adults will compound the problem. Where anxiety is a significant factor in the presentation of symptoms, it is essential that the interaction of anxiety and symptoms is understood and that the child is assured that the adults understand. Medical approaches to assessment and treatment need to take account of iatrogenic anxiety. Some conditions such as migraine and recurrent abdominal pain seem to be triggered by stressful experiences. Stresses arising as a result of a condition may compound the problem as seen in the following case.

CASE STUDY

A child misses school because of abdominal pain and finds it difficult to return because of the work and social contact that have been missed. School return creates further stress, which triggers further pain, compounding the difficulty in managing school. A psychophysiological cycle leads to a psychiatric problem 'school phobia'.

The diagnostic problems of pain and fatigue

Both pain and fatigue syndromes may be classified within the psychiatric section of the International Classification of Diseases (ICD) (F Codes) (World Health Organization (WHO), 1992) but these symptoms are also found elsewhere in the classification (R52 – pain not elsewhere classified; and R53 – malaise and fatigue). The ICD expects practitioners to distinguish between pain and fatigue of physical or psychological origin but this is not always possible. A psychophysiological approach to pain and fatigue in childhood may be preferable to a dualist model. This holistic approach may be difficult to sustain in the face of entrenched positions within our culture, exemplified in discussion about chronic fatigue syndrome. Whereas some physicians argue for a purely organic aetiology for this condition, others insist on the importance of psychological factors; this may be a false dichotomy. The limitations of the current diagnostic framework for pain syndromes and fatigue disorders mean that symptoms are best understood in a biopsychosocial context. This is a useful approach in all childhood disorders. Treatment planning depends upon the relative significance of factors precipitating and maintaining symptoms. Diagnostic certainty is valuable but it is not helpful to provide definite statements about matters that are not definitely understood.

Family factors

The meaning of illness is defined in the context of culture and family. Family history may alter the psychological impact of symptoms, e.g. a child who develops asthma in the context of a relative having died in status asthmaticus will be likely to be a focus for family anxiety. Where a child's condition has a strong genetic basis there is likely to be a family culture in relation to the disease, which may determine the child's adaptation. Behavioural phenotypes associated with some disorders may affect adjustment as in Huntington chorea. A child's presentation may be particularly shocking because it uncovers genetic disease not previously recognized in the family.

CASE STUDY

A child collapses with a dissecting aortic aneurysm, he is the first member of his family to be diagnosed with Marfan syndrome. Family members are screened for aortic dilatation, with much attendant anxiety.

Genetic advances provide opportunities to predict the risk of disease prior to conception. Genetic counselling and appraisal of risks may support healthy adjustment. On the other hand a child born following particular effort to ensure health may have to carry the burden of adult expectations. There is a particular difficulty where a healthy child is born following the death of an infant, if the new baby is seen as a 'replacement child'.

Consent and related issues

UK law recognizes the responsibility of parents to give consent to medical procedures on behalf of young children. It is good practice that even the youngest children should be given some explanation of procedures and a child's consent should be sought where possible. This may be the first stage in a doctor–patient relationship that can be helpful in subsequent illness episodes. Adolescents have increasing autonomy in decision making. In some families there may be high levels of conflict in relation to the young person's desire for autonomy and this may focus on a medical condition. Young people with chronic illnesses such as diabetes and cystic fibrosis need to face many personal adjustments to illness in adolescence, which they will not have considered earlier in development. Parents may be anxious about handing over responsibility for aspects of treatment to rebellious adolescents. Paediatricians have an important role in educating young people and supporting parents in recognizing young people's developing responsibility for their own illness and treatment.

Within the UK, young people aged 16 years and over generally have the same rights to consent or refuse medical treatment as adults. In Scotland there is a legal framework for dealing with adults who are incapable of these decisions but in England and Wales the problem of obtaining medical consent for the treatment of incapable adults is still subject to review. Children under 16 years have the right to give consent for medical treatment if certain circumstances are fulfilled. In England and Wales the tests include a consideration of the child's understanding of the benefits, risks and alternatives, and the consequences of not having the treatment, the child should be able to retain information for long enough to make an effective decision and be in a position to make a choice, free from pressure. In Scotland, the Age of Legal Capacity Act 1991 states that a child may consent if the medical practitioner attending them 'considers the child capable of understanding the nature and possible consequences of the procedure or treatment' and if a child has capacity, the child's consent should be sought rather than that of the parent. Parents may be surprised to find that where the child is capable they lose the right to consent on the child's behalf. Where the child is not capable, parental consent must be sought. It is good practice to involve the parent in helping the child to reach a decision, unless there are particular concerns about confidentiality.

Where there is conflict about consent and children or parents are deemed not capable of giving or withholding consent to treatment, three important legal frameworks may be invoked. The Common Law is relevant in emergency situations where there is an expectation that practitioners will act in the best interests of patients. Children's legislation is useful when parents are perceived as not acting in their child's best interests. Mental health legislation is relevant where consent is not obtained for the assessment and treatment of mental disorder. In decisions regarding treatment of children, doctors should proceed in the child's best interests with due regard to the law. Practice based upon this principle is likely to lead to the best chance of engaging children and young people in meaningful discussion of consent and improved treatment adherence. Where the doctor–patient relationship has broken down, both doctor and patient factors may be important and the involvement of another clinician may be helpful. The significance of stress and anxiety in child, family and medical staff should not be underestimated. Adolescents are at greater risk than children of developing psychiatric illness and the presence of physical illness can make the recognition of psychiatric disease particularly difficult. Mental health professionals may have a significant role in supporting paediatric teams where there are concerns about possible psychiatric disorder or family factors affecting capacity to consent or adhere to treatment.

KEY LEARNING POINTS

- Psychosocial factors play an important role in how the child and family manage illness and treatment.
- The interaction between stress and physical illness is mediated by a psychophysiological cycle involving anxiety and autonomic arousal.
- A biopsychosocial approach to all childhood disorders is useful, particularly with pain and fatigue syndromes.
- Paediatricians require knowledge and understanding of law governing consent issues and its application to children and adolescents.

BEHAVIOURAL PROBLEMS AND PSYCHIATRIC DISORDERS

CONCEPTS OF NORMALITY AND DIAGNOSIS

Difference is not necessarily disorder. It is good practice to think of a profile of strengths and weaknesses. Factors such as overactivity or disorders of attention may be on a continuum. Normality may be defined according to the significance attributed to individual deviations from a population norm. Some patterns of behaviour are recognized as normal responses to experience. Oppositional behaviour may be an understandable reaction to stress. A child who appears overactive in a high-rise flat may function well on a farm. Transient depressive states, labile moods and thoughts of suicide in adolescents are common and have little diagnostic significance unless there are associated signs of disturbance.

It is important to distinguish between normal adjustment to stress and disorders where adjustment processes have broken down to the extent that an individual is experiencing symptoms which interfere with healthy development and social functioning. Adjustment disorders may involve emotional and behavioural symptoms and may progress into specific disorders, such as needle phobia or depression. Supporting the emotional task of

Table 2.1 International Classification of Diseases (ICD)-10 multiaxial classification

Axis 1	Psychiatric disorder
Axis 2	Specific disorders of psychological development (e.g. motor coordination disorder)
Axis 3	Intellectual level (mental retardation)
Axis 4	Medical conditions (diagnoses from non-psychiatric sections of the ICD-10)
Axis 5	Associated abnormal psychosocial situations
Axis 6	A global assessment of psychosocial disability

adjustment to stress may relieve disorder but more specific treatment may be required.

A distinction may be drawn between common, uncomplicated **behavioural problems** and **psychiatric disorders**, which justify diagnosis within the ICD (WHO, 1992), or an alternative system, such as the *Diagnostic and Statistical Manual* (DSM) of American Psychiatric Association (1994). Psychiatrists in the UK use a multiaxial version of the ICD which draws together biopsychosocial factors (Table 2.1).

Many child psychiatric disorders are common and child mental health services are sparse. Paediatricians should have sufficient expertise to deal with common psychiatric disorders. Understanding of the multiaxial classification can help decisions about referral. A range of psychosocial stressors contributes to the impact of psychiatric disorder and may define the need for child psychiatric intervention. Symptom severity is also important in deciding whether or not a child requires specialist referral.

COMMON BEHAVIOURAL PROBLEMS

The crying baby

Infants differ in temperament and some seem to spend most of their waking hours crying (Black and Cottrell, 1993). Mothers usually know what their baby's cry means but for inexperienced parents it can be an exhausting puzzle. Doctors should investigate likely medical causes of persistent crying (e.g. pain) while being alert to potential problems in the parent–child relationship. Management involves treating underlying causes, practical advice and support, and regular review until the situation resolves.

Sleep disorders

Most infants and young children develop a settled sleeping routine with 85 per cent of 6-month-old infants sleeping through the night and only 10 per cent of 1-year-olds waking regularly.

> Sleep disorders
>
> - Dyssomnias include settling problems and night waking
> - Parasomnias include nightmares, night terrors and sleep walking
> - Hypersomnias include narcolepsy and the Klein–Levin syndrome

Difficulties in going to sleep and night waking are the commonest sleep disorders in pre-school children. They may be due to biological factors, e.g. serious illness, psychosocial factors, e.g. stressful life events, or a combination of both.

Nightmares are disturbing dreams which may be triggered by exposure to frightening events. They reach a peak at 5–6 years and usually diminish in frequency thereafter. If they occur more than twice a week, they may be part of an anxiety disorder and require treatment. Night terrors cause the child to sit up, scream as if in distress, although unresponsive, with no recollection the next day. If they persist, a behaviour management programme involving waking the child up just before the onset of symptoms has been shown to be effective.

Feeding problems

Feeding difficulties, poor appetite and, later, food fads are common in infants and young children. They may reflect temperamental difficulties in the child, medical conditions, learning disability, parental overanxiety or disturbed parent–child interaction. Management will therefore require physical examination of the child, assessment of the child–parent relationship and family's social circumstances.

Non-organic failure to thrive

This can be diagnosed only after exclusion of any underlying medical conditions. Sometimes, the reason for a child to fail to put on weight and grow satisfactorily is due to a combination of organic and non-organic factors. Management needs to address the salient issues and input from a dietitian in establishing a successful eating programme is invaluable. Often many agencies will need to work together for a successful outcome.

CASE STUDY

A 4-year-old girl was referred to a paediatrician with failure to thrive. All investigations were normal and during admission her weight increased. She was the third of four children to a single mother who appeared depressed. Management involved input from social services to support the mother and a referral to the adult mental health services.

Toddler training

For parents the toddler years can be both immensely rewarding and challenging (Green, 1992). Difficulties may reflect the quality of family relationships. Paediatricians will frequently be asked about the management of behavioural problems. They are common, especially temper tantrums and overactivity, but tend to be short lived. For most parents reassurance is all that is needed. Behavioural management approaches to challenging behaviour in toddlers help the parents to:

- avoid predictable difficult situations, e.g. by distraction or diversion
- consistently praise positive behaviour
- ignore negative behaviour as much as possible
- establish firm, consistent limits to the child's behaviour.

Parenting groups are effective in providing alternative ways of managing children's difficult behaviour in addition to providing mutual support.

Enuresis

This is defined as the involuntary passing of urine after the age of 5 years with no organic cause. It is helpful to think of it as a developmental delay although there is a non-specific association with emotional and behavioural problems (Green, 1992; Royal College of Psychiatrists, 1999). Enuresis may be diurnal, nocturnal or both. Secondary enuresis occurs after being dry for at least six months and is primary if never dry.

Associations of enuresis

- Family history (70 per cent)
- Stressful life events
- Social disadvantage
- Other developmental problems

Most cases are managed in primary care. Referral may be for exclusion of underlying organic causes or where problems persist. Information about waterproof bedding protection and useful literature can be purchased from Education and Resources for Improving Childhood Continence (ERIC) (website: www.eric.org.uk). Assessment requires a detailed history of the wetting, enquiry about other urological symptoms, faecal soiling or other problems. Urinary microscopy and culture is essential to rule out infection, with other investigations as clinically indicated.

The choice of treatment will depend upon the main concerns expressed by the family, e.g. the child being able to spend nights away from home without embarrassment and the motivation of the child and parents to participate in a programme. A combination of a behaviour management programme and medication is most effective. Most children with enuresis do not need psychiatric help but a few may need referral to CAMHS.

Encopresis

Encopresis, a developmental disorder, is defined as a disorder of bowel function and control over the age of 4 years in the absence of underlying physical pathology and is about three times more common in boys than in girls.

CASE STUDY

A 6-year-old girl is referred to a paediatrician for management of soiling. Her parents had separated when she was 3 years old. She had never been toilet trained and examination revealed chronic constipation with overflow.

Reasons for faecal soiling

- No habit of sitting on the toilet
- Constipation with overflow
- Fear of pain passing stools
- Toilet phobia
- Stress-induced loss of control
- Provocative soiling

Some children have two or more of the difficulties listed in the box above. Each needs to be addressed within the overall management plan. Successful behavioural programmes depend upon engaging the child and family and providing adequate support, monitoring medication and bowel functioning as required. In severe, complex cases encopresis is best dealt with by joint working between paediatricians, CAMHS and primary care.

KEY LEARNING POINTS

- The success of toileting programmes will be determined by initially resolving underlying physical problems, e.g. constipation.
- Underlying difficulties need to be identified and addressed, e.g. an anal fissure causing the child to retain faeces.
- Encopresis may occur as part of a more generalized emotional disorder in the context of significant family dysfunction.
- Sexual abuse should always be considered.

Where children smear faeces on walls or furniture, there are usually multiple significant difficulties within the child and family. Successful management may require input from education and social services in addition to paediatrics and CAMHS.

DISORDERS CHARACTERIZED BY BEHAVIOURAL DISTURBANCE

Oppositional behaviour and conduct disorder

Behaviour disorders may arise in children where adverse temperamental characteristics have been identified from birth. Environmental factors such as parental behaviour may be a primary aetiological factor in the child's difficulties (for example, maternal depression or excessive criticism). Parenting styles may develop as a reaction to the child's behaviour, which in turn lead to further difficulties. Some parents who are capable of effective parenting of a temperamentally easy child may have serious difficulties in parenting an oppositional sibling. Family processes may contribute to difficulties, for example a tendency to blame the identified child as a way of avoiding other problems within the family.

In children under the age of 10 years, the label **oppositional defiant disorder** may be used where there is repetitive or persistent, markedly defiant, disobedient and provocative behaviour without more severe dissocial or aggressive acts. Around 3–4 per cent of pre-school children may fulfil criteria for this diagnosis. There is continuity between early oppositional defiant behaviour and subsequent conduct disorder although progression is not inevitable. Interventions for such children should be based upon behavioural principles. It is important to involve both parents in counselling where possible. Behavioural advice and family counselling may be supported by social interventions including the provision of good pre-school care or family support.

Conduct disorder is defined by the presence of repetitive and persistent patterns of dissocial, aggressive or defiant conduct, violating age-appropriate social expectations to a severe degree and violating the law or the rights of others. This includes behaviours such as excessive fighting or bullying, cruelty to animals or other people, severe destructiveness, fire-setting, stealing, truancy and other persistent, severely disobedient or provocative behaviours. Presenting behaviours change with age. Conduct disorder should not be diagnosed in the presence of serious underlying psychiatric disorder, such as **pervasive developmental disorder**. The label **hyperkinetic conduct disorder** describes children where constitutional hyperkinesis accompanies severe social disturbance. The diagnosis of conduct disorder although clear within the ICD is not accepted in all professional groups and concepts of behavioural disturbance and delinquency may be used as alternative ways of thinking about difficult behaviour. Conduct disorder is common with prevalence rates of between 3 and 5 per cent in general population studies, increasing in the inner cities. It is markedly more common in boys and dysfunctional families. Social class is a less important factor than associated social conditions, such as overcrowding, neighbourhood unemployment and crime rates. Factors within schools can reduce rates of truancy and other forms of delinquency among their pupils. The influence of ethnicity on recognition of conduct disturbance confounds attempts to identify associations with this factor.

CASE STUDY

James, age 13 years, lives with his mother who is single and unemployed with an alcohol problem. Undiagnosed dyslexia has led to school failure and truancy with older boys involved in shoplifting. Police refer him for social services assessment. Social intervention does not address his educational difficulty and the outcome is poor.

Conduct disorder is rooted in social factors but individual variables are also important. Children with aggressive tendencies may seek out exposure to violent images which in turn may increase the risk of violent behaviour amongst boys. Fire-setting behaviour generally occurs as part of conduct disorder, but in a few cases arson is related to more profound psychopathology.

There is evidence for a genetic contribution to aggressive behaviour and temperamental factors, particularly hyperactivity, predict development of conduct disorder. Children with physical problems such as epilepsy are more likely to develop conduct disorder. There is interaction between conduct disorder and educational failure. Clinical assessment of these children should pay attention to remediable medical and developmental conditions although overemphasis of medical factors may reduce the child's sense of responsibility for behaviour. There is debate about the degree to which medical assessment can contribute to good management and limited evidence of benefit from drug treatment. The key professionals in most treatment programmes will be those with specific skills in psychological treatments relating to harm reduction, parenting skills and social and educational interventions. Multisystemic therapy combines family and individual counselling with social and educational interventions. To date the evidence may not support such complex and costly programmes but social and financial benefits come if the well recognized progression from conduct disorder to adult criminality is interrupted.

Sexual promiscuity may be defined as indiscriminate sexual activity with several partners and carries the risk of sexually transmitted diseases and unwanted pregnancy. Promiscuity may be associated with attentional problems, hyperkinetic disorder and hyperkinetic conduct disorder.

Promiscuity may be associated with:

- adolescent exploration of sexuality
- rebellion against parental and societal mores
- intoxication from drugs or alcohol
- psychiatric disorders, e.g. hypomania
- child sexual abuse.

Hyperkinetic disorder (ADHD)

The symptom triad of impulsivity, overactivity and attentional problems occurring in younger children in more than one setting is characteristic of a constitutionally based disorder described in around 5 per cent of American children, using the DSM diagnosis of **attention deficit disorder with hyperactivity** (ADHD). A further sub-group whose problems are primarily due to difficulties in sustaining attention are described using the DSM category of **attention deficit disorder**. In the UK, these DSM categories are increasingly replacing the ICD diagnosis of hyperkinetic disorder (Hk D), which requires the same triad of symptoms with a more severe and pervasive presentation. **Hyperkinetic disorder** is found in around 1 per cent of children. As with ADHD there is an increased prevalence in boys. The NICE (2000) and SIGN (2001) guidelines recognize the validity of the ADHD concept as a basis for treatment. ADHD is often co-morbid with developmental vulnerabilities (such as specific developmental disorders), which may be sufficient to justify specific intervention, and there is an increased prevalence of tics amongst children with ADHD. A picture like ADHD may be found in children with learning disability or pervasive developmental disorders.

Most children with ADHD have no underlying physical disorder and clinic assessment will only lead to laboratory investigation in a minority of cases where history or physical signs are suggestive. Assessment should include screening for remediable factors, e.g. hearing problems, with audiometry as indicated. School or nursery reports are essential for reliable diagnosis and may highlight co-morbid conditions. Standardized rating scales, such as Conner's Teacher Rating Scale are a valid way of obtaining information. There may be progression from ADHD to conduct disorder. There is genetic loading for ADHD and other family pathologies are often found in children with these difficulties.

CASE STUDY

Kieran is 6 years old and has always been very active, with difficulty settling to play. In school, he is disruptive and teachers relate his problems to those shown by his father (age 24 years) who was excluded from the same primary school. Both parents are drug users and are seeking a stimulant prescription for Kieran. The community paediatrician finds normal hearing and no sign of neurodevelopmental disorder. She involves other agencies in work with child and family prior to considering the parents' request for medication.

Treatment for ADHD without co-morbid disorder is best considered as a multimodal process. Children may benefit from group programmes that address the core symptoms of the disorder. Training in parenting skills and classroom strategies can enhance attentional skills and support impulse control. Stimulant medication has a good evidence base and should be initiated by a specialist with arrangements for its monitoring. Methylphenidate is generally the drug of first choice, with dexamphetamine as a second line. Atomoxetine and a range of non-stimulant drugs are available for non-responding children, under more specialist supervision. Self-help groups can be helpful but may differ in their advocacy of various assessment and treatment methods. Dietary restriction may be useful in some cases.

Emotional disorders

Children may present with a range of emotional symptoms that do not always fulfil criteria for adult-type psychiatric diagnoses. A category of emotional disorder of childhood is recognized in ICD-10, although it is not unusual to find adult disorders in children. Anxiety is a psychophysiological trait that may become extreme or persistent in anxiety disorder. Anxiety is found in association with panic in panic disorders and with fear in phobic disorders.

Symptoms of both anxiety and depression are on a continuum being part of normal experience, but when severe, persistent and interfering with normal functioning they become disorders.

Anxiety disorders

These present differently according to the child's developmental stage and age-related concerns, e.g. fears about school. Separation anxiety characterizes a specific disorder of childhood. Generalized anxiety manifests in all areas of life and is associated with expressed fears, unexplained physical complaints, regressed behaviour and deterioration in schoolwork. Aetiology is usually a combination of genetic predisposition, parental anxiety, traumatic events and ongoing stressors. There may be co-morbidity, e.g. with depression. Management requires reducing stresses and improving coping skills (e.g. relaxation training), often working with the child individually and the family.

Phobias

Fears and phobias are common in childhood. Phobias are unrealistic and inappropriate fears of specific objects or situations. About 2 per cent of children have phobias (e.g. animal phobia). Problems arise when the phobia interferes with normal functioning, e.g. needle phobia. Management involves desensitization to the feared stimulus, modelling normal behaviour and relaxation training.

Post-traumatic stress disorder

A severe and frightening life experience may constitute a trauma that leads to breakdown of normal adjustment processes with a consequent anxiety disorder, characterized by intrusive recollections and images of the event. Children may show sleep disturbance and nightmares. Avoidance of situations that trigger symptoms may become disabling and lead to disruption of school and social activities. Older children may try substance abuse to block symptoms and frequently find it difficult to express their difficulties. Hospitalization, especially with intensive care, can trigger this disorder. Symptoms may be maintained by family anxieties. Specialist treatment may include individual and family psychological interventions, as well as attention to social and environmental factors.

Depression

Depression occurs throughout life, with its incidence rising significantly in adolescence, especially in girls. Symptoms can manifest in all areas of a child's life (Table 2.2), but often they do not seek help and depression goes unnoticed. Many children and adolescents will report feeling unhappy, especially those with other emotional and behavioural disorders. It can be difficult to distinguish such misery from depression but it is described as qualitatively different, in addition to its severity and persistence. For a **depressive disorder** to be diagnosed the core symptoms must be present on most days for two

Table 2.2 Symptoms of depression

Emotional	Behavioural	Physical	Cognitive
Low mood	Regression	Somatic symptoms	Negative view of self, the world and future
Hopeless/helpless	Social withdrawal	Poor appetite/overeating	Low self-esteem
Suicidal	Educational failure	Poor concentration	
Anhedonia/bored	Self-harm	Poor sleep/reduced energy	
Angry/irritable			

weeks and associated with social impairment. In rare cases severe depression is complicated by psychotic symptoms.

Unlike adolescents and young adults, children with depression are more likely to have behavioural and physical problems. Depressive thoughts and feelings will become apparent on careful, sensitive questioning. Co-morbidity is common, most often with anxiety and conduct disorders. Depression is common in children and young people with eating disorders and/or chronic physical conditions. Depression is often familial, and is associated with dysfunctional families, adverse life events and disordered monoamine neurotransmitters.

CASE STUDY: Adolescent depression

A 14-year-old girl has a history of irritability, frequent complaints of headaches and deterioration in her schoolwork. On questioning, she admits to feelings of sadness, disturbed sleep, weight loss and thoughts of self-harm. Her parents separated the previous year after several violent incidents. Clinical psychology referral for cognitive–behavioural therapy is helpful.

Assessment requires exploration of personal and family strengths and difficulties. Collateral information should be sought. Other disorders need to be considered and excluded. In children and adolescents with depression there is a high rate of spontaneous remission, but there is also a high rate of relapse, both in treated and untreated groups. Specialist mental health practitioners can provide psychosocial interventions and advise on medication, if deemed necessary (Wolpert *et al.*, 2002).

Mania and bipolar affective disorder

Mania is characterized by an excessively elated mood with grandiosity, overactivity, reduced sleep and disordered appetites. Often the mood is irritable and labile, rather than elated. Delusions and hallucinations may be present. In childhood, mania is rare and often organically based. It occurs in adolescence as part of a bipolar disorder, which features both depression and mania. The milder form of mania is termed hypomania.

Deliberate self-harm

Completed suicide is rare in children and adolescents, but over the past 30 years the rate has increased, especially in young men. Deliberate self-harm (DSH or attempted suicide, parasuicide) is about 100 times commoner than completed suicide in children and adolescents and is five times commoner in females. Self-poisoning is the commonest method, others include self-cutting and strangulation. The challenge is to identify those young people at risk of significant self-harm and successful suicide.

Risk factors for suicide

Young men 15–25 years (or men over 50 years)

Highest and lowest socioeconomic groups

Early summer

History of depression, alcohol and drug abuse, chronic painful illness and epilepsy

Lack of supportive family relationships

A family member with a psychiatric disorder

A history of physical or sexual abuse

School or work problems

An episode of DSH is often precipitated by a disciplinary or relationship crisis. Children and young people have little knowledge of toxicology and the medical seriousness of an overdose will not reflect suicidal intent. Children and young people who have deliberately harmed themselves require a mental health assessment. Hospital admission provides an opportunity to assess the reasons for DSH. A history of advanced planning, precautions to avoid discovery, no attempt to gain help, dangerous method, suicide note left and preparations in anticipation of death suggests serious suicidal intent. Assessment includes establishing risk and protective factors for repetition of DSH with a management plan formulated and implemented.

Eating disorders

Eating disorders in younger children take a variety of forms, consistent with their mixed aetiology. Some children develop food avoidance as an expression of distress and disordered eating may reflect conflict or chaos within the family. Adult-type disorders generally evolve with adolescent development. **Bulimia nervosa** is characterized by near-normal weight, overeating in 'binges' followed by self-induced vomiting and/or laxative abuse. **Anorexia nervosa** can be associated with a fatal outcome and early detection improves prognosis. Although onset of anorexia nervosa is usually in mid to late teens, children as young as 7 years can present. It occurs 10 times more often in girls, but in prepubertal children this ratio falls to 4:1. Eating disorders are commoner in 'Western' societies.

Aetiology of anorexia nervosa

- Genetic basis
- Excessive dieting
- Low self-esteem
- Perfectionist tendencies
- Family difficulties with autonomy

Diagnosis of anorexia nervosa requires:

- <85 per cent of expected body weight for age and height
- deliberate dietary restriction, purging, vomiting, excessive exercise or use of appetite suppressants
- an intense fear of fatness and body image distortion
- amenorrhoea or delayed puberty in girls, lack of sexual interest and potency in boys.

Physical examination in anorexia may reveal little other than signs of starvation. There may be lanugo or coarse skin. Dental erosions are pointers to concealed vomiting. Blood pressure may be reduced and in severe cases there will be hypothermia. Investigations may reveal disruption of the hypothalamic–pituitary–gonadal axis, electrolyte imbalances, anaemia, starvation-induced electrocardiographic changes, immature ovaries on ultrasound scan and loss of bone density in chronic cases.

Whereas bulimia nervosa often improves with education and support, anorexia requires input from skilled mental health professionals and paediatric colleagues. Most cases will be managed on an outpatient basis with the initial focus being on gradual weight restoration using advice from a dietitian. This is managed by a combination of family therapy, behavioural techniques and individual therapy. Hospitalization can be unhelpful and is rarely required. Of those with anorexia, 25 per cent do badly and significant long-term sequelae include growth restriction, infertility and osteoporosis.

Conversion disorders

Symptoms or deficits affecting motor or sensory functioning in the absence of underlying organic pathology and with evidence of underlying psychosocial distress may be part of conversion disorder. Children and young people present with symptoms (e.g. paralysis) which correspond with their idea of illness and not to known patterns of organic disease. Their symptoms are viewed as an unconscious enactment of illness in response to an unbearable predicament and may be maintained by the way in which the child is treated by family members and professionals (e.g. gaining attention and being relieved of duties). The term 'abnormal illness behaviour' describes the prolongation of symptoms after an illness or injury without demonstrable organic reason. These disorders are related to **somatoform disorders** (e.g. pain disorders) and psychosomatic disorders. The clinical picture is often complex with a mixture of symptoms, some of which have a recognized organic aetiology, for example, a child with known epilepsy presenting with psychological seizures. Suspicion of conversion disorder should not distort the diagnostic process as serious underlying organic conditions may be overlooked. The unbearable predicament in which children are communicating through their symptoms may be sexual abuse.

Conversion disorders rarely present before the age of 7 years. In mid-childhood they occur equally in boys and girls but there is female preponderance in adolescence. This presentation is thought to be commoner in developing countries.

CASE STUDY

A 12-year-old girl was admitted to hospital with a history of acute onset blindness. Neurological and eye examination and magnetic resonance imaging (MRI) brain scan found no abnormality. The girl, viewed as highly intelligent by her parents, was struggling at school and had been due to sit a test the following day. With the involvement of a child psychiatrist she was discharged home with follow-up individual and family meetings. Over the course of two weeks the blindness resolved and no new symptoms presented.

Paediatric, primary care and mental health staff should work together in assessing and treating this group of patients. It is helpful to complete physical investigations quickly and to ensure that as far as possible the child is free of pressures that may have precipitated their symptoms. Management is most successful when it involves both physical and psychological treatments, enabling progress without 'loss of face', e.g. physiotherapy and psychotherapy sessions with both the child and family. The aim is to reduce the secondary advantages of the sick role and increase the rewards of healthy behaviour, while facilitating the expression of emotions.

Table 2.3 Key features of school refusal and truancy

	School refusal	Truancy
Peak age (years)	5, 11-12, 14	14+
Socioeconomic group	All	Lower
Association with anxiety	Yes	No
Association with conduct disorder	No	Yes

School refusal and truancy

Children may not attend school for different reasons, the commonest one being physical illness. Other reasons include truancy and school refusal. The latter is a symptom rather than a diagnosis and may reflect a variety of problems in the child, family or school system (Table 2.3). Paediatricians may become involved in assisting a child to return to school after a prolonged illness or in clarifying the diagnosis of underlying medical conditions or anxiety disorders presenting with somatic symptoms. A combination of difficulties is not uncommon.

Unlike school refusers, truants conceal their school non-attendance from their families, usually meeting up with friends and being involved in antisocial activities. Often these are children and young people, usually male, from deprived and dysfunctional families and are struggling with schoolwork.

School refusal is equally common in boys and girls. The core symptom is an irrational fear of attending school, which may be based partly or fully on difficulty separating from home. Often the problem presents after an absence from school, e.g. due to illness or holiday or at a transition time (nursery to primary, primary to secondary). The child may openly express reluctance to attend school or may present with anxiety-based symptoms, e.g. abdominal pain. These symptoms are usually absent at weekends or school holidays. Attempts to force the child to go to school will be met with tears or tantrums and often the parents are unable or unwilling to make them go. Mothers are often anxious or depressed and there is often a past history of difficulty separating, e.g. on starting nursery. Successful school return requires close working between health and education services. When children present with physical symptoms, investigations should be carried out rapidly to exclude any underlying condition. For those with a recent onset of school refusal, return to school is usually managed by primary care practitioners and school. Prolonged cases are often more entrenched and underlying depressive or anxiety disorders may require input from a CAMHS team. Rarely, a residential placement is required.

CASE STUDY

An 11-year-old boy had a six-month history of poor school attendance since starting secondary school. Most days he complained of abdominal pain and had been referred by his general practitioner for investigations, which were negative. His father had died the previous year and his mother was still overwhelmed by grief. His two younger siblings attended school without difficulty. Progress was rapid once a diagnosis of school refusal led to increased family support from grandparents.

Substance abuse

Paediatricians will encounter substance abuse in children and their parents, either of which may be associated with detrimental effects to both. By mid-adolescence, the consumption of tobacco, alcohol and cannabis is widespread. There is particular cause for concern when alcohol and drug use is associated with physical and psychological harm.

Alcohol and drug misuse associated with significant damage needs to be addressed using psychological therapies and social support, working within a family-based model. The scale of substance abuse reflects social and economic trends that are not easily influenced by medical practitioners.

THE CHILD WHO IS SEEN AS STRANGE

Any professional working with children will recognize a few that stand out as 'different' but sometimes it is difficult to identify why. A group of children might be categorized as 'strange' because of disturbances in the capacity to relate, not explained by neurological or special sense disorders. Difficulties range from extreme shyness and elective mutism through to severe developmental disorders and major psychiatric disorders such as schizophrenia. Social anxiety is common and major psychiatric disorder is rare. This section will highlight some disorders that may be underlying such presentations.

Disorders of social functioning in childhood

Mutism is characterized by an emotionally determined selectivity in speaking, not derived from other significant psychiatric disorder and so marked that a child who may be competent in verbal communication in some settings will present no verbal language in others. It may be associated with speech and language or other learning difficulties and is likely in children who are anxious, obsessional or socially fearful. There may be associated parental difficulties and secondary overprotection. Prolonged mutism may require considerable effort to support the child and avoid entrenching difficulties. A stepwise approach to support in communication is often beneficial but medication may be considered in a small number of cases presenting to psychiatry.

Attachment disorders are serious disturbances of social functioning, seen in children with an experience of seriously disrupted early relationships, presenting with unusual patterns of behaviour in social situations, being excessively clingy and/or aloof and avoidant. They show extreme distress or rage for relatively minor triggers and can be difficult to reassure. Such children may develop attentional disturbance, overactivity and impulsivity as well as disturbances of language, suggestive of constitutional disorder. There may be disturbances of appetite and failure to thrive in young children. If deprivation continues through childhood, the prognosis is poor. Adoptive placements can offer a way forward but adoptive parents require considerable support. This category of disorder is a subject of debate among professionals and the evidence in relation to epidemiology is uncertain. Children with attachment disorders are commoner in populations who have experienced early privation, such as looked after and accommodated children.

CASE STUDY

Donna was adopted at age 5 years from a mother whose recurrent hospitalizations with acquired immune deficiency syndrome (AIDS)-related illness had disrupted her early childhood. The adoptive parents could not form a loving bond with Donna, whose angry outbursts led to adoption breakdown at age 11 years. A chaotic experience of the care system followed and she became involved in prostitution at the age of 15 years, recapitulating her mother's history.

Tic disorders and obsessionality

Tic disorders are classified according to the nature and duration of the tic with transient motor tic disorders occurring commonly, particularly in children around the of age 4–5 years. Chronic disorders are identified when symptoms persist for more than 12 months and may involve motor or vocal tics. Motor and vocal tics together for a prolonged period lead to a diagnosis of Tourette syndrome. Tourette syndrome may commence in childhood and worsen in adolescence but around 50 per cent of adolescents will be symptom-free in adulthood. Tic disorders often do not require treatment but it is important for children and families to understand the problem. Parents may be more distressed by seeing their child tic than the child feels. Children who appear to be ticking quite markedly at home and in the clinic may manage to limit the expression of symptoms in school to the extent that teachers do not even notice. In some cases, tics are misunderstood and children identified as disruptive. Where reactions to tics are increasing stress for the child, explanation of the problem may reduce stress and symptom frequency. Children with persistent or severe difficulties may require psychological intervention. Drug treatment has a place in the management of severe and complex tic disorders but the risks may outweigh the benefits. Where tic disorders are associated with obsessional compulsive disorder or hyperkinetic disorder, it may be more appropriate to treat the associated disorder first.

CASE STUDY

Stephen, 6 years old, developed a facial tic when his father was hospitalized after an accident at work. The symptom resolved when his father discussed the changes in the workplace that would reduce the risk of a similar occurrence.

Obsessionality is a normal feature of early childhood, when magical thinking can lead children to unusual repetitive patterns of behaviour, driven by ideas of causation which although age appropriate are not shared by adults. Rigid and obsessional behaviour is a characteristic of children with developmental disorders and brain injuries and may provide a defence against the anxiety that such children experience in relation to their lack of flexibility in dealing with unpredictable factors in their environment. Obsessional traits are often inherited.

Obsessional compulsive disorder is characterized by repeated driven or compulsive behaviours and obsessions, which are repetitive thoughts or mental images that the individual usually finds distressing. Children may become so preoccupied by obsessional thoughts and caught up in compulsive behaviours that they are quite disconnected from day-to-day activities. The child will have a sense that their thoughts and compulsions come from within his or herself. Both obsessional and tic disorders may be found together and it may be difficult to establish the boundary between obsessionally driven and compulsive behaviours and complex tics.

Obsessional compulsive disorder or tic disorders may occur together with other developmental disorders. Once the presentation has been understood, the child's anxiety levels may come down, with a reduction in symptom frequency and also reduction in the apparent severity of developmental vulnerabilities. Streptococcal infection may trigger tics and obsessional compulsive disorder.

Treatment for obsessional compulsive disorder is best undertaken after a multidisciplinary assessment involving psychological expertise and an understanding of individual and family issues that may increase stress and symptom frequency. Obsessional compulsive disorder is particularly responsive to cognitive-behavioural interventions but in some cases drug treatments may be required. The specific serotonin reuptake inhibitor sertraline is now licensed for this purpose, along with the older antidepressant clomipramine. Obsessional compulsive disorder has a remitting and relapsing course, although it is to be hoped that intervention will modify the course of the disease.

CASE STUDY

Mark, 14 years old, spends an hour washing his hands before every meal. His concern for hygiene has developed from the start of school and become increasingly disabling. He refuses treatment as he is afraid that his habits will be challenged with the result that he may catch an infection. Mark's father is a successful accountant, who recognizes the value of his own obsessionality. His general practitioner keeps contact and as Mark becomes anxious prior to exams his symptoms worsen to the extent that he accepts referral to CAMHS.

Autistic spectrum disorders and the pervasive developmental disorders

A triad of communication disorder, disorders of social functioning and behavioural rigidity with deficits in imagination is characteristic of classical **autism** but also found in other developmental disorders (Rapin, 2002). Autism as described by Kanner is accompanied by learning disability in over 70 per cent of cases. Learning disability syndromes may have underlying physical causes and specific disorders such as tuberous sclerosis may be found underlying the autistic presentation in a small minority of cases even when there is no generalized learning disability. The severely autistic child will have presented some difficulties by the age of 2–3 years, with abnormalities of eye contact, lack of stranger anxiety and a failure to develop interest in shared attention. As the child develops, behavioural rigidity, a lack of symbolic play, with a lack of interest in shared activities and unusual patterns of communication are striking. A limited repertoire may include stereotyped behaviours or mannerisms, with a lack of awareness of the impact of their behaviour on others. Autistic children desire sameness in their environment. They react catastrophically and are vulnerable to disturbances in routine. Verbal and non-verbal communication impairments may be severe, 50 per cent of autistic children may not be producing any verbal language at school entry. Abnormalities include unusual patterns of voice production with a lack of expressive variation in volume and tone and concrete use of language with repetition of stereotyped phrases. Echolalia is the mechanical repetition of sounds or words. Together with these disturbances are striking problems with language pragmatics, which mean that these children have great difficulty in understanding social rules and engaging in conversational strategies. Many children with autism fail to develop useful verbal communication.

CASE STUDY

Tanya, 9 years old, sits under the table if she can. She loves music and sings advertising jingles but has no useful verbal language. She points for what she wants and screams if it is not provided. Her level of learning disability has not been established as her understanding seems to be in advance of her social functioning. She has been diagnosed autistic from age 3 years. There are no markers of an underlying disorder. She recently developed a difficult-to-treat epilepsy and an MRI scan, under anaesthesia, was normal. Her family benefits from respite support and she attends a special school.

Asperger syndrome is characterized by the same triad of difficulties that are found in autism with the difference that disturbances of speech and language are less marked in early childhood. These children have an impaired capacity to understand the point of view of others and difficulty in social relationships despite normal IQ. They are rigid and lack symbolic play and narrow interests can be all consuming. Motor difficulties may be part of the syndrome. The concept of Asperger syndrome has been widened to include children with **schizoid disorder of childhood** who have more imaginative capacities.

Asperger syndrome is increasingly frequently diagnosed and there is much discussion about the overlap of this condition with other disorders, particularly **semantic and pragmatic disorders of language** and other mixed or complex developmental disorders which include features of the autistic triad. There is also debate about the value of applying a lifetime diagnosis to children with difficulties at the mild end of the spectrum. Children who do not fulfil criteria for autism or Asperger syndrome may be diagnosed with 'atypical autism', a term generally used with more severe generalized learning disabilities or identified specific language disorders.

CASE STUDY

Peter, 11 years old, has no friends. He loves to draw and designs unusual farm machinery. His father is a hill farmer and met his mother through a dating agency. Both parents appreciate the isolation of their home and saw little difficulty with their son's limited social contacts. He was only recently diagnosed but now is receiving additional support to prepare him for secondary school where he will have a part-time placement in a unit for pupils with Asperger syndrome.

The concept of the autistic spectrum has become increasingly prevalent and the boundaries of this spectrum of disorders vary in different areas of literature. It is generally accepted that autism, Asperger syndrome and atypical autism lie within the **autistic spectrum**, but other conditions may be considered to be part of this spectrum. These include the **pervasive developmental disorders** (PDDs), which also present with features of the autistic triad. Rett syndrome is a genetically based PDD occurring in girls caused by mutations of the MECP2 gene on Xq28. This disorder has a characteristic onset with near-normal early development followed by a striking loss of acquired hand skills and speech and a deceleration of head growth after 6 months of age. Very rarely children present with a late-onset progressive loss of skills and impairment of social function and communication together with rigid and repetitive behaviours that have no clear organic basis and may be described as a **childhood disintegrative disorder** (Heller syndrome).

Schizophrenia and psychotic disorders

Psychosis is defined by a breakdown of the ability to recognize the boundaries of reality. In younger children it generally signifies organic disorder. Adult type psychotic illnesses are very rare in prepubertal children, arising with increasing frequency in adolescence. Schizophrenia is characterized by delusions and hallucinations that may be ill defined in cases with early onset. Diagnosis of psychosis can be difficult in the younger age range. Schizophrenia may be preceded by developmental difficulties and children with PDD may appear psychotic when distressed. Early diagnosis and treatment can significantly reduce chronic disability and specialist advice should be sought if this disorder is suspected. Bipolar affective disorders may cause psychosis in small numbers of adolescents.

REFERENCES

Ainsworth M, Blehar M, Waters E, Wall S (1978) *Patterns of Attachment: A Psychological Study of Strange Situations.* Hillsdale, NJ: Lawernce Erlbaum.

American Psychiatric Association (1994) *Diagnostic and Statistical Manual of the Mental Disorders*, 4th edn. Washington, DC: American Psychiatric Association.

Black D, Cottrell D (ed) (1993) *Child and Adolescent Psychiatry.* London: Gaskell.

Bowlby, J (1988) *A Secure Base: Clinical Applications of Attachment Theory.* London: Routledge.

Carr A (1999) *Handbook of Child and Adolescent Clinical Psychology.* London: Routledge.

Chess S, Thomas A (1995) *Temperament in Clinical Practice.* New York: Guildford.

Goodman R, Scott S (1997) *Child Psychiatry.* Oxford: Blackwell Science.

Graham P, Turk J, Verhulst F (1999) *Child Psychiatry – A developmental approach.* Oxford: Oxford University Press.

Green C (1992) *Toddler Taming.* London: Vermilion.

Kutcher SP (1997) *Child and Adolescent Psychopharmacology.* Philadelphia: WB Saunders Company.

Lask B, Fosson A (1989) *Childhood Illness: The Psychosomatic Approach.* Wiley: Chichester.

National Institute for Clinical Excellence (2000) *Guidance on the use of Methylphenidate (Ritalin/Equasym) for Attention Deficit/Hyperactivity Disorder (ADHD) in childhood.* www.nice.org.uk (accessed 1 December 2004).

National Health Service (NHS) Health Advisory Service (1995) *Together We Stand: A Thematic Review of the Commissioning, Role and Management of Child and Adolescent Mental Health Services.* London: The Stationery Office, 1995.

Rapin I (2002) The autistic spectrum disorders. *N Engl J Med* **347**:302–303.

Ross C, Davies P, Whitehouse W (2002) Melatonin treatment for sleep disorders in children with neurodevelopmental disorders. *Dev Med Child Neurol* **44**:339–44.

Royal College of Paediatrics and Child Health (2000) *Medicines for Children; Information for Parents and Carers.* London: Royal College of Paediatrics and Child Health. Available at www.rcpch.ac.uk (accessed 15 November 2004).

Royal College of Psychiatrists (1999) *Mental Health and Growing Up. Fact sheets for parents, teachers and young people.* 2nd edn. London: Gaskell; Royal College of Psychiatrists. Also available from the College website (www.rcpsych.ac.uk).

Scottish Intercollegiate Guidelines Network (2001). *Attention Deficit and Hyperkinetic Disorders in Children and Young People.* Edinburgh: SIGN. Available from the SIGN website (www.sign.ac.uk).

Wolpert M, Fuggle P, Cottrell D, *et al.* (2002) *Drawing on the Evidence.* Leicester: The British Psychological Society.

World Health Organization (1992) *The ICD-10 Classification of Mental and Behavioural Disorders.* Geneva: WHO.

Chapter 3

Clinical genetics

John Tolmie

Trainee paediatricians already foster the two most important skills that are required to make genetic diagnoses: family history taking and competence in clinical examination. These skills are also essential for correct interpretation of all genetic laboratory tests that are employed to investigate all types of genetic disease (Figure 3.1).

In the genetic clinic, drawing the family tree or pedigree may take anything from 5 to 25 minutes. However, in the case of the acute admission (or during a professional examination), much less time is available and only essential data are recorded.

The symbols used in the genetic clinic to record a three-generation family tree with details of relatives who may be at risk of developing a genetic disorder are illustrated in Figure 3.2. Note that geneticists frequently do not get all the information they need from one consultation. Anyway, many if not most individuals have patchy knowledge of more distant relationships or health problems within their extended family. Going over the family tree at a second consultation is usual, just as repeating the physical examination is good practice.

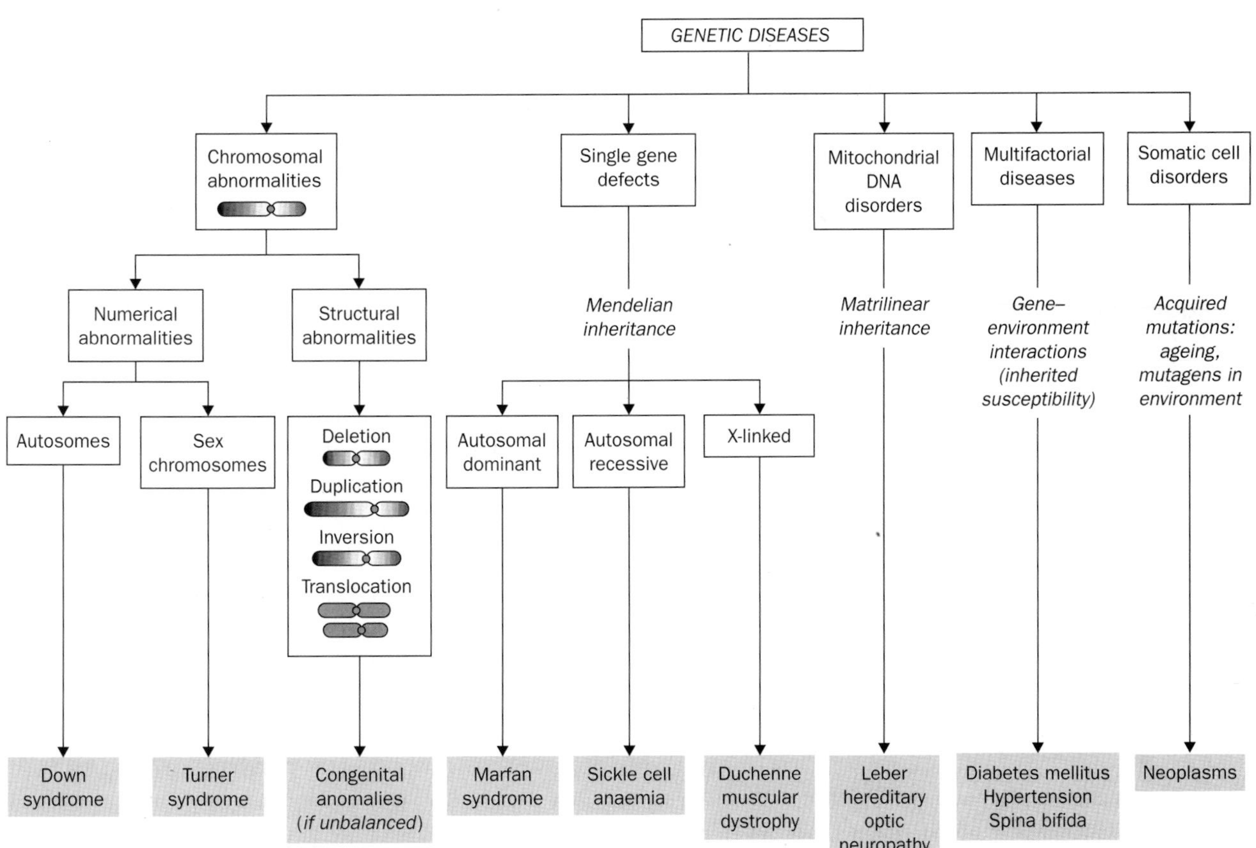

Figure 3.1 Types of genetic disease

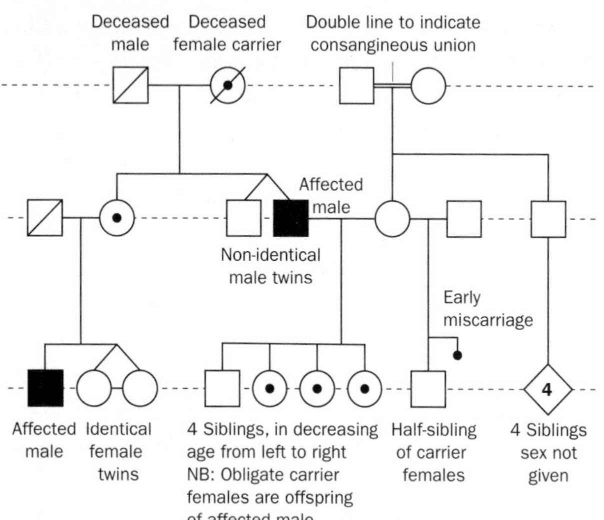

Figure 3.2 Sketching the family tree. Example: X-linked recessive inheritance of haemophilia A. *Arrow indicates proband who first brought the family to medical attention

> Drawing the family tree
>
> Start on a fresh page, orientated in landscape style. The patient or affected child who first brings the family to medical attention is the **proband**. Place the parents of the proband (the **consultants**) in the middle of the page.
>
> Conventionally, the male partner is placed on the left, female on the right, enquiring whether they are blood relatives. If a consanguineous union is difficult to draw, it is quite acceptable to write a description of the relationship (e.g. second cousins).
>
> Place the proband's siblings from oldest on left to youngest on the right. Enquire about stillbirths and miscarriages.
>
> Extend the family tree upwards, outwards and downwards to include uncles, aunts, cousins, nephews and nieces.
>
> Phrase enquiries carefully and tactfully, e.g. when asking about relatives' intellectual attainments, enquire first about their schooling.
>
> Ask if relatives will communicate with each other about illnesses that run in the family. With written permission, confirmatory medical records may be sought.

The family history may supply evidence that identifies a disorder's particular mode of inheritance, even when the precise diagnosis is not known. Remember, however, not everything that runs in the family is genetic. Families share their environment as well as their genes and mimicry of a genetic condition (**phenocopy**) is well described. For example, hereditary spastic paraplegia in a child may be mistaken for birth injury if the parents are not questioned and examined; the radiology of inherited vitamin D-dependent rickets is indistinguishable from radiology of dietary deficiency of vitamin D.

Interpreting the significance of family history information requires knowledge of mechanisms of heredity. Although Gregor Mendel's discovery of the particulate nature of inheritance and his introduction of the terms **dominant** and **recessive** predated the discovery of meiosis and chromosomes, this chapter first describes the chromosomal basis of Mendelism.

CHROMOSOMES AND CLINICAL CYTOGENETICS

Chromosomes are the visible structures into which genes are packaged. A gene may be defined as a specific sequence of DNA that occupies a specific position or locus on a chromosome.

There are 23 pairs of chromosomes in the cell nucleus. Pairs 1–22 are designated **autosomes**, each pair comprising two identical chromosomes, one inherited from the mother and the other from the father. Each pair of autosomes is identified by size and banding pattern. The twenty-third pair comprises the sex chromosomes. This pair is non-identical in males, comprising one X chromosome and one Y chromosome. In females, there are two X chromosomes and no Y. Boys receive their X chromosome from their mother and the solitary Y chromosome from their father. The Y chromosome harbours genes that are essential for male sex determination and fertility.

The **diploid** number of chromosomes is 46 in somatic cells, but only one copy of each pair is present in ova and sperm and 23 is the **haploid** number.

Meiosis is the specialized type of cell division that achieves reduction in chromosome number from diploid number (46) to the haploid number (23) of chromosomes in mature eggs and sperm. At the same time, meiosis generates new combinations of genes by genetic recombination between homologous chromosomes (Figure 3.4). Essentially, there are two meiotic cell divisions, but only the first division is preceded by DNA replication. During the first meiotic division, homologous chromosomes pair and exchange genetic material before separating, one homologue into each daughter cell. During the second meiotic cell division, each of the two sister chromatids that make up a single chromosome separate into the haploid gametes.

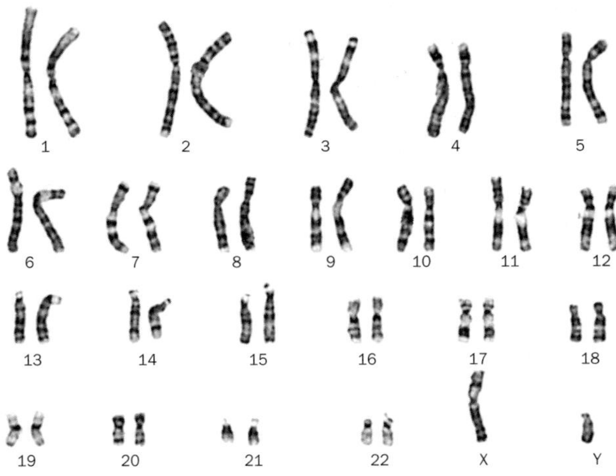

Figure 3.3 Normal male karyotype. The two chromosomes that comprise each identical pair of autosomes are called homologues

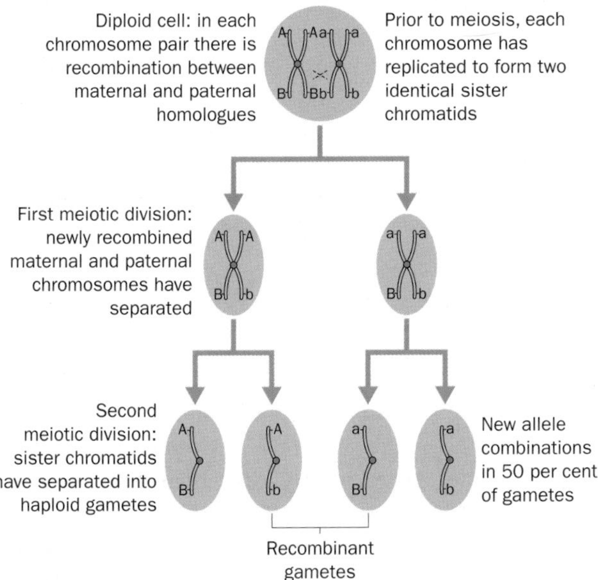

Figure 3.4 Meiosis: the production of haploid gametes with new genetic combinations

KEY LEARNING POINT

Meiosis reduces the diploid number of chromosomes in somatic cells, 46, to the haploid number in gametes, 23. Meiosis generates new genetic variation by the following mechanisms: exchange of genetic material between the maternal and paternal derived copies of each homologous chromosome pair; segregation of the recombined, homologous chromosomes; independent assortment of non-homologous chromosomes.

Clinical cytogenetics studies chromosome number and structure. A karyotype is a formal description of an individual's chromosome constitution, given after a systematic examination by the cytogeneticist. Chromosome analysis is carried out on 2–3 mL of heparinized blood. Results are usually available within three weeks but rapid reporting of urgent samples, for example, from a neonate who is affected by congenital malformations, can be obtained in one week.

TYPES OF CHROMOSOME ABNORMALITY

Numerical abnormalities and uniparental disomy

Numerical abnormalities are called aneuploidies and involve having any number of chromosomes other than the usual euploid number, 46. Aneuploidies are more frequent among spontaneous abortions, only a minority of aneuploid conceptions survive to term. Severe developmental abnormalities (congenital malformations) are often present in the aneuploid embryo or fetus.

An extra chromosome 21 (trisomy 21, Down syndrome; Figure 3.5) is the commonest aneuploidy and occurs in about 1 in 700 births. Trisomy 21 usually results from failure of separation of the two chromosome 21s (non-disjunction) at the first meiotic cell division in the mother; consequently there is an extra chromosome 21 in her egg. Such non-disjunction events are more liable to happen with advanced maternal age. Trisomy 18 (1 in 6000 births; Figure 3.6) and trisomy 13 (1 in 6000 births; Figure 3.7) are also more common in babies of older mothers. In each of these conditions the baby's facial features and characteristic pattern of congenital malformation permits early clinical diagnosis. In every case, including fetuses and stillbirths, chromosome analysis should be performed to confirm the clinical diagnosis.

Trisomy 16 is the commonest chromosome abnormality at conception, occurring in up to 5% of all clinically recognized pregnancies. Trisomy 16 embryos spontaneously abort but, rarely, a trisomic conceptus is 'rescued' if the extra chromosome is lost in very early development, leading to **mosaicism** with an admixture of normal diploid cells and trisomic cells in different tissues.

Note that trisomic rescue with loss of the additional chromosome in the very early embryo is one cause of **uniparental disomy** (UPD) (Figure 3.8). Uniparental disomy is present if both members of a pair of homologous chromosomes are derived from one parent, with no copies of that chromosome from the other parent.

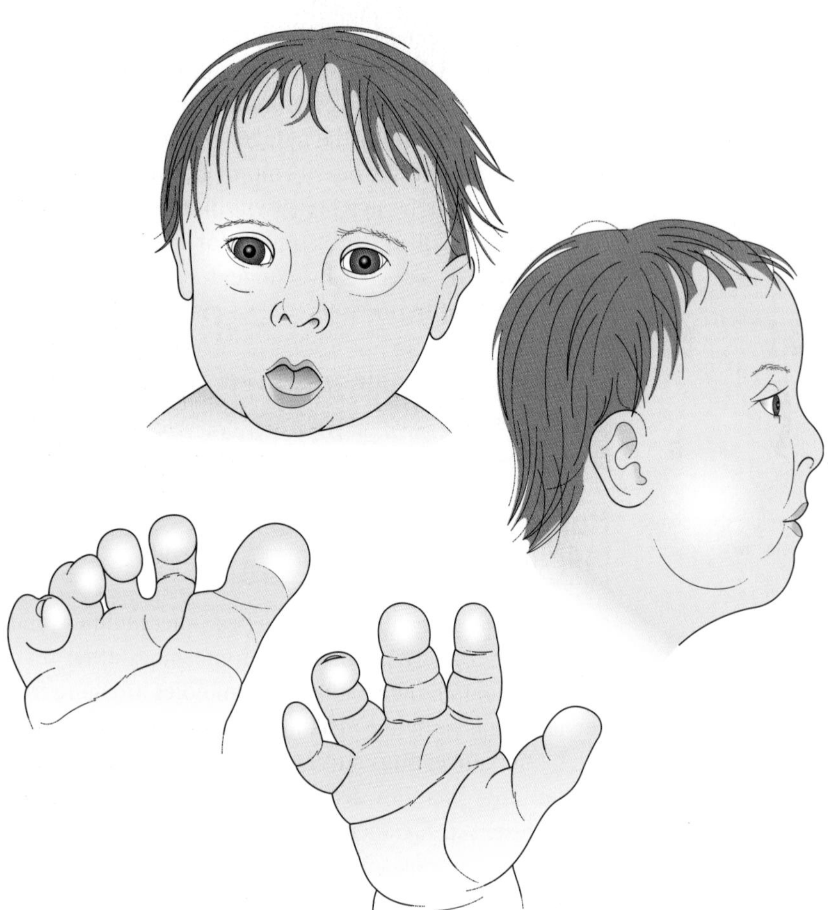

Figure 3.5 Common clinical signs in trisomy 21. Note the recognizable facial appearance ('gestalt' diagnosis), sandal gap between the first and second toes, single palmer crease and fifth finger clinodactyly with single flexion crease

Uniparental disomy may cause disease or malformation through a **genomic imprinting defect** if one maternal derived and one paternal derived copy of a chromosomal region or gene are required for normal development. This may happen if particular maternal or paternal derived genes require switching on or, alternatively, silencing during gametogenesis and in the embryo. Imprinted genes are few in number but conditions that may result from UPD or genetic imprinting defects include Prader–Willi and Angelman syndromes, Russell–Silver syndrome, transient neonatal diabetes mellitus and Beckwith–Weidemann syndrome.

KEY LEARNING POINT

An aneuploidy such as trisomy 21 Down syndrome is usually a sporadic occurrence in families although the risk of recurrence may be slightly increased in subsequent born siblings of an affected child. Families who have questions about risks of recurrence of chromosome disorders should be offered a genetic clinic appointment.

The main **sex chromosome aneuploidies** are 47,XXY, 47,XXX, 47,XYY and 45,X. The Y chromosome is small with important genes mainly concerned with male sex determination and fertility. In females (and in men with Klinefelter syndrome or 47,XXY), the second X chromosome is visibly condensed in non-dividing cells (the sex chromatin body or **Barr body**), giving correspondence between the number of Barr bodies and the number of X chromosomes in excess of one. Thus, 45,X Turner syndrome females have no Barr bodies and 47,XXX females have two Barr bodies in their cells. The Barr body reflects a genetically inactive X (see lyonization, page 69). This also means the adverse clinical effects of additional X chromosomes are minimized.

47,XXY, 47,XYY and 47,XXX each have a birth incidence of about 1 in 1000, but diagnosis at birth is exceptional since the babies generally appear normal. Occasionally, sex chromosome aneuploidies are diagnosed at school age following chromosome analysis in children with mild learning disability and behavioural problems. Tall stature, hypogonadism and infertility occur in 47,XXY Klinefelter syndrome and most individuals are diagnosed in adulthood. The majority of XXX females

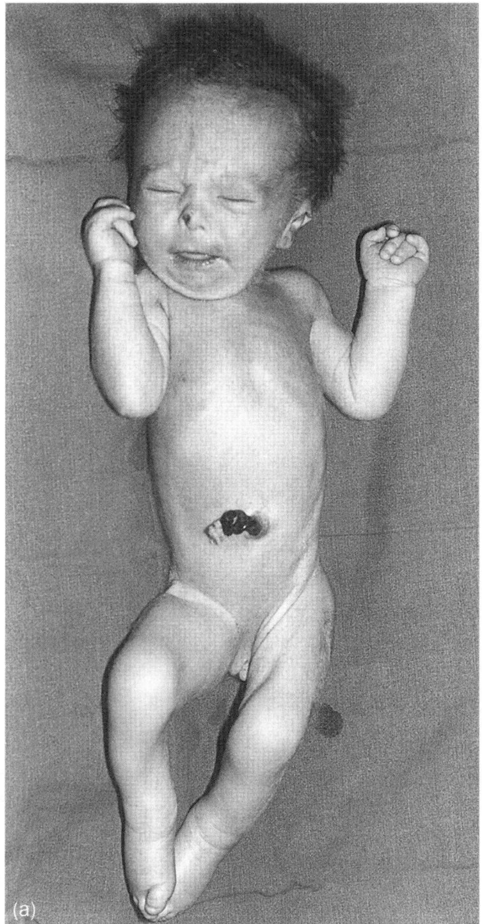

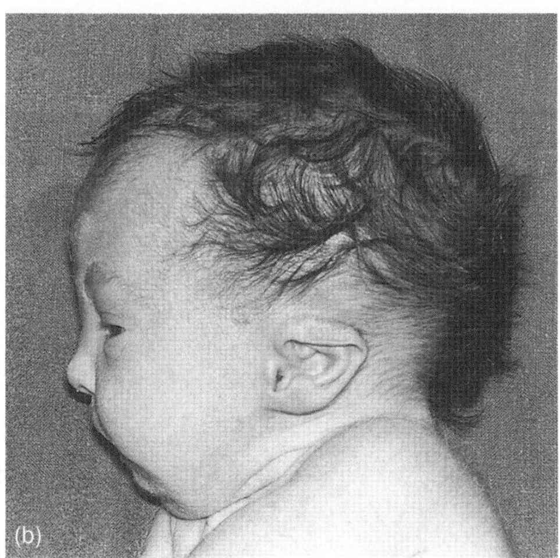

Figure 3.6 (a, b) An infant with trisomy 18. Note the flexed overlapping fingers

and XYY males go undiagnosed, but about one-third of XXX females have significant learning difficulties. A smaller proportion of XXY and XYY boys have mild learning difficulties, emotional and behavioural problems in addition to tall stature.

Turner syndrome (Figure 3.9), most commonly due to 45,X karyotype, affects 1 in 3000 girls but its somatic complications – including neck webbing, dysplastic nails, coarctation of aorta, short stature, hypogonadism and hypertension – mean that it is diagnosed more often than other sex chromosome aneuploidies. Learning difficulties are not so prominent in Turner syndrome but complex psychological impairments occur in many girls who often underachieve.

KEY LEARNING POINT

Sex chromosome aneuploidy syndromes are less likely to be associated with congenital malformations and severe learning disability. Apart from girls with Turner syndrome, most children with sex chromosome aneuploidy are not diagnosed.

Structural abnormalities

These are classified as 'balanced' rearrangements without visible gain or loss of chromosome segments, or 'unbalanced' rearrangements with visible evidence of extra or missing material on individual chromosomes. Nearly all unbalanced chromosomes cause clinical abnormalities whereas balanced chromosomal rearrangements seldom cause harm.

Examples of apparently balanced rearrangements in normal individuals include the reciprocal **chromosome translocation** where there is exchange of chromosome material between non-homologous (i.e. non-identical) chromosomes. As balanced chromosome rearrangement carriers are healthy, these rearrangements are often inherited unnoticed in families, but they may disturb meiosis and generate chromosomally unbalanced eggs and sperm.

KEY LEARNING POINT

In the family tree, a history of miscarriages, stillbirths, neonatal deaths, or of congenital abnormalities and learning disabilities are clues to disturbed chromosome segregation in a balanced rearrangement carrier.

Chromosome abnormalities nomenclature

The laboratory report employs formal shorthand nomenclature (termed ISCN) to describe each chromosome abnormality. Reports may be difficult

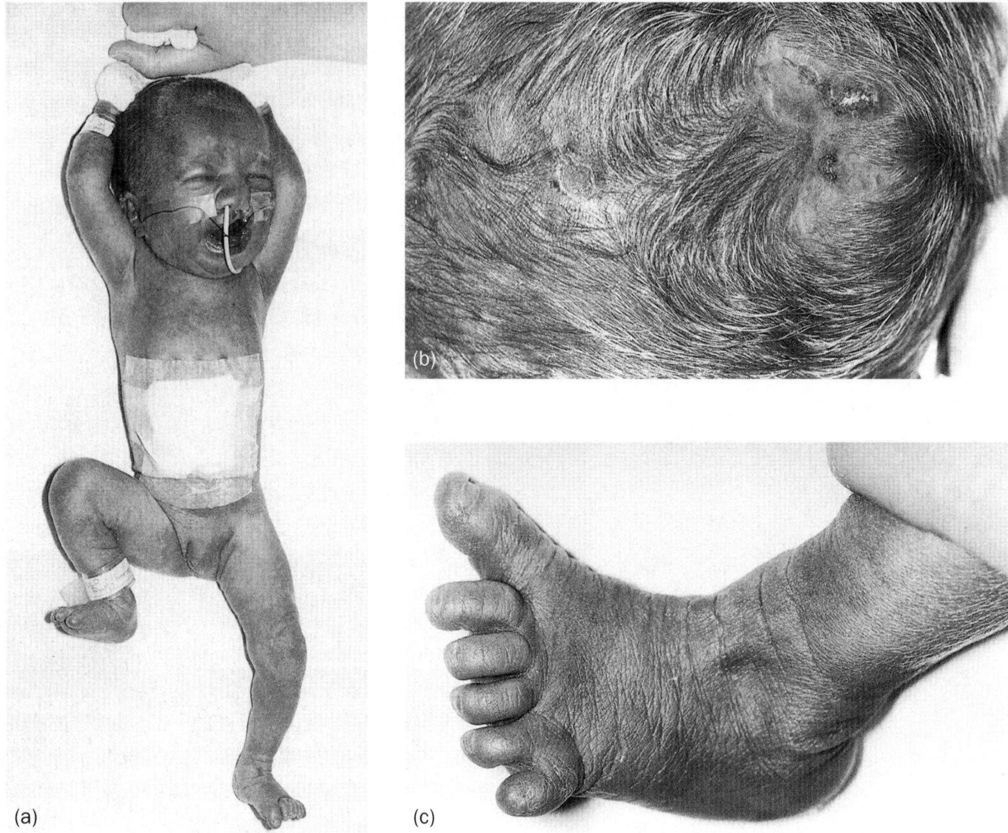

Figure 3.7 (a–c) An infant with trisomy 13. The scalp defect (b) is characteristic. Note the repaired abdominal wall defect in (a)

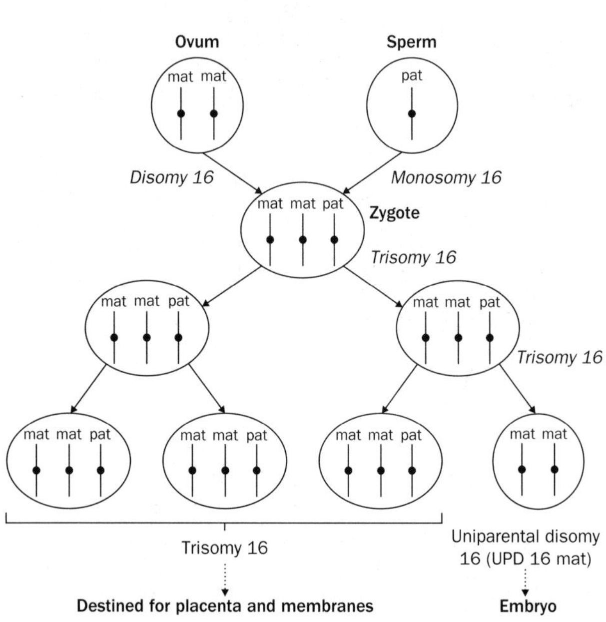

Figure 3.8 Possible origin of confined placental mosaicism and maternal uniparental disomy of chromosome 16

to decipher and complex cases are best discussed with the cytogeneticist.

A method for basic description of the chromosome constitution or karyotype is as follows:

1 the number of chromosomes in each cell is given, normally 46
2 the sex chromosome complement: usually XY or XX
3 expand on the abnormality noted, e.g. a numerical abnormality, 47,XX + 18; or, locate the chromosome arm, bands and sub-bands involved in a structural abnormality, e.g. 15q11-q13 deletion in Prader–Willi syndrome.

Structural abnormalities are described using abbreviations:

t	translocation
del	deletion
dup	duplication
inv	inversion
r	ring chromosome

p	chromosome short arm (above the primary constriction or centromere)
q	chromosome long arm (below the primary constriction or centromere)
p21;q34	landmark bands on chromosome arms are located by their specific number

Examples

47,XY + 21	trisomy 21, Down syndrome
47,XY + 21/ 46,XY	mosaic Down syndrome with admixture of chromosomally normal and trisomic cells
47,XYY	extra Y chromosome
45,X	Turner syndrome
45,XX,t(14q;21q)	balanced carrier of a Robertsonian (centromere fusion) translocation
46,XX,t(14q;21q)	female with translocation Down syndrome
46,XX,del(5p)	female with chromosome 5 short arm deletion
69,XXY	male triploid (spontaneous abortion likely)
69,XXX/46,XX	diploid/triploid mosaicism (more likely to survive to term)

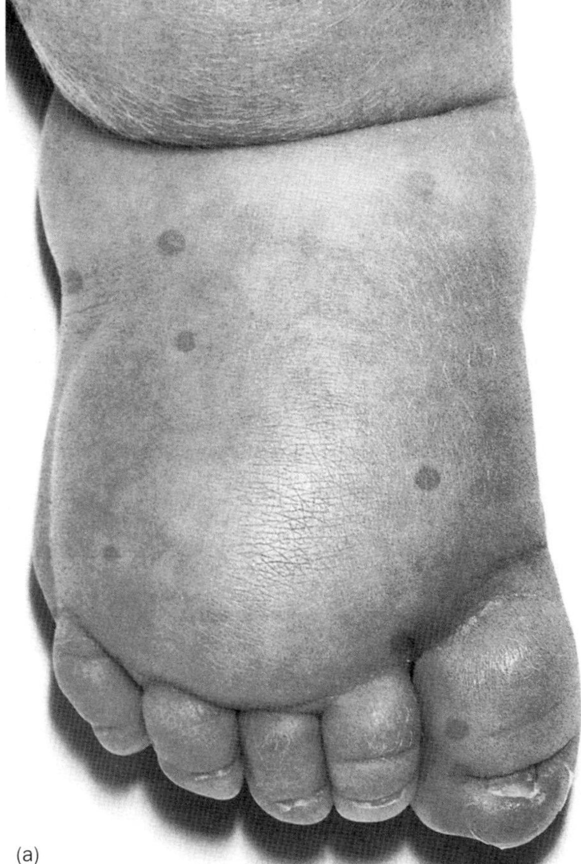

(a)

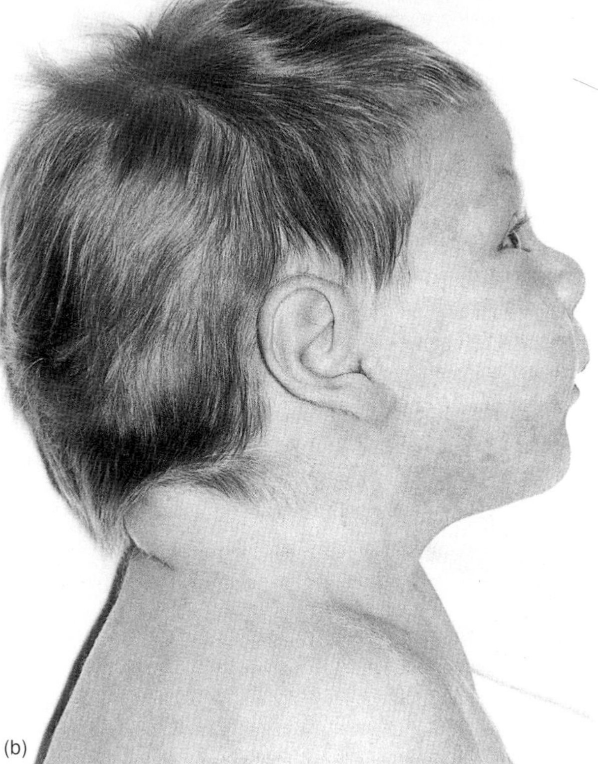

(b)

Figure 3.9 Turner syndrome. Note the puffy feet and nail dysplasia (a) and redundant skin at the neck (b)

KEY LEARNING POINT

Always contact the laboratory that has reported an unfamiliar result to ask the cytogeneticist or clinical geneticist for an explanation in plain English of the abnormal finding and its clinical implications.

Robertsonian translocations occur when two of the smallest chromosomes fuse at or near the centromere. The chromosome short arms (p) are lost without any phenotypic effect. A healthy Robertsonian carrier has only 45 chromosomes. Commonly, 13 and 14 fuse, less commonly 14 and 21, rarely 15 and 21. A rare but important Robertsonian translocation is the 21q;21q fusion chromosome. Carriers of the 21q;21q chromosome have 100 per cent chance of Down syndrome in their offspring.

If one parent is a balanced 14q;21q Robertsonian translocation carrier, there is also increased risk of Down syndrome in the offspring. However, the chance of translocation Down syndrome when the mother is a carrier is 15 per cent, whereas if the father carries the same chromosome there is 5 per cent chance of a baby affected by translocation Down syndrome. The chance of translocation trisomy 13 (Patau syndrome) arising in the baby of a Robertsonian 13q;14q carrier is much lower, at no more than 1 per cent.

KEY LEARNING POINT

Long chromosome segment imbalances, typically representing a length of chromosome greater than 5 per cent of the total length of all 23 chromosomes, lead to early miscarriage. Smaller chromosome segment imbalances are associated with viable pregnancy and have high risks (10 per cent or more) of causing malformation, dysmorphism and mental retardation. Carriers of structural chromosome rearrangements should be referred to the genetic clinic.

Indications for cytogenetic analysis

Neonates

- Confirm a clinical diagnosis (e.g. trisomy 21, trisomy 18, trisomy 13)
- Exclude chromosome imbalances as the cause of major congenital malformations
- Investigation of ambiguous genitalia

Childhood

- Investigation of learning difficulties (also request fragile X gene DNA analysis)
- Investigation of growth retardation and short stature
- Recheck previous 'normal result' study in cases where chromosome imbalance is strongly suspected
- Specific fluorescence in situ hybridization (FISH) studies, e.g. Williams syndrome, Prader–Willi syndrome (see below)

Adults

- Infertility
- Recurrent miscarriages
- Family history of chromosome abnormality or 'Down syndrome' (karyotype unknown)
- Family history of congenital malformations/ mental retardation of unknown cause

Special investigations undertaken by arrangement with the laboratory

- Chromosome breakage syndromes (e.g. Fanconi anaemia)
- Investigation for chromosome mosaicism (skin fibroblast chromosomes)
- Chromosome telomere studies (in selected cases with unexplained dysmorphism and mental retardation)

Chromosome microdeletion syndromes

The smallest abnormality of chromosome structure that may be visualized after a routine chromosome banding study represents a change affecting several genes (about 5 000 000 base pairs (bp) or 5 megabases (Mb) of DNA). The largest human gene is 3 Mb in size and codes for the muscle protein called dystrophin that is absent in boys who are affected by X chromosome-linked Duchenne muscular dystrophy.

Nearly 20 years ago, several boys with Duchenne muscular dystrophy were noted to carry a barely visible cytogenetic deletion at Xp21. This deletion removed the dystrophin gene and several neighbouring genes, including the glycerol kinase and adrenal hypoplasia genes. It was realized that this caused a complex phenotype with muscular dystrophy, glyceroluria and adrenal insufficiency, sometimes called a contiguous gene syndrome, by deletion of three adjacent genes.

Several eponymous syndromes are now known to be caused by 3 Mb or slightly larger size deletions at other chromosomal locations (Table 3.1). These tiny chromosome deletions may be missed by traditional monochrome chromosome banding studies, but they are readily demonstrated by cytogenetic methods on immobilized chromosomes that employ DNA probes, each tagged with a fluorescent dye specific to the syndrome's deleted chromosome region. This methodology is called **chromosome fluorescence in situ hybridization** (FISH) (Figure 3.10).

KEY LEARNING POINT

Since each FISH probe is chromosome specific, the cytogeneticist must first be informed that there is clinical suspicion of the particular syndrome in order to carry out the appropriate FISH test.

Table 3.1 Commoner microdeletion syndromes associated with learning disability

Syndrome	Chromosome locus	OMIM no.†	Main clinical features
Miller-Dieker syndrome	17p13.3	247200	Lissencephaly, epilepsy
Smith-Magenis syndrome	17p11.2	182290	Self-mutilation, appearance may suggest trisomy 21
Williams syndrome	7q11.2	194050	Congenital heart disease, hypercalcaemia
Prader-Willi syndrome	15q11-q13	176270	Hypotonia, obesity, short stature
Angelman syndrome	15q11-q13	105830	Hypotonia, ataxia, epilepsy, absent speech
DiGeorge syndrome/velocardiofacial syndrome	22q11.2	188400/192430	Thymus hypoplasia, congenital heart disease, hypocalcaemia, palatal incompetence
Rubinstein-Taybi syndrome	16p13.3	180849	Broad thumbs and hallux, congenital heart disease

† The OMIM number refers to the specific catalogue entries in Online Mendelian Inheritance in Man (see page 74).

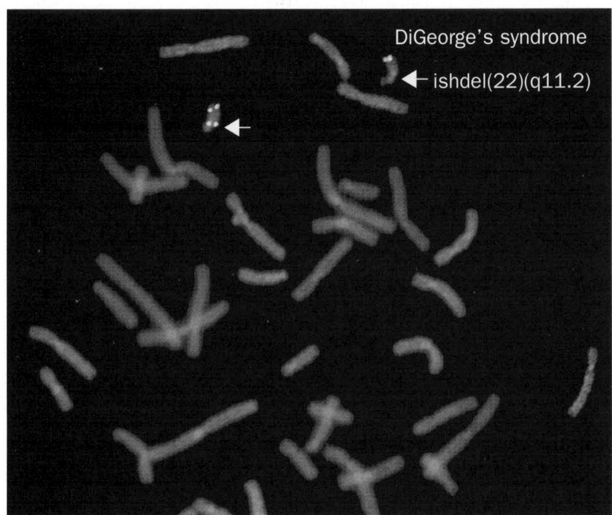

Figure 3.10 Microdeletion of chromosome 22q11.2 associated with DiGeorge syndrome/velocardiofacial syndrome

Chromosomes, somatic cells and cancer

A chromosome abnormality is described as constitutional if it is present in all tissues from conception, for example trisomy 21 Down syndrome. In contrast, a somatic chromosome abnormality arises at a mitotic cell division some time after fertilization.

The best known somatic chromosome abnormality is the small, abnormal chromosome 22 or **Philadelphia chromosome** in chronic myeloid leukaemia (CML) cells. This chromosome results from translocation or exchange of chromosome material between chromosome 9 and chromosome 22 – t(9;22)(q34;q11). In the hybrid chromosome 22 at the site of union with chromosome 9 material, fusion of BCR gene from chromosome 22 and the ABL gene from chromosome 9 creates a new gene and gene product, a fusion protein tyrosine kinase. This molecule gives leukaemic cells with the Philadelphia chromosome a growth advantage. Recently, a small molecule inhibitor of the BCR-ABL protein has been developed and has proved an effective initial treatment for CML although patients' responses have been short lived due to emergence of drug resistance.

KEY LEARNING POINT

Somatic cytogenetic abnormalities are important events in the multistep process that leads to cancer. Different tumour types tend to be associated with particular chromosome abnormalities, therefore chromosome analysis of cancer cells is an important diagnostic test. In some haematological malignancies the disappearance of chromosomally abnormal clones of malignant cells from the bone marrow is an important indicator of response to treatment.

The important relationship between development, chromosomes and cancer was illustrated by the discovery of a cytogenetic abnormality in a few individuals who had both retinoblastoma and congenital malformation due to deletion in the long arm of chromosome 13. This confirmed the location of the retinoblastoma gene on chromosome 13 and detailed analysis of the family histories of individuals with retinoblastoma led Knudson to develop a general model for the development of cancer – the 'two hit' hypothesis (see case study on Retinoblastoma, page 89).

Retinoblastoma is the classic example of inherited cancer caused by mutation in a **tumour suppressor gene.** The retinoblastoma gene Rb1 was the first tumour suppressor gene to be isolated. Normally, tumour suppressor genes act to restrain the rate of cell division, or to promote DNA repair or programmed cell death (**apoptosis**) when appropriate. Rb1 mutations have been detected in eye, breast and colon cancer.

Oncogenes are different because excess activity of the encoded protein causes cells to become cancerous. The normal version of an oncogene is called a proto-oncogene and it mutates to become overactive. The mutant oncogene causes cancerous change by suppressing the normal proto-oncogene allele on the other chromosome.

In contrast, tumour suppressor gene mutations are usually recessive at the cellular level as both copies of the gene have to be inactivated before unrestrained cell growth ensues. Dominance and recessiveness are key features of Mendelian (single gene) inheritance and this is discussed next.

PATTERNS OF INHERITANCE

Autosomal dominant

Affected individuals may be identified in more than one generation, leading to a vertical inheritance pattern in the family tree. Males and females are affected generally with equal frequency and severity. Transmission of the condition from a father to his son is an important clue since this observation excludes the possibility that the gene mutation is located on the X chromosome. If there is no family history prior to the birth of an affected child, the disease may have arisen by a fresh mutation in the germ cells of either parent. Different genes have different rates of mutation and there is a weak positive association with increased paternal age.

How might a dominant gene mutation cause its clinical effect? A **dominant-negative mutation** is when the abnormal product of the mutant gene interferes with the normal copy's functioning product, this can occur in dimeric or multimeric proteins, for example in collagen molecules to produce osteogenesis imperfecta. **Haploinsufficiency** occurs if half-normal quantity of the normal gene product results in the mutant phenotype. Haploinsufficiency is observed in developmental genes that have gene dosage-sensitive functions, for example, haploinsufficiency of PAX2 gene causes eye and kidney malformations.

KEY LEARNING POINT

Autosomal dominant diseases often display **variable clinical expression.** In other words, mildly affected individuals may suffer no ill health and their diagnosis is overlooked until they have an affected child. In some individuals there are no signs that he or she carries an autosomal dominant mutation, in such individuals the mutation is said to be **non-penetrant.** Penetrance and expressivity are aspects of genetic variation. Penetrance is an all-or-none phenomenon whereas expressivity reflects variation in severity of a genetic condition or trait.

Autosomal recessive

A gene mutation is recessive when there is no phenotypic effect in the individual who is carrying one mutant copy or allele, and one normal functioning copy of the gene in question. The unaffected carrier of one mutant allele is called a **heterozygote** or heterozygous carrier. Two common autosomal recessive conditions in the UK are cystic fibrosis (carrier frequency of 1 in 22) and haemochromatosis (carrier frequency of 1 in 10).

A typical autosomal recessive pedigree shows one or more affected siblings born to unaffected carrier parents (horizontal inheritance pattern). Males and females are equally likely to be affected. In the case of very rare recessive disorders, parental consanguinity is more likely to be observed.

KEY LEARNING POINT

Each child of two parents who are heterozygous for the same recessive mutation has a 1 in 4 chance of inheriting two mutant alleles and being homozygous affected. In the case of a fertile, affected homozygote, his or her children are most likely to be unaffected heterozygotes, for it would be rare to encounter a unrelated carrier of the same gene mutation in the general population.

In the past, certain recessive gene mutations for serious disorders such as cystic fibrosis, Tay–Sachs disease and the haemoglobinopathies may have become more common in the population if carriers of these mutations had advantages in health and reproduction. Possible mechanisms are through relative immunity to cholera, tuberculosis or malaria in populations exposed to these infections.

X-chromosome linked inheritance

Genes located on the X chromosome are present in two doses in females and are single copy in the male. Female heterozygotes carry a mutation on one X chromosome and a second, normal functioning allele on the other X. In contrast, males with a mutant gene on their solitary X chromosome (**hemizygotes**) are affected by recessive mutations located on the X. One exception to this rule is the man with Klinefelter syndrome (47,XXY) who would be an unaffected heterozygous carrier.

KEY LEARNING POINT

X-linked inheritance is suggested in pedigrees with several affected males who are related through unaffected females. Absence of male-to-male transmission is an important supporting observation since each son of an affected father inherits the Y chromosome and is therefore unaffected. On the other hand, each daughter of an affected father is always a carrier since she inherits the solitary paternal X chromosome that carries the mutant gene (see Figure 3.2).

Note that a form of gene dosage compensation occurs with X-chromosome linked inheritance. The biological mechanism for this is **X-chromosome inactivation**, also called lyonization after the scientist, Mary Lyon, who discovered the phenomenon. Lyonization ensures there is only one active X per cell regardless of the number in the karyotype. Males with 47,XXY inactivate one X, and 47,XXX females inactivate two Xs. The number of inactive Xs corresponds to the number of Barr bodies observed in the nucleus of non-dividing cells.

Lyonization occurs in each female cell in the embryo at about the blastocyst stage. At this stage, one or the other X chromosome is rendered genetically inactive or silent. Which X is inactivated is usually determined randomly and, overall, a 50:50 ratio is expected so that females heterozygous for an X-linked character are mosaics of cells that express one or the other allele.

KEY LEARNING POINT

Skewing of the 50:50 ratio with preferential activation of one X chromosome that carries a mutation may lead to signs and symptoms of the X-linked disease in the carrier female.

Although a single functioning X chromosome is sufficient for normal development in males, this is not the case in females, otherwise there would be no phenotypic consequence of the 45,X karyotype in Turner syndrome. The importance of the second normal X for female development is evident from the observation that over 95 per cent of Turner syndrome conceptions either fail to develop or spontaneously miscarry. Two active copies of genes at the tip of the X chromosome short arm are required for normal female development.

Polygenic inheritance

Polygenic traits are influenced by several or many genes with neutral, deleterious or protective effects. Continuous traits like body weight and height, and diseases such as morbid obesity and hypertension, are influenced by interaction between polygenes and environment, so-called **multifactorial conditions.**

Polygenes may also cause discontinuous traits such as spina bifida and other congenital malformations if there is a genotype 'threshold' beyond which genetic susceptibility is increased sufficiently for the malformation to occur. In the multifactorial model, the threshold may be raised by beneficial measures such as folic acid supplements given to the mother in the periconceptual period to protect against occurrence of spina bifida. Alternatively, drugs like sodium valproate may lower the threshold leading to increased incidence of spina bifida in offspring of mothers who take this medication. These observations are examples that illustrate contributions of genetics and environment to origins of health and disease.

KEY LEARNING POINT

Most common single congenital malformations are unexplained and occur sporadically in families. However, risks to first-degree relatives of patients are increased and are mostly in the range of 2–5 per cent. If two siblings are affected by a congenital malformation, the risk of recurrence rises further but always offer to refer the parents to the genetic clinic for more specific advice.

Table 3.2 Mitochondrial disorders

Disorder	Mitochondrial gene(s)
Lactic acidosis, encephalopathy, stroke-like episodes (MELAS)	tRNA leucine
Diabetes with sensorineural deafness	tRNA leucine
Neuropathy, ataxia, retinitis pigmentosa (NARP)/Leigh syndrome	mtATPase subunit 6
Myoclonic epilepsy, myopathy (MERFF)	tRNA lysine
Leber hereditary optic neuropathy	ND1, ND4, ND6
Pearson marrow-pancreas syndrome	Various (deletions and duplications)

Mitochondrial inheritance

Mitochondria are intracellular organelles that are pivotal in energy metabolism and adenosine triphosphate (ATP) production. Each mitochondrion has its own circular DNA molecule, 16 569 nucleotide pairs that encode genes for ribosomal RNA, transfer RNA and protein subunits of oxidative phosphorylation enzymes. Since mitochondria are passed on in the cytoplasm of the egg, diseases caused by mutation in mitochondrial DNA (mtDNA) show **matrilinear inheritance** and are never transmitted by the father.

The symptoms and signs of mitochondrial disorders are from tissues with high energy requirements: problems in the nervous system include encephalopathy, regression, ataxia, retinopathy, neuropathy; in muscle include weakness especially ptosis and ophthalmoplegia, dilated cardiomyopathy and heart rhythm disturbances. Such diverse symptomatology is sometimes described as mitochondrial cytopathy.

About 100 000 mitochondria are passed on in the cytoplasm of the egg and mutations in mtDNA can be present in a proportion of these mitochondria (**heteroplasmy**) or in 100 per cent (**homoplasmy**). In heteroplasmic disorders, the mitotic cell divisions after fertilization provide many opportunities for daughter cells in different somatic tissues to inherit different proportions of normal and mutant mitochondria. This partly explains why symptom complexes in mtDNA disorders are so varied (Table 3.2).

KEY LEARNING POINT

mtDNA mutations are always present in at least some tissues of the mother and siblings of each affected child. However, the chance that a close relative may show signs and symptoms of mitochondrial disease is often low. Egg donation from an unrelated donor is one option to avoid recurrence of mitochondrial cytopathy in a family.

DNA STRUCTURE AND PROTEIN SYNTHESIS

Figure 3.11 gives an overview of the organization of genetic material within the cell. Most important are the nucleic acids deoxyribose nucleic acid (DNA) and ribose nucleic acid (RNA). Each nucleic acid contain four bases comprising two purine bases, adenine (A) and guanine (G), and two pyrimidine bases, cytosine (C) and thymine (T). In RNA the thymine is replaced by another pyrimidine, uracil (U).

A **nucleoside** consists of a base covalently bonded to the 1-prime (1′) position of a pentose sugar ring. In RNA, the sugar molecule is ribose, in DNA it is 2′-deoxyribose in which the hydroxyl group at the 2′-position is replaced by a hydrogen.

A **nucleotide** is a nucleoside with one or more phosphate groups bound covalently to the 3′ or 5′ position. In the case of the 5′ position, up to three phosphate groups may be attached. For example adenosine 5′ triphosphate is ATP. Nucleoside 5′ triphosphates, chemically phosphate esters, are the building blocks of the DNA or RNA chain.

In DNA and RNA chains, deoxyribonucleotides and ribonucleotides, respectively, are joined into a polymer by covalent bonding of a phosphate group between the 5′ hydroxyl of one ribose and the 3′ hydroxyl of the next – a phosphodiester bond. This gives the nucleic acid strand a direction, from a free 5′ end to a free 3′ end. The acidity of the molecule comes about from the phosphate group's single negative charge at neutral pH. The repeating monomers of the nucleic acid strands, designated A, G, T, C and U are conventionally described in sequence starting from the 5′ end at the left, for example 5′ CATAAGCCTA 3′.

The DNA double helix is two separate strands of the polymer wound around each other in a helical path. The sugar-phosphate backbone is negatively charged on the outside of the helical structure. The DNA base pairs are stacked within the double helix. There is specific H-bond pairing of adenine with thymine (two hydrogen bonds) and guanine with cytosine (three hydrogen bonds) and the strands of the double helix are complementary. The two strands run in opposite directions in terms of their 5′ to 3′ directions. The sequence of one strand uniquely specifies the sequence of the other, this is central to the faithful replication of the DNA prior to meiosis and mitosis.

Gene transcription is the synthesis of a single-stranded RNA molecule from the double-stranded DNA template. RNA synthesis runs in the 5′ to 3′ direction and, with U in place of T, its sequence is the same as the sequence of deoxynucleotides in the DNA strand known as the **sense** strand. The other DNA strand, the actual template strand, is known as the **antisense** strand.

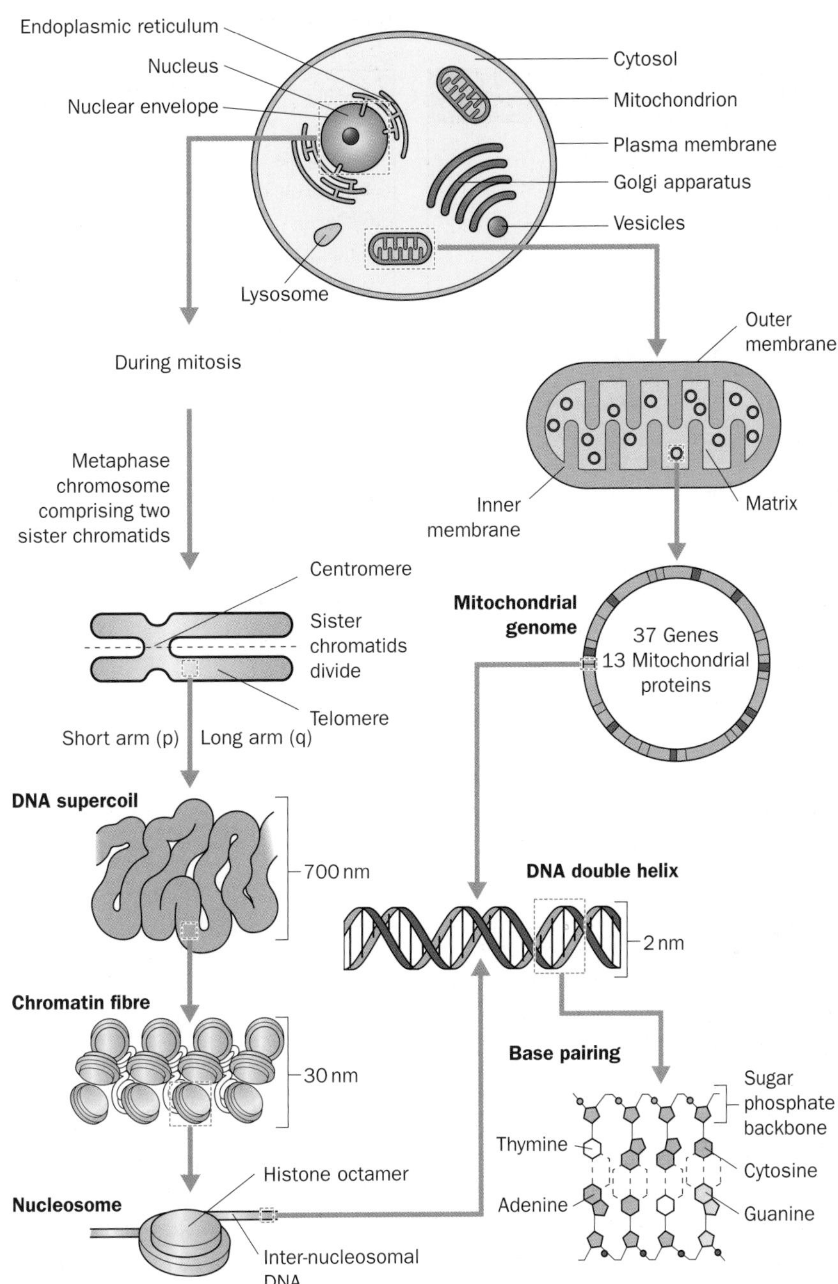

Figure 3.11 Organization of genetic information

The transcription complex includes an RNA polymerase molecule and co-factors that, together, add ribonucleotides to the growing 3′ end of the RNA strand. A specific DNA promoter sequence initiates transcription. Another short DNA sequence, the terminator sequence, signals cessation of transcription.

The **genetic code** (Table 3.3) reveals how the sequence of nucleotides in nucleic acid specifies the sequence of amino acids in protein. Groups of three adjacent nucleotides called **codons** each specify the 20 amino acids (Table 3.4) as well as three stop codons that terminate transcription. Since four bases allow 4^3 or 64 possible codons, most amino acids are specified by more than one codon. The code is consequently said to have redundancy, one effect of which is to decrease the chance of a harmful effect from some types of DNA sequence change, especially point mutations (see below), that would otherwise alter the amino acid composition of the protein.

Gene **transcription** in the cell nucleus produces a **messenger RNA** molecule (mRNA) (Figure 3.12). The initial message, called a pre-mRNA, is processed by removal of the intervening sequences or **introns** that interrupt the coding regions of genes or **exons**. Excision of mRNA intervening sequences is called **splicing** and this occurs in the nucleus. A feature of mRNA processing in higher

Table 3.3 The genetic code

1st position	2nd position				3rd position
	T	C	A	G	
T	Phe	Ser	Tyr	Cys	T
	Phe	Ser	Tyr	Cys	T
	Leu	Ser	STOP	STOP	A
	Leu	Ser	STOP	Trp	G
C	Leu	Pro	His	Arg	T
	Leu	Pro	His	Arg	C
	Leu	Pro	Gln	Arg	A
	Leu	Pro	Gln	Arg	G
A	Ile	Thr	Asn	Ser	T
	Ile	Thr	Asn	Ser	C
	Ile	Thr	Lys	Arg	A
	Met	Thr	Lys	Arg	G
G	Val	Ala	Asp	Gly	T
	Val	Ala	Asp	Gly	C
	Val	Ala	Glu	Gly	A
	Val	Ala	Glu	Gly	G

Description of mutations uses shorthand nomenclature: e.g. 1 in 10 individuals carry a single C282Y haemochromatosis gene mutation. This means cysteine (C) is substituted by tyrosine (Y) at codon 282. This amino acid change is due to a single base substitution G → A at position 845 changing the codon from TGT (cysteine) to TAT tyrosine. See the genetic code table above.

organisms is that not all exons within a gene are retained. Rather than specifying just one protein, several proteins may be specified by one gene as different combinations of exons undergo **alternative splicing** from unprocessed mRNA.

KEY LEARNING POINT

Genotype does not always predict phenotype: due to differences in patient selection and study methodologies, the proportion of all C282Y homozygotes that develop clinical haemochromatosis remains unknown – current estimates range from 1 per cent to 70 per cent.

Table 3.4 Amino acid shorthand

Alanine	Ala	A
Arginine	Arg	R
Asparagine	Asn	N
Aspartic acid	Asp	D
Cysteine	Cys	C
Glutamic acid	Glu	E
Glutamine	Gln	Q
Glycine	Gly	G
Histidine	His	H
Isoleucine	Ile	I
Leucine	Leu	L
Lysine	Lys	K
Methionine	Met	M
Phenylalanine	Phe	F
Proline	Pro	P
Serine	Ser	S
Threonine	Thr	T
Tryptophan	Trp	W
Tyrosine	Tyr	Y
Valine	Val	V

The mature mRNA specifies the sequence of amino acids in the polypeptide chain by a process called **translation.** There are three stages in protein synthesis:

- **Initiation:** when the translation apparatus or ribosome is assembled on the mRNA.
- **Elongation:** of the polypeptide occurs from the fixed start point (an AUG) in the message. Each codon or group of three bases in the mRNA is recognized by a complementary anticodon located on a particular transfer or tRNA molecule, leading to serial addition of amino acids to the growing chain.
- **Termination:** occurs when the completed polypeptide chain is released into the cytoplasm.

For many years, the central dogma of molecular biology was 'DNA makes RNA makes protein'. Exceptions to this flow of genetic information are now known. Retroviruses, including human immunodeficiency virus (HIV), each comprise a single-stranded RNA molecule. Using an enzyme called **reverse transcriptase**, the single-stranded RNA is converted within the cell to double-stranded DNA and, in turn, is inserted into the host genome. Another exception concerns RNA molecules that are not themselves translated but function in gene expression, e.g. in RNA processing and in translation.

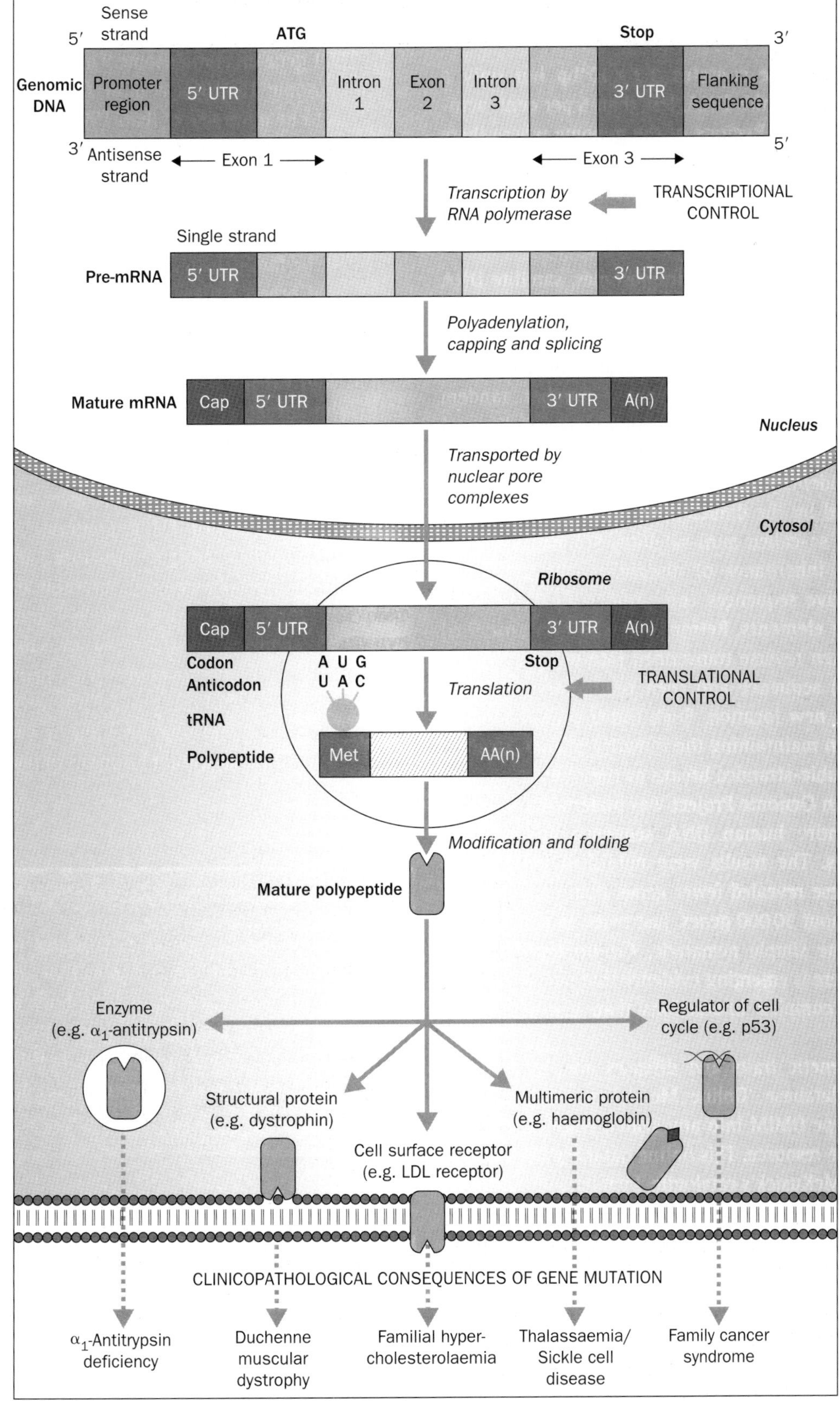

Figure 3.12 Gene expression. A(n), polyadenylated tail; AA(n) nth amino acid; LDL, low density lipoprotein; Met, methionine; UTR, untranslated region

THE HUMAN GENOME

The human genome contains 3.3×10^9 bp but only a small proportion of this DNA, less than 5 per cent, actually encodes genes. Regions of the genome where there are no genes contain different classes of **repetitive sequence DNA** that, as well as having unknown functions, may have had a role in evolution of the human genome.

Near the centromeres of chromosomes, satellite DNA consists of very large numbers of short (<30 bp) tandem repeats. In different healthy individuals, the number of repeat sequences may vary quite markedly. These size differences are hereditary. Variable number tandem repeats (VNTRs) are useful in genetic linkage studies and also in forensic science to establish or disprove paternity and genetic identity. Another variable size type of DNA is represented by the dinucleotide repeats, for example (CA)n; these so-called mini-satellites are also useful in tracking the inheritance of disease genes in families. Other repetitive sequences come under the heading of **transposable elements.** Retroposons can be transcribed into RNA, then reverse transcribed into complementary DNA (cDNA) sequence and then reintegrated into the genome at a new location. Such transposable elements have a role in maintaining the integrity of DNA strands, repairing double-stranded breaks as they arise.

The **Human Genome Project** was undertaken to determine the entire human DNA sequence and identify human genes. The results were published in February 2001 and these revealed fewer genes than expected. We each have about 30 000 genes, just twice as many as are present in the simple nematode, ***Caenorhabditis elegans***, but there is emerging evidence that our genes have many more complex interactions than genes in lower organisms.

Human genetic traits and diseases are listed in the web-based database 'Online Mendelian Inheritance in Man' (just type OMIM into any search engine), which is an invaluable resource. This online database has evolved from Victor McKusick's catalogue, Mendelian Inheritance in Man, which listed known disease genes and phenotypes allocating each one a unique number along with an expert, referenced review. In total, these reviews aim to provide a description of the 'morbid anatomy of the human genome'.

OMIM is the core reference for information on genetic diseases. OMIM emphasizes genetic heterogeneity and this has important implications for clinical diagnosis, genetic advice and the predictive value of genetic tests. Genetic heterogeneity means that a single disorder may be caused by disease genes located on different chromosomes. For example, tuberous sclerosis may be caused by a mutation in the TSC1 gene on chromosome 9 or a mutation in TSC2 on chromosome 16. TSC2 is more frequently diagnosed and tends to be more severe than TSC1.

Heterogeneity has consequences for gene-based diagnosis. Only 5 per cent of breast cancers are caused by mutations in single genes. There are two major breast cancer genes, BRCA1 and BRCA2. Both genes are large and when the family history indicates there is a high risk of inherited breast cancer, both genes may be screened for mutations. However, other genes and non-genetic factors influence susceptibility to breast cancer. Thus, a woman who carries a BRCA1 or BRCA2 mutation may not develop breast cancer. Conversely, a negative BRCA1 or BRCA2 gene test result is not totally reassuring.

In **bioinformatics**, computer databases of assembled DNA sequences from higher and lower organisms are compared and searched using programs that identify genes and predict protein structure and function. **Proteomics** is the name given to the study of all the proteins that different cell types produce. Proteins are more complicated than nucleic acids and are subject to many different chemical modifications (e.g. phosphorylation, glycosylation, acetylation). Protein production varies in health and disease and proteins bind to many different molecules in different cellular locations in response to different signals.

KEY LEARNING POINT

New technologies such as microarray techniques or DNA chip technology are tools that are used for high-throughput chemical assays. Such assays are required to map patterns of gene mutation, gene expression and protein production in different cell types. Proteomics will be important for drug development in the future.

DNA sequence variations

Shorthand nomenclature for the description of DNA (and RNA and protein) sequence variations is daunting. Usually a description in plain English is the easiest to understand. The term 'sequence variation' is often employed alongside or instead of the older terms 'mutation' and 'polymorphism' that were introduced long before the chemistry and function of DNA were discovered.

Alternative forms of a gene found at one specific gene locus are termed **alleles**. For example, at the ABO blood group locus on chromosome 9, the three common alleles result in A, B and O blood groups. The ABO system is a good example of a **polymorphic system**, reflecting DNA sequence variants that occur at measurable frequency (>1 per cent individuals). The commonest, non-disease causing allele at a gene locus is called the **wild-type** allele.

Alleles occur at equal frequency in different populations in the presence of migration and contact (interbreeding). In contrast, relatively small populations that are isolated for geographic, ethnic or religious reasons often display allele frequencies that are quite different. An allele may be fixed at high frequency in a population that is derived from a few ancestors (founder effect). Populations that were originally sizeable but diminished before expanding may exhibit an ancestral or genetic bottleneck that can also fix unusual allele frequencies.

KEY LEARNING POINT

Knowledge of allele frequencies in different populations may lead to targeted genetic screening tests or increased clinical suspicion when diagnosing rare diseases, e.g. β-thalassaemia gene in Mediterranean peoples, Tay–Sachs disease gene in Ashkenazi Jews.

Ultimately, DNA sequence changes are caused by physical or chemical agents (sunlight, X rays, cytotoxic drugs) damaging DNA, or by non-fatal errors in biological processes of DNA replication or meiotic recombination. Cells have DNA repair systems but disease-causing mutations are inevitable. Everyone carries potential disease-causing recessive mutations including at least one recessive gene mutation that, if homozygous, is lethal.

Single nucleotide polymorphisms (SNPs) are common DNA sequence variants occurring at 1 per 1000 bp in the human genome. They occur within genes as well as in non-coding DNA sequences. Increasingly, SNPs are being used to study complex inheritance: for example, certain SNPs may influence gene expression and protein function. Even if an SNP does not directly do this, it may lie close to and thus act as a marker for another unknown deleterious sequence change. SNPs are easily detected in high-throughput sequence analyses and are therefore valuable in studies of common diseases such as hypertension, autism and schizophrenia. SNPs are also used in pharmacogenomics to map genetic backgrounds that make individuals more or less prone to side effects of drugs, or responsive to different therapies.

Different types of mutation

Point or single-nucleotide mutation

Single base substitutions include transitions where one purine or one pyrimidine is exchanged for another purine or pyrimidine, respectively, or transversions where a purine is replaced by a pyrimidine or vice versa. If the point mutation does not result in a change in the amino acid sequence in the protein it is termed 'silent'.

A **missense** mutation results in a changed codon that specifies a different amino acid in the protein. Single base substitution may also create a new 'stop' codon: a **nonsense** mutation results in a shortened protein. Point mutations may also affect regulation of gene transcription (causing too much or too little) or intracellular processing of the mRNA product (e.g. splice site mutations).

Insertion or deletion mutations

Insertion or deletion mutations commonly cause a shift in the codon reading frame. A 3 bp deletion can cause omission of a single amino acid molecule from an otherwise intact protein, but if the amino acid has a crucial function, e.g. the phenylalanine residue at position 508 in the cystic fibrosis gene, the clinical effect is severe. Insertions or deletions that add/remove 1, 2, 4, 5, 7 bp, etc., are termed out-of-frame and result in a completely changed amino acid sequence, usually terminating with a new 'stop' codon and a shortened abnormal protein.

Trinucleotide repeats

Different trinucleotide repeat sequences are found throughout the genome. Certain repeats may undergo abnormal expansion and this mutation mechanism underlies several neurological and neuromuscular diseases (Table 3.5). Some trinucleotide repeat disorders exhibit unusual pedigree features. For example, in myotonic dystrophy there is tendency to have more severe disease with younger age of onset in successive generations. This is called **anticipation** and it is due to progressive increases in the repeat size as it passes from parent to child.

Submicroscopic or cryptic structural chromosome abnormalities

Limited resolution of conventional chromosome studies means very small chromosome rearrangements, typically

Table 3.5 Common trinucleotide repeat disorders

Disease	Trinucleotide repeat and chromosome location	Normal range of repeats	Premutation range (unstable but without clinical effect)	Affected range of repeats
Fragile X syndrome	CGG Xq27	5-54	60-200	200-1000
Myotonic dystrophy	CTG 19q13	5-37	38-49	50-3000
Huntington disease	CAG 4p16	10-35	36-39	40-120
Friedreich ataxia	GAA 9q13	6-34	80	112-1700

3–5 Mb, cannot be seen, but the resulting syndromes are suspected on clinical grounds and family history evidence. Diagnosis is by molecular cytogenetic (FISH) or DNA techniques.

Visible cytogenetic abnormalities

Disorders of chromosome number (aneuploidies) and disorders of chromosome structure such as translocations have also been classed as mutations.

THE MOLECULAR GENETICS LABORATORY

In the 1970s, recombinant DNA research permitted manipulation of small segments of DNA and the first diagnostic molecular genetics laboratories were established in hospitals. Since that period, the three main methodologies in molecular genetic diagnostics have been Southern blotting, polymerase chain reaction (PCR) and DNA sequencing (Figure 3.13). Polymerase chain reaction is used to detect point mutations and other types of mutation that are already known. DNA sequencing is a method employed to detect mutation that may not have been described previously. Southern blotting is required to detect some special types of mutation such as large genomic rearrangements.

To obtain DNA, anticoagulated blood is ideal. Very small samples of 1 mL or less may be used for some but not all tests and sufficient DNA might be obtained from a mouth wash or buccal scraping. Care should be taken not to contaminate the sample. DNA is also obtained from solid tissues and tumour but previous pathological processing may make this more difficult.

In **Southern blotting**, intact strands of nuclear DNA from blood lymphocytes are cut into fragments using microbial restriction enzymes. The resulting short segments of DNA sequence are separated by electrophoresis, transferred to a solid membrane (the blot) and then visualized using autoradiographic methods. Radiolabelled DNA sequences are made to probe the fragmented DNA mix for the sequence of interest. Southern blotting takes several weeks and was named after its inventor, Professor Ed Southern. Variations of the Southern technique are **northern blotting** which uses RNA instead of DNA, and **western blotting**, where proteins are examined in place of nucleic acids.

Polymerase chain reaction is now much more commonly employed than Southern blotting. The PCR gives rapid results by direct examination of short DNA sequences after their selective amplification in the test tube without any use of radioactivity. Polymerase chain reaction involves rapid copying of a short stretch of target DNA selected by an oligonucleotide primer DNA sequence specifically synthesized for this purpose. The target DNA in a mix is first made single stranded by heat denaturation. The oligonucleotide primer is added and it binds to DNA at the location containing its complementary sequence. DNA polymerase and added nucleotides permit extension of the synthesized DNA sequence from the primer sequence until the reaction is stopped by heat denaturation. The cycle is then repeated many times but on each occasion more newly synthesized template strands are available for the primer to bind to. The net result is selective amplification and exponential increase in concentration of the targeted sequence.

DNA sequencing reveals the sequence of bases in DNA and comparison of results with reference sequence data locates unknown mutations or confirms the presence of a mutation detected by another method. Neutral or non-pathological sequence changes may substitute one amino acid in a protein with another amino acid that has similar chemical properties. Yet other DNA sequence changes may be examples of rare polymorphisms.

DNA amplification by the polymerase chain reaction (PCR)

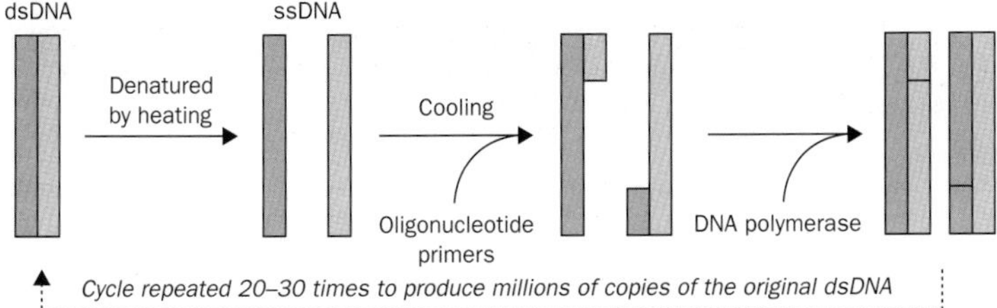

DNA sequencing

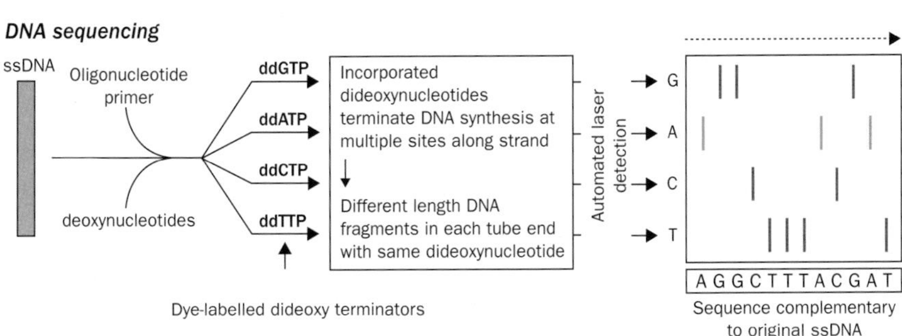

Restriction fragment length polymorphism (RFLP) analysis

Example: sickle cell disease

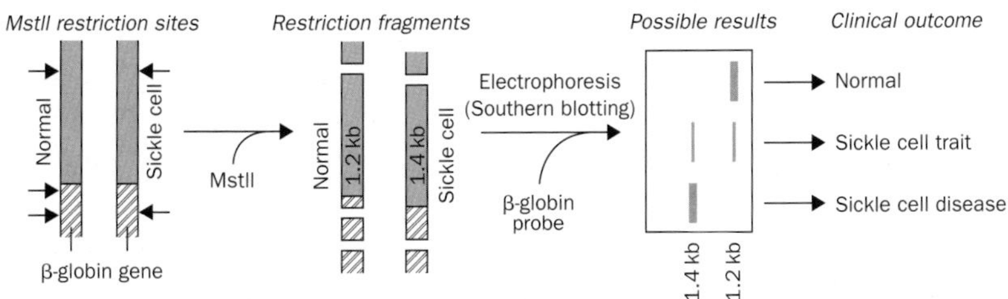

Figure 3.13 Molecular genetic techniques

KEY LEARNING POINT

A single mutation is pathological if it is found in many patients who suffer the same disease. If a mutation is novel, its presence in affected relatives in one family, but not in the unaffected relations, indicates that it causes disease. Mutation databases and OMIM catalogue entries should be consulted for details of pathological and non-pathological DNA sequence changes, but expert advice may be required to establish the pathogenicity of some DNA sequence changes.

THE GENETIC CLINIC AND GENETIC COUNSELLING

Genetic counselling

The term 'genetic counselling' was first employed to describe the activities undertaken by the clinical geneticist at the genetic clinic. The term 'counselling' has also come to be associated with talking therapy that seeks to repair psychological damage. This is not the primary purpose of a consultation at the genetic clinic, although provision of information to patients and relatives who are at risk of a genetic disorder may have therapeutic consequences.

Activities undertaken at the genetic clinic

- Family history taking, clinical examination, ordering genetic laboratory tests.
- Formulating a diagnosis.
- Giving information on clinical consequences to patients and relatives.
- Assessing the probability of developing or transmitting genetic disease.
- Discussing prevention, avoidance and amelioration.
- Arranging ongoing psychological support, where appropriate.

In essence, the geneticist seeks to make or confirm a precise diagnosis, explain the origin or hereditary mechanism of genetic disease and discuss hereditary implications for relatives. Information on additional genetic investigations, including prenatal diagnosis and presymptomatic tests may also be given.

Who should be offered referral to the genetic clinic?

Basically, any individual who either seeks or who may benefit from a genetic professional's opinion should be offered referral to the genetic clinic. In the UK, up to half of all referrals to the genetic clinic concern family history of cancer. Of the remainder, approximately equal numbers of referrals come from specialists in paediatrics, obstetrics and general practice. Among unscreened referrals, there are a few apparently trivial problems, but even these may have an unexpected twist and pitfall for the unwary counsellor.

KEY LEARNING POINT

Every genetics centre encourages phone calls to discuss patient and family referrals.

Providing non-directive advice

The aim of non-directive genetic counselling is to equip individuals to make their own informed choices. Once the family tree has been drawn and the genetic diagnosis made, issues raised by the patient and family are addressed. Good communication skills are essential. It is often difficult to provide families with information about uncertain genetic diagnoses. Frequently, advice based upon past experience (**empirical**) is all that can be offered.

Families and individuals are never instructed to undergo or avoid predictive genetic tests or prenatal diagnosis. All available options are explained and discussions cover topics such as the predictive value of tests, the chance of test error and the chance of serious side effects, such as miscarriage after amniocentesis. Several appointments at the genetic clinic may be required. A typical genetic counselling session might last 45 minutes. Complex situations may require two or more sessions to discuss inheritance, availability of tests and risks to relatives. In many centres, a jargon-free written summary is sent to the patient after the final session. A home visit by a genetic co-worker may be arranged to provide psychological support after bad news is given.

KEY LEARNING POINT

At the genetic clinic, families should not be told what course of action to take, but they should leave the consultation more informed and able to weigh up relative merits and drawbacks of different options.

ETHICAL ISSUES IN MEDICAL GENETICS

Beneficence is the medical ethics principle that commits the physician to practise medicine for the benefit of his or her patient. A second medical ethical principle states that there should be respect for each patient's autonomy. Like all doctors, the geneticist encounters many ethical challenges in diagnosis and management of diseases but, more than most, the geneticist will feel obligations that extend to patients' relatives who may be unaware of their risk of developing hereditary disease, or the chance of transmitting such diseases to their own children.

To assist doctors, the discipline of bioethics has emerged to provide the framework and tools for ethical medical practice that uses new technologies in medicine. Ethical practice has the power to dispel lingering suspicion about eugenic motives in medical genetics. This suspicion has been fuelled by history of abuse of genetics, developments in biotechnology ('genetic engineering') and some unique characteristics of clinical genetic information. Gene test results may not alter clinical care, they seldom open avenues for treatment, even time of onset of genetic disease or the severity of symptoms may not be predictable from positive gene test results. Test results on one person often have direct health implications for unsuspecting or asymptomatic relatives, including revelation of undisclosed non-paternity.

Since the benefits of gene tests may not always outweigh adverse consequences, it is no surprise that the uptake of predictive genetic tests is low: only 10 per cent of adults who are at 50 per cent risk of developing Huntington disease choose to have a predictive gene test. For conditions such as breast cancer or colon cancer where early diagnosis and better treatment are options, the uptake of gene testing is higher.

Consent and confidentiality

Genetic advice is unreliable if it is given without opportunities to examine patients and consult records. Yet relatives may not wish to inform each other about genetic

KEY LEARNING POINT

Issues of consent and confidentiality are best resolved by relatives within families. Guidelines on consent and confidentiality issues in clinical genetics are available on the British Society of Human Genetics (BSHG) website (www.bshg.org.uk).

risks. Consent may not be given to examine medical notes to establish or refute diagnoses. Genetic testing may reveal unsuspected non-paternity. Such ethical problems are encountered regularly in clinical genetic practice.

Testing children for genetic disorders

Many adults choose not to undergo genetic tests and routine testing of children breaches autonomy and confidentiality. Clear advice from the American Academy of Pediatrics is that unless there is anticipated benefit to the child, paediatricians should decline requests from parents to obtain predispositional genetic testing until the child has the capacity to make a choice. Despite such advice being published, a recent survey revealed that many paediatric residents in the USA are either unaware or hold a different opinion, suggesting a problem in the realm of education about ethics in genetics.

One example of clear-cut benefit to the child from genetic testing is presymptomatic testing for mutation in the RET gene on chromosome 10 that causes medullary thyroid carcinoma. Prophylactic surgery should be carried out on children who test positive. Another example concerns testing for the polyposis coli gene on chromosome 5 prior to undertaking colonoscopy on an at-risk child.

KEY LEARNING POINT

In general, children should not undergo predictive or presymptomatic genetic testing unless there are medical interventions to treat or prevent complications in the event of a positive test result.

Consanguinity

Consanguineous marriage, customary in many societies, does lead to slight increase in childhood morbidity, largely from rare autosomal recessive disorders. However, discouraging consanguineous unions on medical genetics grounds is unethical and overlooks the social importance of consanguineous marriage. In many communities where there is consanguinity, access to accurate, understandable information on genetics and disease prevention is appreciated.

Abortion

In England and Wales, 0.2 per cent of all terminations are carried out for a genetic diagnosis or serious congenital malformation. Ethical issues inevitably arise when a genetic disorder is diagnosed in the fetus. Medical science alone cannot answer questions such as how serious a disorder needs be to justify request for pregnancy termination, or how trivial it needs be to warrant refusal of such a request. The courts may be asked to rule in difficult or controversial cases. For individuals and families in such cases, high-profile legal arguments are awful to endure but, inevitably, medical ethicists, politicians and lay individuals who represent special interest groups, all wish to contribute to open debate on ethical issues.

Assessing the seriousness of a genetic condition (the likely clinical burden)

- Parents' view of the condition
- Likely degree of suffering associated with the condition
- Availability of effective therapy or treatment
- Speed of degeneration in progressive disorders
- Extent of any intellectual impairment
- Individual circumstances of the family or woman, including other siblings

Preimplantation genetic diagnosis

Embryo biopsy and genetic analysis of a single cell is performed on a 6–8 cell cleavage stage embryo in culture at three days post insemination. The majority of couples seeking preimplantation genetic diagnosis (PGD) will have either had a previously affected child or pregnancy or a close relative affected by a serious genetic condition. Through use of PGD, couples have the opportunity of having an unaffected child without repeated antenatal diagnosis and possible termination of pregnancy. Preimplantation genetic diagnosis has been accomplished in spinal muscular atrophy, cystic fibrosis, Tay–Sachs disease, Marfan syndrome, Duchenne muscular dystrophy and fragile X syndrome, as well as chromosome disorders such as Down syndrome and the Wolf–Hirschhorn del 4(p) syndrome.

More controversially, PGD has also been used to provide an immunologically matched sibling for a child who is affected by a disorder such as Fanconi anaemia, which might be cured by bone marrow or umbilical stem cell transplantation. In the UK, PGD is tightly regulated and may only be performed under licence, considered on a centre by centre and condition by condition basis. In England, more than several hundred cycles have been completed to egg collection since PGD was introduced about 10 years ago. The numbers are growing each year but PGD is not more widely used because it is a complex technique incorporating the physical, emotional and financial problems of *in vitro* fertilization. The safety of PGD is a concern. Initial evaluation of babies born worldwide after this procedure has not indicated increased risk of congenital malformation. There may, however, be increased risk of disorders such as Beckwith–Weidemann syndrome caused by disturbance of genetic imprinting. Other reservations about the use of PGD tend to be general in nature – concerns that PGD should not be used to deliberately choose 'desirable' characteristics and worries that new genetic technology might disadvantage disabled people now or in the future. At present, the complexity of PGD operates as an effective protection against its misuse.

GENETIC SCREENING

Antenatal screening for Down syndrome

Antenatal screening for Down syndrome is an established part of antenatal care in many countries but there is great variation in the type of screening offered. The ideal screening test identifies all true carriers (maximum sensitivity) and only true carriers (maximum specificity).

In practice, 5 per cent of all pregnancies fall into a 'high-risk' category that is set to place a ceiling on the number of diagnostic amniocentesis performed. In the UK, most but not all couples choose to have screening tests for Down syndrome and the maximum potential impact is 80 per cent reduction in the number of affected babies born.

Table 3.6 gives details of some statistics used to measure the performance of a screening test. In assessing performance, numbers do not tell the whole story, the aim of the test and the psychological consequences of false positive and false negative results must also be considered.

> Antenatal screening practices for trisomy 21
>
> **Maternal age-based mid-trimester screening:** Women over the age of 35 years are offered an invasive diagnostic test such as amniocentesis. The risk of miscarriage after amniocentesis is 1 per cent.
>
> **Combined mid-trimester screening with biochemical markers and age:** Individual risk assessment based upon maternal serum α-fetoprotein level, maternal serum human chorionic gonadotrophin (hCG) level and the maternal age.
>
> **First trimester screening with combined fetal nuchal thickness measurement, biochemical markers and age:** This protocol has greatest sensitivity.

Neonatal screening

Neonatal screening for genetic disorders aims to decrease the morbidity and mortality attributable to

Table 3.6 Measuring the performance of a screening test

	Disease +	Disease −		
Test +	True positive (TP)	False positive (FP)	All with positive test TP + FP	Positive predictive value = TP/(TP + FP)
Test −	False negative (FN)	True negative (TN)	All with negative test FN + TN	Negative predictive value = TN/(FN + TN)
	All with disease	All without disease	All = TP + FP + FN + TN	
	Sensitivity = TP/(TP + FN)	Specificity = TN/(FP + TN)	Pretest probability = (TP + FN)/(TP + FP + FN + TN) (sometimes = prevalence)	

Sensitivity: The proportion of people with disease who have a positive test result.

Specificity: The proportion of people free of a disease who have a negative test.

Positive predictive value (PPV): The percentage of people with a positive test result who actually have the disease.

Negative predictive value (NPV): The percentage of people with a negative test who do NOT have the disease.

Likelihood ratio: The likelihood that a given test result would be expected in a patient with a disease compared to the likelihood that the same result would be expected in a patient without that disease.

selected diseases. Certain principles govern the introduction of new tests and the maintenance of established tests:

- the identification of the genetic condition must provide a clear benefit to the child
- a system must be in place to confirm the diagnosis
- treatment and follow-up must be available for affected neonates.

The effects of false-positive results on parents has to be considered as well.

The treatment clause causes greatest difficulty. Screening tests for phenylketonuria and hypothyroidism are established as early diagnosis leads to treatment and improved outcomes. Neonatal screening for cystic fibrosis is not so widespread. Long-term studies are in progress to answer whether detection of cystic fibrosis in the neonatal period improves life quality and expectancy by improving pulmonary and nutritional status. In some regions there is neonatal screening for Duchenne muscular dystrophy, mainly instigated to prevent late diagnosis in families who would otherwise be unaware of their young child's genetic diagnosis until after the birth of a second affected boy.

Carrier screening

DNA tests permit identification of individuals who are carriers of mutations in certain single genes. Examples include **targeted screening**, e.g. Tay–Sachs disease in Ashkenazi Jews, and **cascade screening** in relatives of patients with, e.g. Duchenne muscular dystrophy or cystic fibrosis, after identification of an index case.

Population-based carrier screening for genetic disorders is more problematic. A salutary example was targeted population screening for the sickle cell trait in America in the 1970s. This experience illustrated how lay people are confused by the difference between being an asymptomatic heterozygous carrier (sickle cell trait) and homozygous affected (sickle cell disease).

Sickle cell disease is caused by homozygosity for a point mutation at codon 6 (GAG to GTG) leading to substitution of a glutamic acid residue by valine. This substitution alters the chemical properties of the heteromeric $\alpha_2\beta_2$ globin molecule. Aggregation of haemoglobin S (Hb S) in hypoxic conditions causes deformed, sickle-shaped red cells that block microvascular networks. Affected homozygotes have diverse symptoms and repeated, painful acute crises that cause infarction and infection in extremities and bones especially. Repeated blood transfusions cause iron overload. In contrast, heterozygous carriers are healthy. In America, targeted screening and insufficient education led to healthy heterozygous carriers being stigmatized and discriminated against by employers, insurance companies and government agencies.

In the UK, only a minority of pregnancies affected by haemoglobinopathies are diagnosed. There is antenatal screening but with late recognition of genetic risk, the uptake of prenatal testing is low. Suggestions for improvement have involved simultaneously screening both partners when a woman in an at-risk group reports a pregnancy, or opportunistically offering screening in primary care before a woman becomes pregnant.

Predictive genetic tests for late-onset disorders

Myotonic dystrophy, haemochromatosis, polycystic kidney disease, Huntington disease, and some cancers are examples of diseases that may be diagnosed before the onset of symptoms. A positive test result simply means the disease gene is present. Predictive genetic diagnosis may have health benefits, for example, avoiding unguarded general anaesthesia in the unconscious patient with myotonic dystrophy. Psychological benefits are gained from learning that a mutation is not present. Some individuals argue that they gain benefit from reduction in uncertainty if a mutation is identified. But diagnostic or predictive testing for late-onset disorders should always be considered carefully: for example, if a child with vague symptomatology and a distant family history of Huntington disease is tested for the gene, a positive test result in the child automatically means the intervening parent carries the gene mutation too.

DNA may be examined for sequence changes that influence the risk of common, adult-onset disorders such as coronary artery disease, diabetes, stroke and Alzheimer disease. Mostly, however, these tests have low predictive value and are only ever carried out on consenting adults in research programmes.

KEY LEARNING POINT

Presymptomatic or predictive genetic tests should not be undertaken without careful prior discussion at the genetic clinic.

CONGENITAL MALFORMATIONS, SYNDROMES AND DYSMORPHOLOGY

Congenital malformations account for about 20 per cent of all infant deaths. Malformation of the nervous, cardiovascular and respiratory syndromes account for most malformation deaths. Congenital malformations are a leading cause of infant mortality and morbidity. Overall, about 1 in 50 infants will have a serious congenital malformation.

The child with dysmorphism

Where are dysmorphisms most readily identified?
- Structures with complicated form – face, hands, feet, genitalia

How are dysmorphisms best described?
- Plain English is preferred; jargon is least helpful
- Photographs
- Measurements and comparison with growth charts

Causes of dysmorphism
- The effects of single, pathological gene mutations
- The effects of chromosome imbalance
- Non-pathological effects of multiple genes (children do resemble their parents)
- Teratogenic effects
- Effects of abnormal fetal growth and/or lack of movement

Clinical significance of dysmorphism
- Multiple dysmorphisms indicate increased chance of major malformation
- Patterns of dysmorphism may lead to diagnosis of specific syndromes

What are the advantages of syndrome diagnosis?
- A 'name' can help, for example, on medical certificates
- Clarification of genetic implications for the family
- Psychological – the relief from 'not knowing'; abolition of guilt

There are many causes of congenital malformations: these range from single gene causes such as autosomal recessive Zellweger syndrome to environmental causes such as thalidomide embryopathy. Probably, in most cases, the malformation arises from combinations of genetic susceptibility, environment factors and random chance. A definite example of gene–environment interaction is reduction in the incidence of spina bifida due to better maternal diet and periconceptional folic acid supplementation; possible examples include varying genetic susceptibilities to fetal alcohol syndrome and fetal anticonvulsant syndrome.

A very useful tool that aids syndrome diagnosis is the computerized database of dysmorphic syndromes. This may be used to provide a list of candidate diagnosis for the child or adult who has an unusual pattern of congenital malformations. The database is compiled by extracting details (clinical features) of all known syndromes from the literature. The database may then be asked to list all syndromes that have a specified combination of features. Efficient syndrome searching is a skill developed by the dysmorphologist who is aware that the results of each search must always be used cautiously. Original sources must be checked before judging the likelihood that a suggested diagnosis is correct.

Useful definitions

Primary malformation: An abnormality of differentiation of a specific body part; examples include atrioventricular canal defect, holoprosencephaly, polydactyly.

Secondary malformation or disruption: Initial normal differentiation but subsequent abnormality in development and growth due to an extrinsic cause. A poorly understood example might be amniotic bands that are considered a cause of bizarre facial clefts, constriction bands and *in utero* amputations of digits.

Dysplasia: A development abnormality of tissue structure, for example cystic dysplasia of the kidneys. Dysplasia of the lymphatic system probably causes cystic hygroma, lower limb oedema and toenail dysplasia in Turner syndrome.

Deformity: A misshapen but normally differentiated structure, e.g. some cases of club foot. Deformations often arise *in utero* due to extrinsic compression associated with oligohydramnios or uterine malformation. Deformations generally have a good prognosis.

Syndrome: A loose definition is 'a clinically recognizable pattern of congenital abnormalities'.

Dysmorphism: Less common appearance or form in a normally differentiated part of the body, for example anteverted nares, clinodactyly of the fifth finger, a single palmer crease.

Although recognisable patterns of dysmorphism are the sole basis for diagnosis of many rare syndromes, such patterns of dysmorphism are neither 100 per cent specific or sensitive. Down syndrome is the most easily recognized dysmorphic syndrome and the trisomy 21 facial 'gestalt' is the most important clue, but it is not so obvious in African babies, hence their older age at diagnosis. Table 3.7 gives some features of selected syndromes.

Table 3.7 Genetic and dysmorphic syndromes

Typical presenting scenario	Consider	Clinical clues/helpful tests
Multiple malformations presenting in newborn period	Trisomy 18	Congenital heart disease, flexed overlapping fingers, short great toe
	Trisomy 13	Polydactyly, micro-ophthalmia, scalp defects, facial clefts, cystic kidneys
	Meckel syndrome	Encephalocele, cystic kidneys, polydactyly, liver fibrosis
	Smith-Lemli-Opitz syndrome	2/3 toe syndactyly, polydactyly, 7-dehydrocholesterol estimation
	VATER association	*V*ertebral, *a*nal, *t*racheo-oesphageal fistula, *r*enal abnormality; diagnosis by exclusion
Cardiac defect/short stature/learning disability	Noonan syndrome	Pulmonary stenosis, facial gestalt, some with DNA mutation
	Deletion 22q.11 syndrome	Short palpebral fissures, small mouth, palatal insufficiency, low threshold for ordering FISH 22 studies
	Fetal alcohol syndrome	Take history from multiple sources. Exclude 22q11 deletion
	Williams syndrome	Hypercalcaemia, supravalvular aortic stenosis, FISH for chromosome 7 deletion
	Poorly controlled maternal diabetes	Confirm poor diabetic control during embryonic period
	Turner syndrome	Learning difficulties usually not apparent, look for naevi and nail dysplasia
Very short stature (not skeletal dysplasia)		
With severe learning difficulties, microcephaly	DeLange syndrome	Synophrys with typical facial gestalt, limb defects
With cognitively normal or near normal, normocephalic	Russell-Silver syndrome	IUGR, pseudohydrocephalic appearance, limb asymmetry, UPD 7 in some cases
Coarse features, regression	Hurler syndrome	Regression in infancy, corneal clouding (do urinary glycosaminoglycans)
	Hunter syndrome	Boys only, no corneal clouding (do urinary glycosaminoglycans)
	Sanfilippo syndrome	Deteriorating behaviour, regression after infancy, little/no coarsening of appearance (do urinary glycosaminoglycans)
Learning disability		
Delayed walking	Duchenne muscular dystrophy	Creatine kinase
Macrocephaly	Fragile X syndrome	DNA confirmation
Macrocephaly, large stature	Sotos syndrome	DNA mutation in most cases
Normocephalic boy, tall	XYY, XXY	Cytogenetics
Normocephaly, hypoglycaemia, ear pits, organomegaly, body asymmetry	Beckwith-Weidemann syndrome	Clinical diagnostic criteria published, DNA studies sometimes helpful
Reduced OFC, epilepsy	Angelman syndrome	Electroencephalogram helpful, request DNA studies
Reduced OFC, regression, epilepsy	Rett syndrome	Clinical diagnostic criteria published, DNA studies helpful in some cases
Minor facial and limb dysmorphism	Fetal anticonvulsant syndrome	Always take maternal drug history
Macrocephaly, café-au-lait macules	Type 1 neurofibromatosis	Examine siblings and parents
Seizures, hypopigmented macules	Tuberous sclerosis	Ultraviolet light examination (parents too), fibrous forehead plaque, brain calcification

FISH, fluorescent in situ hybridization; IUGR, intrauterine growth retardation; UPD, uniparental disomy; OFC, occipitofrontal circumference.

KEY LEARNING POINT

When first assessing an infant with congenital malformations, remember that an atypical presentation of a relatively common condition (e.g. an autosomal trisomy) is more likely than the discovery of a second case of an extremely rare diagnosis.

In summary, rare syndrome diagnosis poses the same challenges that any medical diagnosis may pose. The list of questions that parents of the dysmorphic child ask are predictable and include: What is the diagnosis? Why did it happen? What is the outlook? Will it happen again in my family? What may be done to prevent recurrence? Although for many conditions the responses are much more complete than those given just a few years ago, in everyday clinical genetics practice, answers to these fundamental questions are frequently still clouded by uncertainty.

PROBLEMS

CASE STUDY: A baby with multiple congenital abnormalities

A newborn baby boy is admitted to neonatal intensive care with cyanosis from birth, failure to pass a nasogastric tube and hypoplastic right thumb. Pregnancy was complicated by polyhydramnios. Investigations show oesphageal atresia in conjunction with other congenital abnormalities.

In this case, urgent cytogenetic analysis should be arranged to rule out trisomy 18. If the chromosomes are normal, oesphageal atresia with radial limb defect is suggestive of the VATER association (vertebral abnormalities, anal abnormality, tracheo-oesphageal fistula, renal abnormality). As a rule, assessment of the newborn or stillborn baby affected by a multiple congenital abnormality syndrome should be systematic.

1 Obtain detailed family history, specifically ask about infant deaths and consanguinity.
2 Review prenatal history, mother's health and medications.
3 Complete physical examination including measurements of length, weight and occipitofrontal circumference (OFC).
4 Document and photograph dysmorphisms.
5 Check eyes, heart, kidneys, brain (cranial ultrasound) and hearing.
6 Order radiographs if skeletal dysplasia suspected.
7 Check blood has been sent for chromosome analysis.
8 Consult clinical geneticist colleagues.
9 When the malformations are lethal, check tissue samples are stored for future diagnostic studies and request consent for post-mortem examination.

KEY LEARNING POINT

Clinical examination is most important to seek dysmorphic signs that may suggest a serious chromosome imbalance syndrome. Examination is best carried out immediately after lifesaving measures and before application of tapes and masks.

In many cases, there is no definite diagnosis. It is unwise to speculate as this can lead to an incorrect diagnosis becoming fixed. It is better to offer repeat diagnostic assessments. At the genetic clinic, advice about risk of recurrence and prenatal diagnosis may still be possible in such cases.

CASE STUDY: Cleft palate in the mother of a healthy neonate

At discharge examination, the mother of a healthy neonate asks that her baby's palate is checked thoroughly as she herself underwent repair of cleft palate. The newborn baby is well and the mother is aware that isolated cleft palate has genetic implications.

Cleft lip with or without cleft palate is one of the commonest congenital abnormalities, affecting approximately 1 in 1000 neonates. Isolated cleft palate affects 1 in 2000 neonates and this malformation is more frequently associated with other congenital malformations.

Although the majority of individuals who have cleft lip and palate do not have a similarly affected relative, family studies indicate increased risk (1 in 20) of cleft lip and palate in siblings and offspring of an affected individual. Sibling recurrence risk is slightly greater after an affected male baby. Candidate genes for orofacial clefting have been identified but in most cases the genetic origin of this common malformation is unknown.

KEY LEARNING POINT

All individuals with cleft palate or cleft lip or both should have family history taken and be examined carefully for signs of a rare autosomal dominant condition called van der Woude syndrome. This condition shows variable expression and lip pits in the vermilion border may be the only minor sign that is detected.

Orofacial clefts may be diagnosed in the fetal period by detailed ultrasound examination. In the future, *in utero* surgery might offer repair with minimal scarring. Folic acid supplementation of the mother's diet in the periconceptional and embryonic period may reduce the chance of recurrence of cleft lip and palate (as the chance of neural tube defects is decreased by folic acid supplementation).

CASE STUDY: Type 1 spinal muscular atrophy (SMA1 or Werdnig–Hoffmann disease)

A 7-week-old neonate was admitted to hospital with poor feeding and floppiness. The mother reported that the baby never kicked when bathed. Areflexia was noted on clinical examination and the diagnosis was confirmed by discovering electromyographic evidence of anterior horn cell loss.

The incidence of the most severe type 1 SMA is between 1 in 10 000 and 1 in 20 000. There is symmetrical weakness of the trunk and limbs with proximal muscles being affected more severely than distal muscles and the lower limbs being affected more severely than the upper limbs. Tongue fasciculation is usually evident at the time of presentation, this ranges from birth to 6 months, with most infants presenting by 2 months. In type 1 SMA, an affected infant is never able to sit unaided. Weakness progresses from the trunk and limbs to bulbar and respiratory muscles. Affected infants usually die before the age of 2 years. In a few cases of type 1 SMA there is slower progression of generalized weakness and slightly longer survival.

Type 2 SMA (chronic childhood SMA) may present as early as type 1 SMA but infants acquire sitting balance although they fail to pass later motor milestones because of proximal weakness and hypotonia. Progression is slower and survival into adulthood is the rule. The mildest form of proximal SMA is type 3 or juvenile SMA (Kugelberg–Welander disease). Onset is from the first year of life but cases may present at any time during childhood and early adult life. Children with type 3 SMA learn to walk without support, distinguishing this variant from type 2 SMA.

Homozygous deletions of the survival motor neurone (SMN) gene on the long arm of chromosome 5 are present in 98 per cent of patients with SMA. The frequency of heterozygous carriers of deletion of SMN is approximately 1 in 50. Correlations between genotype and phenotype in the milder forms of SMA are emerging with understanding of genetic modifiers of the SMN gene mutation.

KEY LEARNING POINT

Each sibling has 25 per cent chance of inheriting SMA. Parents of an affected baby may be offered first-trimester, DNA-based prenatal diagnosis. Usually, this is uncomplicated if the gene mutation was confirmed in the firstborn affected child. When termination of an affected pregnancy is unacceptable, preimplantation genetic diagnosis may be an option.

CASE STUDY: Juvenile Huntington disease

The mother of a 10-year-old boy was summoned to meet his school teacher. The estranged father of the boy is known to have a family history of Huntington disease. The boy's teacher reports that she has observed a pattern of deteriorating schoolwork, poor concentration and, latterly, disinhibited sexual behaviour.

The triad of Huntington disease is chorea, dementia and autosomal dominant inheritance in families. George Huntington described the condition in 1872. The prevalence of the disorder is approximately 1 per 10 000. About 5–10 per cent of cases of Huntington disease have childhood onset. A diagnostic genetic test confirms the boy has juvenile Huntington disease with a CAG expansion numbering 63 repeats.

Huntington disease brain pathology is widespread with changes in pyramidal and extrapyramidal systems, especially involving the caudate nucleus, causing choreiform movements or rigidity. Personality change, seizures and dementia result from cerebral cortex atrophy. Brain atrophy is related to cell death with accumulation of an abnormal protein produced by the mutated gene.

KEY LEARNING POINT

Confirming this boy's clinical genetic diagnosis has also established that the estranged father carries the Huntington disease gene although he may not wish to know this. Genetic test results usually have implications for other family members.

Huntington disease often shows earlier age of onset in successive generations of a family (**anticipation**). The youngest age of onset occurs when the affected parent is the father. The mutation is abnormal expansion of a CAG codon near the start of a gene. The increased repeat size leads to an expanded polyglutamine tract in the Huntington protein. In unaffected individuals, CAG is repeated fewer than 27 times (CAGCAGCAGCAG ... CAG, $n < 27$). Forty or more CAG repeats always lead to adult-onset Huntington disease; 36–39 CAG repeats may lead to Huntington disease during patient's lifetime; and 27–35 CAG repeats do not cause the disease in the lifetime of the carrier although this size repeat is unstable and may expand in a subsequent generation leading to symptoms.

Juvenile-onset Huntington disease is associated with the largest repeat number, typically greater than 60. Age of onset is 3–9 years and presenting features are deterioration in academic work and behaviour, plus seizures in 50 per cent. Rigidity and dysarthria are more prominent than chorea. An eye movement disorder (oculomotor apraxia) may be present. Caudate and cortical atrophy may be evident from imaging. The duration of illness to its terminal phase is variable – eight years on average. There are no effective drug treatments but haloperidol, levodopa, diazepam, carbamazepine and sodium valproate are used to try to ease symptoms. New drug treatments and embryonic stem cell treatment are under investigation.

CASE STUDY: Cystic fibrosis

A $2\frac{1}{2}$-year-old boy was admitted to hospital for failure to gain weight. In the past he had suffered respiratory infections that were treated by his general practitioner. Investigations included a sweat test and the result showed elevated chloride concentration. DNA investigations revealed the boy was homozygous for the cystic fibrosis mutation known as δ-F508.

Cystic fibrosis is an autosomal recessive condition that results from defective function of the cystic fibrosis transmembrane conduction regulator (CFTR). The CFTR acts as a chloride channel, regulating exocrine secretion and electrolyte composition. Mutant CFTR causes raised concentration of sodium and chloride in sweat. The CFTR gene is located on chromosome 7. Many different mutations within it cause a range of clinical conditions from meconium ileus in the neonate to bilateral absence of the vas deferens in an otherwise healthy adult. In the UK, homozygosity for δ-F508 (delta for deletion of three base pairs at codon 508 leading to loss of an F or phenylalanine molecule from the protein) accounts for 50 per cent of cystic fibrosis cases. A multiplex PCR is used to screen for this mutation and about 30 less common cystic fibrosis gene mutations that make up 90 per cent of the total.

KEY LEARNING POINT

Severe respiratory disease and pancreatic insufficiency tend to occur in δ-F508 homozygotes. Compound heterozygosity with one δ-F508 allele and a second less common (or unidentified) mutation accounts for most other genotypes, often associated with milder respiratory disease and pancreatic sufficiency. Rare cystic fibrosis gene mutations are also present in adults with bilateral absence of the vas deferens.

There is evidence that early diagnosis of cystic fibrosis in the neonatal period, prior to the development of symptoms, improves prognosis. Neonatal screening programmes for cystic fibrosis employ a combination of immunoreactive trypsinogen assay and DNA tests on dried blood spots.

When one child in a family is affected by cystic fibrosis, unaffected siblings have 2/3 chance of carrying one cystic fibrosis mutation. Parents of an affected child are obligate carriers of a cystic fibrosis gene mutation and aunts and uncles of an affected child each have 1/2 chance of being a cystic fibrosis gene carrier. Prenatal diagnosis of cystic fibrosis at 10 weeks gestation by DNA analysis may be offered when both parents are cystic fibrosis gene carriers. When termination of an affected pregnancy is unacceptable, PGD may be an option. 'Cascade screening' is the term used when genetic screening is offered to relatives who are identified through an index (affected) case. Healthy children who are too young to give informed consent are usually not tested just to discover whether they carry a single mutation in the cystic fibrosis gene. Given a negative DNA test result in a healthy person with no family history of cystic fibrosis, the chance of being a cystic fibrosis gene carrier is reduced from 1 in 22 to less than 1 in 140.

Many attempts have been made to treat cystic fibrosis with gene therapy. The technical challenges of transferring functional CFTR genes into the lungs have proved difficult to overcome. Recent efforts using an adenovirus vector in an aerosol have reported inflammatory complications in the lungs.

CASE STUDY: Neurofibromatosis

An 8-year-old boy with short stature was referred to the paediatric clinic. General enquiries revealed that extra tuition had been required in reading and number work. His height was 2 standard deviations below the mean and OFC was 2.5 standard deviations above the mean. The rest of examination was unremarkable except 12 variable-sized café-au-lait spots were counted on the trunk and lower limbs.

The likely diagnosis is type 1 neurofibromatosis (NF1), a common autosomal dominant disorder, incidence 1 in 3000. In children, café-au-lait spots are evident, adults often have soft, subcutaneous neurofibromas. Many affected individuals are not diagnosed. Lisch nodules are harmless iris hamartomas; short stature, macrocephaly and mild learning difficulties are also common but the rarest complications are most serious. These include congenital pseudarthrosis, progressive scoliosis and central nervous system tumours. Children with NF1 should be kept under medical surveillance. Parents may be educated about the condition with information from the Neurofibromatosis Association, but it is important to emphasize that serious complications are rare.

The NF1 gene is located on chromosome 17 and encodes a protein called neurofibromin. The NF1 gene has a complex structure and many different mutations may cause the disease. The gene functions as a tumour suppressor with tumour development resulting from loss of wild-type alleles.

KEY LEARNING POINT

Over 50 per cent of NF1 index cases arise as a result of a new mutation. In the above case, the boy's parents and siblings should be examined for clinical signs of neurofibromatosis. If one parent has signs of NF1, other at-risk relatives on that side of the family should be offered a genetic clinic appointment.

Note that type 2 or central neurofibromatosis (NF2) is a different autosomal dominant disorder caused by mutations in the gene on chromosome 22 that encodes the protein called schwannomin. Neurofibromatosis 2 typically causes bilateral acoustic neuromas with onset in early- to mid-adult life. Other central nervous system tumours may develop and close follow-up of gene carriers is important. Although young children are rarely affected, they may have lenticular opacities, a helpful diagnostic clue.

CASE STUDY: Duchenne muscular dystrophy

A 3-year-old boy was referred because his parents were concerned that he was clumsy and fell excessively. The boy had started to walk at 20 months of age. At 3 years his speech development was limited to single words only. On examination, he had prominent calves and a positive Gower sign. Serum creatine kinase level was 9000 IU/L.

X-chromosome-linked Duchenne muscular dystrophy is by far the most likely diagnosis. Traditionally, this is confirmed by muscle biopsy, which shows evidence of dystrophy with death and regeneration of fibres. Specific immunochemical staining of muscle fibres reveal absence of the Xp21 gene product, dystrophin, from its location close to the muscle fibre membrane. Dystrophin is a component of the dystrophin-glycoprotein complex that spans the muscle cell membrane and is essential for fibre contractility. Absence of dystrophin leads to muscle fibre degeneration.

Some paediatric neurologists do not undertake muscle biopsy in familial Duchenne muscular dystrophy cases. Nearly 70 per cent of boys with Duchenne muscular dystrophy carry a dystrophin gene deletion in blood lymphocyte DNA. The remaining affected boys have a variety of mutations. Older boys and men who present with milder, allelic Becker muscular dystrophy have dystrophin gene mutations that produce a shortened dystrophin molecule. It is not clear why a third of boys with Duchenne muscular dystrophy have learning disabilities but it is known that the dystrophin gene is expressed in the brain. Life expectancy for boys with Duchenne muscular dystrophy has nearly doubled in recent years due to improved supportive care and judicious use of ventilatory support. Gene therapy is not yet a treatment option.

Provision of genetic counselling is essential. About a third of all cases represent a new mutation. There is two-thirds chance that the mother of an affected boy is herself a Duchenne muscular dystrophy gene carrier. This risk may be adjusted by pedigree analysis, measurement of serum creatine kinase and by DNA studies. If a mutation within the dystrophin gene is identified, carrier detection and prenatal diagnosis are straightforward. Where no mutation is identified, gene tracking studies with linked DNA markers can identify the particular Xp21 haplotype in the extended family that tracks with the Duchenne muscular dystrophy gene.

KEY LEARNING POINT

Note that the mother of an isolated case cannot ever be reassured about the chance of recurrence of Duchenne muscular dystrophy in her future children. The risk remains substantial (around 10 per cent) because the mother could be mosaic with a mutation confined to her ovaries. This phenomenon is called **gonadal mosaicism.**

CASE STUDY: Phenylketonuria

A 15-month-old child was referred with a heart murmur and slow development. Examination revealed a non-dysmorphic child with height and weight on the tenth centile and OFC 3 standard deviations below the mean. Cardiac examination revealed a small ventricular septal defect. The father was unemployed and mother, aged 39 years, had had two miscarriages. Several genetic investigations were performed on the child, each gave a normal result, but a spot measurement of the maternal blood phenylalanine level was grossly elevated at 1100 mmol/L.

Congenital heart defects with microcephaly and learning disability are common problems caused by teratogenic effects of untreated maternal phenylketonuria (PKU). In the above case, the child is likely to be a heterozygous carrier of the PKU gene and does not have elevated blood phenylalanine. Although undiagnosed or untreated maternal PKU is now rare, older mothers, who were born before neonatal screening for PKU became available, mothers who were born in countries without universal neonatal screening and mothers who were treated for PKU but then lost to follow-up, are all at risk.

A prescribed dietary regimen that reduces maternal blood phenylalanine levels below 360 mmol/L is effective at preventing mental retardation in babies of mothers with PKU only if the restrictive diet starts prior to conception and continues during gestation. However, many pregnancies are unplanned and compliance with the diet is often poor in young affected adults.

KEY LEARNING POINT

There is over 90 per cent chance of neurological impairment in the child of a mother with PKU who has not been on dietary restriction at the time of conception and during early gestation. It is essential that affected teenagers, especially girls, are given advice about family planning and the hazards of unplanned pregnancy.

Classic phenylketonuria is an autosomal recessive condition caused by mutations in the phenylalanine hydroxylase gene on chromosome 12. In families with an affected child, both parents are unaffected carriers and there is 25 per cent chance of recurrence in siblings. In western Europe the disease is common and an incidence of 1 in 5300 gives a carrier frequency of 1 in 36. Biochemical tests to detect heterozygotes in the general population are imprecise.

The risk of a treated, affected parent having an affected child may be calculated as follows:

1 (=chance the affected parent transmits the mutation) × 1/36 (=chance of affected parent encountering a carrier parent in the general population) × 1/2 (=chance of the mutant gene being transmitted by a carrier parent) = 1 in 72.

CASE STUDY: Myotonic dystrophy

A baby was born prematurely at 34 weeks gestation and required prolonged ventilatory support. The pregnancy had been complicated by polyhydramnos. Once weaned from the ventilator the baby fed poorly. Hypotonia and bilateral club foot deformity were noted. When the mother visited the baby, it was noted that mother had myopathic facies and grip myotonia.

Myotonic dystrophy is common in adults (1 in 10 000) but it is not always diagnosed. Families with several affected adult relatives may only come to medical attention following the birth of a baby who is affected by congenital myotonic dystrophy. In such cases, the mother is nearly always affected, as are other relatives in her family. Provision of detailed genetic advice to the extended family is essential.

In congenital myotonic dystrophy, modern neonatal care has reduced mortality and morbidity from problems of prematurity and respiratory failure. Myotonia is absent in early childhood but evidence of myopathic facial appearance with 'tenting' of the mouth is present, usually with mild-to-moderate learning disability. Affected adults have muscle weakness, myotonia, early onset cataract, cardiac conduction abnormality, frontal balding and, in males, testicular atrophy.

KEY LEARNING POINT

General anaesthesia given without knowledge that the patient has myotonic dystrophy is hazardous. Provision of a medic-alert or 'care card' to gene carriers can prevent serious complications such as postoperative respiratory failure.

Myotonic dystrophy is an autosomal dominant condition, the mutant DMPK gene is on chromosome 19. Nearly all affected individuals have an expanded CTG trinucleotide repeat sequence and a DNA test detects its presence, confirming clinical diagnosis. The CTG repeat size is normally 5–37 repeats; expansion is greatest (up to 3000 repeats) in the congenitally affected infant. Moderately expanded repeats are present in adult-onset myotonic dystrophy and smallest expansions are present in older individuals who have minimal clinical signs. As with Huntington disease (see above) anticipation may be evident in the family tree, but in myotonic dystrophy there is maternal transmission of the largest expansions, contrary to paternal transmission in Huntington disease.

CASE STUDY: Retinoblastoma

A 3-year-old boy presented with a squint. A recent photograph taken at a party showed a white reflex in one eye and a red reflex in the other. Examination under anaesthesia confirmed solitary retinoblastoma in one eye only.

Retinoblastoma is a malignant cancer of retinal cells that usually presents before the age of 5 years. Sporadic cases with no family history of an affected relation usually have solitary tumour in one eye and slightly later age of onset. In familial cases, one or both eyes contain tumour, or one eye might have several tumours. Familial cases are inherited in an autosomal dominant fashion but apparent non-penetrance of the disease is sometimes observed in the case of the unaffected parent who, on family tree evidence must be an obligate gene carrier. Sometimes, examination of the eyes of the apparently unaffected parent reveals signs of spontaneously regressed retinoblastoma.

Knudson analysed family history data and deduced that retinoblastoma results from two separate mutational events that inactivate both functioning copies of the retinoblastoma gene. Knudson's 'two hit' hypothesis proposed that in cases of familial retinoblastoma, a single mutant allele is passed through the generations in the germ line. Tumour occurs when the second normal allele is inactivated in a somatic retinoblast cell during prenatal or early postnatal life. In cases with a single constitutional mutation, the chance of a second independent mutation occurring in one retinoblast is high since there are 10^7 cells retinal cells in each eye. Note that even if a second hit does not occur in the retinoblast, in later life a second somatic hit or mutation may occur in another tissue. This accounts for the high incidence of second cancers including sarcomas in individuals with familial or bilateral retinoblastoma.

KEY LEARNING POINT

The chance of occurrence of retinoblastoma in the offspring of the familial case, or of any parent treated for bilateral retinoblastoma, is high. Ophthalmic screening under anaesthesia is undertaken from birth in such neonates. If a germ-line mutation can be identified in the retinoblastoma gene of the affected parent, this can be tested for in the infant, and only infants who carry the mutation need undergo regular examinations under anaesthesia.

Most individuals with retinoblastoma have no family history, nor do they harbour a germ-line mutation. In such individuals, both mutations or 'hits' occur in a single retinal cell. The chance of two independent hits involving one cell is correspondingly much lower, hence the preponderance of single tumours. There is a low risk of recurrence of retinoblastoma in siblings and in offspring of the sporadic case who has a solitary tumour. However, even given the low chance that a child with a solitary tumour in one eye might carry a germ-line mutation, it is also worth undertaking DNA studies in such cases.

ACKNOWLEDGEMENTS

The author would like to thank Dr Lia Paton and Dr Marianne Scott for illustrations in this chapter.

FURTHER READING

Jones KL. (1997) *Smith's Recognizable Patterns of Human Malformation*, 5th edn. Philadelphia: WB Saunders.

Rimoin DL, Connor JM, Pyeritz RE, Korf BR, eds. (2002) *Principles and Practice of Medical Genetics*, 4th edn. Edinburgh: Churchill Livingstone.

Chapter 4

Acute illness, injuries, and ingestions

Jack Beattie and David Hallworth

INTRODUCTION

In the UK, children under the age of 14 years make up 25–30 per cent of all attendances at general Accident and Emergency (A&E) departments, with around 40 per cent of the child population seen yearly. A substantial proportion of these are under 5 years old. Two broad categories of attendance are seen:

- injuries, poisoning and medical emergencies (70 per cent)
- non-acute medical, surgical or orthopaedic conditions (30 per cent).

There are significant seasonal variations in presenting problems, with trauma much more common in the long days of summer and a marked rise in medical respiratory problems in the winter, especially bronchiolitis (Figure 4.1).

Much paediatric injury is of minor-to-moderate severity. Approximately 10 per cent of children require admission following their injury, usually for observation after head injury, repair of wounds or lacerations under general anaesthesia, treatment of fractures, and removal of foreign bodies from body orifices and the skin. Increasingly, such procedures are carried out under sedation in A&E, and the children discharged after a period of observation.

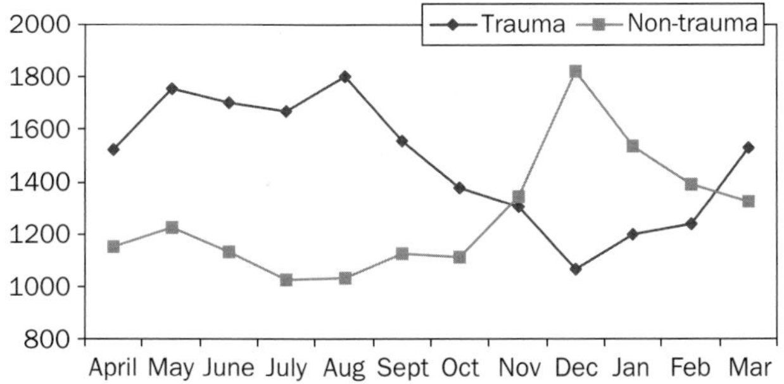

Figure 4.1 Seasonality of trauma and non-trauma attendances at the Accident and Emergency Department, Royal Hospital for Sick Children, Glasgow

SERIOUS CHILDHOOD INJURY

Road vehicle crashes, including passenger, bicycle, and pedestrian injuries are responsible for most deaths and acquired disability among children and adolescents, principally from head injury. These events represent an incalculable burden of individual personal tragedies, reflect a considerable loss of future potential and productivity, and are a significant drain on healthcare resources.

Other significant causes of unintentional injuries in children include drowning, burns and scalds, choking, falls, poisoning and participation in sport. Child abuse and neglect account for significant harm in pre-school children.

CHILDHOOD INJURY AND SOCIAL DEPRIVATION

There is a clear link between childhood death or significant injury and social deprivation. Risk factors for early childhood injury include low birth weight, young maternal age, single parenthood, high parity and low maternal educational attainment.

There is evidence of a widening socioeconomic gap in deaths from unintentional injury, with the rate of decline least in the most deprived children. Worldwide, children in low-income countries are about six times more likely to die from road traffic injuries than in high-income countries. In developing countries, death rates and morbidity are rising significantly as motor vehicle use increases.

INJURY PATTERNS

Age

Pre-school children

Infants admitted to hospital for any reason during the first three months of life are 50 per cent more likely to have a subsequent serious injury than infants who are not hospitalized early. Pre-school children are usually injured in the home since they spend most of their time there. Between the ages of 15 months and 2 years, one in four toddlers sustain a significant injury (major falls, burn or scald injury or ingestion) and one in six experiences multiple events.

By the age of 2 years, almost one in 10 pre-school children will have had a long-term injury or be permanently scarred. Many of these events arise from poor supervision or inadequate domestic 'childproofing'. Falls down the stairs in baby walkers or placement of baby chairs on high surfaces are prime examples. Young children are especially vulnerable in house fires because they depend on adults to escape.

Pre-school children are also at much increased risk of being hospitalized because of intentional injury before their second birthday. While this may partly be explained by improved detection, there is an apparent rise in true incidence of severe injury and death attributed to maltreatment and abuse in young children.

School-age children

In school-age children, pedestrian injuries from motor vehicles are the leading cause of death and serious injury, with around one child death from this caused daily in the UK. Sports injuries are also a very common reason for hospitalization at this age. Protective devices such as mouth guards (rugby) or helmets (horse riding) are well proved to be useful, but some protective sports equipment (rugby shoulder pads/padded helmets) may give a false sense of security and more risk of trauma.

Gender and injury

Until the third birthday, the overall incidence of fractures, burns, foreign body ingestion and poisoning is the same in boys and girls. Intentional injury related to child abuse remains a significant issue in this age group.

With increasing age, a clear male predominance for unintentional injury emerges. This is partly explained by different activity patterns such as more sport activity, walking to school and bicycle use in boys, but also reflects gender differences in (risk-taking) behaviour and the use of protective equipment such as cycle helmets. However, deliberate self-harm events such as poisoning/self-cutting are a much more prominent feature in older girls than boys.

INJURY PREVENTION

The traditional concept of 'accidental' death and injury implies unavoidable events. This fatalistic view is wrong. Most of these deaths and injuries are not inevitable, many are preventable, or their effect reduced.

Injury prevention strategies generally involve passive environmental modifications such as device redesign to prevent injury (the development of childproof drug containers) or active prevention strategies to enhance parental vigilance (cooking safety) or change in individual behaviour.

> Interventions that reduce child deaths and morbidity from injury
>
> Home
> - Child-resistant closures to prevent poisoning
> - Use of domestic smoke alarms
> - A window guard to prevent falls
> - Domestic product designs, e.g. latch-type freezer and refrigerator doors
>
> Roads
> - Traffic speed reduction
> - Car seat belt and child restraint legislation
> - Bicycle helmets

Active strategies are much more difficult to introduce and maintain. Many, such as bicycle helmet use, are known to be highly effective – 85 per cent reduction in risk of head injury, 88 per cent reduction in brain injury – yet only a small proportion of school-aged cyclists in the UK use them. Similarly, despite proof that seat belts protect school-age children at least as well as adults in motor vehicle crashes, many school-age children still travel unbelted in cars.

Around one-half of child motor vehicle deaths are due to pedestrian–motor vehicle collisions and are commonest among primary school children; very few survivors of such events escape significant injury, with many sustaining serious head trauma. Pedestrian injuries have a complex causation and multiple interventions are needed to prevent them. These include environmental changes (railings at school gates. road humps), road skills training for children, reflective clothing use and vehicle redesign.

KEY LEARNING POINTS

- There is a close link between social deprivation and the risk of accidental death and injury.
- Patterns of injury vary significantly with age.
- Most 'accidental' deaths and injuries are preventable.

The recent fall in pedestrian fatalities to children in the UK and other industrialized countries is probably due to a reduction in walking by children.

ACCIDENTAL INGESTIONS AND POISONING

Almost 40 000 children attend A&E departments each year in the UK because of potential poisoning. Almost all are under 5 years old, most do not need admission, and few need specific treatment. However, around 10 children die each year in the UK from poisoning.

Cases generally fall into three categories:

- unintentional ingestions in pre-school children (children under 5 years of age)
- self-harm events in older children, usually 9 years or older
- factitious illness (uncommon).

Unintentional ingestions in pre-school children

Toddlers have an insatiable curiosity, and this, coupled with increasing skill in exploring their environment, means that unintentional ingestions by pre-school children (especially boys) are common. Such events are more frequent in stressed or disadvantaged households, or linked to situations such as moving house or visiting relatives, where 'childproofing' is not established. They usually involve ingestion of non-toxic plants, household cleaning products, over-the-counter medications and cosmetics. Although ingestion of some substances such as paracetamol (acetaminophen) suspension is potentially dangerous, most of these events are benign, significant clinical effects are uncommon and deaths very rare. However, some exposures are potentially very toxic.

Drugs causing most risk to toddlers

- β-blockers
- Digoxin
- Calcium antagonists
- Tricyclic antidepressants
- Oral hypoglycaemics
- Opioids – pain relief (codeine), drug-habit management (methadone) or antidiarrhoeals (diphenoxylate (Lomotil®))

Ingestions in school-age children

By school age, a change in the pattern of poisoning emerges. With progressive maturity, the frequency of intentional poisoning rises, and the gender ratio of those involved reverses with a higher proportion of girls involved in intentional pharmaceutical product overdose.

The National Poisons Information Service

In the UK, clinical toxicology advice for health professionals is organized on a national integrated basis. The National Poisons Information Service (NPIS) comprises six poisons centres (Belfast, Birmingham, Cardiff, Edinburgh, London and Newcastle). These NPIS centres are for the use of National Health Service (NHS) professionals only, and provide specialized advice on the treatment and management of more complex clinical cases. This advice is accessed by a single national telephone number (0870 600 6266) and callers are automatically routed to their local centre.

TOXBASE

TOXBASE (www.spib.axl.co.uk) is the internet/NHS web-based clinical toxicology information database of the NPIS. It is available to all medical practitioners and other healthcare professionals within the NHS as the primary source of information about routine diagnosis, treatment and management of patients suffering from exposure to a wide range of substances and products.

Telephone advice about possible poisoning for the public

In the USA, parents are encouraged to call a poison control centre for advice. More than half such calls are about children under 6 years of age. The use of poison control centres to triage patients is said to significantly reduce unnecessary visits to emergency departments, with around one in three children able to remain at home. In the UK, non-professional contact with NPIS centres is neither routine nor encouraged, and calls are redirected to family doctors or A&E departments.

The recent development of the nurse-led NHS health telephone advice service in England and Wales (NHS Direct; 0845 46 47) and Scotland (NHS 24; 08454 24 24 24) allows carers to obtain advice from nurse advisers who can access TOXBASE or a poison centre on their behalf. How this new service might influence present emergency attendances of children to hospital remains to be seen.

Informal telephone triage and advice in such circumstances is complex and fraught with medicolegal risk. In most circumstances, callers should be redirected to NHS Direct/NHS24 or invited to bring their child to hospital for face-to-face evaluation. If children are to attend hospital, it is important to ask their parents to bring along the medication or other container in which the ingested substance was stored together with any remaining contents, or any plants/berries that have been eaten.

MANAGING THE CHILD WITH POTENTIAL POISONING

Pathophysiology of common poisonings: elimination and reduction of absorption

There are seven phases in the management of the poisoned child.

1 – Initial stabilization

Most children who present to hospital with suspected poisoning are well, but sometimes they arrive seriously ill. Start with the basics: assess the airway, breathing and circulation (ABC). Give oxygen if there is any doubt about the child's general condition. Intubate if the child has depressed respirations. Obtain intravenous access if ill or if there is a potentially serious toxic exposure.

Add 'D' for disability: establish the level of consciousness using the AVPU system (*A*lert, responds to *V*oice, responds to *P*ain or *U*nresponsive), perform a brief neurological exam and determine pupil size and reactivity. If reduced conscious level, check finger prick glucose. Seizures may occur with a number of ingestions. Start drug therapy: oxygen, dextrose, naloxone or lorazepam as indicated.

2 – Obtain an accurate history

Some children present before toxicity has developed but they still need a rapid but systematic clinical risk assessment. Significant paracetamol poisoning, for example, will cause no symptoms initially but is potentially fatal if early intervention is delayed. An accurate history is essential.

WHAT HAS BEEN INGESTED?

Containers brought with the child may offer more detailed information than carers can provide. Strength of medication, when it was dispensed and how much may have been left or details of the dispensing pharmacy may be on the label, where more information may be obtained.

HOW MUCH HAS BEEN TAKEN?

Reports of amounts ingested are insecure especially in intentional ingestions. Volumes of liquid products taken are often overreported by parents but cannot be assumed to be wrong.

WHEN WAS IT TAKEN?

Knowledge of the time gap between ingestion and presentation or onset of symptoms allows more reliable decisions to be made about specific investigations or the need for treatment. Again, paracetamol provides a prime example of this, where plasma level at a known time after ingestion defines the need or otherwise for treatment.

WHAT SYMPTOMS OR SIGNS HAS THE CHILD SHOWN?

A child who was sleepy and ataxic after swallowing grandfather's benzodiazepine tablets for insomnia but is now lively and walking steadily is in a different situation from a child who was lively and active but is now difficult to wake.

3 – Check the clinical management guidelines

With the above information available, TOXBASE can be accessed to guide potential risk, specific clinical signs to search for and appropriate laboratory or other investigations.

4 – Clinical evaluation

A general examination should be completed, focusing on the cardiopulmonary, respiratory and neurological systems. Look for signs of secondary trauma.

ARE THERE FEATURES TO SUGGEST A TOXIDROME?

A toxidrome is the constellation of signs and symptoms that suggest a specific class of poisoning. Knowledge of toxidrome syndromes is essential for the successful recognition of poisoning patterns (Table 4.1).

5 – Laboratory investigations

In an ill child consider some routine laboratory investigations – urea and electrolytes (UEs), liver function tests (LFTs), full blood count (FBC), glucose, blood gases. In some situations it may be useful to screen for toxins. Urine and blood samples can be taken and stored for future analysis. Such situations include investigation of unexplained confusion or coma, concern about possible factitious illness or ingestion of illegal substances. If possible, these cases should be discussed with the laboratory in advance of sampling.

6 – Treatment after poisoning

Most children need nothing other than simple supportive therapy and may be discharged after a period of observation. Some need specific and aggressive intervention.

Table 4.1 Some common toxidromes

Sympathomimetics	
Dopamine Ephedrine Aminophylline Amphetamine	CNS: agitated, psychoses, hallucinations, seizures, dilated pupils CV: tachycardia, dysrhythmias, hypertension GI: nausea, vomiting, abdominal pain Other: fever, sweating
Tricyclics	
Amitriptyline Clomipramine	CNS: agitation, coma, dilated pupils, seizures CV: tachycardia, hypo- or hypertension, prolonged QRS interval, ventricular arrhythmias Other: fever
Sedative-hypnotics	
Benzodiazepines	CNS: sedated, coma, miosis, ataxia, nystagmus CV: hypotension Respiratory: decreased respiratory rate, shallow breathing Other: slurred speech, hypothermic
Opiates	
Heroin Methadone	CNS: euphoria, coma, seizures, miosis CV: bradycardia, hypotension Respiratory: shallow respirations, decreased respiratory rate
Anticholinergics	
Atropine Scopolamine Phenothiazines	'Mad as a hatter, red as a beet, blind as a bat, hot as a hare, dry as a bone' CNS: delirium, disorientation, agitation, hallucinations, psychosis, loss of memory, extrapyramidal movements, ataxia, picking or grasping movements, seizures, coma, dilated pupils CVS: tachycardia, dysrhythmias, hypertension, hypotension (late) GI/GU: urinary retention, decreased bowel sounds Other: dry and flushed skin, dry mucous membranes, fever

CNS, central nervous system; CV, cardiovascular; GI, gastro-intestinal; GU, genitourinary.

7 – Reducing absorption/enhancing excretion

The goal of decontamination is to minimize absorption of a toxin by removing it from the gastrointestinal tract or by binding it to a non-absorbable agent. After many years of controversy about the indications for ipecac-induced vomiting, gastric lavage, activated charcoal (single dose only), cathartics and whole bowel irrigation, an international consensus on use of these interventions has emerged.

Emetics such as Syrup of Ipecac are of no value. **Gastric lavage** or **activated charcoal** should only be considered in specific situations; even here, the benefit is uncertain. Airway protection is essential if there is alteration in conscious level. Gastric lavage is contraindicated after ingestion of corrosive substances or volatile hydrocarbons. There is a limited role for this technique to promote active elimination of toxic substances. Repeated doses of activated charcoal may be used to remove toxins such as barbiturates, carbamazepine or theophylline that undergo enterohepatic circulation.

Although **forced diuresis** is now no longer recommended, excretion of weakly acidic drugs such as salicylates may be enhanced by urinary alkalization. Intravenous sodium bicarbonate is given (1–2 mEq/kg per dose IV over one hour) to keep urine pH >7.5. This technique is contraindicated with cerebral oedema or impaired renal function. Electrolytes need to be carefully monitored.

For **whole bowel irrigation**, polyethylene glycol and electrolytes (GoLYTELY®) can be administered by nasogastric tube when large amounts of a toxic substance are ingested, a slow-release substance is involved or the substance is not absorbed by charcoal. Patients must be able to protect their airway.

Extracorporeal techniques have been used when other treatment methods have failed. Each technique is limited to certain toxin characteristics: **dialysis** (low molecular weight, high water solubility: polyethylene glycol, salicylates), haemoperfusion (low water solubility: carbamazepine) and **haemofiltration** (high molecular weight: aminoglycosides, theophylline, lithium).

SPECIFIC ANTIDOTES

Selected specific antidotes for some ingested toxins are shown in Table 4.2.

Paracetamol ingestion

Paracetamol is one of the most commonly used medications during childhood. It has been available over the counter for many years and is produced in a variety of dosage formulations. Toddler ingestion of children's liquid paracetamol preparations is very common and rarely serious. Not all poisonings are the result of accidental ingestions by curious toddlers.

Table 4.2 Some ingested agents have specific antidotes

Agent	Antidote
Benzodiazepines	Flumazenil
β-Adrenergic blockers	Glucagon, adrenaline infusion
Carbon monoxide	Oxygen 100% inhalation, consider hyperbaric oxygen for severe cases
Digoxin	Fab antibodies (Digibind®)
Iron	Desferrioxamine
Isoniazid	Pyridoxine
Opiates	Naloxone
Paracetamol (acetaminophen)	*N*-Acetylcysteine (NAC)

CASE STUDY

An otherwise well 12-year-old girl presented to A&E at 11 pm with her elder sister. She claimed she had taken 12 × 500 mg paracetamol (158 mg/kg) five hours earlier following an argument with her mother. Clinical evaluation was normal and she was asymptomatic. Paracetamol level was measured immediately. Her plasma paracetamol level was 0.55 mmol/L (84 mg/mL). Urgent LFTs, plasma glucose and coagulation study were normal. *N*-Acetylcysteine was not given but she was observed overnight to allow emotions to defuse. An assessment next morning by the child and family psychiatry service considered this as an impulsive act on a background of multiple family stressors.

Unintentional therapeutic overdose by carers

Most parents exhibit a degree of 'fever phobia' and are used to administering paracetamol when their child is suffering from minor febrile illness. Some carers administer inappropriate doses. If the illness persists for some days, it is easy to develop excessive and sustained paracetamol exposure with the potential for severe liver injury. Parents of young children should be given specific instructions about the use of calibrated measuring devices for liquid preparations.

Management of paracetamol ingestion

If only paracetamol has been taken, gastric lavage is not helpful. Activated charcoal may be useful if:

- more than 150 mg/kg body weight of non-liquid preparations of paracetamol is thought to have been taken
- it can be given without difficulty and within an hour of ingestion.

Figure 4.2 presents a structured approach to decision making in children presenting with paracetamol ingestion.

1 Assess if the child is at enhanced risk of developing severe liver damage: underweight children with 'failure to thrive' whatever the cause; eating disorders; cystic fibrosis or established liver disease; those on anticonvulsant or barbiturate treatment, or those taking St John's Wort; those who abuse alcohol; and those with a recent high intake of therapeutic paracetamol.
2 Take blood for urgent estimation of the plasma paracetamol level as soon as possible after four hours or more from the time of ingestion.
3 Use the treatment graph (Figure 4.3) to assess need for specific treatment with *N*-acetylcysteine (NAC) (see box below). If the plasma paracetamol level is above line A of the paracetamol overdose treatment graph or above line B for 'at enhanced risk' patients, treatment should be started with NAC by IV infusion. Measure activated partial thromboplastin time (APTT)/international normalized ratio (INR) and baseline LFTs on insertion of IV line.
4 When NAC is started within eight hours of the overdose, it is reasonable to expect the child to be declared fit for discharge from medical care on completion of its administration. However, the INR, plasma creatinine and alanine aminotransferase (ALT) should be checked for normality on completion of the treatment and before discharge. Advice should be given for the child to return to hospital if vomiting or abdominal pain develop or recur.

Dosage for NAC infusion – children <12 years

From Royal College of Paediatrics and Child Health (2003) *Medicines for Children*. Consult the original document for full details of administration and alternative routes of administration

- Body weight 20 kg or more
  1 150 mg/kg IV infusion in 100 mL 5 per cent dextrose* over 15 minutes, then
  2 50 mg/kg IV infusion in 250 mL 5 per cent dextrose over four hours, then
  3 100 mg/kg IV infusion in 500 mL 5 per cent dextrose over 16 hours
- Body weight under 20 kg
  1 150 mg/kg IV infusion in 3 mL/kg body weight 5 per cent dextrose over 15 minutes, then

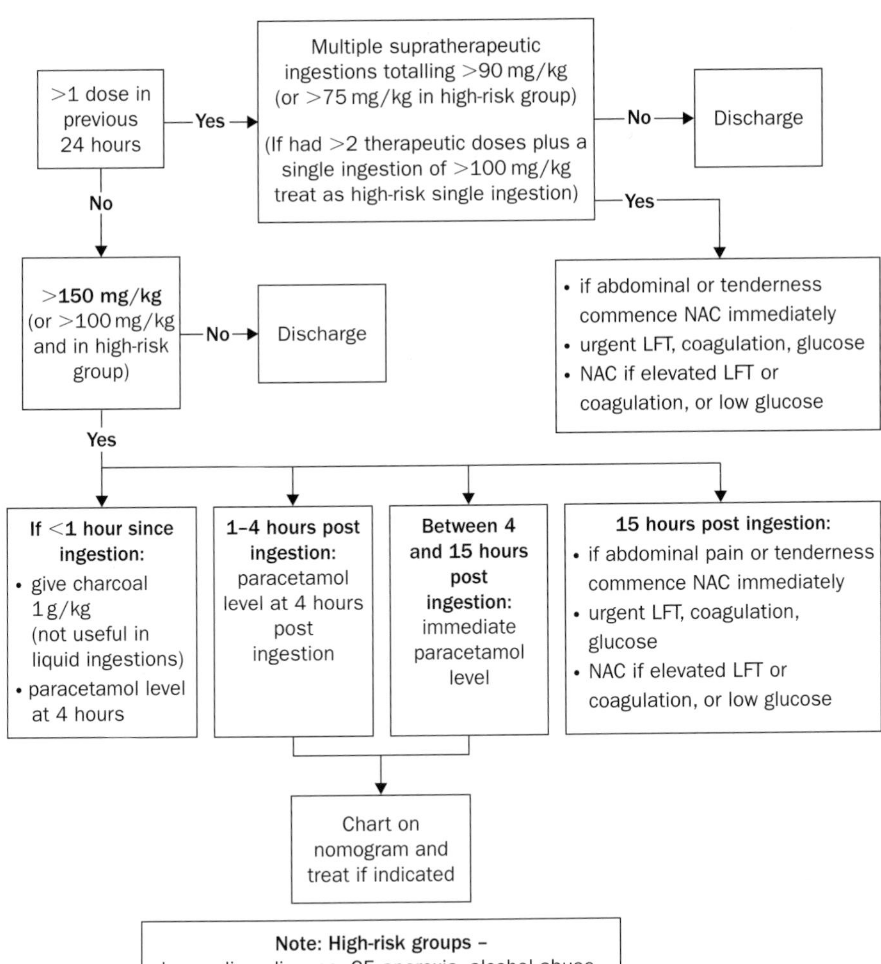

Figure 4.2 Decision making flowchart for management of paracetamol ingestion (courtesy Dr M South and colleagues, Melbourne). LFT, liver function test; NAC, *N*-acetylcysteine; CF, cystic fibrosis

2 50 mg/kg IV infusion in 7 mL/kg 5 per cent dextrose over four hours, then
3 100 mg/kg IV infusion in 14 mL/kg 5 per cent dextrose over 16 hours

*If dextrose is unsuitable, use 0.9 per cent sodium chloride solution.

CARDIOPULMONARY RESUSCITATION SKILLS

In Europe, the European Paediatric Life Support Course (EPLS) has replaced the US-based Pediatric Advanced Life Support (PALS) course. For paediatric practitioners EPLS and Advanced Paediatric Life Support (APLS) courses are widely available, and APLS provider status is mandatory to enter specialist paediatric training. True emergency situations in paediatric practice are relatively rare (<1 per cent of A&E attendances) so these skills should be regularly refreshed by recertification and regular reference should be made to the internet-based Resuscitation Council guidelines or their publications. Current procedures for resuscitation in the main clinical scenarios encountered are detailed below.

Rapid and effective assessment and resuscitation of the seriously injured child needs clear priorities and a coordinated team approach. One person should assume overall responsibility for directing care. Parents are now generally encouraged to stay with their child if they wish during resuscitation; they should be supported by a senior nurse, who may also collect some background medical or incident history.

Before the child arrives

Use this time to organize the resuscitation team, inform other staff (e.g. radiology), check the resuscitation equipment, and prepare IV lines and fluids. Predict the

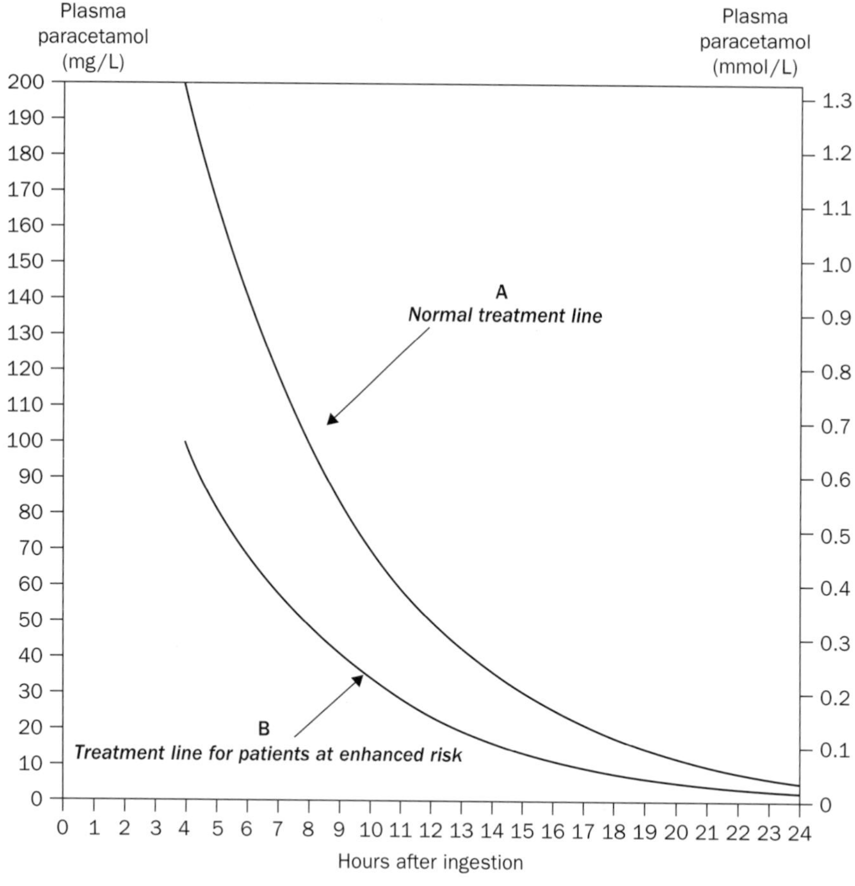

Figure 4.3 *N*-Acetylcysteine therapy treatment lines after paracetamol ingestion (reproduced with permission of Dr G Brandon, Paracetamol Information Centre)

child's weight using the formula: (age + 4) × 2. Then estimate:

- amount of fluid bolus at 20 mL/kg
- endotracheal tube size: (age/4) + 4 or relevant infant sizes
- dose of any drugs that may be used.

When the child arrives, this estimate should be reviewed with the Broselow tape method. Obtain a rapid history of the injury (or illness) circumstances.

Cardiac arrest

1 Quickly establish diagnosis (10 seconds):
 a no response to verbal or physical stimulation
 b no palpable carotid (1 year +) or brachial (<1 year) pulse
 c no audible or visible respiration or agonal gasps only.
2 Oxygenate and ventilate:
 a clear airway
 b ventilate with high-concentration oxygen using self-inflating bag and mask or mouth-to-mouth or nose and mouth.
3 Commence external cardiac massage while maintaining ventilation (two operator):
 a Figure 4.4 illustrates hand positions for different age groups.
4 a Secure airway with endotracheal tube
 b Start electrocardiogram (ECG) monitoring
 c Obtain vascular access – attempt for one minute only, if unsuccessful insert intraosseous needle (see page 102).
5 Observe cardiac rhythm:
 a asystole or pulseless electrical activity – common in children
 b ventricular fibrillation or ventricular tachycardia with no palpable pulses – uncommon in children.

Treatment of asystole or pulseless electrical activity:

1 Give adrenaline (epinephrine) 10 μg/kg (0.1 mL/kg of 1:10 000 solution) IV or intraosseous.
2 If no access give 100 μg/kg (1 mL/kg of 1:10 000 solution), i.e. 10 × dose via the ETT with a narrow-bore suction catheter and flush with saline.
3 Continue ventilation and external cardiac massage for three minutes.
4 If no response give further 10 μg/kg dose of adrenaline followed by three minutes massage.

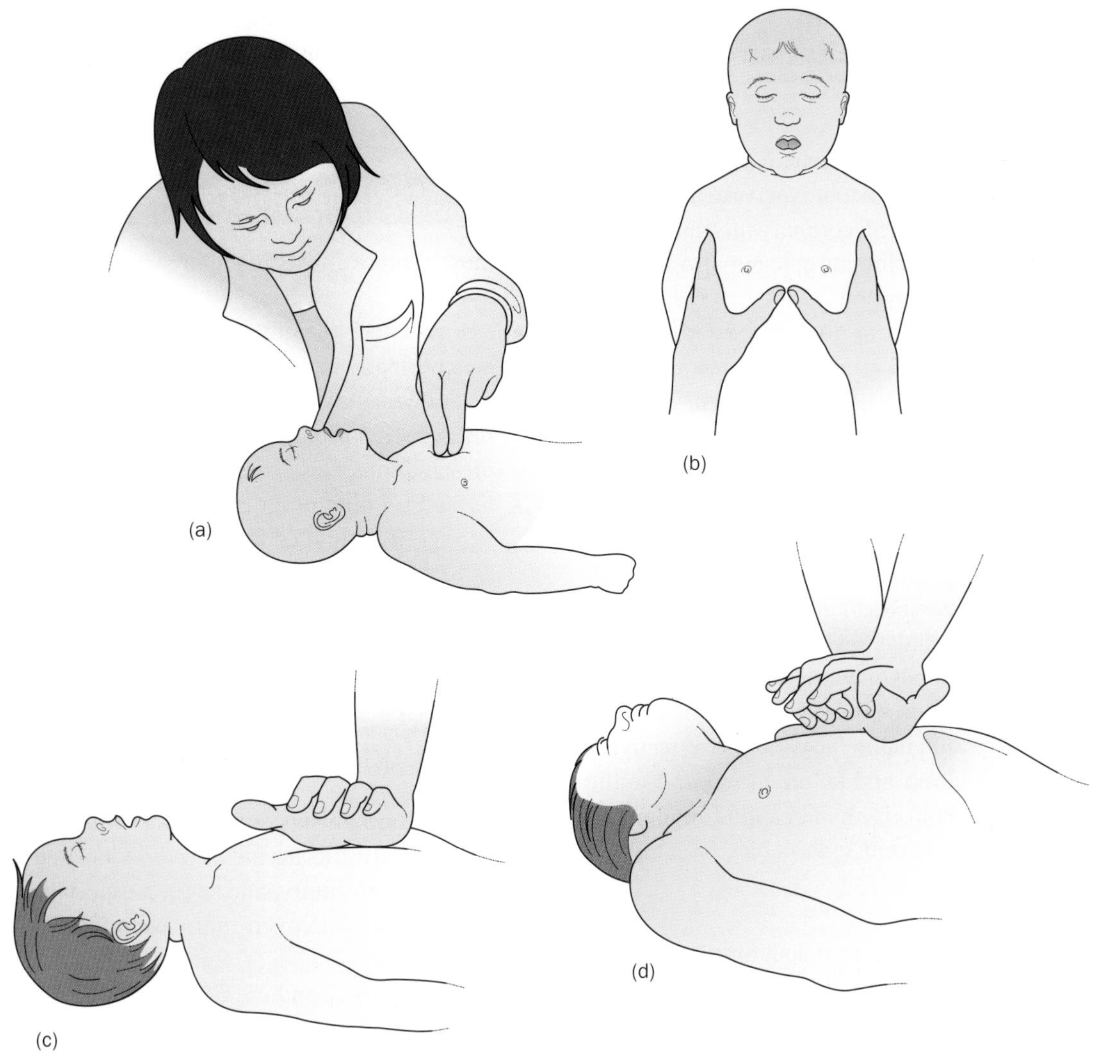

Figure 4.4 (a and b) Two techniques for cardiac compression in infants. Chest compression technique for (c) younger and (d) older children (modified with permission from Philips *et al.*, 2004)

5 Consider possible causes of arrest and treat appropriately (e.g. fluid loss, electrolyte disturbance, tension pneumothorax, pericardial tamponade – see later).
6 Continue cycles of adrenaline and massage until response obtained or resuscitation abandoned.
7 Children usually revert to sinus rhythm or sinus tachycardia – if ventricular fibrillation ensues defibrillate as below.
8 If arterial pressure monitoring is available adrenaline dose may be titrated against effect.
9 For prolonged arrest or asystole refractory to adrenaline, consider the use of alkalizing agents such as sodium bicarbonate.

Ventricular fibrillation or pulseless ventricular tachycardia is uncommon.

1 Place defibrillator pads on the chest wall, one just below the right clavicle, the other at the left anterior axillary line.
2 Use a sequence of three direct current (DC) shocks: 2 joules (J)/kg, 2 J/kg, 4 J/kg, observing the effect after each shock.
3 Persistence of dysrhythmia requires continuation of cardiac massage and administration of 10 μg/kg adrenaline.
4 Three further shocks of 4 J/kg are then administered, again observing effect.
5 Repeat defibrillation and one minute cardiac massage until stable rhythm and cardiac output is achieved.
6 Consider the use of antiarrhythmic agents for resistant ventricular dysrhythmias.
7 Treat known problems, e.g. hyperkalaemia.

Pharmacological agents in cardiopulmonary resuscitation

Adrenaline (epinephrine)

Adrenaline is a mixed α and β sympathomimetic agent. It causes peripheral vasoconstriction, increase in diastolic pressure and hence increased coronary perfusion. The β effects are inotropic and chronotropic but also increase myocardial oxygen consumption.

Dosage in cardiac arrest is 10 μg/kg by the IV or intraosseous route. Second and subsequent doses of adrenaline may be increased 10-fold if desired.

Alkalizing agents

Cardiac arrest in children is usually precipitated by hypoxia so most victims are profoundly acidotic. However, routine use of alkalizing agents has not proved beneficial. Sodium bicarbonate dissociates to produce carbon dioxide, thus increasing intracellular pCO_2 and paradoxically worsening acidosis. It should only be given if ventilation is established, allowing carbon dioxide clearance.

Despite the above, adrenaline does not act effectively in the presence of acidosis, and failure to respond to the second or subsequent bolus is an indication for administration of 1 mL/kg 8.4 per cent sodium bicarbonate.

Antiarrhythmic drugs

Recent experience has shown that amiodarone is the agent of choice for shock-resistant ventricular dysrhythmias. The dose is 5 mg/kg given by rapid IV injection. One minute should be allowed for circulation and defibrillation repeated. Lidocaine is an alternative at a dose of 1 mg/kg or an infusion of 20–50 μg/kg per minute. Bretylium is no longer considered appropriate for use in children.

Fluids

Hypovolaemia due to acute fluid loss should be treated with bolus fluid administration (20 mL/kg 0.9 per cent saline solution or 10 mL/kg colloid).

Stopping resuscitation

The prognosis for out-of-hospital cardiac arrest is dismal in terms of both survival and quality of survival. A possible exception is the child who is profoundly hypothermic.

As with all severely injured patients, a policy decision must be made at some point during resuscitation concerning the duration and extent of resuscitative efforts. This decision must be agreed by all present. Quality of survival as well as potential survival must be considered. It is generally agreed that failure to respond to three cycles of adrenaline and cardiac massage for the normothermic child who arrives in asystole to the emergency department is a suitable point to reconsider further resuscitation efforts. Persistence beyond this period is unlikely to result in long-term survival and will certainly result in severe disability.

KEY LEARNING POINTS

- Most cardiac arrests in children arise from hypoxia.
- Always check the glucose level if mental state is abnormal.
- Ensure you stay up to date on specific resuscitation protocols for common emergency presentations.
- Formal training programmes such as APLS are strongly encouraged to develop and maintain skills and confidence.

ASSESSMENT AND MANAGEMENT OF THE SERIOUSLY INJURED CHILD

Some injury mechanisms such as falls from significant height or road traffic accidents are associated with a high risk of serious injury, and suggest especially careful clinical evaluation for covert injury even if the child initially appears well.

Children's anatomy and physiology produce a different injury pattern from adults (e.g. serious internal injuries with minimal external signs because of the elastic skeleton and soft-tissue compliance) and altered physiological response. These differences mean they need child-specific care, but they often have a better prognosis than adults.

The outcome of the child with serious trauma depends on the mechanism and severity of injury, and the success of initial resuscitation. The structured approach to the seriously injured child is subdivided into:

- Primary survey and resuscitation
- Secondary survey.

The primary survey

The primary survey aims to diagnose and treat life-threatening conditions and to recognize and reverse abnormal physiology to avoid secondary damage. It begins, as usual, with the *A*irway, *B*reathing and *C*irculation sequence.

A – Airway with cervical spine control

All seriously injured children should have the cervical spine immobilized initially using in-line bimanual stabilization before fitting a hard cervical collar of correct size with sandbags and adhesive tape strapping of the head and trunk to a spinal board. If necessary open the airway by jaw thrust and gently clear any blood or other secretions by suction under direct vision with the insertion of a suitably sized oropharyngeal (Guedel) airway if necessary.

B – Breathing

All should all receive high-flow supplemental oxygen by facemask. Assess breathing by noting:

- the work of breathing (rate, recession, accessory muscle use)
- the effectiveness of breathing (oxygen saturation, chest expansion, breath sounds)
- the effects of inadequate breathing (heart rate, conscious level).

If respiration is inadequate, check for evidence of a tension pneumothorax and start bag/valve/mask ventilation using 100 per cent oxygen. If ventilation remains inadequate the patient should be intubated, using an assistant to stabilize the head and neck in a neutral position with the cervical collar temporarily loosened. Correct tube placement is confirmed by good symmetrical bilateral chest expansion and breath sounds, perhaps supplemented by end-tidal carbon dioxide monitoring.

Gaseous gastric dilatation may be released by passing an orogastric tube.

C – Circulation

Poor circulation (pale, cold peripheries with prolonged capillary refill time) in an injured child suggests hypovolaemia. Assess circulation by noting:

- the pulse rate (brachial or femoral arteries), skin colour, capillary refill time, blood pressure
- the effects of an inadequate circulation (breathing rate, conscious level).

Since blood pressure and cerebral perfusion are maintained until terminal collapse, a child confused or unresponsive as a result of blood loss is close to decompensation and death. Obtain IV access (preferably two cannulae, as large as possible) and take blood for blood sugar, FBC, cross-match and amylase. If there is any difficulty in vascular access, insert an intraosseous needle, avoiding a fractured limb.

If circulation is inadequate, give boluses by syringe or rapid infusion of isotonic crystalloid (0.9 per cent saline or lactated Ringer solution) at 20 mL/kg or colloid (human albumen) at 10 mL/kg depending on local protocol. Use direct pressure to control any continuing external bleeding. If the circulatory failure has not responded to three boluses of resuscitation fluid, blood should be infused and urgent surgical assessment requested for possible internal bleeding. Non-surgical causes of resistant circulatory failure include tension pneumothorax or cardiac tamponade (chest injury) or spinal shock. The latter should be treated with vasopressors.

D – Disability

Rapidly assess the neurological status by noting the mental state (using the AVPU system), posture and pupillary reactions.

E – Exposure

Full exposure is important to examine fully the child with major trauma. There is a serious risk of significant heat loss, so the exam should be as brief as possible. Minimize the risk of hypothermia by using warmed fluids, a heating mattress, bubble wrap and space blanket all within a warm environment.

Radiology

It is usual to order cervical spine, chest and pelvis radiographs with ongoing cervical spine protection until injury can be excluded. Cervical spine injury (CSI) is uncommon (1–2 per cent) in children with major trauma but if missed the consequences for the child may be catastrophic. Children present particular challenges in clinical assessment and interpretation of cervical spine radiographs. The cervical spine can be cleared if a high-quality cervical spine radiograph series is normal, the child is alert and cooperative without a painful distracting injury, there have been no peripheral neurological symptoms or signs at any time and there is no pain or limitation on movement of the neck with the collar removed.

Normal radiographs in a child with altered conscious level or distracted by other significant painful injury do not rule out cervical spinal cord damage because of the spectre of SCIWORA – spinal cord injury without radiological abnormality. The choice here may lie between computed tomography (CT) scanning and prolonged neck immobilization.

The primary survey is a dynamic process and continues with frequent reassessment until the patient is stable, with regular monitoring of respiratory rate, heart rate, blood pressure, oxygen saturation, rectal temperature, conscious level and pupillary reflexes. A good outcome after initial resuscitation is suggested by improvement in initial tachycardia (<130 beats per minute (bpm)), normal skin colour with warming extremities, normal mental state, rising blood pressure (>80 mmHg) and pulse pressure (>20 mmHg) and adequate urine production (1–2 mL/kg hourly).

The secondary survey

Continue resuscitation and monitoring

The secondary survey should not begin until the primary survey has been completed and the child is stable and treatment is ongoing. Continue to monitor:

- airway, breathing rate, oxygen saturation
- heart rate, blood pressure, capillary refill time
- conscious level.

The primary survey must be repeated immediately if any of these variables worsen, and action taken to correct the problem.

History

A more detailed history should be obtained at this stage, both of the incident and any relevant previous medical history using the 'AMPLE' mnemonic:
A – Allergies
M – Medications
P – Past illnesses
L – Last meal; Last tetanus
E – Event details.

Head-to-toe examination

This should be conducted systematically, sympathetically and efficiently. Minimize unnecessary exposure to maintain warmth and dignity. This must include a front-and-back exam by log-rolling the child and a detailed neurological examination. If rectal examination is necessary, the most senior member of the attending surgical team should perform this once.

Investigations

Investigations should be limited to those essential for immediate management. **Laboratory investigations** should include FBC, electrolytes, LFTs, blood cross-match and blood glucose. If immediate treatment has involved significant blood transfusion (>20 per cent blood volume), clotting factors should be requested. Correction may require the administration of fresh frozen plasma and platelet concentrate. Blood gas analysis should be done initially every 30 minutes or so in the ventilated patient. The frequency of analysis may be reduced once stability has been achieved. Any urine obtained should be tested for the presence of blood or myoglobin. **Imaging** in the emergency room should be limited to those investigations which are immediately helpful and will usually include a baseline chest radiograph, cervical spine views and pelvic radiographs. Repeat chest radiograph is usual in the multiply injured or ventilated child at the time of the secondary survey to exclude pathological changes and to check the positioning of the endotracheal tube. Look for pneumothorax, haemothorax, rib fractures, pulmonary contusion and mediastinal widening. Other areas should be radiographed where clinically appropriate. If the patient is stable, these views are best taken in the radiology department. Any significant head injury requires early CT scan, especially if associated with persistent changes in conscious level or focal neurological signs. It is sensible to image other areas of concern in addition to the head. An ECG should be obtained in children with chest trauma and possible myocardial contusion.

Referral and transfer to definitive specialty care

Referral and transfer to definitive specialty care depends on each child's spectrum of clinical problems. It is essential that an adequate handover takes place between the resuscitation team and those taking over responsibility for further management. This should include the information already given to the parents about the child's present status and prognosis. Children should not be moved until the new care area confirms they are ready to receive them.

TECHNICAL SKILLS

Emergency vascular access

Intraosseous infusion

Intraosseous infusion is a temporary emergency measure indicated in life-threatening situations when IV access fails (three attempts or >90 seconds). Usually the anteromedial aspect of the tibia is used, 1–2 cm below the tibial tubercle unless there is an ipsilateral fracture or local infection. The iliac crest has been used in older children. The specially designed trocar and cannula is inserted slightly caudally to avoid the epiphyseal growth plate using an aseptic technique with local anaesthesia if the child is conscious. A sudden loss of resistance occurs as the marrow cavity is entered, often with a 'pop'. It should be well fixed to avoid displacement. Crystalloids, colloids, blood products and drugs can be infused. Fluid can be infused under gentle pressure manually by using a 50 mL syringe or by inflating a blood-pressure cuff around the infusion bag. The needle is removed as soon as the child has been resuscitated and IV access has been established.

Potential complications include extravasation, tibial fracture, osteomyelitis, epiphyseal injury and lower extremity compartment syndrome, but all are rare.

Venous cut down and central venous cannulation

Venous cut down and central venous cannulation are not procedures to be attempted without experience and training as there is a risk of serious damage. Attempts to obtain venous access by these means should not delay intraosseous needle placement. Sites for cut down include the saphenous vein at the ankle or the antecubital fossa. Central venous cannulation sites include the femoral, internal jugular and subclavian veins.

Emergency needle thoracocentesis

Clinical suspicion of a tension pneumothorax in a critically ill child is an indication for immediate release of extrapleural air using needle thoracocentesis. It can be life-saving and should be performed immediately without waiting for radiological confirmation. The minimum equipment includes alcohol swabs, a large over-the-needle IV cannula (18 G or larger for older children; 20 G or 22 G for infants), a 10 or 20 mL syringe and a three-way stopcock.

Identify the second intercostal space in the mid-clavicular line of the affected side (hyperresonant; tracheal deviation to opposite side) and swab the area. Assemble the cannula and syringe together and insert the cannula vertically through the chest wall just above the rib, gently aspirating during insertion. Free flow of air confirms correct placement, at which point the cannula is advanced off the needle. The needle is removed and replaced by a three-way stop tap. Air is allowed to escape under pressure or taken out by syringe. When airflow ceases or cardiovascular stability is achieved, drainage is stopped and a formal chest drain inserted as soon as possible.

Chest drain

Guidewire-directed chest drains are most suited to the occasional user. This procedure should be carried out under sterile conditions with gown, gloves, full skin prep and good local anaesthesia. The needle of the device is inserted into the fifth intercostal space in the mid-axillary line. The syringe attached to the needle should be constantly aspirated until free flow of air, blood or pleural fluid is obtained. The syringe is removed from the needle and the guidewire inserted until it is reliably inside the pleural cavity. At this stage, the skin incision should be enlarged with a scalpel to allow easy passage of the dilators and drain. The passage through the tissues is then enlarged with a series of dilators of increasing size, each passed over the guidewire, until it is large enough to admit the drain. The drain is then advanced until all the side-holes lie within the pleural space. An underwater seal system is then connected. Drain position should be confirmed by chest radiograph.

Pericardiocentesis

Pericardiocentesis is used for emergency treatment of cardiac tamponade caused by a pericardial effusion. ECG monitoring is essential and ultrasound guidance if available. A 20-G cannula-over-needle IV device, attached to a syringe, is inserted in the notch between the xiphisternum and the costochondral cartilage on the left side of the chest. The needle is advanced towards the left scapular tip at an angle of 45° to the horizontal, with constant suction applied until fluid is aspirated. If the needle is advanced too far and touches the myocardium an injury pattern will appear on the ECG – marked ST changes and a widening of the QRS complex. Ventricular ectopic beats may occur. If blood is aspirated from the right ventricle it will appear thick and dark and will coagulate quickly in the syringe; a blood stained pericardial effusion is less viscous and does not clot. The catheter is then advanced over the needle and the needle withdrawn. A three-way tap is attached to the catheter and fluid is aspirated by syringe. The cannula should be left in place until it is certain that the underlying problem has resolved.

The surgical airway – needle cricothyroidotomy

This procedure is reserved for an extremely rare emergency situation when the airway cannot be maintained by bag and mask and intubation proves impossible. It involves the aseptic placement of an over-the-needle cannula through the cricothyroid membrane that lies between the lower edge of the thyroid cartilage and the upper edge of the cricoid cartilage. When air is aspirated, the cannula is advanced over the needle into the trachea. A 3-mm connector is attached to the cannula and ventilation attempted by bag and positive pressure with 100 per cent oxygen. Observation and auscultation will reveal adequacy of ventilation. The cannula should be carefully secured to prevent displacement until a more secure airway can be obtained.

PARTICULAR PROBLEMS

Anaphylaxis

Anaphylaxis is a relatively common clinical syndrome of severe systemic hypersensitivity reaction typically mediated by immunoglobulin E (IgE), leading to the classic features of urticaria and angioedema, bronchoconstriction and hypotension. Reactions may follow exposure to a variety of agents, especially insect stings, drugs or vaccinations, contrast media and some foods such as peanuts. Treatment of this potentially lethal condition is often suboptimal. Early recognition and treatment of anaphylaxis is vital.

CASE STUDY

A 10-year-old boy from a local Scouts camp is brought to A&E after being stung by a bee. He had been well until he was stung on his left forearm. He initially complained of pain and swelling around the sting site. After 20 minutes, he began to complain of difficulty breathing and was noted to be wheezing. He said that he felt very shaky and dizzy. His vital signs are: temperature 37.2°C, pulse rate 118, respiratory rate 38, blood pressure 68/46, SaO_2 92 per cent. He has mild respiratory distress. He appears sleepy and pale but responds appropriately when spoken to. His voice sounds normal. He has generalized urticaria but his lips and tongue are not swollen. He has reasonable peripheral pulses. Chest examination reveals mild wheezing and reasonable air entry with minimal indrawing. Abdominal examination is normal. There is localized redness and swelling at the bee sting site on his forearm.

Recognition of anaphylactic reactions

The mode of presentation and the range and severity of clinical features is very variable, so recognition may be difficult. The rate of progression is also unpredictable, some patients are critically ill within minutes of onset and in others the reaction evolves over several hours. A previous benign course does not guarantee a similar outcome next time.

Initial symptoms can include sneezing, coughing, itching or a tingling sensation of the skin, and significant anxiety – a feeling of impending doom. There may be flushing or pallor, facial swelling, urticaria, breathing difficulties, progressing to hypotension, and collapse. Simple fainting (vasovagal syncope) or panic attacks may cause diagnostic confusion. With fainting, the patient changes from a normal to an unconscious state within seconds; in anaphylaxis, features usually evolve over several minutes, usually involve multiple body systems (skin, breathing, circulation) and unconsciousness only develops later on in severe cases. The pulse rate is a key distinguishing feature: a tachycardia usually occurs with anaphylaxis and bradycardia with syncope. A panic reaction in an individual who has previously experienced true anaphylaxis presents particular problems.

Clinical assessment and treatment

As usual, an initial structured response is important, following the usual *A*irway, *B*reathing and *C*irculation sequence. Give high-flow oxygen with a mask. A brief history of previous reactions is important as well as that of the recent episode. During examination key features are the vital signs, including blood pressure, the skin (flushing, pallor, urticaria), the upper airway (oral swelling, stridor, dysphonia), and the chest (accessory muscle use, indrawing, wheeze). Peak flow should be recorded where possible. Inspiratory stridor, wheeze, cyanosis, pronounced tachycardia and delayed capillary refill time are features of a severe reaction.

Treatment should follow the algorithm produced by the Resuscitation Council of the UK (Figure 4.5).

Adrenaline given early is the key to effective treatment for any severe allergic reaction. Its α-receptor agonist activity reverses peripheral vasodilatation and reduces oedema, and its β-receptor activity opens the airways, improves myocardial contractility and suppresses histamine and leukotriene release. Adrenaline should be given intramuscularly to all patients with clinical signs of shock, airway swelling, or definite breathing difficulty. Intravenous adrenaline is only indicated in profound life-threatening shock. Antihistamines (chlorpheniramine) and corticosteroids should also be given routinely. However, antihistamines alone will be insufficient except in the mildest cases. Parenteral hydrocortisone has a slow onset of action (four to six hours), but is particularly valuable in those cases with a significant asthma component.

At the time of gaining IV access it is worthwhile taking samples for specific IgE antibody levels and mast cell tryptase (10 mL clotted blood will cover both). This may help retrospective investigation and aid diagnostic certainty.

Children with significant events should be followed up at a specialist allergy clinic.

KEY LEARNING POINTS

- Intramuscular adrenaline is the key therapy in anaphylaxis.
- Intravenous adrenaline is dangerous and reserved for life-threatening collapse.
- Follow-up is important to ensure future safety.

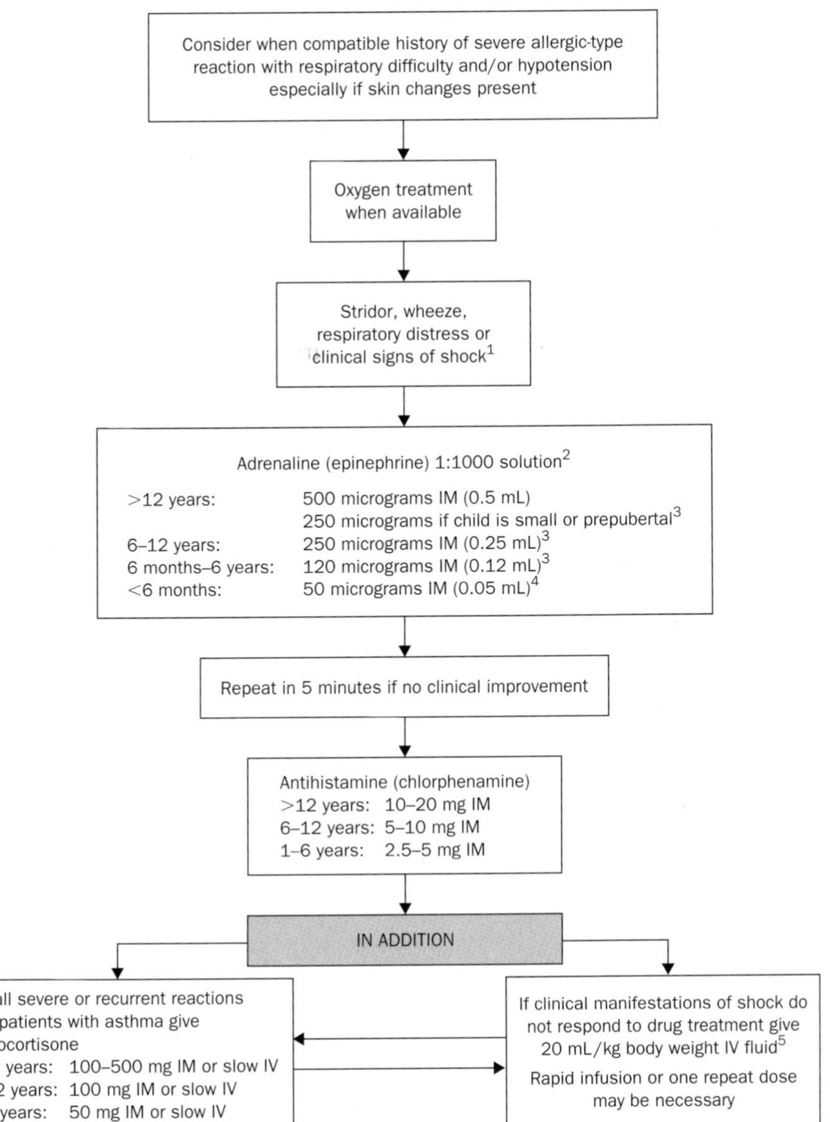

1 An inhaled β_2-agonist such as salbutamol may be used as an adjunctive measure if bronchospasm is severe and does not respond rapidly to other treatment.

2 If profound shock judged **immediately** life threatening give CPR/ALS if necessary. Consider **slow** intravenous (IV) adrenaline (epinephrine) 1:10 000 solution. This is **hazardous** and is recommended only for an experienced practitioner who can also obtain IV access without delay. Note the different strength of adrenaline (epinephrine) that may be required for IV use.

3 For children who have been prescribed Epipen, 150 micrograms can be given instead of 120 micrograms, and 300 micrograms can be given instead of 250 micrograms or 500 micrograms.

4 Absolute accuracy of the small dose is not essential.

5 A crystalloid may be safer than a colloid.

Figure 4.5 Algorithm for the treatment of anaphylaxis in children (reproduced with permission of UK Resuscitation Council). ALS, advanced life support; CPR, cardiopulmonary resuscitation; IM, intramuscular; IV, intravenous

Burns

Burns are common in children; injury severity and secondary metabolic response is directly related to the depth and surface area of the burn. Scalds are the commonest injury, often caused by hot water spillages from cooking pots, hot drinks or even immersion in a hot bath. Some burns (especially immersion injuries) are non-accidental; the history and pattern of injury should provoke further investigation.

Burns caused by flame or direct heat usually results from house fires or motor vehicle accidents. There may be associated traumatic injuries from being thrown from a window or high velocity fall. Any fire in an enclosed location will produce smoke and carbon monoxide. Hydrogen cyanide is also produced by combustion of some soft furnishings. Exposure to these agents can be lethal; many individuals who die as a result of fire have no direct thermal injury.

> **CASE STUDY**
>
> A 19-month-old boy dislodged a fresh mug of coffee from the kitchen table while reaching for a piece of toast. His mother soaked a towel in cold water and held it on his chin and chest and then a neighbour drove them quickly to the hospital. On arrival, he is screaming and is agitated, his mother is distraught. There are obvious areas of erythema and blistering scattered over his lower face, neck and upper chest.

Electrical burns can cause severe injury. An apparent minor skin wound may have extensive hidden deep tissue injury. Damage is related to the current passed, which follows the path of least resistance – preferentially through nerves and blood vessels. Much of the injury following electrical burns is due to vascular coagulation and distal ischaemia. Early surgical exploration is usually indicated to determine the extent of damage and relieve compartment swelling due to muscle damage. Myocardial damage may also occur; cardiac enzymes and a 12-lead ECG should be obtained. ECG monitoring should be continued for 24–48 hours following a significant electrical injury as late death due to cardiac arrhythmia has been described.

Strong acids or alkalis such as caustic cleaning solutions can cause chemical burns. If accidentally drunk, they may cause serious injury to the mouth, pharynx and oesophagus. Major airway problems may develop early and later oesophageal stricture may develop. Chemical burns should be irrigated for long periods – up to an hour – with tepid water to dilute and neutralize the agent. Care must be taken with small children to avoid hypothermia during this process.

Classification of burn injuries

The extent of damage (depth of injury) is related to temperature and duration of exposure. Other factors directly influencing final burn depth are:

- thickness of the skin (thin on eyelids, thick on back) and age of the patient – younger children have thinner skin
- vascularity of the affected area (facial skin has high blood flow that conducts away heat)
- nature of the burning agent (oil boils at a higher temperature than water and runs off more slowly)
- effective first aid treatment (cooling reduces the amount of heat transmitted to the deeper tissues).

The appearance of the burn enables an estimate to be made of the degree of tissue damage, although this can be difficult in the early stages and the severity of injury may vary.

- **Superficial burns** involve only the epidermis. Sunburn is a common example. These burns are red, dry and painful, do not blister and blanch with pressure. They do not scar and need only local wound care.
- **Partial thickness burns** involve the dermis, with some residual dermis remaining viable and are further subdivided into superficial and deep partial-thickness burns.
- **Superficial partial-thickness** burn injuries involve the papillary dermis, containing pain-sensitive nerve endings. Blisters may be present, and the burns usually appear pink and moist. These areas usually heal spontaneously without significant scarring.
- **Deep partial-thickness burns** also involve the papillary and reticular dermis. Some areas are painless and often appear white or mottled pink. These lesions eventually heal, often with scarring. Debridement and grafting may be required.
- In **full thickness burns** the entire dermis is destroyed leaving subcutaneous tissue exposed (full thickness). They appear white, mottled or charred and are dry and may be firm or leathery. Full thickness burns do not blanch and are not painful since the nerve endings are destroyed. They always need surgery.

Estimating the area of a burn

The rule of nines is a well-established system used to evaluate the extent of a burn injury. The body is divided into multiples of nine (Figure 4.6). Small areas of damage can be calculated using the principle that the palmar surfaces of the hands of the patient represents approximately 1 per cent. In making this calculation, only areas of partial- and full-thickness burns are included. Superficial burns are NOT included.

For children, estimates of involved area are better with a Lund and Browder chart (Figure 4.7). In this system, the patient's age, weight and degree of burn are all factored into the total burn picture. The Lund and Browder chart divides the body into smaller proportions giving a more precise measure of burn damage.

Burns triage

Partial-thickness burns of less than 10 per cent body surface area (BSA) and full-thickness burns of less than

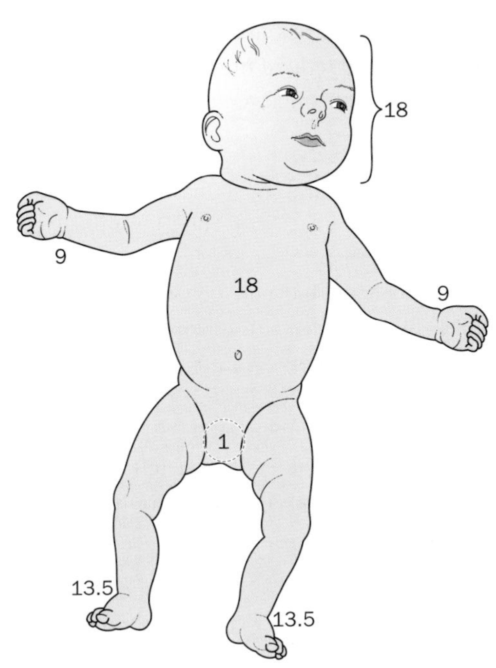

Figure 4.6 Rule of nines - infant proportions

2 per cent BSA can usually be managed in an outpatient setting if there is no involvement of critical areas (hands, face, eyes, ears, feet or perineum), no smoke inhalation, no electrical injury and no suspicion of non-accidental injury. All other patients require admission.

Analgesia

Partial-thickness burns are very painful. Occlusive dressings help, but adequate analgesia is essential. Adequate IV morphine should be given, taking care to avoid respiratory depression.

General management of the burned child

A child with burns may have other injuries so a detailed history of the incident should be obtained.

PRIMARY SURVEY

As with all injuries, the *A*irway, *B*reathing and *C*irculation resuscitation scheme is followed. Particular airway and

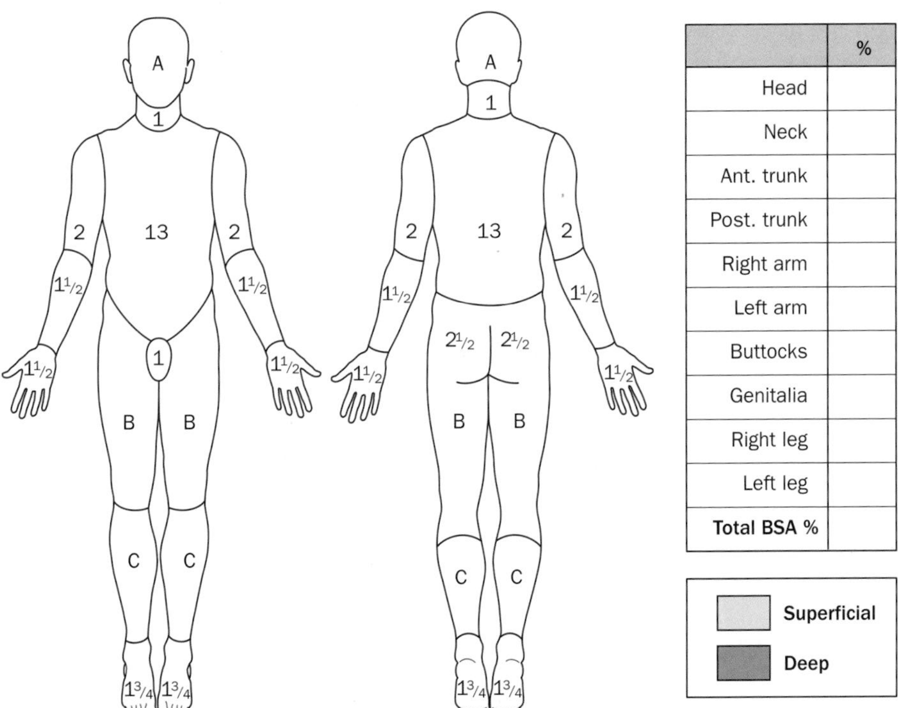

	%
Head	
Neck	
Ant. trunk	
Post. trunk	
Right arm	
Left arm	
Buttocks	
Genitalia	
Right leg	
Left leg	
Total BSA %	

Relative percentage of areas affected by growth

Age (years)	0		5	10	15	Adult
A – 1/2 of head	$9\frac{1}{2}$	$8\frac{1}{2}$	$6\frac{1}{2}$	$5\frac{1}{2}$	$4\frac{1}{2}$	$3\frac{1}{2}$
B – 1/2 of one thigh	$2\frac{3}{4}$	$3\frac{1}{4}$	4	$4\frac{1}{4}$	$4\frac{1}{2}$	$4\frac{3}{4}$
C – 1/2 of one leg	$2\frac{1}{2}$	$2\frac{1}{2}$	$2\frac{3}{4}$	3	$3\frac{1}{4}$	3

Figure 4.7 Modified Lund and Browder chart for estimating areas in children with burns

breathing issues arise. Soot contamination, especially round the mouth and nose, suggests smoke inhalation and facial or pharyngeal burns indicate a high risk of airway obstruction. Damaged tissue will swell rapidly in the hours following injury and intubation may be extremely difficult if delayed. An altered state of consciousness or combative behaviour may be due to hypoxia, as a result of either smoke inhalation and pulmonary damage, or carbon monoxide poisoning. Give 100 per cent oxygen through a close fitting facemask with reservoir bag. Intubation is indicated if there is early airway, respiratory or neurological compromise, severe facial burns, inhalation injury seen on laryngoscopy or bronchoscopy, or extensive thoracic burns restricting chest wall movement.

In all but the most trivial burn injury rapid vascular access is mandatory, avoiding burnt areas because of the risk of infection. If IV access is not obtained quickly, the intraosseous route should be used. Shock due to hypovolaemia is common when the burn exceeds 12 per cent BSA. Until fluid/electrolyte needs are calculated give normal saline at 20 mL/kg per hour.

FLUID AND ELECTROLYTE MANAGEMENT

Fluid therapy includes normal maintenance plus replacement of burn losses. Denuded skin produces a sixfold increase in evaporative loss and exudative losses (blisters) have a protein content half of the serum protein level.

The Parkland formula using Ringer Lactate (see below) is a well-established method to calculate fluid replacement, determined from the time of injury, not the time of arrival at hospital as stated above.

In infants and young children, maintenance fluids should be given over 24 hours in addition to these replacement fluids. Potassium is not added to the fluids for the first day because injured cells release potassium into the extracellular fluid.

> **The Parkland formula**
>
> Total volume of Ringer Lactate = patient weight (in kg) × per cent burn area (as a number)
>
> Half of this volume is given over the first eight hours, the remainder over the subsequent 16 hours.

Clinical and physiological variables must be assessed to avoid excess or inadequate fluid administration. These include monitoring heart rate, blood pressure, peripheral perfusion, urine output and regular urea and electrolyte assays. In severe cases, central venous pressure measurement allows direct assessment of circulating volume. Signs of fluid overload include development of pulmonary oedema, liver enlargement and triple rhythm.

WOUND MANAGEMENT

Burns should be covered as soon as possible to reduce evaporative fluid and heat loss and to minimize contamination by environmental organisms. Clingfilm provides a transparent barrier that will not stick to the damaged skin. Pain is also reduced if the wound is covered.

Circumferential lesions around digits, the limbs or torso may impair distal blood flow or restrict chest movement. These may require incision (escharotomy) to relieve constriction. This procedure is best left to an expert. A careless escharotomy may result in serious haemorrhage.

SPECIFIC MANAGEMENT ISSUES

Electrical burns should always be treated with caution; they are often much more extensive than they initially appear. They may need urgent surgical exploration to relieve compartment pressure caused by extensive muscle damage. Myocardial damage can occur as a result of electrical injury. A 12-lead ECG should be obtained and continuous ECG monitoring maintained for at least 24 hours after high voltage electrocution, but is unnecessary after domestic electrocution if the initial ECG is normal.

Skeletal muscle damage may result in myoglobinuria, and require alkaline diuresis to protect against renal tubular damage. Serum potassium levels are also often elevated following electrical burns. Blood should be sent for cardiac enzyme assay, and blood and urine examined for the presence of myoglobin.

INVESTIGATIONS

Baseline investigations should include FBC, platelet count, clotting screen, blood glucose, UEs and, depending on the severity of injury and the need for surgery, blood should be cross matched or grouped and saved. If the injury sustained was due to fire, particularly in an enclosed environment, carboxyhaemoglobin level should be obtained and arterial blood gas analysis carried out. Both these investigations should be done if any respiratory distress is evident.

A baseline chest radiograph should be obtained in severe cases. This helps in assessment of possible pulmonary oedema during resuscitation and evolution of lung injury following smoke inhalation. Other radiographs are required as dictated by other potential injuries.

OTHER FACTORS

Early enteral nutrition has been shown to be of benefit during the hypercatabolic phase of burn injury, which lasts several days. It also protects against stress ulceration and reduces bacterial translocation across the gut wall, which may be a significant source of sepsis in these vulnerable patients. Passage of a nasogastric tube reduces the risk of aspiration in the acute phase and enteral feeding can be commenced within the first 24 hours.

Inhalation injury

Soot produced in enclosed fires can mechanically clog and irritate the airways, causing reflex bronchospasm. Noxious gases released during thermal decomposition include carbon monoxide and hydrogen cyanide.

Inhalation injury can occur in three ways:

- direct lung damage by irritants
- hypoxia from interruption of oxygen delivery by asphyxiants (carbon monoxide)
- end-organ damage by systemic absorption through the respiratory tract.

Lung damage can be broadly categorized as the result of thermal or chemical damage to the epithelial surfaces of the intrathoracic and extrathoracic airways. Secondary insult with bacterial pneumonia may occur days after inhalation, causing further injury. Impaired ciliary function leads to accumulation of airway debris.

Carbon monoxide poisoning is a potentially fatal complication of smoke inhalation. Fortunately, carbon monoxide can be displaced from haemoglobin by high-inspired oxygen concentrations. The half-life of carboxyhaemoglobin can be reduced to around 90 minutes compared with five hours in room air by giving 100 per cent oxygen via a facemask or ventilator. Hyperbaric oxygen at 3 atmospheres (atm) pressure reduces this further to around 25 minutes. There is some evidence that late treatment (days) with hyperbaric oxygen produces significant improvement in neurological symptoms following carbon monoxide poisoning.

KEY LEARNING POINTS

- The depth, extent and body areas involved define the need for admission.
- Use adequate analgesia as soon as possible.
- Remember the possibility of child abuse.

Child abuse

It is a sad reality that some of the two million children who attend hospital accident and emergency departments in the UK each year have been deliberately injured. Audit figures suggest 1.5 per cent (at least) of child attendances merit referral for investigation of suspected intentional injury. If such cases go unrecognized, the children are at significant risk of future injuries. At least one child is killed as the result of abuse, usually by a parent or carer, every week in the UK. In the face of this reality, all clinical staff working in A&E departments or acute care areas must be aware of the possibility of child abuse and be able and prepared to act appropriately if they are concerned. Child protection fails not just because of failure of recognition. It also fails because of problems of record keeping, communication and failure to follow procedures. Recent reviews of fatal child abuse cases (notably the Victoria Climbié Inquiry) have highlighted significant system failures in the child protection process, and severely criticized the clinical competencies and behaviour of doctors involved. The Climbié case

CASE STUDY

A mother brought her 17-month-old daughter to the A&E department. She had been shopping with a friend while her boyfriend looked after her children from a previous relationship. She found the girl crying uncontrollably. The boyfriend explained to her that he had left a hot iron on the floor to cool, and the girl had 'shuffled into it' while he was preparing to change her nappy. There was a significant burn injury on the inner thigh and vulva (Figure 4.8). The child was admitted for treatment and a child protection investigation was initiated because of concern about the circumstances of injury.

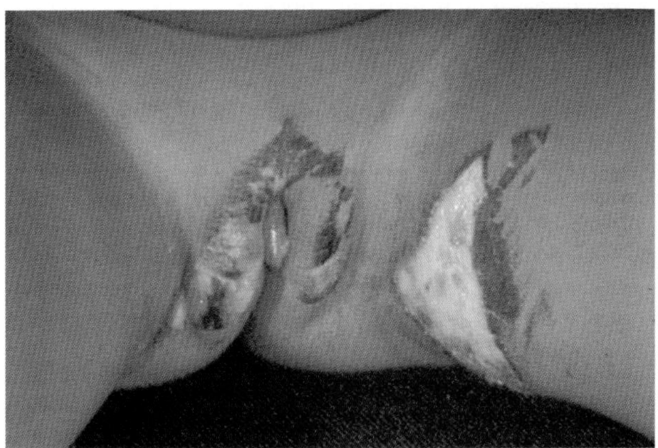

Figure 4.8 Extensive partial-thickness burns of vulva and inner thigh

also highlighted inadequate communication between individual professionals (health or otherwise), failure to follow agreed protocols and poor awareness of child protection issues.

There are four overlapping categories of abuse.

- **Physical abuse** is any action that causes physical injury to a child, such as hitting, shaking, poisoning, burning or scalding, drowning and suffocation. This also includes factitious illness (Munchausen syndrome by proxy) when a parent or carer feigns illness symptoms, or deliberately induces symptoms, in a child they are responsible for (see later).
- **Emotional abuse** involves behaviour towards a child that impairs their emotional development so they feel unloved, worthless or inadequate. Some degree of emotional abuse is involved in all types of maltreatment.
- **Neglect** arises when parents/carers consistently fail to meet a child's needs. These include adequate shelter, clothing, nourishment and medical care, as well as emotional security and developmental stimulation.
- **Child sexual abuse** includes situations where children are forced to take part in activities for the sexual gratification of adults; this may include both physical contact as well as non-contact activities (e.g. genital touching, orogenital contact and sexual intercourse).

Recognition of child abuse

The factors described below are often found in cases of child abuse. They do not prove that abuse has occurred but indicate the need for careful assessment and discussion with the designated child protection lead or at least an experienced colleague. The absence of such indicators does not mean that abuse or neglect has not occurred. The following features (not exhaustive) must generally be regarded as indicators of concern:

- unexplained delay in seeking treatment
- parents are absent without good reason when their child is presented for treatment
- an explanation inconsistent with an injury or the developmental stage of the child
- multiple explanations provided for an injury
- the parents are uninterested or unperturbed by an accident or injury
- family use of different doctors and A&E departments
- reluctance to give information or mention previous injuries.

Use of a checklist in the case record of all injured young children may improve detection of child abuse (Figure 4.9).

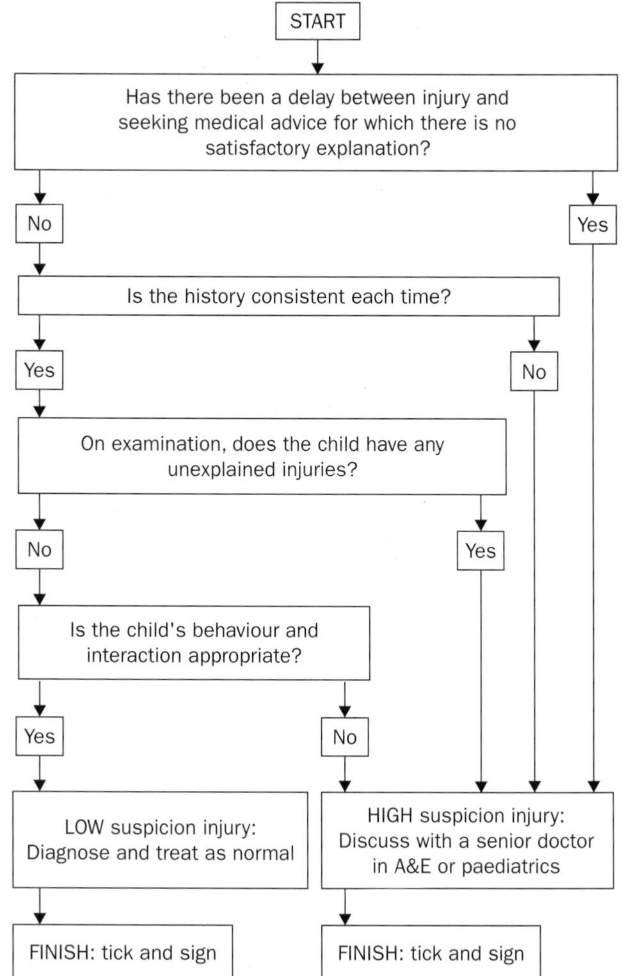

Figure 4.9 Accident and emergency record label to improve detection of child abuse (from Benger JR, Pearce AV. Quality improvement report: simple intervention to improve detection of child abuse in emergency departments. *BMJ* 2002;**324**:780–2, with permission)

There is no gold standard diagnostic tool for diagnosing non-accidental injury. Each case must be assessed individually and the circumstances of the injury, the clinical presentation and other individual features of the scenario that make up the full picture must be taken into account. Some clinical and investigative features, however, are very suggestive. For example, rib fractures in children less than 3 years of age are highly predictive of non-accidental injury, the likelihood of non-accidental injury decreasing with increasing age. Children with disability are at greater risk of abuse than their peers, but some are also more prone to accidental injury – children with severe mobility problems are liable to fracture osteoporotic bones during passive physiotherapy. Assessment needs care and tact.

For most doctors in training, the issue is not subtle forensic assessment but the critical importance of passing on any concern to more experienced senior colleagues.

Fabricated or induced illness (Munchausen syndrome by proxy)

The fabrication or induction of illness in children by a carer has been referred to by a number of different terms, usually Munchausen syndrome by proxy, factitious illness by proxy or illness induction syndrome. The key issue is not what term to use to describe this type of abuse, but the impact of fabricated or induced illness on the child's health and development and consideration of how best to safeguard the child's welfare.

The fabrication or induction of illness in a child by a carer is uncommon. On the basis of 128 cases notified to the British Paediatric Surveillance Unit from the UK and Republic of Ireland over a two-year period, researchers have estimated that the combined annual incidence in the British Isles of these forms of abuse in children under 16 years was at least 0.5 per 100 000 and for those under 1 year of age at least 2.8 per 100 000. The age range of children in whom illness is fabricated or induced extends throughout childhood but most are under 5 years old, with a median age of 20 months. In those identified, retrospective symptoms were often present for more than six months, with some for much longer. Mothers are usually involved, but passive collusion by fathers is well recognized. A personal background of organic illness and a history of assessment for mental health problems are not uncommon.

Fabrication or illness induction can simulate almost any disorder and there is a danger in thinking of 'typical scenarios'. Some have grouped cases into 'clinical categories':

- verbal fabrications including fabrication of records or tests but no direct illness induction: symptoms reported commonly included bleeding, apnoea, seizures, diabetes, recurrent infections, etc.
- withholding nutrients
- production of signs and symptoms other than by poisoning or smothering (other inductions): children with fevers, rashes, bleeding, renal stones, etc.
- poisoning of low toxicity: children presented with diarrhoea, vomiting, dehydration and failure to thrive that was due to administration of emetics, laxatives and diuretics
- poisoning of high toxicity: insulin-induced hypoglycaemia, salt poisoning, drugs, e.g. sedatives
- apparent life-threatening events (ALTE; see later) that includes smothering to produce signs.

There is clearly a need to distinguish 'normal' overanxiety in carers about minor illness. Some children may have a background of illness from early life, such as prematurity; some may have a history of feeding problems and poor growth progress.

Mortality and morbidity in factitious illness is significant. In the study referred to above, 8/128 (6 per cent) children died as a direct result of abuse. A further 15 (12 per cent) required intensive care and an additional 45 (35 per cent) suffered major physical illness.

Clearly, doctors dealing with acute emergencies in children need to be aware of this issue, which lies within the broader context of child protection. Perhaps the most important practical point is to be alert to ensuring that the history (including that of the child if possible), clinical features and progress are concordant, and admit the child for further assessment if there are emerging concerns. Training grade doctors should have a low threshold to discuss concerns with senior staff, and clinical supervisors must ensure that the working environment they lead encourages uncertainties to be aired. The reader is referred to the document *Fabricated or Induced illness by Carers* (Royal College of Paediatrics and Child Health; see Further reading) for a much more indepth review of this topic.

KEY LEARNING POINTS

- Early recognition of the abused child is essential to minimize future harm.
- Certain historical and clinical features should alert you to the possibility.
- Any concern about possible abuse should be discussed at once with more senior colleagues.

Drowning

In the UK, drowning or near-drowning occurs most commonly when young children are unsupervised near open water, usually garden ponds and rivers. Home accidents also occur in baths, and infants may even topple head first into a bucket of water. Older children and adolescents, often encouraged by alcoholic bravado, usually get into difficulties outdoors. Pool diving accidents may also result in cervical spine or head injuries and consequent drowning due to paresis or coma.

Pathophysiology

Osmotic differences between fresh water and salt water produce injury by different effects after immersion. Fresh

CASE STUDY

A 15-month-old infant arrived in the A&E department by ambulance in full arrest. His mother had left him playing with older children in her friend's garden while she helped prepare lunch. He was found lying face down in the neighbour's garden pond 20 minutes later. A gate leading to a shared rear lane was found to be open. He was cold, blue and limp. The ambulance crew performed CPR en route to the hospital. The infant is intubated and adrenaline administered via a tracheal tube. An intraosseous line is inserted and adrenaline given by this route as well. After 45 minutes of full resuscitation in A&E, the infant is pronounced dead.

water (especially soapy) causes dilution and destruction of surfactant with consequent atelectasis and ventilation–perfusion mismatch, whereas salt water draws fluid into the alveoli producing pulmonary oedema. In practice, the relatively small volumes of water aspirated make the distinction between fresh and salt water drowning irrelevant. The end result of both processes is hypoxia and intrapulmonary shunting. The response to immersion in water can be divided into three stages:

1 struggle – small aspiration resulting in laryngospasm
2 increasing hypoxia – larger volume of water swallowed
3 laryngospasm relaxes:
   a large volume of water aspirated (85 per cent)
   b small aspiration leading to further laryngospasm with hypoxia – 'dry drowning' (15 per cent).

The laryngospasm group have little or no pulmonary damage and outcome depends on the duration and severity of the hypoxic insult.

Significant aspiration leads to variable pulmonary damage due to surfactant loss and destruction of the alveolar membrane. These cases may develop adult respiratory distress syndrome. In most cases the lung injury is reversible. All organs may be affected by the hypoxia.

Management

On arrival, rapidly assess *A*irway, *B*reathing, *C*irculation and conscious level. Immobilize the spine if there is any question of cervical spine injury. If the child is in cardiorespiratory arrest, standard resuscitation should begin. If the child is breathing spontaneously, give 100 per cent oxygen by facemask. A child whose breathing is inadequate, with a persistently reduced conscious level or deteriorating arterial oxygen despite high-inspired oxygen level, needs intubation and ventilation. There is a significant risk of regurgitation of swallowed water, so airway protection by cricoid pressure is required during rapid sequence induction and endotracheal intubation, before the stomach contents can be removed with a large-bore gastric tube.

Severe pulmonary oedema may result in copious pink, frothy secretions in the endotracheal tube, which may require repeated suctioning. The application of positive end-expiratory pressure (PEEP) will reduce oedema production. If oxygenation cannot be maintained without high positive-pressure ventilation, high-frequency oscillation may prove beneficial. Extracorporeal oxygenation may be considered if gas exchange remains poor and a good neurological outcome is likely.

If the initial circulation is inadequate, give fluid bolus of 20 mL/kg. Inotrope support should be considered early to maintain circulation. Once a stable circulation is established, secondary brain injury (and pulmonary oedema) will be minimized by avoiding hypoxia and hypercarbia, restricting maintenance fluids to around two-thirds of the calculated requirements and close monitoring of haemodynamic and biochemical status, including regular blood gas measurement and continuous saturation monitoring.

Submersion in cold water can cool the core body temperature much more rapidly than exposure to cold air, because thermal conductivity of water is 32 times greater than that of air. Thus significant hypothermia may be seen in near-drowning children (see below).

KEY LEARNING POINTS

- Toddler drowning is an increasing problem in the UK, often associated with garden ponds.
- Cervical spine precautions are important if there is a possibility of associated trauma.
- Hypothermia is a common associated problem.

Hypothermia

Moderate hypothermia is defined as 32–35°C and severe hypothermia <32°C. The physiological immaturity, large surface area relative to body mass and lesser subcutaneous tissue, especially in young babies, puts them particularly at risk of hypothermia. The effects of hypothermia are global since all the body's enzyme systems operate most efficiently over a narrow temperature range of about 36–38°C.

> **CASE STUDY**
>
> A Canadian toddler wandered outside wearing only her nappy in subzero weather and was found virtually frozen face down in the snow some hours later. She had a core temperature of 15°C and was in asystole when she was found. After prolonged resuscitation and gradual rewarming, she appeared to have survived the ordeal neurologically intact. The A&E paediatrician said, 'We don't declare somebody dead here until they're warm and dead.'

Hypothermia increases peripheral vasoconstriction, worsens acidosis, and decreases oxygen delivery to the tissues. Progressive hypothermia leads to slowing of conduction in both nerve fibres and cardiac conduction tissue. The heart rate slows and the QT interval is prolonged. Atrial arrhythmias (<32°C), ventricular tachycardia, ventricular fibrillation and asystole (30°C) may occur. Respiratory drive falls significantly and initial tachypnoea is replaced by a significant reduction in breathing rate and effectiveness.

Initial central nervous system features include confusion and disorientation. Hypoglycaemia is often seen in hypothermic children, so a rapid plasma glucose check is mandatory. As the temperature falls there is progressive weakness, onset of coma and loss of pupillary and deep tendon reflexes. The electroencephalogram (EEG) is silent at about 20°C.

Management

Hypothermia can be treated by active or passive techniques. The evidence base for their use comes from adult patients.

Passive peripheral warming involves the application of insulating materials (usually blankets) to prevent further heat loss. This is most effective in older children with core temperatures above 32°C but may not be effective in very ill children – children in shock do not generate heat.

Active warming techniques include radiant heat, warmed fluids and humidification and heating of inspired gases. These measures are slow to produce an effect in the profoundly hypothermic patient and multiple methods may be required. Various techniques have been employed, including warm peritoneal and pleural lavage, warm bladder irrigation and heat exchanging oesophageal tubes. If available, the most effective method is to establish extracorporeal circulation and warm the circulated blood.

After primary ABC has been completed, wet clothing should be removed, the skin dried and the child wrapped in insulating material such as warm blankets, bubble wrap and a space blanket to conserve body heat. Core body temperature should be recorded by measuring rectal temperature with a low-reading thermometer. The usual variables for assessment of circulation may be difficult to use because of vasoconstriction, etc. Pulse oximeters do not work well in hypothermic patients with vasoconstriction and will not accurately reflect oxygenation. Volume depletion is a common clinical finding in severe hypothermia and IV fluids are indicated.

Mild hypothermia may be managed by the use of radiant heaters and a warm environment, free of draughts. Careful monitoring of urine output and circulatory status is required to prevent hypovolaemia during the rewarming process and to prevent circulatory overload while the vasoconstriction persists. Fluids should be warmed. The aim is to achieve a 1°C temperature rise per hour.

Severe hypothermia is more challenging. There is a high risk of dysrhythmias and external stimulation may provoke fibrillation. If there is an organized rhythm on ECG monitoring, despite a barely detectable cardiac output CPR should not be instituted. The apnoeic patient should be intubated and ventilated with careful observation of the ECG, as this may also precipitate dysrhythmias. If ventricular fibrillation is evident CPR should be commenced. At low temperatures this rhythm may be refractory. Cardioversion should be attempted but limited to two or three shocks. Persistence is unlikely to be successful and will cause more myocardial damage. Drugs given at this stage are unlikely to be effective and probably should be given in lower doses at increased intervals. Active and/or invasive warming and CPR should be continued until the usual dysrhythmia threshold is passed (around 32°C). Cardioversion is more likely to be successful above this temperature.

> **KEY LEARNING POINTS**
>
> - Even in the UK, hypothermia is a significant risk especially in outdoor accidents.
> - During resuscitation of any child, minimize heat loss as much as possible.
> - Resuscitation should not be abandoned until hypothermia has resolved.

Head injury

Head injury is a leading cause of childhood death and disability worldwide, and is one of the commonest reasons for children to attend A&E departments in the UK. Although most head injuries are minor and require

CASE STUDY

A 6-year-old boy chased a football into the road and was struck by a car travelling at 25 mph, throwing him some distance along the road. Bystanders provided CPR and paramedics transferred him to hospital. On arrival pulses were present but he had a depressed Glasgow Coma Scale (GCS) of 8. He had a significant head injury with basal skull fracture; a moderate right haemothorax; fractured right femur and iliac crest; and multiple abrasions and lacerations. Initial resuscitation was successful and he was transferred to the paediatric intensive care unit. He survived but has moderate disability.

outpatient management or a brief stay in hospital, some of these children will require prolonged hospitalization.

Most of the head injuries in children under 10 years of age are caused by falls, and motor vehicles cause most in adolescents. Long-term follow-up of children with head injuries shows that although most make a full recovery, a significant number experience long-term neurological or psychological effects. Some children with apparently trivial head injuries develop significant intracranial complications. The clinical challenge is to recognize these cases early and provide appropriate treatment, while avoiding over-investigation and overtreatment of the uncomplicated majority.

The first step in the management and resuscitation of children with head injuries is the assessment and management of the ABCs together with cervical spine protection. Seriously ill children may need ventilatory support and treatment of shock. A child with a minor head injury can be classified into low, medium and high risk for associated brain injury on the basis of the history and the findings on physical and neurological examination. This offers a structured approach to decisions about imaging and admission.

Risk classification after apparently minor head injury

Low risk

- Low-risk mechanism of injury
- Transient loss of consciousness (<5 minutes)
- Glasgow Coma Score (GCS) of 15
- Asymptomatic
- Mild or absent headache and vomiting (<3 episodes)
- Scalp injury – minor bruise or superficial laceration
- Age >2 years

Medium risk

- Multiple trauma/high-risk mechanism of injury
- Loss of consciousness (>5 minutes)
- Post-traumatic amnesia or seizure
- GCS of 13–14
- Serious facial injury or signs of basal skull fracture
- Suspicion of penetrating injury or depressed skull fracture
- Progressive lethargy or headache
- Persistent vomiting (>3 times) or associated with other symptoms
- Possible child abuse
- Significant co-morbid conditions
- Aged <2 years

High risk

- GCS score of 12 at any time or drop of 2 points or more during observation
- Focal neurological signs
- Penetrating skull injury
- Palpable depressed skull fracture
- Compound skull fracture

History

WAS THERE A HIGH-RISK MECHANISM OF INJURY?

Examples include road traffic accidents, falls from a significant height, high-velocity focal injuries (golf club) or possible penetrating injury.

DID THE CHILD'S INITIAL RESPONSE SUGGEST SIGNIFICANT RISK OF BRAIN INJURY?

More than a few minutes' loss of consciousness or any associated neurological dysfunction (focal paralysis, loss of vision) or seizure suggests significant injury. Headaches, nausea, vomiting and lethargy are common and rather non-specific symptoms often reported after minor head injury. In the absence of high-risk features, they are unlikely to be significant and usually settle after a few hours. Persistent vomiting may lead to dehydration and may be an independent reason for admission to hospital.

ARE THERE ANY CO-MORBID CONDITIONS THAT INCREASE THE RISK OF INTRACRANIAL INJURY?

Children with established medical conditions such as coagulation disorders (e.g. haemophilia) or pre-existing intracranial problems (e.g. shunted hydrocephalus) are obviously at greater risk of complications.

Examination

WHAT IS THE LEVEL OF CONSCIOUSNESS?

The GCS (Table 4.3) is a classification of the degree of coma and is fundamental to the triage, initial management and ongoing assessment of a child with head injury. Serial measurements allow early recognition of deterioration or response to treatment. The standard GCS works well for adults and older children and a paediatric version is used for younger children (<4 years).

ARE THERE ANY EXTERNAL INJURIES THAT SUGGEST A HIGH RISK OF INTRACRANIAL DAMAGE?

Examine the face and scalp for lacerations, bruising and deformity and look in the ears. Bleeding or leak of cerebrospinal fluid from the ear or haemotympanum suggests a base of skull fracture. Other signs are periorbital bruising (raccoon or panda eyes), bruising behind the ear (Battle sign), and leak of cerebrospinal fluid from the nose (rhinorrhoea).

Exploration of cranial lacerations with a gloved finger may reveal a depressed fracture, and a marked localized boggy swelling (often not present initially) suggests an underlying fracture. In practice, a detailed head examination is often difficult because of anxiety and distress.

Infants and toddlers present particular challenges. It is often very difficult to get a clear history of loss of consciousness. Associated apnoea, pallor and failure to cry immediately after the injury, perhaps with brief limb jerking all suggest a significant risk of brain injury but may simply reflect a benign brief reflex anoxic event. Anterior fontanelle tension should be recorded in infants. This age group is also at particular risk of non-accidental injury. They justify a cautious approach with a low threshold for imaging and admission.

Well children with minor head injury in the low-risk group do not require skull radiographs or other imaging and can be discharged home with a reliable carer, but clear written advice must be given to parents/carers when to seek further clinical evaluation.

Selection for imaging or admission

No clinical evaluation and selective imaging strategy has been shown to be fully reliable in predicting traumatic brain injury in children with apparently minor head injury. Direct generalization of the experience with adults to children is inappropriate because of the differences in anatomy and physiological response to cerebral trauma. Despite numerous clinical studies of various management strategies no unanimous opinion has emerged about the indications for skull radiographs, CT, observation and neurosurgical consultation. Two head injury clinical guidelines produced in the UK in recent years provide a (somewhat conflicting) framework for clinical decision making (SIGN 2000; NICE 2003). Neither has a primary focus on childhood head injury but makes some effort to acknowledge specific childhood issues.

Cranial CT scanning is the accepted standard for diagnosis of traumatic brain injury and in recent years there

Table 4.3 The original Glasgow Coma Scale and the modified paediatric version

Glasgow Coma Scale (GCS)		Score	Paediatric modification of GCS
Activity	Best response		Best response
Eye opening	Spontaneous	4	Spontaneous
	To speech	3	To speech
	To pain	2	To pain
	None	1	None
Verbal	Oriented	5	Social smile, follows, oriented to sounds
	Confused	4	Cries, consolable, inappropriate interactions
	Inappropriate words	3	Inconsistently consolable, moaning
	Non-specific sounds	2	Inconsolable, agitated
	None	1	None
Motor	Follows commands	6	Spontaneous, obeys commands
	Localizes pain	5	Localizes pain
	Withdraws to pain	4	Withdraws to pain
	Flexion to pain	3	Flexion to pain (decorticate)
	Extension to pain	2	Extension to pain (decerebrate)
	None	1	None

has been a significant rise in the number of children undergoing post-traumatic cranial CT scanning. Recent UK guidelines have encouraged that trend. However, the vast majority of scans prove to be normal, and very few children with positive findings need surgical intervention. A low threshold for childhood CT scanning poses significant logistical and clinical challenges, including the need for transfer if CT scanning is not available locally, the need for sedation in some children, and the individually low but potentially important risks around significant childhood radiation exposure.

Isolated plain X-ray imaging is of relatively limited value. Skull radiographs may be useful to exclude underlying fracture in well younger children with an associated boggy scalp swelling, full-thickness scalp lacerations, or where there is uncertainty about a possible depressed fracture or penetrating injury. Simple linear parietal fractures are a relatively common finding and usually benign. In such children, a period of observation (at least six hours) may be all that is required. In areas where CT scanning is not available this may offer an alternative to transfer for some children. They may be useful as part of possible child abuse investigation. In children with palpable/visible skull deformity or signs of base of skull fracture, radiographs add little unless there will be significant unavoidable delay in CT access. Children in the medium-risk groups will need CT scanning and skilled observation for at least six hours. There should be a low threshold for more prolonged observation and clear written instructions should be given to carers on discharge.

In practice, most children in the moderate- or high-risk group will undergo cranial CT scanning and admission for observation. Children transferred for CT should be accompanied and monitored by appropriately trained clinical staff.

Neurointensive care of the child with a head injury

Head injury management primarily involves attention to detail and effective primary resuscitation. The brain is highly vulnerable to hypoxia and ischaemia so the first priority is to establish adequate respiratory and circulatory functions. For the patient with a GCS of 9–12, oxygen administration and volume resuscitation if required will probably be adequate, unless airway or thoracic injuries necessitate mechanical ventilation.

Neurosurgical advice should be sought at an early stage for those patients with GCS of 8 or less, any penetrating injury and any lesion discovered on CT scan. If transfer is required, the child must be closely monitored and the transfer team must include an anaesthetist with the necessary airway skills in case of deterioration in transit.

A discussion of the details of neurointensive care in severe intracranial injury in childhood is beyond the scope of this chapter. Raised intracranial pressure (ICP) is a common problem in such children whether or not they have a mass lesion, and control includes several components.

- Establish controlled ventilation (partial pressure of CO_2 35–40 mmHg; normocarbia).
- Elevate head of bed 30–45° and minimize stimuli such as suctioning.
- Ensure head and neck in midline position.
- Restrict fluids to 60 per cent of normal intake (except in circulatory failure).
- Prescribe diuretics (mannitol, 0.5–1 g/kg IV, or frusemide (furosemide), 1–2 mg/kg IV) in cases of documented deterioration despite above measures.

KEY LEARNING POINTS

- Head injury is a significant cause of death and long-term morbidity in children but most children with minor head injuries are at low risk of traumatic brain injury.
- Careful history and examination guides the need for imaging and observation.
- Young children pose particular problems in evaluation – have a low threshold for admission for observation.
- The carers of discharged children need clear written guidance on home observation and actions if concerned.

Sudden unexpected death in infancy

One baby in every 1500 live births dies suddenly and unexpectedly between the ages of 1 week and 2 years. There are about 350 of these deaths each year in the UK, accounting for half of all deaths in this age group. Babies die unexpectedly for many reasons. Autopsy may reveal an unsuspected abnormality or a severe disease such as meningitis, and with evolving pathological and laboratory techniques other causes are increasingly recognized. In most cases, however, the cause of death remains unexplained and these are attributed to sudden infant death syndrome (SIDS). Several risk factors for SIDS are recognized, including prone sleep position (the basis for the 'Back to Sleep' campaign), parental smoking, and bed sharing. Post-mortem evidence of minor infection, which probably contributed to death, is sometimes found and may be mentioned as the registered cause of death with SIDS as an associated cause. In others nothing significant

CASE STUDY

A 5-month-old infant is brought to A&E by emergency ambulance. He was reported to have taken a normal feed around 10 pm and was settled in his cot by his mother. The mother awoke at 7 am and thought it strange that he had not woken for a feed earlier. She found him pale and unresponsive in the cot and ran with him to a neighbour next door, who was a nurse. She began CPR and an ambulance was called. On arrival he was pale, lifeless and in asystole. Resuscitation was continued but he did not respond to intubation, ventilation and endotracheal adrenaline. Post-mortem livido was evident. Resuscitation was abandoned after 10 minutes.

is found. Sudden infant death syndrome is now accepted as a natural cause of death that can be registered.

Typically, an apparently normal baby, perhaps with trivial symptoms of illness, is put to rest and found dead sometime later. Sudden infant death syndrome deaths are commoner in the winter months, among boys and babies of low birth weight, with a peak incidence at 2–5 months of age. Associated socioeconomic disadvantage is a common feature. Specific mechanisms remain unclear.

Initial assessment of the infant presenting unexpectedly dead or moribund to A&E

Most sudden unexpected deaths in infancy (SUDI) are natural tragedies, but a minority result from ignorance, neglect or abuse. Recently, a multidisciplinary working party of the Royal College of Paediatrics and Child Health and the Royal College of Pathologists have developed a detailed multiagency protocol for the care and investigation after the sudden unexpected death of an infant or child – the Kennedy Report. This provides a framework for the investigation and care of families after all unexpected deaths in infants and children up to the age of 2 years.

The success of the 'Back to Sleep' campaign to reduce the risk of SIDS means that there have been marked changes in the socioeconomic distribution of SUDI, with proportionately far more deaths occurring in the most deprived families, often single mothers without immediate family support. For such isolated and vulnerable parents immediate skilled professional support is likely to be particularly helpful (see below).

The fall in numbers of SIDS also means that fewer healthcare professionals now have personal experience of dealing with such cases, of the needs of the families involved and the need to collect relevant information in such circumstances.

The immediate response

Almost all infants found apparently dead or collapsed will be brought immediately to an A&E department. The initial response must always be to continue or begin resuscitation, following the APLS protocol, until an experienced doctor (usually the consultant paediatrician on call) decides that further efforts are futile. Sometimes it is clear immediately on arrival that the infant has been dead for some time.

The care of the family and the investigation of the cause of the death should follow a similar process whether or not resuscitation has been attempted.

After death is confirmed

If resuscitation has been attempted, any IV and intra-arterial lines inserted for this reason should be removed (after carefully documenting for the pathologist all such sites of access). Other sites of attempted vascular access should also be carefully recorded. If an IV cannula has been inserted and it is thought that it may have contributed to failed resuscitation (e.g. by causing a pneumothorax), then it should not be removed. If an endotracheal tube has been inserted, this should also be removed after its correct placement in the trachea has been confirmed by direct laryngoscopy (preferably by someone other than the person who inserted it).

A consultant in paediatrics or accident and emergency medicine should carefully examine the infant as soon as possible after resuscitation has ceased. It is important to record any marks, abrasions, skin rashes, evidence of dehydration or identifiable injuries at this time. An enlarged liver should be checked for and noted. Any discoloration of the skin, particularly dependent livido should be precisely documented. Skin livido and pallor from local pressure (e.g. on the nose in a child who has been lying face down) may help in estimating the time of death, as well as the position in which the child was lying. It usually fades rapidly and may be absent when the pathologist sees the baby. Recording this using a police photographer should be considered if available. Frothy, bloodstained fluid is often evident around the nose and/or mouth on arrival, and its presence should be documented, although it does not indicate the cause or mode of death.

Any stool or urine passed by the infant, together with any gastric or nasopharyngeal aspirate obtained should be carefully labelled and frozen after samples have been sent for bacterial culture and for virology. If the nappy is wet or soiled it should be removed, labelled and frozen also.

During resuscitation, various samples may have been taken, including blood samples for blood gases, urea and electrolytes, full blood count, blood sugar and blood culture. Blood and, if possible, urine samples should also be taken at this time for metabolic investigations. If resuscitation is not initiated, then in most cases such investigations should be taken as soon as possible after the arrival of the infant. A lumbar puncture should also be performed and a sample of cerebrospinal fluid sent for microscopic examination and culture. If possible, a further sample of cerebrospinal fluid should also be frozen for future metabolic investigation.

Remember: once death has been declared the coroner (or Procurator Fiscal in Scotland) assumes immediate responsibility for the body and no further samples for investigation may be taken without his or her permission. However, in many parts of UK, there is a clear understanding with the coroner that certain samples may be taken immediately after the end of resuscitation in order to support appropriate investigation and in particular to identify the presence of metabolic conditions, increasingly recognized as causes of unexpected death in infancy. Details of the recommended samples to be taken and the purposes for which they are intended are given in Table 4.4.

It may be difficult to obtain blood samples from an infant after death. In general samples should not be taken by cardiac puncture since this may damage intrathoracic structures and confuse the interpretation of findings at autopsy. If the autopsy is to be conducted within 24 hours, it may be more appropriate for the pathologist to take most of the blood samples at the beginning of the procedure. Some additional samples may be taken after discussion with senior staff if the post-mortem examination is to be delayed by more than 24 hours.

- Liver biopsy – frozen section for fat – if history suggestive of metabolic disorder and liver enlarged.
- Skin biopsy for fibroblast culture.
- Muscle biopsy – if history suggestive of mitochondrial disorder.

Details are likely to vary in different hospitals, so it is important to be aware of local arrangements.

Care of the parents after the loss of a child

This process should be followed initially whenever any critically ill child is admitted. Immediately on arrival at the hospital, the parents should be allocated a member of staff to care for them, to explain what is happening, help them to contact friends, other family members and cultural or religious support. This staff member should ensure that the family are kept fully informed during any resuscitation and, with the approval of the medical staff involved, the parents should be given the option to be present during the resuscitation and treatment. The allocated member of staff should stay with the parents throughout this period to explain what is going on, especially the procedures which may look alarming, such as cutting off

Table 4.4 Routine samples to be taken immediately after sudden unexpected deaths in infancy

Sample	Send to	Handling	Test
Blood (serum) 0.5 mL	Clinical chemistry	Normal	Urea and electrolytes
Blood (serum) 1 mL	Clinical chemistry	Spin, store serum at −20°C	Toxicology
Blood (lithium heparin) 1 mL	Clinical chemistry	Spin, store plasma at −20°C	Inherited metabolic diseases
Blood (fluoride) 1 mL	Clinical chemistry	Spin, store plasma at −20°C	3-hydroxy butyrate, sugar, free fatty acids, lactate
Blood (EDTA) 0.5 mL	Haematology	Normal	Full blood count
Blood cultures: aerobic and anaerobic 1 mL	Microbiology	If insufficient blood, aerobic only	Culture and sensitivity
Blood: syringe to completed Guthrie card	Clinical chemistry	Normal (do not put into plastic bag)	Inherited metabolic diseases
Blood (lithium heparin) 5 mL	Cytogenetics	Normal (keep unseparated)	Chromosomes (if dysmorphic)
CSF (a few drops)	Microbiology	Normal	Microscopy, culture and sensitivity
CSF 0.5 mL	Clinical chemistry	Store at −20°C	Inherited metabolic diseases
Swabs from any identifiable lesions	Microbiology	Normal	Culture and sensitivity
Urine (if available)	Clinical chemistry	Spin, store supernatant at −20°C	Toxicology, inherited metabolic diseases
Urine (few drops)	Microbiology	Normal	Microscopic examination, culture and sensitivity

CSF, cerebrospinal fluid.

clothing, attempts at vascular access including the use of intraosseous needles or intubation.

Staff will need to make an assessment of the capacity of the parents to engage in the processes unfolding around them. For some the shock of the situation will inhibit their understanding, and for others there may be issues of language, health or mental capacity that need to be taken into account.

Immediate responsibility for providing information and coordinating appropriate care and support to the family should rest with the paediatric team on call (almost always led by the consultant paediatrician on call). Although senior staff from the disciplines of emergency medicine and/or intensive care may have been involved in the resuscitation, it is generally more appropriate that the consultant paediatrician on call takes responsibility for the continuing pastoral care of the family and liaising with the primary care team or other agencies.

The consultant paediatrician on call should, as part of the initial assessment, take a detailed and careful history of events leading up to and following the discovery of the infant's collapse. This requires sensitivity and time. A checklist of the relevant information to be obtained is available from the original SUDI protocol document. As far as possible the parents' or carers' account of events should be recorded verbatim. At an early stage of the process the paediatrician on call should make contact with the paediatrician with designated responsibility for SUDI locally and agree precise arrangements and timing for the SUDI paediatrician to meet the family. Whenever possible this should be before the family leave the A&E department.

The parents and other close relatives should normally be given the opportunity to hold and spend time with their baby. Such quiet time is very important for families and professional presence at such times should be discreet. Many parents value photographs of their baby taken at this time, along with hand or footprints and a lock of hair. Only in very exceptional circumstances should such mementos not be taken.

When the baby has been pronounced dead, the consultant paediatrician on call should break the news to the parents, having first reviewed all the available information. This interview should be in the privacy of an appropriate room. The member of staff allocated to care for the family should also be present. The family must also be informed at this time that because the baby has died suddenly and unexpectedly the coroner or Procurator Fiscal must be informed and that, as a matter of routine practice, the police also have to investigate the death. The paediatrician must explain that possible medical causes of the infant's death will also be very carefully and thoroughly sought.

Unless the cause of death is immediately apparent to the paediatrician (e.g. the typical rash of meningococcal septicaemia), it is important to explain to the parents that the cause of the death is not yet known, and that the aim of the investigation is to establish the cause of death. If the cause of death is unclear, however, it is also inappropriate to tell them the cause is SIDS. That label must only be applied after subsequent investigations have been completed. The parents must be informed that the coroner will order an autopsy examination and that a pathologist with special expertise in diseases of children will carry this out. This may require transport of the child some distance from home, but arrangements will be made for the child to be returned to the local hospital or funeral director as soon as possible. The nature and purpose of the post mortem should be explained to the parents in understandable terms and they should be given a copy of the NHS leaflet on the post-mortem examination ordered by the coroner or Fiscal. It is important that the family know where the post mortem will be carried out, what will be the approximate timescale, and when they will be able to see their child again.

If the mother is breast-feeding, she will need advice on suppression of lactation. Sometimes parents will be immediately very anxious about risks to surviving siblings. It is certainly reasonable to offer admission and observation for a surviving co-twin of the dead infant.

Apparent life-threatening events

An apparent life-threatening event (ALTE) occurs in around 1 in 50 healthy infants, often around 2 months of age. These are frightening events for families, and usually involve a combination of apnoea (central or obstructive), colour change (pallor or cyanosis), alteration in muscle tone (usually floppiness) and choking or gagging. ALTE is a symptom complex that needs careful evaluation rather than a final diagnosis. At least half of such infants have no specific findings on clinical examination and despite various investigations the episode remains unexplained. Some may reflect parental misinterpretation of physiological events such as periodic breathing.

The infant's birth and medical history may give useful clues. For example, recent pertussis immunization might suggest a vaccine-related hypotonic hyporesponsive episode. A detailed review of the event should include whether or not the infant was awake or asleep, the position, when they were last fed and any preceding regurgitation or cough. The duration, associated colour change, breathing difficulties or apnoea and unusual movements, and any resuscitation manoeuvres should all be recorded.

Where an underlying cause is defined, it is usually attributed to infection, especially serious bacterial sepsis, pertussis, respiratory syncytial virus (RSV) (up to 40 per cent in the appropriate season), and, rarely, underlying cardiac or neurological disease. Many infants have their events explained by gastro-oesophageal reflux (GOR) but a causal association is often uncertain.

It is often difficult to decide how aggressive the investigation should be, especially in a well-looking infant without any significant medical history or symptoms suggestive of acute or chronic disease. Infants with no previous history of similar episodes, transient self-limiting symptoms and who are clinically well on assessment are at low risk and do not justify aggressive investigation. Those with transient self-limiting choking or gagging episodes associated with feeding need simple parental reassurance. Even if well, most others justify at least a period of observation and some simple screening tests that would probably include a period of cardiorespiratory monitoring, FBC, plasma glucose, capillary blood gases for acidosis, urine culture and ECG (to exclude arrhythmia or conduction disorder).

Given the level of parental anxiety such events generate, it is reasonable to offer all parents and carers training in infant resuscitation before discharge. This should at least improve their confidence about going home.

Those who present later in infancy, have a previous or family history of similar events or SIDS, who needed resuscitation, who appeared unwell on arrival or are febrile need much more aggressive investigation and observation.

ALTE and SIDS

Previously, such events were often labelled 'near-miss cot deaths' but the relation between ALTE and SIDS is unconvincing and this expression has been abandoned. Experience suggests that the overall risk for subsequent death among infants experiencing an ALTE is 1–2 per cent, similar to the normal population. This risk doubles in infants whose ALTE is linked with RSV infection and is even higher if the ALTE occurred during sleep or if they needed resuscitation or vigorous stimulation. However, only 5 per cent of SIDS infants have a previous history of an ALTE. Neither home apnoea monitoring nor any other intervention after ALTE has influenced the incidence of SIDS.

KEY LEARNING POINTS

- Resuscitation should begin on any child brought to A&E apparently dead, unless it is explicitly clear that this is inappropriate.
- Once declared dead, the most senior paediatrician available should discuss the situation with the parents and coordinate investigations with other agencies.
- Ensure you are fully familiar with local protocols for such a situation.
- ALTE events cause great carer concern; a period of observation helps diffuse anxiety.
- Detailed clinical evaluation and judicious investigation should detect any underlying causes.

REFERENCES

National Institute for Clinical Excellence (NICE) (2003) *Clinical Guideline 4. Head injury. Triage, assessment, investigation and early management of head injury in infants, children and adults.* London: NICE. Available at www.nice.org.uk/pdf/cg4niceguideline.pdf (accessed 26 October 2004).

Phillips B, Mackway-Jones K, Wieteska S, eds. (2004) *Advanced Paediatric Life Support: The Practical Approach*, 4th edn. London: BMJ Books.

Royal College of Paediatrics and Child Health (2002) *Fabricated or Induced illness by Carers.* Report of the Working Party of the Royal College of Paediatrics and Child Health. London: RCPCH.

Royal College of Paediatrics and Child Health (2003) *Medicines for Children.* London: RCPCH and the Neonatal and Paediatric Pharmacists Group.

Scottish Intercollegiate Guidelines Network (SIGN) (2000) *Early Management of Patients with a Head Injury.* Summary of Paediatric Practice Points. SIGN Publication no 46. Edinburgh: SIGN Executive. Available at www.sign.ac.uk/guidelines/fulltext/46/paediatric.html (accessed 26 October 2004).

Chapter 5

Fetal and neonatal medicine

J Coutts, JH Simpson and AM Heuchan

INTRODUCTION: BASIC DEMOGRAPHICS

Over the past half century, neonatal mortality (death in the first 28 days) has almost halved from around 15 per 1000 to 7 per 1000 live births. This is mainly due to improvements in maternal health and obstetric care, although advances in neonatal intensive care have contributed. Mortality in the most immature neonates remains high. The EPICure study examined outcome in all live births <26 weeks' gestation in the UK and Ireland in 1995. This demonstrated overall survival of 6, 26 and 43 per cent in infants of <23, 24 and 25 weeks, respectively. The Confidential Enquiry into Stillbirths and Deaths in Infancy (CESDI) was established in 1992 to collect information on all late fetal losses (>20 weeks), stillbirths and infant deaths in England, Wales and Northern Ireland. This information is analysed regularly to try to establish ways in which these deaths might be prevented. CESDI project 27/28 reported patterns of practice or service provision that might have contributed to the deaths of premature babies at 27–28 weeks' gestation over the period 1998–2000. This report recommended a number of changes for future practice including improved communication, documentation and staff training.

THE PLACENTA AND FETUS: PHYSIOLOGY, GROWTH AND MONITORING DURING PREGNANCY

Placenta

Growth of the fetus is dependent on placental function. Most placental growth occurs in early pregnancy when its rate of growth exceeds that of the fetus. Placental development begins one week after conception, when the developing blastocyst sinks into the endometrial lining. The outer layer, the syncytiotrophoblast, invades the endometrium as villous processes. These are bathed by maternal blood and nutrients are transferred into the villous trophoblast. Extravillous trophoblasts then migrate into the myometrial arteries. They replace the arterial endothelium and smooth muscle coat transforming them into dilated thin-walled vessels known as the uteroplacental vessels.

The ability of the placenta to invade the decidua and the myometrium depends on some unique immunological features. Villous trophoblasts do not exert human leucocyte antigen (HLA) class I or class II surface antigens and are immunologically inert. Extravillous trophoblasts exhibit unusual HLA class antigens, which are not recognized by T cells. Additionally, the decidua contains few T cells and virtually no B cells, limiting the possibility of the production of trophoblast antibodies.

Uteroplacental vascular remodelling continues until mid-trimester and effects a marked decrease in resistance to blood flowing into the uteroplacental vessels. This process is essential to the development of a healthy fetal–placenta unit and is adversely affected by maternal smoking. Failure of placental growth and trophoblast invasion of the uterine arteries underlie many cases of intrauterine growth retardation (IUGR) and the hypertensive disorders of later pregnancy.

KEY LEARNING POINTS

- Placental growth is most rapid in the first trimester.
- Myometrial arteries are extensively remodelled during placentation.
- IUGR and hypertensive disorders of pregnancy are associated with abnormal placental development.

Embryonic development

Following implantation of the blastocyst there is an intense period of cellular differentiation (weeks 3–8 *in utero*) during which the skeletal system, facial structures and organs are formed. Interruption of normal embryogenesis may result in major and minor abnormalities. The aetiology is poorly understood but is associated with, genetic factors, increasing maternal age, maternal diabetes and teratogen exposure. Genetic factors may be polygenic, reflect single chromosomal abnormalities or aneuploidies. Epidemiological studies suggest that many common defects such as congenital heart disease, cleft lip and neural tube defect have multifactorial modes of inheritance and can be influenced by environmental factors such as folic acid consumption. Preconceptual supplementation of 0.4 mg/day can reduce neural tube defects two- to five-fold. Doses of 4 mg/day are recommended in high-risk situations.

Autosomal aneuploidies not only cause major congenital malformations but also result in early fetal loss (70–90 per cent) in the first trimester. Teratogen exposure may cause 7 per cent of all abnormalities. Maximum teratogen damage occurs in the early embryonic phase and preconception counselling is important. The most common teratogens are listed in Table 5.1.

Fetal development

After 12 weeks the fetus grows rapidly. Length increases steadily with gestation but organ weight increases most rapidly in the third trimester. Growth is dependent on maternal nutrition, placental function and the oxygen transferring capacity of fetal haemoglobin (Hb F). Fetal haemoglobin ($p50 = 19$ mmHg) aids the transport of oxygen across the placental villi into the placental circulation. Blood from the umbilical vein crosses the ductus venosus to the inferior vena cava and the right atrium. Oxygenated blood is directed via the foramen ovale or the arterial duct to the arch of the aorta with little blood passing through the pulmonary vasculature. The steep slope of the oxyhaemoglobin dissociation curve of Hb F facilitates oxygen release to the hypoxic fetal tissues. When fetal demands cannot be met by the placenta, growth restriction may follow. The commonest causes of growth failure are maternal smoking and pregnancy-induced hypertension which are associated with abnormal placental vasculature. The most severe cases result in severe growth failure, fetal cardiac decompensation and fetal death. Abnormal fundal height may be the first indication of a fetal problem. Table 5.2 lists some causes of abnormal fundal height patterns.

Despite the rapid growth and maturation of organs in the second and third trimesters the only major structural changes are the return of the physiologically herniated midgut to the abdominal cavity by week 12 and the descent of the testes to an extra abdominal position. However, temporary interruption in the vascular supply to an organ may contribute to developmental anomalies such

Table 5.1 Classification of teratogens

Infectious agents	Drugs	Physical
Rubella	Thalidomide	Radiation
Cytomegalovirus	Warfarin	Heavy metals
Herpes simplex virus	Ethanol	
Toxoplasmosis	Retinoic acid	
Varicella zoster	Cocaine	
Syphilis	Valproic acid*	
	Immunosuppressants†	

*Sodium valproate is no longer recommended for use in epilepsy in women of childbearing age but if necessary high-dose folic acid supplementation is recommended preconception.

†Many are safe in pregnancy but there are only limited data on newer agents. Recent data should always be checked. Suggested source: www.perinatology.com/exposures/druglist.htm

Table 5.2 Causes of abnormal fundal height presentation

Abnormality	Diagnosis
Small for gestational age	Constitutional Maternal cigarette smoking Uteroplacental dysfunction Chromosomal abnormality Structural malformation Congenital infection
Large for gestational age	Constitutional Macrosomic infant of a diabetic mother Fetal hydrops
Polyhydramnios	Fetal hydrops Renal dysfunction Oesophageal atresia Neuromuscular abnormality
Oligohydramnios	Prolonged rupture of the membranes Placental dysfunction Renal dysfunction/agenesis Posterior urethral valves

as bowel atresia or cystic brain lesions. Environmental abnormalities such as amniotic bands can cause major limb defects, and oligohydramnios before the third trimester will cause severe pulmonary hypoplasia. Fetal organ failure may result in fetal compromise but placental function often maintains fetal viability. Rarely severe cardiovascular decompensation results in fetal hydrops. Conversely, many deaths *in utero* have occurred in apparently normal fetuses. The majority remain unexplained but are thought to be due to disruptions of the fetal placental circulation. Possible causes of fetal compromise, presentation and investigation are outlined in Table 5.3.

Organ maturation is essential if the fetus is to adapt to the extrauterine environment and is usually achieved by the 37th postconceptual week. Adequate surfactant production, gut maturation and coordinated neurological responses such as sustained breathing, sucking and swallowing are essential.

The normal onset of labour from 37 to 41 weeks is in part a response to fetal catecholamines and steroids produced when the uterine environment can no longer sustain fetal demands. These agents also enhance surfactant production and fetal lung maturation. Administration of maternal glucocorticoids prior to premature delivery promotes

Table 5.3 Possible causes and investigations of fetal compromise

Aetiology	Clinical presentation	Investigation
Placental insufficiency		
Idiopathic	PIH	Ultrasound
Abnormal placental development	Small for dates	Serial fetal growth measurements
Maternal smoking	Fetal distress	Umbilical Doppler ultrasound
Chronic maternal disease	Meconium stained liquor	Maternal (PIH, chronic disease)
	Death *in utero*	Placental pathology (postnatal)
Interrupted fetal circulation		
Placental abruption	Abdominal pain	Fetal ultrasound
Umbilical cord compromise	APH	Kleihauer test
prolapse	Reduced fetal movement	Vaginal examination for cord prolapse
knots	Fetal distress	Placental and cord pathology
entanglement	Meconium stained liquor	
rupture	Death *in utero*	
Fetal maternal haemorrhage		
Massive maternal haemorrhage		
Ruptured vasa previa		
Hydrops fetalis		
Immune hydrops	Polyhydramnios	Maternal blood
Congenital infection	Fetal cardiac arrhythmia	Gp/AB titres/serology
Fetal heart block/arrhythmais	Maternal mirror syndrome	Fetal blood sampling
Twin to twin transfusion	Dealth *in utero*	FBC/blood group
Structural cardiac malformation		PCR/serology
Arterio-venous malformations		Acid/base
Hydrothorax		Karyotype/cytogenetics
Cystic lung malformation		Fetal heart rate
Chorioangioma		Fetal anomaly scan
Metabolic disease		Serial ultrasound monitoring
Aneuploidy		
Abnormal uterine environment		
Structural uterine abnormalities	Fundal height	Ultrasound
Oligohydramnios/polyhydramnios	PPROM	Vaginal examination
Multiple pregnancy	Maternal fever	Maternal infection markers
Chorioamnionitis	Abdominal pain	
Uterine rupture		

APH, antepartum haemorrhage; CRP, C-reactive protein; FBC, full blood count; IUGR, intrauterine growth retardation; PCR, polymerase chain reaction; PIH, pregnancy-induced hypertension; PPROM, preterm premature rupture of membranes.

lung maturation and significantly reduces RDS, IVH and perinatal mortality.

Labour is less likely to be well tolerated by the IUGR fetus with increased rates of fetal distress, meconium staining of the liquor and perinatal mortality and morbidity.

KEY LEARNING POINTS

- Maximum effect of teratogens is in weeks 3–8 of embryonic life.
- Preconceptual folic acid reduces the risk of neural tube defects.
- Most major structural abnormalities can be detected by ultrasound at 16–18 weeks' gestation.
- Maternal smoking is strongly associated with IUGR.
- Many cases of sudden death *in utero* remain unexplained.
- Maternal glucocorticoids significantly reduce mortality and morbidity in infants delivered prematurely.

Monitoring in pregnancy

The emphasis of current antenatal care is to identify the fetus with significant congenital abnormalities and the fetus at risk of death or intrapartum morbidity.

Routine assessment

The following methods of screening are employed in early pregnancy:

- Dating scan at 8–12 weeks (important when estimating later fetal growth)
- Maternal blood group, antibody titres and serology for syphilis, rubella, hepatitis B and HIV. Hepatitis C screening is offered to all at-risk women.
- Multiple serum screening: Maternal serum α-fetoprotein (AFP) and β-human chorionic gonadotrophin (βHCG) routinely offered in all Scottish centres at 16–18 weeks to screen for spina bifida and trisomy 21 respectively. Interpretation of results depends on gestation and maternal age. Ultrasound and/or amniocentesis should be offered if results are abnormal.
- Combined ultrasound (nuchal translucency measurements) and biochemical screening (βHCG and PAPP-A) (CUB screening) between 11 and 14 weeks detects trisomy 21 with much greater sensitivity than serum βHCG alone at 16–18 weeks. This has replaced biochemical screening alone for trisomy 21 in certain centres but is not yet universally available.
- Chorionic villus sampling (CVS) is available until 15 weeks of pregnancy. This provides DNA for molecular analysis and early karyotype results when there is a high risk of chromosomal or genetic abnormality.
- Amniocentesis for fetal chromosomal analysis is available if indicated from 15 weeks of pregnancy.
- Detailed anomaly scans are ideally performed between 16 and 18 weeks and can detect most major fetal malformations. These are routinely offered in some centres but only in high-risk pregnancies in many UK centres.

Monitoring of the uncomplicated pregnancy during the second and third trimesters is based on clinical assessment of fundal height and maternal screening for gestational diabetes and pregnancy-induced hypertension.

When the pregnancy is complicated at any stage a detailed fetal medicine assessment is required.

Fetal medicine assessment

- *Ultrasound*
  Detailed anomaly scanning is optimal at 16–18 weeks but can be performed later. Fetal growth can be assessed by taking standardized measurements of the head and the abdominal circumference which are compared with standard reference charts. Liquor volume can be assessed by measurement of the deepest pool or other indexes of liquor volume.
- *Doppler ultrasound*
  Umbilical artery Doppler studies can contribute to the assessment of fetal wellbeing. A fall in umbilical/artery end diastolic velocity suggests increased resistance to perfusion. These changes are consistent with impaired placental function and possible fetal hypoxia. Reversed end diastolic umbilical flow is abnormal and has been associated with fetal demise and increased rates of postnatal necrotizing enterocolitis.

  Middle cerebral artery (MCA) Doppler studies may detect falling MCA resistance. This may reflect brain sparing redistribution of blood flow in the hypoxic fetus. Umbilical vein Doppler studies can detect abnormal flow indicative of cardiac decompensation in the extremely compromised fetus.
- *Antenatal cardiotocograph (CTG)*
  CTG changes consistent with chronic placental failure have been recognized and may allow delivery

of the IUGR infant before decompensation into acidaemia occurs.

- *Biophysical profiles*
  Cardiotocograph plus ultrasound measurements of fetal breathing, movement, tone and amniotic fluid volumes in the high-risk pregnancy are useful for predicting fetal distress in labour.
- *Fetal blood sampling*
  This is possible from 20 weeks and can provide information on fetal serology and viral load by polymerase chain reaction (PCR), blood group, haematocrit, platelets, biochemistry, acid/base balance and cytogenetics.

Fetal medicine assessment may result in therapeutic fetal intervention, decisions to deliver prematurely, decisions on the mode of delivery and possibly the need for delivery in a specialist centre. Whenever premature delivery is anticipated maternal glucocorticoids should be administered.

KEY LEARNING POINTS

- Detailed anomaly scans and CUB screening are not yet routinely offered as antenatal screening in many parts of the UK.
- Optimal management of the compromised fetus requires communication between obstetricians and neonatologists.
- Antenatal maternal glucocorticoids should be administered if premature delivery is anticipated.

Monitoring in labour

Monitoring in labour remains a controversial area. The fetus responds to hypoxia produced by uterine contractions by transient changes in the fetal heart rate. Continuous CTG monitoring may reveal abnormal responses such as loss of baseline variability, abnormal heart rates and late decelerations in response to contractions. Evidence suggests that intervention based on these changes may improve outcome in the high-risk pregnancy or where there is other evidence of fetal distress, e.g. meconium-stained liquor. However, there is no evidence that routine CTG monitoring reduces adverse outcome in uncomplicated pregnancies and labour. Current monitoring techniques in regular use during labour include:

- *Fetal heart rate monitoring*
  - Intermittent only – appropriate for low-risk pregnancies.
  - Continuous as CTG – may be difficult to interpret and should be focused on high-risk pregnancies. May reduce adverse outcomes in high-risk deliveries (IUGR, meconium-stained liquor) but is not of proven benefit in the uncomplicated pregnancy. Certain CTG patterns such as progressive bradycardia and sinusoidal traces are particularly ominous.
- *Fetal scalp blood sampling*
  This may provide useful additional information if other assessments raise concerns.
  - A scalp pH of <7.2 is generally an indication for urgent delivery.

Any decisions regarding intervention should only be made after consideration of other risk factors and progress in labour.

CARE OF THE NEONATE: GENERAL PRINCIPLES

Temperature regulation

Maintenance of normal temperature is an important aspect of neonatal care. Hypothermia is associated with several problems including increased oxygen requirements, decreased surfactant production and reduced survival. Neonates should be nursed in an environmental temperature that maintains their intrinsic heat production at a minimum and at which their temperature is normal. This is known as a neonate's thermoneutral environment and it varies with gestation, weight, postnatal age and environment (e.g. under a radiant heater versus in a double-walled incubator).

Heat loss occurs mainly as a result of convection, evaporation and radiation, with minimal loss via conduction. Convection is influenced by the temperature difference between the neonate and the surrounding air. It is an important source of heat loss due to the large surface area to volume ratio of a neonate and can be minimized by the use of incubators and the avoidance of drafts. Radiant heat loss depends on the difference in temperature between the neonate and the surrounding surfaces. It can be minimized by the use of double-walled incubators and the maintenance of a high temperature within the neonatal unit. Evaporation is predominantly a problem in premature infants who have high transepidermal water losses through their poorly keratinized skin, although the use of overhead radiant warmers and phototherapy can increase evaporative heat loss in any infant. Drying all neonates at delivery and the routine use of humidification in those <1000 g effectively reduce evaporative heat loss. Conduction depends on the difference between the infant and objects he or she is in contact with and the conductance of those objects.

Fluid and electrolyte balance

Water

In a term neonate water comprises 80 per cent of body weight; this is even greater in premature infants. Following delivery increased renal perfusion and glomerular filtration rate (GFR; see Chapter 12) produce diuresis, with reduction in total body water and weight loss of around 5 per cent. Water loss also occurs via transepidermal evaporative loss, via the respiratory tract and in gastrointestinal fluids. In healthy term neonates water intake increases gradually to around 150 mL/kg by day 5. Fluid management in unwell or premature infants varies considerably between neonatal units but can generally be guided on an individual basis by assessing weight, urine output, insensible and measured fluid losses and plasma electrolytes.

Sodium

Renal tubular function and therefore sodium homoeostasis are influenced by gestational age (see Chapter 12). Hyponatraemia, plasma sodium of $<$130 mmol/L, can occur as a result of water overload, sodium loss or inadequate sodium intake (Table 5.4). Treatment involves fluid restriction, sodium replacement or a combination of both based on the underlying cause. Hypernatraemia, plasma sodium of $>$145 mmol/L, can occur as a result of water loss or sodium excess (Table 5.4). Treatment involves cautious rehydration or sodium restriction depending on the underlying cause.

Potassium

The causes of hypokalaemia, plasma potassium $<$3.0 mmol/L, and hyperkalaemia, plasma potassium of $>$7.0 mmol/L, are listed in Table 5.4. Treatment of hypokalaemia involves increased potassium intake and treatment of hyperkalaemia, especially if life threatening, includes calcium infusion, sodium bicarbonate, intravenous (IV) salbutamol or glucose/insulin infusion.

Acid–base balance

The kidney and lungs maintain neonatal acid–base homoeostasis (see Chapter 12). Acidosis may be respiratory, metabolic or a mixture of both. Neonates with chronic lung disease often retain carbon dioxide, which in turn produces carbonic acid. This can be compensated for over a period of days by an increase in renal hydrogen ion excretion and bicarbonate regeneration. A metabolic acidosis occurs due to an increase in acid (most commonly lactic acid due to tissue hypoxia) or a reduction in base. In a neonate with normal lungs this may stimulate increased carbon dioxide elimination via hyperventilation.

Drug therapy

Neonatal pharmacokinetics differs from those of older infants and children. Apparent volumes of distribution are increased, particularly in the premature neonate, and larger weight-related drug doses are required to achieve therapeutic drug levels. Lower availability of plasma protein binding results in an increased free fraction of drug in neonates compared with older children. This free fraction may lead to greater pharmacological activity at lower total plasma levels. Drug level monitoring may help to guide treatment, especially in drugs with a narrow therapeutic index.

Neonates may be exposed to drugs via maternal breast milk, although very few drugs are contraindicated in breast-feeding mothers. If doubt exists, advice should be

Table 5.4 Causes of electrolyte imbalance

Electrolyte abnormality	Cause
Hyponatraemia	Water overload (excess intravenous fluid, oliguric acute renal failure, inappropriate antidiuretic hormone) Sodium loss (renal loss in premature infants, bowel loss during obstruction) Inadequate sodium intake (inadequate intravenous sodium, unfortified breast milk or term formula in premature infants)
Hypernatraemia	Water loss (transepidermal, gastrointestinal, osmotic diuresis associated with glycosuria) Sodium excess (generally iatrogenic)
Hypokalaemia	Inadequate intravenous/enteral intake, gastrointestinal losses, diuretics, alkalosis (pushes potassium into cells)
Hyperkalaemia	Acute renal failure, acidosis (pushes potassium out of cells), congenital adrenal hyperplasia

sought from a paediatric clinical pharmacist or a drug information reference source.

Pain management

It is only within the past 15 years that pain and discomfort in the neonate have been seen as a priority. Before this, neonates were operated on with little or no anaesthesia and no analgesia in the belief that they differed from older children in their perception of pain. It is now well recognized that even premature neonates have similar behavioural, endocrine and metabolic responses to painful stimuli as older children. Intravenous opiates are the mainstay of pharmacological analgesia in the neonatal unit although non-pharmacological interventions, including oral glucose, are useful alternatives during minor procedures.

Care and support for parents

Modern neonatal care is designed to support the social and emotional needs of the parents as well as the physiological needs of the infant. A close parent–child relationship is encouraged from the outset and is facilitated by open-door visiting policies, parental involvement in neonatal care (such as nasogastric feeding) and availability of rooms for parents within the neonatal unit. Parental visiting may be difficult for financial reasons or due to issues regarding childcare of older siblings and social work input can be useful.

The birth of a premature or sick baby is often associated with grief and anxiety, and parents require adequate support and information. This involves regular updates, given in a clear and sensitive manner, on their baby's progress and prognosis. Many neonatal units now adopt a multidisciplinary approach involving psychologists, social workers, physiotherapists and speech therapists in addition to medical and nursing staff. This family-centred approach is useful in not only the neonatal unit but also following discharge, particularly if an infant is discharged on oxygen or requiring nasogastric tube feeding. The availability of a liaison neonatal nurse or midwife who can visit parents at home following discharge is particularly helpful not only for parental support but also to facilitate earlier discharge from hospital.

KEY LEARNING POINTS

- Maintenance of normal temperature is an important aspect of neonatal care.
- In a term neonate water comprises 80 per cent of body weight; this is even greater in premature neonates.
- Renal tubular function and therefore sodium homoeostasis is influenced by gestational age.
- Neonatal acid–base homoeostasis is maintained by the kidney and lungs.
- Neonatal pharmacokinetics differs from those of older infants and children.
- Neonates have similar behavioural, endocrine and metabolic responses to painful stimuli as older children.
- Modern neonatal care is designed to support the social and emotional needs of the parents.

ASSESSMENT OF THE NORMAL NEONATE

A detailed physical examination of every neonate is established as good practice and is required as part of the child health surveillance programme in the UK. This examination should be performed by an appropriately trained doctor or nurse, with recent evidence suggesting that specifically trained advanced neonatal nurse practitioners are more likely to identify an abnormality than inexperienced doctors. There is no optimal timing for this examination but it is generally carried out between six and 72 hours. Before beginning the examination, the family, maternal, pregnancy, fetal and birth histories should be reviewed and specific risk factors identified. These risk factors include, e.g. family history of deafness or developmental dysplasia of the hip, maternal history of diabetes or systemic lupus erythematosus (SLE), abnormal antenatal serum screening or ultrasound scans, shoulder dystocia or other difficulties at delivery. It is often worthwhile to start by identifying any parental concerns and the opportunity should be used to provide specific health education (e.g. sudden infant death syndrome) and parental reassurance.

The baby's colour, behaviour, posture and respiration should be observed prior to a hands-on structured systemic examination. Even the most detailed examination cannot exclude all abnormalities; however, particular attention should be given to examining the eyes, hips and cardiovascular system (see below and Table 5.5).

Eyes

Congenital cataract is the commonest form of preventable childhood blindness, and the red reflexes must be

Table 5.5 Some of the commoner abnormalities identifiable during the routine neonatal examination

System	Important clinical findings	Key investigations	Differential diagnoses
Skin (see Chapter 18)	Petechiae	Examine for signs of congenital infection, FBC (mum and baby)	Maternal ITP, NAIT, congenital infection, venous congestion associated with delivery
	Bruising	FBC and coagulation screen	Traumatic delivery, coagulopathy
Head and skull	Third fontanelle	Examine for associated dysmorphism, consider karyotype	Trisomy 21
	Ridged suture line	Skull radiograph	Craniosynostosis
	Scalp defect	Examine for associated dysmorphism, consider karyotype	Trisomy 15
	Small head (compared to parents)	Examine for associated dysmorphism, consider karyotype, investigation for congenital infection and cranial ultrasound	Syndrome, congenital infection, isolated abnormality
	Large head (compared to parents)	Examine for signs of hydrocephalus, cranial ultrasound	Syndrome, hydrocephalus, familial megalencephaly
Ears	Abnormal shape or position	Examine for associated dysmorphism	Syndrome
	Preauricular pits, skin tags or accessory auricles	Hearing screen	Can be associated with inner ear malformations. May be associated with renal tract abnormalities although the literature on this subject is conflicting.
Eyes (see Chapter 17)	Purulent discharge	Examine for associated conjunctival inflammation, routine eye swabs, consider gonococcal and chlamydial eye swabs	Infection with *Staph aureus*, *Strep pneumoniae* or Group B streptococcus Rarely can be due to *Neisseria gonorrhoeae* or *Chlamydia trachomatis*
Mouth (see Chapter 10)	Cleft palate	Examine for associated abnormalities, hearing screen	Isolated abnormality, syndrome
Neck	Short, webbed neck	Examine for associated dysmorphism, karyotype, cervical spine radiograph	Turner syndrome, abnormalities of cervical vertebrae (Klippel–Feil syndrome)
	Redundant skin	Examine for associated dysmorphism, karyotype	Trisomy 21
	Swelling	Investigations directed by examination findings	Cystic hygroma, sternomastoid tumours, goitre, subcutaneous fat necrosis
RS/CVS	Persistent tachypnoea (>60 breaths/minute)	Examine for murmurs, altered pulse volume, organomegaly, Chest radiograph, FBC, CRP, blood cultures, CBG and consider cardiology assessment	Infection, lung pathology (pneumothorax, congenital diaphragmatic hernia), cardiac disease, metabolic abnormality
	Weak/absent femoral pulses	Urgent cardiology assessment	Coarctation, interrupted aortic arch, LHHS

Abdomen (see Chapter 20)	Abdominal distension	Ask about vomiting, delayed passage of meconium, examine for signs of sepsis or abdominal obstruction, abdominal radiograph	Gut atresias, volvulus, meconium plug, Hirschsprung's disease, necrotizing enterocolitis, generalized infection
Genitalia (see Chapter 14)	Hydrocele	Reassure and follow up as an outpatient	
	Unilateral undescended testis	Reassure and follow up as an outpatient	
	Ambiguous genitalia	Karyotype, 17OH progesterone, urinary steroid profile, urinary sodium	Female virilization (congenital adrenal hyperplasia), Incomplete male virilization (testosterone deficiency, androgen insensitivity syndrome)
Spine	Midline swelling, dimple, hairy patch, naevus	Examine for associated neurological abnormality, spinal radiograph, consider spinal ultrasound/MRI	May be associated with underlying vertebral/spinal cord abnormality
	Sacrococcygeal dimples or pits		Usually no associated underlying abnormalities
Upper limbs	Absent/reduced movement	Examine for associated fracture (clavicle or humerus)	Fracture, brachial plexus injury
	Polydactyly/syndactyly	Examine for associated dysmorphism	Syndrome, isolated finding
Lower limbs	Puffy feet	Examine for associated dysmorphism, karyotype	Turner's syndrome
	Talipes	Examine whether this is fixed or correctable, assess hips	True talipes equinovarus (requires urgent orthopaedic review), positional talipes, generalised neuromuscular abnormality
	Abnormal shaped feet (rocker bottom)	Examine for associated dysmorphism, karyotype	Trisomy 18
CNS	Hypotonia	Examine for associated dysmorphism, evidence of neuromuscular abnormality, karyotype	Central (trisomy 21), neuromuscular disease
	Jittery	Blood glucose, calcium, magnesium	Normal, drug withdrawal, hypoglycaemia, hypocalcaemia, HIE

CBG, capillary blood gas; CRP, C-reactive protein; FBC, full blood count; HIE, hypoxic ischaemic encephalopathy; ITP, idiopathic thrombocytopenic purpura; LHHS, hypoplastic left heart syndrome; NAIT, neonatal alloimmune thrombocytopenia.

visualized. In some neonates this may be facilitated by holding the baby upright or the use of a mydriatic; however, if any uncertainty remains an urgent ophthalmological review is indicated.

Hips

Clinical outcomes for developmental dysplasia of the hip (DDH) improve with early detection and treatment. For this reason screening for DDH by clinical examination was introduced in the 1950s. Unfortunately, this did not reduce the incidence of late presentation of hip abnormalities and alternative screening programmes, using selective hip ultrasonography, are now recommended as best practice. Guidelines vary slightly according to local service provision but generally recommend hip ultrasonography for neonates with specific risk factors for DDH or an abnormal clinical examination. These risk factors include breech presentation, a family history of DDH and clinical deformities suggestive of intrauterine compression or oligohydramnios.

Cardiovascular system

Cardiac murmurs are relatively common following delivery; up to 60 per cent of neonates have a systolic murmur at 2 hours and the majority of these are innocent. Clinical features that support the diagnosis of an innocent murmur include: a grade 1–2/6 systolic murmur at the left sternal edge, no associated ejection clicks, normal pulses and an otherwise normal examination. Although recent research supports the early investigation of all babies with cardiac murmurs, preferably by echocardiogram, to clarify if there is a significant cardiac anomaly this may depend upon the expertise available locally. Examination by an experienced colleague, with prompt referral of suspicious murmurs, is an acceptable alternative. Parents should be reassured that 80–90 per cent of murmurs identified in the neonatal period will disappear within a year, the majority within three months, at which time the baby will be discharged from outpatient follow-up. It is very important to remember that the absence of a murmur does not exclude a cardiac anomaly.

The femoral pulses must be palpated. If they are absent or difficult to feel coarctation should be suspected. Four-limb blood pressure may demonstrate a differential between the upper and lower limbs but can also be normal and urgent cardiology assessment is required irrespective of blood pressure readings.

KEY LEARNING POINTS

- Detailed physical examination of every neonate is required as part of the child health surveillance programme in the UK.
- There is no optimal timing for this examination although it is generally undertaken between six and 72 hours.
- Particular attention should be given to the eyes, hips and femoral pulses.

EARLY POINTERS TOWARDS SIGNIFICANT ILLNESS

Neonatal jaundice

Jaundice is extremely common in the newborn and generally reflects immaturity of the liver's excretory pathways for bilirubin at a time of increased haem degradation. Two-thirds of healthy term neonates and almost all preterm neonates are affected.

Following delivery, haem is released in increased quantities from the destruction of erythrocytes. Production is increased in the neonate because of the short lifespan of the erythrocyte (70–90 versus 120 days in the adult), degradation of haematopoietic tissues which cease to function shortly after birth, and enhanced enterohepatic absorption. Haem is catabolized in two stages initially to the water-soluble product biliverdin and then to bilirubin. Bilirubin is not water-soluble and circulates bound to albumin in a molar ratio of 3:1. Carrier proteins assist in its transfer across the hepatocyte membrane where conjugation with glucuronic acid occurs in the smooth endoplasmic reticulum. The hepatic enzyme uridine diphosphate glucuronosyltransferase (UDPGT) catalyses conjugation. Levels of UDPGT are initially very low in the neonate although they increase rapidly over the first few days of life. This rate-limiting step is responsible for the vast majority of neonatal jaundice. Water-soluble conjugated bilirubin is then transported out of the hepatocyte into the biliary canaliculi and is excreted, predominantly in the diglucuronide form, as a component of bile.

Most neonatal jaundice is unconjugated and harmless but high serum levels of unconjugated bilirubin can be neurotoxic and result in kernicterus. Three phases of kernicterus have been described clinically:

- Phase 1 – this is marked by poor suck, hypotonia and lethargy. If treated these changes are transient.

- Phase 2 – fever, hypertonia and opisthotonus may be present.
- Phase 3 – this is marked by high-pitched cry and athetosis.

These changes may evolve over 24 hours. Long-term sequelae include choreoathetoid cerebral palsy, upward gaze palsy and sensorineural deafness. Cognitive impairment is unusual except in preterm survivors. Many factors contribute to the degree of neurotoxicity associated with a high serum bilirubin level. These include gestational age, pathological breakdown of erythrocytes, metabolic acidosis, low albumin levels and free fatty acids.

In the presence of hepatic cell injury and/or biliary obstruction, hepatic excretory transport is exceeded resulting in conjugated hyperbilirubinaemia. Causes of conjugated hyperbilirubinaemia are expanded on in Chapter 10 but biliary atresia must always be excluded.

KEY LEARNING POINTS

- Most neonatal jaundice is a physiological adaptive process.
- The main aim of early assessment is to identify neonates at risk of kernicterus.
- Prolonged jaundice needs to be carefully investigated to exclude extrahepatic obstruction, cholestasis and other disease processes.
- Term infants with peak serum bilirubin (SBR) >400 μmol/L should have early audiology review.

Measurement and imaging

NON-INVASIVE ASSESSMENT OF JAUNDICE

Visual assessment

Jaundice becomes apparent visually at SBR levels of 80–90 μmol/L. Clinical jaundice in the first 24 hours of life suggests a non-physiological cause. Visual assessment is unreliable under artificial light and, in particular, phototherapy lights. However, in term neonates, assessment by dermal zones (Kramer's) has been validated and is a useful screening test. Jaundice limited to the head and neck has an average value of 100 μmol/L, beyond the elbows and knees but not as far as the hands and feet an average value of 250 μmol/L and jaundice on the hands and feet 300 μmol/L.

Icterometer

This provides estimation of the bilirubin level by visual comparison with yellow coloured panels. This has been validated against serum levels in term neonates.

Transcutaneous bilirubinometry

This utilizes a handheld spectrophotometer and has a role in screening well term and near term neonates, provided a threshold is established beyond which formal serum bilirubin levels must be measured.

INVASIVE MEASUREMENTS

Serum bilirubin levels

Serum bilirubin levels are plotted against time on standard phototherapy charts, which reflect normal physiological trends. Phototherapy thresholds vary, but tend to be conservative with lower thresholds for the preterm infant.

Umbilical cord bilirubin levels

This is a useful investigation when there is an antenatal suspicion of isoimmunization. Cord full blood count (FBC), blood group and direct Coombs' test (DCT) may also be checked. In cases of previous intrauterine transfusion (IUT) these results may be misleading.

IMAGING

Ultrasound

This may be useful in the evaluation of cholestasis. The presence of a gall bladder is usually indicative of intrahepatic cholestasis but cannot reliably exclude biliary atresia.

HIDA (hydroxyiminodiacetic acid) scan

This compound is extracted by hepatocytes and excreted with bile into the intestine. A negative scan indicates biliary atresia. Pretreatment with phenobarbital for seven days promotes excretion and reduces the chance of mistaken diagnosis of extrahepatic biliary obstruction in neonates with severe cholestasis.

Clinical approach to the assessment of neonatal jaundice

The challenge is to identify those neonates with an abnormally rapid rise and abnormally high levels of serum bilirubin and those with features that suggest a pathological cause. This is done by identifying the at-risk neonates, clinical assessment and laboratory investigations (Tables 5.6 and 5.7).

Clinical features that suggest a pathological cause for jaundice in the newborn

- Early jaundice <24 hours
- Total serum bilirubin >250 μmol/L day 2
- Rapidly rising serum bilirubin >100 μmol/L/ 24 hours
- Prolonged jaundice (>14 days term babies; >21 days in preterm infants)

- Conjugated serum bilirubin >25 μmol/L
- Pale stools and dark urine
- Jaundice in a sick neonate

Management of neonatal jaundice

Phototherapy

Phototherapy detoxifies bilirubin and facilitates its excretion in an unconjugated form. Light energy causes three photochemical reactions:

- Photo-oxidation
- Configurational isomerization
- Structural isomerization.

Structural isomerization is now recognized to be the most important. This creates the structural isomer lumirubin, a stable molecule that is efficiently excreted in bile and urine.

Optimal phototherapy depends on the appropriate light wavelength, dose and exposure. Most lights produce mixed blue and white light with blue light at a wavelength of 450 nm, which is the maximal absorbance of bilirubin. There is a dose–response relation between energy output or spectral irradiance and the production of lumirubin, which is saturated at a spectral irradiance of 25–30 μW/cm^2/nm. The distance from the infant is inversely related to the effective spectral irradiance. Recently, lamps have been manufactured that produce blue/green light to maximize the production of lumirubin.

Phototherapy is generally well tolerated. Common side effects are skin rashes, fluid loss, poor temperature control. Potential serious adverse effects (DNA damage, retinal damage) remain unsubstantiated.

Table 5.6 Investigation of jaundice in the neonate

Early/onset jaundice (<24 hours)	Prolonged jaundice
Blood group and DCT Full blood count Blood film and reticulocytes Infection screen Serology for congenital infection Urine for cytomegalovirus Stool for virology Glucose 6-phosphate dehydrogenase screen Red cell enzyme assays	Total and conjugated bilirubin Thyroid function Urine culture Urine reducing substances α_1-Antitrypsin assay and phenotype Cystic fibrosis DNA screen Immunoreactive trypsinogen Plasma cortisol Serum amino acids

DCT, direct Coombs' test.

Exchange transfusion (indications and complications)

All neonatal units will have bilirubin charts with guidance for exchange transfusion and these should be used for reference. However, since the advent of *in utero* transfusions and phototherapy the indications for exchange transfusion in the management and prevention of severe hyperbilirubinaemia are less certain.

Suggested indications are:

- Cord Hb <10 g/dL at birth in the presence of haemolytic disease
- Clinical signs of hydrops at delivery
- Sick jaundiced infants
- Rapidly rising SBR despite phototherapy (>17 μmol/L per hour)
- SBR >400 μmol/L at 25–48 hours
- SBR >500 μmol/L at 49–72 hours.

Table 5.7 Pathological causes of jaundice in the neonate

Unconjugated	Conjugated
Haemolysis *Isoimmunization* e.g. Rhesus, ABO *Other* e.g. spherocytosis, glucose 6-phosphate dehydrogenase deficiency, pyruvate kinase deficiency, sepsis Polycythaemia e.g. small for dates, delayed cord clamping, infant of diabetic mother Extravasated blood	Intrauterine infections Bacterial sepsis Severe haemolysis Prolonged parenteral nutrition Biliary atresia Intrahepatic biliary hypoplasia α_1-Antitrypsin deficiency Cystic fibrosis Cryptogenic hepatitis Choledochal cyst

When indicated, exchange transfusion has the advantage of correcting anaemia, removing red cell antibodies and reducing levels of serum bilirubin.

Local protocols for exchange transfusion should be followed but a double volume transfusion (180 mL/kg) to maximize antibody removal is recommended. Potential problems include cardiac arrhythmia, hypocalcaemia, hypomagnesaemia and hypoglycaemia. Vital signs, electrocardiogram (ECG), biochemical and haematological monitoring are required throughout. Other complications include portal vein thrombosis, portal vein perforation, necrotizing enterocolitis and infection.

Other therapies

High-dose IV immunoglobulin in conjunction with phototherapy has been demonstrated to reduce the need for exchange transfusion in haemolytic disease of the newborn (HDN) in several randomized controlled trials. This approach has not been studied in the UK, which has a much lower rate of exchange transfusion than the study populations. Further research is required and at present, the use of high-dose IV immunoglobulin in the management of HDN is not routinely recommended.

The administration of IV albumin prior to exchange transfusion has been described. This may promote the transfer of bilirubin from the extravascular to the intravascular space to facilitate its removal. However, there is insufficient evidence to support its use at present.

Phenobarbital and other hepatic-enzyme-inducing agents can reduce serum unconjugated bilirubin levels. Phenobarbital has a role in the diagnosis and occasionally management of Crigler–Najjar syndrome.

Metalloporphyrins inhibit the activity of haem oxygenase and can reduce peak bilirubin levels in human neonates. However, further studies are required.

KEY LEARNING POINTS

- Phototherapy is the mainstay of the management of unconjugated hyperbilirubinaemia.
- Exchange transfusion requires careful monitoring but is usually well tolerated.
- The roles of albumin and immunoglobulin transfusions in the management of hyperbilirubinaemia have not been substantiated.

INFECTION IN THE NEONATE

Infection remains a significant cause of neonatal mortality and morbidity and should be considered in the differential diagnosis of any unwell baby. An inverse relation exists between birth weight and sepsis. Rates of culture-proven sepsis of up to 30 per cent, with similar mortality, are seen in neonates <1500 g.

There are a variety of reasons why neonates, particularly those <1500 g are at risk of infection. These include both impaired host defences, especially humoral and phagocytic, and environmental factors. Transplacental passage of immunoglobulins from mother to fetus occurs mainly after 32 weeks' gestation and effective endogenous synthesis does not begin for several months thereafter. Neonatal neutrophils exhibit both quantitative and qualitative abnormalities. Immature granulopoiesis is manifest by a low neutrophil cell mass and a reduced capacity for increasing progenitor cell proliferation. Neutropenia is often found in small for gestational age babies and also occurs as a consequence of sepsis. In addition, neonates, especially those <1500 g, have less effective mucosal and cutaneous barriers and are subject to more invasive procedures. Finally, babies in the neonatal intensive care unit (NICU) are exposed to environmental pathogens, which often show resistance to antibiotics.

Timing and causes of infection

The majority of neonatal infections present within 48 hours of birth (early onset) and are vertically transmitted or perinatally acquired from organisms colonizing the maternal genital tract. These classically present as fulminating septicaemia, often complicated by pneumonia or meningitis. The commonest causative organisms are group B streptococcus, *Escherichia coli*, *Haemophilus influenzae*, and *Listeria monocytogenes*.

Infections occurring after 48 hours (late onset) are generally nosocomial or environmentally acquired. The spectrum of late-onset infection ranges from minor skin infection to fulminating septicaemia. The commonest causative organisms are coagulase-negative staphylococci, Gram-negative bacilli (such as *Klebsiella*, *E. coli*, *Serratia marcescens* and *Pseudomonas*), *Staphylococcus aureus*, and *Candida*.

Group B streptococcus

Group B streptococcal (GBS) infection accounts for approximately a third to half of early-onset neonatal infections. Approximately 20 per cent of pregnant women harbour GBS in the lower genital tract, and vertical transmission from mother to baby during delivery occurs in around half. Only 1–2 per cent of these colonized neonates will develop invasive disease and neonatal sepsis. Ninety per cent of cases of early-onset GBS infection present within 12 hours with a fulminating septicaemia. Late-onset

GBS infection generally presents with focal disease, typically meningitis or pneumonia.

Controversy exists about the prevention of GBS disease. Intrapartum antibiotic prophylaxis (IAP) has been shown to significantly reduce the incidence of early-onset GBS disease but not late-onset disease. In the USA, it is now recommended that all pregnant women undergo bacteriological screening, with vaginal and rectal swabs taken for GBS culture at 35–37 weeks' gestation. Extrapolation of practice from the USA to the UK may be inappropriate given that variations in both the vaginal carriage rate and the incidence of early-onset GBS infection exist between populations. Currently in the UK, clinical practice with respect to antenatal screening and IAP varies, with most units adopting a risk-factor-based approach; IAP is offered to all women with risk factors for early-onset GBS disease. The risk factors are: previous baby affected by GBS, GBS bacteriuria, preterm labour, prolonged rupture of the membranes and fever in labour. Although both approaches reduce the incidence of early-onset GBS disease neither is without disadvantages to both mother and baby, including fatal anaphylaxis and infection with resistant organisms.

Investigations

Blood culture is the definitive diagnostic test for neonatal bacterial sepsis, although false-negative results can occur if small blood samples (<0.5 mL) have been collected. Other samples worth collecting when early-onset infection is suspected include ear and throat swabs and a maternal high vaginal swab. Collection of urine and cerebrospinal fluid (CSF) should also be considered in both early- and late-onset infections. The neutrophil count may be low or high in bacterial infection and the platelet count falls to $<100 \times 10^9$/L in 50 per cent of babies with bacterial infection. Acute-phase proteins such as C-reactive protein (CRP) and interleukin (IL)-6 rise in response to infection, but there is often a delay of 10–12 hours between the onset of infection and the rise in CRP. Serial measurements of CRP are useful in monitoring the progress of infection.

Treatment of neonatal infection

Appropriate antibiotics remain the mainstay of treatment of neonatal infection; their selection is guided by the timing of onset of infection combined with knowledge of the commonly occurring local pathogens. Antibiotics should be started empirically when infection is suspected.

The observation that neutropenic septic neonates have increased mortality compared with those who are septic but not neutropenic prompted studies of adjunct treatments to improve neutrophil count. These have included the transfusion of granulocytes and colony-stimulating factors such as granulocyte-macrophage colony-stimulating factor. These therapies are effective in increasing neutrophil counts but do not improve overall mortality. There is some evidence that granulocyte colony-stimulating factor may be effective in the prevention of infection in small for gestational age preterm infants and this is being explored further in a large multicentre study (PROGRAMS (PROphylactic GRAnulocyte-Macrophage colony-stimulating factor to reduce Sepsis in preterm neonates) trial). The effect of IV immunoglobulin on mortality and morbidity in infants with infection has also been assessed by meta-analysis. In infants with confirmed infection, there is a small but statistically significant reduction in mortality. A further large randomized study of the role of IV immunoglobulin is currently in progress (INIS (International Neonatal Immunotherapy Study) trial).

Congenital infections

Rubella

High rates of immunization have reduced the incidence of congenital rubella in the UK to less than 2 cases per 100 000 births. The risk of rubella-induced congenital abnormalities decreases with advancing gestation. Malformations occur in 90 per cent of infants whose mothers are infected in the first two months of pregnancy, but in only 20 per cent of those infected in the fourth and fifth months. Infants with congenital rubella typically present with jaundice, petechiae and hepatosplenomegaly at birth. Further clinical examination may reveal microcephaly, cataracts, microphthalmia and a murmur. Over two-thirds of these infants will have sensorineural deafness and at least half will show profound developmental delay at long-term follow-up. Diagnosis is confirmed by culturing the virus from a throat swab or urine, and by demonstrating rubella-specific IgM in plasma.

Cytomegalovirus

Cytomegalovirus (CMV) is the commonest cause of congenital infection worldwide. In the UK, just over half of all women presenting at antenatal clinics are seropositive for CMV. Congenital infection can occur as a consequence of both recurrent and primary infection. Over 90 per cent of infants with congenital CMV are asymptomatic at birth, although about 10 per cent will subsequently develop sensorineural deafness. The minority with symptoms at birth can present with multisystem disease similar to congenital rubella. Cytomegalovirus hepatitis results in intrahepatic and extrahepatic bile duct destruction. Central nervous system (CNS) infection results in microcephaly with periventricular calcification and occasionally hydrocephalus. Eye involvement occurs in 10–20 per cent and includes chorioretinitis, cataracts and blindness. The diagnosis is confirmed by culturing CMV from a throat swab or urine, and by demonstrating CMV-specific IgM in plasma. Treatment with ganciclovir has been reported but its efficacy is uncertain.

Toxoplasmosis

In the UK, the number of women developing toxoplasmosis in pregnancy is in the range of 1–6 per 1000. Infection can involve the fetus at any gestation, with the highest risk of infection in the third trimester but the greatest risk of damage to the fetus in the first or second trimesters. A quarter of infected fetuses develop subclinical disease affecting only their eyes and 5–10 per cent have widespread infection. Widespread infection classically presents with hydrocephalus, epilepsy, diffuse cerebral calcification and chorioretinitis, although these babies can also present with jaundice, hepatosplenomegaly and petechiae. Diagnosis is confirmed by demonstrating toxoplasma-specific IgM in plasma; this can be negative initially and should be repeated after four weeks. This is a potentially treatable condition. Pregnant women should be treated antenatally to reduce the risk of fetal infection and the congenitally infected neonate, even if asymptomatic, should be treated postnatally. The prognosis for asymptomatic neonates is good although they should continue to be followed up until early adult life for the development of chorioretinitis. The majority with neurological involvement are severely handicapped at follow-up.

Herpes simplex virus

Neonatal herpes simplex virus (HSV) infection is a rare but serious condition with a significant mortality and morbidity. In three-quarters of cases, infection is due to HSV type 2, with the remainder due to type 1. In 85 per cent of cases, infection is acquired perinatally via delivery through an infected birth canal or secondary to ascending infection following rupture of membranes. Infection may also be present at birth as a result of transplacental intrauterine infection in 5 per cent of cases and in the remaining 10 per cent infection is acquired postnatally. Often there is no history of maternal infection and a high index of suspicion is necessary.

Neonatal HSV infection usually presents in the first month, with two-thirds of cases presenting within the first week. Infection is categorized clinically into three types according to the site(s) of infection: localized disease of the skin, eyes and mouth (SEM), localized CNS disease and disseminated disease. Of the clinical presentations, SEM disease is the least severe. Central nervous system disease includes focal encephalitis and meningoencephalitis, usually presenting with fever, altered consciousness and seizures, which may be focal and difficult to control. Disseminated disease usually involves several organs, including liver, lung, brain, skin and adrenals. Clinical findings in neonates with disseminated disease can be similar to those associated with fulminant bacterial sepsis.

Congenital or intrauterine HSV infection is characterized by the presence of vesicles or scarring at birth, or chorioretinitis, microphthalmia and microcephaly. Atypical presentations of neonatal HSV infections include herpetic whitlow, supraglottic ulceration and fulminant hepatic failure.

Women with clinical signs of genital infection with HSV at the time of delivery should be delivered by caesarean section. Neonatal management depends upon establishing risk factors, particularly evidence of active maternal genital infection, the type of infection (primary versus recurrent) and mode of delivery. In high-risk situations, prophylactic aciclovir is indicated. In babies with symptoms prompt investigation and treatment with high-dose IV aciclovir is required. Investigations should include cerebrospinal fluid analysis (cell count, protein, glucose, polymerase chain reaction for HSV DNA), viral culture of oropharynx, nasopharynx, stool, blood and CSF, immunofluorescent antibody staining of cutaneous lesions, electroencephalography and magnetic resonance imaging (MRI).

Human immunodeficiency virus (HIV)

The vast majority of children with human immunodeficiency virus (HIV) are infected in the perinatal period. In the USA, HIV is now the commonest congenital infection, and in the UK, the prevalence of HIV seropositivity in the childbearing population remains relatively low but is increasing. With appropriate antiretroviral treatment of mothers during pregnancy and labour, carefully considered management of delivery and avoidance of breastfeeding, the risk of vertical transmission of HIV is reduced from 25 per cent to around 2 per cent. The risk to the baby varies with maternal viral load, duration of rupture of membranes, mode of delivery and gestational age. In general HIV-infected neonates are normal at delivery but very occasionally they may present with hepatosplenomegaly, lymphadenopathy or thrombocytopenia (see Chapter 6).

Infection control in the NICU

The risk of nosocomial infection increases exponentially with prolonged duration of hospital stay and multiple carers. The very low birth weight infant who spends weeks in NICU attached to various tubes, needles and catheters is therefore at very high risk of such infection. Although early detection and treatment of infection is important in the management of these infants equal attention should be given to the prevention of infection. The principles of infection control in hospitals are well established and should be adhered to. There should be adequate space, ideally 3 m^2, for each incubator and single rooms should be available for the isolation of sick babies. Ideally, each infant should have their own dedicated equipment, and where this is not possible equipment should be thoroughly cleaned between patients. Equipment coming into contact with infectious body fluids should be disposable. There should be enough sinks so that handwashing protocols can be adhered to. The hands of the medical and nursing staff are the main potential routes of cross-infection and, of all the measures for preventing nosocomial infection, hand washing is by far the most important. Finally, antibiotic use influences the pattern of nosocomial infection by influencing the colonizing flora and predisposing to antibiotic resistance. Close liaison with the local microbiologist is important in the rational use of antibiotic in the NICU.

KEY LEARNING POINTS

- Infection is a significant cause of neonatal mortality and morbidity.
- Group B streptococcal infection is the commonest cause of early onset infection.
- Handwashing is the most important measure in the prevention of nosocomial infection in the NICU.

HYPOGLYCAEMIA IN THE NEONATE

Intrauterine growth retardation with asymptomatic hypoglycaemia

CASE STUDY

A term baby boy is born at 37 weeks' gestation weighing 1800 g (<0.4th percentile) and length measurement on the 50th percentile. He is admitted to the neonatal unit and given an early feed. Blood sugar is checked fours hours later and is low (1.5 mmol/L). He is well on examination and after a second feed the blood sugar increases, but before the next feed four hours later it is low again.

Neonatal hypoglycaemia is defined as a true blood glucose (TBG) level below 2.6 mmol/L. Most infants with low blood glucose levels are asymptomatic, although symptoms attributable to hypoglycaemia include jitteriness, apnoea, floppiness, irritability and convulsions. Transient low blood glucose levels are physiological in the first few hours following delivery in the majority of healthy term neonates. These occur until the appropriate metabolic adaptations to extrauterine life are established. These adaptations involve the activation of gluconeogenic counterregulatory hormones such as adrenaline, cortisol, growth hormone and glucagon, which overcome the hypoglycaemic influence of residual fetal insulin. Appropriately grown, well, term babies should not be screened for hypoglycaemia and intervention is only required if they are symptomatic.

Certain groups of infants are less able to make the appropriate metabolic adaptations to extrauterine life and are at risk of long-term neurological sequelae from prolonged or recurrent hypoglycaemia. These include infants with growth retardation, premature infants, infants of diabetic mothers and infants of mothers on labetalol. These 'at-risk' babies should be kept warm and offered an early feed or started on an IV dextrose infusion if enteral feeding is not possible. All cot-side blood sugar screening tests are inaccurate at low readings, therefore a confirmatory TBG should be sent to the biochemistry laboratory.

Management of the 'at-risk' infant

- Commence three-hourly enteral feeds (60–90 mL/kg per day) or IV 10 per cent glucose infusion at 60–75 mL/kg if unable to feed
- Check sugar before second feed or after one hour of IV infusion
- Check four-hourly for 12 hours then 6–8 hourly for 24 hours if normoglycaemic
- Continue to check sugars until stable if episodes of hypoglycaemia

Approach to moderate hypoglycaemia (1.5–2.5 mmol/L) in infant able to feed:

- Initially increase feed volume up to 120 mL/kg or until feed intolerance develops
- Add additional glucose (e.g. Maxijul™) to feeds if continued hypoglycaemia
- Commence IV 10 per cent glucose (continue feeds) at 2 mL/hour

- Increase IV glucose up to 50 mL/kg and check plasma electrolytes because of large fluid intake
- If continued hypoglycaemia change concentration of infusion to 12.5 per cent dextrose
- If continuing hypoglycaemia increase infusion to 15 then 20 per cent glucose via central line
- Consider glucagon and hydrocortisone

Approach to moderate hypoglycaemia in infant unable to feed:

- Intravenous 10 per cent glucose solution at 90 mL/kg
- Increase IV glucose up to 150 mL/kg and check electrolytes because of large fluid intake
- If continued hypoglycaemia change infusion to 12.5 per cent dextrose
- If continuing hypoglycaemia change to 15–20 per cent glucose via central line
- Consider glucagon and hydrocortisone

Any child with persistent or refractory hypoglycaemia despite a glucose intake of >10 mg/kg per minute needs investigation to exclude a pathological basis, notably hyperinsulinaemia (see Chapter 15).

Emergency treatment of symptomatic or significant hypoglycaemia (TBG <1.5 mmol/L)

- If able to feed use Hypostop and give early feed
- If unable to feed give bolus of 2 mL/kg of 10 per cent dextrose over 5 minutes. Start 10 per cent glucose infusion at 2 mL/hour following bolus to prevent rebound hypoglycaemia

KEY LEARNING POINTS

- Certain 'at risk' babies need screening for hypoglycaemia.
- If possible continue enteral milk feeds in hypoglycaemic infants.
- Persistent or refractory hypoglycaemia requires investigation.

NEONATAL SCREENING PROGRAMMES

Biochemical screening

Since February 2003, biochemical screening for congenital hypothyroidism, phenylketonuria and cystic fibrosis has been available for all neonates delivered in Scotland and a number of regions in England and Wales. Dried blood spots (formerly known as the Guthrie test) are collected around day 5 after written, informed parental consent has been obtained. This should be delayed for 72 hours after a blood transfusion.

Screening for cystic fibrosis involves the measurement of immunoreactive trypsinogen (IRT) combined with DNA analysis. DNA analysis (which covers about 86 per cent of the commonest mutations in the native UK population) is performed on those above a cut-off point of IRT. There is evidence that the more severe mutations of the cystic fibrosis transmembrane regulator gene are the ones most likely to cause an increase in IRT. This combined analysis reduces the number of false-positive tests that arise if IRT alone is measured but inevitably leads to the identification of some healthy carrier infants. This has significant ethical implications. Immunoreactive trypsinogen levels are influenced by enteral feeding and false-negative results can occur in parenterally fed infants.

Screening for congenital hypothyroidism involves the measurement of thyroid stimulating hormone (TSH). An initial result of <5 mU/L is reported as normal, intermediate results of 5–24 mU/L are repeated and reported as normal if <8 mU/L, and results of >25 mU/L are immediately notified to the referring paediatrician. This system identifies thyroid agenesis and problems with thyroid hormone biosynthesis but may miss rare cases of hypothalamic/pituitary hypothyroidism.

Screening for phenylketonuria was the original Guthrie test and involves the measurement of phenylalanine (see Chapter 15). For this to be accurate, the neonate should have been fully enterally fed for 48 hours.

Hearing screening

Universal neonatal hearing screening is likely to be implemented in all National Health Service (NHS) Boards by October 2005. This will replace the current targeted neonatal hearing screening programme. Otoacoustic emissions are low-amplitude sound waves produced by the inner ear that occur spontaneously as well as in response to a click stimulus. The measurement of OAE is a screening test only and auditory brainstem response testing is required for a definitive diagnosis of hearing loss.

KEY LEARNING POINTS

- Biochemical screening exists for hypothyroidism, phenylketonuria and cystic fibrosis.
- Universal neonatal hearing screening should be implemented by October 2005.

MECHANISMS OF NEONATAL ADAPTATION

A neonate needs to make the change from collapsed fluid-filled lungs to effective gas exchange. At the start of labour the fetal lung switches from fluid secretion to fluid absorption. After delivery there is a rise in the systemic vascular resistance when the cord is clamped, removing the low resistance placental circulation from the system. There is also a rapid fall in the pulmonary vascular resistance caused by expansion of the lungs. The oxygen present in the inspired gas will enter the circulation, increasing the oxygen saturation above that seen in fetal life and further decreasing pulmonary vascular resistance by relaxing pulmonary vascular tone. By these mechanisms the fetal shunting of blood away from the pulmonary circulation is changed to allow effective gas exchange.

Transient tachypnoea of the newborn (or 'wet lung')

CASE STUDY

A baby is delivered by elective caesarean section at 38 weeks' gestation because of previous maternal caesarean section. The baby develops an audible expiratory grunt, has a respiratory rate of 70/min and is cyanosed. He is admitted to the neonatal unit and oxygen therapy is commenced. A chest radiograph shows a 'streaky' appearance of the lungs and there is fluid in the horizontal fissure.

Transient tachypnoea of the newborn (TTN) is a failure of normal respiratory adaptation to birth. It is characterized by a failure of adequate lung expansion and a delay in the normal clearance of lung fluid. It is commoner in babies delivered by elective caesarean section prior to the onset of labour who may be depressed at birth due to maternal sedation. The incidence is significantly higher in babies delivered by lower uterine segment caesarean section before 39 weeks. The affected baby presents with tachypnoea (respiratory rate >40/min). A chest radiograph shows pulmonary plethora with fluid in the transverse fissure. Treatment is to provide respiratory support as required, IV fluids and antibiotics. The natural history is for slow resolution over the first day, though it can take several days in unusual circumstances.

Persistent pulmonary hypertension of the newborn

CASE STUDY

A baby is delivered by forceps at 41 weeks because of a non-reassuring CTG. There is old meconium present in the amniotic fluid. The baby requires some resuscitation with bag/mask ventilation. Following the onset of normal respiration he develops grunting and marked recession, the respiratory rate is 65/min and he is deeply cyanosed. He is admitted to the neonatal unit and oxygen therapy is commenced. A chest radiograph shows oligaemic lung fields and a blood gas shows low pCO_2 and pO_2.

Persistent pulmonary hypertension of the newborn (PPHN) is a failure of the normal cardiovascular adaptation to birth. It is characterized by right-to-left shunts through the ductus arteriosus and foramen ovale caused by the pulmonary vascular resistance either remaining high or becoming greater than the systemic vascular resistance. Mixing of oxygenated and deoxygenated blood occurs in the aorta and left atrium and there is lung hypoperfusion due to the shunting of blood away from the pulmonary arteries. Persistent pulmonary hypertension of the newborn is not simply a description of raised pulmonary vascular resistance, as this will occur in a variety of lung diseases but a combination of decreased pulmonary blood flow and physiological shunting of blood from right to left. It can occur for a variety of reasons such as prenatal hypertrophy of pulmonary arteriolar muscles (seen in congenital diaphragmatic hernia), or primary failure of pulmonary vascular resistance to fall following birth (idiopathic PPHN), or due to hypoxia or acidosis from various respiratory diseases or as a combination of several factors.

Clinically, a baby with PPHN will have hypoxaemia on a post-ductal gas (e.g. from the umbilical arterial catheter) with a relatively normal or low carbon dioxide. A saturation monitor can be placed on the right hand and compared to a reading from a lower limb. A difference of >5 per cent in these readings is characteristic of ductal shunting. In the situation of persistent foramen ovale (PFO) shunting alone there will be no difference. Cardiac ultrasound with Doppler is now the investigation of choice for the diagnosis of PPHN. This also excludes cyanotic heart disease (which can mimic PPHN). The chest radiograph may show pulmonary hypoperfusion in idiopathic PPHN, or the changes from the pre-existing respiratory problem in secondary PPHN.

Treatment of PPHN is aimed at reducing the shunt by dropping the pulmonary vascular resistance relative to the systemic vascular resistance. Additional inspired oxygen will encourage pulmonary vasodilatation. Intubation and ventilation will often be required along with sedation. Correction of acidosis may rapidly vasodilate the pulmonary arteries, though prolonged alkalinization by hyperventilation or bicarbonate infusion has not been shown to be helpful and may cause significant side effects such as air leak or deafness. Systemic blood pressure should be maintained (mean 45–55 mmHg) to prevent damage to organs by poor perfusion in additional to the hypoxia. Apart from oxygen the only selective pulmonary vasodilator currently available is inhaled nitric oxide. This has been shown to reduce the need for extracorporeal membranous oxygenation. In a baby with PPHN secondary to lung disease, surfactant and high-frequency oscillatory ventilation may be useful.

KEY LEARNING POINTS

- Normal labour prepares the fetus for extrauterine life.
- Elective LUCS should be performed after 39 weeks.
- Cardiac echocardiography (ECHO) will distinguish PPHN from cyanotic congenital heart disease.

HOMOEOSTATIC SUPPORT FOR THE VERY IMMATURE OR SICK NEONATE

Extreme prematurity

Babies born at <27 weeks' gestation are a special group with regard to management and possible complications. They are at the highest risk of all problems resulting from prematurity. Often they will have minimal ventilatory requirements initially but may suffer from a pulmonary haemorrhage in the first few days of life. They have a higher incidence of both periventricular haemorrhage and periventricular leukomalacia. Their kidneys are immature, compounding their large transepidermal fluid losses. If their IV fluids are increased to account for this fluid loss the resultant increased sugar load can cause hyperglycaemia and glycosuria, which will further increase renal water loss. Water intake should be increased separately from sugar to normalize fluid balance, possibly using additional 5 per cent dextrose, rather than increasing any standard total parenteral nutrition (TPN) solution. Retinopathy of prematurity and chronic lung disease are often inevitable for these very immature babies.

Hypoxic ischaemic encephalopathy

CASE STUDY

A mother presents at 41 weeks with reduced fetal movements. A CTG recording is non-reassuring and there is meconium staining noted at artificial rupture of membranes (ARM). A sudden profound fetal bradycardia develops and emergency caesarean section is carried out. A baby boy is born in poor condition and requires intubation for apnoea. Following admission to the NICU an arterial blood gas shows a base deficit of 20. He remains apnoeic, anuric and develops generalized convulsions.

A baby who experiences perinatal oxygen deficiency will develop multiorgan damage. Renal failure causes reduced urine output with subsequent hyponatraemia, hyperkalaemia and acidosis combined with increased urea and creatinine. Myocardial ischaemia causes hypotension from reduced cardiac output. Liver damage causes coagulopathy and gastrointestinal ischaemia leads to an increased risk of NEC when feeds are started. Most organs have the potential for full recovery if supportive measures such as ventilation and IV fluids are maintained. Any damage to the central nervous system is permanent, however, cerebral protective measures such as selective head or systemic cooling are undergoing evaluation. A scoring system developed by Sarnet quantifies cerebral involvement. Minor ischaemia causes a hyperalert state. Moderate-to-severe ischaemia leads to cerebral depression, apnoea and seizures. Muscle tone may be low at first then becomes increased. It is difficult to predict long-term outcome. Magnetic resonance imaging after day 4 and EEG provide useful prognostic information but long-term outpatient follow-up is essential.

Sepsis

Significant sepsis causes multiorgan failure from tissue hypoperfusion despite increased tissue metabolic requirements. Maintenance of myocardial, renal and central nervous system oxygen delivery is vital. Improvement in systemic blood pressure will overcome reduced cerebral autoregulation and maintain renal function.

Metabolic disease

CASE STUDY

A baby girl collapses on the fifth day while on the postnatal ward. Her parents are first cousins and previously lost a baby in the first week of life. She is ventilated and admitted to the NICU. Blood sugars are low and she has a moderate metabolic acidosis. She has palpable femoral pulses and a cardiac ECHO is normal.

Neonates with a significant metabolic illness will present in a similar fashion to infants with sepsis or congenital cardiac disease. In the absence of risk factors for sepsis and a normal cardiac examination one should suspect an inherited metabolic illness. Immediate management is to stop oral feeds, provide IV glucose and obtain blood and urine for investigation of hyperammonaemia or an abnormal amino acid or organic acid profile in urine or blood. See Chapter 15 for further investigation and management.

KEY LEARNING POINTS

- Premature infants born before 28 weeks are at the highest risk for neonatal complications.
- In hypoxic ischaemic encephalopathy damage to the brain may be reduced by cooling techniques.
- Inherited metabolic disease should be excluded in a collapsed neonate.

NUTRITION IN WELL AND SICK BABIES

Enteral nutrition

Breastfeeding

Breast milk provides the optimal nutrition for term babies. The benefits of breast milk include improved gastrointestinal tolerance and reduced NEC, anti-infective properties, reduced allergenicity and improved neurodevelopment. Most maternity hospitals have baby-friendly feeding policies that aim to promote breastfeeding in healthy term babies. These policies encourage rooming-in of mothers with babies, demand feeding, the avoidance of supplementary feeds and accessibility of trained staff who can provide consistent support and advice. Sick or premature babies often have an even greater need to receive breast milk and it is important to actively encourage their mothers to express breast milk from an early stage. Breast milk generally requires fortification with additional calories, protein, sodium, calcium and phosphate to meet the nutritional requirements of low birth weight infants (Table 5.8).

Problems with breastfeeding can occur because of both maternal (poor technique, mastitis, etc.) and/or infant (cleft lip and palate, reluctant feeder, etc.) reasons. These can usually be overcome by good, midwifery-led breastfeeding support. Hypernatraemic dehydration, although uncommon, can be a devastating consequence of inadequate breastfeeding. Babies usually present with marked weight loss (>15 per cent) 5–21 days after birth. They often look very well but may progress rapidly to seizures or coma. Weighing babies helps to identify inadequate breastfeeding but may undermine maternal confidence if performed too regularly. A balance between the protection of breastfeeding and the early detection of feeding problems can generally be achieved by weighing at around 72 hours old, on days 5–7 and at 2 weeks.

Formula feeding

Modern infant formula milks have been extensively modified to resemble human milk. Many milks are available that are designed to meet the nutritional requirements of both term and preterm babies (see Table 5.8). Long-chain polyunsaturated fatty acids (LCPs), derived from essential fatty acids, are important cell membrane constituents, especially in the brain and eye. Formula milks containing LCPs have been demonstrated to enhance short-term visual maturation, studies of their long-term effect on visual performance are still ongoing. A beneficial effect of LCPs on neurodevelopment has also been shown in both preterm and term babies. Most preterm and many term formula milks now contain LCPs.

Weaning

Data from animal models and large, retrospective, epidemiological studies support the concept that dietary manipulation in infancy may influence cardiovascular risk, bone health, learning and memory in adult life. Barker has shown that birth weight, and weight at one year, is correlated with a reduced death rate from cardiovascular disease and a reduction in the incidence of non-insulin-dependent diabetes mellitus. Despite this increasing evidence of a link between fetal and infant nutrition and long-term morbidity, very little evidence exists regarding the optimal timing for the introduction of solid foods (weaning). Increased body fat, higher body

Table 5.8 Average daily nutritional requirements and nutrient content of various milks

Nutrient	Requirements per kg		Milk content per 100 mL			
	Birth weight (<2.5 kg)	Birth weight (>2.5 kg)	Term formula	Preterm formula	Term breast milk	Fortified breast milk
Energy (kcal)	110–150	105–115	65–70	80	70	80
Fat (grams)	3.0–4.0	3.0	3.5–4.0	4.5	4.0	4.0
Protein (grams)	3.0–4.0	2.0	1.5	2.0–2.5	1.0–1.5	2.0–3.0
Sodium (mmol)	1.0–10.0	2.0–3.0	1.0	1.5–2.0	0.5	3.0
Potassium (mmol)	2.0–5.0	2.0–3.0	1.5–2.0	2.0	2.0	2.0
Calcium (mmol)	2.0–6.0	1.5	1.0–2.0	2.0–2.5	1.0	2.0
Phosphate (mmol)	2.0–5.0	1.5	1.0	1.5	0.5	1.5

mass index and a greater incidence of wheezing have been associated with weaning before 4 months and the Department of Health currently recommends the introduction of solids at 4–6 months. More recently, the World Health Organization (WHO) recommended exclusive breastfeeding for at least 6 months as the optimal mode of infant feeding, with the introduction of solids thereafter. It is, however, well recognized that many parents do not adhere to these professional recommendations and introduce solids before 4 months.

Current weaning recommendations apply to preterm, low birth weight and healthy, term infants although a recent study demonstrated improved growth velocity and iron status in preterm infants weaned earlier with higher energy foods. Further research into this subject is required before clear evidence-based guidance can be given to parents.

KEY LEARNING POINTS

- Breast milk provides the optimal nutrition for term infants.
- Breast milk generally requires fortification to meet the nutritional requirements of low birth weight infants.
- Formula milks containing LCPs enhance visual maturation and neurodevelopment.
- Diet in infancy may influence cardiovascular risk, bone health, learning and memory in adult life.
- Minimal enteral feeding in premature infants enhances gut motility, gut hormone secretion and a less pathogenic gut flora.

Parenteral nutrition

Parenteral nutrition facilitates nutritional adequacy and reasonable postnatal growth in babies in whom enteral feeding is impossible (e.g. intestinal atresia), inadequate (e.g. immaturity) or unsafe (e.g. NEC). The risks associated with parenteral nutrition include infection, hyperglycaemia, metabolic acidosis, cholestasis and cardiac tamponade related to central venous lines. Parenteral nutrition solutions are available commercially although many neonatal units use solutions that are customized in their own pharmacy. Even when a baby's nutritional requirements are met by TPN it is important to introduce enteral feeding as early as possible. Enteral feeding, even in small volumes, enhances gut motility, gut hormone secretion and a less pathogenic gut flora. These changes have been shown to reduce the incidence of feed intolerance, nosocomial infection and cholestatic jaundice.

Problems with feeding: necrotizing enterocolitis

CASE STUDY

A baby girl born at 28 weeks is now 10 days old. She has been on full enteral feeds of formula for two days. Overnight she develops a distended abdomen with bilious aspirates. A radiograph shows bowel wall thickening and intramural gas.

Necrotizing enterocolitis affects 2–5 per cent of very low birth weight infants with significant mortality and long-term sequelae. Major risk factors are prematurity, IUGR and asphyxia. Most affected babies are on enteral feeds and it is thought that the stress of feeding superimposed on a damaged immature intestine causes mucosal ischaemia. Gut translocation from the gut lumen leads to the classic 'bubbly' pattern of intramural gas on abdominal radiographs. Treatment is gut rest, antibiotics and general support. Perforation can occur and this is an indication for laparotomy as is continued evidence of sepsis with abdominal signs. The terminal ileum and ascending colon are most commonly affected. Gut resection may lead to significant long-term morbidity with short gut syndrome.

Problems with feeding: bile-stained vomiting

> **CASE STUDY**
>
> A term breastfed baby boy has an episode of bilious vomiting on day 3 in the postnatal ward. He is otherwise well, has passed meconium and has a normal abdominal examination.

Most reports of 'bile' vomiting are inaccurate. Often a yellow colour in the vomit is thought to be bile, though this may be from breast milk. However, a dark-green coloured vomit is of concern and even if the examination is normal a plain abdominal radiograph must be taken. If this is abnormal or if the bile vomits continue, a contrast study should be performed to exclude a malrotation or intestinal atresia. It is important to exclude anal atresia even if there is a history of meconium. A baby girl can present with anal atresia combined with a rectovaginal fistula.

COMPLICATIONS AND OUTCOME OF INTRAUTERINE GROWTH RETARDATION

Intrauterine growth retardation is defined as a birth weight less than the tenth percentile for gestational age and can be either symmetrical (length, weight and OFC all decreased) or asymmetrical (length and OFC preserved). A growth chart appropriate for the local population must be used. Investigation of symmetrical IUGR aims to identify an intrinsic fetal cause such as a chromosomal abnormality (trisomy 18, 21, ring chromosome 5), other congenital anomalies or intrauterine infection. Asymmetrical IUGR is caused by abnormal placental function following pre-eclampsia, placental infarcts, abruptio placenta, multiple gestation, substance abuse or cigarette smoking. The stressed fetus has increased levels of circulating catecholamines. This causes loss of fat and muscle mass and reduced glycogen stores, and increased flow to essential organs leading to the head-sparing pattern of asymmetrical IUGR. Oligohydramnios is frequently associated with asymmetrical IUGR due to decreased renal blood flow and urine output. Umbilical artery Doppler flow studies will demonstrate absence of end-diastolic blood flow. Biophysical profiles may lead to a decision for early delivery. The risks to the fetus of continued compromise and possible death *in utero* are weighed against any risk from premature delivery. Babies with IUGR are prone to hypoxaemia during labour and delivery from cord compression due to oligohydramnios in addition to any pre-existing placental insufficiency and meconium aspiration is more common. Prolonged fetal hypoxia leads to polycythaemia, reduced glycogen stores and increased insulin-like factors that promote hypoglycaemia. Hypothermia is increased because of reduced subcutaneous fat combined with an increased surface/volume ratio. Initial management is to maintain temperature and prevent hypoglycaemia. In mild cases, this can be achieved by providing high-calorie enteral feeds, though in more severe IUGR prolonged redistribution of blood flow away from non-essential organs leads to gastrointestinal compromise with an increased risk of NEC. Avoidance of early enteral feeds with cautious introduction of feeds is indicated. Follow-up after discharge is essential to document catch-up growth. Babies with IUGR have an increased risk of developmental problems (see section on long-term outcome, page 155) reflecting the abnormal fetal environment, with possible perinatal asphyxia and postnatal hypoglycaemia.

> **KEY LEARNING POINTS**
>
> - Intrauterine growth retardation reflects a hostile uterine environment and careful fetal assessment is essential.
> - Babies with IUGR are at risk from early and late complications and require long-term follow-up.

NEONATAL CARDIAC DISEASE

Cyanotic congenital heart disease

This is dealt with in detail in Chapter 9. In the face of a cyanosed baby with or without respiratory distress congenital heart disease should be considered. A hyperoxic test or nitrogen washout will show a failure to improve saturations with 100 per cent oxygen because of the presence of a right-to-left shunt. The placement of pre- and post-ductal saturation monitors may show a decrease of 5–10 per cent, which is significant. If the post-ductal saturation is greater transposition of the great arteries should be suspected.

Differential diagnosis of the blue baby

Cyanotic heart disease

Children with right-to-left shunts without obstruction to flow often present in the postnatal ward with cyanosis and mild tachypnoea without other signs of respiratory distress. A murmur may not be present although the second heart sound will often be loud. An unwell baby with persisting hypoxia and a metabolic acidosis on blood gas should be assumed to have significant sepsis, metabolic disease or an obstructed cardiac abnormality. Prostin should be commenced to open the duct while awaiting a definitive diagnosis.

Persistent pulmonary hypertension of the newborn

There is usually a presenting problem such as meconium aspiration. In contrast to the majority of structural heart disease, these babies are unwell and acidotic as well as cyanosed.

Polycythaemia

Babies with a high haematocrit will often appear cyanosed as cyanosis will be clinically apparent when there is 5 g/dcl of desaturated haemoglobin, which can occur more readily in polycythaemia. The cyanosis will tend to be present in the extremities (acrocyanosis) and not centrally. A normal saturation and an FBC will confirm the diagnosis. There is controversy as to when a partial exchange should be performed; this should only be done if the venous haematocrit is greater than 75 per cent or if it is >70 per cent and associated with hypoglycaemia.

Methaemoglobinuria (rare)

A well baby who is centrally cyanosed with a normal saturation may have methaemoglobinaemia. Levels above 10 per cent require treatment with methylene blue. Care should be taken as this can itself precipitate methaemoglobinuria.

Cardiac failure

Cardiac failure is unusual in the immediate neonatal period. In the clinical situation of early-onset cardiac failure an arteriovenous malformation, arrhythmia or cardiomyopathy should be suspected. A cerebral bruit will be present in failure due to a vein of Galen's malformation with the large abnormal vessel easily seen on cranial ultrasound. It is more common for cardiac failure to occur in the presence of a left-to-right shunt (e.g. patent ductus arteriosus (PDA), ventricular septal defect (VSD)), which increases in size as the pulmonary vascular resistance decreases over the first few weeks of life. A ventilated baby will fail to wean and non-ventilated babies will become more tachypnoeic, sweat on feeding and may fail to thrive.

Persistent ductus arteriosus with cardiac failure

CASE STUDY

An baby is born at 26 weeks' gestation and requires ventilation for eight days. Oxygen requirements have been decreasing after the first week, but over the next 24 hours there is a need to increase the fraction of inspired oxygen (FiO_2) and pressure settings on the ventilator. There is no evidence of sepsis. Examination reveals a long systolic murmur with full femoral pulses, and a chest radiograph shows a large heart with increased pulmonary markings.

Premature babies often develop a symptomatic duct as pulmonary vascular resistance (PVR) decreases and increased shunting occurs from left to right through the ductus arteriosus. This produces high-output cardiac failure and pulmonary oedema with decreased lung compliance. Examination initially reveals a short systolic murmur. This increases in length as the PVR continues to drop and eventually presents as a continuous murmur when there is left-to-right flow during the whole of the cardiac cycle. In addition, a right ventricular impulse develops and the femoral pulses become easily palpable. A chest radiograph shows an enlarged heart with pulmonary plethora and a cardiac ECHO shows a large left atrium, a PDA with left-to-right flow and reverse flow in the descending aorta during diastole. Initial treatment in most neonatal units is with indometacin, although this has side effects from renal, mesenteric and cerebral arterial constriction. Alternatives are other non-steroidal drugs or operative ligation.

Congenital vascular rings

Congenital vascular rings cause rare problems in neonates and a high index of suspicion is required. The symptoms include stridor, feeding difficulty and apnoea. A chest radiograph is often normal, and barium swallow will show only lateral or posterior aberrant vessels and will miss an anterior tracheal compression such as an aberrant innominate artery. Cardiac ECHO may be normal, as it is difficult to see all the vessels. Angiography will define any abnormal vessels but will not show the extent of tracheal compression. Bronchoscopy will show the narrowing with associated arterial pulsation. New computed tomography (CT) scanners with three-dimensional reconstruction will demonstrate both the vessels and airways and are the most useful single investigation.

KEY LEARNING POINTS

- Congenital heart disease should be excluded in all cyanosed babies.
- Cardiac failure is unusual in the immediate postnatal period due to the high PVR.
- Congenital vascular rings are a rare cause of stridor, poor feeding or apnoea.

NEONATAL RESPIRATORY DISEASE

The lung bud in the fetus develops in stages (see Chapter 8). By about 24 weeks' gestation gas exchange can occur although true alveolar formation does not start until about 36 weeks. Before this time terminal branching of the airways occurs with the development initially of saccules, which then form alveolar ducts. After alveolar development, septation continues to occur increasing lung surface area for the first two years of life. This process ensures that there is great potential for lung growth and recovery, but any insult to the lungs during this critical period can lead to the failure of the lung to achieve its full size. In the term neonate surfactant is produced to help lower surface tension and maintain a functional residual capacity. This improves the compliance of the lung by preventing atelectasis.

Idiopathic respiratory distress syndrome

Idiopathic respiratory distress syndrome (IRDS) is due to a relative deficiency of surfactant and most commonly occurs in premature neonates. The lack of surfactant causes atelectasis and subsequent respiratory failure. Although it is commonest in premature neonates, term neonates can be affected in certain situations such as a diabetic mother or in cases of elective caesarean section (especially before 39 weeks). Surfactant can also be inactivated by meconium, infection or hypoxia. It is possible to stimulate surfactant production via maternal steroid injection (usually betamethasone) 12–48 hours before birth. The pathophysiology of IRDS is due to an inadequate amount of active surfactant. This leads to alveolar collapse at the end of expiration and increased work of breathing. Respiratory failure occurs due to the atelectasis compounded by apnoea, presenting as hypoxia and then hypercapnia. The hypoxia and acidosis cause increased pulmonary vascular resistance, which in a near term neonate can lead to PPHN. The shear forces acting on the fragile lung lead to capillary leak of proteinaceous material (which is noticeable on histology as a hyaline membrane).

CASE STUDY

A baby boy is born at 31 weeks' gestation following a placental abruption. He requires bag/mask ventilation and following this is noted to have marked sternal recession. An arterial blood gas shows high pCO_2 and low pO_2. A chest radiograph shows bilateral diffuse opacification.

Management of idiopathic respiratory distress syndrome

Prevention of IRDS is the preferable option and optimal antenatal care has reduced the severity in developed countries. Preventing premature birth or recognizing the need to administer maternal steroids reduces the incidence and severity of IRDS. Delaying planned delivery by caesarean section to 39 weeks is also important. Prompt resuscitation of high-risk neonates to prevent hypoglycaemia and cold injury is vital.

In established IRDS exogenous surfactants are available for treatment. Curosurf (porcine surfactant) and Survanta (bovine surfactant) are the two natural surfactants available in the UK. Exosurf is an artificial surfactant, which is slower to act due to the lack of surfactant proteins. It is now established that prophylactic surfactant given at or shortly after birth to intubated premature neonates is superior to rescue administration of surfactant given only to those babies who develop increasing oxygen requirements. However, it is not clear if all premature neonates should be intubated on a resuscitaire in order to give them surfactant.

Increased inspired oxygen should be given to all babies who are hypoxaemic. Early use of nasal continuous positive airways pressure (CPAP) should be considered if the oxygen requirement is rising, the pCO_2 is raised or there is moderate respiratory distress. Nasal CPAP recruits collapsed alveoli and increases the functional residual capacity, increasing lung compliance and reversing the changes seen in RDS. If nasal CPAP fails, the baby will need intubation and ventilation.

Air leak

CASE STUDY

A term baby boy is noted to have an increased respiratory rate shortly after birth. He is not cyanosed and a capillary blood gas is normal. A chest radiograph is taken and this shows a moderate right-sided pneumothorax.

Air leak (pneumothorax, pulmonary interstitial emphysema, mediastinal emphysema) is much less common since the introduction of surfactant therapy. Previously the combination of stiff lungs and high-pressure ventilation would often lead to rupture of the delicate lung with subsequent air leak. Pneumothorax is now more commonly seen in larger babies with moderate respiratory distress who generate marked negative inspiratory pressure. In this situation there is often a dilemma regarding treatment. Even when there is associated mediastinal shift a conservative 'wait and see' approach is often best. Inhaling a high oxygen content can encourage the shrinkage of a pneumothorax (by removing the nitrogen down a concentration gradient) and avoid the need for a chest tube.

Pneumonia

Infection should always be considered as the cause of respiratory distress in a neonate. It is impossible to rule out sepsis and therefore antibiotics against the normal neonatal pathogens should be commenced in any neonate with respiratory distress that does not resolve rapidly (<4 hours).

Pulmonary haemorrhage

Pulmonary haemorrhage will usually occur in the most immature babies. It often occurs at days 3–6 of life and can be severe. The resultant hypotension and coagulopathy may cause intracerebral bleeding. Following a haemorrhage, ventilation requirements will increase. Treatment involves correcting coagulopathy and increased positive end-expiratory pressure (PEEP) to prevent further bleeding. In mature infants unusual causes such as an inherited coagulopathy should be considered.

Meconium aspiration syndrome

Acute or chronic hypoxia *in utero* may cause the meconium to be passed before birth. Infants may aspirate meconium either *in utero* or at the time of delivery due to the deep gasping breaths that occur from hypoxia. The majority of meconium aspiration is mild but in severe cases it causes marked respiratory distress. Two forms of lung pathology can result:

- emphysema resulting from partial obstruction of the airway causing a ball valve effect
- atelectasis resulting from total obstruction of the airway.

Both processes are usually present in the same case making the management of these babies difficult. Artificial ventilation can cause significant air leak if standard IRDS settings of short inspiratory times and fast rates are used. In addition, meconium aspiration syndrome (MAS) can be complicated by PPHN.

Initial management of MAS consists of nursing the baby in high-inspired oxygen to reduce the hypoxia caused by ventilation–perfusion (V/Q) mismatching and to prevent the development of PPHN. Higher pCO_2 levels are acceptable in an effort to avoid intubation and ventilation. If a baby needs ventilation then sedation and/or paralysis should be used to enable the use of slow rates and long inspiratory/expiratory times. Meconium inactivates surfactant and frequent dosing with surfactant has been shown to be helpful. If a baby is failing, standard ventilation high-frequency oscillatory ventilation can be used, but is often unsuccessful due to the non-homogeneous nature of MAS. Nitric oxide may reduce the need for extracorporeal membrane oxygenation (ECMO). If a baby does require ECMO the survival in most units is >90 per cent, therefore transfer to an ECMO centre should be considered early in the neonate failing conventional therapy.

KEY LEARNING POINTS

- A neonate with respiratory distress must be treated with antibiotics.
- Early surfactant use is advantageous in IRDS.
- Severe MAS should be referred to an ECMO centre.

Chronic lung disease

Premature lungs are easily damaged even if there is little in the way of IRDS. Chronic lung disease (CLD) is now the preferred term for this damage rather than bronchopulmonary dysplasia (BPD). The damage to the lungs of babies is less severe now than in the pre-surfactant, pre-antenatal steroids era. However, some severely affected babies may still behave in a fashion similar to those with 'old style' BPD. Chronic lung disease is a complication of any neonatal lung injury, though this is virtually exclusively IRDS with ventilator-induced damage. It is defined as oxygen dependency at 28 days with clinical evidence of respiratory distress and an abnormal chest radiograph. High inspired oxygen and lung damage from over-distension of the surfactant deficient lung by ventilation are the most important causes. Infection, persistent ductus arteriosus and the poorly developed antioxidant system of the premature baby are important contributing factors. As more smaller babies are surviving, the incidence of CLD is increasing.

There is a lack of clear evidence about treatment of established CLD. It is important to ensure that a normal oxygen saturation is obtained using oxygen therapy, usually by low flow oxygen cannulae. In these older infants a saturation of greater than 93–95 per cent is optimal. Nutrition is vital to ensure ongoing growth as the babies will effectively outgrow their illness while in the neonatal unit in most cases.

Medical treatment with steroids has been shown to have short-term benefits of weaning from ventilation or decreasing oxygen need. This is at the expense of inducing a catabolic state that can interfere with growth and there are concerns about the long-term effects on brain development. Postnatal steroids should therefore be reserved for the most severe cases where there is concern about death from CLD. Inhaled steroids do not carry the same concerns regarding short- or long-term effects, but have not been shown to be useful. Diuretics have been shown to have short-term beneficial changes on lung function measurements but, again, not to affect long-term outcome. There are increased risks of nephrocalcinosis in babies treated with diuretics.

Bronchodilators (either inhaled or in the form of high-dose theophylline) have been advocated as histological examination of severe CLD demonstrates bronchial smooth muscle hypertrophy and these babies often wheeze when unwell. Again there is no established evidence. The wheeze is likely due in part to the small airway size.

In summary, optimal nutrition and adequate oxygenation are the most effective treatments for CLD. Most infants will outgrow their oxygen requirement before they are ready to be discharged. A small number will continue to need oxygen after they are sucking all their feeds and it is now established practice to send these babies home with domiciliary oxygen.

In the long term, these infants will have good respiratory function. In the first few years they are at risk of decompensating with lower respiratory infections. Respiratory syncytial virus (RSV) is the most often identified pathogen but influenza A and parainfluenza viruses and adenovirus will often cause similar problems. All these children should be protected in the winter months with parental education to avoid risks and influenza vaccination if older than 6 months. The roles of pneumococcal vaccination and passive immunization against RSV are not yet established.

KEY LEARNING POINTS

- Limiting ventilator-induced lung damage is the optimal approach to CLD management.
- Medical therapy produces short-term effects but may have significant side effects.
- Avoidance of hypoxaemia and growth failure are the primary medical goals in CLD.

Congenital malformations

Congenital diaphragmatic hernia

CASE STUDY

A male infant is born at term and immediately develops respiratory distress and cyanosis. He is intubated and ventilated. On examination he has reduced breath sounds on the left and his apex displaced to the right. He has a scaphoid abdomen. A chest x-ray shows a left diaphragmatic hernia. He remains hypoxic with a high pCO_2 and his ventilator pressures are increased. A short period of improvement follows before he collapses. A repeat chest x-ray shows a left pneumothorax which is drained.

Congenital diaphragmatic hernia (CDH) affects 1 in 2000 pregnancies. The cause of the defect is unknown. Thirty per cent of affected babies have other abnormalities such as cardiac defects, chromosomal abnormalities (trisomy 13, 18 and 21) or the CDH can be part of a dysmorphic syndrome such as Fryns. Eighty per cent of defects are on the left side. There is significant lung hypoplasia on the affected side, but the contra-lateral lung is also affected due to mediastinal shift. In both lungs there is a decrease in the number of bronchiolar and arteriolar divisions and excessive muscularization of the pulmonary vessels. This leads to a decreased lung surface area and an increased pulmonary vascular resistance with hypoxia, hypercarbia and PPHN. Antenatal diagnosis is possible though it may be difficult to distinguish a CDH from a CCAM. Clinical presentation varies, large defects may present with mild respiratory distress or a newborn can become moribund immediately after delivery and die in labour suite on the resuscitaire. Antenatal treatment either by repairing the defect early in pregnancy or obstructing the trachea to stimulate lung growth has now been abandoned. Current management aims to identify cases antenataly, offer planned delivery in a tertiary centre (possibly only in a centre offering ECMO), use low ventilator pressures (permissive hypercapnia from gentle ventilation) designed to reduce the risk of pneumothorax, and to commence iNO and other measures for PPHN if indicated. Surgical repair of the hernia is delayed until the pulmonary vascular resistance has decreased. Large defects may require the placement of a gortex patch at operation, and in this situation as the child grows, re-herniation through the repaired diaphragm may occur. Research into postnatal stimulation of lung growth with perflurocarbon liquid is ongoing.

Congenital cystic adenomatous malformation

Congenital cystic adenomatous malformation (CCAM) is the commonest congenital lung malformation. *In utero*, it appears as an isolated lung opacity that can expand, causing mediastinal shift and hydrops in extreme cases. After birth there is an initial failure of lung fluid to clear but this may be followed by a rapid expansion of the lesion due to a ball valve effect. Subsequent mediastinal shift may cause cardiac and respiratory compromise. After the immediate neonatal period it is unlikely that the lesion will expand significantly but it is recommended that the lesion be removed electively as there have been reported cases of later cancerous change.

Congenital lobar emphysema

Congenital lobar emphysema may be diagnosed *in utero* as a lung opacity. After birth the affected lobe will expand and cause respiratory compromise. Treatment is surgical removal.

Sequestration

Sequestration can be confused with CCAM *in utero*. However, after birth there will not be a problem with lung expansion. These lesions tend to present with repeated infections rather than lobar inflation. Investigation will show a separate arterial supply to the sequestered lobe.

Pulmonary hypoplasia

Pulmonary hypoplasia can be caused by a congenital abnormality or be due to oligohydramnios. A common cause is diaphragmatic hernia where the lung on the affected side will be hypoplastic. Often there will be associated pulmonary hypertension and PPHN. In cases of oligohydramnios there may be bilateral lung hypoplasia, which can be severe. Neuromuscular disease with reduced fetal breathing will also cause bilateral hypoplastic lungs.

Choanal atresia

CASE STUDY

You are asked to see a term neonate in the delivery suite. Pregnancy and delivery were uncomplicated. Following birth, the baby girl has blue episodes. When you examine the baby, she is active, crying and pink with no respiratory or cardiac abnormality. As she settles and stops crying she goes blue, following this she cries and goes pink. You are unable to pass a feeding tube down either nares.

Choanal atresia is a failure of the posterior nares to form. There may be a complete membrane causing obstruction. More often there is severe stenosis causing a functional obstruction. Most neonates are obligate nasal breathers and so are only able to breath when crying through their mouth. If choanal atresia is suspected a feeding tube should be passed. If this is impossible a CT scan should be performed to identify the degree of obstruction. Treatment involves surgical drilling of a nasal airway followed by placement of a bilateral nasal stent for several weeks. Restenosis can occur.

Pierre–Robin sequence

CASE STUDY

A male infant is noted to have a small mandible and a cleft palate shortly after birth. He has moderate sternal recession and a high pCO_2 on blood gas estimation. Positioning the infant prone reduces his recession and normalizes his pCO_2.

The Pierre–Robin sequence is a triad comprising a midline posterior cleft palate, a hypoplastic mandible and upper airway obstruction caused by the subsequent posterior positioning of the tongue. The obstruction can worsen over the first week, and if it is not treated the hypoxaemia and hypercapnia will lead to pulmonary hypertension and failure to thrive. Mild cases respond to positioning to enable the tongue to fall forward. Passage of a long nasopharyngeal tube (Figure 5.1) to sit above the larynx is an effective means of providing an airway and parents can be taught to pass this at home. If the airway obstruction is severe a tracheostomy may be required. Long-term outcome is good with jaw growth occurring. The cleft palate will need surgical repair.

KEY LEARNING POINTS

- Congenital malformations causing neonatal respiratory problems are rare.
- Detailed investigation may be required following an abnormal chest radiograph.
- If a congenital malformation is identified *in utero*, delivery should be in a specialist unit.

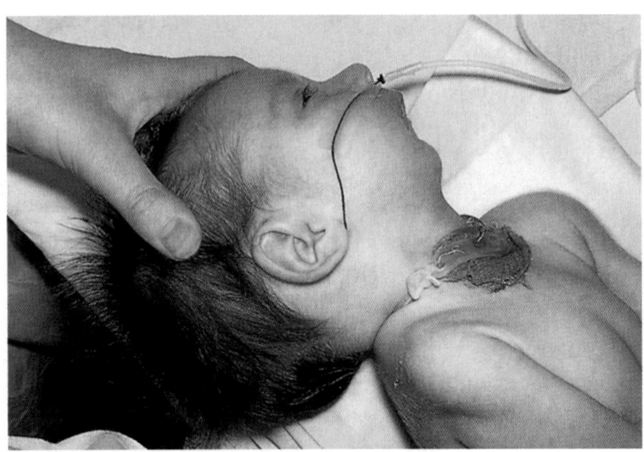

Figure 5.1 A case of Pierre–Robin syndrome

NEONATAL RESPIRATORY SUPPORT

Oxygen therapy

Oxygen is a highly reactive molecule that, although essential for life, is toxic in excess. Increasing evidence suggests that premature babies exposed to excess oxygen are more likely to develop chronic lung disease (CLD) and retinopathy of prematurity (ROP). Research has shown ROP rates may be reduced by lowering saturation limits. There is no consensus as to the 'optimal' oxygen saturation and wide variations in practice exist among NICUs. We suggest that in premature neonates in the first week of life saturations should be in the range 85–92 per cent. At some point this could be increased to 92–95 per cent. Whatever limits are set, large swings in saturation from low to high should be avoided as this is a risk factor for the development of retinopathy. Larger term babies are less likely to develop retinopathy and in the clinical situation of PPHN saturation targets should be >95 per cent to encourage a fall in pulmonary vascular resistance. Babies with congenital cardiac disease will often have oxygen saturations in the range of 70 per cent. There are three methods of providing additional FiO_2 (Table 5.9).

Continuous positive airways pressure

Continuous positive airways pressure splints the upper airway preventing pharyngeal collapse caused by increased respiratory effort. It prevents end-expiratory alveolar collapse increasing compliance. It is now accepted that early CPAP is effective in preventing atelectasis caused by surfactant deficiency. Continuous positive airways pressure should be commenced shortly after delivery at 4–6 cmH_2O, increasing by 1–2 cmH_2O if the baby continues to show recession. CPAP may cause gastric distension and diaphragmatic splinting. Irritation of the nostril and nasal septum can occur.

Table 5.9 Methods of providing additional fraction of inspired oxygen (FiO_2)

	Advantages	Disadvantages
Incubator oxygen	No need for equipment No need for tape to skin	Need closed incubator FiO_2 changes if ports open to access infant
Head box	Less oxygen flow than above Able to measure FiO_2 accurately No need for tape to skin	Occludes infant's face from parents Prevents facial care from nurse Not portable
Nasal cannula	No barrier to parent or nurse Portable	Tape to skin Unable to measure FiO_2 accurately

Intubation

Shouldered endotracheal tubes (ETTs) were developed to prevent low insertions. However, the wide portion of the tube can be pushed down with force on the larynx, causing damage, and therefore straight ETTs are preferable. A chest radiograph should be taken to ensure that the tip of the ETT is not misplaced. Ideally the tip should be just beyond the clavicles. Long-term damage to the nares, nasal septum or palate can occur from pressure. Subglottic stenosis is rare now since babies are ventilated for shorter periods.

Intermittent positive pressure ventilation

Several modes of intermittent positive pressure ventilation (IPPV) are available on modern neonatal ventilators, which also have graphic displays and volume measurements. It has not yet been shown that the use of synchronized ventilation leads to improved respiratory outcomes, although short-term physiological benefits have been demonstrated. The three commonest ventilator modes are described in Table 5.10.

Ventilation weaning

Weaning using a synchronized mode is beneficial compared with conventional mandatory ventilation (CMV). And patient-triggered ventilation (PTV)/synchronized IPPV (SIPPV) leads to shorter weaning times than synchronized intermittent mandatory ventilation (SIMV). Endotracheal tube (ET) CPAP increases the work of breathing, leading to atelectasis, which explains the benefit of PTV/SIPPV. When weaning on SIMV the baby spends increasing periods of time on ET CPAP as the rate is decreased. In general, the peak inspiratory pressure should not be reduced below 12 cmH_2O if using SIPPV/PTV, or 15 cmH_2O on SIMV with a low rate. The modes of ventilation are summarized in Table 5.10.

Table 5.10 Modes of ventilation

Abbreviation	Description	Established role
CMV (conventional mandatory ventilation) IMV (intermittent mandatory ventilation)	Non-synchronized standard time cycled pressure limited (TCPL) ventilation. Rate, inspiratory time, peak and end expiratory pressure are set Baby can take additional breaths with no support from ventilator	All roles if older ventilator used *or* In apnoeic/paralysed/heavily sedated baby with no respiratory effort
SIMV (synchronized intermittent mandatory ventilation)	Synchronized triggering of ventilator delivering positive pressure support up to a set number of breaths using TCPL ventilation as above Baby can take additional breaths with no support from ventilator	All roles if initial high back-up rate used *or* When moving to a weaning strategy and staff more comfortable with reducing rate and pressure rather than pressure alone.
SIPPV (synchronized intermittent positive pressure ventilation) *or* PTV (patient-triggered ventilation)	Every breath taken by baby results in triggered positive pressure support with a back-up number of breaths set in case of apnoea using TCPL ventilation	Initial mode with possible switch to SIMV for weaning as above *or* Initial mode and weaning if staff comfortable with pressure reduction alone

High-frequency oscillatory ventilation

High-frequency ventilators use high mean airway pressures to maintain lung volumes, but deliver small tidal volumes, reducing injury to lungs. High-frequency oscillatory ventilation is accepted as rescue therapy for near term neonates failing maximum conventional ventilation and it is very effective in hyaline membrane disease as the high mean airway pressure keeps the surfactant deficient lung open without the need to use high peak pressures. It may have a role as the initial form of ventilation in very preterm babies with minimal lung disease, reducing their risk of pulmonary injury.

Strategy for use in IRDS

In IRDS lung inflation may be poor for a given mean airway pressure (MAP) as the surfactant deficient lung is poorly compliant and is on the inflation limb of the pressure/volume curve (Figure 5.2). A high MAP is required

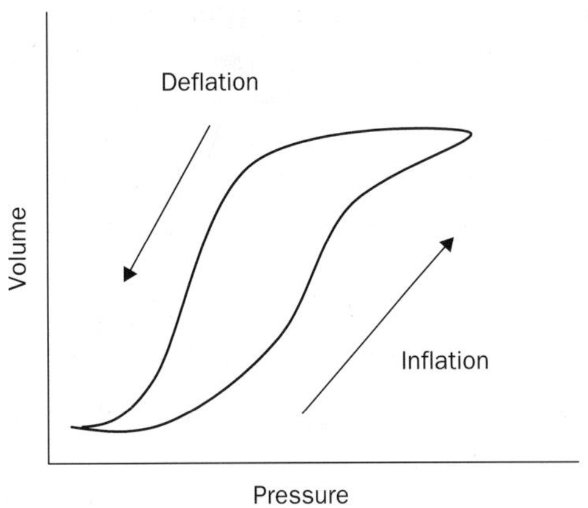

Figure 5.2 Pressure/volume curves

initially (increase MAP on CMV by 2 cmH_2O). As the lung inflates, the compliance improves and tidal volumes increase for the same settings, and as the lung approaches optimal inflation the FiO_2 decreases. Optimal lung inflation seen in a chest radiograph usually correlates with obtaining an 8–9 posterior rib level expansion of the right hemidiaphragm with decreased lung opacification. A flattened diaphragm, narrow heart or intercostal lung bulging are signs of overdistension. Once the lung is at optimal inflation with an FiO_2 of 25–30 per cent the MAP can be reduced without significant loss of lung volume. Failure to reduce the MAP will lead to overdistension.

The pCO_2 is affected by the amplitude and frequency settings. Initially the amplitude should be varied to control pCO_2. Increasing the amplitude lowers pCO_2. Changes in frequency can be made though 10 Hz is the normal setting. Decreasing the frequency lowers pCO_2.

Issues relating to high-frequency oscillatory ventilation

POOR OXYGENATION

The FiO_2 is a guide to lung inflation. If the lung is optimally inflated the FiO_2 will be less than 30 per cent. It may not reach such a low level if the lung pathology is not IRDS. Generally, however, an increased FiO_2 reflects atelectasis or overdistension. A chest radiograph is essential for diagnosis though decreased blood pressure and perfusion may occur in overdistension. It may be necessary to empirically decrease or increase the MAP to see what effect this has on oxygenation. Secretions can cause problems by increasing the resistance in the ETT, which will dampen the high-frequency oscillatory ventilation waveform and make ventilation less effective.

AIR LEAK

High-frequency oscillatory ventilation is the preferred mode of ventilation in established air leak due to the small in tidal volumes promoting resolution. There is a compromise between attaining optimal lung inflation and causing overdistension or continued air leak. Look for overdistension early with a chest radiograph.

> Initial settings
>
> - MAP equal to, or slightly lower than on, CMV
> - Frequency of 10 Hz, but consider increasing to 12–15 Hz
> - Amplitude set to produce minimal chest wall movement
> - Allow the pCO_2 to rise if the pH is >7.20

CONGENITAL DIAPHRAGMATIC HERNIA

There is usually one severely affected hypoplastic lung and one less severely affected. Management is aimed at ensuring optimal inflation of the better lung without causing overinflation of the smaller lung. Use the initial settings for air leak as above. The aim of increasing MAP is not to lower the FiO_2 to 30 per cent but rather to produce an improvement in oxygenation. Once this happens the MAP should be left constant and the lung will slowly inflate as the compliance changes and improves with increasing inflation.

MECONIUM ASPIRATION SYNDROME

Babies with MAS are often less responsive to high-frequency oscillatory ventilation as the disease tends to be patchy and is associated with air-trapping. There is often an associated degree of cardiac impairment caused by hypoxia, which leads to hypotension when the MAP is increased. Babies with MAS who have been ventilated for several days will often have a chest radiograph suggestive of diffuse homogeneous lung disease and may then respond better to the high-frequency oscillatory ventilation.

EXTUBATION

> End-points for weaning MAP:
>
> - MAP at 6 cmH_2O and FiO_2 <40 per cent then extubate
> - Problems with weaning MAP to 6 cmH_2O: change to CMV
> - Problems with excessive secretions: change to CMV

If after changing to CMV the baby develops increasing FiO_2 or increasing MAP, consider changing back to high-frequency oscillatory ventilation.

KEY LEARNING POINTS

- Ventilator strategies vary with lung pathology.
- Optimal inflation and avoidance of volutrauma are key goals.

Inhaled nitric oxide therapy

Nitric oxide is an endogenous vasodilator derived from L-arginine by several nitric oxide synthetases. It has an extremely high affinity for haemoglobin and rapidly binds to it, becoming inactive as it does so. In the clinical setting inhaled nitric oxide exerts only a vasodilator effect in the lung. Treatment with inhaled nitric oxide aims to decrease shunting caused by pulmonary hypertension. It is mainly used as a rescue therapy in near term neonates with hypoxic respiratory failure. Ventilation should be optimized prior to starting treatment because inhaled nitric oxide (iNO) is effective only in ventilated lung units. It may be best to recruit the lung first with high-frequency oscillatory ventilation. Nitric oxide interferes with platelet function and is relatively contraindicated in thrombocytopenia, coagulopathy, periventricular haemorrhage and other active bleeding (e.g. pulmonary haemorrhage). A response to iNO is defined as an increase in post-ductal oxygenation of 10 mmHg or an increase in SaO_2 by 10 per cent within one hour.

Extracorporeal membrane oxygenation

A near term neonate with reversible respiratory failure unresponsive to ventilation should be placed on extracorporeal membrane oxygenation (ECMO). This is not in itself a treatment but rather a method of providing respiratory support while any reversible lung pathology such as MAS improves. Heparinization and alterations in cerebral blood flow created by ECMO cause a significant increase in the risk of cerebral haemorrhage – this risk is greatest in premature infants.

Current indications for neonatal ECMO are:

- Weight >1500 g, 35 weeks completed gestation
- No significant coagulopathy or uncontrollable bleeding
- No major intracranial haemorrhage (>grade I)
- Mechanical ventilation <10–14 days
- No reason to question continuing conventional care or major congenital malformation

Before consideration of ECMO infants should be failing conventional therapy, which now includes therapies such as HFOV and iNO. The use of an oxygenation index (OI) >30 should act as the trigger for contact with an ECMO centre since an OI >40 carries a 60 per cent mortality with present conventional treatment.

KEY LEARNING POINTS

- Optimal ventilation is essential before using inhaled nitric oxide.
- Extracorporeal membrane oxygenation provides temporary respiratory support, enabling resolution of acute problems.

NEONATAL CENTRAL NERVOUS SYSTEM DISEASE

Periventricular haemorrhage

Despite advances in neonatal care periventricular haemorrhage (PVH) remains a significant cause of morbidity and mortality in premature babies. A premature baby has a vascular area around the ventricles known as the subependymal germinal matrix. This is an area of neuronal proliferation, which is present until about 32 weeks' gestation. Capillary bleeding in this area is the cause of PVH. Bleeding occurs in sick premature babies who lose the ability to control cerebral blood flow. A lack of cerebral autoregulation combined with acute changes in cerebral blood flow due to events such as pneumothorax, asynchrony between spontaneous and ventilator breaths, suction, seizures, or rapid changes in pH, pCO_2, or pO_2 can lead to an acute bleed. This vascular germinal matrix involutes as gestation advances.

Periventricular haemorrhage is generally classified into four grades of severity according to work by Papille which is useful for prognostic reasons. The original classification was based on CT findings, but the grades have been adopted to describe ultrasound findings, which remains the standard method of diagnosis of PVH (Table 5.11).

Major sequelae of PVH are due to either destruction of cerebral parenchyma or to the development of posthaemorrhagic hydrocephalus.

Porencephalic cysts

An area of the brain parenchyma involved in a grade 4 haemorrhage will evolve into a porencephalic cyst. Healing in areas of the brain destroyed by PVH results in

Table 5.11 Standard methods of diagnosis of periventricular dilation

Grade 1	Germinal matrix bleed	Good outcome
Grade 2	Intraventricular blood but no ventricular dilatation	Good outcome
Grade 3	Intraventricular blood and ventricular dilatation	Less good outcome (depends on dilatation)
Grade 4	Intraventricular blood and parenchymal blood	Poor outcome

the formation of fluid-filled spaces that communicate with the adjoining ventricle. This contrasts with the cysts of periventricular leukomalacia (PVL, see below) which are adjacent to but do not communicate with the ventricle. The pattern of long-term injury depends on which area of the brain is involved, with motor handicap being common as the cortical spinal motor tracts are present in this region.

Posthaemorrhagic hydrocephalus

Blood present in the ventricle will not by itself cause any problem unless the volume is large enough to cause hypotension. However, subsequent obstruction caused by inflammation affecting the arachnoid villi and debris obstructing drainage channels can lead to the development of hydrocephalus (grade 3 PVH). It is common for mild ventricular dilatation to occur. In the face of increasing hydrocephalus defined by an increasing ventriculo-cerebral ratio on ultrasound, increasing OFC and clinical signs of separated sutures and a tense fontanelle surgical intervention should be considered (see Chapter 7). Medical treatment with diuretics, acetazolamide and isosorbide are still used but it is controversial if they are beneficial or even harmful in the long term. Irrigation of the ventricular system with artificial CSF following fibrinolysis is still an experimental technique (the DRIFT trial).

Prevention of periventricular haemorrhage

Modern neonatal care is aimed at reducing acute changes in cerebral blood flow. The reduced incidence of pneumothorax has helped to decrease the incidence of severe PVH. Drug therapy with indometacin in the first few days of life is effective in the prevention of PVH. However, it does not reduce long-term neurological disability and is therefore not an established therapy.

KEY LEARNING POINTS

- Optimizing obstetric and neonatal care reduces PVH.
- There is no effective medical treatment for established PVH.
- Prediction of handicap is difficult and affected babies require neurodevelopment follow-up.

Periventricular leukomalacia

Periventricular leukomalacia is an ischaemic brain injury occurring in the watershed areas of the deep penetrating branches from the middle cerebral artery that supply the white matter adjacent to the lateral ventricles. Damage to the descending corticospinal tract leads to impairment of motor function such as diplegia. The visual and acoustic radiations can also be involved. Damage can occur *in utero* if there is poor placental function or fetal blood loss. Other antenatal events such as chorioamnionitis with cytokine production have also been implicated in cerebral white matter damage possibly due to free radical damage. Following delivery hypotension may cause reduced cerebral perfusion due to impaired cerebral autoregulation. Cerebral artery vasoconstriction may occur secondary to hypocarbia and persistent ductus arteriosus may cause poor perfusion due to the 'steal' of blood through a large duct. Periventricular leukomalacia tends to be bilateral compared to the unilateral changes often seen in PVH. It occurs most commonly in babies less than 32 weeks' gestation. Most babies with PVL will develop motor handicap and cerebral palsy. The commonest pattern is one of spastic diplegia, although if the injury is severe the child may have quadriplegia. There may be no intellectual impairment even in those with significant motor disability, but the smallest survivors may have associated PVH and marked global disability.

Investigation

Initial head ultrasound shows a white periventricular flare. In some infants this will fade, with subsequent cyst formation two to four weeks later in those with significant ischaemic damage. Some do not develop cystic changes but show mild irregular ventriculomegaly. If the initial scan already shows cyst formation the insult can be assumed to have occurred antenatally. A CT scan will show ventriculomegaly and loss of white matter.

KEY LEARNING POINTS

- Delivery of a compromised fetus may prevent PVL.
- Avoiding hypotension and hypocarbia may reduce PVL.
- Medical treatment with free radical scavengers has not been proved.

In addition MRI will show abnormal signal intensity of the deep white matter and thinning of the posterior body and splenium of the corpus callosum.

Neonatal seizures

Most neonatal seizures occur as a reaction to an acute neonatal problem such as hypoxia, electrolyte imbalance, infection or intraventricular bleed. Therefore, most seizures occur early rather than later in the neonatal period. It may be difficult to distinguish the 'jittery' baby from one having a seizure and observation of an otherwise well baby reported as having a seizure in the postnatal ward is preferred to initiating investigations. Jitteriness resembles a tremor, is stopped with holding the limb affected and is not associated with ocular deviation or other physiological changes.

Metabolic causes

Metabolic causes of seizures may occur early or late. The most important early cause is hypoglycaemia, with hyponatraemia or hypocalcaemia occurring less frequently. Both hypocalcaemia and hypomagnesaemia can cause later seizures. It is less likely that any inborn errors of metabolism will be the cause of a neonatal seizure but this should be excluded in a baby who is older than 72 hours, is feeding and has associated lethargy or acidosis.

Hypoxic-ischaemic encephalopathy

This may be suspected from the delivery and resuscitation history. Significant hypoxic-ischaemic encephalopathy will lead to seizures in the first 72 hours of life. Some of these seizures may be subtle, consisting of lip smacking or cycling movements of the limbs on a background of an irritable, anxious looking baby. Otherwise focal clonic or generalized seizures may occur. These children are at risk of renal and hepatic impairment and these should be excluded.

Neonatal stroke

This is increasingly recognized and the initial presentation is with early seizures in an otherwise normal baby. Magnetic resonance imaging reveals changes most typically associated with a middle cerebral artery infarction. Inherited clotting disorders (protein C or S deficiency, antithrombin 3) must be excluded by performing a thrombophilia screen on the parents.

Periventricular haemorrhage

Significant PVH can cause seizures. Often these babies are extremely immature and have associated pathology. It can be difficult to diagnosis the subtle seizures which are seen in this situation. More commonly the PVH will be identified on head ultrasound examination.

Meningitis

Meningitis should be excluded in all babies with seizures and no identified cause.

Neonatal abstinence syndrome

Drug withdrawing infants/babies can suffer seizures. This can be precipitated by the use of naloxone at delivery. Most children will have a relevant history and associated features.

Benign idiopathic neonatal seizures

Benign idiopathic neonatal seizures are also known as 'fifth day fits'. They can occur between days 4 and 6. The seizures are often short lasting and multifocal.

Myoclonic jerks

Myoclonic jerks can be thought initially to be seizures. The presentation is one of rhythmic movements that occur only during sleep.

Outcome of seizures

The outcome depends on the aetiology. In the situation when no abnormality has been identified despite full investigation outcome is usually good with normal developmental progress.

KEY LEARNING POINTS

- Check blood glucose in any neonatal seizure.
- Investigation is required in most babies to establish a diagnosis (Table 5.12).

AFTERCARE OF HIGH-RISK BABIES

Immunizations

In the neonatal period

Hepatitis B vaccine is recommended in all babies whose mothers have a history of hepatitis B infection. In particularly high-risk situations (i.e. where there is a history of maternal infection during pregnancy or where maternal hepatitis B surface antigen is positive) hepatitis B immunoglobulin should also be administered shortly after birth.

Varicella zoster immunoglobulin is recommended as soon as possible after birth for all babies born to women

Table 5.12 Approach to a child with seizures

History	Initial approach to investigation	Treatment
Useful in hypoxia-induced encephalopathy and neonatal abstinence syndrome	Exclude jitteriness or myoclonic jerks Measure glucose and electrolytes Septic screen including lumbar puncture Cranial ultrasound	Correct any metabolic disturbance and treat sepsis if present Phenobarbital is still the initial drug of choice. A stepwise approach of loading with 20 mg/kg followed by another 10 mg/kg is preferred. Measure drug levels if seizures continue with further 5–10 mg/kg to achieve therapeutic levels. If seizures persist despite therapeutic levels add phenytoin. Failure to control seizures with adequate phenobarbital and phenytoin levels is a poor prognostic sign. Benzodiazepines either as a clonazepan infusion or midazolam bolus can be added at this stage. In most children seizures will be controlled with phenobarbital. Common clinical practice is to discharge a baby on phenobarbital and allow them to simply grow out of the dose prescribed and discontinue it at 3–4 months
	Investigation if no cause identified from above Electroencephalogram Cranial MRI or CT Urine amino and organic acids Serum amino acid assay	

who develop chicken pox in the five days before or two days after delivery. It should also be considered following postnatal exposure to chicken pox either in premature infants where the mother is susceptible, or in infants < 1000 g irrespective of maternal immunity.

Bacille Calmette Guérin (BCG) vaccine is recommended either in the neonatal period or with the primary immunizations at 2 months in high-risk infants. These include infants with one or both parents of Asian, African or Central/South American origin or where there is a current or past history of tuberculosis in the household.

Beyond the neonatal period

PRIMARY IMMUNIZATIONS – DTP, HIB, MENINGITIS C AND POLIO

These are given in three doses at monthly intervals starting at 2 months (i.e. 2, 3 and 4 months) with no correction for prematurity. Infants who have received recent steroids or IV immunoglobulin may have impaired seroconversion and immunization should be delayed. Apnoeas are well described in premature infants following their first immunization, particularly if they have a history of apnoea or chronic lung disease.

INFANTS WITH CHRONIC LUNG DISEASE

Pneumococcal vaccine should be considered in infants with CLD, particularly if they required prolonged respiratory support or home oxygen therapy. Until recently the only vaccine available against invasive pneumococcal disease was a polysaccharide vaccine, which did not stimulate an adequate immune response in infants. Prevenar® is a conjugated pneumococcal vaccine that effectively stimulates the immune system of infants and creates immune system memory. It can be given in three doses at monthly intervals simultaneously with the DTP, HIB and meningitis C vaccines.

Palivizumab (Synagis®) is a humanized monoclonal antibody, which prevents entry of RSV into host cells. It is licensed for use in premature infants with CLD and has also been shown to be both safe and effective in infants with congenital heart disease. It is given as a series of monthly intramuscular injections throughout the RSV season. A course of five injections costs between £2000 and £3500, depending on the infant's body weight; opinions regarding cost effectiveness vary among paediatricians.

Influenza A vaccine is also recommended in these infants in their first winter season.

KEY LEARNING POINTS

- Commence routine immunizations at usual postnatal age.
- Infants with CLD may require additional vaccinations in the winter months.

FOLLOW-UP AND LONG-TERM OUTCOME

Many complications arising from the neonatal period do not become apparent until the child is much older (Table 5.13). For the very preterm infants a follow-up programme of at least two years is essential to ensure that the children are walking and speaking. However even children who appear 'normal' at 2 years old are at risk of significant problems at school (see below). Close liaison with local child developmental clinics facilitates a smooth transition for infants who require long-term community care.

Cerebral palsy

Cerebral palsy is a term describing the end result of damage to the developing brain resulting in problems with movement, tone and posture. Children with cerebral palsy may also have cognitive, visual and/or hearing difficulties. Major causes of cerebral palsy in premature babies are PVH and PVL, which may lead to hemiplegia, diplegia or quadriplegia. Most children with cerebral palsy will leave the SCN with no apparent movement disorder, but as the CNS matures, changes in tone become obvious. No treatment will restore the damaged neural tissue, but early developmental physiotherapy is vital. This encourages good posture, enabling the infant to progress though each stage of normal motor development. The use of folded sheets as boundaries (similar to a nest) and side lying to bring the neonate's hands together in the midline near the face are measures that are routinely practised in most neonatal units. Speech and language therapists can help with the feeding problems that can cause later speech delay. Occupational therapists can help provide aids for sitting, walking etc. Many children will be able to go to mainstream school, but educational needs may favour placement in a special needs school.

Visual problems

Visual problems in premature babies may be due to retinopathy of prematurity (ROP), PVL, or direct damage to the visual cortex. Retinopathy of prematurity affects the blood vessels growing out of the optic disc to supply the retina. When a baby is born prematurely the peripheral retina is incompletely vascularized. During the first few weeks of life the vessels will continue to grow and will, in most infants, complete the normal supply to the whole

Table 5.13 Long-term outcome

Problem	Cause	Detection	Treatment
Cerebral palsy	Prematurity PVH PVL	Cranial ultrasound in NICU Cranial CT or MRI later Neurodevelopmental follow-up	Prevention of prematurity General good NICU care CDC with therapist input
Retinopathy of prematurity Other visual problems	Prematurity PVL PVH	Screening in NICU Neurodevelopmental follow-up	Laser photocoagulation Visual aids Behavioural
Learning problems	Prematurity PVL PVH	Long-term neurodevelopmental follow-up School	Psychology Teaching support
Bronchopulmonary dysplasia or chronic lung disease Small stature	Prematurity Ventilator lung damage *In utero* growth failure Poor nutritional support	Saturation monitors Chest radiograph Follow-up clinic	Oxygen Nutrition to allow for growth Dietitian support Growth hormone injections
Hearing loss	PVH PVL Drug toxicity	Targeted screening Repeat at follow-up clinic	Hearing aids Cochlear implants

NICU, neonatal intensive care unit; CDC, child development clinic; PVH, periventricular haemorrhage; PVL, periventricular leukomalacia.

retina. However, if this process is interrupted there is a risk that the avascular retina will cause vascular proliferation with increased risk of bleeding and retinal detachment. Retinopathy of prematurity is multifactorial with extreme prematurity and periods of hypoxia or hyperoxia recognized as important risk factors. Infants at risk of ROP should be screened until either the retina is fully vascularized or retinal ablation treatment is needed. Laser therapy is used to destroy the peripheral retina, preventing blindness from retinal detachment but causing a reduction in the peripheral visual fields. Even in the absence of ROP the visual pathways and cortex can both be damaged by either PVH or PVL. Any concern about sight should prompt ophthalmic assessment of the visual pathway. Cortical damage can cause blindness in an extreme case, but may also cause 'processing problems'. The child may see single objects well but, as the amount of information received increases, the visual processing system fails to cope. At school, reading aids (such as using a ruler under the sentence while reading) can help the child from getting lost while reading a page of a book.

Hearing problems

Sensorineural hearing loss can occur due to damage from drugs (e.g. gentamicin), hypoxia, PVH and PVL. The cause in a single child is probably a combination of mechanisms. All neonatal unit graduates should be screened for hearing loss. All neonatal units should aim to minimize ambient noise levels. Simple measures to reduce noise include not placing objects onto the incubator roof (may result in a magnified thump if they fall onto the roof), not clicking the incubator door shut, and providing ear protection during episodes of predicted high noise such as helicopter transfer.

Learning problems

There is a 'hidden' risk of learning problems that may only become apparent as the children start school. Early identification of learning problem allows prompt intervention. Children with cerebral palsy, visual impairment and deafness are at obvious risk of cognitive dysfunction. However, even more mature infants (32–34 weeks' gestation), who are passed as 'normal' at 2 years may end up with subtle but significant learning difficulties.

Short stature

Premature infants will mostly attain their expected adult height with catch up growth during the first 1–2 years if adequate nutrition is provided. Some infants remain small despite adequate calorie and protein intake and may respond to human growth hormone treatment by increasing their height velocity. However, it is not yet clear if final adult height is affected, but even if this is not changed the increase in a child's height during school years will be beneficial.

Barker's hypothesis

The 'thrifty phenotype' hypothesis was popularized by Professor Barker who suggested that children with IUGR have increased risk of developing some types of adult-onset disease. Diabetes, hypertension, myocardial events and stroke are all increased in infants with IUGR when they become adults. *In utero* fetal adaptation associated with IUGR can re-set normal physiological systems as a survival technique, which then becomes a problem when the child encounters different nutritional circumstances after birth. The concept of a 'thrifty phenotype' is one that will store fat when offered to protect against future famine.

KEY LEARNING POINTS

- Neurodevelopmental handicap may only become apparent after discharge.
- Visual problems are underrecognized in PVL.
- Adult disease may be a consequence of fetal and neonatal illness.

TECHNICAL SKILLS

Basic life support

All neonatal units delivering babies need to have personnel skilled in providing basic life support. In many

Any delivery unit should provide the following:

- Safe environment: resuscitaire; warm towels; clock
- Immediate care: assessment; stimulation; dry and replace wet towel
- If persisting apnoea: airway management (open, position, suction); facial oxygen; bag/mask IPPV

cases the need for neonatal resuscitation can be predicted. Premature birth, significant IUGR and when there has been passage of meconium or non-reassuring signs from fetal monitoring warn the labour ward staff that the neonate may be compromised. However, there is always a chance that a baby will be born apnoeic without any prior warning signs.

Most apnoeic neonates will respond to the measures outlined above. A baby who is bradycardic despite adequate ventilation should receive cardiac compressions. Neonatal resuscitation can be learnt from the Newborn Life Support course (provided by the Resuscitation Council in the UK) or the Newborn Resuscitation Programme course. Some neonates require special resuscitation measures from birth (Table 5.14).

SPECIFIC PROBLEMS

Babies of diabetic mothers

Up to 10 per cent of pregnancies occur in women with abnormal glucose control, mostly due to gestational diabetes, increasing the risk to the fetus and neonate. Glucose crosses the placenta while insulin is unable to do so, and the fetus is subjected to high levels of glucose whenever maternal diabetic control is poor. A subsequent increase in fetal insulin production and islet cell hyperplasia results in increased growth of the fetus *in utero*. There is a subsequent increase in birth injuries and caesarean section delivery in these large babies. After birth the increased insulin production continues with

Table 5.14 Some infants require special measures from birth

Problem at birth	Complication it can cause	Approach to resuscitation
Congenital diaphragmatic hernia	Severe respiratory failure and airleak Persistent pulmonary hypertension of the newborn	Antenatal diagnosis Intubate Nasogastric tube and drainage Paralyse to control ventilation Low pressure ventilation No antenatal diagnosis Suspect if concave abdomen Check for mediastinal shift As above
Gastroschisis	Increased fluid and heat loss Gastrointestinal tract (GIT) ischaemia from traction to mesentery	Wrap at birth with clingfilm or other occlusive dressing Do not use saline soaked towels as these cool rapidly After wrapping lie on side supporting exposed GIT
Exomphalous	Increased fluid and heat loss	Wrap at birth with clingfilm or other occlusive dressing Do not use saline soaked towels as these cool rapidly After wrapping lie on side supporting exomphalous
Pierre-Robin sequence	Airway obstruction	Lie on side or prone Nasopharyngeal airway Intubate if possible if severe distress
Cystic hygroma	Airway obstruction	Nasopharyngeal airway Intubate if possible if severe distress
Congenital heart disease	Usually none at delivery Absent pulmonary valves can cause severe bronchial obstruction	If well but cyanosed assess cardiac status Ventilate with long (1 s) inspiratory time
Hydrops	Severe respiratory failure due to pleural effusions and/or ascitis	Intubate Paracentesis in LIF before draining pleural fluid Pleural drainage only if continued respiratory difficulty

consequent risk of neonatal hypoglycaemia. There are often problems achieving suck feeding and some babies will require tube feeding. There is an increase in congenital malformations such as cardiac defects and most have a hypertrophic cardiomyopathy. The children are more likely to have hypocalcaemia and polycythaemia (with secondary thrombocytopenia) and an increased risk of developing hyaline membrane disease. All the complications are related to the degree of diabetes control.

Drug withdrawal syndromes

CASE STUDY

You are asked to review a 3-day-old baby boy on the postnatal ward because of poor feeding, irritability, diarrhoea and vomiting. On further questioning it transpires that his mother was taking methadone and diazepam throughout pregnancy.

Neonatal abstinence syndrome (NAS) can affect babies delivered to mothers who are dependent on physically addictive drugs. Signs (in addition to those above) include sleeplessness, tremors, sneezing, yawning and seizures. Hypoxic ischaemic encephalopathy, hypoglycaemia, hyponatraemia, hypocalcaemia and meningeal irritation should be considered in the differential diagnosis. The incidence of NAS is increasing both nationally and internationally although there is little consensus on the optimal management. Non-pharmacological treatment includes the use of swaddling, dummies and frequent feeds. Pharmacological options include oral morphine, methadone and phenobarbitone. Treatment can be guided by the use of a validated scoring system (e.g. the Lipsitz score). An integrated multiagency approach is needed to meet the social and medical needs of these infants and their families and discharge planning involving the primary care team is imperative.

Hydrops fetalis

CASE STUDY

Antenatal review at 33 weeks' gestation of a mother with systemic lupus erythematosus (SLE) reveals that the fetus is bradycardic and developing heart failure. Steroids are given and delivery planned for the following day. At delivery the neonate is difficult to intubate and ventilate. Drainage of 50 mL of peritoneal fluid relieves abdominal distension and improves ventilation.

Hydrops fetalis describes a fetus or neonate with generalized oedema combined with fluid collections in pericardial, pleural and/or peritoneal spaces. The causes of hydrops fetalis are divided into immune (maternal–fetal blood group incompatibilities) or non-immune (Table 5.15). With the advent of anti-D immunization of rhesus-negative mothers, immune hydrops is rarely seen and non-immune causes account for the majority (>85 per cent) of cases of hydrops fetalis. This neonate had non-immune hydrops fetalis secondary to congenital heart block.

Hydropic infants are often in poor condition at birth and ideally two experienced members of staff should be present at the delivery. Oedema of the vocal cords makes intubation difficult and pulmonary hypoplasia is often present. Drainage of pleural and peritoneal effusions may improve respiratory compromise and aid resuscitation.

Neonatal SLE occurs in infants of asymptomatic mothers as well as in those with established disease (as in this case). It occurs as a result of transplacental passage of maternal autoantibodies, particularly Ro or La autoantibodies. It is characterized by one or more of the following: congenital heart block, cardiomyopathy, cutaneous lesions, hepatobiliary disease and thrombocytopenia.

Table 5.15 Commoner causes of non-immune hydrops fetalis

Causes	Per cent	Examples
Genetic and chromosomal	10–35	Trisomies, Turner syndrome
Haematological	10–27	Severe fetal anaemia (e.g. feto-maternal bleed, parvovirus)
Cardiovascular	19–26	Any cause of heart failure (e.g. supraventricular tachycardia, heart block, structural heart disease)
Twinning	4–8	Twin-to-twin transfusion syndrome
Idiopathic	15	

Apnoea of prematurity

The definition of significant apnoea has changed with time. Currently, it is accepted that a pause in breathing of 20 seconds is abnormal and this is the limit set on apnoea monitors. In reality an apnoea is only significant if it is part of a general physiological upset with desaturation and bradycardia. There are many causes of significant apnoea. Sepsis, anaemia, respiratory failure and gastro-oesophageal reflux can cause apnoea, but it may also occur as a normal physiological symptom of prematurity. Treatment is confined to excluding predisposing factors and then treating with respiratory stimulants (caffeine, aminophylline, theophylline).

Gastro-oesophageal reflux

CASE STUDY

A baby girl born at 31 weeks is now 3 weeks old. She is nursed in special care and has frequent desaturations, some accompanied with apnoea. She has four to six significant episodes per day. She is receiving three-hourly tube feeds and the nursing staff comment that most episodes follow after a feed. She has an occasional non-bilious vomit.

Gastro-oesophageal reflux (GOR) is difficult to diagnose in the neonatal period. A suggestive history may lead to investigation with a barium swallow or pH study. There is little information on normal reference values for pH studies in premature infants and some neonates may not produce enough acid to show a positive result in a pH study. Yet despite this it is clear that some babies with reflux on pH study will have lung disease suggestive of recurrent aspiration or will have significant apnoea. A trial of therapy, either postural or using thickened feeds with Gaviscon® or ranitidine may produce a decrease in episodes of desaturation.

Coagulopathy and thrombocytopenia

CASE STUDY

A baby boy is born at 25 weeks' gestation by emergency LUCS following significant antepartum haemorrhage. Following stabilization routine bloods are taken. The platelet count is normal but the coagulation screen shows a prolonged prothrombin time and activated partial thromboplastin time (APPT) with normal fibrinogen.

It is common to have a coagulopathy in preterm babies. In this clinical situation where there is a high risk of PVH or pulmonary haemorrhage the coagulopathy should be corrected. No further investigation is needed. However if the coagulation is persistently abnormal, or if an abnormality is identified in a near term neonate then further investigation of coagulation factors is required. Haemophilia should be suspected in males with excess bruising or bleeding.

CASE STUDY

A baby girl is born by spontaneous vaginal delivery (SVD) at term. After birth, the midwife notices a generalized petechial rash and minor bruising. Examination is otherwise normal. A coagulation screen is normal, but the platelet count is very low.

Thrombocytopenia in a well neonate is usually due to alloimmune thrombocytopenia. An affected neonate is platelet antigen positive and the mother is platelet antigen negative and has a normal platelet count. Sensitization of the mother occurs during pregnancy and the antibodies produced cross over the placenta and cause thrombocytopenia, which may be severe enough to cause fetal intracerebral haemorrhage. The platelet count will continue to fall in an affected neonate after birth and if it is <20 000 (or <50 000 in the presence of bleeding) urgent transfusion of platelet antigen negative platelets should be given. In subsequent pregnancies IV immunoglobulin infusions will prevent significant sequelae.

An alternative diagnosis of maternal idiopathic thombocytopenia should be considered if the maternal platelet count is low. If the mother had chronic idiopathic thombocytopenia requiring a splenectomy this may normalize the mother's platelet count while leaving the baby at risk. Congenital viral infections will cause IUGR and hepatitis. Thrombocytopenia due to infection or disseminated intravascular coagulation should be obvious clinically.

FURTHER READING

Rennie JM and Roberton NRC, eds. (1999) *Textbook of Neonatology*. Edinburgh: Churchill Livingstone.

Stephenson T, Marlow N, Watkin S, Grant J, eds. (2000) *Pocket Neonatology*. Edinburgh: Churchill Livingstone.

Chapter 6

Problems of infection, immunity and allergy

Rosie Hague

CLASSIFICATION OF PATHOGENS

Bacteria

Bacteria are classified according to their morphology (spherical bacteria are cocci and rod-shaped are bacilli), the properties of their cell walls (which determines ability to take up Gram stain) and by the conditions required for growth (aerobic or anaerobic).

Table 6.1, which is intended to be used for reference, lists the major pathogens in each category, together with the antibiotics to which they are likely to be sensitive while acknowledging that resistance to first-line agents is increasing.

Viruses

Viruses are classified on the basis of their genome into either DNA or RNA viruses. Each group is further distinguished by the possession (or not) of an envelope (Table 6.2) consisting of protein, lipid, and glycoprotein. Further classification is based on the capsid architecture.

Fungi

Fungi can be divided into two basic groups: yeasts and moulds (Table 6.3). Yeasts exist as single cells that reproduce by budding or fission. Moulds are multicellular and produce hyphae, which develop reproductive spores. Some fungi can exist in both forms.

WHY DO SOME CHILDREN GET MORE INFECTIONS THAN OTHERS?

Despite being surrounded by microorganisms, most children escape overwhelming infection. The risk of infection is determined by:

- the characteristics of the microorganism (virulence, or pathogenicity)
- the characteristics of the host
  - efficiency of defence mechanisms
  - behavioural characteristics
- the characteristics of the environment.

Established infection requires the following.

1 Contact with the host:
   - Overcrowding enhances transmission by direct contact, droplet or aerosol. Pre-school daycare is a risk factor for recurrent otitis media, respiratory and gastrointestinal infections.
   - Other environmental risks include exposure to animals that harbour potential human pathogens, insect vectors, contaminated water, inadequately cooked or contaminated food or exposure to blood or body fluids.
   - Behaviours increasing risk include low standards of personal hygiene inherent in young children, sexual behaviour, smoking and intravenous (IV) drug use.

2 Adherence to the host. This is assisted by:
   - pili on the surface of the Gram-negative pathogens such as *Escherichia coli*, which determine the virulence
   - lipoteichoic acid and M protein produced by Gram-positive organisms such as *Streptococcus*
   - the number and arrangement of binding sites on the host epithelium.

3 Local proliferation and tissue damage.
   - Potentially invasive organisms compete with the normal non-pathogenic flora by:
     - inhibiting the competition by producing antibiotic-like toxins (bacteriocins)
     - chelating ferric iron necessary for bacterial growth
     - producing IgA proteases which act against secretory IgA.
   - They spread by:
     - producing hyaluronidase which acts on hyaluronic acid in connective tissue, allowing

Table 6.1 Classification of bacteria

Class	Chief pathogens	Source	Clinical manifestations	Treatment of choice	Alternatives
Aerobic Gram-positive cocci	*Staphylococcus aureus*	Skin, nasal; GI carriage; environmental	Impetigo; soft tissue and deep abscess; wound infection; conjunctivitis; lymphadenitis; pneumonia; endocarditis/ pericarditis; osteomyelitis/arthritis Toxin mediated: food poisoning; scalded skin syndrome; toxic shock syndrome	Flucloxacillin	Cephalexin; cefuroxime; clindamycin; erythromycin; vancomycin* (MRSA only)
	Coagulase-negative staphylococcus	Normal skin flora	Bacteraemia in: immunocompromised; neonates Associated with foreign body, e.g. central venous line; shunt ventriculitis	Vancomycin	Teicoplanin; clindamycin if sensitive
	Group A streptococcus	Carried on skin and nasopharynx	Pharyngitis/tonsillitis; peritonsillar abscess; scarlet fever; impetigo; erysipelas; pneumonia; myositis/ fasciitis; osteomyelitis; puerperal sepsis	Penicillin	Ampicillin; erythromycin; clindamycin
	Group C, G streptococcus	Carried on skin and nasopharynx	Pharyngitis/tonsillitis adenitis	Penicillin	Erythromycin; clindamycin
	Group B streptococcus	GI and GU tract; skin and nasopharynx	Bacteraemia; neonatal meningitis; pneumonia; arthritis/osteomyelitis; cellulitis/adenitis	Penicillin + gentamicin	Ampicillin + gentamicin; cefotaxime
	Enterococcus (Group D streptococcus)	GI tract; environmental	UTI; endocarditis; bacteraemia; ?GI/biliary infection	Ampicillin + gentamicin for *E. faecalis*	* Vancomycin for resistant organisms Note emergence of vancomycin resistant enterococci
	Streptococcus viridans	Oral mucosa	Bacteraemia in immunocompromised; neonatal sepsis; dental caries; endocarditis; deep abscess, e.g. liver	Penicillin	Penicillin + gentamicin; vancomycin + gentamicin in immunocompromised
	Pneumococcus	25–30 per cent children Nasopharyngeal colonization	Bacteraemia; pneumonia; meningitis; otitis media; endocarditis/pericarditis; osteomyelitis/arthritis	Penicillin	Cefotaxime; ceftriaxone; ampicillin; erythromycin
Gram-negative cocci	*Moraxella catarrhalis*	URT colonization	Otitis media; sinusitis; pneumonia	Erythromycin	Augmentin; azithromycin; co-trimoxazole; cefuroxime; cefotaxime
	Neisseria meningitidis	10 per cent nasopharyngeal carriage	Septicaemia; meningitis; conjunctivitis; (pneumonia)	Cefotaxime; ceftriaxone; penicillin; rifampicin or ciprofloxacin for prophylaxis	
	Neisseria gonorrhoeae	GU tract-infected individuals	Ophthalmia neonatorum; scalp abscess; vaginitis; PID; urethritis; pharyngitis	Ceftriaxone	

Gram-positive bacilli	*Corynebacterium diphtheriae*	URT of carriers	Diphtheria	Penicillin; antitoxin	Erythromycin
	Bacillus anthracis	Domestic herbivores	Anthrax	Penicillin Ciprofloxacin	Erythromycin; tetracycline
	Bacillus cereus	Soil; food	Food poisoning	Supportive	
	Listeria	Animals; food-borne	Neonatal sepsis; meningitis; enterocolitis	Ampicillin + gentamicin	
	Mycobacterium tuberculosis	RT-infected individuals	Tuberculosis	Isoniazid + rifampicin + pyrazinamide + ethambutol	Dictated by sensitivities Note emergence of multidrug resistance
	Mycobacterium other spp.	Soil; water	Lymphadenitis; pulmonary (IC); disseminated disease (IC)	Excision Clarithromycin + ethambutol + rifampicin	Dictated by sensitivities
	Mycobacterium leprae	?? nasal;? fomites	Leprosy	Dapsone; clofazimine; rifampicin	
	Nocardia	Soil; dust	Pneumonia; CNS infection	Sulfisoxazole	Co-trimoxazole
Gram-negative bacilli – enterobacteria	*Citrobacter*	GI tract (rare)	Neonatal sepsis; neonatal meningitis	Cefotaxime	Meropenem
	Enterobacter	Soil; water; sewage	Central line infection; respiratory; UTI; biliary; neonatal meningitis	β-lactam + aminoglycoside	Often multi-resistant
	Escherichia coli	GI tract	Diarrhoeal disease Sepsis; UTI	Supportive Cefotaxime; trimethoprim/ augmentin	 Other β-lactams; aminoglycoside
	Klebsiella	Hand carriage; environment	Neonatal sepsis; neonatal meningitis; neonatal pneumonia	β-lactam + aminoglycoside	May have extended-spectrum β-lactamase resistance (ESBL)
	Morganella morganii	Faeces	UTI	Aminoglycoside	Dictated by sensitivities
	Proteus	Soil; sewage; manure	Neonatal sepsis; meningitis; osteomyelitis UTI	Ampicillin + gentamicin	
	Providencia	Faeces	UTI	β-lactam + aminoglycoside	Usually multiresistant
	Shigella	Faeces	Dysentery	Cefotaxime; ceftriaxone	Co-trimoxazole; ciprofloxacin
	Serratia	Hands; environment	Neonatal sepsis; neonatal meningitis; UTI	Amikacin	Dictated by sensitivities
	Salmonella	Animals; food	Typhoid; gastroenteritis	Cefotaxime; ceftriaxone	Co-trimoxazole ciprofloxacin
	Yersinia pestis	Rat fleas	Plague	Doxycycline	Chloramphenicol
	Yersinia enterocolitica	Animals; water; faeces	Enteritis; mesenteric adenitis; reactive arthritis	Cefotaxime + gentamicin	Co-trimoxazole; ciprofloxacin
Others	*Aeromonas*	Water sources	Septicaemia; gastroenteritis; skin infection	Tazocin; cefotaxime	Dictated by sensitivities
	Pasteurella	Animals oral flora	Local infection post-bite; respiratory infection	Penicillin	Augmentin; cefotaxime
	Vibrio cholerae	GI tract man; water	Cholera	Doxycycline; furazolidone	Ampicillin; erythromycin
	Vibrio parahaemolyticus	Water, sediments; shellfish	Gastroenteritis; dysentery	Supportive; doxycycline	

(*Continued*)

Table 6.1 *(Continued)*

Class	Chief pathogens	Source	Clinical manifestations	Treatment of choice	Alternatives
	Vibrio vulnificus	Water; shellfish	Wound infection; sepsis	Ampicillin; cefotaxime	
	Acinetobacter	Soil; fresh water; sewage	Suppurative infection; cerebral abscess	β-lactam + aminoglycoside	Dictated by sensitivities
	Alcalagenes	Water	Neonatal sepsis; meningitis	Cefotaxime + aminoglycoside; co-trimoxazole	Extended-spectrum β-lactam + aminoglycoside
	Eikenella	Mouth, GI/GU tract Normal flora	Periodontitis; pleuropulmonary infection; endocarditis	Incision and drainage; penicillin	
	Flavobacterium	Fresh water; salt water	Neonatal sepsis; meningitis	Erythromycin; vancomycin; co-trimoxazole; rifampicin	Combination of these required
	Pseudomonas	Soil; water; vegetation	Wound infection; dermatitis/otitis externa; chronic suppurative osteamyelitis; neonatal sepsis; skin infection in burns; Pulmonary infection in CF	Tazocin; ceftazidime; aminoglycoside; ciprofloxacin; meropenem	β-lactam or ciprofloxacin + aminoglycoside advisable
	Stenotrophomonas maltophilia	Water; soil	Catheter-related sepsis	β-lactam and aminoglycoside	Dictated by sensitivities
Gram-negative cocco-bacilli	*Bartonella bacilliformis*	Man + primate host; sandfly vector	Bartonellosis	Chloramphenicol	Penicillin; tetracycline
	Brucella abortus	Cattle	Brucellosis	Tetracycline	Ciprofloxacin + rifampicin
	Brucella melitensis	Goat		Gentamicin	
	Brucella suis	Pig		Co-trimoxazole + gentamicin	
	Bordetella	Respiratory tract infected individuals	Whooping cough	Erythromycin	Co-trimoxazole
	Calymmatobacterium granulomatis	Sexual transmission	Granuloma inguinale	Tetracycline; erythromycin	Co-trimoxazole
	Campylobacter jejuni	Animals	Enteritis; perinatal infection	Clarithromycin; azithromycin	
	Francisella tularensis	Tick-borne	Tularaemia	Erythromycin; streptomycin; gentamicin	
	Haemophilus influenzae	Respiratory tract	Bacteraemia; meningitis; pneumonia; epiglottitis; arthritis/osteomyelitis; cellulitis; pericarditis	Cefotaxime; ceftriaxone	Cefuroxime; augmentin; chloramphenicol
	Haemophilus ducreyi	STI	Chancroid	Azithromycin; ceftriaxone	
	Helicobacter pylori	Gastric mucosa	Peptic ulcer disease; gastritis	Bismuth + amoxicillin + metronidazole	
	Kingella	Oral flora	Suppurative arthritis; osteomyelitis; endocarditis	Penicillin	Ampicillin
	Legionella	Warm water	Legionnaire's disease	Erythromycin; azithromycin	Co-trimoxazole; doxycycline
	Streptobacillus moniliformis	Rat oropharynx	Rat bite fever	Penicillin	Cefuroxime/cefotaxime
	Bartonella henselae	Cat oropharynx	Cat scratch fever	Azithromycin; clarithromycin	Co-trimoxazole + gentamicin

Treponemataceae	*Borrelia recurrentis*	Body lice vector	Relapsing fever	Macrolides	Tetracycline
	Borrelia burgdorferi	Deer ticks	Lyme disease	Early: amoxicillin; Late: ceftriaxone	Cefuroxime; high-dose penicillin
	Leptospirosis	Rodents and other animals	Leptospirosis	Doxycycline	Penicillin
	Spirillum minus	Rat oropharynx	Rat bite fever	Penicillin	
	Treponema pallidum	STI; endemic	Syphilis Yaws	Penicillin	
	Treponema carateum	Skin contact	Pinto	Penicillin	
Anaerobic bacteria	*Clostridium botulinum*	Food-borne wound	Botulism; infant botulism	Supportive; penicillin	
	Clostridium perfringens	Faeces	Gas gangrene; soft tissue infection; septic abortion; food poisoning	Surgery; penicillin	
	Clostridium difficile	Faeces	Pseudomembranous colitis	Metronidazole	Vancomycin
	Clostridium tetani	Soil; animal faeces	Tetanus	Antitoxin; wound toilet; metronidazole	
	Actinomyces	Oral flora	Actinomycosis	Surgery; penicillin	Tetracycline; clindamycin
Chlamydia Obligate intracellular pathogen; Gram-negative envelope; no peptidoglycan; relies on host ATP for protein synthesis	*C. trachomatis*		Urethritis; cervicitis; neonatal; conjunctivitis; pneumonia in infancy	Erythromycin; clarithromycin	Tetracycline
	C. psittaci		Psittacosis	Tetracyclines; new macrolides	Erythromycin
	C. pneumoniae		Atypical pneumonia	Erythromycin; new macrolides	Tetracycline; ciprofloxacin
Rickettsia Obligate intracellular pathogen; multiplies by binary fission; contains RNA and DNA	*R. rickettsii*		Rocky mountain spotted fever	Tetracycline	Chloramphenicol
	R. conorii		Mediterranean spotted fever		
	R. akari		Rickettsial pox		
	R. prowazekii		Louse-borne relapsing fever		
	R. mooseri		Murine typhus		
	R. tsutsugamushi		Scrub typhus		
	Coxiella burnetii		Q fever		
	Ehrlichia		Ehrlichiosis		
Mycoplasma Free living small organism; lacks cell wall	*M. pneumoniae*		Atypical pneumonia	Macrolides	Tetracyclines
	Ureaplasma urealyticum		Urethritis; chorioamnionitis; neonatal penumonia	Tetracyclines	Macrolides
	M. hominis		Urethritis; PID; cervicitis	Tetracyclines	

CF, cystic fibrosis; CNS, central nervous system; GI, gastrointestinal; GU, genitourinary; IC, immune complex; MRSA, methicillin-resistant *Staphylococcus aureus*; PID, pelvic inflammatory disease; URT, upper respiratory tract; UTI urinary tract infection.

Table 6.2 Classification of viruses

Virus type	Family	Genus	Common species	Human disease
Non-enveloped				
RNA – single strand	*Picornaviridae*	*Enterovirus*	Polioviruses	Polio
			Coxsackie	Hand, foot and mouth Pleurodynia
			Echovirus	URTI, conjunctivitis Exanthem Myocarditis Aseptic meningitis
		Hepatovirus	Hepatitis A	Hepatitis
		Rhinovirus	Rhinovirus types	URTI
	Caliciviridae	*Norovirus*	Norwalk agent	Gastroenteritis (winter vomiting disease)
RNA – double strand	*Reoviridae*	*Reovirus*	Types 1,3	RTI, exanthem, diarrhoea
		Orbivirus	Colorado tick fever	Colorado tick fever
		Rotavirus	Various types	Vomiting and diarrhoea
DNA – single strand	*Parvoviridae*	*Erythrovirus*	Erythrovirus B19	Fifth disease (erythema infectiosum)
DNA – double strand	*Papovaviridae*	*Papillomavirus*	Human papillomavirus	Warts
		Polyomavirus	JC and BK viruses	Progressive multifocal leukoencephalopathy
	Adenoviridae	*Mastadenovirus*	Human adenoviruses	Bronchiolitis, pneumonia, Diarrhoea, hepatitis
Enveloped RNA – single strand	*Togaviridae*	*Alphavirus*	Various arboviruses	Equine encephalitis
		Rubivirus	Rubella	Rubella
	Flaviviridae	*Flavivirus*	Arboviruses	Yellow fever Dengue Japanese, Murray Valley, St Louis encephalitis West Nile Fever
			Tick-borne viruses	Tick-borne encephalitis
			Hepatitis C	Hepatitis
	Orthomyxoviridae	*Influenzavirus*	Influenza A Influenza B Influenza C	Influenza
	Paramyxoviridae	*Paramyxovirus*	Parainfluenza viruses	'Flu-like' illness Bronchiolitis Croup
			Mumps virus	Mumps
		Morbillivirus	Measles virus	Measles
		Pneumovirus	Respiratory syncytial virus	URTI, bronchiolitis
	Rhabdoviridae	*Lyssavirus*	Rabies virus	Rabies
	Filoviridae	*Filovirus*	Marburg virus	Viral haemorrhagic fever
			Ebola virus	Viral haemorrhagic fever
	Coronaviridae	*Coronavirus*	Human coronavirus	URTI
	Bunyaviridae	*Hantavirus*	Hantaan virus	Haemorrhagic fever with renal syndrome
		Bunyavirus	California encephalitis virus	California encephalitis
		Phlebovirus	Rift valley fever virus	Rift valley fever
			Sandfly fever virus	Sandfly fever
		Nairovirus	Crimean-Congo haemorrhagic fever virus	Viral haemorrhagic fever

(*Continued*)

Table 6.2 *(Continued)*

Virus type	Family	Genus	Common species	Human disease
	Retroviridae	HTLV-BLV group	HTLV 1 and 2	Adult T cell leukaemia
		Lentivirus	HIV	AIDS
	Arenaviridae	*Arenavirus*	Lassa fever virus	Viral haemorrhagic fever
DNA – double strand	*Hepadnaviridae*	*Hepadnavirus*	Hepatitis B	Hepatitis
	Alphaherpesvirinae	*Simplexvirus*	Human herpes simplex (HSV) 1, 2	Stomatitis, vesicular eruption 'cold sores', encephalitis
		Varicellovirus	Varicellazoster virus	Chicken pox, shingles
	Betaherpesvirinae	*Cytomegalovirus*	CMV (herpes virus type 5)	Congenital syndrome, glandular fever, hepatitis
		HSV 6 and 7	HSV 6 and 7	Exanthem subitum (roseola)
	Gammaherpesvirinae	*Lymphocryptovirus*	Epstein–Barr virus (HSV 4)	Glandular fever, lymphoma
	Poxviridae	*Orthopoxvirus*	Vaccinia	Cowpox
			Variola virus	Smallpox
		Parapoxvirus	Orf virus	Orf
		Molluscipoxvirus	Molluscum contagiosum virus	Molluscum

AIDS, acquired immune deficiency syndrome; CMV, cytomegalovirus; HIV, human immunodeficiency virus; HTLV, human T-lymphotrophic virus; URTI, upper respiratory tract infection.

Table 6.3 Classification of fungi

Fungus	Type	Tissues affected	Treatment
Aspergillus	Mould	Lung, sinuses, CNS, bone, skin, heart	Amphotericin B; itraconazole, voriconazole
Blastomyces dermatitidis	Dimorphic	Lung, dissemination in IC	Itraconazole
Candida	Yeast	Mucous membranes, GI, GU tracts, eye, disseminated disease, central line	Nystatin, clotrimazole, fluconazole, amphotericin B, 5 flucytosine
Coccidioides immitis	Dimorphic	Lung, skin, bone and joint, meninges	Amphotericin B
Paracoccidioides braziliensis	Dimorphic	Mucocutaneous, visceral, lymphatic, mixed	Sulfadiazine, co-trimoxazole, amphotericin B
Cryptococcus neoformans	Yeast	CNS, lung	Amphotericin B + 5 flucytosine
Histoplasma capsulatum	Dimorphic	Lung, skin, disseminated	(None), itraconazole, amphotericin B
Sporothrix schenckii	Dimorphic	Cutaneous sporotrichosis, disseminated	Potassium iodide, itraconazole
Zygomycetes (Mucor, Rhizopus)	Mould	Rhinocerebral, cutaneous, lung	Surgery, amphotericin

CNS, central nervous system; GI, gastrointestinal; GU, genitourinary; IC, immune complexes.

invasion through tissue planes (group A streptococci)
  - destroying tissue by producing proteases such as elastase (*Pseudomonas aeruginosa*)
  - producing locally (e.g. *Vibrio cholerae*) or systemically (e.g. *Clostridium botulinum, Staphylococcus aureus*) acting toxins.
- Host factors inhibiting this process include:
  - physical barriers of intact skin and mucous membranes. Injury to these barriers, by wounds, burns, smoke inhalation predisposes to invasion
  - lactoferrin, which limits the availability of ferric iron
  - secretory IgA on mucosal surfaces, which inhibits bacterial adherence
  - specific immune mechanisms.

4 Invasion and dissemination through immune evasion. Characteristics which enable bacteria to evade the immune system and spread include:

- a polysaccharide cell wall which is poorly antigenic and poorly opsonized, thus inhibiting phagocytosis, e.g. *Streptococcus pneumoniae*

- lipopolysaccharide of Gram-negative organisms such as *E. coli*, which resists complement activation
- M protein of group A streptococcus, which has antiphagocytic properties.

KEY LEARNING POINTS

- A successful pathogen is easily transmitted, has a mechanism to adhere to host surfaces, can compete with established flora, invade underlying tissues, and evade the immune system.
- A vulnerable host frequents the environment where there is risk of exposure, takes no precautions to remove pathogens from surfaces, has damaged skin or mucosal surfaces, has available binding sites for the pathogen and has poor innate and specific immunity.

HOST DEFENCES

Immune function can be divided into innate (non-specific) and adaptive (specific) components, as outlined in Table 6.4. The processes involved in eliminating bacteria and viruses are illustrated in Figures 6.1 and 6.2, respectively.

The innate immune system

Physical barriers

Physical barriers include the skin and mucous membranes.

SKIN

In addition to providing a mechanical barrier, sebum inhibits bacterial growth and the normal skin flora inhibits other species. In preterm neonates, the barrier is thinner, there is no sebum, and abnormal skin flora is often acquired.

MUCOUS MEMBRANES

Although the physical barrier is thin, surfaces are protected by washing by secretions, ciliary movement of debris, and

Table 6.4 Components of the immune system

Innate		Acquired	
Humoral	**Cellular**	**Humoral**	**Cellular**
Acute phase proteins	Macrophages	Antibody	T-cells
Lysozyme	Neutrophils		Other effector cells
Complement	Natural killer cells Mast cells Basophils Eosinophils		

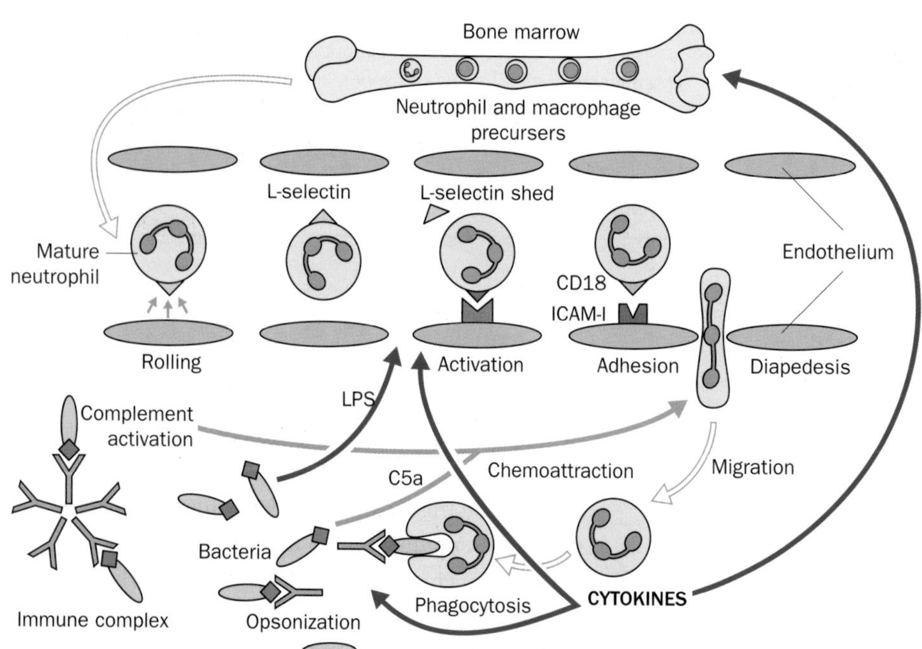

Figure 6.1 (a) Bacterial killing, the role of the phagocyte. LPS, lipopolysaccharide

lysozyme, surface antibody, and phagocytes. The gut is also protected by gastric acid and by the chemical environment and bacteriocins produced by normal flora. These may all be lacking in the preterm baby.

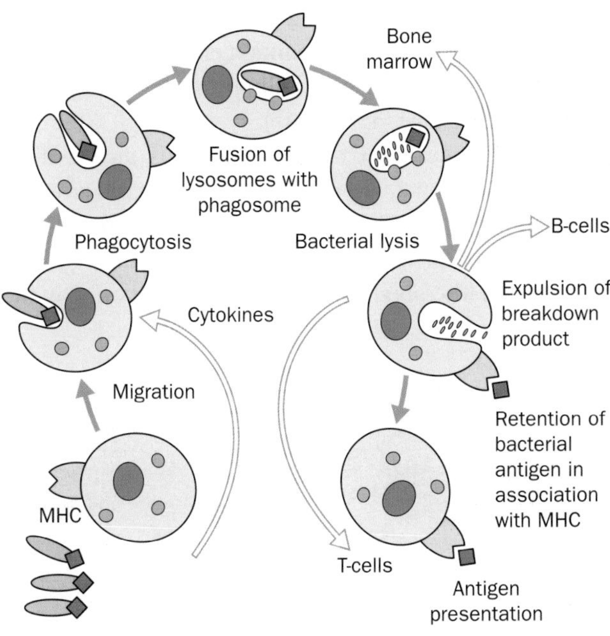

Figure 6.1 (b) Phagocytosis and antigen presentation

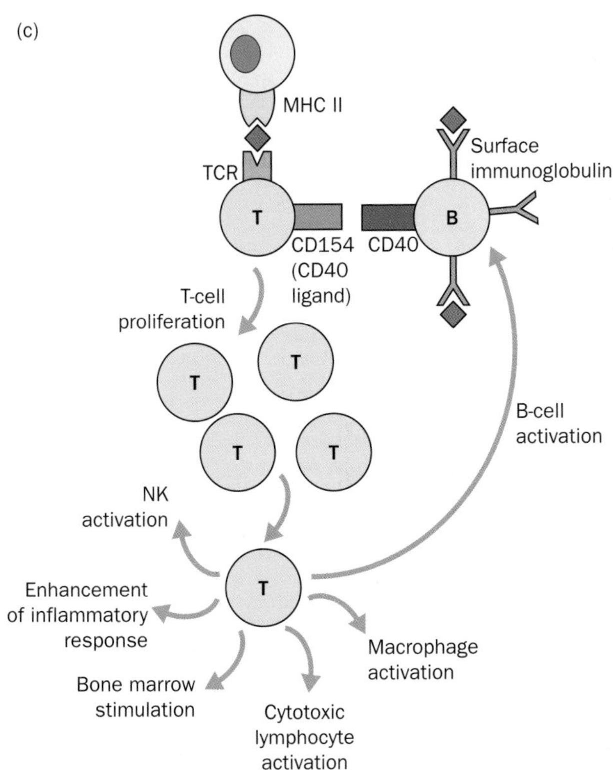

Figure 6.1 (c) Antigen presentation

Complement

This is a series of heat-labile proteins that lead to lysis of bacteria. The complement cascade is illustrated in Figure 6.3. Activation of the classical pathway requires bacterial antigen to be bound to antibody. IgM is the most efficient C1 activator. The alternate pathway is activated directly by bacterial oligosaccharides, endotoxins, yeast-cell walls and immunoglobulin aggregates. As well as bacterial lysis, activation of complement leads to anaphylactoid responses. Complement components are important for chemoattraction, opsonization, and clearance of immune complexes.

Neonates have reduced alternate pathway activity, slightly reduced classical pathway activity and decreased activity of C8 and C9, resulting in deficient opsonization. By 6–18 months of age, however, function is equivalent to adults.

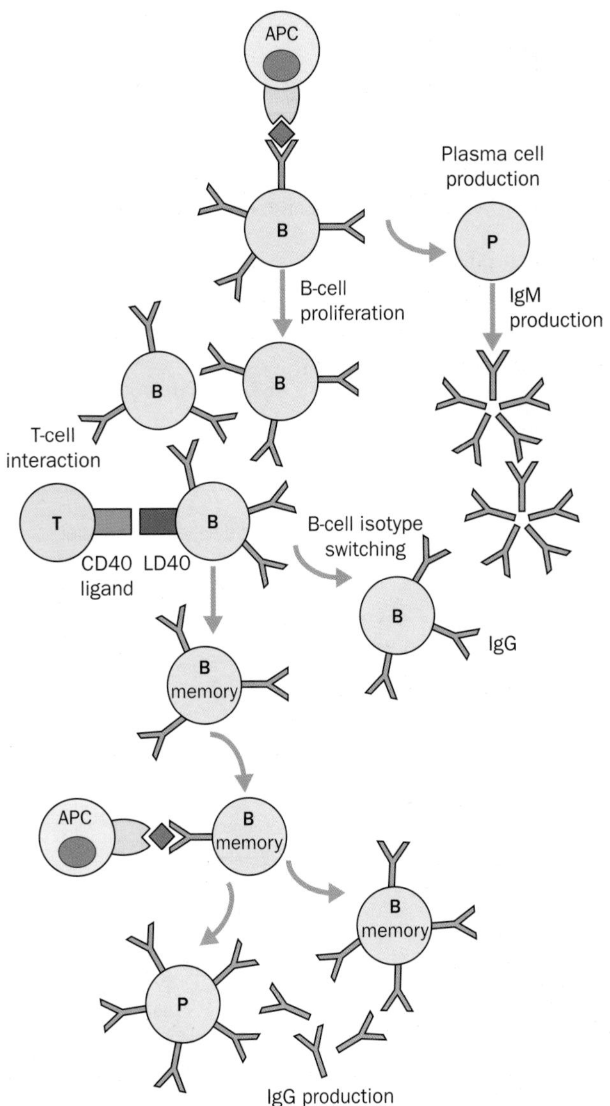

Figure 6.1 (d) B-cell activation and immunoglobulin production. APC, antigen presenting cell

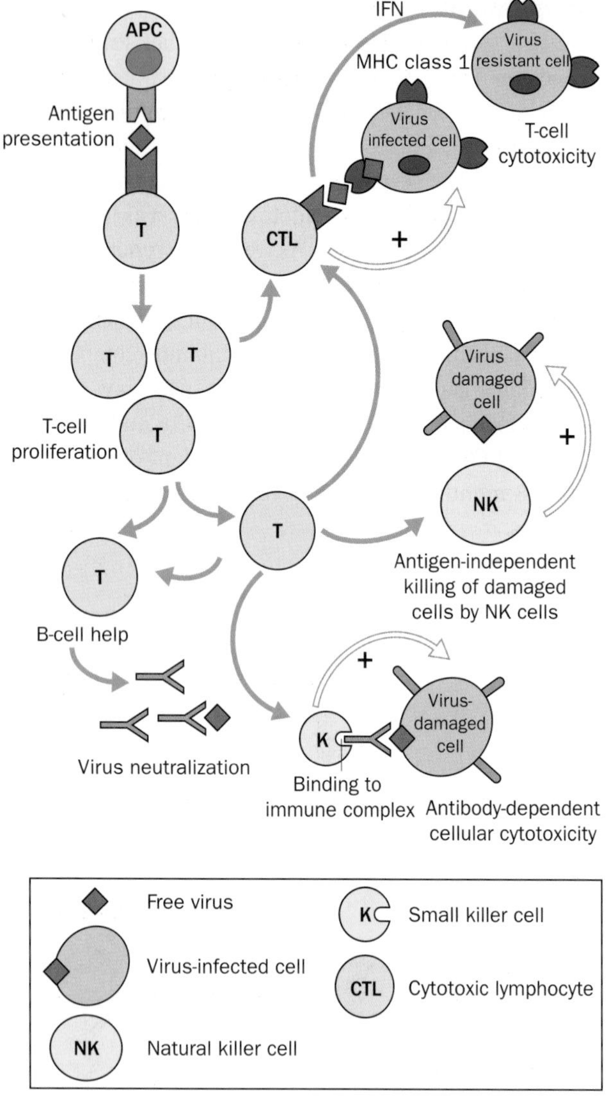

Figure 6.2 Mechanisms of cell mediated defence against viral infection. IFN, interferon

Cells of the innate immune system and their functions

PHAGOCYTES: NEUTROPHILS, MONONUCLEAR PHAGOCYTES (MACROPHAGE, MONOCYTE)

Phagocytosis involves the attachment of opsonized microorganisms to specific receptors on the cells surface, leading to engulfing of the organism. Neutrophil granules and macrophage lysosomes contain enzymes and chemicals that mediate bacterial killing and then digest the microorganism (see Figure 6.1b).

The major means of bacterial killing is mediated by the oxidative burst, in which oxygen is converted to superoxide via the nicotinamide adenosine dinucleotide phosphate (reduced form) (NADPH) oxidase system (Figure 6.4). Microbial killing is mediated not only by the

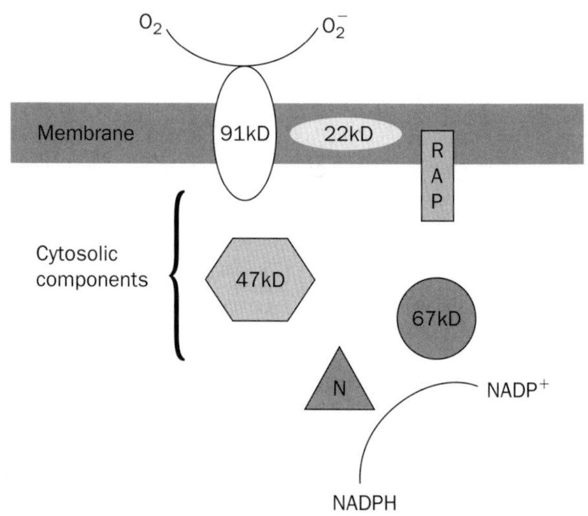

Figure 6.4 Respiratory burst in neutrophils. NADPH, nicotinamide adenosine dinucleotide phosphate (reduced form)

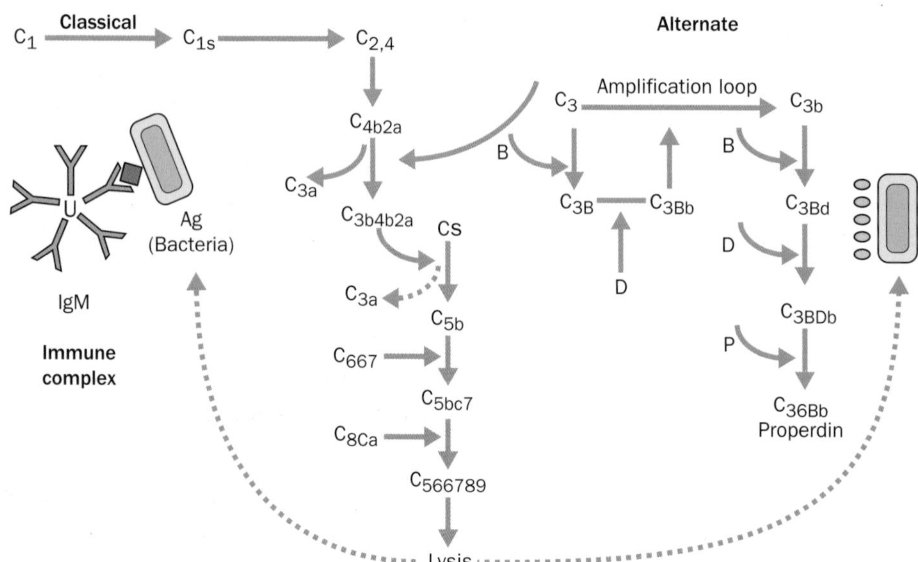

Figure 6.3 The complement cascade

oxygen radicals, but also by reactive oxygen intermediates, e.g. hydrogen peroxide and hydroxyl ions, generated during superoxide metabolism.

Other mechanisms of killing include:

- incarceration in the phagosome leading to accumulation of toxic microbial waste
- enzymes which disrupt bacterial cell walls, e.g. bacterial permeability increasing protein (BPI) and cationic antibacterial proteins (CAP)
- antibiotic-like molecules called defensins
- activity of lactoferrin
- alteration of the pH of the phagosome.

The neutrophil

The chief function of this cell is bacterial killing. It is therefore required to move rapidly to the site of infection, and chemotaxis is the most efficient method of movement. The neutrophil can sense a 1 per cent gradient in concentration of chemoattractant and migrates towards the higher concentration. Chemoattractants include:

- C5a (generated during complement activation)
- secretory products from inflammatory cells (e.g. cytokines)
- arachidonic acid metabolites derived from other neutrophils
- proteins of the coagulation pathway
- components of microorganisms.

Migration into the extravascular space is illustrated in Figure 6.1a. Selectins prevent neutrophils from their usual rolling along the endothelium. Leucocyte adhesion molecules on the surface of the neutrophil and endothelial intercellular adhesion molecule 1 (ICAM-1) interact, so they stick to the endothelium. They then squeeze between endothelial cells (diapedesis).

Less than 10 per cent of white cells in the second trimester fetus are neutrophils, compared with 50–60 per cent at term. At any gestation, within hours of birth the numbers increase rapidly. However, a common neonatal response to sepsis is neutropenia. In neonates, neutrophils adhere poorly to the endothelium, and all phagocytes have limited migration in response to chemotactic stimuli. Phagocytosis is suboptimal, but bacterial killing within the phagosome is normal compared with that of adults.

Antigen-presenting cells

Macrophages

Macrophages have the following features:

- Antigen presentation
  - In the process of bacterial killing, a portion of protein escapes proteolysis and is recognized as antigen. This is presented in association with major histocompatibility complex (MHC) class II on the cell surface. The T-cell receptor binds to the site resulting in T-cell activation (see Figure 6.1c).
- Antibody-independent cytotoxicity
  - Defence against tumour cells
- Secretion of inflammatory mediators
  - Cytokines leading to T- and B-cell activation
  - Haematopoietic colony stimulating factors
  - Macrophage pyrogens
  - Growth factors
  - Regulatory anticytokine molecules
- Tissue remodelling and wound healing

Dendritic cells

- These do not adhere to tissue or act as phagocytes.
- They capture antigen and present it to T-cells.
- They transport captured antigen to lymphoid tissue in which T-cells are activated and proliferate.

The function of most antigen-presenting cells at birth is equivalent to that in the adult.

The adaptive immune system

T-cells

These are the cells which coordinate and regulate the adaptive immune response. They:

- support and regulate immunoglobulin production by B-cells
- can be cytotoxic
- mediate delayed hypersensitivity
- regulate the size of immune response by balanced helper and suppressor functions.

They do this by:

- Cellular interactions
  - between T-cells and antigen-presenting cells (see Figure 6.1c)
  - between T- and B-cells (see Figure 6.1d). When the protein CD40 ligand is expressed on the T-cell surface, it binds a receptor (CD40) on the B-cell. This leads to:
    - B-cell proliferation
    - B-cells switching from expression of IgM and IgD to production of IgG, IgM and IgA
    - suppression of B-cell apoptosis
- Cytokine production

Cytokines are the regulatory proteins of the immune system. They can be divided into four groups based on their functions and interactions.

1 Cytokines regulating lymphocyte growth and development
   - Interleukin (IL)-2, IL-4, IL-7, IL-10, transforming growth factor (TGF)-β
2 Cytokines activating effector cells
   - IL-5 – eosinophils
   - IL-12 – NK and cytotoxic T cells
   - interferon (IFN-)γ – macrophages, antigen-presenting cells
   - tumour necrosis factor (TNF-)β – T- and B-cells
3 Cytokines mediating innate immunity and inflammation
   - IL-1, IL-6, IL-8, TNF-α, IFN-α, IFN-β
4 Cytokines regulating haematopoiesis
   - IL-3, IL-11, stem cell factor, granulocyte colony stimulating factor (GCSF), granulocyte–macrophage colony stimulating factor (GM-CSF), macrophage colony stimulating factor (M-CSF), erythropoietin

ROLE OF THE THYMUS IN DEVELOPMENT OF ADAPTIVE IMMUNITY

Immature T-cells enter the thymus early in gestation. Here, there is sequential rearrangement of the genes encoding the T-cell receptor (TCR). T-cell receptors are composed of either αβ chains, or γδ chains, each of which has a variable joining and a constant region. By this rearrangement process, receptors recognizing thousands of different antigens are produced. There is positive selection of αβ TCRs which recognize self-MHC bound to non-self-antigen. T-cell receptors that recognize self antigens are eliminated by apoptosis.

As T-cells mature they acquire CD3, CD4 and CD8. In the thymic medulla, cells differentiate either to become T helper (Th) cells, bearing CD4, or to become T suppressor/cytotoxic cells, bearing CD8. These are then released into the circulation.

T HELPER CELLS

Under cytokine influence, these differentiate into either Th1 or Th2 (Figure 6.5).

- Th1 cells stimulate cytotoxic T-cells and activate cells of the innate immune system.
- Th2 cells stimulate differentiation of B-cells.

CYTOTOXIC/SUPPRESSOR T-CELLS

These bear CD8 and bind to MHC class I. They are cytotoxic for virus-infected cells (see Figure 6.2).

From the second trimester to until 6 months after birth the number of circulating T-cells increases, after which there is a gradual decline to adult levels. The ratio of CD4:CD8 is about 3.5:1 in fetal life, declining to the adult

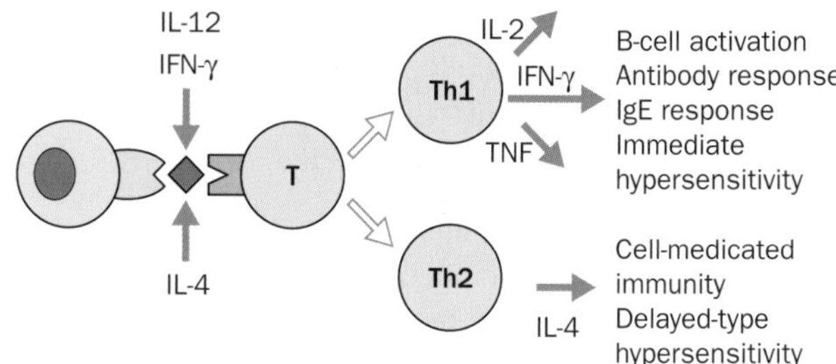

Figure 6.5 Factors influencing the differentiation of T helper cells into Th1 and Th2.

ratio of 2:1 by the age of 4 years. Only a small number are γδ T-cells, which do not bear CD4 or CD8 markers.

In adults, 40 per cent of T-cells are 'primed' by previous exposure to antigen, and are capable of rapid proliferation following repeated antigen exposure. In neonates, the vast majority are naive. Compared to adult T-cells, those in neonates have diminished cytokine production, cytotoxicity, delayed hypersensitivity and help for B-cell differentiation.

B-cells

B-cells have immunoglobulin on their surface which binds to antigen. Once binding occurs, with the help of T-cells, the B-cell proliferates to produce a clone, which can be activated by exposure to the antigen (see Figure 6.2). From this clone, some become plasma cells which secrete IgM during the primary immune response. Others persist with immunological memory, which is passed to subsequent generations of B-cells. Further exposure to antigen then leads to development of plasma cells secreting large amounts of IgG in the secondary antibody response. Some antigens, such as polysaccharides, can activate B-cells without T-cell help. The primary response is with IgM, and the secondary response is also chiefly IgM, with little IgG production and poor immunological memory.

The 'free' immunoglobulin released by plasma cells combines with antigen. This leads to bacterial killing by opsonization, neutralization, complement fixation, and immune complex formation. Each immunoglobulin molecule consists of polypeptide chains: two heavy and two light, joined by disulphide bridges (Figure 6.6). IgG is monomeric, whereas IgM is a pentamer joined with a J chain. Secretory IgA is dimeric.

Although neonatal B-cells can differentiate into IgM secreting plasma cells, B-cells do not differentiate into IgG secreting plasma cells until the age of 2 years, and IgA by 5 years. B-cell response involving T-cell help matures in the first months of life. T-cell independent responses do not mature until the age of 2–3 years. The neonate is protected by passive transfer of IgG from the placenta. The baby starts to produce its own IgG over the first

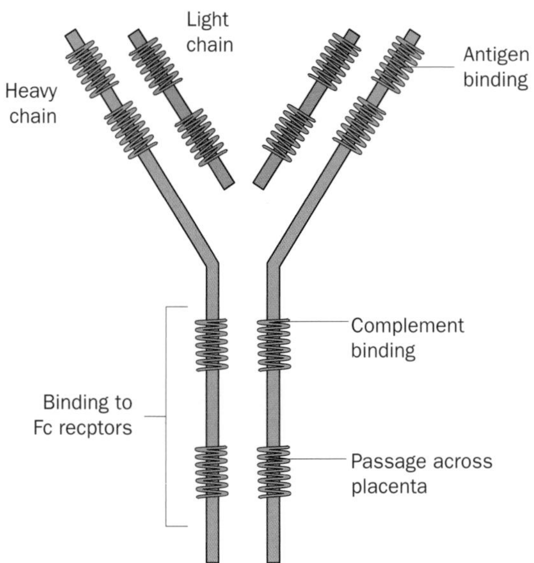

Figure 6.6 Structure of immunoglobulin

months of life, so that at 1 year the levels are 60 per cent those of adults. After birth, IgM rises rapidly in the first month, then more slowly, reaching 60 per cent adult levels by a year. IgA production is the last to develop, and levels are still only 20 per cent of adult levels by 1 year.

KEY LEARNING POINTS

- Defence against attack by pathogens involves the interplay of complex cellular and chemical systems.
- T-cells are the main coordinators.
- Bacterial killing is mediated by phagocytes and complement, after opsonization with specific antibody produced by B-cells.
- Viral defence is mediated by cytotoxic T-cells, and the innate immune system.

INFECTIOUS DISEASES: AN APPROACH TO DIAGNOSIS

The diagnosis of infectious disease is based on the recognition of patterns of symptoms and signs, supported by investigations of the pathology.

History

The entire course of the illness should be documented, including the presence and pattern of fever, associated symptoms, localizing symptoms and the following:

- prevalence of infectious disease within local community
- past exposure and susceptibility to infectious disease
- contact, including nature and length, with an infected person (or a person with similar symptoms)
- exposure to domestic animals/farm animals/birds
- insect or tick bites
- exposure to possibly contaminated food or water (e.g. unpasteurized milk)
- pica
- foreign travel
- contact with visitors from abroad
- history of blood transfusion
- history of IV drug use (personal or maternal)
- sexual contact
- immunization history
- drug history
- family history of infection (e.g. tuberculosis) or susceptibility to infection.

Clinical findings

The commonest manifestation of systemic infection is fever. The febrile child should be assessed for signs of shock. Examination should include the skin for signs of a rash, neck, axillae and groin for lymphadenopathy, and abdomen for hepatosplenomegaly. A full examination may reveal focal signs indicating the infected system or site.

Laboratory investigations

Microscopic examination and culture

Direct microscopy of fluid may reveal white cells (indicating inflammation) and organisms, which can be identified by Gram staining. Specific staining techniques, such as acid-fast stain for mycobacteria and periodic acid-Schiff (PAS) or silver stain for fungus and protozoa, should be used if these pathogens are suspected.

Fluid or swabs are plated onto media designed to support the growth of suspected pathogens. Fluid or blood can be inoculated into broth and incubated. If any delay is anticipated, swabs should be placed in transport medium, and urine should be refrigerated. If infection with fastidious organisms such as *Gonococcus* is suspected, swabs should always be plated out directly onto appropriate media. Some specimens may be cultured in selective media to encourage growth of pathogens, but suppress commensal growth, e.g. in stool. Growth patterns around antibiotic discs determine sensitivity. This process usually takes between eight and 48 hours, but sometimes longer. Biochemical tests, phage typing and serotyping allow further identification. Antigen detection, for example, by latex agglutination, can assist diagnosis of bacterial meningitis. Sensitivity and specificity of these tests is poor compared with molecular techniques.

A definitive diagnosis of infection can be made when an organism is isolated from a specimen taken from a sterile site, such as blood, cerebrospinal fluid (CSF) or urine. However, contamination can occur. Isolation of *S. epidermidis* in blood culture may represent skin contamination during venepuncture, or a true bacteraemia in a child with a central venous line. Coliforms may be isolated from urine left at room temperature. Culture should always be interpreted in the knowledge of how the specimen was obtained and in the light of the clinical presentation. Isolation of organisms from a normally non-sterile site can represent infection or colonization, so other clinical features need to be assessed to determine significance.

Viral infections can be diagnosed by culture in tissue media. The virus may take many days to show a cytopathic effect on the tissue. Direct immunofluorescence is rapid and available for respiratory viruses, such as respiratory syncytial virus (RSV) and influenza viruses. Enzyme-linked immunosorbent assays (ELISAs) are available for common gastrointestinal viruses such as rotavirus and adenovirus. Polymerase chain reaction (PCR) is playing an increasing role, particularly when culture techniques are difficult and lack sensitivity. The technique is based on the amplification and subsequent detection of a sequence of nucleic acids specific to the organism.

Other investigations

DIFFERENTIAL WHITE COUNT

In infants presenting with fever with no apparent source, those with leucocyte counts between 5 and 15 $\times$ 10^9/L are at low risk of bacterial infection compared with those with lower or higher counts.

- Neutrophilia is associated with bacterial infection and neutrophil chemotactic of phagocytic disorders.
- Lymphocytosis is associated with pertussis.
- Neutropenia or lymphopenia may indicate severe sepsis, viral suppression or immunodeficiency.
- Blood film is required for diagnosis of malaria.

BIOCHEMISTRY

C reactive protein (CRP) is useful in distinguishing bacterial sepsis from other causes of collapse and shock in critically ill or immunocompromised children and can be used to monitor response to therapy. In fulminant infection, such as meningococcal disease, the CRP may not have risen by the time of initial presentation, and a low level can be falsely reassuring. Cerebrospinal fluid protein and glucose are abnormal in bacterial meningitis, and levels correlate with the degree of meningeal inflammation. Liver function tests should be done if hepatitis is suspected.

Urinalysis

- Leucocytes and nitrites are predictive for urinary tract infection (UTI).
- Blood and protein are less specific.

KEY LEARNING POINTS

- A careful history and examination is the key to diagnosis.
- A positive culture result does not necessarily indicate infection.
- Culture relies on presence of viable organisms – PCR detects dead ones too.

CLASSIFICATION OF ANTIBIOTICS

Antibiotics are classified according to their structure and mechanism of action. If given in adequate quantities, some kill bacteria (bactericidal) whereas others prevent multiplication (bacteriostatic) (Table 6.5).

Penetration of antibiotics into infected tissue

Intracellular

- Rifampicin
- Erythromycin
- Clindamycin
- Doxycycline
- Metronidazole
- Ciprofloxacin

Urine

- Penicillins
- Cephalosporins
- Carbapenams
- Aminoglycosides
- Glycopeptides
- Quinolones
- Nitrofurantoin
- Trimethoprim
- Sulfamethoxazole
- Fusidic acid

Bile
- Amoxicillin
- Cephalosporins
- Sulfamethoxazole
- Trimethoprim
- Ciprofloxacin

CSF – if meningeal inflammation
- Penicillins
- Amoxicillin
- Cefotaxime
- Ceftriaxone
- Imipenem
- Meropenem

CSF – if no meningeal inflammation
- Chloramphenicol
- Rifampicin
- Co-trimoxazole
- Ciprofloxacin
- Metronidazole

Mechanisms of antibiotic resistance

Some bacteria are naturally resistant to some classes of antibiotics. Resistance can result from spontaneous mutation, or from acquisition of resistance genes from other bacteria, via transposons or plasmids. Administration of antibiotics may select out resistant organisms, which continue to multiply while other bacterial flora is suppressed. Resistant organisms can spread between hosts by direct contact or via fomites or aerosols.

Mechanisms of antibiotic resistance are summarized in Table 6.6. There may be more than one mechanism of resistance to a given antibiotic, and each requires different counter-strategies. For instance, clavulanic acid is effective against organisms resistant to penicillin because of β-lactamase production but has no effect if the penicillin-binding protein is altered.

Rational antibiotic use

Before any antibiotic is prescribed, the answer to the following questions should be 'yes'.

Table 6.5 Mechanism of action of antibiotics

Bactericidal				**Bacteriostatic**		
Mechanism	**Class**	**Examples**		**Mechanism**	**Class**	**Examples**
Inhibit cell wall synthesis	β-Lactams	Penicillins	Penicillin G	Inhibit protein synthesis	Tetracyclines	Doxycycline
		Aminopenicillins	Amoxicillin		Macrolides	Erythromycin
		Penicillinase-resistant	Flucloxacillin			Clarithromycin
		Extended-spectrum	Ticarcillin			Azithromycin
			Piperacillin		Lincosamides	Clindamycin
		Cephalosporins				
		1st generation	Cephalexin			Fusidic acid
			Cephradine			Chloramphenicol
		2nd generation	Cefuroxime	Inhibit nucleic acid synthesis	Trimethoprim	
		3rd generation	Cefotaxime		Sulphonamides	Sulfamethoxazole
			Ceftriaxone			Sulfadiazine
			Ceftazidime			
		Carbapenems	Imipenem			
			Meropeneam			
	Glycopeptides		Vancomycin			
			Teicoplanin			
Inhibitors of protein synthesis	Aminoglycosides		Gentamycin			
			Netilmicin			
			Tobramycin			
			Amikacin			
Inhibitors of nucleic acid synthesis	Quinolones	Ciprofloxacin				
		Metronidazole				
		Rifampicin				
Inhibition of cytoplasmic membrane function		Polymyxins				

Table 6.6 Mechanism of bacterial resistance to antibiotics

Antibiotic	Altered target	Altered uptake	Inactivation	Efflux pumps	Evasion of blocked pathways
β-Lactams	Altered PBP	Decreased cell wall permeability	β-Lactamase production	–	–
Glycopeptide	Altered binding site				Autolysin deficiency
Aminoglycoside	Altered 30S in streptomycin	Reduced cell wall permeability	Bacterial enzyme production		
Quinolones	Altered binding site	Reduced cell wall permeability			
Rifampicin	Altered binding site				
Tetracyclines	Altered ribosomal target		? Enzymatic deactivation by *E. coli*	Most common	
Macrolides	Altered ribosomal target	Gram negative impermeable outer membrane	Enzymatic modification	**Can occur**	
Lincosamides	Altered ribosomal target		**Can occur**		
Chloramphenicol	Occasional	Occasional	Acetylation leading to failure to bind to ribosomal target		
Sulphonamides	Altered dihydropteroate synthetase		Hyper production of PABA: competitive inhibition		
Trimethoprim	Resistant dihydrofolate reductase	Occasional	Overproduction of dihydrofolate reductase		

PBP, penicillin binding protein; PABA, para-aminobenzoic acid.

- Does the child have an infection?
- If so, is it a bacterial infection?
  - most respiratory tract infections in the pre-school child are viral.
- If it is bacterial, is the natural history significantly altered by antibacterial treatment?
  - most cases of streptococcal pharyngitis and bacterial otitis media resolve with symptomatic treatment only.

If antibiotics are started before culture results are available, choice of agent should depend on answers to the following questions.

- What are the likely causative organisms?
- Which antibiotic or combination will be active against them?
- Which antibiotics best penetrate into the infected tissue?
  - see box on page 174.
- Which of the possible choices has the narrowest spectrum?

Other factors to consider include:

- history of drug sensitivity
- underlying disease, e.g. hepatic or renal impairment, glucose 6-phosphate dehydrogenase (G6PD) deficiency
- toxic side effects of the drug
- ease of administration (including taste)
- cost.

Where possible, a single agent should be chosen. A combination may be required:

- where there is established synergism, e.g. trimethoprim/sulfamethoxazole, or penicillin and gentamicin
- where no one antibiotic covers all the possible pathogens adequately, e.g. ceftazidime and amikacin in febrile neutropenia
- to prevent the emergence of drug-resistant mutants, e.g. therapy for tuberculosis.

The disadvantages of combinations include:

- antagonism, e.g. clindamycin/chloramphenicol
- alteration of pharmacokinetics, e.g. rifampicin and fluconazole
- broader spectrum cover, with greater effect on commensal flora
- selection of multidrug resistant organisms.

Once culture results are obtained, the narrowest spectrum antibiotic with adequate penetration should be chosen.

Although guidelines exist for the length of treatment of particular infections, e.g. meningitis, the supporting evidence is frequently lacking. Too short a course may enable the organism to persist and infection to be re-established, whereas too long a course may select out drug-resistant commensal flora. In general, short courses of high-dose antibiotics are effective and less likely to lead to drug resistance than longer lower-dose courses. For infections in relatively avascular tissue, where antibiotic penetration is likely to be poor, such as endocarditis, long courses are necessary. Long courses are also needed when bacterial multiplication is slow, as in mycobacterial infection.

Antibiotic prophylaxis

Antibiotics should only be given to prevent infection when there is clear evidence of benefit, the risk of infection is high, and its consequences potentially severe. Agents used should be well tolerated and have the minimal effect on the commensal flora. For example

- penicillin – pneumococcal sepsis in hyposplenism/functional asplenia
- co-trimoxazole – *Pneumocystis carinii* pneumonia in the immunocompromised
- trimethoprim – urinary tract infection
- perioperative antibiotic – high-risk surgical procedures
- flucloxacillin – pulmonary infection in cystic fibrosis.

Antibiotic prescribing policies

The emergence of multidrug-resistant organisms, the morbidity due to side effects of therapy and the cost burden of antibiotic prescribing have led many hospitals to introduce prescribing policies or guidelines. Guidelines should be evidence based and use data from local surveillance of prevalent flora and patterns of resistance.

KEY LEARNING POINTS

- Do not treat viral infections with antibiotics.
- Treat with the agent with the narrowest spectrum possible.
- Choose an antibiotic that penetrates well into the infected tissue.
- If no initial response, check the dose is adequate.
- If no response, do not add more drugs – change the regimen.

INFECTIONS IN THE FETUS AND NEONATE

The fetus is protected from many infectious agents by physical isolation and also by the placental barrier. Infection can occur, however, as a result of spread from the maternal circulation, usually during maternal viraemia, or due to placental infection or to ascending infection from the birth canal.

Infection during intrauterine life can result in:

- Abortion – the risk of death *in utero* is related to the severity of the systemic illness in the mother, and to the stage of gestation at which infection occurs, the risk being greatest earlier in gestation.
- Fetal damage – infection may interfere with the development of organs (e.g. rubella, varicella zoster), or lead to damage or destruction of already formed organs (e.g. cytomegalovirus (CMV), herpes simplex virus (HSV)).
- Ongoing infection with effects on the neonate and beyond (e.g. CMV, hepatitis B (HBV)).

At the time of birth, the baby is exposed for the first time to a non-sterile environment. Perinatal infection can occur because of:

- exposure to pathogens in the maternal genital tract, e.g. HSV, HIV, *Chlamydia*, group B streptococcus
- exposure to faecal organisms, e.g. coliforms, *Listeria*, group B streptococcus, enterovirus
- direct exposure to maternal blood, e.g. HIV, HBV, HBC.

Postnatal infection may result from:

- horizontal transmission from mother, or other contacts (including nosocomial infection in the nursery)
- transmission via breast milk (e.g. HIV, human T-lymphotrophic virus 1 (HTLV1))
- transmission via blood transfusion (e.g. CMV).

CASE STUDY: Congenital infections

A neonate, born at term after an uneventful pregnancy, weighs 2.2 kg. He is floppy, fails to establish feeding, and on examination is noted to have hepatosplenomegaly.

This history is suggestive of congenital infection referred to by the mnemonic TORCH (*T*oxoplasmosis, *O*ther infections, *R*ubella, *C*ytomegalovirus, *H*erpes simplex). Table 6.7 gives details of fetal and neonatal infections.

CASE STUDY: Perinatal infection

A neonate born by vaginal delivery at term develops sticky eyes on day 6, which progresses to swelling of both eyelids and a mucopurulent discharge. Treatment with fusidic acid, and then chloramphenicol eye drops is not beneficial. At 6 weeks he becomes breathless during feeds and then at rest. Chest radiograph shows diffuse interstitial pneumonitis.

Chlamydia trachomatis is an intracellular pathogen, which often causes asymptomatic infection in the mother and is sexually transmitted. Of neonates born to infected mothers, 50–60 per cent will become colonized after vaginal delivery, and around 20 per cent after caesarean section. Diagnosis is by direct immunofluorescence of conjunctival scrapings or nasopharyngeal aspirate. The neonate should be treated with erythromycin or clarithromycin for 14–21 days. The mother and her partner should receive azithromycin or doxycycline.

KEY LEARNING POINTS

- Consider congenital infection in babies with signs of intrauterine multiorgan damage.
- Infection can sometimes be avoided if women receive appropriate advice and screening during pregnancy.
- Some organisms causing congenital infection are sexually transmitted. Do not forget to screen and treat mother's partner(s).

EXANTHEMATA AND OTHER INFECTIONS OF CHILDHOOD

CASE STUDY: Fever and rash

A previously well 3-year-old develops fever, runny nose and then a widespread macular erythematous rash. He recovers after five days.

Although fever and rash are still common presenting symptoms in childhood, many of the previously common infectious diseases are now prevented by immunization (Table 6.8).

CASE STUDY: Paroxysmal cough

A 4-month-old infant develops coryza but has no fever. A few days later, he begins to cough and is admitted as an emergency with apnoea. He is successfully resuscitated but continues to have frequent episodes of cough with cyanosis, vomiting and apnoea. His mother has had a persistent cough for four weeks.

Pertussis

Bordetella pertussis is transmitted by droplets from infected individuals; there is no carrier state. Its toxin leads to paralysis of cilia and cell destruction, with disruption of the mucociliary blanket, and accumulation of thick secretions. This predisposes to secondary bacterial infection. Most cases now are incompletely vaccinated infants exposed to older children or adults with atypical disease.

The classis clinical course has four stages:

1. incubation – during which antimicrobials may affect course
2. coryzal – non-specific symptoms in afebrile child
3. paroxysmal – severe cough with vomiting, cyanosis, apnoea, leading to weight loss and exhaustion
4. convalescent – decreased frequency and severity of paroxysms.

Complications of pertussis include:

- Pneumonia and subsequent bronchiectasis
- Otitis media
- Seizures
- Encephalopathy
- Subconjunctival, subarachnoid and intraventricular haemorrhage
- Rectal prolapse
- Umbilical and inguinal hernia
- Rupture of diaphragm.

Treatment is mainly supportive. Macrolides modify the course of early disease and later reduce infectivity and secondary bacterial complications.

Table 6.7 Fetal and neonatal infections

Organism	Source	Infectivity in pregnancy	Damage in pregnancy	Clinical features	Diagnosis	Treatment	Prevention
Toxoplasma gondii	Cat, undercooked meat	25 per cent first trimester 65 per cent third	Maximum in first trimester	Chorioretinitis; intracranial calcification; hydrocephalus; fever; hepatosplenomegaly; lymphadenopathy; jaundice, anaemia; maculopapular rash	Neonatal toxoplasma; IgM in blood and CSF; maternal IgM and IgG	Pyrimethamine + sulfadiazine with folinic acid for one year; new macrolides have some efficacy	Avoid sources during pregnancy; antenatal screening and treatment (not UK)
Rubella	Human direct contact/droplet infection	Throughout	Greatest first 14 weeks: no damage after 20 weeks	IUGR; thrombocytopenia; hepatitis; hepatosplenomegaly; congenital heart disease (PDA, pulmonary artery stenosis, aortic stenosis, abnormal subclavian vessels, ventriculoseptal defect); interstitial pneumonitis; cataracts; retinopathy; deafness; developmental delay	Maternal seroconversion (IgM and IgG) Neonatal IgM (can be negative)	None	MMR × 2 during childhood
Cytomegalo virus	Human, direct contact, 60–70 per cent of adults have been infected. Fetal infection due to primary infection or reactivation	Throughout pregnancy, perinatal via contact with cervical secretions, and postnatal (horizontal transmission or via blood)	Greatest in primary infection in the first trimester; later infection asymptomatic	IUGR; microcephaly, intracranial calcification; chorioretinitis; hepatosplenomegaly; hepatitis, purpura	Virus isolation from nasopharyngeal secretions or urine in first three weeks; IgG and IgM in mother; IgM in infant, PCR	Ganciclovir or foscarnet in severe symptomatic disease	Screening of blood transfused in pregnancy and in neonates
Herpes simplex	Human direct (type 1) or sexual contact (type 2)	*In utero* infection can occur, but risk is greatest perinatally	Throughout pregnancy and neonatal period	Congenital: IUGR; microcephaly; seizures; intracranial calcification; chorioretinitis; microphthalmia; vesicles, or bullae Perinatal: sepsis-like fever; lethargy,	Isolation of HSV in culture from vesicles or CSF HSV PCR	Aciclovir	Caesarean section in women with active lesions; screening of high-risk women

(*Continued*)

Table 6.7 (*Continued*)

Organism	Source	Infectivity in pregnancy	Damage in pregnancy	Clinical features	Diagnosis	Treatment	Prevention
				respiratory distress; vomiting; disseminated: hepatitis; adrenal infection; pneumonitis; encephalitis Localized: encephalitis; vesicular lesions in skin, eye or mouth			
Other: Syphilis	Human sexual contact	*In utero* or perinatal	Mortality 25 per cent *in utero*, 25–30 per cent perinatally	Early (1–12 weeks rhinitis) Later (1–6 months) Macular-papular rash fissures and mucous patches; meningovascular disease; pneumonia; hepatosplenomegaly; ectodermal changes; anaemia; thrombocytopenia; leucopenia, or leucocytosis; epiphyseal changes; osteochondritis; periosteitis Late: (variable) Hutchison's teeth (notched biting edge of incisors); interstitial keratitis; neurosyphilis; sensorineural deafness usually around age 8–10 years; keratitis (can progress despite treatment); sclerosing bone lesions; saber shin; frontal bossing; saddle nose; Clutton's joints (painless arthritis of the knee)	Anti-treponemal IgM; maternal VDRL, RPR or ART (indicate acute infection) FTA-ABS or TPHA (acute or past infection)	Benzyl penicillin IV for 2 weeks	Antenatal screening and treatment of infection
Erythrovirus B19	Human? Direct contact	Throughout	Throughout	Hydrops fetalis Spontaneous abortion ? Myocarditis	Maternal Parvovirus IgM	Serial Ultrasound and fetal blood transfusion	None

Hepatitis B	Human: perinatal, sexual, direct contact with blood or body fluids	Perinatal	Postnatal; risk 95 per cent if unimmunized; 5 per cent/year spontaneous seroconversion	Asymptomatic transient hepatitis with seroconversion to antiHBs; asymptomatic persistent carriage, with fluctuating transaminases; clinical hepatitis, with clearance of antigen; clinical hepatitis, progressing to chronic hepatitis; acute fulminant hepatitis; asymptomatic carriage, with progression to chronic hepatitis, cirrhosis, and hepatocellular carcinoma	Hepatitis B surface antigen and e antigen	Interferon alfa or lamivudine in HBeAg positive children with abnormal transaminases and liver histology, aiming to promote seroconversion to anti HBe	Antenatal screening; immunization of infants born to hepatitis B surface antigen positive women; WHO recommends universal vaccination (not yet in UK)
Hepatitis C	Human sexual or blood contact	Perinatal	Risk 2–5 per cent	Asymptomatic carriage, chronic hepatitis and cirrhosis	Hepatitis C antibody at one year, confirmed with PCR	Interferon alfa and ribavirin (no established criteria for treatment in childhood)	Maternal avoidance of high-risk behaviour
Varicella zoster virus (VZV)	Human, aerosol or droplet	Throughout and perinatally	5–10 per cent risk of damage in first trimester; severe varicella in neonate if maternal chicken pox five days before to two days after delivery; maternal zoster: no risk	IUGR; cutaneous scars; eye abnormalities; limb hypoplasia; cortical atrophy; developmental delay Neonatal varicella: disseminated fulminant infection; hepatitis; pneumonitis; encephalitis	Isolation of VZV from vesicle by culture or PCR; Maternal VZV; IgM	Aciclovir	Zoster immune globulin to at-risk neonates ? Vaccination of seronegative teenagers Universal immunization (USA not UK)

ART, automated reagin test; CNS, central nervous system; CSF, cerebrospinal fluid; FTA-ABS, fluorescent tryponemal antibody-absorption (test); HSV, herpes simplex virus; IV, intravenous; MMR, measles, mumps, rubella; PCR, polymerase chain reaction; PDA, patent ductus arteriosus; RPR, rapid plasma reagent; TPHA, *Tryponema pallidum* haemagglutination (test); VDRL, venereal disease research laboratory (test).

Table 6.8 Childhood exanthemata

Disease	Organism	Transmission	Incubation period	Infectivity period	Clinical features	Complications	Treatment	Prevention
Measles	Measles virus	Aerosolized droplets	8–12 days (10 years for SSPE)	1–2 days before symptoms to four days after appearance of rash	Fever; coryza; conjunctivitis; cough; Koplik spots; maculopapular rash spreading from head + neck downwards	Pneumonia; otitis media; croup; lymphadenitis; myocarditis; encephalitis; SSPE	Supportive	Vaccine as MMR
Rubella	Rubella virus	Droplet/direct contact	14–21 days	1–2 days before to seven days after rash appears	Maculopapular discrete rash; lymphadenopathy slight fever; transient arthralgia	Encephalitis (rare); Thrombocytopenia (rare)	Supportive	MMR vaccine
Scarlet fever	Group A streptococcus	Droplet/direct contact/fomites	2–5 days	Variable 24 hours post-antibiotics	Red, finely punctate rash; desquamation; pharyngitis; lymphadenopathy; strawberry tongue	Toxic shock; otitis media; pneumonia; empyema; fasciitis; myositis; osteomyelitis; rheumatic fever	Penicillin or clindamycin	(penicillin prophylaxis if high risk)
Chicken pox	Varicella zoster virus	Aerosolized droplets	14–21 days	Two days before until five days post-rash (while new lesions erupting)	Pruritus; vesicular rash in crops; mild fever	Secondary bacterial infection (Group A strep, *S. aureus*); pneumonitis; encephalitis; progressive disseminated varicella; haemorrhagic varicella; cerebellar ataxia; shingles	Supportive; aciclovir in high-risk patients	Post-exposure prophylaxis with varicella zoster immunoglobulin; varicella vaccine
Erythema infectiosum (fifth disease)	Erythrovirus B19	Droplet Blood contact	4–21 (usually 4–14) days	Not infectious once rash appears	Mild fever; 'slapped cheek' lace-like rash on trunk; arthralgia/arthritis	Aplastic anaemia in immunocompromised and if increased red cell turnover (e.g. sickle cell)	Supportive	None
Roseola infantum (exanthema subitum)	HHV6 Enterovirus Adenovirus Parainfluenza	Droplet/direct contact	9–10 days	Until fever subsides	Fever for 3–5 days, then rash – discrete macular/maculopapular for 24–48 hours	Convulsions; encephalitis	Supportive	None
Mumps	Mumps virus	Droplet/direct contact	12–25 days	1–2 days after parotid swelling to nine days after	Salivary gland swelling; fever; meningism	Meningitis; encephalitis; deafness; orchitis; pancreatitis; arthritis; thyroiditis; mastitis; nephritis	Supportive	MMR

MMR, measles, mumps, rubella (vaccine); SSPE, subacute sclerosing panencephalitis.

KEY LEARNING POINTS

- The impact of most childhood exanthemata is reduced by immunization rather than treatment.
- Assessment of risk to non-immune contacts requires knowledge of mode of spread, infectivity period, and incubation period.
- Late sequelae may be due to secondary bacterial infection, or immune-mediated disease.
- Many result in more severe disease if contracted in adolescence or adult life.

Meningitis

CASE STUDY

A 9-month-old infant develops fever and coryza with some cough. He is diagnosed as having upper respiratory tract infection. Forty-eight hours later, he re-presents with a right-sided focal seizure. Since the last review he has continued to be pyrexial and has been vomiting and irritable. On examination, he is hot centrally with cool peripheries, flexing to pain with normal posture but poorly responsive. The fontanelle is bulging, and he screams on handling. Cerebrospinal fluid contains 1200 white cells and numerous Gram-positive cocci, identified as *Pneumococcus* on culture.

Inflammation of the meninges may be caused by infection with bacteria, viruses, fungi or parasites, or by non-infective processes such as malignancy, immune mediated diseases and drugs.

Bacterial meningitis is commonly caused by organisms which colonize the respiratory tract. Organisms then invade the blood stream, leading to bacteraemia, which can be associated with clinical sepsis. The child may be asymptomatic until infection causes meningeal inflammation.

Table 6.9 outlines the causative organisms in the neonatal and postneonatal age groups, their identification and treatment and outcome as compared with a control population. Sequelae include learning difficulties, neuromotor disorders, seizure disorders, deafness, visual disorders, speech and language disorders, and behavioural problems.

Postneonatal meningitis

Infants between 6 and 12 months of age are at greatest risk, and 90 per cent of cases occur in the under 5s. Prior to the introduction of vaccination, *Haemophilus influenzae* caused 50 per cent of cases. Vaccine failures still occur.

CLINICAL FEATURES

These include fever, nausea, vomiting, irritability, headache, neck stiffness, and reduced conscious level. Younger babies may present with less specific signs. Signs of raised intracranial pressure, such as bulging fontanelle, tonic seizures, abnormal posture and coma may ensue. Papilloedema is uncommon. Twenty per cent will either present with seizures or develop them in the first two days of the illness.

DIAGNOSIS

A lumbar puncture should be performed except in the following circumstances:

- signs of raised intracranial pressure
- focal neurological signs
- clinical coagulopathy
- fulminant sepsis with shock.

Typical findings are:

- raised CSF white cell count (polymorphs in bacterial meningitis, lymphocytes in viral)
- raised protein and decreased glucose concentrations (bacterial meningitis)
- organisms on Gram staining, on culture, latex agglutination tests or PCR.

Neonatal bacterial meningitis

A quarter of episodes of sepsis in neonates are associated with meningitis.

CLINICAL FEATURES

Babies present with non-specific signs of sepsis, such as temperature instability, poor feeding, vomiting, lethargy, irritability and reduced responsiveness. The classic signs of meningitis are less common.

DIAGNOSIS

- Up to 45 white blood cells (WBC)/mm^3 in CSF (60 per cent polymorphs) is normal in neonates.
- By 4 weeks of age the cell count drops to less than 10.
- Higher numbers can persist in the preterm.
- At term, normal range for CSF protein is 0.4–0.88 g/L.
- Normal CSF protein in preterm is up to 1.7 g/L.
- The ratio CSF:plasma glucose is normally 60–70 per cent but can be over 100 per cent.

Table 6.9 Bacterial causes of meningitis

Period	Organism	Per cent cases	Identification	Treatment	Length of treatment	Mortality (per cent)	Severe disability (per cent) (control 0.07)	Moderate disability (per cent) (control 1.5)	Any disability (per cent) (control 21)
Neonatal	Unknown		Micro + culture	Ampicillin + gentamicin; ampicillin + cefotaxime	2-3 weeks	15-30	7	18	50
	Group B streptococcus	50-60	Micro + culture	Penicillin + gentamicin OR cefotaxime	14 days	20	13	17	51
	E. coli	20	Micro + culture	Cefotaxime	21 days	30	6-20	20	50
	S. aureus		Micro + culture	Flucloxacillin	14 days	30	Not studied	Not studied	Not studied
	S. faecalis	<5		Ampicillin/vancomycin	14 days	20	Not studied	Not studied	Not studied
	S. pneumoniae			Cefotaxime	14 days	20	Not studied	Not studied	Not studied
	Listeria monocytogenes	5	Micro + culture	Ampicillin + gentamicin	14 days	10-30	<5	20-25	44
Post-neonatal	Unknown		Micro + culture	Cefotaxime/ceftriaxone + ampicillin <3 months	14 days	1-5	5	8	44
	N. meningitidis	60-70	Micro + culture; PCR; serology	Cefotaxime/ceftriaxone	7 days	7.5 (includes sepsis)	3	6	40
	S. pneumoniae	30	Micro + culture; latex	Cefotaxime/ceftriaxone + vancomycin in areas of high resistance	14 days	15	10	14	50
	Haemophilus influenzae	1	Micro + culture	Cefotaxime/ceftriaxone	10 days	4	3	7	43
	Mycobacterium tuberculosis	<1	Micro + culture; Mantoux's; ?PCR	Isoniazid; rifampicin; ethambutol; pyrazinamide	9 months	1 early; 25 late	Data not available in developed world		
	Enterovirus	2-5	PCR; culture	None		<1	0	6	40
	Group B streptococcus	10 <3 months	Micro + culture	Penicillin + gentamicin; cefotaxime	14 days	20	13	17	51

PCR, polymerase chain reaction.

- It is possible to have normal CSF white cell counts or biochemistry results in the presence of meningitis, but unusual for all parameters to be normal.

TREATMENT

Antibiotics, which penetrate the inflamed meninges, are required in adequate dosage. Studies have shown that steroids given prior to or with the first dose of antibiotics reduces the risk of deafness in *H. influenzae* type B (HIB) meningitis. The same effect is assumed in pneumococcal disease but there is no evidence for efficacy in meningococcal disease. A two-day course should be given. A longer course may result in rebound pyrexia, and may also reduce meningeal inflammation sufficiently to inhibit antibiotic penetration.

If there is raised intracranial pressure, all possible measures should be taken to optimize cerebral oxygenation and perfusion. Seizures should be controlled promptly with anticonvulsants.

KEY LEARNING POINTS

- A definitive diagnosis of meningitis cannot be made without a lumbar puncture.
- Empirical antibiotics should be commenced while culture results are awaited.
- If steroids have not been given with the first dose of antibiotics, there is no evidence to support them being given at all.
- Cerebrospinal fluid results in the preterm neonate should be interpreted with care.

THE PATHOPHYSIOLOGY OF SEPSIS

CASE STUDY: Meningococcal septicaemia

A 2-year-old boy presents with a history of fever for the last eight hours. Over the last two hours, he developed an irregular macular erythematous rash. On initial examination he is alert and playing with toys, and he is pink and well perfused. Closer inspection of the rash reveals a largely blanching rash, but occasional non-blanching lesions.

This is the presentation of early meningococcal disease. If recognized and treated at this stage, outcome is likely to be good. It untreated until there is widespread purpura and established shock, there is significant mortality and long-term morbidity from organ damage and limb ischaemia. A poor outcome can be predicted from a high score on systems such as the Glasgow Meningococcal Prognostic Score (Table 6.10).

Table 6.10 The Glasgow Meningococcal Prognostic Score

Criteria	Score
Systolic blood pressure <75 if <4 years <85 If >4 years	3
Skin/rectal temperature gradient >3°C	3
Glasgow Coma Score <8 at any time OR deterioration of >3 points in one hour	3
Extent of purpura: widespread ecchymoses or extending lesions on review	1
Parental questioning: has your child's condition become worse over the past hour? YES	2
Base deficit (capillary sample) >8	1
Absence of meningism	2
Total	**15**

PATHOPHYSIOLOGY

When bacteria gain access to the bloodstream, they are usually eliminated effectively by the monocyte-macrophage system after opsonization by antibody and complement. In some cases, however, the infection results in a systemic inflammatory response, which then progresses independently of the original infection.

Sepsis: A systemic inflammatory response to possible infection.

Severe sepsis or **sepsis syndrome**: This occurs when sepsis is associated with hypoperfusion resulting in organ dysfunction. It may be associated with altered conscious level or confusion.

Septic shock: This ensues when the patient develops hypotension (blood pressure lower than 5th centile for age) or prolonged capillary refill (>2 s).

In **early septic shock** the patient will respond to parenteral fluid and drug administration.

Refractory septic shock: This ensues if hypotension persists for over an hour despite these measures, and requires vasopressor support.

Multiple organ failure: This is the result of organ hypoperfusion and is manifested in disseminated intravascular coagulation, adult respiratory distress syndrome, renal, hepatic and neurological dysfunction.

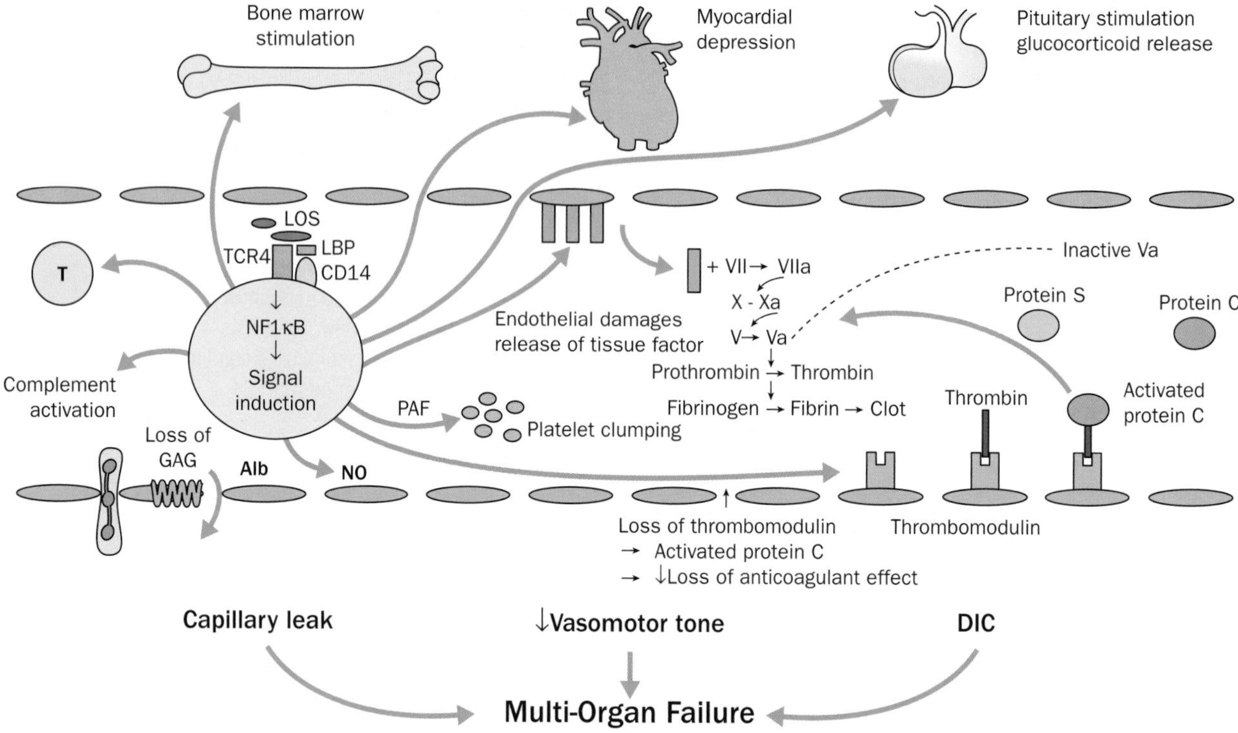

Figure 6.7 Development of septic shock. DIC, disseminated intravascular coagulation; GAG, glucose aminoglycan; LBP, lysobisphosphatidic acid; LOS, lipooligosaccharide; NO, nitric oxide; NF, nuclear factor; TLR, toll-like receptor

The mechanisms involved in the development of septic shock are illustrated in Figure 6.7. The inflammatory cascade is activated by local release of bacteria or toxins, such as the lipo-oligosaccharide endotoxin of Gram-negative bacteria.

Role of the macrophage

The macrophage has receptors such as toll-like receptors (TLRs) on its surface. These bind components of pathogens such as endotoxin, resulting in production and release of cytokines.

Proinflammatory cytokines

TNF:

- promotes macrophage, neutrophil and cytotoxic cell activation
- induces leucocyte and endothelial adhesion molecules
- induces pyrexia
- stimulates production of acute phase proteins
- is procoagulant.

IL-1:

- has TNF-like effects
- induces CD4+ T-cell proliferation and B-cell proliferation and differentiation
- is a chemotactic factor for neutrophils and macrophages.

Anti-inflammatory cytokines

- These cause depression of immune responsiveness after the initial episode of septic shock, e.g. IL-10 inhibits Th1 cytokines and inhibits procoagulant activity.

Nitric oxide

- This is produced by macrophages during acute sepsis.
- It is bactericidal when combined with oxygen radicals.
- It may cause cellular injury.
- Excess leads to reduced vascular resistance.
- It may mediate cytokine-induced myocardial depression and increased intestinal permeability.

Endothelial changes

The normal roles of the endothelium include:

- prevention of coagulation by:
  - expression of thrombomodulin and activation of protein C

- surface heparan sulphate
- tissue plasminogen activator
- production of nitric oxide and prostacyclin, inhibiting platelet aggregation

- facilitation of migration of cells from the blood to the tissues by adhesion molecule expression
- production of chemoattractants
- regulation of arteriole tone, and hence blood pressure
- regulation of vascular permeability.

Endothelial damage by inflammatory cytokines leads to:

- platelets aggregation
- loss of heparan sulphate and exposure of tissue factor leading to activation of the extrinsic coagulation pathway
- loss of thrombomodulin, with loss of negative feedback to activation
- enhancement of leucocyte migration.

Haemodynamic changes

- Decreased arteriolar tone leading to systemic hypotension.
- Decreased venous tone leading to venous pooling.
- Loss of the normal autoregulatory mechanisms in the microvasculature.
- Vascular obstruction and shunting due to reduction in the deformability of red cells and leucocytes, endothelial swelling and increased neutrophil adherence.
- Hypovolaemia: 'third spacing of fluid' due to loss of negatively charged molecules from the endothelial cell surface and leakage of albumin into the tissues.
- Depression of myocardial function.

Management of septic shock

- Treat the underlying infection:
  - appropriate antibiotic at optimal dosage
  - surgical drainage of closed infection.
- Ensure optimal oxygenation:
  - high flow oxygen via face mask
  - intubate and ventilate if inadequate oxygenation despite above OR >40 mL/kg fluid resuscitation required OR signs of development of acute respiratory distress syndrome (ARDS).
- Treat hypovolaemia:
  - initial 10–20 mL/kg crystalloid or colloid. There remains debate as to which is the fluid of choice
  - if failure to respond, further boluses of 10–20 mL/kg colloid.
- Support the circulation:
  - intropes – dopamine, dobutamine, noradrenaline
  - consider adrenaline if hypotension persists despite above.
- Treat anaemia:
  - transfuse if haemoglobin <8 g/dL
  - resist treating borderline anaemia as transfusion may exacerbate sludging in the microvasculature, and encourage apoptosis.
- Treat coagulopathy:
  - Fresh frozen plasma
  - Cryoprecipitate
  - Vitamin K
  - Platelets
- Look for and correct metabolic derangement
  - Hypoglycaemia
  - Acidosis
  - Hypocalcaemia
  - Hypomagnesaemia
  - Hypokalaemia
  - Hypophosphataemia
- The value of using steroids, either in high doses or adrenal replacement dose remains unproven.
- Consider experimental treatment as part of randomized controlled trial
  - Anticytokine preparations
  - Activated protein C and tissue plasminogen activator (tPA)
  - Bactericidal/permeability increasing protein (BPI)
  - Early haemofiltration

KEY LEARNING POINTS

- Early recognition of sepsis is the key to successful treatment.
- Septic shock is the result of complex cellular and chemical interactions: inhibition of a single cytokine or cellular response is unlikely to affect outcome significantly.
- Children requiring over 40 mL/kg fluid replacement should be ventilated and given inotropic support – do not just give more fluid.

PYREXIA OF UNKNOWN ORIGIN

Pyrexia of unknown origin (PUO) was traditionally defined as fever with documented temperatures of >38.3°C on several occasions, persisting more than three weeks and uncertain diagnosis after intensive study during hospital admission for at least a week. With improvements in diagnostic tests, a PUO could now be defined as the presence of fever for eight days or more in a child in whom

CASE STUDY: Pyrexia of unknown origin

A 2-year-old boy presents with a history of fever for seven days. On examination, he is pink, well perfused, flushed, and extremely irritable, with a temperature of 40°C. Examination fails to reveal a focus. Full septic screen, including lumbar puncture, repeated blood culture and viral screen, is negative. While under observation in hospital, he spikes similar fevers once or twice/day, during which he is irritable and sometimes has a faint macular rash but no localizing signs. When apyrexial he is bright and playful.

a thorough history and physical examination, and preliminary laboratory data, fail to reveal a probable cause.

There are reports of over 200 causes of PUO. Some of the causes in children are listed below. Infection accounts for 40 per cent of cases, collagen vascular disease for 12–15 per cent and malignant disease, chiefly leukaemia and lymphoma, for 5–13 per cent of cases. The above case history is suggestive of systemic onset juvenile idiopathic arthritis.

Examples of causes of PUO in children

Infectious diseases

Bacterial – generalized
- Brucellosis
- Leptospirosis
- Lyme disease
- Salmonellosis
- Tuberculosis

Bacterial – localized
- Bacterial endocarditis
- Liver abscess
- Mastoiditis
- Osteomyelitis
- Pelvic abscess
- Perinephric abscess
- Pyelonephritis
- Sinusitis
- Subdiaphragmatic abscess

Viral
- CMV
- Hepatitis
- HIV
- Epstein–Barr virus

Chlamydial
- Psittacosis

Rickettsial
- Q fever

Fungal
- Blastomycosis (non-pulmonary)
- Histoplasmosis (disseminated)

Parasitic
- Malaria
- Toxoplasmosis
- Toxocariasis

Unclassified
- Sarcoidosis
- Chronic recurrent multifocal osteomyelitis

Collagen vascular disease
- Juvenile idiopathic arthritis
- Polyarteritis nodosa
- Systemic lupus erythematosus
- Behçet disease
- Kawasaki disease

Malignancy
- Hodgkin disease
- Leukaemia/lymphoma
- Neuroblastoma

Others
- Diabetes insipidus
- Thyrotoxicosis
- Drug fever
- Factitious fever
- Ectodermal dysplasia
- Crohn disease
- Ulcerative colitis
- Periodic fever
- Serum sickness

Diagnostic approach

A PUO is usually an uncommon presentation of a common disorder, rather than a sign of rare disease, and a systematic approach will often reveal the diagnosis. Fever should be confirmed on multiple occasions while the child is being observed. If possible, all medication, particularly antibiotics and antipyretics, should be stopped.

A full history should be taken (see section on Diagnosis, page 173). It should also include details of the fever itself, maximum (and minimum) temperature, the method of measurement used, any association with location, or with time of day, and whether there are afebrile periods and if so, how long they last. Some diseases have characteristic fever patterns, such as malaria and juvenile idiopathic arthritis. A history of weight loss should be sought. All drugs should be documented, including over-the-counter preparations, herbal/alternative remedies, etc.

Examination

Observation of the child's general demeanour will differentiate, for example a child with Kawasaki disease who is typically acutely miserable and impossible to engage in play, from a child with systemic juvenile arthritis who looks quite well except at the peak of fever. A child who looks completely well despite a documented high temperature may raise the suspicion of factitious fever. Height and weight should be measured and nutritional status assessed. Thereafter, a careful examination including all areas of possible localized infection should be done.

Laboratory investigations

Investigations should be directed by the clues generated by the history and examination. Some basic tests are listed below. A diagnosis is more likely to be achieved in children with a high continuous fever, a high erythrocyte sedimentation rate (ESR) and low haemoglobin. In those with low or episodic fever and normal ESR and haemoglobin, less than 10 per cent will have a definitive diagnosis, but the prognosis for this group is good. Apart from the chest radiograph and abdominal ultrasound, imaging should not be performed routinely.

Basic investigations in PUO

Full blood count and differential white count
ESR
Urea and electrolytes, liver function tests
Lactate dehydrogenase, creatine kinase
Antinuclear antibodies
Rheumatoid factor
Blood cultures × 3
Urinalysis and urine culture
Faecal occult blood and stool culture
EBV serology/heterophile antibody (Monospot)
CMV IgM or virus detection in blood or urine
HIV antibody (if risk factors)
Mantoux test
Chest radiograph

After these investigations, the majority of patients will have potentially diagnostic clues which should guide the further work-up. The pace at which further investigations will need to be performed will largely be dictated by the general condition of the patient. Empirical treatment should be not be started unless the disease is becoming life-threatening.

Further laboratory investigations which may be helpful if the diagnosis remains obscure are given below. Individual risk factors will determine which of these may prove useful. Although the diagnosis remains obscure in most PUOs, those with serious pathology eventually declare themselves, and the prognosis for undiagnosed cases is good. The temptation to overinvestigate should therefore be resisted.

Second line laboratory investigations in PUO

Calcium, phosphate, urate, amylase
Thyroid function (T4, TSH)
C-reactive protein
Angiotensin-converting enzyme (ACE), antineutrophilic cytoplasmic antibodies (ANCA), anti-ds DNA
Immunoglobulins, IgD
Lymphocyte cytometry
C3, C4, CH50
Vanellylmandelic acid (VMA)/homovanillic acid (HVA)
Sweat test
Bone marrow culture and cytology
Throat swab for bacteriology and virology
Blood culture with prolonged incubation
Lumbar puncture – CSF microscopy, culture, and biochemistry
Urine and sputum/gastric aspirate for acid-fast bacilli
Serology

- Antistreptolysin O titre (ASOT)
- *Borrelia* (Lyme)
- Hepatitis A, B, C
- Venereal disease research laboratory (VDRL) test
- *Toxoplasma*
- *Bartonella* (cat scratch)
- *C. psittaci*
- *Coxiella burnetii* (Q fever)
- *Brucella*
- *Leptospira*
- *Salmonella*
- *Mycoplasma*
- *Yersinia*

Radiological investigation

- Chest radiograph
- Sinus radiograph
- Abdominal and pelvic ultrasound
- Computed tomography (CT) scan: abdomen and pelvis
- Barium meal and follow through
- Echocardiography
- Micturating cystourethrogram
- Intravenous urethrogram (IVU)
- Cranial CT/MRI
- Sinus CT
- Chest CT
- Barium enema
- Angiography
- Bone scan
- Nuclear imaging

KEY LEARNING POINTS

- A careful history and examination is the key to diagnosis.
- Target investigations to clinical findings.
- If no cause is obvious after this process, repeat the history and examination.
- Do not overinvestigate and be patient – serious illness will declare itself.

TOXIC SHOCK SYNDROME

CASE STUDY

A 3-year old girl, recovering from chicken pox, develops pain in her right buttock. Twenty-four hours later she becomes delirious, with a temperature of 40.5°C, is covered with a diffuse erythematous rash, with blue, cold extremities, and is screaming with pain in all limbs. Her buttock is acutely tender swollen and fluctuant, and she has profuse watery diarrhoea. After initial resuscitation, incision and drainage of the buttock abscess reveals pus containing numerous Gram-positive cocci.

Toxic shock syndrome (TSS) is due to a toxin produced by an organism (usually TSST 1 produced by *S. aureus*) causing localized infection, rather than dissemination of the infecting organism itself. Most cases in prepubertal children are associated with focal infection, surgical wound infection, burns, varicella, and surgical foreign body placement. The toxin acts as a super-antigen, leading to dramatic T-cell proliferation and cytokine release. Group A streptococcal toxic shock has also been described.

Clinical case definition

1 Fever: T > 38.9°C
2 Rash: diffuse macular erythroderma
3 Desquamation: One to two weeks after onset of illness, particularly extremities
4 Hypotension: systolic blood pressure (BP) <5th centile for age; orthostatic diastolic BP drop >15 mmHg lying to sitting; orthostatic syncope or dizziness
5 Involvement of three or more or the following organ systems
   a Gastrointestinal – vomiting or diarrhoea
   b Muscular – severe myalgia/creatine kinase (CK) >2 × upper limit normal (ULN)
   c Mucous membrane – vaginal, oropharyngeal, conjunctival hyperaemia
   d Renal: urea or creatinine >2 × ULN: >5 WBC per high power field on urine microscopy in absence of UTI
   e Hepatic – transaminases, or bilirubin >2 × ULN
   f Haematological: platelets <100 000/mm^3
   g CNS: disorientation or altered consciousness in absence of focal neurological signs when fever and hypotension absent
6 Negative results on the following
   a Blood, throat, CSF cultures (blood cultures may be positive for *S. aureus*)
   b ± Serological tests for measles, leptospirosis, Rocky Mountain spotted fever

- Probable case – five out of six of the above criteria
- Definite case – six out of six (including desquamation if patient lives for long enough to manifest signs).

Management

- Identify focus of infection – debride, irrigate, and remove any foreign material.
- Intravenous antibiotics to:
  - eradicate organism (flucloxacillin)
  - inhibit toxin production (clindamycin).
- Support shock (see previous section).
- Consider IV immunoglobulin to provide antitoxin antibodies.

- Consider early use of steroids to turn off inflammatory cytokine production.
- Anticipate multiorgan failure.

KEY LEARNING POINTS

- Infection-related shock may occur in the absence of bacteraemia.
- Identification and elimination of the focus of infection is the key to treatment of TSS.

TUBERCULOSIS

CASE STUDY

A 4-year-old boy presents with an acute onset of fever and cough. Chest radiograph reveals right upper lobe collapse and consolidation. He improves following a course of amoxicillin. However, five weeks later, he relapses with cough and fever. Chest radiograph shows persistent right upper lobe changes and hilar lymphadenopathy. At bronchoscopy, there is compression of the right main and segmental bronchi and purulent secretions distally. Microscopy is negative. Culture reveals mixed respiratory flora only. Mantoux test reveals 20 mm induration.

Agent

Mycobacterium tuberculosis is non-motile, non-spore forming and pleomorphic. It stains weakly positive with Gram stain and is acid and alcohol fast due to the high proportion of lipid in its cell wall.

Epidemiology

Tuberculosis is a disease of poverty and overcrowding. In the UK, incidence fell until the 1980s, since when rates have been stable but with a recent increase around London.

Transmission

The source is usually an infected adult with sputum-positive disease. Children rarely transmit tuberculosis because of sparse organisms in endobronchial secretions, lack of cough in primary and miliary disease, and a less forceful cough compared with adults. The organism is spread in droplet nuclei generated during coughing and talking. As few as 1–10 organisms can cause infection; 3000 are produced during an episode of coughing in an adult. The commonest portal of entry is the respiratory tract. Rarely, infection can result from ingestion, or direct contact with infected material.

Incubation period

Around 30 per cent of exposed healthy adults become infected but the risk is greater for infants and children. The skin test becomes positive two to eight weeks (median three to four weeks) after exposure. Risk of developing disease is highest in the first six months, but remains high for two years. Many years may elapse between infection and disease. Infection progresses to disease in around 10 per cent of cases.

Clinical features

Asymptomatic primary tuberculosis

This usually arises about eight weeks after exposure. The primary focus is the area of initial inflammatory reaction around a tubercle bacillus inhaled into the alveolus. The site is commonly subpleural. Bacteria then spread via the lymphatics to the regional lymph nodes. Inflammation, caseation and calcification then occurs, which can be detected on chest radiograph.

Endothoracic lymphadenopathy and endobronchial disease

Enlargement of the peribronchial lymph nodes leads to compression of the adjacent regional bronchus, inflammation within the wall and may progress to bronchial obstruction. This may rarely lead to sudden death due to asphyxia but more commonly causes obstructive emphysema or collapse/consolidation of the affected lung segment. These changes may resolve, but calcification of the lymph nodes, or scarring of the lung or bronchiectasis, may cause permanent changes.

Pleural effusion

This is uncommon in children under 5 years, and results from the spread of bacilli from a subpleural primary focus to the pleural cavity, usually between three and six months after infection. It may present with sudden onset of fever, pleuritic pain, and shortness of breath. The fluid is characterized by high protein, low glucose, high white cell count, but is usually smear-negative. There may be seeding of the pericardium and rarely the myocardium.

Progressive primary tuberculosis

This occurs when the primary complex enlarges. The caseous centre liquefies and there is spread to other parts of the lung. Symptoms include fever, weight loss, malaise and cough.

Reactivation tuberculosis

Reactivation TB is caused by endogenous spread of organisms in a previously sensitized individual. It accounts for only 6–7 per cent of childhood disease and usually occurs in children infected over the age of 7 years. Symptoms are similar to progressive primary disease. Haemoptysis and supraclavicular lymphadenopathy can occur.

Disseminated tuberculosis

Tubercle bacilli may spread via the lymphatics or blood stream to develop foci in bone, skin, superficial lymph node, eye, gastrointestinal tract, or later, renal disease. Widely disseminated lesions are found in miliary tuberculosis. Miliary disease may present insidiously with low-grade fever, lethargy and weight loss or acutely with high fever, lethargy, anorexia, lymphadenopathy, hepatosplenomegaly, progressive weakness, shortness of breath and cyanosis. Chest radiograph shows tubercles throughout the lung fields. Choroidal tubercles may be seen.

Tuberculosis meningitis

Tuberculosis meningitis presents with gradual onset over one to two weeks of lethargy, anorexia, apathy, and personality change. Symptoms and signs of raised intracranial pressure follow, together with signs of meningism and cerebral damage, such as cranial nerve palsies, altered reflexes, and convulsions. Untreated, the child becomes comatose, with loss of brain stem function. Cerebrospinal fluid may be normal in early disease apart from pleocytosis, (predominantly neutrophils) but later glucose drops, protein rises, and lymphocytes predominate. Diagnosis by microscopy and culture, and Mantoux test are both only 50 per cent sensitive. Computed tomography may reveal tuberculomas.

Diagnosis

Microbiological diagnosis

Because of low organism numbers and inability to produce sputum, samples are smear positive in only 5 per cent of clinical cases of childhood pulmonary tuberculosis. The yield is even lower for extrapulmonary disease. Older children may produce sputum, either directly or following induction. Early morning fasting gastric aspiration is unpleasant and invasive but can be diagnostic in younger children who commonly swallow their sputum. Alternative techniques include cough swab, nasopharyngeal aspirate or bronchial lavage. Organisms may also be isolated from biopsy tissue, pleural fluid, urine, CSF, or other normally sterile body fluid.

Ziehl–Neelsen or fluorescent auramine staining will identify mycobacteria. However, microscopy does not distinguish *M. tuberculosis* from other mycobacterial species. Culture on traditional solid media takes from three to six weeks but yield is higher than microscopy – between 25 and 75 per cent. Newer liquid media techniques may produce results in 10–21 days. The role of PCR is yet to be established.

Skin testing

Tuberculin skin testing can be performed using intradermal tuberculin 10IU (Mantoux test), or by multiple skin puncture techniques, such as Heaf test. The test depends on the ability to mount a delayed hypersensitivity reaction and is therefore unreliable in immunodeficient patients. See Table 6.11 for interpretation of positive Mantoux test.

Table 6.11 Interpretation of positive Mantoux test

Induration >5 mm	Induration >10 mm	Induration >15 mm
Children in close contact with known or suspected infectious cases of tuberculosis	Children at increased risk of disseminated disease: Age <4 years Medical risk factors, e.g. Hodgkin, diabetes, chronic renal failure, malnutrition	All children >4 years without risk factors
Children suspected to have tuberculous disease: Consistent chest radiograph Clinical evidence of tuberculosis	Children with increased environmental exposure to tuberculosis: Children or parents born in countries of high prevalence Frequent exposure to high-risk adults	
Children with HIV infection Immunocompromised children		

Radiology

Chest radiograph shows lymphadenopathy in over 90 per cent of cases of pulmonary tuberculosis; the frequency of parenchymal changes is variable and inversely proportional to the child's age. Tuberculous infection is defined as positive skin test, with normal chest radiograph and no symptoms.

Treatment

See Table 6.12. Maintenance drugs may be taken daily or three times weekly in directly observed therapy schedules. Adjuvant therapy, such as surgery for bone disease, and steroids for pericarditis and severe meningitis may be required.

Contact tracing

One in 10 cases of tuberculosis are diagnosed by contact tracing. One per cent of contacts traced will prove positive. Infection is more likely if the index case is smear positive, the child is a close contact of the case, and the child has not had bacille Calmette Guérin (BCG) vaccination. Children are rarely the source for tuberculosis transmission, so diagnosis in a child should prompt a search for the adult index case. Household contacts should be screened and close child contacts identified. Children should be screened if they are close or casual contacts of a smear positive case or if they have had close contact with a smear negative case.

An initial chest radiograph should be taken. If normal, it should be repeated at two to three months after possible exposure together with a tuberculin test. Those who are negative should be offered BCG.

Table 6.12 Treatment of tuberculosis

Disease	Drugs	Duration
Tuberculous infection	INH RIF	3 months
Respiratory tuberculosis	INH RIF	6 months
3 drugs may be used in areas of low resistance	+ PZI + ETH	2 months
Meningitis	INH RIF	12 months
	+ PZI	2 months
	+ Strep or ETH	2 months
Other extrapulmonary tuberculosis	INH RIF	6 months
	+ PZI + ETH	2 months
Multidrug-resistant tuberculosis	Five drugs	Until smear negative
	Three drugs	>9 months

ETH, ethambutol; INH, isoniazid; PZI, pyrazinamide; RIF, rifampicin; strep, streptomycin.

Atypical mycobacterial infection

Organisms such as *M. avium/M. intracellulare* are ubiquitous in soil and water. They rarely cause disease in the immunocompetent, but they may cause disseminated disease in those with severe T-cell immunodeficiency, or defects in IFN-γ and IL-12. Normal children may present with chronic lymphadenitis and with sinus formation, particularly if incision and drainage is attempted. Treatment of choice is gland excision. If this proves impossible, antituberculous drugs may be used. These organisms are resistant to isoniazid.

KEY LEARNING POINTS

- Children with persistent lung consolidation or hilar lymphadenopathy should be investigated for tuberculosis.
- Diagnosis in a child should always trigger the search for an adult source of infection.
- If the child is immunocompromised or has meningitis, a positive skin test is useful, but a negative does not exclude the diagnosis.

HUMAN IMMUNODEFICIENCY VIRUS (HIV) AND ACQUIRED IMMUNODEFICIENCY SYNDROME (AIDS)

CASE STUDY: HIV and AIDS

A 3-year-old child presents with fever, weight loss and difficulty swallowing. Examination reveals oropharyngeal candidiasis, parotid enlargement, significant cervical lymphadenopathy, with palpable nodes in the axillae and groin. His liver and spleen are enlarged. A chest radiograph shows hilar lymphadenopathy with reticular shadowing throughout, compatible with lymphoid interstitial pneumonitis. His mother is well, but his father, whose job involves annual business trips to Thailand, reports a six-month history of chronic diarrhoea and weight loss.

Agent

The human immunodeficiency virus is a single stranded RNA virus which can transcribe its genome into double stranded DNA (reverse transcription). Viral DNA is then integrated into the host cell DNA, allowing the virus to cause lifelong infection and evade the usual immune mechanisms. After a latent period, which may be prolonged, viral gene expression leads to assembly of new virions within the host cell, and budding from the surface, with destruction of the host cell.

Pathogenesis

The human immunodeficiency virus is particularly trophic for cells bearing the CD4 receptor. CD4+ lymphocytes become depleted and dysfunctional due to mechanisms including direct destruction, the formation of syncytia, and the induction of apoptosis. Glial cells within the CNS are also affected, resulting in encephalopathy.

Transmission

Vertical transmission accounts for most cases in children. Other mechanisms include exposure to contaminated needles or infected blood products, and sexual contact. Maternal–fetal transmission can occur *in utero* but most infections occur around the time of birth. The risk in the absence of antiretroviral therapy ranges from 12 to 33 per cent in the developed world and up to 40 per cent in the developing world. Transmission via breast milk accounts for the additional 10–15 per cent risk in breastfed babies.

Factors increasing risk of transmission

- Advanced maternal disease
- High maternal viral load
- Low maternal CD4 count
- Vaginal delivery (compared with caesarean section)
- Prolonged rupture of membranes
- Maternal chorioamnionitis
- Maternal sexually transmitted diseases

Clinical features

Early symptoms and signs include:

- generalized lymphadenopathy
- hepatosplenomegaly
- dermatitis (usually candidal)
- parotitis
- recurrent upper respiratory tract infection.

Those with moderate immune deficiency may develop:

- blood abnormalities, e.g. thrombocytopenia, neutropenia, anaemia
- persistent candidal infection
- bacterial sepsis (meningitis, pneumonia, etc.)
- recurrent or chronic diarrhoea
- cardiomyopathy
- hepatitis
- recurrent or severe herpes simplex infection
- recurrent or disseminated herpes zoster
- severe chicken pox
- lymphoid interstitial pneumonitis.

AIDS-defining conditions include:

- Recurrent invasive bacterial infection
- Opportunistic infections, e.g. pneumocystis, CMV, candidal oesophagitis
- Encephalopathy
- Malignancy, e.g. lymphoma, Kaposi sarcoma (rare in children)
- Wasting syndrome.

Diagnosis

Informed consent should always be obtained from the child, if competent, or if not, the parent. The HIV antibody test in an infant is a test of maternal infection, from whom consent should therefore specifically be sought. In children older than 18 months and children, the presence of HIV antibody in serum is diagnostic. False negatives occasionally occur in late disease or in hypogammaglobulinaemia.

Because of transplacental passage of antibody, all babies born to HIV seropositive women have detectable antibody at birth. Diagnosis under the age of 18 months depends on viral detection, now achieved through PCR. An infant can be assumed to be uninfected after two negative PCR results in the first six months (after six weeks and three to four months). Blood should be tested at 18 months to confirm loss of HIV antibody. If PCR is positive, the test should be repeated, together with viral load and CD4 count. Infection is not confirmed in an asymptomatic child until a second test proves positive.

Natural history

Before specific therapy was available, 20 per cent of infected infants died or progressed to AIDS in the first 18 months. The median age of onset of symptoms was 3 years. However, 40–50 per cent of vertically infected children survived to the age of 10 and a few remained asymptomatic into adolescence.

Management

Prevention of perinatal transmission

The risk of vertical transmission can be reduced to 1 per cent if measures aimed at minimizing viral load and fetal exposure to the virus are taken during pregnancy and delivery. These are:

- combination antiretroviral therapy for women requiring treatment
- zidovudine throughout the third trimester of pregnancy and labour for asymptomatic women with lower viral loads
- treatment of the neonate with the same drug(s) for four weeks after delivery
- delivery by caesarean section
- treatment of sexually transmitted diseases
- no exposure of the baby to breast milk.

P. carinii pneumonia prophylaxis

Co-trimoxazole should be commenced at 1 month of age unless a negative PCR result has been obtained. Infected infants should continue on co-trimoxazole until 1 year of age, when it can be discontinued if the CD4 count remains adequate.

Treatment of infected children

Prognosis in HIV has been dramatically improved with the introduction of highly active antiretroviral therapy (HAART). This involves use of a combination of drugs including the following.

REVERSE TRANSCRIPTASE INHIBITORS

These prevent the elongation of proviral DNA, and thus act on the replicating virus. There are two types:

- Nucleoside analogues (NRTI):
  - Zidovudine
  - Didanosine
  - Lamivudine
  - Stavudine
  - Tenofovir
  - Abacavir
- Non-nucleoside inhibitors (NNRTI)
  - Nevirapine
  - Efavirenz

PROTEASE INHIBITORS

These prevent cleavage of gag-pol polyproteins.

- Nelfinavir
- Saquinavir
- Ritonavir
- Lopinavir
- Atazanavir

The indications for treatment are:

- severe clinical disease
- high HIV viral load
- low CD4 count.

Treatment of infants and children may be complicated by:

- the variable pharmacokinetics of the drugs in this age group
- the limited paediatric formulations
- unpalatable formulations
- the requirements of the drugs to be taken at a specific time in relation to food, which is difficult to achieve in children with unreliable eating habits
- social background and chaotic lifestyles
- concern regarding long-term side effects in the developing child.

The initial treatment regimen will include two NRTIs, and either an NNRTI or a protease inhibitor. Regular monitoring of clinical status, HIV viral load and CD4 count is required to determine response to treatment. Failure to respond may indicate poor compliance, or the development of drug resistance.

KEY LEARNING POINTS

- Most perinatal HIV infection can be prevented if the mother's diagnosis is known antenatally.
- In infancy, HIV antibody is a test of maternal HIV status: PCR is the test of choice.
- Early symptoms and signs of infection are non-specific.
- Effective treatment requires long-term combination therapy, with regular monitoring.

HEALTHCARE-ASSOCIATED INFECTION AND PRINCIPLES OF INFECTION CONTROL

Approximately one in 10 patients admitted to hospital in the UK develop infection as a result of their stay. This problem is escalating in severity with the development of antibiotic resistance in organisms found particularly in the hospital environment. Increasing foreign travel allows the spread of organisms across national boundaries and the increasing numbers of immunocompromised children in hospital provide a particularly susceptible population for infection due to environmental organisms not normally considered to be pathogenic.

Spread of infection

This requires the following:

A source – an infected or colonized person, animal, or environmental reservoir, e.g. soil.

An exit route from the source – e.g. respiratory secretions, contaminated water.

A mode of transmission – e.g. droplet spread, direct contact, use of contaminated water, insect bite.

A portal of entry – e.g. respiratory mucosa, gastrointestinal tract, direct inoculation.

In order to produce infection, the organism needs to enter a susceptible host. Factors influencing susceptibility have been discussed previously. The aim of infection control is to interrupt this process.

Standard precautions

These are practices designed to prevent the spread of infectious agents, and should be applied to all patients. These include:

- Handwashing, which should be performed:
  - before and after direct patient contact
  - before and after aseptic or invasive procedures
  - after contact with body secretions
  - after handling contaminated laundry or equipment
  - after removing protective clothing
  - before serving or eating meals or drinks
  - at the beginning and end of each span of duty.

Clean hands can be decontaminated using alcohol gels, but soiled hands should always be washed with soap.

- Use of protective clothing:
  - Gloves – non-sterile gloves should be worn when contact with blood or body fluids, or articles contaminated with them is anticipated. Sterile gloves should be worn for aseptic and invasive procedures.
  - Masks, eye protectors, face shields should be worn to protect mucous membranes during procedures likely to generate splashes or sprays of blood or body fluids.
  - Disposable aprons protect clothing from soiling or splashing.
- Protection of open wounds using waterproof dressing.
- Safe disposal of clinical waste and sharps.
- Prevention of sharps injury.
- Safe handling of contaminated linen.
- Environmental cleaning.
- Decontamination of medical equipment.

Source isolation

This is necessary to interrupt the transmission of organisms that are spread by direct contact, droplets or aerosols. It involves nursing in a single room, the use of gloves and aprons for any patient contact and hand decontamination after glove and apron removal. Patients infected with organisms that can be transmitted by aerosol, such as measles, chicken pox and tuberculosis, should ideally be nursed in a cubicle with negative pressure ventilation with external exhaust or HEPA-filtered air. Such isolation can be frightening for younger children and boring for older ones. Parents should be encouraged to stay with their child to keep them entertained while contact with other children is restricted. Hospital play specialists have a particularly important role. Toys should be washable or be able to be wiped clean and should not be shared with other children on the ward.

Protective isolation

This is required for children who are particularly susceptible to infection. Before entering the single cubicle, hands should be decontaminated with antimicrobial agent, and a clean apron worn. Extra precautions for exceptionally vulnerable children, e.g. post bone marrow transplant, may include HEPA-filtered positive pressure ventilation or laminar flow ventilation cubicles, full surgical scrub, and protective clothing.

KEY LEARNING POINTS

- To prevent spread of infection, it is important to know the mechanism of transmission.
- Handwashing is the most important practice in preventing spread of infection.
- Children should only be isolated when there is evidence to do so.

Notification of infectious diseases

It is a legal requirement in the UK for medical practitioners to notify the consultant in public health responsible for communicable disease control if they are aware of, or suspect that a patient is suffering from certain infectious diseases or food poisoning.

The following are notifiable diseases:

- Acute encephalitis (England and Wales)
- Anthrax

- Cholera
- Diphtheria (membranous croup)
- Bacillary dysentery (amoebic dysentery (England and Wales))
- Erysipelas (Scotland)
- Food poisoning
- Legionellosis (Scotland)
- Leprosy (England and Wales)
- Leptospirosis
- Lyme disease (Scotland)
- Malaria
- Measles (Scotland)
- Meningitis (England and Wales)
- Meningococcal disease
- Mumps
- Ophthalmia neonatorum (England and Wales)
- Paratyphoid
- Plague
- Poliomyelitis
- Puerperal fever (Scotland)
- Rabies
- Relapsing fever
- Rubella
- Scarlet fever
- Smallpox
- Tetanus
- Toxoplasmosis (Scotland)
- Tuberculosis
- Typhoid fever
- Typhus fever
- Viral haemorrhagic fever
- Viral hepatitis
- Whooping cough
- Yellow fever

IMMUNIZATION

Active immunization

This is the process by which an active immune response can be stimulated without the risk of infection or harm to the host. In response to vaccine antigens, and stimulated by T-cells, B-cells proliferate and produce specific immunoglobulin (see Figure 6.2). T lymphocytes also mediate cellular immune responses. B- and T-cell memory is induced so that re-exposure leads to a rapid response of greater magnitude (anamnestic response).

Inactivated vaccines require repeated doses to achieve this response. Live vaccines have the potential to induce longlasting immunity after one or two doses. Table 6.13 gives examples of both.

Herd immunity

Vaccination programmes are designed both to protect the individual and prevent infection within the population. Herd immunity is achieved when enough people are protected to prevent circulation of the organism within that population. For any infection, the proportion which needs to be protected is determined by:

- contagiousness of the organism
- immune response engendered by the infection
- percentage of the population vaccinated
- efficacy of the vaccine.

Contraindications to vaccination

Any vaccine is contraindicated in presence of:

- acute febrile illness
- anaphylaxis to previous dose or constituent of the vaccine.

Live vaccines are contraindicated in:

- pregnancy
- immunodeficiency
- immunosuppression.

A live vaccine should not be given within three weeks of another live vaccine. If the child has received immunoglobulin, vaccination should be postponed for three months. Vaccination is NOT contraindicated if:

- the child has already had disease (only true for BCG)
- personal or family history of atopy
- personal or family history of epilepsy
- upper respiratory tract infections in the absence of significant fever (38.5°C)
- significant reaction to another vaccine.

Vaccine failure

Vaccine may fail to protect the individual because of:

- failure to store and prepare the vaccine properly
- faulty administration
- poor initial immune response to vaccine
- initially adequate immune response which wanes with time.

Failure to vaccinate

Reasons why health professionals may be reluctant to vaccinate and parents unwilling to accept vaccination for their children include:

- underestimation of severity of the disease
- underestimation of the risk of exposure to the disease

Table 6.13 Examples of vaccines

Vaccine	Type	Schedule	Indications	Side effects	Contraindications	Efficacy (per cent)	Comments
Cholera	Inactivated bacteria	None	None	Local		50	Control of disease depends on public health measures, not vaccine
BCG	Live bacteria	One dose following negative tuberculin test	10–14 years; neonatal (high risk or on request); following contact tracing and screening; health service, veterinary and prison staff; immigrants from countries of high endemicity and their infants; travel to endemic areas >1 month	Vertigo, dizziness, allergy; local abscess formation; lymphadenitis; keloid scarring; disseminated BCG in immunocompromised	Previous BCG scar; positive tuberculin test; fever; septic skin conditions	0–80	No live vaccines within three weeks (oral polio excepted); no vaccination in same arm for three months
Diphtheria	Toxoid	2, 3, 4 months as DTapHib/IPV/ 4–5 years as DTaP/ IPV 14–15 years as dT/IPV	Universal	Local redness and swelling; malaise, transient fever, headache; anaphylaxis		87–96	
Hepatitis A	Inactivated virus	One dose vaccine (720 ELISA units of HM175 strain) with booster at 6–12 months	Travel to endemic areas; hepatitis B, C or other chronic liver disease; haemophilia; during outbreaks	Local reactions; fever, malaise rare		80–90	
Hepatitis B	Inactivated viral antigen	0, 1, 6 months 0, 1, 2, 12 months	Infant of infected mother; infected household member; at-risk profession; high-risk activity, e.g. drug use; families adopting children from high prevalence area;	Local reactions; fever, malaise, flu-like symptoms, arthritis, arthralgia, myalgia; link to Guillain–Barré not established		80–90	Do not give in buttock

			haemophilia; chronic renal failure; residents of homes for severe learning disability; post-exposure prophylaxis				
Hib conjugate	Polysaccharide protein conjugate	2, 3, 4 months as DTaPHib/IPV One dose after one year	Universal; splenectomy/ asplenia; HIV-infected	Local redness and swelling		94–100	
Influenza	Inactivated virus and components	Two doses one month apart – yearly boosters	Immunosuppression; cardiac disease; chronic lung disease including asthma; diabetes mellitus; haemoglobinopathies; long-term aspirin therapy; chronic renal disease; chronic metabolic disease; close contacts of above; including potential carers	Fever (unusual); local redness and swelling; allergy and anaphylaxis; Guillain–Barré syndrome – unproved	Anaphylactic hypersensitivity to egg	50–95	May be given universally in epidemic/pandemic
Measles	Live virus	15 months and 4–5 years as MMR; 6–9 months as single vaccine in endemic areas (not UK)	Universal	Fever; rash, febrile convulsion; thrombocytopenia		90	Side effects less common after second dose; children with egg allergy who have had severe difficulty breathing or shock as a result, or who also have asthma should be immunized under hospital supervision
Meningococcal	Polysaccharide	Single dose after two months	Travel to endemic area; asplenia; HIV; contacts of cases; local outbreaks	Fever rare; local reactions		90: much less under 18 months group C; <3 months in group A	Only available for groups A, C, W135, Y
Meningococcal group C	Polysaccharide protein conjugate	2, 3, 4 months (two doses at 6–12 months)	Universal	Fever rare; local reactions		98	

(Continued)

Table 6.13 *(Continued)*

Vaccine	Type	Schedule	Indications	Side effects	Contraindications	Efficacy (per cent)	Comments
		(One dose >1 year)					
Mumps	Live virus	15 months, 4–5 years as MMR	Universal	Fever; parotid swelling; aseptic meningitis with Urabe strain		90	No license for single vaccine
Whole cell pertussis	Inactivated bacteria	2, 3, 4 months as DTP-Hib	Not used in UK	Local reactions common; fever, crying screaming; hypotonic hyporesponsive episodes; ?? encephalopathy		80	
Acellular pertussis	Purified toxoid and proteins	4–5 years as DTaPIPV 2, 3, 4 months as DTaPHiBIPV	Universal	Local reactions (less common than whole cell); general reactions as above (less common)		70–80	
Pneumococcus	Polysaccharide protein conjugate	<6 months: three doses one month apart with booster in year 2 7–11 months: two doses one month apart, booster year 2 >12–23 months: two doses two months apart	Chronic respiratory; disease; diabetes mellitus; chronic heart disease; chronic renal disease; chronic liver disease; asplenia; immunosuppression; immunodeficiency, particularly HIV; haemoglobinopathies	Local reaction; fever rare		98	Licensed vaccine covers seven serotypes; 9 and 11 valent vaccines are being developed
Pneumococcus	Polysaccha-ride	One dose age >2 years	As above	Local reactions		60–70	Antibody wanes after about five years; covers 23 serotypes
Oral polio vaccine	Live virus	2, 3, 4 months, 4–5 years, 14–15 years	Not used in UK	Vaccine-associated poliomyelitis	Vomiting or diarrhoea Extreme hypersensitivity to penicillin, neomycin, streptomycin, polymyxin	95	May spread to contacts: good hygiene practices recommended
Inactivated polio vaccine	Inactivated virus	2, 3, 4 months as DTaPHiBIPV 4–5 years as DTaPIPV 14–15 years dTIPV	As substitute for OPV in: immune compromised; household contacts of immune	Local reaction	Extreme hypersensitivity to polymyxin B	95	Combined DTPHibIPVHepB vaccine licensed in the USA

			compromised; neonatal nursery/ hospital inmates				
Rabies	Inactivated virus	Post-exposure: 0, 3, 7, 14, 30 days	After exposure	Local reactions in 24–48 hours; Fever, headache; muscle aches; urticaria	None	98 in pre-exposure	If high risk, also give specific immunoglobulin
Rubella	Live virus	12–15 months, 4–5 years	Universal; non-immune women; immigrants to UK	Fever; sore throat; lymphadenopathy; rash; arthralgia; arthritis; thrombocytopenia		95	
Tetanus	Toxoid	2, 3, 4 months as DTaPHiBIPV 4–5 years as DTaPIPV 13–18 years as Td Prophylaxis for tetanus prone wound as Td	First five doses universal; further dose if tetanus prone wound and >10 years since last dose	Local reactions; headache; lethargy; malaise; myalgia; fever; anaphylaxis and urticaria rare			Acute febrile illness not a contraindication in presence of tetanus-prone wound
Typhoid	Inactivated bacteria	Two doses, 4–6 weeks apart	Travellers to endemic areas where hygiene may be poor	Local reactions common; malaise; nausea; headache; pyrexia		70–80	Not recommended for outbreaks in UK
Typhoid	Polysaccharide	Single dose – repeat at 3 years if still at risk	As above	Mild local reaction		70–80	Not effective in children <18 months
Typhoid	Live attenuated bacteria	One capsule alternate days for Three doses by mouth	As above	Nausea, vomiting, abdominal cramps, diarrhoea, urticaria	Children <6 years Concurrent antibiotic use; persistent diarrhoea or vomiting	70–80 for about a year	If taking mefloquine, leave 12 hours between mefloquine and vaccine
Varicella	Live attenuated virus	One dose: 1–12 years Two doses one month apart: >13 or immunocom-promised	13 years with no history of chicken pox and negative serology Available on named patient basis for immunosuppressed children and those at increased risk of severe varicella	Maculopapular/ varicelliform rash in 7–8 per cent; local pain and tenderness; Zoster-like illness in years following vaccination (rare)	Corticosteroids >2 mg/kg per day Severe immunocompromise; allergy to vaccine components; within five months of intravenous immunoglobulin	97 in childhood 99 after two doses in adolescence	Do not give salicylates for six weeks after vaccination

- underestimation of vaccine efficacy
- overestimation of the risk of adverse effects
- overestimation of the severity of likely side effects
- overestimation of efficacy of alternative methods of protecting the child, e.g. homoeopathy
- health professionals' fear of litigation.

Passive immunization

This involves administering preformed antibodies to the child in order to prevent or modify infectious disease. Protection lasts only for a few weeks. It is indicated in the following circumstances:

- when a person is unable to make antibody, e.g. primary antibody deficiencies, T-cell immune deficiencies
- when a susceptible person is exposed to the infectious agent, and is at risk of severe disease
- when a disease is already present, to suppress the effect of a toxin, or to suppress the inflammatory response.

Examples of products used in this way can be found in Table 6.14.

Table 6.14 Products used in passive immunization

Product	Indication	Adverse effects	Comments
Intravenous immunoglobulin (IVIG)	Replacement therapy in antibody deficiency disorders Chronic parvovirus B19 infection Kawasaki disease Paediatric HIV Hypogammaglobulinaemia in CLL Post-bone marrow transplantation Low birth weight infants Immune thrombocytopenic purpura	Fever, chills Headache, myalgia, anxiety, light-headedness, nausea, vomiting Flushing, blood pressure changes, tachycardia Aseptic meningitis Hypersensitivity reactions	Caution if history of adverse reactions to IV or IM immunoglobulin Adrenaline should be available in case of cardiovascular reactions Reduce rate if adverse reaction occurs Children with poor cardiac function at high risk of vasomotor/cardiac complications
Human normal immunoglobulin	Replacement therapy in antibody deficiency disorders (given subcutaneously) Prophylaxis for hepatitis A: within 14 days post-exposure; during outbreaks; as alternative to vaccine for short trips to endemic areas Post-exposure prophylaxis for measles in immunocompromised or those <1 year at risk of severe disease	Local reactions Less common systemic effects as in IVIG Anaphylaxis rare	Caution if history of adverse reactions Adrenaline should be available
Antitetanus immunoglobulin	Prophylaxis for tetanus prone wound if patient partially immunized, last vaccine >10 years age, or immunocompromised	As above	As above
Antihepatitis immunoglobulin	Infants born to hepatitis BsAg-positive women. Given at birth if: HBeAg +ve HBsAg +ve no e markers available Mother had acute hepatitis during pregnancy Post-exposure prophylaxis in non-immune Within 48 hours, not later than one week	As above	As above
Antirabies immunoglobulin	Post-exposure to high-risk animal in partially or non-immune		
Varicella zoster (VZ) immunoglobulin	Infants whose mothers develop chicken pox seven days before to 28 days after delivery VZ antibody-negative infants exposed to chicken pox in first 28 days of life Post-exposure during pregnancy Post-exposure in patients at risk of severe varicella		

Current vaccination schedules in UK

Immunization schedules vary between countries. The current UK schedule is given below.

2, 3, 4 months - DTacPHibIPV, Men C
12–15 months - MMR
4–6 years - DTacPIPV, MMR
12–13 years - BCG
14–15 years dT, IPV

The World Health Organization (WHO) recommends universal hepatitis B immunization, but at the time of writing, this has not been implemented in the UK. A Hib booster may be recommended in the second year of life.

KEY LEARNING POINTS

- Vaccination programmes have reduced the burden of disease due to many infections for which there is still inadequately effective treatment.
- Programmes are designed to benefit not only those vaccinated but also the vulnerable in the population.
- Risk of side effects should be balanced against risks of sequelae from exposure to the disease.
- Passive immunization gives temporary, less effective protection but may benefit those unable to mount an effective immune response.

DISORDERS OF THE IMMUNE SYSTEM

Diagnosis and recognition

Immunodeficiency manifests clinically in an increased susceptibility to infection. It should be suspected in children with:

- frequent episodes of infection
- recurrent episodes of infection with particular organisms
- unusual clinical course of disease with known pathogen
- unusual pathogen.

Many factors influence the frequency of infective episodes in children. These include:

- Breast feeding
- Parental smoking
- Overcrowding
- Exposure to other children (particularly day care/nursery)
- Underlying medical condition (sickle cell, nephrotic syndrome, cystic fibrosis)
- Atopy
- Foreign bodies
- Breech of physical barriers (e.g. skull fracture, burns)
- Exposure to resistant organisms
- Recurrent pathogen exposure, e.g. infected water supply.

Immune dysfunction may also be secondary to:

- Malnutrition/protein or vitamin deficiencies
- Prematurity
- Immunosuppressive infections, e.g. HIV, EBV
- Infiltrative and malignant diseases
- Surgery, e.g. splenectomy
- Immunosuppressive agents.

Immunodeficiency may be diagnosed by:

- Recognition of syndromic features
  - DiGeorge syndrome: These children have dysmorphic features (hypertelorism, downward slant to eyes, low-set abnormal ears, micrognathia), and most commonly present because of hypocalcaemia due to hypoparathyroidism, or as a consequence of cardiac abnormality such as interrupted aortic arch. Thymic aplasia or hypoplasia can lead to severe T-cell immunodeficiency. Those less severely affected may develop autoimmune disease.
  - Ataxia telangiectasia: This is characterized by oculocutaneous telangiectasia, progressive ataxia, drooling, and later muscle weakness. Those affected show increased sensitivity to ionizing radiation. They suffer recurrent sinopulmonary infection. IgA deficiency is seen in 70 per cent, and antibody response to viral and bacterial antigens may be reduced. T-cell immunity is abnormal in 60 per cent. Inheritance is autosomal recessive, the gene defect being located on chromosome 11q.

Symptoms may first appear in other systems:

- Neurological symptoms
  - Ataxia telangiectasia
  - HIV: primary encephalopathy, CNS infection or CNS malignancy
  - Purine nucleoside phosphorylase deficiency. This is a defect of purine metabolism resulting in developmental delay, muscle spasticity, and mental retardation. The progressive T-cell immunodeficiency may not present until a few years of age.

- Skin manifestations
  - Wiskott–Aldrich syndrome: Affected boys most frequently present with petechiae or bleeding in the first 6 months of life, followed by a typical eczematous rash. There is a T-cell immune defect, presenting as recurrent bacterial and viral infections, particularly otitis media, pneumonia, and severe or recurrent herpes virus infections. Death occurs due to bleeding, infection, or malignancy. Investigation reveals low IgM, high levels of IgA and IgE, and defective antibody response to polysaccharide antigens. There is defective CD43 expression. Bone marrow transplantation can be curative, but for those with no human leucocyte antigen (HLA) matched sibling, treatment consists of IV immunoglobulin, splenectomy and antimicrobial prophylaxis.
  - Hyper-IgE (Job) syndrome: Affected children have an eczematoid dermatitis, but with a distribution and appearance not typical of atopic eczema. Characteristic features are recurrent staphylococcal abscesses and pneumonia, with formation of pneumatocoeles. IgE and IgD levels are markedly elevated, with normal IgA, IgG and IgM. There is marked eosinophilia, and reduced specific antibody responses.
  - Graft-versus-host disease: This may occur in undiagnosed severe T-cell immunodeficiency, either due to engraftment of maternal T-cells acquired transplacentally, or due to blood transfusion with non-irradiated blood. It arises as a blotchy erythematous rash, involving palms and soles, can become bullous, but in the chronic form, develops into erythroderma.
- Skin sepsis
  - Antibody deficiency
  - Neutrophil disorders
  - Disorders of complement.

Children can be identified before they become symptomatic if the possibility of inheritance is recognized (Table 6.15).

Suspicion may be aroused because of an abnormal laboratory result, such as leucopenia in T-cell immunodeficiency. A chest radiograph may show the rib and vertebral abnormalities of adenosine deaminase deficiency (SCIDS, severe combined immunodeficiency syndrome).

Testing immune function

Immune function testing should be considered in the following circumstances:

- history of two episodes of major infections (e.g. meningitis, osteomyelitis, pneumonia)
- history of six or more episodes of minor infection/year, particularly if there is also watery diarrhoea, failure to thrive, chronic lung changes
- relative of a patient with immunodeficiency who genetically could have the same defect
- non-infective feature of classic immunodeficiency
- *P. carinii* pneumonia unrelated to drugs
- lymphopenia unrelated to drugs.

Table 6.15 Immunodeficiency syndromes

X-linked	Autosomal recessive	Other
Bruton agammaglobulinaemia	Adenosine deaminase deficiency (SCIDS)	Job syndrome (AD with partial penetrance)
CD40 ligand deficiency (hyper IgM)	IL-7 receptor deficiency (B-cell NK cell SCIDS)	DiGeorge (AD with high spontaneous rate)
Wiskott-Aldrich	PNP deficiency	Common variable immunodeficiency (various)
Common γ-chain deficiency (B-cell SCIDS)	MHC class II deficiency	
Chronic granulomatous disease	Chronic granulomatous disease	
Properdin deficiency (complement)	Leucocyte adhesion defect	
X-linked lymphoproliferative disease		

AD, autosomal dominant; IL, interleukin; NK, natural killer; PNP, purine nucleoside phosphorylase; MHC, major histocompatibility complex.

Which tests?

Full blood count, differential and blood film

- Haemoglobin may be reduced in chronic infection.
- Neutrophil count will identify neutropenia. Serial measurements over a three-week period may be required to diagnose cyclical neutropenia.
- Neutrophilia is often seen in phagocytic or chemotactic disorders, e.g. chronic granulomatous disease (CGD).
- Lymphocyte count is commonly reduced in T-cell immune deficiency. In infants, a persistent count of $<2.8 \times 10^9$/L should prompt further investigation.
- Platelet count and platelet size is reduced in Wiskott–Aldrich syndrome.
- Blood film may show Howell–Jolly bodies in asplenic patients.

Tests of cell-mediated immunity

Skin tests

These are performed by intradermal injection of an antigen to which the individual has already been exposed (e.g. candida, tetanus toxoid, purified protein derivative (PPD)) and recording erythema and induration at 24 and 48 hours. They are of limited use in young children under 2 years because of lack of prior sensitization.

T-cell subset enumeration

This is performed using fluorochrome tagged monoclonal antibodies against markers on the lymphocytes. The results are expressed as percentages of total lymphocyte count. The ratio of CD4:CD8 cells is normally >1 and reverse in this ratio may signify HIV infection. Children with common variable immunodeficiency may have an increased ratio due to relative loss of CD8 cells (Table 6.16).

Lymphocyte proliferation

In this assay lymphocytes are incubated with mitogens (e.g. phytohaemagglutinin (PHA), pokeweed mitogen (PMA), concanavalin A (conA)) or antigens and reactivity measured by uptake of tritiated thymidine to give a stimulation index that is compared to a normal control.

Table 6.16 Lymphocyte subsets

Antigen	Normal numbers <1 year	Comments
Lymphocytes	2.8–8.8 $\times 10^9$/L	
CD3	55–78 per cent	Mature T-cells
CD4	40–60 per cent	Helper T-cells
CD8	16–35 per cent	Cytotoxic-suppressor T-cells
CD19	19–31 per cent	B-cells

Cytokine and receptor assays

These are not so routinely available but may be useful in diagnosis of rare immunodeficiencies.

Tests for humoral immunity

IMMUNOGLOBULINS

Levels are age related. As IgG at birth is largely maternally acquired, levels may be normal initially despite profound immunodeficiency. Hypogammaglobulinaemia occurs in:

- SCIDS
- T-cell immunodeficiency
- X-linked agammaglobulinaemia (XLA)
- Common variable immunodeficiency (CVI)
- CD40 ligand deficiency
- MHC class II deficiency

Raised immunoglobulins are associated with chronic infection, autoimmune conditions, CGD and HIV. Raised IgE is associated with atopy, and also with phagocytic and chemotactic disorders.

SPECIFIC ANTIBODY LEVELS

Measurement of antibody titres against antigen to which the child has previously been exposed is the best functional assay of humoral immunity. Children under 2 years who have been immunized against HIB and tetanus should show protective antibody levels. If initial levels are low, a booster dose can be given and the response measured. There is no clinical value in estimation of IgG subclasses.

Children over the age of 2 years should be able to mount a T-cell independent antibody response to polysaccharide antigen. Measuring response to the pneumococcal polysaccharide vaccine, Pneumovax® tests the ability to do so. As younger children normally do not make adequate response, their titre of pneumococcal antibody, even following invasive infection, is typically low.

TEST OF PHAGOCYTIC FUNCTION

Nitroblue tetrazolium test (NBT)

During phagocytosis, the colourless NBT is reduced to formazan, which is purple. Failure of reduction indicates an inability to generate superoxide, as is the case in CGD.

TESTS OF COMPLEMENT FUNCTION

CH50

This is a test of total haemolytic complement, and will be reduced if there is deficiency of any component of the classical pathway. High levels are found in inflammatory conditions.

C3

Levels of C3 mirror those of total haemolytic complement. Low levels can also be seen in conditions associated with protein loss, e.g. glomerulonephritis, and in systemic lupus erythematosus (SLE), immune complex diseases, and Coombs' positive haemolytic anaemia.

C4

Levels are reduced in complement deficiency and in protein-losing conditions. Levels are also low in C1 inhibitor deficiency (hereditary angio-oedema).

The presentation of immune deficiency

CASE STUDY: T-cell immunodeficiency

A baby boy born at term weighing 3.75 kg develops severe oral candidiasis at 2 weeks of age, followed by candidal dermatitis around the napkin area. At 6 weeks he develops loose watery stools, after which he fails to thrive. At 4 months he develops a cough, becomes breathless and unable to feed. Chest radiograph shows interstitial changes. *P. carinii* is identified and rotavirus is isolated from stool.

This is compatible with SCIDS or HIV. Other features of SCIDS are congenital graft-versus-host disease, chronic respiratory viral infection or disseminated CMV infection. If recognized early, the prognosis following bone marrow transplantation is excellent, with over 95 per cent survival in matched sibling donor transplants, and over 90 per cent in mismatched. A poorer prognosis is associated with being over 6 months at diagnosis, or already having chronic respiratory infection at the time of diagnosis.

Pneumocystis carinii pneumonia is the commonest opportunistic infection in infancy. In the UK, primary T-cell immunodeficiency should be considered, but in countries of higher prevalence, HIV is by far the commonest underlying cause. Others at risk include those with severe DiGeorge syndrome, T-cell activation defects, MHC class II deficiency and CD40 ligand deficiency (hyper IgM).

Early-onset chronic or recurrent sinopulmonary infection is suggestive of **X-linked agammaglobulinaemia** (XLA), which is due to failure of development of mature peripheral B-cells from pre-B-cells, with lack of antibody production. Lymphocyte cytometry demonstrates lack of CD19-bearing cells, and levels of IgG, A and M are very low or undetectable. Specific antibody responses are absent. Children with XLA may also present with sepsis, but only rarely with invasive infections such as meningitis. Treatment is with immunoglobulin replacement.

CASE STUDY: Antibody deficiency

An 18-month-old infant presents with his second episode of lobar pneumonia. He was perfectly well until his first episode at 8 months of age. Thereafter he developed a purulent nasal discharge and conjunctivitis. He has had repeated courses of antibiotics for otitis media with chronic discharge. He is now failing to thrive.

CD40 ligand deficiency can present similarly, but *P. carinii* pneumonia can occur. In this condition, B-cell immunoglobulin isotype switching fails, so that B-cell numbers are normal, IgM levels are high or normal, but there is absence of IgG, A and E. These children need immunoglobulin replacement and co-trimoxazole prophylaxis. They are susceptible to cryptosporidiosis and long-term risk of sclerosing cholangitis. They should be advised to drink boiled water and avoid swimming in public baths or pools. Although most children survive until adolescence, the mortality is high thereafter due to liver disease and malignancy. Bone marrow transplantation should be offered to those with a matched donor.

Common variable immunodeficiency presents similarly but later than XLA. Autoimmune features or granulomatous disease may be prominent features. In this condition, B-cells are present, but immunoglobulins low, with specific antibody responses reduced or absent. Treatment is with IV immunoglobulin.

IgA deficiency may be asymptomatic, but can be associated with recurrent respiratory and gastrointestinal infection. Some may also fail to respond to polysaccharide antigens such as *Pneumococcus*. Management is with additional vaccination and prophylactic antibiotics.

CASE STUDY: Neutrophil disorders

A 15-month-old infant develops fever and abdominal pain. He has had two previous episodes of lymphadenitis requiring incision and drainage. Ultrasound reveals two abscesses in the liver.

In **chronic granulomatous disease** (CGD), there is failure to produce oxygen radical in the phagosome (see Figure 6.4, page 170). Those affected are vulnerable to infection with catalase-positive organisms, e.g. *S. aureus*,

Klebsiella, *Salmonella*, and fungi, e.g. *Candida* and *Aspergillus*. X-linked disease is due to lack of the 91 kD protein (see Figure 6.4, page 170). Deficiency of the other components has autosomal recessive inheritance. Gastrointestinal complications include gastric outflow tract obstruction and a Crohn-like colitis. Management of acute episodes is by aggressive high-dose cidal antibiotics which have good intracellular penetration and with drainage of abscesses. Leucocyte infusions are sometimes necessary. Chronic management is with long-term antibiotics and antifungals (co-trimoxazole and itraconazole). The role of rIFN-γ is debated, but has been shown to reduce frequency of infective episodes. Bone marrow transplantation has been successful in a few cases. Most children now survive into adolescence. Thereafter, mortality increases due to *Aspergillus* infection and chronic lung and gastrointestinal disease.

CASE STUDY: Complement deficiency

A 10-year-old boy develops meningococcal meningitis. He had meningococcal septicaemia at the age of 4 years with no adverse sequelae. In the interim, he has been well apart from an episode of pneumococcal pneumonia a year ago.

Defects of **complement** activation, e.g. properdin deficiency, present with recurrent infection with encapsulated organisms. Although episodes can be recurrent and long-term morbidity from meningitis can result, the septicaemia is typically not fulminant. Management is with prophylactic antibiotics and immunization.

Autoimmune disease

Pathogenesis

Disease results from the failure of tolerance, which is the process by which autoreactive cells are eliminated or neutralized.

CENTRAL TOLERANCE

During the maturation of T-cells in the thymus, anti-self lymphocytes are deleted by apoptosis (negative selection).

PERIPHERAL TOLERANCE

Not all anti-self lymphocytes are eliminated centrally. A small number migrate peripherally, where their activity is controlled by:

- Ignorance – T-cells ignore the antigens because:
  - the level of antigen is below that needed to induce activation
  - the T-cell is physically separated from the antigen, e.g. by the blood–brain barrier
  - the T-cells require co-stimulatory factors for activation which are not present.
- Deletion – presence of antigen in absence of co-stimulation leads to deletion due to:
  - lack of necessary growth factors
  - activation of Fas receptor, which induces apoptosis.
- Anergy – T-cells do not produce IL-2 on encountering the antigen.
- Inhibition of T-cell activation.

Failure of tolerance

These mechanisms may fail due to environmental or genetic factors.

- Environmental factors include:
  - Damage to physical barriers by infective, chemical or physical agents (e.g. sunlight in SLE).
  - Cell death by necrosis rather than apoptosis.
  - Infective agents causing a 'bystander effect' with activation of macrophages and T lymphocytes.
  - Bacterial products acting as superantigens.
  - Molecular mimicry by microorganism or food antigens resembling self-antigen.
  - Expression of self-antigen which is normally hidden intracellularly on the cell surface, as in some malignancies.
  - Internal environment, e.g. hormonal influences.
- Genetic factors: variation in genes influencing tolerance mechanisms.

Mechanisms of autoimmune damage

The following mediate the resulting cellular damage.

CIRCULATING AUTOANTIBODIES

- Complement lysis (e.g. autoimmune haemolysis)
- Interaction with cell receptors (thyrotoxicosis)
- Toxic immune complexes (SLE)
- Antibody-dependent cellular cytotoxicity (? organ-specific diseases)
- ? Intracellular penetration.

T LYMPHOCYTES

- CD4+ cell Th1 responses via proinflammatory cytokines (rheumatoid arthritis, type 1 diabetes).
- Cytotoxic CD8+ T-cells causing direct cytolysis.

NON-SPECIFIC CAUSES

- Recruitment of inflammatory cells into autoimmune lesions, e.g. synovitis.

KEY LEARNING POINTS

- Early recognition and diagnosis of immunodeficiency can markedly improve outcome.
- Immunoglobulin measurement is often unhelpful under 3 months of age.
- Remember to look at the lymphocyte count if a differential white count has been done.
- The pattern of infection can indicate the nature of the immunodeficiency.
- T-cell dysfunction not only leads to infection, but also to autoimmunity.

ALLERGY

CASE STUDY

A 7-month-old is given scrambled egg for lunch. After the second spoonful, he becomes distressed, spits the food out, and develops a rapidly spreading blotchy erythematous rash. His lips are swollen and he claws at his face. He then vomits profusely. The rash gradually settles over the next hour.

Allergy is a clinical event or disorder mediated by an **immune response** whose consequence is **detrimental** to the host. Some allergic stimulants produce a reaction in all individuals. These include the systemic reaction caused by mismatched blood transfusion, or the urticaria produced by nettle stings.

Atopic individuals are those who develop such responses after exposure to substances that are common in the environment, such as pollen, house dust, animal dander, leading to eczema, asthma, and hay fever.

Pathophysiology of allergic disorders

Traditionally, four types of hypersensitivity have been described.

- Type I – mediated by IgE, leading to immediate hypersensitivity responses (within hours of exposure), e.g. anaphylactic reactions, hay fever, allergic asthma
- Type II – due to antibody-mediated destruction of cells or tissues, e.g. autoimmune haemolysis
- Type III – due to circulating immune complexes, which deposit on or around blood vessels, e.g. serum sickness, glomerulonephritis
- Type IV – mediated by sensitized T-cells, leading to delayed hypersensitivity (several hours after exposure). e.g. tuberculin skin reaction, contact dermatitis

Pathophysiology of atopy and mechanism of immediate hypersensitivity

Atopy is often, but not always associated with high levels of circulating IgE, positive skin prick tests to two or more common environmental allergens, and hyperresponsiveness of the end organ to the chemical mediators involved.

Immediate hypersensitivity reactions and anaphylaxis

Characteristic symptoms of an acute allergic reaction (mild to moderate) include:

- Urticarial rash
- Itch
- Sneezing
- Numbness/tingling of lips/metallic taste in mouth
- Lip and facial swelling
- Hoarse voice
- Sensation of a 'lump in the throat'
- Coughing, choking
- Wheeze
- Nausea, vomiting, diarrhoea
- Abdominal cramps

Anaphylaxis is characterized by:

- Sense of 'impending doom'
- Palpitations (tachycardia)
- Cold, clammy peripheries
- Severe difficulty breathing (stridor or wheeze)
- Sudden feeling of weakness
- Collapse/shock
- Unconsciousness

Common precipitants include:

- Food, e.g. peanuts
- Insect venom
- Plants, e.g. strawberry, latex
- Drugs, e.g. penicillin

Anaphylaxis and anaphylactoid reactions

True anaphylaxis is due to type I or III hypersensitivity. Reactions resembling anaphylaxis (anaphylactoid) may be due to release of vasoactive agents by other mechanisms. Drug interactions and reactions to aggregates caused by infusion of plasma substitutes can mimic anaphylaxis. Occasionally, symptoms may be psychosomatic.

Management of reactions

For mild-to-moderate symptoms:

- give an oral antihistamine (chlorphenamine)
- repeat dose if further progression
- bronchodilator (salbutamol or terbutaline via spacer or nebulizer) for mild to moderate wheeze.

For severe respiratory distress (stridor or wheeze) or signs of shock:

- give oxygen if available
- give **intramuscular** 1:1000 adrenaline
- repeat dose after five minutes if no improvement
- give intramuscular or IV chlorphenamine if venous access established

ALSO

- hydrocortisone if reaction involves wheeze or patient has a history of severe asthma
- if shock unresponsive to the above, give IV fluid bolus of 20 mL/kg
- bronchodilator for persistent wheeze
- **In profound shock only**: IV adrenaline 0.1 mg/mL (1 in 10 000) given slowly.

Investigation of possible anaphylaxis

Plasma mast cell tryptase is indicative of mast cell degranulation. Serial samples showing rise and fall over six to 12 hours is indicative of true anaphylaxis. Abnormality in full blood count, differential white count and complement levels may indicate alternative diagnoses. Specific IgE titres may assist diagnosis of the precipitating allergen.

Diagnosis of allergy

The most important diagnostic tool is a careful history. A detailed description of the reaction should be obtained, including the symptoms and their duration. Details of food ingested and possible exposure to other allergens in the one to two hours before the onset of symptoms should be obtained. Previous reactions, or lack of reaction to suspected or related allergens, should be noted. The environment in which the reaction occurred may be relevant, as may an association with exercise.

No further testing is required if typical symptoms and signs consistently occur shortly after exposure to a single allergen. Tests which may be useful if the diagnosis remains unclear include the following.

Skin prick testing

This involves pricking the skin to a depth of a couple of millimetres only through a drop of standard solution containing the allergen. Foods like fruits can be pricked, and then the skin pricked directly. The diameter of the resulting weal is measured after 15–20 minutes. The test is quick and cheap. Wheals of 8 mm to milk, 7 mm to egg and 8 mm to peanut have 95 per cent positive predictive value for clinical reactions. Wheals to inhaled allergens, e.g. pollen, are characteristically of similar size to the positive control in sensitive children. Children under 2 years do not develop such large wheals, reducing the negative predictive value. Skin prick test should not be done if there is a history of recent ingestion of an oral antihistamine or dermographism.

Serological testing (specific IgE cap RAST)

Testing blood is more invasive and more expensive, and there is a delay before results become available. It is useful if the child is taking regular antihistamines, if they have severe eczema, or if appropriate solutions for skin testing are not available. The specific IgE titre does not correlate with the risk of anaphylaxis. Children can have positive serology without developing symptoms on exposure, but a titre of 15 IU/L to peanut correlates well with a positive oral challenge.

Provocation test

This involves controlled exposure to increasing amounts of the potential allergen until a reaction is observed, or there has been sufficient exposure to rule out the possibility of allergy. This may be an open challenge, or double blind with a placebo arm. The double blind challenge is particularly useful for non-IgE-mediated or delayed reactions. Oral challenge can be useful when skin tests or serological tests have suggested sensitivity to an allergen to which there is no history of exposure. It can be used to verify clinical history if other tests are unsupportive or to determine whether a child with a history of sensitivity has developed tolerance. If there is a risk of an acute allergic reaction, IV access should be established prior to commencement. The test should only be performed in settings where resuscitation facilities are immediately available.

Management

This usually consists of avoidance of the allergen, and the use of antihistamine in the event of exposure. Those at risk of anaphylaxis may carry adrenaline. Children, particularly those old enough to be independent, should be advised to wear a MedicAlert® or similar locket or bracelet indicating their diagnosis. Immunotherapy is available for venom allergies (wasp and bee) and for isolated pollen allergy. However, venom desensitization involves weekly injections followed by less frequent maintenance injections over a total of three years. This is usually tolerated only by older children and adults with significant symptomatology. It should be offered only in centres experienced in the management of anaphylaxis with resuscitation facilities immediately available.

Allergic rhinitis (hay fever)

This is the commonest chronic disease in childhood. As well as morbidity due to symptoms of itching, sneezing, nasal discharge, nasal blockage and allergic conjunctivitis, affected children have a high incidence of anxiety, depression, fatigue and reduced learning ability. Sufferers commonly have other atopic symptoms such as asthma. In Britain, hay fever is usually caused by grass pollen (rye or timothy), and symptoms peak in June and July. Spring symptoms are usually due to tree pollen and autumnal symptoms due to weed pollens and moulds. It takes two seasons to become sensitized, thus hay fever is uncommon under the age of 3 years.

Diagnosis

This is usually based on history. Examination reveals pale, bluish, swollen nasal mucosa. Testing for specific allergen sensitivity may help to reinforce advice regarding avoidance.

Management

In addition to pollen avoidance and the use of oral and topical antihistamines, topical cromoglycate can be used for eye symptoms and cromoglycate or topical steroids can be used to treat nasal symptoms. In severe cases, a short course of oral steroids or immunotherapy may be considered.

Food allergy

The prevalence of food allergy in Western society is between 2 and 6 per cent. Rates up to 28 per cent are quoted in some series depending on the definition. There is a marked geographical variation, both in prevalence and in the foods implicated.

Adverse reactions to food include:

- IgE-mediated immune reactions, e.g. peanut allergy
- non-IgE-mediated immune reactions, e.g. cows' milk protein intolerance
- non-allergic food intolerance
  - pharmacological, e.g. caffeine in soft drinks
  - metabolic, e.g. lactose intolerance, galactosaemia
  - toxic, e.g. scombrotoxic shellfish poisoning, botulism
- food aversion.

In the UK, the foods commonly causing allergy include cows' milk and eggs in infants and toddlers, and peanuts and tree nuts in older children. Allergies to wheat, fish, shellfish, strawberry, kiwi fruit, pulses and other seeds are also seen frequently. Some children with peanut allergy will also be sensitive to pulses, tree nuts and seeds. Latex allergy may be associated with allergy to fruits, particularly banana, chestnut, and avocado. The oral allergy syndrome is the combination of birch pollen allergy and reactions to fruits such as apple.

Management

Allergen avoidance will involve the dietitian, who will provide information regarding products to be avoided. They will advise about substitutes and ensure that the diet is nutritionally replete.

Families should be educated on the management of reactions. If there is a history of immediate hypersensitivity, all should carry antihistamine syrup, which is easier to administer in the presence of oropharyngeal swelling than tablets or capsules, even in older children. Family members should be taught to recognize early symptoms and signs and give the medication immediately.

Those at significant risk of anaphylaxis should also carry adrenaline in an auto-injector, e.g. EpiPen®. These individuals include:

- those with a history of a previous reaction with respiratory or circulatory symptoms
- those who also have asthma. The risk of anaphylaxis is particularly high in those with severe uncontrolled asthma.
- adolescents frequently fail to appreciate risk, experiment with alcohol, frequent pubs where nuts may be offered and have oral contact with others who may have just eaten the allergen.

Schools, nurseries and clubs also require training. Care needs to be taken in the school canteen, in domestic science lessons, and with the practice of sharing food and treats around the class.

Prognosis

Of the children allergic to cows' milk, 90 per cent will become tolerant by the age of 3 years, and most children allergic to eggs develop tolerance by school age. Less than 5 per cent of children allergic to peanuts become tolerant. Those who do usually have a history of a small number of urticarial reactions early in life, with a long reaction-free period thereafter. Tolerance is less likely to develop in those with multiple allergies.

KEY LEARNING POINTS

- Allergy cannot be diagnosed on the basis of tests without a clinical history.
- Anaphylaxis does not occur without exposure.
- Early recognition of symptoms of acute allergy and prompt treatment can prevent progression to anaphylaxis.
- Steroids have no place in the management of immediate hypersensitivity in the absence of wheeze.

FURTHER READING

Feigin RD, Cherry J, Demmler GJ, Kaplan S (2004) *Textbook of Pediatric Infectious Diseases*, 5th edn. Philadelphia: Saunders.

Stiehm ER, Ochs HD, Winkelstein JA (2004) *Immunologic Disorders in Infants and Children*, 5th edn. Philadelphia: Saunders.

Chapter 7

The nervous system

R McWilliam and Iain Horrocks

BASIC KNOWLEDGE

EMBRYOLOGY AND DEVELOPMENT

Neurulation: complete by three weeks

The nervous system develops from a group of ectodermal cells extending the entire length of the embryo along the dorsal midline. The central core of this 'neural plate' folds inwards to form a tube – the basic neuraxis – while the more laterally placed 'neural crest' cells migrate inwards to form the main sensory elements of the central, peripheral and autonomic nervous systems (Figure 7.1). The remainder of the central nervous system (CNS) and the motor elements of the peripheral nervous system develop from the neural tube.

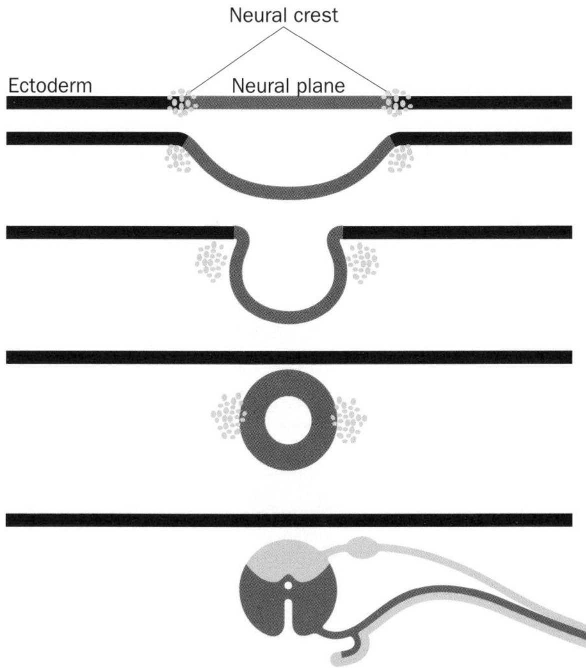

Figure 7.1 Neurulation. The dorsal neural plate folds inwards to form the neural tube followed by the neural crest cells which form the dorsal sensory columns, peripheral sensory neurones and peripheral autonomic nervous system. The remainder of the central nervous system and motor neurones are formed from the neural tube

KEY LEARNING POINT

Failure of normal neurulation gives rise to spina bifida (Figure 7.2) and, in extreme cases, anencephaly.

Encephalization: complete by five weeks

The rostral end of the primitive neuraxis undergoes a process of enlargement and organization to form pairs of vesicles (Figure 7.3 and Table 7.1) from which the main structures of the mature brain will develop.

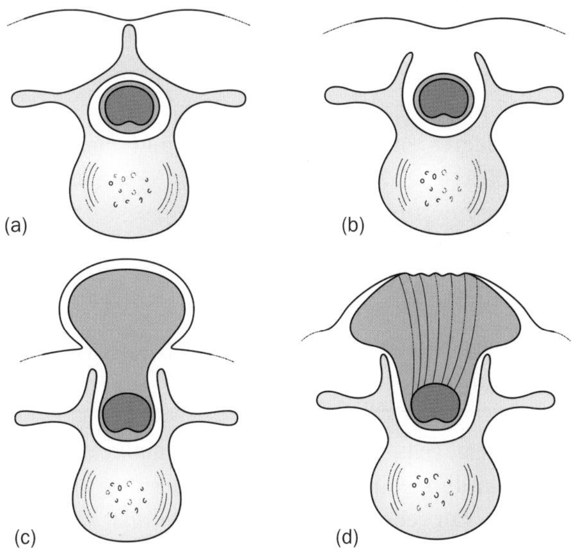

Figure 7.2 Neural tube defects. Cross-sectional representation of varying degrees of neurulation failure: (A) normal, (B) spina bifida occulta (failure of complete mesodermal closure), (C) meningocele (failure of mesodermal and ectodermal closure) and (D) myelocele (failure of complete neural tube closure)

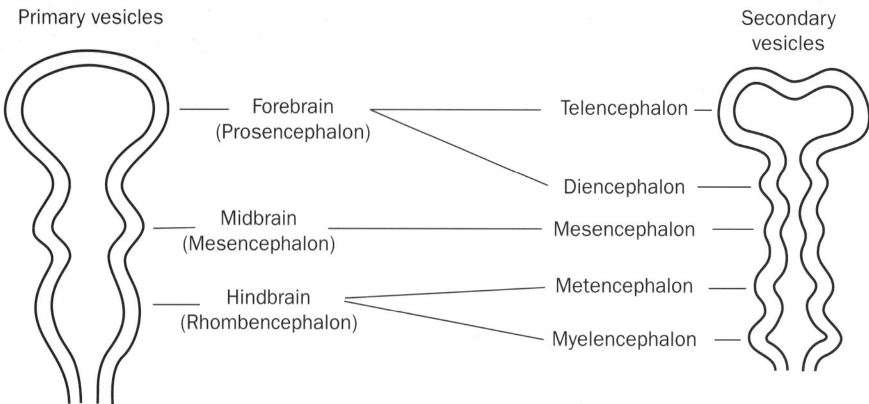

Figure 7.3 Encephalization. The rostral end of the neural tube enlarges to create a series of vesicles from which the major structures of the mature brain develop

Table 7.1 Encephalization and functional differentiation

Three vesicle brain	Five vesicle brain	Adult brain	Function
Forebrain (prosencephalon)	Telencephalon	Olfactory lobes	Smell
		Hippocampus	Memory, emotion
		Cerebral hemispheres, basal ganglia	Cognition, volition, motor coordination
	Diencephalon	Retina	Vision
		Pineal gland	?
		Thalamus	Sensory relay to cerebral hemispheres
		Hypothalamus	Vegetative functions
Midbrain (mesencephalon)	Mesencephalon	Midbrain	Tracts between forebrain and hindbrain, cranial nerve nuclei
Hindbrain (telencephalon)	Metencephalon	Pons	Tracts between forebrain and hindbrain, cranial nerve nuclei
	Myelencephalon	Cerebellum	Motor coordination

KEY LEARNING POINT

Failure of encephalization results in incomplete development of the cerebral hemispheres and a variable degree of associated motor and cognitive disability. Facial dysmorphism and hypothalamic/pituitary dysfunction may also be present – holoprosencephaly (Figure 7.4).

Proliferation and migration: complete by 20 weeks

Neural stem cells surrounding the primitive ventricles divide and differentiate to form neurones and glial cells. The number of cells is greatly in excess of that which will be needed in the mature brain. Simultaneously, neuronal migration begins and continues for some time after proliferation is complete. Oligodendrocytes begin this process, leaving behind 'glial tubes' which guide the following neurones and will eventually form the myelin sheaths of the developing axons. By this process neurones become concentrated in the cortex and central grey matter while their interconnecting axons form the commissures and tracts of the white matter. The characteristic 'wrinkled' appearance of the mature cortex is a consequence of this migration and subsequent growth and branching of cortical neurones. Involution of redundant neurones takes place throughout subsequent brain development – a process that is influenced by environmental and early learning processes.

KEY LEARNING POINT

Disorders of neuronal proliferation (Figure 7.5) and migration are among the most common prenatal causes of learning disability, particularly when associated with severe epilepsy. The underlying cause may be genetic (for example tuberous sclerosis) or environmental (as in fetal alcohol effects) but is frequently unknown. In severe cases it is readily apparent on brain imaging (heterotopias or abnormal

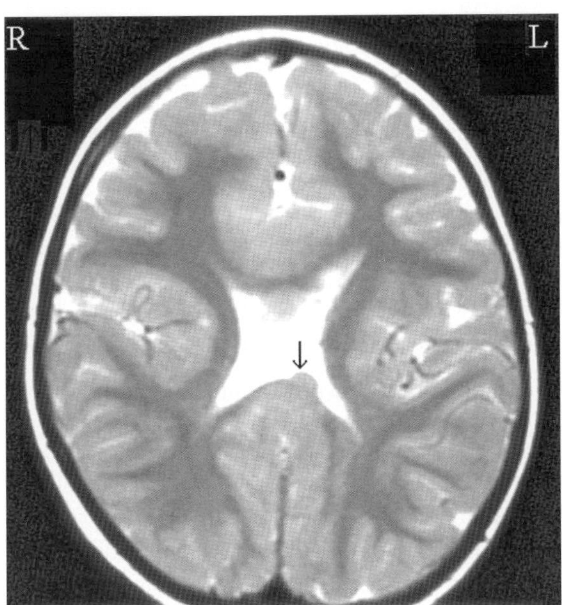

Figure 7.4 Magnetic resonance image – holoprosencephaly. Note the unusually shaped (fused) lateral ventricles, and the continuous band of cortex crossing the midline anteriorly. Note also the small nodule of heterotopic grey matter (arrow) – a neural migration defect

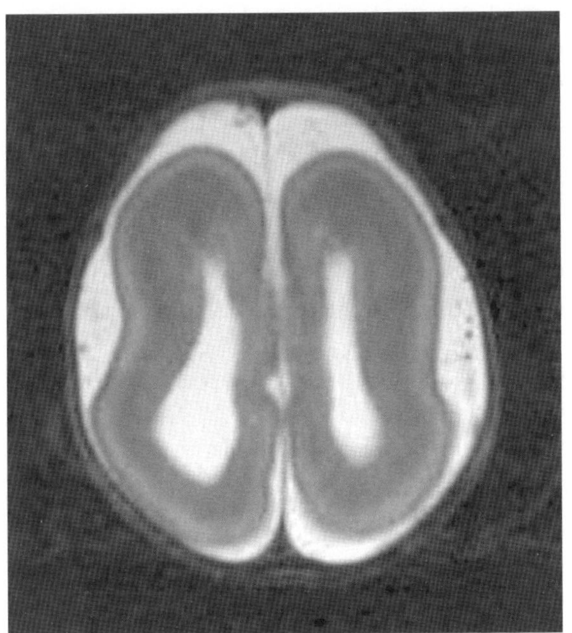

Figure 7.5 Magnetic resonance image – lissencephaly. Note the complete absence of gyri, a consequence of severe disruption to neuronal migration with greatly reduced numbers of cortical neurones. Severe neurological disability results

gyral patterns). In less severe or more diffuse cases imaging may be normal. Abnormal head size (see page 249) in a child with severe learning disability and epilepsy may be an important clue.

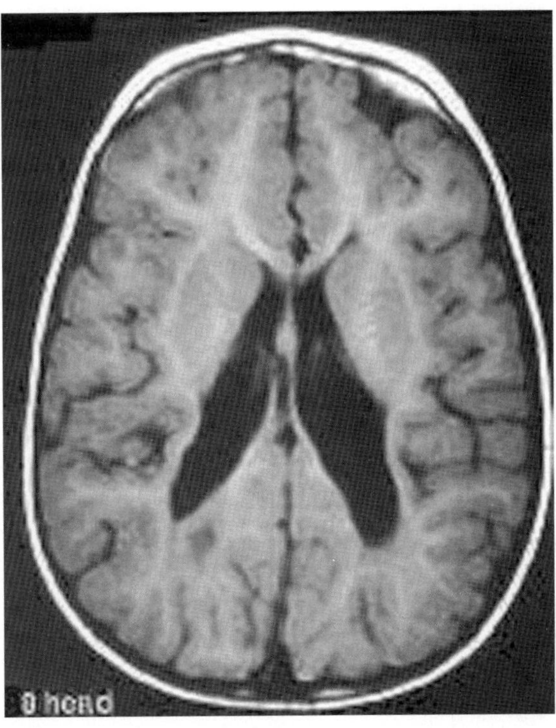

Figure 7.6 Magnetic resonance image – periventricular leukomalacia. Note the selective, *ex-vacuo* dilatation of the posterior horns of the lateral ventricles and the marked reduction in white matter volume posteriorly

Myelination: complete by two years

Most myelination takes place in postnatal life but prenatal events can have a profound influence on its rate and extent of completion. Having blazed a trail for its migrating neurone, each oligodendrocyte remains with its axon processes which it will later invest with its myelin sheath. Oligodendrocytes, being metabolically more active, are vulnerable, particularly to ischaemia or hypoxia. Delayed and incomplete myelination are non-specific effects of a variety of prenatal and postnatal insults.

KEY LEARNING POINT

Because of the vulnerability of oligodendrocytes during prenatal development, disorders of myelination may originate many months before myelination should normally commence. A common example of this is periventricular leukomalacia (PVL; Figure 7.6) – the most frequent cause of diplegic cerebral palsy – which most often results from an insult sustained between five and eight months post conception. The corticospinal tracts do not myelinate until the end of the first year of postnatal life – the time when diplegia is most often first apparent.

Dendritic branching and neuronal pruning: complete by seven years

For much of early childhood two further processes shape ongoing brain development. Neurones that are not used involute, while those which are, grow and increase in complexity. Axonal growth occurs to a limited extent but extensive growth and branching of dendrites results in the increasing 'connectivity' which underpins brain function.

KEY LEARNING POINT

Dendritic branching and neuronal pruning are examples of early 'learning' processes. Common examples of the effect of experience and environment on brain development include visual and motor development. An infant denied normal visual input (for example because of untreated cataracts) will never develop good visual function unless visual input is provided before three months. An infant who sustains a brachial plexus injury will never acquire full function of the affected arm, even if nerve recovery is complete, unless nerve recovery has occurred before six months. In both these illustrations, failure to utilize central neural connections within a critical timescale results in irreversible axonal loss and permanent functional deficit.

NEUROLOGICAL EXAMINATION

There is no such thing as a complete neurological examination. The examination should reflect the information obtained through the history and the aim should be to answer any remaining questions.

In reaching a diagnosis 90 per cent of the information is gained through the history. Of the remainder, 90 per cent can be learned by observation. By observing and interacting non-physically with children you will learn about their mental state, cognitive ability, manipulation skills, gait, muscle strength, any asymmetry of posture, their visual and hearing abilities and any unusual movements.

You may need to clarify specific issues but if you are not reasonably confident about the nature of the problem by this stage you are unlikely to gain anything by, for example, testing the reflexes or examining the fundi. There are some aspects of neurological examination, however, that should always be done and others that should always be done in specific situations.

Things you should always do

In any child

- Measure, record and plot the head circumference.

In an infant

- Look for a red reflex (and examine the fundi if possible; see Chapter 17)

In an ambulant child

- Observe them walking, running, jumping

In a child with a concern about head size

- Measure and plot parental and sibling head size

When raised intracranial pressure (ICP) is a possibility

- Examine upward gaze and convergence
- Examine the fundi – look for venous pulsation (if present ICP is normal) as well as for papilloedema
- Examine the visual fields (binocular and monocular)

When examining the child with suspected weakness

- Observe her getting up from lying to standing
- Test the reflexes
- Look for muscle hypertrophy and tenderness
- Look for joint contractures
- Test vibration sense if peripheral neuropathy suspected
- Look for tongue fasciculation

In a child with a developmental or possible degenerative disorder

- Examine the fundi
- Measure the parent's head size and compare with the child's
- Test the reflexes
- Examine the abdomen
- Examine the skin

In an infant with epileptic spasms

- Examine the skin and hair for depigmented patches
- Examine the fundi (looking for colobomas etc.)

In a child who is having focal seizures

- Look for unusually pronounced (or early expression of) handedness
- Look for asymmetry of gait, posture or limb size

In the child with an acute neurological illness (other than neuromuscular)

- Examine the fundi
- Examine for localized skull tenderness (important clue to possible brain abscess)

- Look for asymmetry of posture, tone or movement
- Observe the respiratory pattern
- Measure and record heart rate and blood pressure

This is not an exhaustive list but should ensure that an appropriate neurological examination is undertaken in most clinical situations you are likely to encounter.

INVESTIGATION

Without a clear idea of the nature of the problem and potential causes gleaned from the history and examination/observation, investigation is at best useless and at worst dangerous (see case study of long QT syndrome (Syncope as a result of a cardiac arrhythmia), page 242). Investigations which may be helpful are indicated within the different subsections of the section on Core system problems.

There are a few circumstances in which specific investigations should always be considered and some investigations that should only be undertaken after careful thought and discussion with the parents (and child).

Always consider:

- Creatine kinase measurement, FRAX studies and urine glycosaminoglycans in a child with delayed development in any domain unless the cause is known.
- Doing multiple invasive or unpleasant investigations (e.g. lumbar puncture, muscle biopsy, rectal biopsy, bone marrow biopsy, liver biopsy, nerve conduction studies) in a child who may need them at some point and is having a general anaesthetic for another reason (e.g. for a magnetic resonance imaging (MRI) scan).
- Always measure blood and cerebrospinal fluid (CSF) glucose levels simultaneously if doing a lumbar puncture for a neurological investigation.
- Undertaking chromosome studies in a child with learning disability or refractory epilepsy not due to a known cause.

Consider very carefully:

- Any painful or unpleasant investigation or one requiring a general anaesthetic.
- Magnetic resonance imaging – up to 3 per cent of the 'normal' population will have an abnormality and the family should be aware of this beforehand. If the scan is being undertaken for 'reassurance' there is a real risk of increasing rather than decreasing anxiety.
- Electroencephalogram (EEG) – for the same reasons as above this should only be undertaken if it is likely to clarify the provisional diagnosis.

CORE SYSTEM PROBLEMS

EVALUATION OF SYMPTOMS

Delayed development

All too often the term 'developmental delay' is misused as a euphemism for a learning disability. Instead, it should viewed as a symptom with many potential causes. Table 7.2 provides a guide to common developmental presentations and their evaluation.

KEY LEARNING POINT

Developmental delay is a symptom, not a diagnosis.

CASE STUDY: Developmental delay

A 18-month-old boy with obvious severe learning disability is seen for a further opinion. He has refractory epilepsy but his mother also wants to know when he will catch up from his 'developmental delay'. Brain imaging revealed lissencephaly (see Figure 7.5). After coming to terms with the implications of the diagnosis his mother says, 'When they told me his development was delayed I didn't think that was too bad – a bit like a bus being late: it will arrive eventually. My son's bus will never come, will it?'

Walking difficulty

The child who has achieved walking may do so with an abnormal gait. Transient gait disturbance is common and usually due to non-neurological causes. A persistent or worsening difficulty may be caused by skeletal (see Chapter 16) or neurological disorders. Systematic

Table 7.2 A guide to the assessment and investigation of the young child with 'developmental delay'

Feature	Post term age by which abnormal	Type of disorder	Potential cause	Key findings and basic investigations
Lack of visual interest	4 weeks	Visual, cognitive or both	Ocular disorder	Possibly abnormal eye movements, possibly impaired pupil light reaction Funduscopy,* ERG
			Visual pathway disorder	Possibly abnormal eye movements Cranial ultrasound,* VEPs
			Learning disability	EEG, chromosomes
Not reaching and grasping	5 months	Cerebral palsy	Various, usually prenatal	Asymmetry, increased/variable tone, retained primitive reflexes MRI
		Cognitive disorder	Learning disability	Chromosomes
Not sitting	7 months	Cerebral palsy	Various, usually prenatal	MRI
		Neuromuscular disorder	Congenital myopathy	Weak, reflexes difficult or absent, alert
			Spinal muscular atrophy	CK, DNA studies
		Cognitive disorder	Learning disability	Chromosomes, urine organic acids, GAGs
Not walking	15 months	'Bottom shuffler'	Benign genetic variant	Family history, early dislike of prone lying
		Cerebral palsy	Various, usually prenatal	MRI
		Neuromuscular disorder	Many	Weakness, CK
		Cognitive disorder	Learning disability	Lack of symbolic play CK*
Not speaking	2 years	Cognitive disorder	Global learning disability	Impaired symbolic play CK,* FRAX,* chromosomes, urine amino acids, organic acids, GAGs*
			Communication disorder	Impaired symbolic play FRAX,* CK,* EEG
			Specific language disorder	Age appropriate symbolic play
		Hearing disorder	Various	Audiometry

*Essential investigation.
CK, creatine kinase; EEG, electroencephalography; ERG, electroretinography; FRAX, fragile X; GAG, glycosaminoglycan; MRI, magnetic resonance imaging; VEP, visual evoked potential.

observation and examination will reveal a neurological cause, if present, and will often indicate a specific diagnosis. Key features are:

- specific difficulty with stairs (up or down) – hip girdle weakness
- specific difficulty rising from sitting/lying – limb girdle and trunk weakness
- needs support (rail, furniture, hand) – central motor disorder – 'cerebral palsy'
- asymmetrical gait – hemiparesis, unilateral skeletal pathology
- toe walking – diplegia/paraplegia, peripheral neuropathy, idiopathic (often familial).

Paroxysmal events

See relevant section (page 238).

School failure

This may manifest in several ways and it is unusual for it to be a specific complaint. More often there will be concern about behaviour which may be overtly challenging and disruptive or the child may simply be 'not paying attention'. Sometimes absence seizures may be suspected and this may, indeed, be the cause of the problem. A child may already be known to be vulnerable to a learning disability, for example because of an acquired brain injury or severe epilepsy. Possible causes include:

- unrecognized learning disability
- emotional disorder (including abusive situations)
- absence epilepsy
- neurological disorder with deteriorating or fluctuating learning ability
- specific neuropsychiatric disorder (attention deficit hyperactivity disorder, Tourette syndrome, Sydenham chorea).

The first two are by far the most likely. Evaluation takes place in stages:

- Identify the main concern and whether it is the school or the parents who are expressing it.
- With parental permission, contact the school for their views on the following questions:
  - Does the child have a learning problem?
  - Has there been a loss of any learning skills?
  - Could the child be having absence seizures?
- Does the developmental history suggest that there may be a learning disability?
- Are there other symptoms suggesting a neurological or a psychiatric disorder?

It should then be possible to form a view on the probable underlying problem although additional assessment by a clinical neuropsychologist may be required if a learning disability or degenerative disorder is suspected.

THE 'FLOPPY INFANT' AND NEUROMUSCULAR DISORDERS

The floppy infant

Neuromuscular disease may well be the first diagnosis to be considered but it is by no means the commonest cause. Even when, as in the following case study, the underlying diagnosis is of a neuromuscular disorder, the hypotonia may be due to CNS mechanisms, often associated with learning disability. The greatest difficulty in the younger infant is differentiating neuromuscular weakness from an evolving cerebral palsy. In the older infant learning disability with 'superficial brightness' provides the greatest challenge.

The main causes of hypotonia and their evaluation are given in Table 7.3. The probability of the various

CASE STUDY: Congenital myotonic dystrophy

A 3-month-old baby girl was seen in the neonatal unit because of hypotonia and poor feeding. The pregnancy had been complicated by polyhydramnios. She had been born at 28 weeks' gestation and had required ventilation for five weeks because of poor respiratory effort but did not have significant lung disease. She was seen with her mother who, when it was explained that family history was often important in this situation, revealed that she had been experiencing stiffness in her hands particularly when cold. She had a normal hand grip and release (in the warm, neonatal environment) but reduced facial expression. Examination of the infant confirmed hypotonia but gave no further clues. DNA studies on the mother and child confirmed the diagnosis. Five years later she has mild learning disability but no neuromuscular symptoms.

KEY LEARNING POINT

A maternal history of symptoms of myotonic dystrophy should always be sought when investigating the hypotonic infant. Polyhydramnios due to impaired fetal swallowing is an important clue to the diagnosis.

CASE STUDY: Prader–Willi syndrome

A 6-month-old girl was seen at the neuromuscular clinic. Gestation and delivery were unremarkable but she required tube feeding for the first month. A DNA test for spinal muscular atrophy had been negative. She presented as hypotonic but would kick and move her arms vigorously when excited. She was alert and interested but still had poor head control and was only beginning to reach and grasp objects. Hand regard was evident. Overall appearance was unremarkable but she had small hands and feet and somewhat hypoplastic genitalia. She had sticky saliva and, when upset gave a somewhat sustained but quiet cry. DNA studies (fluorescence ***in-situ*** hybridization) showed a 15q12 deletion, confirming the diagnosis.

KEY LEARNING POINTS

- Hypotonia and weakness in a child who appears cognitively normal are the hallmarks of neuromuscular disease. Any movements which appear to be strong make neuromuscular disease improbable.
- It is easy to be misled by a 'bright' alert infant into assuming normal cognitive function. Any impaired aspect of development (fine motor control in this case) casts doubt on this assumption.

mechanisms changes with age (for example the infant with evolving cerebral palsy is far more likely to be hypotonic as a neonate than at 1 year) and, in general, the younger the infant the more challenging is the differential diagnosis. Provided that treatable disorders (myasthenic syndromes, some metabolic disorders, hydrocephalus) are excluded, it may be preferable to 'wait and see' rather than embark on a series of sometimes invasive and potentially misleading investigations. Often the clinical picture will become clear with time and the diagnosis confirmed by a few specific and focused investigations. It is important that the parents agree with this expectant approach (and understand the reasons for it).

Table 7.3 The 'floppy infant': causes, assessment and investigation

Underlying mechanism	Key features (not all seen in every condition)	Preliminary investigations
Weakness Congenital myopathy/ muscular dystrophy Congenital myasthenic syndrome Spinal muscular atrophy	No strong movements Ptosis Exclusively diaphragmatic respiration Absent reflexes Alert No developmental delay *not* explicable by weakness Loss of previously acquired motor skills Family history	Plasma creatine kinase (may be raised in the first week, especially if traumatic delivery or 'asphyxia' EMG and nerve conduction studies Trial of pyridostigmine
Evolving cerebral palsy	History to suggest cause, e.g. ex-preterm Abnormal motor patterns Retained primitive reflexes (e.g. asymmetrical tonic neck reflex) Increased tone in any muscle group Marked difference between extensor and flexor trunk tone Inappropriate head growth	Cranial ultrasound if fontanelle patent MRI brain CT brain (avoid if possible as significant radiation exposure) **May be unnecessary if clinical picture conclusive**
Hydrocephalus	Excessive head growth	Cranial ultrasound MRI brain CT brain (if MRI not readily available)
Specific syndrome	Specific dysmorphic features (e.g. Down syndrome) Specific behaviour (e.g. unexplained early feeding difficulty in Prader–Willi syndrome) Inappropriate head size	Chromosomes, depends on suspected syndrome
Learning disability, degenerative and metabolic disorders (see page 235)	Disinterest 'Global delay'	Chromosomes etc. Consider biotinidase deficiency (treatable disorder)
Cervical spinal cord injury	Complete paralysis below level of injury Poor respiratory effort (may be absent or 'intercostals') Normal facial and eye movements Normal gag and suck reflex Reflexes absent initially History of possible injury (except if non-accidental injury)	**Give high dose steroids (prednisolone 2 mg/kg per day) as soon as suspected – within 24 hours of onset** **Immobilize neck if suspected** MRI is best imaging technique
Ill infant	Basic clinical skill	Consider infective, traumatic (non-accidental injury) and metabolic causes

CT, computed tomography; MRI, magnetic resonance imaging.

Table 7.4 Neuromuscular disorders

Structural location	Example	Presentation and key features	Investigation	Treatment and prognosis
Anterior horn cell	Poliomyelitis	Gastroenteritis, aseptic meningitis, focal paralysis	Viral studies	Prevention, supportive Residual disability determined by initial severity
	Spinal muscular atrophy	Floppy infant, progressive weakness Absent reflexes, proximal weakness, legs weaker than arms, diaphragmatic sparing, tongue fasciculation, tremor	DNA studies (EMG and/or muscle biopsy if unavailable)	Supportive Eventually 'static' with severe disability, premature death from respiratory failure in more severe cases
Motor nerves	**Heavy metal poisoning**	Distal weakness; associated behavioural or cognitive difficulties	Nerve conduction studies toxicology	Chelation therapy Excellent with early treatment
Sensory and autonomic nerves	Hereditary sensory neuropathies (at least four types)	Indifference to pain, associated learning disability, autonomic failure	Nerve conduction studies, tests of autonomic function	None Depends on severity of learning disability, risk of hyperpyrexia
	Charcot–Marie–Tooth disease (axonal and demyelinating types) Foot deformity, foot and leg pains, walking difficulty	Pes cavus, absent reflexes, impaired vibration sense, palpably thickened nerves (peroneal and tibial)	Nerve conduction studies, DNA studies	Supportive, relief for neuropathic pain, orthoses, surgery to reduce deformity. Very slowly progressive, a few patients become wheelchair users in adult life
Motor and sensory nerves	**Inflammatory demyelinating polyneuropathy (IDP)** $<$4 weeks progression to maximum weakness Acute – AIDP (Guillain–Barré syndrome) $>$4 weeks progression to maximum weakness Chronic – CIDP	May follow non-specific illness, may have pain/paraesthesia before motor symptoms appear, may seem ataxic rather than weak, reflexes absent – eventually, autonomic dysfunction	May not be needed if AIDP thought clinically definite. Consider MRI if spinal cord compression/myelitis possible, Nerve conduction studies helpful in CIDP, elevated CSF protein without pleocytosis	Intravenous γ-globulin; 2 g/kg – first line treatment, steroids if no response, monitor and support respiratory function, monitor blood pressure, prevent complications of prolonged immobility Complete recovery in most cases of AIDP, CIDP eventually 'burns out' but often with residual weakness

(*Continued*)

Table 7.4 *(Continued)*

Structural location	Example	Presentation and key features	Investigation	Treatment and prognosis
	Toxic neuropathies, e.g. vincristine, mercury	Often asymptomatic, distal weakness, paraesthesia, absent reflexes	Only necessary if toxic agent not apparent	Withdrawal/removal of causative agent if possible Usually good
Neuromuscular junction	**Myasthenic disorders** – genetic and acquired (autoimmune)	Fluctuating (usually) weakness, ptosis, fatigue, acute respiratory failure in infancy	Repetitive stimulation tests, DNA studies, AChR antibodies. Edrophonium (Tensilon) test – if negative or equivocal then one month trial of pyridostigmine	Pyridostigmine (acquired and most genetic types), corticosteroids/azathioprine (acquired), thymectomy (if AChR antibody positive)
Muscle	Congenital, non-progressive myopathies	Floppy infant, respiratory failure in infancy	Creatine kinase level, EMG, muscle biopsy, DNA studies	Supportive, awareness of the risks of malignant hyperpyrexia and respiratory failure in late childhood/early adult life
	Congenital muscular dystrophies	Floppy infant, arthrogryposis, associated severe learning disability may determine presentation		Supportive, awareness of possible respiratory and cardiac implications
	Limb girdle muscular dystrophies (including facioscapulohumeral (FSH) and myotonic (DM) dystrophies)	Global delay (Duchenne), walking difficulty, muscle pain Calf hypertrophy, specific patterns of weakness, e.g. FSH, Emery–Dreifuss		
	Myotonic disorders and periodic paralysis	Fluctuating or intermittent symptoms, exacerbated by cold or immobility	EMG, DNA studies	Carbamazepine and acetazolamide may improve myotonia
	Metabolic muscle disorders (see Chapter 15)	Fluctuating weakness, fatigue, muscle pain during or after exercise, myoglobulinuria	Muscle biopsy	Supportive Generally benign unless part of a generalized metabolic disorder
	Myositis (see Chapter 16)	Muscle pain and weakness with variable rate of progression, may mimic muscular dystrophy	Creatine kinase level, EMG, muscle biopsy	Corticosteroids Outcome generally good

AChR, anti-acetylcholine receptor; EMG, electromyography; MRI, magnetic resonance imaging.

Neuromuscular disorders

Weakness is the cardinal sign of neuromuscular disease although it is rarely the presenting complaint. Delayed motor development and loss of motor skills first cause concern in the young child while, from 2 years onwards, walking difficulty, difficulty running and difficulty climbing stairs are common complaints.

Muscle pain, usually cramping in nature, is a frequent symptom in the older child and may be the presenting feature, particularly in metabolic myopathies. Fatigue without weakness is the classic symptom of myasthenic disorders but a child is far more likely to present with symptoms due to weakness. Fatigue may also be seen in mitochondrial muscle disorders, as may ptosis, another classic feature of myasthenia. Fatigue with tiredness is commonly seen in myotonic dystrophy, especially in older children and adults. It is also seen, often with myriad other symptoms, in the enigmatic disorder chronic fatigue syndrome. Rarely, presymptomatic muscular dystrophy may be the cause of 'unexplained' elevated transaminases.

CASE STUDY: Duchenne muscular dystrophy – presenting as 'occult liver disease'

A 4-year-old boy was seen at the neuromuscular clinic with walking difficulty. Raised levels of aspartate aminotransferase (AST) and alanine aminotransferase (ALT) had been discovered during 'routine' investigation during an acute admission for gastroenteritis in infancy. Apart from mild speech delay he had no developmental difficulties and was in good health. The raised transaminase levels were persistent but extensive investigation, including liver biopsy, had failed to identify a cause. Creatine kinase (CK) level had not previously been checked but was elevated at over 4000 IU/L. DNA studies were unhelpful but the diagnosis was confirmed by muscle biopsy. His 2-year-old brother was also affected.

KEY LEARNING POINT

Transaminase levels are frequently raised concomitantly with CK and do not always imply a hepatic origin.

Neuromuscular disorders may involve any part of the motor unit:

- motor neurone (anterior horn cell) spinal muscular atrophy – poliomyelitis
- motor (and usually sensory) axons – Charcot–Marie–Tooth (CMT) disease type 2; some sensory neuropathies
- myelin sheath (motor and sensory) CMT disease types 1 and 3
- neuromuscular junction myasthenic syndromes
- muscle myopathies and muscular dystrophies.

An outline of various conditions is given in Table 7.4 and a more detailed description of the more common disorders follows.

Duchenne muscular dystrophy

With an incidence of 1 per 3500 male births Duchenne muscular dystrophy (DMD) is the commonest disabling neuromuscular disorder of childhood. Without medical intervention, mean age at death is 18 years but with currently available treatments this can be extended by at least 10 years. It is very much a treatable condition.

In most cases the defective gene is inherited from the mother but a third of cases arise as a result of new mutations. The gene, one of the largest known, is located on the short arm of the X chromosome (Xp21). Most cases result from large deletions or duplications but a third are due to point mutations which are much harder to detect. There is some correlation between severity and the size and location of the gene abnormality. Gene defects causing DMD are 'out of frame' mutations preventing meaningful transcription distally so that a very abnormal gene product – **dystrophin** – results with little functional capacity. 'In frame' mutations which only affect transcription at the site of the defect permit production of dystrophin which retains some (albeit reduced) functional capacity. This results in a much milder, allelic condition – Becker muscular dystrophy. This is illustrated below.

Take the following simple sentence to represent a simple 'gene' of 12 triplets:

'The one who was big was far too big for the job.'

Delete the first 'e', keeping the same word spacing (out of frame deletion) and a meaningless sentence (gene) results:

'Tho new how asb igw asf art oob igf ort hej ob.'

Delete three consecutive letters (in frame deletion) and little sense is lost:

'The who was big was far too big for the job.'

Presentation

Duchenne muscular dystrophy is associated with a variable degree of cognitive impairment with the result that the IQ distribution among affected individuals is shifted downwards. Around a third have a degree of learning disability and few have above average cognitive ability. Developmental delay, particularly speech delay, is consequently the commonest presenting symptom. It is also frequently overlooked. Delayed walking, also a frequent presenting feature, is due not to weakness but to cognitive impairment. Measurement of **plasma CK** should always be considered in boys presenting with delayed speech or walking.

Typically the diagnosis is only considered when there is an obvious walking difficulty – usually between 3 and 4 years – by which time a second affected child may have been conceived.

Diagnosis

Limb girdle weakness can be confirmed by observation of the child walking and rising from lying supine. Duchenne muscular dystrophy is highly likely if this is associated with calf hypertrophy and a CK level over 1000 IU/L but this should be confirmed by DNA studies (blood for this should be taken when the CK level is checked). Muscle biopsy with detailed histochemical studies is required if DNA studies are negative. Autosomal recessive and dominant limb girdle dystrophies are 10 times less common in boys than DMD and are not associated with cognitive problems. They will usually present in a similar way although the CK level may be lower.

Progress

The natural course leads to loss of ambulation between 7 and 12 years followed by progressive loss of upper limb function. Cardiomyopathy may become clinically significant and death (usually from respiratory failure) occurs in the late teens/early twenties.

Management

Many professional disciplines may be involved with the following key aims:

- Providing accurate and appropriate information, verbal, written and web-based.
- Prevention/limitation of complications (ankle contractures, scoliosis).
- Appropriate exercise and nutrition.
- Aids to mobility and personal care.
- Adequate home/school access.
- Treatment of complications (scoliosis, respiratory failure cardiac failure).
- Appropriate medical and surgical interventions:
  - Corticosteroids – prednisolone 0.75 mg/kg per day. There is increasing evidence for the effectiveness of steroids in slowing the rate of deterioration. It is not yet clear whether a continuous or intermittent regimen offers the more favourable risk/benefit balance.
  - Spinal fusion – this is the only effective intervention for control of progressive scoliosis which affects 80 per cent of DMD patients.
  - **Non-invasive ventilation** (NIV). The introduction of NIV, using a simple, transportable, ventilator and a mask, enhances quality of life and has increased life expectancy by at least five years.
  - Treatment of cardiomyopathy – with the expectation of living well beyond 20 years, symptomatic left ventricular failure has become more common. Treatment with diuretics, β blockers and or angiotensin-converting enzyme (ACE) inhibitors is effective.
- Transition to adult services. Another consequence of increasing longevity is the need for ongoing, multidisciplinary care into adult life.

KEY LEARNING POINTS

- Always consider measuring the plasma CK level in a boy presenting with delayed speech or walking.
- Corticosteroids delay progression in DMD.

Spinal muscular atrophy

The gene for spinal muscular atrophy (SMA) is located at 5q12. Different mutations (usually deletions) produce an illness of different severity – types I, II, and III (see Table 7.4). The three types differ only in their age of onset and rate of progression. Weakness is the only manifestation and cognitive function is not affected.

There is a characteristic pattern with proximal and trunk muscles most severely affected, the legs more severely than the arms, and relative sparing of the diaphragm, facial muscles and eye movements. The distribution and severity of weakness associated with an alert, animated facial expression is unmistakable.

Particularly in SMA II, deterioration slows or ceases after an initial progressive phase (lasting from between six and 12 months) and the disorder becomes static. Secondary deterioration may arise as a result of contractures and deformity – especially scoliosis – and prevention of this is an important aspect of management.

Presentation and diagnosis

Types I and II present as a 'floppy infant'. The much rarer type III usually first manifests as walking difficulty. The ready availability of DNA testing means that this will be the preferred initial diagnostic test if the diagnosis seems probable clinically. In more challenging situations such as type III or type I with prenatal onset (presenting with a picture of arthrogryposis, more usually associated with congenital myopathic disorder) it may be necessary first to determine whether weakness is due to a neuropathic or a myopathic process with electrophysiological studies or even muscle biopsy.

Management and prognosis

There is no specific treatment for SMA. The approach should be identical to that for DMD except that steroids are not helpful and there is no cardiac involvement. Prognosis, in many ways, defines the classification of SMA:

- Type I – onset before 6 months, never able to sit, death by 2 years.
- Type II – onset before 1 year, never able to stand, life expectancy depends on degree of respiratory muscle involvement (early teens to middle age).
- Type III – onset at any age, may progress to loss of walking, life expectancy may be normal.

Respiratory failure and contractures, including scoliosis, are the main complications.

Peripheral neuropathies

CASE STUDY: CMT disease type 1a

A 4-year-old girl was referred because of walking difficulty and leg pain. Examination showed pes cavus, absent reflexes and impaired vibration sense. Nerve conduction studies showed a motor velocity of 14 m/s (normal 45–40). DNA studies confirmed the diagnosis. Her father, a professional footballer, observed that he had similar shaped feet. He too had slow motor conduction and a positive DNA test.

This family is typical of CMT 1a, which is responsible for 70 per cent of all hereditary neuropathies. It is seldom a severely disabling disorder in childhood but may result in loss of walking in middle age and is a frequent cause of mild walking difficulty and foot deformity. Asymptomatic cases are common.

CASE STUDY: Acute inflammatory demyelinating polyneuropathy – Guillain–Barré syndrome

A 10-year-old boy was admitted with abdominal pain, leg pain and inability to walk (attributed to pain). Reflexes were present on admission. At laparotomy his (normal) appendix was removed. Post operatively he was still unable to walk or move his legs. Reflexes were absent and he had severe lower limb and mild upper limb weakness. Peak flow rate was half the expected value. He was given intravenous immunoglobulin 2 g/kg and within 48 hours he was noticeably stronger and within a week he could walk. He recovered completely.

This was a slightly unusual case because of the severity of the initial (neuropathic) pain and preservation of reflexes initially is uncommon. Magnetic resonance imaging (to exclude spinal cord pathology) and lumbar puncture were considered but felt to be unnecessary.

CASE STUDY: Polymyositis

A 4-year-old boy was seen three days before Christmas with severe walking difficulty and leg pains. He had limb girdle weakness and CK level was over 5000 IU/L. His parents had been told that he probably had DMD and wished a further opinion. Further enquiry revealed that his symptoms had only been present for a few weeks and that he had no evidence of weakness prior to that. He was of well above average cognitive ability. The time of year precluded rapid muscle biopsy. Prednisolone 1 mg/kg per day was prescribed and within a week he was able to run and climb stairs. A month later his CK level was 500 IU/L. One year later he had recovered completely.

This case illustrates the importance of precision in history taking. Muscular dystrophies seldom produce weakness of such rapid onset. Polymyositis is a rare but treatable disorder. Diagnosis can be difficult, even with muscle biopsy and a therapeutic trial is appropriate if in doubt.

FEBRILE CONVULSIONS

CASE STUDY: Febrile convulsions – severe myoclonic epilepsy of infancy

A 2-year-old girl was seen because of repeated febrile convulsions. Several had lasted for more than 20 minutes and her parents had been given a supply of rectal diazepam for rescue treatment. Two convulsions had been unilateral (one right, one left) and on one occasion transient left-sided weakness had been observed following the seizure. MRI brain scan and EEG were normal. Development was felt to be normal apart from delayed speech. She had begun to have brief absence-like events and myoclonic jerks. Symbolic play was limited to brushing her hair and drinking from a cup. She went on to have refractory epilepsy and severe learning disability with autistic features.

Although usually a benign, age-limited disorder, febrile convulsions (particularly when complex as in this case) can be the first manifestation of an epileptic disorder – thankfully not often such a severe one as this.

Any event involving abnormal movement, posture and/or consciousness associated with a febrile illness may be regarded as a febrile convulsion. There is no generally agreed age range although they occur most frequently between 1 and 3 years and seldom before 6 months or after 6 years.

It is often assumed that febrile convulsions are all epileptic events (see definition of epileptic seizure on page 236 but other mechanisms may be responsible (Table 7.5). It is preferable to adopt the broad definition above at presentation and subsequently to consider the underlying pathophysiology, aetiology and prognosis.

Assessment

After appropriate emergency management the nature and cause of the seizure should be sought. A description of the seizure should give a reasonable indication of its nature. It is then helpful to review the history and examination systematically. Priority should be given to considering the underlying cause of the febrile illness and, in particular, treatable pathology such as infection or raised intracranial pressure (ICP). A child in whom conscious level is not normal or clearly improving 30 minutes after a seizure should be assumed to have increased ICP and managed accordingly (see page 251).

KEY LEARNING POINTS

- The first priority after a child has had a febrile seizure is to establish the cause of the underlying febrile illness.
- The next priority is to determine the nature and mechanism of the seizure itself – it may take a little longer.

Management

Early decisions are required regarding the need for further observation and whether CNS infection should be excluded by CSF examination (which should be preceded by cranial computed tomography (CT) scanning if consciousness is impaired or there are *new* abnormal neurological findings). It is impossible to give precise guidelines, but in general the need for observation will depend on the age of the child, how 'ill' they seem, social circumstances and parental views. The younger and more ill the infant the more likely is lumber puncture necessary. Additional investigations after the acute episode are rarely helpful and there is no place for routine EEG or brain imaging.

KEY LEARNING POINT

Neurodevelopmental follow-up is important to identify children in whom febrile seizures may be symptomatic of underlying brain pathology.

There is seldom a need for prophylactic antiepileptic drugs even in children who have recurrent events and there is no evidence that the long-term outlook is influenced by such treatment. Recurrence risk may be reduced in the short term by treatment with phenobarbital and some parents may prefer this and accept the small risk of adverse effects from treatment.

KEY LEARNING POINT

For children who have had a febrile convulsion lasting longer than 10 minutes, the carers should be offered rescue medication and instructed in its use (see Acute management of convulsive status epilepticus, page 228).

Table 7.5 Febrile seizures: types and mechanisms

Mechanism	Cerebral physiology	Possible aetiology	Clinical description	Prognosis	Historical feature	Implication
Epileptic	Hypersynchronous cortical discharge	Reduced seizure threshold associated with fever Meningeal/cortical inflammation (associated with meningitis/ encephalitis) Underlying predisposition to 'idiopathic epilepsy' Pre-existing brain pathology Metabolic disorder (e.g. hypoglycaemia)	Clonic jerking, face and eye movements often involved. May be lateralized. Any tonic phase is brief and there will usually be superimposed clonic movements. Rarely a complex partial seizure may occur	Depends on underlying cause. Later epilepsy in 10–30 per cent. More likely if lateralized, >20 min duration, family history or pre-existing structural pathology	Abnormal preceding development	Structural brain pathology likely
Anoxic	Transient brain ischaemia	Increased sensitivity of vagal-cardiac mechanism	Tonic seizure possibly followed by a few clonic jerks	Excellent		
Increased intracranial pressure	Brain ischaemia	Brain swelling Acute hydrocephalus (e.g. blocked shunt, secondary to meningitis, tumour, haemorrhage)	Tonic seizures (decerebrate posturing) – usually preceded by drowsiness and/or vomiting	Death or severe brain damage unless rapid intervention		
Rigor	Normal physiological response	Underlying febrile illness	Exaggerated shivering. May be associated with acute delirium	Depends on underlying cause		
'Delirium'	Fever-induced confusional state	Underlying febrile illness, especially meningitis/encephalitis	Confusion and unusual behaviour. May be combative	Depends on underlying cause		

Acute management of convulsive status epilepticus

*A*irway, *B*reathing, *C*irculation. Give high flow oxygen. Measure blood sugar at bedside. Clinically confirm epileptic seizure (consider raised ICP).

Step 1

- Immediate IV access: lorazepam 0.1 mg/kg (over 30–60 seconds)
- No IV access: IV diazepam 0.5 mg/kg PR or midazolam 0.2 mg/kg via buccal or nasal route*

If seizure continuing at 10 minutes

Step 2 (secure IV access if possible)

- Immediate IV access: lorazepam 0.1 mg/kg (over 30–60 seconds)
- No IV access: paraldehyde 0.4 ml/kg

If seizure continuing at 10 minutes call for senior help and use intra-osseous route if still no IV access

Step 3

- Phenytoin 18 mg/kg IV over 20 minutes

or

- Phenobarbitone 20 mg/kg IV over 10 minutes if already on phenytoin

and

- Paraldehyde 0.4 mg/kg PR with same volume of olive oil if not already given in Step 2 above and summon the on-call anaesthetist or intensive care doctor

Seizure continuing at 20 minutes since starting Step 3

Step 4

- Rapid sequence induction of anaesthesia with thiopentone 4 mg/kg IV. Transfer to intensive care unit

*This is appropriate for home use by parents/carers as rescue medication (may be repeated once after 10 minutes if seizure continuing).

HEAD INJURY

CASE STUDY: Head injury (traumatic brain injury) with 'good' outcome

A 12-year-old boy sustained a head injury in a pedestrian road traffic accident. He did not lose consciousness but was confused. Computed tomography showed a frontal fracture and underlying cerebral contusion. He recovered without intervention and returned to school two weeks later. All appeared well and initial school reports were satisfactory. His parents found him a little more moody and impulsive but attributed this to puberty. A year later he had made no academic progress at school and was disruptive. Neuropsychological assessment revealed specific difficulties with memory and planning (executive dysfunction). With appropriate help his behaviour improved and he began to learn again.

KEY LEARNING POINT

Subtle learning problems very frequently follow even minor brain injury.

Traumatic brain injury is the commonest cause of acquired neurodisability in childhood and accounts for a third of all accidental deaths. One seventh of hospital admissions in childhood result from head injury. Boys are three times more likely to be injured than girls and early adolescence is the time of greatest risk. Poverty is an additional risk factor for both sexes and all ages.

Mechanisms of injury

Brain injury results either from direct trauma (penetrating, high velocity injury or depressed skull fracture) or from acceleration/deceleration (linear or rotational) forces (low velocity impact such as road accidents or falls).

PRIMARY INJURY (IN ORDER OF SEVERITY)

- **Lacerations** are usually associated with penetrating injury or severe rotational injury
- **Contusions** are associated with impact and may be coup or, more often, contrecoup in location with the frontal lobes being most susceptible
- **Shearing injuries** are associated with acceleration/deceleration when diffuse shearing of axons occurs throughout the white matter including the corpus callosum. Lesions are frequently associated with petechial haemorrhages, which may be visible on MRI
- **Concussion** results from relatively minor trauma, presumably from transient membrane dysfunction. It is reversible but may be associated with short term deficits, particularly anterograde amnesia.

SECONDARY INJURY

While little can be done to prevent or reduce the severity of primary injury, secondary injury is, to a considerable extent, avoidable by effective early management. Cerebral ischaemia/hypoxia is the final common pathway to all secondary causes of brain injury and it may arise in several ways:

- systemic hypoxia or hypotension caused by extracranial injury
- **increased intracranial pressure** may result from intracranial haemorrhage (parenchymal, subdural, extradural, subarachnoid or intraventricular), acute hydrocephalus or diffuse brain swelling
- **vascular injury/spasm** from stretching associated with shearing or contusion and resulting in focal ischaemic injury
- **loss of cerebral vascular autoregulation** with resultant maldistribution of blood flow
- **uncontrolled epileptic seizures** with resultant imbalance of cerebral metabolism and perfusion.

KEY LEARNING POINT

Primary brain injury cannot be avoided but secondary damage can. Early recognition and correction of potential secondary brain insults is the key to acute brain injury management.

Assessment – Glasgow Coma Scale and Score

Neurological examination should include observation for asymmetry of movement, posture, tone and reflexes. Abnormality or asymmetry of pupil size or eye movement/position should also be sought. Conscious level is assessed using the Glasgow Coma Score (GCS) (Tables 7.6 and 7.7). Any neurological abnormality not known to have been present before the injury, or a GCS <15 should be assumed to be due to focal cerebral pathology or increased ICP and necessitates an urgent CT head scan.

Table 7.6 Glasgow Coma Scale and Score

Score		Eye opening
4	Spontaneous	When the patient is approached their eyes may be open
3	Opening to speech	First speak and, if necessary, shout to see if they open
2	Opening to pain	Administer painful stimuli, e.g. pressure on the nailbed with a pen
1	No eye opening	Neither eye opens to painful stimuli
		Verbal response
5	Orientated	Ask the patient who they are, where they are and what the year and month are. If accurate answers are given the patient is orientated
4	Confused conversation	The patient can produce meaningful sentences but cannot give accurate answers to simple questions
3	Inappropriate words	The patient says only one or two words (often swear words). This usually happens if you touch them Occasionally a patient will call out the names of relatives or friends or shout obscenities for no apparent reason
2	Incomprehensible sounds	Groans, moans or mumblings, no intelligible words
1	No verbal response	Prolonged or repeated stimulation produces no verbal response
		Motor response
6	Obeys commands	Patients can accurately respond to instructions. Tell the patient to perform a number of different movements, e.g. 'Open your eyes', 'Raise your left arm'
5	Localizes pain	The patient can move an arm in an effort to remove a painful stimulus from the head or trunk
4	Withdraws from pain	Pulls away from painful stimulus
3	Abnormal flexion	After painful stimulus is applied at the fingertips the arm bends at the elbow, but does not achieve a localizing response when stimulated at other sites
2	Extensor response	When painful stimulus is applied at the fingertips the elbow straightens. This response is sometimes accompanied by inward rotation of the shoulders with extension of the wrist and fingers (decerebrate rigidity)
1	No response to pain	When repeated pain stimuli causes no detectable motor response

Table 7.7 Glasgow Coma Scale and Score (verbal modification for children <4 years)

Score	Verbal response	
5	Smiles, orientated to sounds, follows objects, interacts	
	Crying	**Interacting**
4	Consolable	Inappropriate
3	Inconsistently consolable	Moaning
2	Inconsolable	Irritable
1	No response	No response

Management

Immediate management of severe injury focuses on airway, respiratory and cardiovascular homoeostasis and is essentially no different from that of any other clinical emergency. Life-threatening extracranial injuries must be excluded or stabilized before detailed assessment of the intracranial injury. Epileptic seizures should be terminated promptly.

New neurological abnormality or GCS <15 are indications for a CT head scan

Worsening neurological abnormality or GCS are indications for intervention if a surgically treatable pathology (haematoma, hydrocephalus) is present and for monitoring ICP. Maintenance of adequate cerebral perfusion pressure (mean arterial pressure minus mean ICP) may improve outcome

In a child with a less severe injury (no neurological abnormality and GCS = 15) CT scanning is not generally indicated but the key decision is whether or not to admit for observation. If in doubt admission is advisable and is mandatory if *any* of the following apply:

- history of loss of consciousness
- persisting headache or vomiting
- clinical or radiological evidence of skull fracture or penetrating injury
- difficulty in making a full assessment
- suspicion of non-accidental injury
- other significant medical problem
- not accompanied by responsible adult or social circumstances considered unsatisfactory.

Rehabilitation

The need for early rehabilitation is dependent on the severity of the neurological deficits. It is best provided by a coordinated team of professionals supporting the injured child in hospital and enabling smooth transition to community-based services by effective discharge planning.

- **Physiotherapy** involvement, directed at maintaining symmetrical posture and avoidance of contractures is important as soon as the patient is physiologically stable.
- **Orthoses** and **botulinum toxin** injection to specific muscles may help prevent contracture development.
- As consciousness is regained **speech and language therapy** input will assist establishment of communication and safe feeding.
- Adequate nutrition should be supervised by a **dietitian.**
- Recovery of skills involved in daily living and self-help activities are assessed with the help of an **occupational therapist.**
- **Neuropsychological and psychiatric** advice may be needed for management of acute behavioural disturbance, often seen during the early recovery stages.
- Social, educational and emotional recovery may be supported and guided by the involvement of a **specialist teacher** and **play coordinator.**

Follow-up

In general terms about 90 per cent of the functional recovery from an acquired brain injury takes place in the first six months with further, more gradual recovery over the following two or more years. Whereas the most apparent, predominantly motor, deficits will often resolve almost completely, more subtle cognitive difficulties may not manifest until some years later. These deficits almost invariably arise from relatively minor frontal or temporal lobe injury – usually contusions. Functional difficulties may include:

- attention and concentration difficulties
- poor planning and organizational skills
- memory difficulties
- impaired impulse control
- emotional lability.

These difficulties, often misinterpreted as behavioural in origin, contribute to progressive educational failure, adjustment and behavioural problems and impaired social integration. Delinquency and even criminal behaviour may be the eventual outcome. Early recognition and appropriate educational and neuropsychological intervention may help prevent this potentially avoidable outcome. It follows that long-term follow-up by a rehabilitation team which includes a neuropsychologist is essential.

Subdural collections and non-accidental injury

Subdural (and subarachnoid) fluid collections may arise through a number of mechanisms.

BENIGN EXTERNAL HYDROCEPHALUS

Increased subarachnoid CSF volume is sometimes seen when a child is investigated for unexplained macrocephaly. It may be associated with motor delay and subsequent minor motor difficulties. Although essentially benign, children may be at increased risk of haemorrhage from overstretched bridging veins as they cross the widened subarachnoid space.

EX-VACUO COLLECTIONS

These occur when there has been relatively rapid reduction in brain volume following, for example, shunt surgery for hydrocephalus. They may also be seen when brain shrinkage results from neurodegenerative disorders such as glutaric aciduria type 1 or Menkes disease.

EFFUSIONS ASSOCIATED WITH CNS INFECTIONS

Subdural effusions may be associated with bacterial meningitis. They may be associated with persisting irritability but generally resolve without specific treatment. Rarely an effusion may become infected with resultant empyema formation requiring surgical evacuation.

CHRONIC SUBDURAL HAEMATOMA IN INFANCY

The mechanisms whereby acute subdural haemorrhage evolves into a persisting fluid collection are poorly understood. Postulated mechanisms include:

- Osmotic influx of fluid from blood breakdown products.
- Cerebrospinal fluid influx from 'ball valve' tear in arachnoid membrane.
- Exudation and repeated small haemorrhages from the inflammatory membrane which evolves from the original bleed.
- Repeated small haemorrhages from stretched bridging veins as they cross the enlarged subdural space.
- Repeated episodes of injury – minor subdural and subarachnoid haemorrhages are frequently seen in normal neonates, particularly following instrumental delivery but generally resolve within a few weeks. It is not known whether such haemorrhages ever evolve into chronic collections.
- Acute subdural haemorrhage, when seen in older infants, is frequently associated with imaging evidence of pre-existing fluid collections and sometimes signs of earlier episodes of bleeding. Suspicion of inappropriate handling or non-accidental injury clearly arises and child protection enquiry is appropriate. The degree and type (shaking or impact) of trauma required to cause such bleeding is unknown and may even be encountered during normal handling, particularly if a predisposing cause, e.g. benign external hydrocephalus, is present. In most cases inappropriate handling seems likely and should be considered highly probable in the following circumstances:
  - other unexplained injuries or bruises
  - signs of an otherwise unexplained acute encephalopathy (seizures, impaired conscious level, focal neurological signs)
  - imaging evidence of parenchymal brain injury (contusions, lacerations, intracerebral/intraventricular haemorrhage)
  - inappropriate or delayed response to symptoms by the carers
  - retinal haemorrhages are frequently seen in infants with subdural haemorrhage. While they may be a consequence of inflicted trauma, they are not pathognomonic of this cause and may be seen following acute increase in ICP from any cause.

KEY LEARNING POINT

Subdural fluid collections in infancy are frequently but *not invariably* due to inappropriate handling (non-accidental injury).

CEREBRAL PALSY

CASE STUDY: Cerebral palsy not due to perinatal factors

A 4-year-old boy was seen for consideration of botulinum toxin to try to improve his walking. He was mildly asphyxiated at birth and was admitted to the special care baby unit for two days because of lethargy and poor feeding. Cerebral palsy (diplegia) was diagnosed at 2 years, when he was still not walking, and attributed to perinatal events. Examination showed a child with mild learning disability and spasticity with a diplegic distribution. His head circumference (see Figure 7.12, page 252) was 1.5 standard deviations above the mean whereas both parents' head circumferences were below the mean. The parents agreed to him having an MRI scan (see Figure 7.4, page 215) which showed that he had holoprosencephaly.

It is uncommon for diplegia to result from a brain insult in the term fetus. Brain damage tends to result in reduced brain growth and smaller than expected head size unless there is associated hydrocephalus.

CASE STUDY: Cerebral palsy due to perinatal factors

A 2-year-old girl was seen because of delayed walking. She had been born at 32 weeks after premature rupture of the membranes and had required ventilation for respiratory distress. There was increased tone in the legs, particularly in the calf muscles and hip adductors. Reflexes were increased in the arms and legs. She had normal cognitive development. Head circumference was just above the mean whereas her parents' head circumferences were 1.5 and 2 standard deviations above the mean (see Figure 7.12, page 252). It was reasonable to assume that she had PVL on the basis of the perinatal history and clinical findings but an MRI (see Figure 7.6, page 215) was done and confirmed the diagnosis.

CASE STUDY: Cerebral palsy due to perinatal factors

A 7-year-old boy was admitted for hip surgery. He had been born at term by emergency caesarean following uterine rupture. He was severely asphyxiated with multiorgan failure. Subsequently he showed severe developmental delay due to total body dyskinetic cerebral palsy. He also had severe pseudobulbar palsy with secondary laryngomalacia requiring tracheostomy and he was fed via a gastrostomy. Fundoplication was required for gastro-oesophageal reflux and he had epilepsy. He had suffered two pathological fractures because of osteoporosis and had recently developed renal failure from nephrocalcinosis (possibly due to perinatal ischaemic damage). Hip surgery was required because of painful arthropathy secondary to dislocation. Although hard to assess, he was not severely cognitively impaired.

This boy's cerebral palsy was due to severe ischaemic damage to the basal ganglia and was clearly perinatal in origin. He has suffered all of the common complications of severe cerebral and several less common ones. Thankfully his story is not typical.

Cerebral palsy (literally, brain paralysis) is defined as 'a persisting, but not unchanging disorder of posture and/or movement caused by non-progressive pathology within the developing brain'. It is not a diagnosis but a clinical description of a group of disorders with a number of underlying causes. The overall prevalence in Western populations is 2.5 per 1000.

KEY LEARNING POINT

Cerebral palsy is not a diagnosis by itself. The history and all the clinical factors must be consistent with the presumed cause.

KEY LEARNING POINT

Although many children with cerebral palsy also have a learning disability this should not be assumed as normal intelligence may coexist with very severe motor disability. Because many people with severe cerebral palsy are effectively 'locked in' by their motor disorder it is wise to assume that cognitive ability exceeds the ability to express it.

The movement disorder

There are three main patterns of movement disorder which may occur discretely or in combination (with usually one predominating). These are outlined in Table 7.8.

Spasticity due to pathology within the corticospinal tracts is defined as 'a velocity dependent increase in tone' as compared to rigidity where resistance to movement is increased regardless of rate of movement. In reality they frequently coexist.

Dyskinesia, which superficially resembles spasticity, results from damage to or disordered development of a relatively small part of the brain, the basal ganglia or extrapyramidal motor system. This system is not involved in the initiation of voluntary movement but serves to facilitate, sustain and regulate activities primarily under voluntary control. The compact structure of the basal ganglia means that dyskinetic cerebral palsy tends to involve the whole body although a degree of asymmetry between the two sides is not unusual. Dyskinesia is characterized by increased muscle tone and abnormal postures which vary spontaneously and more particularly in reflex response to changes in posture elsewhere (the asymmetrical tonic neck reflex for example). Involuntary movements are also seen, mainly provoked by attempted voluntary activity but present to some extent at rest. Various more specific terms have been used to define the involuntary movement (tremor, chorea, athetosis, dystonia) but the inclusive title dyskinesia is preferred.

Ataxic cerebral palsy in its pure form is rare and quite distinct from other types. It results from pathology within the cerebellum or its several neural connections. The control of balance and smooth execution of voluntary motor activity (in this aspect it has important anatomical and

Table 7.8 Patterns of motor disorder in cerebral palsy

	Tone	Posture	Primitive reflexes	Distribution
Spasticity	Increased in affected distribution	'Decerebrate'	Not prominent	Hemiplegia, diplegia
Dyskinesia	Rigidity Which is variable in time and position (commonly reduced trunk tone with increased limb tone)	Variable but tends to reflect primitive reflex patterns	Usually present	Usually total body (quadriplegia)
Ataxia	Reduced	Reflects hypotonia	No	May affect mainly balance (dysequilibrium) or total body

functional connections with the basal ganglia) are its main functions and these are impaired in ataxia (the term dysequilibrium is commonly used to describe disorders of balance without significant limb coordination disturbance). It is nearly always symmetrical and muscle tone is reduced unless spasticity is also present. Abnormal postures are not seen except as a manifestation of reduced tone.

Why does it happen?

This is, perhaps, the question most frequently asked by parents and all too frequently answered inaccurately. Someone must be blamed and all too frequently it is the obstetrician or midwife. In reality, avoidable factors during labour may contribute to the cause of no more than 6 per cent of all cases of cerebral palsy. It is helpful to consider some aspects of normal brain development in order to understand more clearly both abnormal development and the effects of damaging insults on the developing brain.

KEY LEARNING POINTS

- Most cerebral palsies are caused by factors originating outwith the intrapartum period.
- Intrapartum causes account for, at most, 6 per cent of cases.

Myelination of the principal motor pathways takes place between five and eight months post conception. This is, of course, the time when most surviving preterm babies are born and the susceptibility of these pathways to damage as a consequence of premature birth accounts for the very strong association between spasticity and prematurity.

The susceptibility of the motor control mechanisms, particularly the extrapyramidal system, to damage following loss or reduction of their blood supply renders them especially vulnerable in all stages of brain development. During prenatal life any impairment of placental function if sufficiently severe and prolonged may damage the extrapyramidal system. The placenta, as an exclusively fetal organ, is approaching senescence towards the end of pregnancy and premature failure becomes an increasing hazard. While labour itself presents an additional stress for the fetal/placental unit, most instances of damage have occurred in the preceding weeks. The fetus who has already sustained brain damage in late pregnancy is less able to withstand the rigors of labour and so appears 'asphyxiated' at birth. Naturally the asphyxia is blamed for the motor disorder that manifests later although in reality the reverse is true.

The causes so far discussed are generalized 'insults' resulting in widespread motor impairment although a degree of asymmetry is often present. Hemiplegic and monoplegic cerebral palsies on the other hand are the consequence of focal brain damage. There are distinct similarities between the child with a hemiplegia and the older person who has suffered a stroke and this is more than coincidence. Many children with hemiplegia or monoplegia have in fact suffered occlusion of a major blood vessel supplying the motor cortex on one side of the brain usually towards the end of pregnancy. Stroke, while not common, is a unique hazard for the fetus as a consequence of the very different arrangement of the circulation before birth.

Presentation and evolution

Not unexpectedly the child with cerebral palsy presents with delayed or disordered motor development. All delayed motor development is not cerebral palsy however, and severe learning disability, neuromuscular weakness and certain benign developmental variants all present this way. The child with a learning disability may well be thought to be ataxic if 'bright' and floppy; until the failure of symbolic play to appear during the second year clarifies the situation. Provided it is looked for, weakness will not escape detection, but the specific motor disorders found in Prader–Willi and Angelman syndromes may prove more difficult. The benign and more commonplace head turning and bottom shuffling syndromes are easily identified once considered.

An understanding of the evolution of the cerebral palsies within the individual should enable the condition to be diagnosed positively once other disorders are excluded. The pattern of motor abnormality changes with time as the brain abnormality influences the normal course of development. In most cases reduced muscle tone is present initially and may persist after the first birthday (longer in severe dyskinesia, indefinitely in ataxia and where severe learning disability is also present). Abnormal limb and trunk postures either persist or make their appearance (except in ataxia) and are accompanied by unsuppressed reflex activity. Increased muscle tone appears last and reflects the abnormal postures that precede it.

Associated problems

Two types of problem may occur. The first results from brain abnormalities associated with those causing the motor disorder and includes learning disability (global or specific), visual and hearing disorders, impaired sensory function (especially proprioceptive) and epilepsy. The second are consequential and include nutritional and growth difficulties, gastrointestinal disorders (poor swallowing, gastric reflux, constipation), respiratory disorders, and behavioural or psychological problems of which sleep disorders are easily the most troublesome. To these should be added the direct manifestations of the motor disorder itself; reduced independent mobility, manipulation and self-help skills, impaired communication and liability to fixed postural deformities.

Management

With such a catalogue of associated and consequential problems it is hardly surprising that the person with cerebral palsy receives numerous, often conflicting recommendations as to which problems are the most important and what approaches to adopt in order to best overcome them. Least forgivable are those who offer a 'cure' based usually on an untested (and of course untestable) hypothesis involving 'brain reprogramming' and the known (but very limited) 'plasticity' of the nervous system.

Many reasonable and realistic approaches are available (although seldom as available or as accessible as one would like) emphasizing one or more specific aspects of cerebral palsy. Physiotherapists have traditionally been prominent and rightly emphasized the dual goals of prevention of deformity and encouragement of function. The principles and techniques of the Bobath approach exemplify this approach. A somewhat different and arguably more holistic approach is offered by conductive education, which emphasizes motor learning as part of an overall educational curriculum.

From a medical perspective there are limited but important opportunities for intervention in many ways reflecting the same basic goals of the physiotherapist. Prevention of deformity may be helped by reducing increased muscle tone. Appropriate positioning and discouraging unhelpful reflex activity are made easier by using lightweight splints (orthoses) and, in selected cases, muscle tone reducing drugs such as baclofen and L-dopa. Persisting increased muscle tone, not responding to the above measures and affecting specific muscle groups (hamstrings, hip flexors and adductors for example) may merit direct surgical intervention to lengthen or transfer tendons or block its nerve supply. More recently three new techniques have provoked interest.

DORSAL RHIZOTOMY

Dorsal rhizotomy is a neurosurgical procedure involving partially cutting specific sensory (dorsal) roots thereby interrupting the reflex arc (and reducing spasticity). Like all surgical procedures it is permanent but in selected subjects it is effective and the associated sensory loss is of little functional significance.

BOTULINUM TOXIN

Simpler and more widely applicable is the use of botulinum toxin. This drug when injected into a specific muscle causes a dose-dependent degree of paralysis with little if any effect outside the selected muscle. The paralysis lasts for three to six months, the lack of permanent effect permitting a degree of empiricism in treatment although having the disadvantage of repeated treatments being required.

INTRATHECAL BACLOFEN

Intrathecal baclofen treatment, in which the drug is infused by an implanted pump directly into the spinal subarachnoid space is an expensive but highly effective means of reducing tone. It enables the achievement of levels of the drug within the spinal cord which are impossible by oral administration without excessive sedation from cerebral effects.

A disarmingly simple concept, cerebral palsy is anything but simple; in its causes, its presentation, its many manifestations and associated problems it is both challenging and complex. Medical involvement, particularly in diagnosis and some aspects of management remains important, even essential, and all sufferers should have continuing access to medical expertise. Other disciplines are of much greater importance and rightly the gauntlet has been thrown down to the educationalists in their many guises. Are they equal to the challenge?

DEGENERATIVE DISORDERS OF THE CENTRAL NERVOUS SYSTEM

See also sections on neuromuscular disorders and epileptic syndromes, and Chapter 15.

CASE STUDY: Rett syndrome

A 3-year-old girl is referred with a provisional diagnosis of an autistic spectrum disorder (ASD). For the past 18 months her parents have been concerned by her social withdrawal, loss of early vocal communication and poor weight gain. The key examination findings are: microcephaly (having had a 'normal' occipitofrontal circumference (OFC) at birth), hand wringing, an irregular breathing pattern and tiny hands and feet.

Rett syndrome is a genetic neurodevelopmental disorder, affecting mainly females with features as outlined in the case study above, it often presents after an apparently normal developmental period of at least six months from birth. Mutations in the methyl-CpG-binding protein 2 (MeCP2) can be detected in approximately 70 per cent of cases. Amongst the affected female population, the phenotypic presentation is remarkably consistent; the same however is not true of affected males.

Life expectancy is extremely variable with some children dying suddenly in sleep but most progressing to a more stable state of reduced seizure frequency, loss of independent ambulation and gradual deterioration in intellectual function.

CASE STUDY: Neuronal ceroid lipofuscinoses (Batten disease)

A 6-year-old boy in a persistent vegetative state is admitted with a chest infection. He was normal until just beyond 2 years of age when he suddenly presented with catastrophic myoclonic epilepsy that proved drug resistant. He had rapid deterioration in intellectual motor function in the ensuing months and developed optic atrophy.

The term neuronal ceroid lipofuscinoses describes a number of related genetic biochemical abnormalities that all lead to accumulation of lipopigment in neurones as well as other cells. The additional terminology, i.e. infantile, late infantile and juvenile describes differing age and phenotypic presentations. However, features consistent to all groups include **epilepsy**, **dementia**, **motor failure** and **blindness**.

Particularly in young infants and in very slowly progressive disorders, it can be difficult to distinguish a static neurodevelopmental disorder from a degenerative disorder in which deterioration is masked initially by normal developmental progress. The key to establishing the presence of a degenerative disorder at any age is the loss of previously acquired skills, e.g. visual attention, purposeful reaching, and sitting. A specific exception to this is the loss of oral feeding skills in the infant with severe cerebral palsy. For older children, where presentation may be with a behavioural problem, information about educational progress and assessment by a neuropsychologist may be needed. Psychiatric illness at any age may cause regression and, if this is suspected, the opinion of a child psychiatrist should be sought at an early stage.

Having concluded that the child is suffering from a progressive disorder, the search for the cause is daunting with over 60 specific disorders to consider. Initially priority should be given to potentially treatable disorders:

- biotinidase deficiency
- adrenoleucodystrophy
- epileptic encephalopathies (see section on epilepsy syndromes)
- Wilson disease
- amino acid disorders
- some organic acid disorders (e.g. methylmalonic aciduria)
- Glut 1 deficiency
- hypothyroidism
- opsoclonus myoclonus syndrome
- infection (e.g. human immunodeficiency virus (HIV)).

Then consider those disorders that are most commonly reported in the UK. These data originate from the progressive intellectual and neurological deterioration (PIND) surveillance of UK children group, set up by the British Paediatric Neurological Association (BPNA). The top five diagnoses (in order) are as follows:

- San Filippo mucopolysaccharidosis
- adrenoleucodystrophy
- mitochondrial cytopathies
- neuronal ceroid lipofuscinosis (late infantile Batten)
- Rett syndrome.

Tables 7.9–7.12 categorize these, and other clinically relevant neurodegenerative disorders, into age-specific groups. With brief descriptions of each condition we have created a much condensed classification system that should help influence the choice of initial investigation.

Table 7.9 Classification of degenerative brain disorders: disorders of early infancy (1 month to 1 year)

	Clinical presentation	Key investigations
Lysosomal disorders		
Tay-Sachs disease AR	Seizures, startle, hypotonia, visual loss, Cherry red spot on macula	Leucocyte hexosaminidase assay
Mitochondrial disorders		
Leigh's subacute necrotizing encephalomyelopathy AR, mitochondrial	Irritability, nystagmus, feeding difficulty, disordered respiratory pattern, may have acute onset with intercurrent illness	MRI/CT, blood/CSF lactate, muscle biopsy
Amino and organic acid diseases (see Chapter 15)		
Glutaric aciduria (type 1) AR	Predominantly motor impairment - mimics cerebral palsy, macrocephaly, seizures	Urine organic acid analysis
Biotinidase deficiency AR	Hypotonia, seizures, ataxia, developmental delay, skin rash, sparse hair	Urine organic acid analysis, plasma biotinidase assay
Others		
Hypothyroidism	Hypotonia, poor feeding, hoarse cry, coarse features, constipation, prolonged jaundice	Thyroid stimulating hormone (TSH)

Clinical features - to be sought in each case
History - Loss of acquired skills, irritability, seizures, excessive startle, loss of vision, feeding deterioration
Examination - Head growth, visceromegaly, faltering growth, eye movements, dysmorphism (including facial coarsening), hair, fundi, respiratory pattern

AR, autosomal recessive; CT, computed tomography; MRI, magnetic resonance imaging.

Table 7.10 Classification of degenerative brain disorders: disorders of early childhood (1 year to 3 years)

	Clinical presentation	Key investigations
Lysosomal diseases		
Neuronal ceroid lipofuscinosis - (late infantile Batten) AR	Presents before 2 years, loss of hand skills, ataxia, spasticity, optic atrophy, pigmented macula	ERG, rectal biopsy
Mucopolysaccharidoses		
San Filippo syndrome MPS III AR	May appear as static learning disability initially, irritable, hyperactive, mild facial coarsening, frequent ear infections	Skeletal survey, urine glycosaminoglycans
Others		
Rett syndrome XD (usually lethal for males)	6 months - 2 years, loss of hand skills with stereotypies, hyperventilation, ataxia, secondary microcephaly, seizures	DNA analysis (MeCP2 gene)
Opsoclonus myoclonus syndrome Non-genetic	Ataxia, irritability, chaotic eye movements, multifocal myoclonic jerks	Exclude neuroblastoma
Epileptic encephalopathies see section on Epileptic syndromes	Presentation from birth through childhood, seizures, intellectual decline	EEG
HIV dementia	Mental regression, seizures, spasticity	CD4:CD8 count

Clinical features - to be sought in each case
History - Psychomotor regression, behavioural changes, loss of acquired skills, unsteady gait, tremors, visual problems, respiratory pattern, feeding problems
Examination - Posture, tone and reflexes, head growth, visceromegaly, faltering growth, eye examination (including cornea, fundi and movements), dysmorphism (including facial coarsening), respiratory pattern

AR, autosomal recessive; EEG, electroencephalography; ERG, electroretinography; MPS, mucopolysaccharidosis.

Table 7.11 Classification of degenerative brain disorders: disorders of later childhood and adolescence

	Clinical presentation	Key investigation
Lysosomal disorders		
Neuronal ceroid lipofuscinosis – (Juvenile Batten)	Visual failure, seizures, dementia, extrapyramidal and cerebellar signs	ERG, rectal biopsy
Peroxisomal disorders		
Adrenoleucodystrophy	Insidious dementia, hyperactive, gait disorder eventually, skin pigmentation	MRI, plasma cortisol assay, plasma very long chain fatty acid assay
Movement disorders and ataxia		
Wilson disease	Dyskinesia, dysarthria, pseudobulbar palsy, Kayser-Fleischer rings, bone and joint disorders	Urinary copper excretion, blood caeruloplasmin assay
Ataxia telangiectasia AR	Choreoathetosis, oculomotor apraxia, infections, absent lymph nodes, minute tonsils, periocular telangiectasia, and neoplasms	Plasma AFP assay (elevated) **Avoid CT**

History – More insidious and varied presentation, often as a behavioural problem, school failure

AR, autosomal recessive; EEG, electroencephalography; ERG, electroretinography; MPS, mucopolysaccharidosis.

Table 7.12 Early investigations for neurodegenerative conditions

Mode of investigation	Investigation	Examples where relevant
Imaging	CT	(**avoid CT** in ataxia telangiectasia)
	MRI	Adrenoleucodystrophy
	Skeletal radiography	MPS
	Ultrasound scans	Peroxisomal disorders
Electrophysiology	EEG	Epileptic encephalopathies
	EMG and nerve conduction studies	Friedreich ataxia
Ophthalmology	Clinical examination	Opsiclonus myoclonus, Wilson's (KF ring)
	Fundoscopy	Tay-Sachs, MPS
	VEP/ERG	Neuronal caeroid lipofuscinosis
Dermatology	Skin and hair examination	Menkes syndrome
		Biotinidase deficiency
	Biopsy for fibroblasts	'Enzyme deficiencies'
	Wood light	Tuberous sclerosis
Cardiology	ECG/ECHO	Glycogenosis type II, Friedreich ataxia
Genetic studies	Clinical genetic	Dysmorphology
	Chromosomes	Ataxia telangiectasia
	FISH	Angelman syndrome
	DNA	Rett syndrome
Tissue examination	Muscle/rectal/(brain) Conjunctival/nerve	Neuroaxonal dystrophy
Biochemistry: cerebrospinal fluid/urine/plasma	Urine organic acids	Glut 1 deficiency
	Urine GAGs	San Filippo
	Plasma TSH	Hypothyroidism
	Plasma caeruloplasmin	Wilson disease
	Plasma cortisol	Adrenoleucodystrophy
	CSF lactate	Leigh disease

(*Continued*)

Table 7.12 *(Continued)*

Mode of investigation	Investigation	Examples where relevant
Haematology	Marrow trephine Vacuolated lymphocytes Acanthocytes and other red cell abnormalities	Neumann-Pick type C Lysosomal disorders Abetalipoproteinaemia
Immunological and microbiological studies	Refer to Chapter 6	SSPE HIV

CT, computed tomography; ECHO, echocardiography; EEG, electroencephalography; EMG, electromyography; ERG, electroretinography; FISH, fluorescence *in-situ* hybridization; GAG, glycosaminoglycan; HIV, human immunodeficiency virus; KF, Kayses-Fleischer; MPS, mucopolysaccharidosis; MRI, magnetic resonance imaging; SSPE, subacute sclerosing panencephalitis; TSH, thyroid stimulating hormone; VEP, visual evoked potential.

Management

Once a neurodegenerative disorder is suspected a specific diagnosis is often difficult, but the benefits of achieving that diagnosis include:

- advances in treatment options, such as dietary or drug therapies and, occasionally bone marrow transplant
- the genetic implications to other family members as well as the possibility of prenatal screening
- help with management issues including prognosis and the application of more appropriate care plans.

KEY LEARNING POINTS

- An accurate history is the key to recognizing and diagnosing a neurodegenerative process.
- Priority must be given to treatable causes when considering investigation.
- Consider multiple invasive investigations if the child is having a general anaesthetic since the opportunity may not arise again.

PAROXYSMAL DISORDERS INCLUDING EPILEPSY

An epileptic seizure is an event of abrupt onset in which disturbance of consciousness, posture, movement, behaviour, affect and/or sensation is due to abnormally increased electrical activity of cerebral neurones. Epilepsy is a condition in which there is a predisposition to having epileptic seizures. It is usually defined as having had two or more epileptic events.

Non-epileptic paroxysmal events

As many as 40 per cent of children, diagnosed or presumed as having epilepsy, are having events which are due to another mechanism, usually syncopal or behavioural. It is preferable to use the term probable epilepsy rather than such pejorative (and often incorrect) terms such as 'known epileptic'. Non-epileptic events can be divided into the following categories:

- syncope and anoxic seizures
- parasomnias
- paroxysmal movement disorders
- psychological disorders
- migraine related disorders
- gratification (masturbatory) phenomena seen in normal infants
- stereotypies (repetitive, often complex movement patterns seen in people with severe learning disability and autistic disorders).

Syncope and anoxic seizures

Syncope is the result of a sudden reduction in oxygenated blood to the brain, and is a term that encompasses a number of clinical events. Probably best recognized as a classic 'Hollywood' faint, vasovagal syncope is the most common and familiar. Others include **reflex asystolic syncope** (RAS) (previously termed reflex anoxic seizures), breath-holding attacks (prolonged expiratory apnoea), and compulsive Valsalva manoeuvres. Cardiac dysrhythmias are a rare but potentially life-threatening cause of syncope. Syncope, of any cause, can result in anoxic seizures. These classically have:

- a 'seizure' duration of less than 60 seconds
- a non-epileptic EEG (if recorded during event)

- clinical features that may include:
  - tonic stiffening
  - convulsive jerks
  - eye deviation
  - automatisms
  - incontinence
  - post-ictal sleepiness.

This description will be familiar to many as typical of a 'tonic-clonic epileptic seizure'. The key features pointing to the correct diagnosis are the onset (including trigger and setting) and duration.

CASE STUDY: Reflex asystolic syncope

An 18-month-old infant is hit on the head with a wooden spoon by his older brother. He turns suddenly very pale and utters a small scream while dropping to the ground. He then becomes rigid and his eyes roll back. Within 20 seconds he stiffens in tonic extension and has a few convulsive jerks, following which he then relaxes and comes around, the whole event lasting less than 60 seconds. Afterwards he is sleepy and wishes only parental contact.

In young children, RAS are most commonly induced by a fright or a bump to the head. The whole episode is usually brief but prolonged spells with several syncopes clustering due to repeated stimulation are recognized. The ECG shows a period of asystole relating to the onset and resolving prior to the conclusion of clinical features. The important investigation therefore in any patient with cardiogenic syncope is an ECG as convulsive syncope can result from prolonged QT or other cardiac causes.

CASE STUDY: Vasovagal syncope

A 12-year-old girl wakes in the morning to find blood on her pillow from a nosebleed. She calls on her mother and gets out of bed. Her mother runs into her room to find her on the floor pale, stiff and jerking both arms. The episode lasts about two minutes and afterwards the girl goes back to bed for a half-hour sleep. Later the same day she goes to the hairdressers to get her ears pierced for the first time. The next morning on coming down the stairs she looks at herself in the hall mirror and sees her ears covered in pus, she again shouts to her mum and as mum runs to her she collapses to the floor 'like a rag doll', and has a very similar ictal event as the one described above. With each of these episodes the girl remembers a strong abdominal discomfort, dizziness and a gradual blacking out of her vision. Interestingly her mother also suffered from 'faints' during the latter stages of pregnancy.

Vasovagal syncope may be present from early childhood but is more commonly recognized in the older child or adolescent. This girl had been referred as a 'new epileptic' because of the jerking activity during her convulsive syncope. The relatively common 'aura' of abdominal discomfort with vasovagal syncope can be misleading as a focal seizure of temporal lobe origin. Often there is a family history of vasovagal syncope and familial misdiagnosis of epilepsy is by no means uncommon.

Breath-holding attacks differ in that they are respiratory in origin. The exact physiology is poorly understood but in most cases there is a moderate sinus tachycardia. Although widely believed to be a behavioural phenomenon this only applies to the initial crying which initiates a physiological cascade in the genetically susceptible infant.

Parasomnias

Paroxysmal events occurring within sleep (e.g. night terrors, somnambulism) can usually be easily differentiated from epilepsy with good history taking. As a general rule, episodes occurring only once or twice per night are usually non-epileptic, however, when they recur several times during a single sleep period they are usually epileptic.

Migraine and related disorders

There are mechanistic similarities between migraine and epilepsy – they are both the result of disordered ion channel function. A particular difficulty may arise in differentiating some focal epileptic seizures from migraine, e.g. occipital seizures and classic migraine with visual aura. Other migraine-related disorders include:

- cyclical vomiting
- benign paroxysmal vertigo of childhood
- benign paroxysmal torticollis of infancy
- alternating hemiplegia.

Epilepsy

CASE STUDY: Infantile spasms

A 4-month-old girl arrives in accident and emergency with a two-week history of irritability and

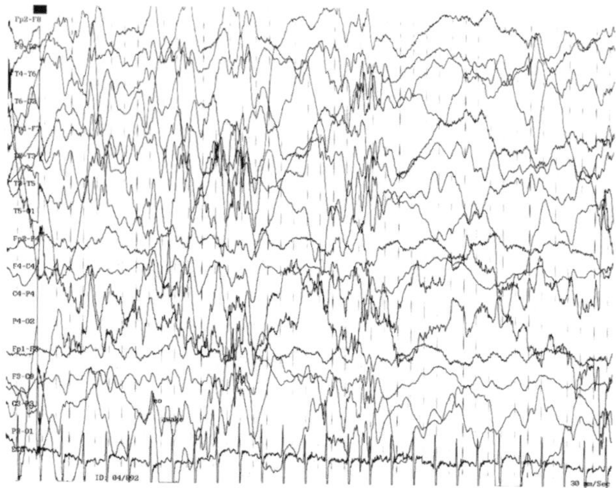

Figure 7.7 Electroencephalogram – hypsarrhythmia

'painful episodes' usually when waking or dropping off to sleep. She has been given colic and antireflux remedies with no improvement. An episode is witnessed and described as repeated brief spasms of head nodding with arms extending during which the girl becoming increasingly drowsy and agitated. The EEG of this case is shown in Figure 7.7.

Infantile spasms can be subtle with a mixed presentation of flexor and extensor spasms occurring most commonly in the same child. Outwith the classic presentation of repeated flexion spasms, any repetitive stereotypical movements in infancy should suggest the possibility of infantile spasms. However, non-epileptic infantile gratification and stereotypies are frequent causes of confusion, and home video recording in these circumstances is of great value. The EEG shows a characteristic chaotic pattern – hypsarrhythmia (see Figure 7.7).

In **West syndrome**, spasms usually occur in clusters with the child becoming increasingly drowsy and often distressed until the cluster ceases. West syndrome is an **epileptic encephalopathy** – a group of conditions in which the epileptic (electrical) disorder contributes to progressive intellectual decline. Some other examples are:

- **Ohtahara syndrome** – unremitting neonatal seizures with minimal developmental progress.
- **Dravet syndrome** – severe polymorphous (myoclonic) epilepsy of infancy; often presenting with prolonged febrile seizures.
- **Lennox–Gastaut syndrome** – in which developmental regression is associated with multiple seizure types (tonic, prolonged absence, myoclonic) and slow spike wave EEG discharge during sleep.
- **Landau–Kleffner syndrome** – a disorder in which loss of language, communication and (sometimes) motor skills is associated with persisting EEG discharge. It may not be associated with actual seizures and skills recover with effective treatment (corticosteroids).

CASE STUDY: Benign childhood epilepsy with centrotemporal spikes

A 10-year-old boy presents with a history of two events. On the first occasion he had walked through to his parents' room within an hour of going to his bed at night. He looked pale, scared, his face was twisted and he was drooling, unable to speak. This lasted less than one minute and afterwards he was upset but able to describe tingling over one cheek. Several days later again while sleeping he had a generalized, brief, clonic seizure, alerting his parents with guttural, grunting noises.

These episodes sound probably epileptic in nature even without a full event history, with the most likely syndromic diagnosis being benign childhood epilepsy with centrotemporal spikes (BCECT), previously called benign Rolandic epilepsy (BRE). An EEG will be extremely valuable in confirming this diagnosis.

The usual onset age of BCECT is around 8–10 years with boys more commonly affected. The syndrome is included in a group of benign partial epilepsies of which occipital epilepsies and benign partial epilepsy of childhood belong and have a generally excellent prognosis. The seizure onset is often missed as they most commonly just occur within an hour of falling asleep or just prior to waking. The typical seizure is brief, lasting seconds to occasionally several minutes. It is a focal seizure with semiology related to the somatosensory and motor areas in the Rolandic region. Often the child is unable to speak, hypersalivates, is frightened due to a feeling of suffocation, and has paraesthesia and motor involvement of one side of the face. Seizures may spread to become secondary generalized seizures.

The prognosis for BCECT is excellent and within two years of the onset of seizures the majority have resolved, over 90 per cent being seizure free by 12 years. Landau–Kleffner syndrome is sometimes associated with BCECT with a poorer outcome.

The EEG shown in Figure 7.8 demonstrates the typical pattern of focal sharp waves seen in the mid-temporal and central regions in BCECT. Of note, however, is that only a fraction of patients with typical Rolandic sharp

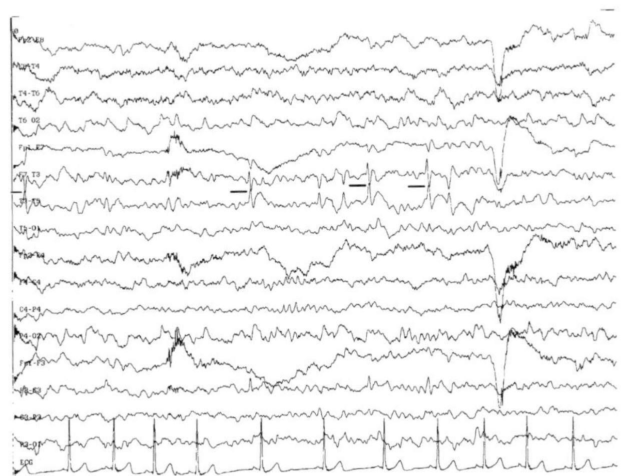

Figure 7.8 Electroencephalogram – Rolandic spikes, indicated by horizontal bars

waves have clinical seizures. With a typical history, and supportive EEG, it is felt by many to be unnecessary to proceed to brain imaging except when the seizures are atypical or particularly persistent.

Classification

Epileptic seizures may be generalized (appearing to involve the entire cortex from the outset) or focal (partial). The various types of focal and generalized seizures may be further classified according to their aetiology:

- **Idiopathic** – a primary, usually genetic, predisposition to inappropriate neuronal discharge.
- **Symptomatic** – where structural brain pathology or metabolic derangement lead to inappropriate neuronal discharge.
- **Probably symptomatic (cryptogenic)** – where structural brain pathology is suspected but cannot be demonstrated using current imaging methods.

A careful description surrounding the event, including the circumstances before, during and following each episode should narrow the classification to:

- non-epileptic
- epileptic
- probably epileptic.

This diagnostic process is best achieved with a structured approach, with both subjective and eyewitness accounts being important and opportunistic video recordings being invaluable. When more than one episode is described it is important to question (within reason) the history surrounding each event. A list of the type of questions to be considered when taking such a history are given below.

Taking a seizure history

Typical questions to in a 'seizure' history

- First ask the child of their recollection and recall of events

Pre-event

- Who was with the child and who saw the event?
- Where did the event occur?
- What time of day was it?
- What was his/her temperament like at that time, and what were they doing?
- Was there any 'trigger', e.g. pain, noise, meals?
- Can you tell if a child is about to have an event?

Event

- What happened first? What happened next, and next, ...?
- If movements or noises are described ask the eyewitness to mimic these.
- Any lateralizing signs –eye deviation, unilateral clonic activity, posturing, facial twisting?
- How long did it last – using a watch and talking through the event with the witness can be helpful?
- Was there any colour change?
- Was there bowel or bladder incontinence?
- Were there vocal automatisms, change in respiratory pattern and excessive salivation?
- Were the eyes open or closed during the event?
- How did they know the event was over, and how did it terminate?

Post-event

- What happened afterwards – did they sleep, cry, eat, ...?
- How long was it until the child was 'back to normal'?
- Did they show any signs of recollection at the time?

If there are several types of event then a history for each should be taken.

The purpose of this careful interrogation of the patient and witness serves to further classify the seizure phenomenon into a **seizure type** (Table 7.13). Identification of seizure type is essential for appropriate management and investigation planning. The importance of correct terminology allows doctors to have an international language that is simple and reproducible. This has allowed the expansion of the science of epilepsy and has resulted in improved management strategies for seizure types and epilepsy syndromes. An EEG is invaluable in the

Table 7.13 Classification of epileptic seizures

Main seizure types	Seizure definition
Generalized seizures	A seizure whose initial semiology indicates, or is consistent with, more than minimal involvement of both cerebral hemispheres
Tonic-clonic seizures	A sequence consisting of a tonic followed by a clonic phase. Variants such as clonic-tonic-clonic may be seen
Clonic seizures	Myoclonus which is regularly repetitive, involves the same muscle groups, at a frequency of about 2–3 cycles/s and is prolonged. Synonym: rhythmic myoclonus
Typical absence seizures	Loss of awareness and responsiveness with cessation of ongoing activities
Atypical absence seizures	Resemblance to typical absence seizures, with incomplete loss of consciousness and, commonly, association with motor phenomenon
Myoclonic absence seizures	A clinical absence seizure accompanied by rhythmical, bilateral myoclonic jerks
Tonic seizures	A sustained increase in muscle contraction lasting a few seconds to minutes
Spasms	A sudden flexion, extension or mixed extension-flexion of predominantly proximal and truncal muscles which is usually more sustained than a myoclonic movement but not as sustained as a tonic seizure, i.e. about 1 s
Myoclonic seizures	Sudden, brief (< 100 ms) involuntary single or multiple contraction(s) of muscles(s) or muscle groups of variable topography (axial, proximal limb, distal)
Eyelid myoclonia	Sudden involuntary jerks of eyelids, often multiple with associated upward eyeball deviation
Negative myoclonus	Interruption of tonic muscular activity for < 500 ms without evidence of antecedent myoclonia
Atonic seizures	Sudden loss or diminution of muscle tone without apparent preceding myoclonic or tonic event lasting one to two seconds or more, involving head, trunk, jaw or limb musculature
Focal seizures	A seizure whose initial semiology indicates, or is consistent with, initial activation of only part of one cerebral hemisphere
Gelastic seizures	Bursts of laughter or giggling, usually without an appropriate affective tone
Secondarily generalized seizures	A seizure that develops from involving only a single hemisphere to involving both hemispheres
Continuous seizure types (generalized or focal)	A seizure which shows no clinical signs of arresting after a duration encompassing the great majority of seizures of that type in most patients or recurrent seizures without resumption of baseline central nervous system function interictally
Reflex seizures	Seizures that are objectively and consistently demonstrated to be evoked by a specific stimulus or by specified patient activity

diagnosis and management of seizures but it has limitations and without an adequate clinical history it can even be dangerous.

CASE STUDY: Syncope as a result of a cardiac arrhythmia

A request was made for an EEG from a peripheral hospital with a history as follows: 'recurrent seizures now four in total of recent onset – family history of seizures in childhood'. The EEG was reported as: 'Rolandic spikes present in both hemispheres – does the history fit benign childhood epilepsy with centrotemporal spikes?' The child was treated by the referring clinician with antiepileptic medication and died subsequently one year later while playing football. On review of the EEG recording and the associated cardiac rhythm strip the **QT interval was prolonged** (Figure 7.9).

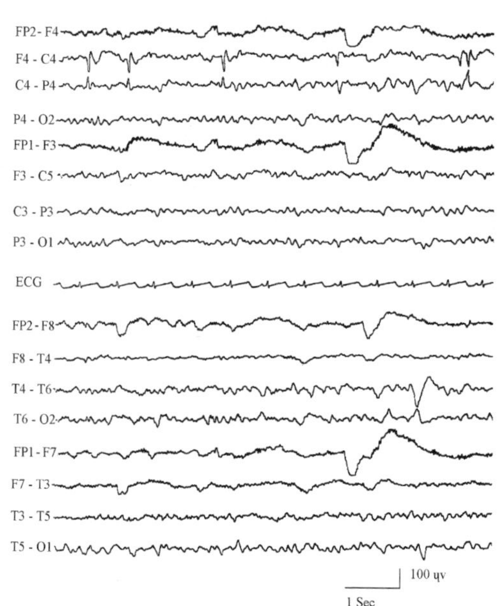

Figure 7.9 Electroencephalogram – Rolandic spikes plus long QT interval on electrocardiogram trace

Electroencephalogram traces can be achieved in most clinical situations without the need for sedative medications. Probably the most challenging group are older children with significant behavioural disturbances. An EEG can be performed in different ways to maximize the information obtained and discussion with the electrophysiology team can allow a more economic use of this service. The non-invasive options available with EEG include:

- **EEG with video** – 30 minute session can be done at bedside or in department.
- **Sleep EEG** – one hour session usually only for those children over 5 years.
- **Ambulatory EEG** – continual 24-hour recording with child in usual surroundings.
- **Video telemetry** – continual 24-hour inpatient recording with video camera and EEG.

The next step in the epilepsy diagnostic hierarchy, once a **diagnosis of epilepsy** has been made and **seizure type** identified, is to consider if the presentation meets the criteria of an **epileptic syndrome** (Table 7.14). The **epileptic syndromes** are defined by a constellation of clinical and electrophysiological features that make up a specific epilepsy condition. It is important to re-visit this concept regularly when reviewing patients with epilepsy, although it must be understood that a syndromic diagnosis will not be possible in all patients.

> **CASE STUDY: Typical absence seizures**
>
> A bright 7-year-old girl presents with a history of 'blank spells' recognized by her teacher at school. Characteristically each episode is short, about 15 seconds in duration, associated with loss of awareness, some lip-smacking and a gradual lowering of her head. After each 'spell' she smiles and continues with her previous task and has no recollection of events. Her EEG is shown in Figure 7.10.

In this case there is a high probability of the diagnosis being epilepsy prior to capturing an event on EEG. The seizure type and the EEG are highly suggestive of an **epileptic syndrome** – typical childhood absence epilepsy (CAE). In this case the prognosis is excellent and the decision regarding management is not a difficult one for the parents.

Other epileptic syndromes have a clinical picture similar to absence seizures and should be differentiated from CAE. These include:

- juvenile absence epilepsy
- atypical absence seizures such as those that occur in Lennox–Gastaut syndrome
- absence seizures that occur in other forms of idiopathic generalized epilepsies such as juvenile myoclonic epilepsy
- some focal epilepsies.

In these conditions the absence seizures may be atypical, e.g. there may be only partial loss of awareness, and often the absence seizures are only one of several seizure types within a polymorphous epilepsy syndrome. It must be acknowledged however that not all CAE is benign and up to a third of cases have demonstrable cognitive decline and slightly more have one or more generalized clonic seizure. For full listings of the new International League Against Epilepsy (ILAE) definitions and classifications visit the website (www.ilae-epilepsy.org).

Aetiology

Consideration should be given to a cause that may be:

- **genetic**, e.g. Angelman syndrome
- **infective or post-infective**, e.g. subacute sclerosing panencephalitis
- **metabolic**, e.g. pyridoxine deficiency
- **a result of brain injury**, e.g. accidental head trauma
- a result of brain developmental abnormalities, e.g. focal cortical dysplasia.

The benefits of achieving as complete a diagnosis of epilepsy as possible are (i) prognostic indications for the patient with possible genetic implications for the family and (ii) with a standardized approach therapeutic advances in the form of international trials or experiences can be shared to improve care.

Management

Unfortunately, the diagnosis of epilepsy still carries with it a significant stigma. Communication is the key to establishing a good relationship that will be repeatedly tested in the future if the epilepsy becomes drug resistant. We suggest that from the initial consultation all medical correspondence should be shared with the family and the primary care team, as crucially, it is often this team that carries out early notification and education of schools or nurseries, unless an epilepsy nurse specialist is employed.

BREAKING THE NEWS

The first few consultations should include:

- The diagnosis of epilepsy, the possible aetiology and the likely prognosis.
- A discussion regarding supervision during potentially life-limiting activities such as swimming

Table 7.14 A selection of syndromic classifications

Syndrome	Description
Ohtahara syndrome (early myoclonic encephalopathy)	Onset within a few hours from birth with clusters of tonic spasms. Prognosis poor EEG shows characteristic suppression-bursts
West syndrome	Onset usually 4–6 months Clusters of spasm EEG – hypsarrhythmia Mental retardation Prognosis poor – <12 per cent are normal
Dravet syndrome (severe myoclonic epilepsy of infancy (SMEI))	Onset within first year Onset often with (focal) febrile seizure or status epilepticus Myoclonic seizures and absences later Psychomotor regression usual
Benign childhood epilepsy with centrotemporal spikes (benign Rolandic epilepsy)	Onset 2–13 years EEG characteristic (Figure 7.8) Partial (hemifacial) seizures with motor and somatosensory signs are common, generalized seizures may be the only ones witnessed 50 per cent only have seizures in sleep No intellectual deficit prior to onset Almost all remit by adolescence
Early onset benign childhood occipital epilepsy (Panayiotopoulos type) (There is also a late onset childhood occipital epilepsy)	Mean age onset 5 years Autonomic manifestations include: nausea, retching and vomiting Eye deviation and head turning Seizures often arise from sleep Often seizures are prolonged and episodes of unexplained unconsciousness or 'ictal syncope' can occur Prognosis excellent
Lennox–Gastaut syndrome	Onset 2–8 years EEG – diffuse slow spike and wave Mental retardation. Poor prognosis Polymorphic epilepsy including: atypical absences, tonic and atonic seizures
Landau–Kleffner syndrome	Onset 3–8 years Aphasia being the prominent feature may never resolve 20 per cent have no seizures
(Typical) Childhood absence epilepsy	Onset 4–10 years Normal neurologically Short duration of seizures (<20 s) EEG – 3 Hz spike and wave
Idiopathic generalized epilepsies with variable phenotypes, for example juvenile myoclonic epilepsy	Onset 12–20 years Myoclonic jerks usually more prevalent in the morning Later generalized seizures occur Lifelong medication is necessary

and advice about safety in the home and contact sports is necessary.

- Lifestyle issues, such as:
  - Keeping a routine with regular mealtimes, sleep, etc.
  - Alcohol and recreational drug advice as these may lower seizure threshold.
  - Contraceptive advice, especially important for adolescent girls on medication, remembering not only the teratogenic effects of medication but also the interaction of the oral contraceptive pill with many antiepileptic drugs. Some centres advocate prescribing folic acid supplementation

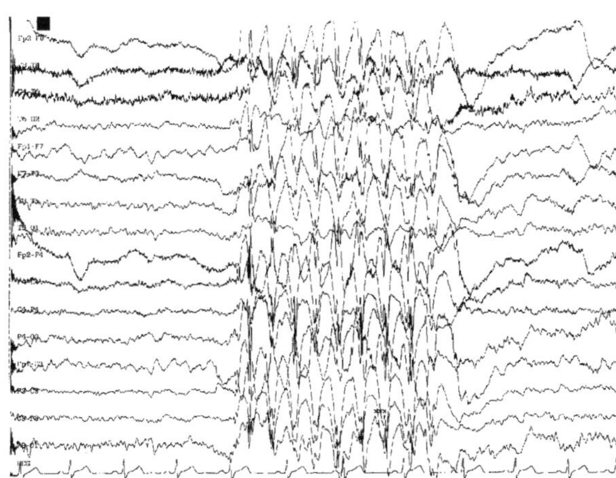

Figure 7.10 Electroencephalogram - burst of 3 Hz spike wave discharge

to all women of childbearing age with epilepsy.
  - Driving and the importance of being seizure free for at least one year prior to applying for a provisional licence – this is particularly important when considering trials off medication.
  - Future employment, e.g. bias against active duty with the armed forces, or welding with photo-sensitive idiopathic generalized epilepsy (IGE).
- An open discussion about medication (Tables 7.15 and 7.16).
  - Whether medication is required or not depends very much on the clinical situation and the wishes of the family. This is not usually resolved on the first consultation and is where written information is invaluable.
  - Consideration must be given to the potential side effects as well as potential benefits of any medication that may be prescribed.

Table 7.15 Suggested treatment schedule for epilepsy

Indication	Medication (in order of preference)
Focal seizures	Carbamazepine Sodium valproate Topiramate Lamotrigine Levetiracetam
Generalized seizures	Sodium valproate Carbamazepine Lamotrigine Topiramate
Absence seizures	Sodium valproate Ethosuximide Lamotrigine
Infantile spasms	Vigabatrin ACTH/Prednisolone Benzodiazepines Topiramate Sodium valproate Pyridoxine
Neonatal seizures	Phenobarbital Benzodiazepines Phenytoin Pyridoxine (always if refractory to others)
Myoclonic seizures	Sodium valproate Topiramate Benzodiazepines
Status epilepticus	Benzodiazepines Paraldehyde Phenytoin Thiopental
Seizure clusters	Benzodiazepines Steroids Phenytoin

Table 7.16 Side effects of antiepileptic drugs

Medication	Selected side effects
Sodium valproate	Hepatotoxicity, thrombocytopenia, neural tube defects in neonates, encephalopathy, pancreatitis, hair loss, weight gain, nausea, vomiting, gastritis
Carbamazepine	Allergic rash, leucopenia, hyponatraemia, ataxia, personality change, vomiting, diplopia, cognitive impairment, may worsen seizures in myoclonic epilepsies
Lamotrigine	Stevens-Johnson type rash especially when combined with sodium valproate, insomnia, nausea, vomiting, tics
Topiramate	Cognitive impairment, nephrolithiasis, weight loss, paraesthesias, drowsiness
Levetiracetam	Somnolence, behavioural problems
Ethosuximide	Gastritis, hiccups
Vigabatrin	Irreversible visual field constriction, agitation, sedation
Phenytoin	Ataxia, gum hyperplasia, hirsutism, allergic reactions, neuropathy
Benzodiazepines	Rapid tolerance to initially therapeutic dose, behavioural and sedative side effects
Phenobarbital	Osteoporosis in the immobile, sedation, aggressiveness, may induce spasms with prolonged neonatal use

- Give an indication of timescale of not only how long it will take for the medication to be effective, but also an indication of how long it will be prescribed for the child, e.g. with the focal benign epilepsies of childhood an initial trial of two years is suggested, whereas with juvenile myoclonic epilepsy medication is usually lifelong.
- Planning of future medications can be done early especially in conditions where refractory epilepsy or combinations of medicines are likely to be necessary with written information supplied.
- The requirement of rescue medication and where, when and how to use it.
- What to do in the event of future seizures.
- Teenage after-school clinics where the children often come themselves promote independence and encourage responsibility. This is a particularly vulnerable time for patients with epilepsy, where peer pressure and curiosity can lead to unsafe sex/drugs and conflict with authority figures leading to the typical epilepsy triggers: late nights, high emotion and poor routine.
- SUDEP (sudden unexplained death in epilepsy) – with the explosion of the internet and the trend of professional liability this type of discussion has become increasingly important and the documentation of such discussions even more so.
- Introduction, in the form of pamphlets or website addresses, to support groups.

KEY LEARNING POINTS

- Forty per cent of those attending first seizure clinics have non-epileptic paroxysmal events.
- It is beneficial to achieve as complete an epilepsy diagnosis as possible, and to re-visit this hierarchical scheme regularly during follow-up.
- There are many issues surrounding the management of epilepsy beyond the scope of medication.

INCREASED INTRACRANIAL PRESSURE, BRAIN HERNIATION SYNDROMES AND HYDROCEPHALUS

CASE STUDY

A 10-year-old girl attends the accident and emergency department several times over a two-week period. She is complaining of abdominal pain and headache and has slight pyrexia. She has normal blood pressure but her heart rate is only 65 bpm despite appearing quite distressed. A simple viral illness is suggested. On the latest visit she seems confused. While being examined she loses consciousness (GCS 8). Urgent CT shows a large frontal abscess with surrounding oedema.

KEY LEARNING POINT

Although this girl's symptoms were predominantly abdominal, she did also complain of headache and the bradycardia was an important clue to the correct diagnosis. Early detection of increased intracranial pressure requires vigilance and awareness.

Raised intracranial pressure (ICP) can result as a consequence of a wide range of neurological disorders and therefore is akin to many of the other sections in this chapter, not a diagnosis in itself, but an indication that one should be sought. The clinical manifestations vary according to the child's age, the aetiology and the rapidity of progression. Early detection of raised ICP with the timely implementation of treatment will improve the prognosis, as delay in appropriate management can be potentially disastrous.

Common causes of raised ICP

Cranial abnormalities
- Primary craniosynostosis

CSF/cerebral blood flow (CBF) abnormalities
- Extradural haemorrhage
- Subdural space lesions
- Subarachnoid space lesions: obstructive hydrocephalus
- CSF dynamics, i.e. endocrinopathies
- Benign intracranial hypertension

Parenchymal involvement
- Neoplasms
- Infection – bacterial meningitis, viral meningoencephalitis, abscess
- Trauma – head injury
- Hypoxic-ischaemic encephalopathy

- Reye syndrome
- Inborn errors of metabolism
- Diabetic encephalopathy
- Hepatic coma

Normal intracranial pressure

In a manner similar to mean arterial pressure (MAP), normal ICP increases with age through childhood from less than 3.5 mmHg in the neonatal period, <7 mmHg throughout childhood to <15 mmHg in adolescence and adulthood. Note that measurement in mmHg is perhaps more appropriate when considering raised ICP to more easily relate pressures to MAP and help with calculation of cerebral perfusion pressure (CPP) (1.36 cmH_2O = 1 mmHg).

In the pre-suture closure age group, chronically elevated ICP will lead to suture separation and excessive cranial enlargement. Serial occipitofrontal circumference (OFC) measurements allude to this diagnosis often before any other clinical signs. Worth mentioning here is the relatively normal tracking of OFC growth across the centiles in the first year of life towards the 'normal' centile for that child. The 'normal' centile is a representation of the OFCs of both genetic parents – in a similar way that final height can be estimated from both genetic parents. As in adults, transient fluctuations in ICP occur with normal daily activities and pressures of up to 75.5 mmHg (100 cmH_2O) are not unusual to record with coughing or sneezing.

Pathophysiology of raised ICP

In the first three years of life the skull vault is compliant (sutures usually closing by 18 months). Re-opening (diastasis) of the sutures can occur with raised ICP and this allows a greater relative volume displacement. Ossification of the sutures is not complete until adolescence, but, after the age of 3 years, the solidity of sutures means that the skull effectively is a rigid container with a fixed volume.

There are three main intracranial components: the brain (80 per cent), blood (10 per cent), and CSF (10 per cent). The intracranial volume is equal to the volume of these components. The CSF volume appears to be the major compensatory mechanism for alterations in ICP, and this is followed by compression of intracranial venous spaces. Cerebrospinal fluid is actively secreted in the colloid plexus and reabsorbed passively through the arachnoid granulations, *the rate of production* decreasing only when CBF begins to decline, and the rate of absorption reducing only when ICP reduces.

This highlights a key management point, that to maintain vital CBF in the presence of increased ICP systemic blood pressure must be actively managed. If CBF drops below a critical level, the resultant ischaemia produces cytotoxic oedema that leads to irreversible cell damage from membrane disfunction. A useful marker of CBF is the CPP. The following equation shows the relation of CPP to systemic blood pressure.

$$CPP = MAP - ICP\ (-CVP)$$

(CPP <40 – increased mortality; CPP >60 – better outcome)

Other pathophysiological mechanisms leading to cell damage by accumulation of intracerebral oedema are well recognized and each has therapeutic implications:

- Vasogenic oedema – from interruption of the dynamics of the blood–brain barrier.
- Interstitial oedema – caused by high-pressure obstructive hydrocephalus.
- Osmotic oedema – resulting from a fall in serum osmolarity and hyponatraemia.
- Hydrostatic oedema – caused by an increase in the transmural vascular pressure.

Intracranial pressure monitoring

Many devices are available for monitoring ICP in children beyond the age of closure of the anterior fontanelle. These devices include:

- fibreoptic intraparenchymal monitor
- subarachnoid screw
- epidural transducer
- subdural catheter
- intraventricular catheter.

The choice of device depends on the clinical situation and the age of the child. Monitoring is usually performed on the same side as any intracranial pathology, and is usually *initiated* when ICP is 10 mmHg greater than expected for the age of the child for duration of at least five minutes.

Hydrocephalus

The literal translation of **hydrocephalus** does not imply raised ICP. Normal pressure hydrocephalus is a controversial term used when ventricular dilatation occurs in the absence of increased pressure.

Increased pressure in CSF spaces is the result of a pathophysiological process with consequences involving the intracranial system. The clinical presentation, therapeutic options available and the potential for recovery depend on factors including:

- the aetiology
- the rate of evolution of the hydrocephalus
- brain compensatory mechanisms.

CEREBROSPINAL FLUID DYNAMICS

In order to understand the pathophysiological process that leads to hydrocephalus it is important to understand the dynamics of CSF production, circulation and reabsorption. The majority of CSF is produced in the choroid plexus system. The majority of the choroid plexus tissue is found in the lateral ventricles with small amounts also residing in the other ventricles. The CSF circulates through the ventricular system and bathes the spinal cord and is reabsorbed by the arachnoid granulations in the superior sagittal sinus.

AETIOLOGY OF HYDROCEPHALUS

There are two main categories when considering the mechanism of blockage to CSF flow:

- **Non-communicating hydrocephalus** denotes a blockage of the CSF pathways proximal to the outlet of the fourth ventricle.
- **Communicating hydrocephalus** denotes a blockage anywhere else in the normal CSF circulation beyond this point.

> Aetiology of hydrocephalus
>
> Non-communicating hydrocephalus
>
> - Aqueduct stenosis
> - Chiari malformation (type 1)
> - Dandy–Walker malformation
> - Atresia of the foramen of Munroe
> - Skull base abnormalities
> - Mass effect from intracranial lesions
> - Inflammatory ventriculitis
>
> Communicating hydrocephalus
>
> - Leptomeningeal inflammation – infection, haemorrhage, iatrogenic agents
> - Congenital anomalies resulting in hydrocephalus for usually unknown reasons
> - Carcinomatous meningitis

The clinical signs are discussed below in the section on clinical manifestations of raised ICP and the expanding OFC is shown in the head circumference charts in Figure 7.12.

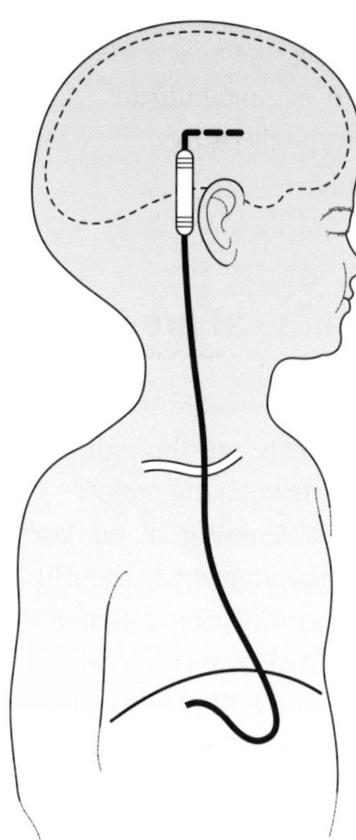

Figure 7.11 A ventriculoperitoneal shunt

MANAGEMENT OF HYDROCEPHALUS

The management of raised ICP is discussed later but the specific management of hydrocephalus and the use of available surgical options is a topic that merits specific discussion.

There are essentially two surgical techniques. A foreign body drainage device usually in the form of a **ventricular shunt** – a plastic tube that is inserted into the ventricle above the obstruction through a burr hole, then threaded down, behind the ear subcutaneously and placed in a cavity of choosing, usually the peritoneum (Figure 7.11). The side effects include lifelong shunt dependency, infection and recurrent failure to name but a few.

As a result there has been the emergence of endoscopic **third ventriculostomy** – a procedure that avoids the use of any foreign material within the cranial vault and therefore reduces morbidity. The main operative risk, although rarely reported is that of basilar artery perforation. It is not always effective.

Clinical manifestations of raised ICP

Unfortunately the early symptoms and signs of raised ICP can be invariably subtle and all too easily missed.

> **CASE STUDY**
>
> A 2-year-old child has been attending community paediatric clinics for a year for constipation. He is

admitted to hospital for several days of nasogastric bowel cleansing prior to restarting his oral laxative agents; there has been concern regarding compliance. The admitting physician notes he has not reached some of his developmental milestones and requests a neurological consult. The child is scrawny, has delayed closure of sutures and an OFC well above that expected by measuring his parents; the crack-pot sign also is demonstrated. The child has retention of upward gaze and no other neurological sequelae can be found. Diencephalic syndrome is suspected and a tumour confirmed later that day on MRI.

This is list of typical symptoms and signs that can be present in patients with ICP, some of these signs are limited to certain age groups.

Impaired upgaze

The classic feature in infants with 'sun setting' is also present in the older child and adult who is unable to maintain or achieve upward gaze. This is caused by pressure over the pretectal region from the effect of a supratentorial mass. An additional feature is retraction of the upper eyelids due to associated mid-brain dysfunction with excessive sympathetic stimulation.

Change in personality – deterioration of nocturnal sleep pattern

The non-specific features of irritability, lethargy, mood swings, deterioration in school performance and the onset of poor nocturnal sleep pattern are common in children with subacute rising ICP. These features are also suggestive of nocturnal seizure activity, electrical status in slow wave sleep (ESES), even in children in whom there is no past history of seizures.

Diplopia

The sixth cranial nerve runs the longest course of all the cranial nerves from its source in the pons, which renders it the most sensitive to supra or infratentorial brain shift. The term 'false localizing sign', coined for a sixth nerve lesion, refers to the unlikely possibility that, in the absence of other cranial nerve involvement, there is a pontine lesion.

Other causes of diplopia due to involvement of the other cranial nerves to the eyes, or due to pressure on the eye itself for example by an invading tumour are less common.

Headache

Headache is a commonly quoted symptom of raised ICP.

CASE STUDY

A 10-year-old girl presents to her general practitioner on two occasions over the past week with a three-week history of headache which is worse in the morning and occasionally leads to vomiting. Her mother has become more anxious about her over the past week saying to the doctor that she seems unsteady at times and on one occasion has complained of diplopia; she is reassured. Her father brings her to hospital, as several days later, while searching through rock pools at the seaside she falls and bumps her head. Afterwards she is ataxic and confused for around six hours.

On attending accident and emergency that evening she is passed as 'neurologically normal' but a neurology consult is requested because of the previous history of headache. On neurological examination there is limitation of lateral movement of the right eye beyond the central point and visual acuity is on bedside testing slightly reduced. The rest of the examination is normal but due to the right sixth nerve involvement emergency imaging is performed which shows a 4 cm lesion in her posterior fossa occluding the fourth ventricle and causing obstructive hydrocephalus. The lesion turned out to be an astrocytoma and proved impossible to resect completely.

More prolonged headache than this above example is unusual, with pain commonly being frontotemporal or occipital in nature. Classically manoeuvres that increase ICP, such as forced Valsalva, or coughing, or squatting to tie a shoelace will increase the pain. Nocturnal wakening or early morning wakening with vomiting or nausea are classic features.

Other signs and symptoms of raised ICP are:

- Seizures
- Papilloedema
- Excessive cranial enlargement
- Full fontanelle
- Decreased sensorium
- Cushing response

Brain herniation syndromes and space occupying lesions (SOL)

Essentially any SOL or focal cause of raised ICP can give rise to a brain herniation syndrome. SOL is typically synonymous with structural lesions such as neoplasms or abscesses but also includes any focal area of increased mass, such as localized inflammation in a post varicella-zoster cerebellitis.

It seems logical when thinking of the compartments within the skull that the presentation of subsequent clinical features of a SOL depends on several factors:

- the compartment(s) in which the lesion is located
- rate of growth (or shrinkage, if for example CSF is removed rapidly) of a lesion
- relative compliance of the compartment(s) involved (suture fusion?)
- underlying parenchymal architecture – is there any underlying structural abnormality.

The falx cerebri runs in the sagittal/vertical plane and divides the two cerebral hemispheres. As it progresses posteriorly the falx divides, forming a roof for the posterior fossa and separating the cerebellum below from the temporo-occipital lobes of the cerebral hemispheres above. This section of dura is known as the tentorium cerebelli. The partitions are not complete allowing parenchymal shift between the different compartments in circumstances of localized pressure increase, which cannot be compensated for by intracranial fluid pool reduction. There are three areas of herniation that give distinct clinical features and can guide the clinician to the compartment involved.

SUBFALCIAL HERNIATION OF THE CINGULATE GYRUS

The part of the cerebral hemisphere that shifts under the falx is the cingulate gyrus. This action may lead to compression of the anterior cerebral artery that runs alongside the free edge of the falx causing infarction. Clinically, this would lead to upper motor neurone paralysis of the contralateral leg.

TRANSTENTORIAL HERNIATION OF UNCUS AND PARAHIPPOCAMPAL GYRUS

Coming up through the tentorial notch (opening) are the mesencephalon, the posterior cerebral arteries and beneath them the third cranial nerves. A classic clinical sequence is observed with transtentorial herniation from a unilateral lesion:

- alteration in conscious state as a result of pressure on the diencephalon and mesencephalon.
- ipsilateral pupil dilatation.
- pupil fixation followed by the contralateral side as both third nerves cease to function.
- Initial contralateral hemiplegia as a result of an expanding lesion, with the subsequent evolution also of an ipsilateral hemiplegia, i.e. a double hemiplegia. With the expanding mass the mesencephalon, and therefore the pyramidal tracts, on the opposite side are compressed against the free edge of the tentorium. This is often called a paradoxical hemiplegia and is of concern since it can develop first giving a false localizing sign.
- Various respiratory dysrhythmias can occur due to compression and displacement of the brainstem.

CEREBELLAR TONSIL HERNIATION

The diffusely swollen brain will herniate through the tentorium as described above but, with continuing pressure caudally, may also herniate through the foramen, with the cerebellar tonsils being forced through the foramen magnum. In addition, cerebellar herniation can result from expanding infratentorial masses, such as a cerebellar bleed, or as a result of decrease in pressure from below, for example when a lumbar puncture is done in the setting of raised ICP.

Clinically compression of the medullocervical junction leads to progressive apnoea and quadriplegia, as pressure on the reticulospinal tracts stops automatic breathing and quadriplegia secondary to pressure-induced ischaemia stops volitional breathing. If there is an expanding infratentorial lesion then upward transtentorial herniation causing midbrain signs may confuse the clinical picture and make the clinician think of a supratentorial lesion.

Management

If there is suspicion of raised ICP then lumbar puncture is contraindicated because of the risk of brain herniation.

Simple management rules are important in managing raised ICP

- Consideration of invasive monitoring of ICP and CVP
- Appropriate fluid management, avoiding hypovolaemia and SIADH
- Head elevation 30° above the heart facilitates venous return
- Considerate nursing and appropriate medication to reduce agitation
- Prompt management of labile temperature

From a pathophysiological viewpoint management of raised ICP is limited to three specific areas

- Decreasing cerebral blood volume
- Decreasing brain and CSF volume
- Increasing intracranial volume

DECREASING CEREBRAL BLOOD VOLUME

Cerebral blood volume constitutes around 10 per cent of intracranial volume with CSF being another 10 per cent. For rapid control of ICP the cerebral blood volume is usually the most malleable compartment. Hyperventilation can manipulate cerebral blood volume within minutes of administration by reducing $PaCO_2$ safely to around 30 mmHg which leads to cerebral vasoconstriction. This is only safe to do for short periods, ideally less than 24 hours as irreversible ischaemic damage can result from more chronic use.

Vasoconstrictive anaesthetic agents, such as thiopental and propofol should be used with caution. They can reduce cerebral metabolic rate but may also induce systemic hypotension.

DECREASING BRAIN AND CSF VOLUME

Diuretics such as mannitol, an osmotic diuretic, and furosemide, a loop diuretic, are effective in controlling acutely raised ICP within 15 minutes of administration. They both work by reducing CSF production, are synergistic when used together, with mannitol having an added mechanism of reducing blood viscosity thereby increasing blood flow and reducing cerebral blood volume. Furosemide is generally safer to use, especially when there are concerns regarding the integrity of the blood–brain barrier or of cardiac and renal function. Acetazolamide, a carbonic anhydrase inhibitor, can reduce CSF production in the acute and chronic situations although can temporarily cause raised ICP by increasing CBV. Cerebral vasogenic oedema can be decreased by administration of glucocorticoids. The efficacy of corticosteroids in the treatment of brain tumours in unquestionable, however, uncertainty remains over their effectiveness in more diffuse brain injuries.

Surgical manipulation of CSF volume can prove to be extremely useful in the form of a ventricular drain, ventriculostomy or tapping the reservoir of a shunt if there is a distal obstruction. Surgical resection of a brain tumour or selected lobectomy has an effect on reducing ICP as well as the obvious benefit of removing abnormal tissue.

INCREASING INTRACRANIAL VOLUME

Acute surgical decompressive craniectomy is not currently widely used in the paediatric population. As a management strategy however, in primary craniosynostosis with chronically raised ICP craniectomy is commonly used.

KEY LEARNING POINTS

- Timely management is the key.
- Management of ICP – maintain systemic blood pressure.

HEAD SIZE AND SHAPE

Occipitofrontal circumference

The OFC is a measure of the greatest circumference around the skull and is the most important measurement in infancy. It should be monitored regularly throughout the first year of life, as it correlates with brain size and growth.

- Microcephaly, so called when the OFC falls below two standard deviations, always represents poor growth.
- Macrocephaly, so called when the OFC is greater than two standard deviations of the mean, does not always represent increased brain size or megalencephaly.
- Hydrocephaly, 'water head', often presents with macrocephaly but not megalencephaly, i.e. the head size is physically large but the brain is not.

Genetic and environmental factors are important in determining 'normal' OFC, it is therefore important that accurate measurement and documentation of parental head circumferences become a routine part of the complete neurological examination (Figure 7.12).

A logical approach should be adopted when seeing a child for the first time with abnormal head size:

- Ask about maternal history especially specific questions surrounding maternal health and medications during pregnancy.
- Ask about the child's development, and any symptoms of raised ICP (poor feeding, irritability, sleep pattern) and neurocutaneous stigmata.
- Enquire about family history and record parents' OFCs as well as any siblings present.
- Measure the OFC and palpate the skull, feeling for size and tension in the fontanelle(s) and the suture lines; are they separated, normal or overriding?
- Are there any features suggestive of facial scoliosis, suggesting unilateral coronal suture synostosis, or a genetic syndrome?
- Examine the child including the cranial nerves and optic fundi.

Head shape

Outwith the neonatal period there are two main reasons why heads are misshapen:

- positional moulding
- craniosynostosis.

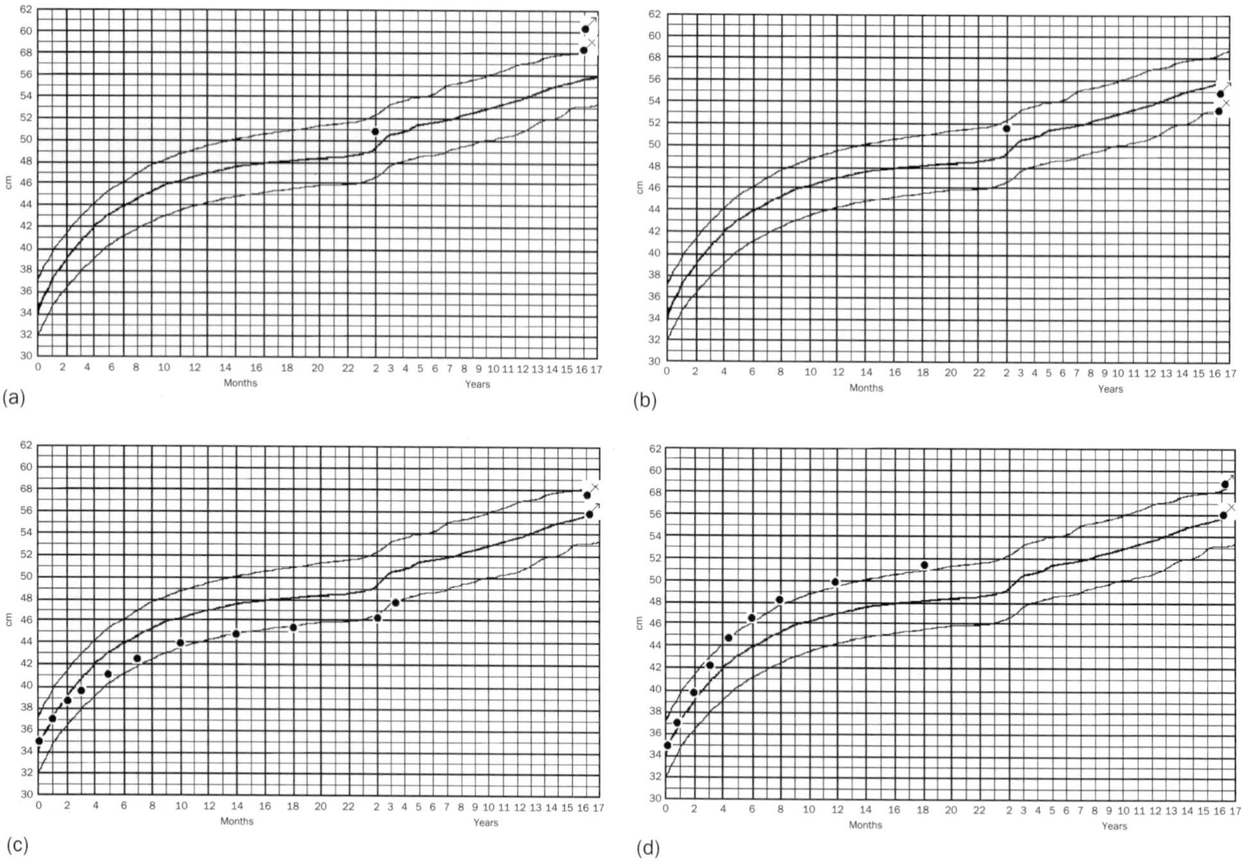

(a)

(b)

(c)

(d)

Figure 7.12 Patterns of head growth (a) Normal head size but comparison with parents reveals relative microcephaly; (b) normal head size but comparison with parents reveals relative macrocephaly; (c) head size deviates progressively further from the mean (and parental centile position), suggesting degenerative disorder or synostosis; and (d) familial macrocephaly, head circumference increases more rapidly than normal in the first six months reaching the same centile position as the father – normal infant, no need for investigation

Positional moulding has become more frequent with the advent of the 'back to sleep' policy in an attempt to reduce cot death. Babies are positioned on their back or side leading to flattening of the calvarium or occipital regions of the skull. This moulding tends to self-correct with time as the infants become more mobile. When the period of relative immobility is prolonged, such as in the neonatal care of premature babies, infants with motor impairments, or torticollis, the results of 'simple' moulding can be quite dramatic. The clinician's role is to monitor head growth and reassure. Techniques employed to improve physical appearance include cot repositioning, head pads for sleep and even specially made skull helmets.

Craniosynostosis is a more serious condition where head shape is altered due to premature closure of the sutures. The main cranial sutures are shown in Figure 7.13.

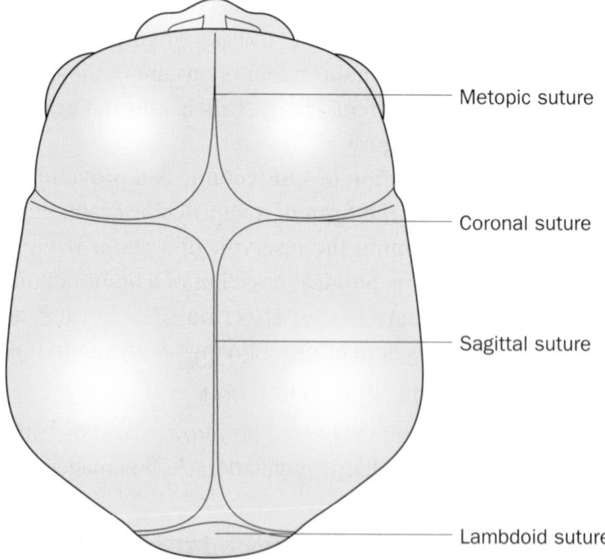

Figure 7.13 The main cranial sutures

When the sutures fuse growth ceases in a perpendicular direction to the suture plane resulting in the head shape shown in Figure 7.14. It is important to note that closure of only one suture is very rarely associated with increased intracranial pressure, however closure of more than one suture restricts vault expansion and therefore brain growth. When this occurs secondary to a genetic syndrome such as in Apert, acrocephalosyndactyly and Crouzon syndromes the coronal suture is usually the first to fuse.

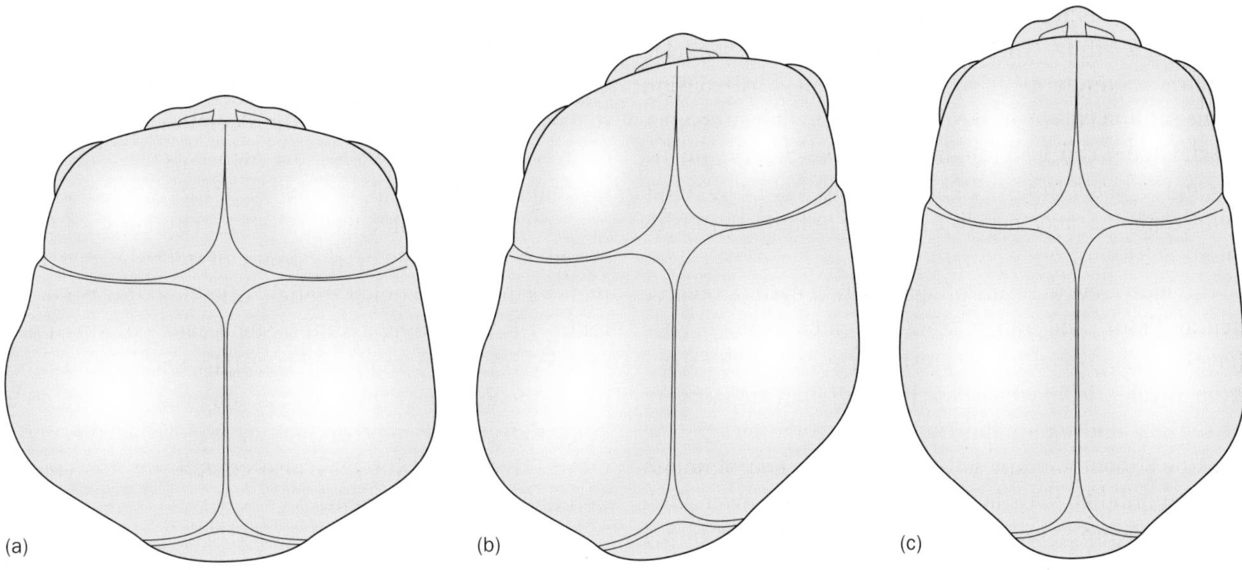

Figure 7.14 The effects of synostosis (a) coronal – brachycephaly; (b) lambdoid/part of coronal – plagiocephaly (c) sagittal – scaphocephaly

SPINA BIFIDA

Neurulation has been discussed earlier in the chapter, and it is an interruption to this process that results in the development of spina bifida. The global term neural tube defect (NTD) is used to describe infants born with spina bifida and meningocele or myelomeningocele defects as well as encephaloceles, iniencephaly and anencephaly and is often associated with hydrocephalus. There is an interesting geographical variation in the incidence of the different types of NTD with the spinal anomaly of meningocele and myelomeningocele constituting 80 per cent of NTD liveborn infants in Europe, North America, Australia and some communities in South Africa. However, defects of the cranial end, particularly encephaloceles, are more common in south-east Asia than in Europe and account for 40 per cent of the NTDs found there.

The incidence of NTD is approximately 1 per 1000 live births and there is a similar frequency of stillbirths or early neonatal deaths due to anencephaly. A couple who have a fetus or child affected by an NTD have an approximately 10-fold increased likelihood of subsequent siblings being affected, and if the couple have two siblings affected there is a further increase by a factor of 3 for subsequent children. In 1992 an expert advisory group of the UK Department of Health recommended the use of daily folic acid supplements until the twelfth week of pregnancy to prevent recurrence. To prevent a first occurrence of NTD, women who are planning a pregnancy should eat more folate-rich foods and take 4 mg folic acid daily from when they begin trying to conceive until the twelfth week of pregnancy. A study from the Medical Research Council study published in 1991 suggested that folic acid offered a protective effect of 72 per cent in the risk of a second affected child.

Detection of elevated maternal serum α-fetoprotein levels and refinement in intrauterine ultrasound diagnosis have resulted in early intrauterine diagnosis and termination of pregnancy in many cases. A genetic predisposition to the development of NTDs may explain the higher incidence in those of Celtic (Irish, Welsh and West of Scotland) extraction than in those of Anglo-Saxon or Norse origin in the UK.

In **spina bifida occulta** there is failure of fusion of the spinous process posteriorly but in the majority of individuals this is a minor deviation from normal. A few children have an associated haemangiomatous or hairy patch over the site of the spina bifida occulta and this may be associated with neurological deficits such as a foot drop or alteration in urinary continence. Tethering of the cord is the most common problem, and if producing neurological signs, merits exploration and freeing of the cord. **Diastomyelia** is an anomaly where a bony spur protrudes from the posterior aspect of the cerebral bodies and results in splitting of the cord and in a few patients this may merit exploration and removal of the bony spur. Spinal imaging has been greatly enhanced with the development of MRI which gives very much better definition of the intraspinal anatomy than was previously possible.

In **spina bifida cystica** the defect may result in a meningocele in which there is simply a protrusion of the spinal cord covering to form a sac that contains CSF. This defect accounts for less than 10 per cent of babies born with spina bifida. There are no neurological sequelae from the meningocele itself and treatment is by excision of the sac and closure of the dura and overlying structures. Fascial flaps can be brought across the defect and no attempt is made to alter the bony structure. Progressive hydrocephalus may develop in these infants before or after excision of the meningocele.

The more severe forms of spina bifida cystica involve neural tissue and range from the meningomyelocele (myelomeningocele) to the most severe end of the spectrum, myelocele, in which case there is severe impairment of sensory and motor function distal to the lesion. The next most common site is the sacral area and although affected infants may have relatively good lower limb function, neuropathic dysfunction of bladder and bowel is present.

In consequence of the intrauterine paralysis that occurs in many of these infants, there may be secondary structural problems and deformities such as loss of the normal lumbar lordosis and kyphosis. These problems may progress as they are secondary to imbalance of muscular activity and similar imbalanced muscle activity may result in dislocation of the hips, deformities of the knees or talipes. Effective management of the baby born with spina bifida depends on an initial detailed clinical examination and assessment of the level of neurological impairment. It is also important to assess upper limb function. This is normal in the majority of babies, but in a small number upper limb problems become apparent as time goes by. A very common accompaniment of spina bifida is hydrocephalus and this will in many infants be progressive and require active treatment.

Treatment of the infant with spina bifida is designed to maximize the potential of the child rather than being in any way curative. The neurological problem has been in existence for six or seven months before birth and the exposed neural tissue is irreversibly damaged. However, in some infants early closure of the back defect may be indicated to prevent infection and fibrosis affecting parts of the spinal cord that were not previously damaged. Also closure of the back has an important cosmetic aspect in that it quickly allows the back to be covered by normal skin and is therefore much easier for the parents to manage. The one drawback of early closure of myelomeningocele is that progression of hydrocephalus requiring active treatment is almost invariable and leaving the larger defects (in which paraplegia is complete) to epithelialize spontaneously can result in the production and reabsorption of CSF becoming balanced so that active intervention is unnecessary. Decisions should be made according to the circumstances of each individual infant and family.

An **encephalocele** is a protrusion at the cranial end of the neural tube, usually in the occipital region. These defects are occasionally simply meningoceles, but more commonly contain neural tissue, either cerebellum or cerebrum, i.e. encephalocele. There is frequently an associated malformation of the brain despite the fact that there is no neurological deficit affecting the trunk or limbs. The protruding neural tissue is rarely of any functional value to the infant and is usually excised and closure of the dura over the defect is achieved. This leaves a bony defect that may or may not close as the child grows. Hydrocephalus may also complicate this condition and require treatment.

HEADACHE

CASE STUDY: 'Tension headache' with recent change in symptoms

A 12-year-old boy had attended the headache clinic two years previously. Chronic daily headache (a pattern seen in 'tension headache') had been diagnosed. A few weeks before admission his headaches had changed in character and become more severe. They were now wakening him at night. His gait was unsteady and his headache was worse if he coughed or sneezed. Urgent CT scan showed a posterior fossa tumour with early hydrocephalus. Surgery was curative. The family complained as they believed his symptoms for the past few years were due to his tumour. Undoubtedly his tumour had been present for a long time – probably from before birth but, because it was very slow growing, it did not cause meningeal stretching until hydrocephalus developed as a result of compression of the cerebral aqueduct. The acute hydrocephalus was also the cause of his unsteadiness, not the tumour. The original diagnosis was correct.

Headache becomes an increasingly frequent symptom as children grow older and during adolescence it may well be commoner than in adults. It is rarely encountered in pre-school children but there is no evidence that it has any more sinister implication for this age group than for any other. It is seldom an indicator of serious underlying pathology but that is nearly always the concern which prompts medical review.

Table 7.17 Headache: mechanisms, features and management

Headache type	Mechanism	Features	Management
Tension	Continous scalp muscle contraction	Often longlasting, sometimes daily, may be made worse by eye movements	Reassurance, explain mechanism, paracetamol
Migraine	Aura mechanism unknown. Scalp artery dilatation?	Throbbing, may be unilateral, sensory intolerance, often incapacitating	Reassurance
Symptomatic (increased intracranial pressure)	Meningeal stretching	Recent onset or change in character. Made worse by coughing/sneezing or bending forward. Made worse by 'physiological' increases in ICP (sleep, minor illness) May be associated with vomiting 'Cushing triad'	Assume due to intracranial pathology and manage accordingly
Facial/scalp tissue pathology	Inflammation (e.g. in frontal sinuses)	Usually localized, local tenderness, blowing nose may make it worse	Diagnose and treat

ICP, intracranial pressure.

Mechanisms and types of headache

The brain itself has no pain receptors but they are plentiful within the meninges, periosteum, extracranial blood vessels and scalp muscles. Most headache originates from extracranial structures but headache of intracranial can arise if the meninges are stretched or inflamed. Table 7.17 outlines the main causes and characteristics.

For discussion of sensory deficits – hearing see Chapter 1, for vision see Chapter 17, for meningitis see Chapter 6 and for the unconscious child see Chapter 4.

FURTHER READING

Aicardi J (ed). (1998) *Diseases of the Nervous System in Childhood.* 2nd edn. London: MacKeith Press.

Stephenson JBP (ed). (1990) *Fits and Faints.* London: MacKeith Press.

Chapter 8

The respiratory system

Neil Gibson

The upper airways, lower airways and lungs present a surface area open to external factors greater than any other organ system. In consequence, they have developed a complex structure and set of mechanisms to provide protection and act as a defence against injury or harm. The bellows function is but a fraction of the utility and there are important functions with regard to acid–base homoeostasis and immunology.

Disorders of the respiratory system constitute a large proportion of illness in children. In primary care this relates mainly to respiratory infections and in secondary care chronic respiratory problems are among the commonest diagnoses.

GROWTH AND DEVELOPMENT

Growth and differentiation of the respiratory tract occurs in four stages, with one merging into another. Three of these stages occur in fetal life and the fourth is primarily a feature of postnatal growth and development. Knowledge of these processes aids explanation of congenital malformations and the effects of premature birth on lung function and health.

Embryonic stage

The respiratory system develops as a ventral growth from the foregut around the fourth week of gestation with the laryngotracheal groove appearing in the endodermal foregut around 26 days, when it evaginates and begins to branch at 26–28 days. This endodermal bud goes on to form the whole lining of the respiratory system.

Pseudoglandular stage

This lasts from five to 16 weeks' gestation and commences with condensing of mesenchyme around the endodermal bud. The mesenchyme forms all the supporting structures of the airways, such as cartilage, muscle and connective tissue, as well as the lymphatics and blood vessels. The essential co-development of mesenchymal and endodermal components is vital for the correct fashioning of the lungs and airways. Airway branching continues until about 16 weeks when all the conducting airways, i.e. trachea to terminal bronchioles, are present as a tree of narrow tubules with thick epithelial walls. No new airway branches form after 16 weeks' gestation.

Canalicular stage

Between 16 and 24 weeks' gestation, there is great mesenchymal proliferation with considerable growth of airways and the establishment of what will become the respiratory bronchioles. At the end of this stage there is the potential for close association of blood vessels and air spaces. This almost certainly explains the apparent limit of viability of preterm neonates to the very end of the canalicular stage.

Terminal sac stage

The alveolar stage from about 22–23 weeks' gestation extends into postnatal life and is characterized by the formation of alveoli and development of the areas of the lung responsible for gas exchange. There is progressive thinning of the blood–gas barrier. Initially saccules, which are larger and more irregular than alveoli, form and these then gradually change into clusters of the smaller, smoother-walled gas exchange areas with a much larger surface area. This process of alveolar creation extends until 5–8 years of age. After this age, the airways and lung tissue undergo no further differentiation but simply increase in size, reaching a peak of function in early adulthood.

Fetal lung fluid and breathing

During the intrauterine period the developing lungs are filled with fluid formed in the lungs. This fluid is vital for lung development and its function seems to be co-dependent on fetal breathing movements, which occur periodically during the middle and later trimesters. There is a change in the composition of the fluid with presence of type II pneumocytes producing surfactant from about 24 weeks and delivering this to the alveolar surface by 30 weeks' gestation. Surfactant consists of a number of phospholipids that together create surface tension within the respiratory portion of the airways and sacs and thereby allow the alveoli and smallest airways to resist collapse at low lung volumes. Large loss of amniotic fluid or oligohydramnios with low production, if associated with scant or absent fetal breathing, is associated with severe lung hypoplasia and failure to adapt to extrauterine life. This is most commonly seen in Potter syndrome. Rarely, genetic mutations can cause failure of normal surfactant production, leading to severe neonatal respiratory failure.

Postnatal lung development

There are 20 million air spaces at birth with ~2.8 m^2 of blood–gas exchange surface. Soon after term the true alveoli form and these rapidly multiply until the adult number of 300 million is reached between 5 and 8 years of age with a surface area for gas exchange of 32 m^2. Thereafter growth occurs only in size and not in complexity, allowing the rise in lung function to mirror somatic growth, leading to an adult male air–tissue interface for gas exchange of 75 m^2.

The pulmonary circulation

There is a close link between growth of the airways and the pulmonary blood vessels. The main pulmonary artery and its two branches develop from the sixth embryonic aortic arch, on its left. This connects with the developing right ventricle. In parallel, the newly formed atrial structures connect with the pulmonary venous system. The pulmonary vessels accompany all the major airway structures by the end of the pseudoglandular stage. Thereafter, there is further development in line with the respiratory portion of the lung, giving rise to the gas exchange areas. Muscle is lost from the arteries, especially peripherally, and this process continues in postnatal life. The neonate has relatively muscular pulmonary arteries, which rapidly decline in muscularity in early postnatal life.

KEY LEARNING POINTS

- Major airways are formed in the middle trimester.
- Air sacs do not appear until 22 weeks *in utero.*
- The lungs develop in complexity until around 8 years of age.

RESPIRATORY TRACT MALFORMATIONS

It follows from the above that many things can go wrong in the developmental processes resulting in varying degrees of malformation. Further, an understanding of lung development helps explain the structure and consequences of the malformations, which can range from the complete failure of differentiation of a lung structure to minor abnormalities of the branching structure of no functional significance, e.g. the so called 'pig's bronchus' in which the apical segment of the right upper lobe originates from the trachea rather than the right main bronchus. Problems giving rise to reduced lung fluid *in utero* and/or diminished fetal breathing will result in varying degrees of lung hypoplasia. Disturbance of lung development by the presence of gut in the chest cavity in diaphragmatic hernia will also result in lung hypoplasia on the affected side as well as consequences for the development on the other side.

A relatively recent clinical challenge has been that of antenatal ultrasound detection of lung abnormalities. Even in the best of units the diagnosis can be imprecise and the outlook very unclear. Such babies should always be delivered in a unit with ready access to expert neonatal care, facilities for investigations and paediatric surgical support.

Congenital overdistension of a lobe

Congenital overdistension of a lobe is also known as congenital lobar emphysema (CLE), a term that implies innate abnormality of the lung tissue or airways causing emphysematous changes to occur in development. However, it seems that the clinical picture of an overdistended lobe developing soon after birth causing compression of other lung tissue leading to respiratory distress may also be caused by an abnormality of the airway, partial blockage of the airway or compression of the airway (e.g. by a pulmonary artery sling). This mechanism causes overdistension of normal lung because of pressure effects (due to a ball valve effect). Cartilage and elastic tissue abnormalities are described in CLE when the supplying airways are anatomically normal and not obstructed.

Investigation must include visualization of the airways by bronchoscopy and radiological assessment of the lungs, most likely by high resolution computed tomography scanning (HRCT). Treatment is almost always surgical with relief of the airway compression if this is found or removal of the abnormal lobe if that is the primary problem.

Pulmonary sequestration

Pulmonary sequestration occurs when a part of the lung develops without normal airway or vascular connections. It very often has a separate systemic supply suggesting that it probably arises as a separate outgrowth in very early embryonic life and undergoes development parallel to the normal lung tissue. Venous drainage is normally by the pulmonary venous system. The sequestration can be intralobar or extralobar with its own pleural cover. There are poorly developed bronchial and alveolar tissue structures within the sequestration. The majority are in the left lower lobe with most others in the right lower lobe. They are most likely to present when they become infected, resulting in a protracted and unusual clinical course with poor resolution of a 'cystic pneumonia'. Alternatively, they can be an incidental finding. Surgical removal is recommended if they cause clinical problems. Investigation must delineate the vascular arterial supply in order to avoid a nasty shock for the surgeon!

Pulmonary cysts

Pulmonary cysts are uncommon and variously classified. Single cysts normally arise because of abnormal differentiation of lung tissue giving rise to a cyst in relation to the trachea or major bronchi – a bronchogenic cyst. They may present clinically when they result in infection, compression of an airway or in pneumothorax.

Congenital cyst adenomatoid malformation

Congenital cyst adenomatoid malformation (CCAM) is a more problematical cystic lesion, which is likely due to abnormal differentiation of the developing lung. They can be quite large and contain prominent abnormal vascular elements as well as abnormal bronchial and cystic structures. They can present with neonatal high-output cardiac failure or respiratory distress due to space occupation and are often diagnosed antenatally or in the neonatal period. They also have a propensity for infection. Most clinicians believe that all CCAMs should be removed as they have an unquantified but definite risk of subsequent malignant change.

Malformations of the conducting airways

Bronchial atresia is associated with abnormal development of the distal lung and consequent dysfunction and should be treated by lobectomy. **Tracheal and bronchial stenoses** can occur as isolated findings or in association with complete tracheal rings or a tracheo-oesophageal fistula (TOF). Tracheal stenosis may have a poor outcome as surgical treatment is often of limited benefit. Rarely, a whole lung will fail to develop. This is usually due to early disturbance in development in the embryonic stage.

Various lesions can occur due to incomplete separation of the foregut structures that become the trachea and oesophagus. These range from a small cleft of the posterior larynx to tracheal agenesis, which may be associated with a distal TOF. By far the commonest lesion is the association of oesophageal atresia with distal TOF (Chapter 10). The severity of the malformation and the availability of specialized surgical expertise determine the outcome of these lesions.

Malformations of the chest wall

Localized depressions or prominence of the chest wall are common and usually of no functional significance. Pectus carinatum can be a personal oddity but is more often associated with chronic respiratory failure and increased work of breathing. Pectus excavatum is usually only a cosmetic problem, but if severe it can be associated with restrictive lung abnormalities. Surgical treatment seldom has a significant effect on lung function and should be carried out only with expectations of change of appearance. Many surgeons will wait until children themselves can give informed consent. Two approaches are possible; either movement forwards of the sternum in a process involving mobilization of the sternum and anterior rib ends following fracturing of ribs; or a procedure known as the Nuss bar, in which a curved bar is inserted under the ribs concave to the front and then rotated through 180° to push the sternum forward. The relative value and success of these two procedures is controversial, although there is agreement that both can have significant morbidity.

Malformations of the upper airways

The commonest lesions affecting the upper airway are the cleft lesions that involve the soft and hard palates.

These are often associated with a cleft lip. They present in the neonatal period if there is a visible cleft lip or with difficulties in feeding associated with nasal regurgitation. A more severe problem with upper airway obstruction is Pierre–Robin syndrome where there is a small mandible, retrognathia, a relatively large tongue and often a cleft palate. The children frequently have quite significant obstruction with hypoxia and great difficulty feeding. All should have breathing assessed, especially during sleep. Those with significant obstruction may be treated with a nasopharyngeal airway that remains *in situ* until sufficient jaw growth has occurred to relieve the obstruction. Nowadays, rarely, a tracheostomy may be required for very severe obstruction. Choanal atresia occurs when the nasal airway is not patent through to the upper nasopharynx and severe obstruction results. It is treated surgically.

KEY LEARNING POINTS

Congenital abnormalities may present with:
- neonatal tachypnoea
- chest asymmetry
- stridor
- mass or cyst on a chest radiograph
- poorly resolving pneumonia
- pneumothorax.

EFFECTS OF CIGARETTE SMOKE EXPOSURE

The results of cigarette smoke exposure represent the single largest theoretically avoidable cause of respiratory morbidity in childhood as well as in adulthood. This problem has been exacerbated by the trends in smoking, i.e. with much greater take up by females, especially adolescent girls and young women, over the past three decades. The problem starts *in utero* with effects on the developing airways. There are good data from animal studies to support the view that passive prenatal exposure to maternal cigarette consumption causes abnormalities of the smallest airways with increased tortuosity and smaller size. There may also be effects that result in increased bronchial responsiveness. Several studies of infant lung function have shown decreased lung function measured very early in life suggesting abnormalities of the smallest conducting airways. Prospective cohort studies show that this group of infants with high maternal smoking continue to show lung function impairment at least into adolescence. This is associated clinically with a greater incidence of asthma and more severe asthma. The chances of sudden infant death syndrome (SIDS) and of admission to hospital with viral lower respiratory tract infection in infancy are increased manyfold in those with ongoing passive smoke exposure.

The effects of antenatal exposure are clear, but the subsequent effects of postnatal exposure are more difficult to ascertain because of the difficulty of recruiting children to studies who have only antenatal or postnatal exposure. There is good evidence that current exposure to smoke from parents is associated with more asthma admissions in those already known to have asthma.

Clinicians should also be aware that early experimentation with smoking might begin as young as 8 years of age and that respiratory illness may be complicated by the take up of smoking by the child. There is depressingly little evidence that children with pre-existing respiratory disease are very much less likely to become smokers themselves.

Adverse effects of cigarette smoke exposure

- Worse neonatal lung disease
- Abnormal small airways development
- Increased risk of SIDS
- Increased risk of hospitalization with wheezing illness
- Reduced lung function
- Increased risk of certain cancers

RESPIRATORY NOISES

Central to a good history is the careful characterization of the abnormal sounds produced in respiratory disorders. It is useful to remember that in health inspiration is the active phase of gas movement. Stridor is a harsh sound usually in inspiration that is characteristic of upper airway obstruction. The presence of biphasic stridor implies pathology below the thoracic inlet. Wheeze is a term that is often used indiscriminately, especially by parents. When used correctly, wheeze is a high-pitched continuous sound heard over the lungs, most noticeable in expiration. Classically, wheeze is thought to reflect air movement through narrowed small airways. Crackles are lower-pitched discontinuous sounds, which are harsh and biphasic in suppuration, such as in bronchitis and bronchiectasis, or fine and late inspiratory in interstitial lung disease. Pleural rubs are relatively uncommon in childhood.

Various squeaky and popping sounds can also be heard on auscultation, especially in the resolution phase of respiratory infection. A respiratory noise without a consensus name is the upper airway rattle so characteristic of the first couple of years of life. This sound is often palpable and heard particularly during viral upper respiratory infections. It is seldom associated with significant respiratory distress but is often misclassified as 'wheeze'. Some clinicians describe it as 'transmitted sounds' denoting that these are probably originating in the large airways but the sound may disseminate over the chest wall. Characteristically they sound the same everywhere you listen, whereas lung and small airway noises tend to be more localized or vary over the chest wall.

Cough

Cough is a universal respiratory symptom that occurs in very many diseases. It is the sound produced from the forced expulsion of air from behind a closed glottis. It is principally a method of airway clearance. The acoustic nature of the cough is determined by the resonant qualities of the upper airway (as is the timbre of the voice). The cough may be dry or moist, productive of secretions or unproductive and may have particular patterns such as the characteristic paroxysms of cough heard and seen in pertussis infection. Isolated cough without other significant problems can be a very difficult clinical problem to investigate and manage. A threshold of cough response to stimuli can be determined by measuring the response to capsaicin. There is evidence that this cough threshold can be altered in various disease states, especially after recent viral infection. This is analogous to changes in bronchial reactivity.

At all ages, cough is an infrequent complaint in the absence of disease or infection. It is almost always absent in active or rapid eye movement (REM) sleep. Patterns of cough and the nature of the cough can help greatly in the differential diagnosis.

Differential diagnosis of cough

Acute cough is most often associated with acute viral upper respiratory tract infection and is also a major feature of viral infection of the lower respiratory tract.

Chronic cough is a fairly common cause of referral to paediatric clinics. Very often the cough is due to asthma and/or rhinitis. However, the cough is often not significantly accompanied by wheeze or breathlessness and the referral is made because of a lack of response to asthma therapy. A careful history and examination must include the response to bronchodilators and steroids, which are frequently tried in primary care. Particular emphasis should be placed on the early history of the cough. A choking episode and sudden onset is suggestive of foreign body. A relation with meals or a pattern of worsening when lying down, perhaps associated with vomiting, may suggest gastro-oesophageal reflux as a cause. Chronic cough that is moist sounding raises the possibility of chronic respiratory suppuration from conditions such as cystic fibrosis, ciliary dyskinesia or other causes of bronchiectasis. Chronic cough may also be associated with an airway abnormality, most strikingly in the chronic 'bovine' TOF cough of those with repaired TOF and accompanying tracheomalacia.

A pattern to look out for is that of an acute infection precipitating cough followed by a persistence of bizarre or unusual coughing for many months of even years. This type of cough may often be associated with odd movements and have a throat-clearing quality. A cardinal feature of the history is that the cough only occurs when the patient is awake. The cough has a habit or psychogenic basis. Exploration of psychological triggers is important, although often the cough is in the nature of a habit. Breathing exercises with the help of a speech therapist or physiotherapist usually allows the child to learn how to suppress the desire to cough and allows resolution. Rarely, there is significant psychopathology and treatment to alleviate this is indicated.

Another common cause of persisting cough is the lingering cough of the resolution phase of pertussis or parapertussis infection. This may last many months. In immunized children pertussis infection may go unrecognized, as there are no physical signs when the child is not coughing and an inadequate history of the coughing spasms has been taken. This seems to happen particularly in children with a diagnosis of asthma in whom the cough is misinterpreted as an exacerbation of the asthma and referral follows lack of response to steroids and bronchodilator. The cough of the pertussis syndrome may take three to six months to settle.

Stridor

This is a harsh squeaky sound produced on inspiration, normally accompanied by increased inspiratory effort and associated with narrowing of the upper airway. It may be biphasic in airway narrowing situated below the thoracic inlet. In chronic cases chest wall deformity may result from chronic obstruction. Mild cases of chronic infantile stridor may not require investigation but most chronic cases should result in flexible bronchoscopy of the upper and lower airway – this has largely replaced radiological investigation. In cases of acute stridor securing a safe airway takes precedence over discovering the precise cause.

KEY LEARNING POINTS

Causes of acute stridor:
- Foreign body inhalation
- Laryngotracheobronchitis (croup)
- Anaphylaxis
- Airway trauma
- Epiglottitis
- Diphtheria

Causes of chronic stridor:
- Laryngotracheomalacia
- Foreign body aspiration
- External airway compression – tumour, cyst, aberrant vessel
- Tracheal stenosis
- Complete tracheal rings

PHYSIOLOGICAL FUNCTIONS OF THE RESPIRATORY SYSTEM

The respiratory system carries out two main functions:

- ventilation – the transfer of gas to the respiratory bronchioles and alveoli,
- respiration – the transfer by diffusion of oxygen from alveolar air to capillaries and the diffusion of carbon dioxide in the opposite direction.

The lung has less prominent roles in metabolism, heat control and host defence.

In health, ventilation is a process with active contraction of the diaphragm and intercostal muscles to lift the ribs, articulating from the spine in an upward and outward direction, accompanied by downward movement of the diaphragm to create an increase in negative intrathoracic pressure and thereby draw air in through the upper airway. Exhalation is passive, allowing deflation and a rise in pressure. Increased effort may be necessary to overcome airway obstruction or stiffer (less compliant) lungs or chest wall, which necessitates use of the accessory muscles of respiration such as the neck muscles and more vigorous intercostal muscle action.

Measurement of pulmonary function

Pulmonary function is commonly assessed by measurement of clinical variables such as respiratory rate, signs of respiratory distress (indrawing, sternal heave, use of accessory muscles) and observing for cyanosis, which is unlikely to be clinically apparent until the arterial saturation of oxygen (SaO_2) is below 90 per cent. The SaO_2 is commonly assessed by a photometric technique in a finger. The normal value is >94 per cent. The technique is unreliable in the presence of a poor arterial signal because of movement, although most modern monitors have good artefact rejection. More detailed assessment of gas exchange come from arterial or capillary gas measurement, which allows assessment of carbon dioxide and oxygen levels and the acid–base balance.

Measurement of the mechanical aspects of lung function is dependent on the patient, the observer and the equipment used. These assessments rely on the measurement of characteristics of the following manoeuvre. The patient takes a maximum breath in and then exhales as hard and fast as possible until they can exhale no more. A typical graph of flow against volume is shown in Figure 8.1 along with definitions of the main variables.

The simplest equipment is the peak expiratory flow (PEF) meter, usually a cheap, simple device of poor accuracy, which gives a value for the maximum velocity of expired air expelled with maximum force from total lung capacity. Measurements of forced expiratory volume 1 (FEV1), forced expiratory flow (FEF), forced vital capacity (FVC) and peak expiratory flow (PEF) can all be made by an accurate spirometer. Lung volumes can be assessed by the use of gas dilution techniques or by plethysmography. The details of these tests can be found in the texts given in the Further reading section. Sophisticated devices can also assess the pressures

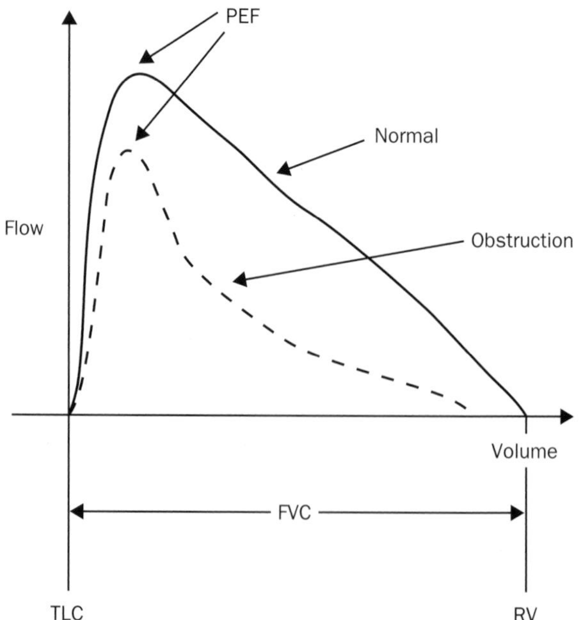

Figure 8.1 A typical flow–volume graph. PEF, peak expiratory flow; FVC, forced vital capacity; TLC, total lung capacity; RV, residual volume

generated during forced inspiration and expiration, allowing monitoring of respiratory muscle function.

The reactivity of the bronchi to stimuli can be assessed by repeated measurements of lung function while the stimulus is increased or the absolute response to a given stimulus, such as administration of histamine. In this way the bronchial responsiveness can be measured to assess the provocative concentration of histamine that causes a 20 per cent reduction in FEV1 (PC20) or the percentage drop in PEF following a standardized six-minute exercise test.

Abnormalities of lung function

There now exist good data on normal ranges of various lung function parameters from about 5 years of age. The normal ranges show small sex differences in childhood but are most closely aligned to the child's height. For most of the values the normal range lies between 80 and 120 per cent of the mean for sex and height.

Obstruction is demonstrated by a reduction in the flow achieved at various lung volumes. Peak expiratory flow reflects mainly the flow early in an expiratory manoeuvre and, as such, the flow in larger airways. This explains its poor discrimination of airflow obstruction in asthma despite the fact that many advocate routine use of PEF monitoring. In obstruction there will characteristically be a reduction in FEV1/FVC below 80 per cent, with values below 50 per cent signifying severe obstruction. Furthermore, there may be a rise in total lung capacity signifying hyperinflation of the lungs and a rise in the residual volume indicating trapping of air secondary to obstructed airflow. Obstruction most apparent in early expiration is indicative of large airways obstruction, e.g. tracheal stenosis. Reduction in flows at lower lung volumes is characteristic of small airways disease.

In restrictive lung disease there will be reduction in all lung volumes and a preservation of their relative values resulting in a normal FEV1/FVC ratio. This is most often associated with disorders where there is paucity of chest wall movement such as severe kyphoscoliosis, severe obesity or arthropathy or when there is stiffness of the lung parenchyma caused by an alveolitic process or by interstitial lung disease. The other main cause of restriction is muscle weakness. This eventually leads to respiratory failure in serious muscle disease.

Special investigations

Flexible bronchoscopy involves the passage of a thin fibreoptic instrument typically of only 2.8–3.5 mm diameter into the airways for diagnostic or therapeutic purposes. The patient may be sedated or given a general anaesthetic. Flexible bronchoscopy allows visualization of the airways to several generations of conducting airways. Airway anomalies or foreign material can be found and secretions obtained by bronchial washing or tissue by bronchial biopsy for subsequent study. Foreign bodies can normally only be removed with a rigid bronchoscope.

Plain radiology is invaluable in respiratory medicine but increasing use is being made of **HRCT** that gives much more information on airway structure and the pathologies of the interstitium and respiratory zone of the lung. The increasing use of bronchoscopy and HRCT has resulted in a great reduction in the use of bronchography. **Radioisotope scans** can give detailed information on ventilation and perfusion using inhaled and injected tracers, respectively.

Lung biopsy is normally done when there is concern over interstitial lung disease or diffuse radiological change in the immunocompromised subject. The biopsy can be performed with a percutaneous instrument to obtain a core of tissue, normally with CT-guided technique. Alternatively, an open lung biopsy is performed via a minithoracotomy. It is likely that there will be an increase in the use of thorascopic techniques in paediatric practice. However, the choice of method used to obtain lung tissue for histological and histochemical analysis is usually determined by the availability of practitioners skilled in a particular technique.

Other specialist investigations such as the **sweat test** and **ciliary biopsy** are described along with the diseases for which they are diagnostic.

EAR, NOSE AND THROAT PROBLEMS

Otitis media

Otitis media is a common infection in the pre-school child, normally caused by upper respiratory pathogens such as *Haemophilus* and streptococci. The child may experience mild fever and coryzal symptoms followed by pain or discomfort in the ear. Examination of true otitis media will reveal a bright-red inflamed ear drum with loss of anatomical definition. However, lesser infection may simply cause mild erythema with vessel dilatation. Much attention has been paid to the idea that otitis media is overtreated with antibiotics. Most practitioners will reserve them for children with severe local inflammation and systemic upset. Simple broad-spectrum antibiotics are sufficient.

Formerly, chronic middle ear infection was associated with the spread of infection to the adjacent mastoid bone resulting in mastoiditis. In the twenty-first century this is a rare situation in developed countries. Chronic otitis media may also predispose to the build-up of inflammatory material behind the drum causing a cholesteatoma.

Secretory otitis media

Frequently in the pre-school child, a situation develops in which repeated otitis media leads to chronic inflammation in the middle ear with discharge. The drum can perforate and fluid may build up behind the drum resulting in hearing impairment. This is often referred to as 'glue ear'. The drum is surgically incised (myringotomy) with suction drainage of the fluid and the placement of drainage tubes (grommets). This procedure may be augmented by adenoidectomy when large adenoids are obstructing the distal end of the eustachian tube and thereby exacerbating the situation in the middle ear.

Tonsillitis

Many children will experience a few episodes of acute infection of the tonsils. This gives rise to fever, sore throat and a characteristic breath smell. Viruses are a common cause but bacterial infection, particularly with streptococci, is frequent. Broad-spectrum antibiotics are often prescribed. A better approach may be to culture a throat swab, and if this is positive for streptococci the child is treated with penicillin. Adenotonsillectomy is an operation that has waxed and waned in popularity. Recent guidelines recommend that it should be reserved for those with five episodes of sore throat over a one-year period.

Rhinitis

Rhinitis is a common problem, especially in pre-school children. There may be a strong atopic element to the symptom pattern. The child will have recurrent episodes of clear rhinorrhoea with nasal stuffiness. Much sniffing, snorting and snoring may occur. The symptoms are often precipitated by common respiratory viruses. A mild cough often coexists. This is particularly at night and is quiet and moist sounding.

Decongestants are often prescribed but are of limited, if any, help. If there is an atopic element then an oral antihistamine treatment may well be successful. The best therapies are the topical nasal steroids, but many children find the sprays difficult to tolerate. A two-month therapeutic trial will often show benefit. The therapy can be taken seasonally if that is the pattern of the symptoms. Perennial rhinitis is less common in children, often coexisting with asthma and requiring regular topical nasal steroids. Great caution should be exercised in the use of highly potent agents such as betamethasone as the systemic absorption through inflamed mucosa can lead to significant systemic adverse effects.

Haemoptysis/epistaxis

Blood originating in the nose or nasopharynx is relatively common in childhood. Trauma, especially nose picking, is a common precipitant. The blood often leaks from friable surface vessels in Little's area on the nasal septum at times of acute infection. The application of pressure is normally sufficient to abort the bleed. In severe bleeding, specially in the presence of a coagulopathy or severe thrombocytopenia, nasal packing may be necessary.

In the majority of cases that children cough up blood the origin is actually from the upper airway. True haemoptysis is rare but persistence should be investigated by bronchoscopy.

Causes of haemoptysis

- Epistaxis
- Vascular malformations of upper airway
- Bronchiectasis
- Pulmonary arteriovenous malformations
- Pulmonary haemosiderosis
- Rare tumours

ACUTE RESPIRATORY TRACT INFECTIONS

Acute respiratory tract infections constitute the majority of respiratory morbidity in primary care and a large part of that in secondary practice. Acute respiratory infections account for 50 per cent of illnesses in pre-school children and 30 per cent of illness in those 5–12 years of age. Upper respiratory tract infections are the commonest and are normally manifest as mild fever, coryza (red eyes, runny nose with clear secretions) and mild cough. They are caused by many viral agents including picornaviruses, rhinoviruses, and influenza and parainfluenza viruses. They are self-limiting and last three to five days. The only treatment is symptomatic relief with paracetamol or ibuprofen.

Acute sore throat is very common in pre-school and early school-age children. It is usually caused by pharyngitis or tonsillitis. There is fever, lethargy and anorexia but seldom much cough. The typical findings are cervical lymphadenopathy, fever and inflamed tonsils, which may be covered in exudates. Analgesia with paracetamol is usually sufficient. A throat swab can be taken and should be sent for viral and bacterial studies. The evidence base for the use of antibiotics is poor but they are often given for more severe cases with systemic upset. Penicillin is the drug most often used. Practitioners should be wary of infectious mononucleosis (Chapter 6) and avoid using ampicillin-based antibiotic preparations. Tonsillectomy for recurrent sore throat/tonsillitis has waxed and waned over the years. Current recommendations are that it should be confined to those with symptoms for over a year, with at least five episodes of tonsillitis that are disabling and affect function. Tonsillectomy is obviously indicated in other clinical scenarios such as acute peritonsillar abscess and to treat obstructive sleep apnoea hypopnoea syndrome.

Laryngotracheobronchitis (croup) is an acute viral infection commonly caused by parainfluenza viruses and also by respiratory syncytial virus (RSV), influenza virus and rhinoviruses. Croup begins with a coryzal illness which progresses to stridor, respiratory distress and a harsh barking bovine cough. There is marked inflammation of the upper airway structures with resultant laryngeal narrowing. If there is significant stridor or respiratory distress the child should be treated with oral steroids, typically prednisolone 1–2 mg/kg. Obviously, hypoxia should also be corrected and hydration attended to. In the steroid era intubation to relieve upper airway obstruction in croup has become a relatively rare event. The illness settles slowly over a few days. Any child who has recurrent croup should have airway endoscopy to rule out an anatomical airway problem.

Epiglottitis is a severe life-threatening infection usually caused by *Haemophilus influenzae* type B (Hib). Since immunization became common, it has become a rare diagnosis. The child presented with very rapid onset over a few hours of high fever, mild shock, severe airway obstruction with stridor and often drooling due to inability to swallow. Cough was unusual. The treatment consisted of intubation (or tracheostomy) to secure the airway, followed by intravenous (IV) antibiotic therapy. At intubation, a huge inflamed epiglottis would be seen obstructing the upper airway. Intubation was often needed only for a day or so as the obstruction settled quickly with antibiotic treatment. Inhaled foreign body is the other common cause of acute stridor and is often clear from the history. The treatment consists of expert airway examination and removal of the obstruction.

Tracheitis is often caused by *Staphylococcus* and presents with a short history of very harsh barking cough, fever and mild stridor that might be biphasic. The treatment includes administration of broad-spectrum antibiotics including good antistaphylococcal cover. **Acute bronchitis** is often seen in the winter months and is commonest in young children. The infecting organism is mostly viral and there is no specific treatment.

The investigation and management of tuberculosis and diseases due to non-tuberculous mycobacteria are discussed in Chapter 6.

Pertussis infection

CASE STUDY

A 2-month-old infant presents with a seven-day history of cough, poor feeding, vomiting and colour change. There are no focal examination findings. The chest radiograph shows peribronchial thickening. There is a lymphocytosis. The child has a characteristic pattern of being well until he starts coughing in a crescendo fashion with the development of apnoea and cyanosis. He is treated with a 14-day course of erythromycin to try to reduce infectivity.

Pertussis used to be a common problem and then waned in importance due to immunization. Recent poorly substantiated fears about the immunization led to large numbers of children being unimmunized and has allowed a reservoir of infection to exist in the population. The condition is caused by *Bordetella pertussis* and *Bordetella parapertussis* and is at its most damaging when it occurs in the very young infant in whom morbidity is very high and mortality still occurs.

The illness begins with a coryzal phase progressing rapidly to a long stage of several weeks of coughing spasms. These consist of runs of short coughs with progressively diminishing lung volume until the spasm is terminated with a fast intake of breath or 'whoop', which may be followed by further paroxysms. These are particularly common when provoked by exercise and during the night, causing severe sleep disturbance. The chest will usually be normal on examination. The convalescent phase lasts several months until the cough finally subsides.

Young infants may present with central apnoea in response to coughing spasms and may also develop a pertussis pneumonitis. The youngest are also particularly at risk of severe hypoxia with spasms and may rarely have anoxic seizures.

Treatment with macrolide antibiotics may reduce the infectivity if given early in the paroxysmal phase but probably has no effect on the natural history of the condition. The treatment is essentially supportive and only young infants are likely to require inpatient care with oxygen therapy and assistance with feeding and the coughing spasms. Thankfully, long-term sequelae are uncommon unless the infant has required ventilatory assistance for severe pertussis pneumonitis. Post-pertussis bronchiectasis has been described but is probably rare. It does seem that the cough threshold is lowered for many months after pertussis infection.

Bronchiolitis

CASE STUDY

A 3-month-old baby boy presents in December with a six-day history of snuffles, cough and breathlessness with increasing difficulty finishing feeds. On examination he is mildly cyanosed in air, has a respiratory rate of 60 with intercostal indrawing and audible wheeze and crackles. The chest radiograph shows mild hyperinflation with peribronchial thickening. A nasopharyngeal aspirate is positive for RSV. He is treated with oxygen and nursing care.

Bronchiolitis is a common viral infection that primarily affects the smallest conducting airways and also affects later conducting airways. There is a recognizable pattern of occurrence of epidemics every winter in both hemispheres. The main pathogen is RSV, which in epidemics is the causative organism in over 90 per cent of hospitalized infants. Classically, bronchiolitis affects the infant below 6 months of age. A slightly greater number of males are admitted to hospital. Also at increased risk of severe disease are infants who were born prematurely (even without significant neonatal respiratory disease), those with chronic lung disease (CLD) of prematurity, the very young, those with significant cardiac lesions or those with pre-existing respiratory problems or congenital malformations. The severity of the infection may be reduced by monoclonal antibody immunization of high-risk infants. No antiviral therapy is effective *in vivo*.

The illness tends to present with a short history of a few days of coryza followed by a harsh moist cough, increased respiratory rate, intercostal indrawing and poor feeding. Very immature and premature infants classically present with central apnoea. Clinical findings include cough, respiratory distress and hyperinflation. There are always harsh crackles to be heard on auscultation and sometimes also wheezes. Secondary bacterial infection and focal signs probably occur in less than 5 per cent of hospitalized cases. The worst phase of the illness lasts a few days and is followed by slow resolution over one to two weeks.

The treatment of bronchiolitis is supportive – oxygen and care with feeding including the use of nasogastric feeding or IV fluids in those unable to tolerate this. There is no convincing evidence to support the use of steroids or bronchodilator therapy.

Debate has ravaged over several decades about the links between bronchiolitis and asthma. It is clear that those hospitalized with RSV bronchiolitis are more likely to experience future respiratory problems and, in particular, asthma. Some believe that RSV infection causes a change in a normal host or some form of damage that predisposes to subsequent abnormal airway behaviour. Others maintain that those predestined to have a high risk of subsequent asthma due to underlying aspects of airway function are also those most likely to get infection with RSV that results in a need for hospital treatment. The full explanation probably lies somewhere in between.

Pneumonia

CASE STUDY

An 8-year-old girl presents with a five-day history of coryza followed by cough, fever and abdominal pain. She had fever, mild tachypnoea, reduced air entry at the right base and crackles on auscultation. A chest radiograph confirms consolidation of the right lower lobe. She makes a full recovery following antibiotic treatment.

Pneumonia is still a common diagnosis in childhood. Children present with symptoms of cough and fever. The clinical findings in infancy may not show any focal nature. In the older child there may be localized dullness to percussion with bronchial breathing or crackles. The chest radiograph shows focal consolidation of a segment or lobe, often with collapse. The commonest causative organism is *Streptococcus pneumoniae*, with other bacterial organisms less often responsible. Classically staphylococcal pneumonia is associated with a severe illness with toxicity and the formation of pneumatoceles. Viral pneumonia is also common. In atypical pneumonia there may often be more systemic features such as rash, headache and gastrointestinal symptoms and the radiograph may show more a more diffuse pattern of change in the absence of specific respiratory findings on examination. Atypical pneumonia is often caused by *Mycoplasma pneumoniae* or viral infection.

Recent UK guidelines are available on the diagnosis and management of pneumonia. The guidelines recommend the use of amoxicillin, which in most cases can be given orally for seven days. Supportive therapy such as oxygen is given as clinically indicated.

All patients with pneumonia should have clinical follow-up around four to six weeks later. In a patient with uncomplicated lobar pneumonia, if there has been complete clinical resolution of symptoms and signs then no follow-up radiograph is indicated. However, in those with multi-lobe disease, effusions or incomplete clinical resolution a chest radiograph is important. Reasons for persisting problems include an airway anomaly, infection of a pre-existing congenital lung abnormality, foreign body bronchial obstruction or an underlying respiratory disorder such as cystic fibrosis.

Pleural effusion is a complication of pneumonia that has returned in frequency to previous levels, having been less common in the 1980s and early 1990s. This most often occurs with pneumococcal pneumonia. The patient responds poorly to treatment of the pneumonia and develops worsening respiratory distress and chest pain/discomfort. The radiograph shows the presence of fluid in the pleural space, a finding that can be confirmed on ultrasound. Most effusions can be treated conservatively as they are small sterile parapneumonic collections of straw-coloured fluid. Some clinicians advocate a tap of the pleural fluid to assess its consistency and for diagnostic purposes. If the fluid proves to be frankly infected then an empyema has occurred with active infection in the pleural space. The management of empyema is hotly disputed. Options include early surgical intervention with thoracotomy, debridement and removal of infected material, video assisted thoracoscopy to achieve the same by less invasive means or urokinase-assisted pleural drainage by an ultrasound-guided chest drain placement. The end result is unchanged by the choice of approach. Pleural circulation is restored and slow resolution occurs with residual pleural scarring.

Paediatric chronic bronchitis

Paediatric chronic bronchitis is a condition that is said to occur almost exclusively in the socially disadvantaged. There may be an association with passive cigarette exposure. The patient, often a pre-school child, suffers recurring bouts of moist cough and the production of yellow or green secretions from the larger airways. There may be localized crackles on auscultation but there should not be any clubbing or significant chest deformity. Paediatric chronic bronchitis may represent the milder end of the bronchiectasis spectrum. Treatment consists of antibiotics that cover the common respiratory pathogens.

KEY LEARNING POINTS

- Most respiratory infections are viral.
- Respiratory syncytial virus causes epidemics each winter.
- Treatment of croup with steroids is very effective.
- The outlook for most children with pneumonia is good.
- Empyema has become common again in the past decade.

ASTHMA

Asthma is a condition that defies accurate unambiguous definition and is almost a diagnosis of exclusion. It is a disease characterized by inflammation of the small- and medium-sized airways with symptoms of cough, wheeze and breathlessness in particular patterns. Other respiratory conditions, such as recurrent respiratory infection, gastro-oesophageal reflux and aspiration lung disease, cystic fibrosis, chronic foreign body or congenital lung anomaly, require to be excluded on clinical grounds or by investigation. In most patients there is a significant overlap with atopy suggesting that, in part, asthma is a consequence of an abnormal reaction to inhaled allergens. Many features of later twentieth-century life may predispose to atopic reactions such as fewer episodes of serious infant infection, fewer parasites, a diet relatively low in antioxidants, less contact with animals and a more sedentary life in enclosed conditions. Asthma is certainly a disease of the relatively affluent 'western' societies.

In the later twentieth century there was a marked rise which was followed by a small fall in the incidence of asthma. Epidemiological studies suggest that lung function characteristics indicative of poorer small airway function and airway reactivity are present in early infancy in those most likely to develop asthma. These may be further influenced during childhood leading to a degree of irreversibility of airway obstruction over time. The presence of an atopic phenotype probably interacts with these patterns of lung function to produce the clinical disease.

Patterns of asthmatic symptoms

Mild intermittent
- No chronic symptoms
- Episodic cough and wheeze due to viral upper respiratory tract infections or allergen exposure

Mild persistent
- Mild chronic cough
- No limitation of exercise
- Episodic cough, wheeze and breathlessness

Moderate persistent
- Chronic cough, especially at night
- Exercise symptoms may restrict exercise
- Frequent exacerbations of cough, wheeze and breathlessness

Severe persistent
- Troublesome chronic cough and wheeze
- Exercise impairment
- Frequent disabling exacerbations

'Wheezing' in infants

Differential diagnosis of wheezing in infants

- Congenital airway malformation
- Benign airway 'rattle'
- Cystic fibrosis
- Recurrent viral lower respiratory tract infection
- True early asthma

Most of what presents as 'wheezing' in young children is either misreported rattling sounds from the upper and middle airways or is due to acute viral infection of the airways and not associated with subsequent development of classic atopic asthma. It is all too often labelled as asthma and treated unsuccessfully with inhaled steroids and bronchodilators. Only if it is frequent, persistent, associated with focal or fixed signs or present in a child who is truly 'ill' is any action required. The vast majority are children with smaller small airways who have an increased predisposition to wheezing. The largest risk factor is maternal smoking, especially during pregnancy. The mechanism appears to be retardation of the growth of the smaller airways *in utero*.

CASE STUDY

A 5-year-old boy has a past history of eczema, a mother with rhinitis and a history of cough, wheeze and breathlessness precipitated by viral infection, exercise, emotion and colder weather. These symptoms occur several times a week. Examination, including PEF is normal. He is treated with twice-daily inhaled steroids and bronchodilator when required via a large volume spacer. He responds well to treatment.

Making a diagnosis of asthma

A diagnosis of asthma is based on a history of cough, wheeze and breathlessness in a pattern consistent with the diagnosis and the absence of features such as poor weight gain, focal signs, clubbing, etc. that might suggest other disorders. Often there will be a family history of atopic disease and the child will have a history of eczema. Typically, the child has episodes of cough, wheeze and breathlessness for five to seven days following a coryzal illness. This should be responsive to bronchodilator therapy. Additional symptoms classically include a chronic dry cough, worse during the night, first thing in the morning and after exercise. Precipitants of symptoms include viral upper respiratory infections, exercise, emotion or excitement, dust or pet exposure, smoke exposure and colder weather.

Often clinicians will be happy to make the diagnosis on clinical grounds but if there are atypical features then investigation may be necessary, e.g. chest radiograph, sweat test, and/or pH study.

Chronic management of asthma

All children with asthma should be supplied with a β-2 agonist bronchodilator in an inhaled form appropriate for their age and ability. The threshold for starting 'prophylactic' preventive/controller therapy would normally be chronic symptoms requiring bronchodilator three to four days a week or significant monthly exacerbations. Therefore, many with mild intermittent disease do not require regular therapy but anyone with persistent disease should have prophylaxis. All modern guidelines recommend commencing low-dose inhaled corticosteroids (ICS) (100–200 μg betamethasone dipropionate or budesonide twice daily) at this level of symptoms with a therapeutic trial of these agents. An alternative would be to try an oral cysteinyl leukotriene receptor antagonist (LTRA – montelukast or zafirlukast) if the parents have concerns about ICS or have difficulties with inhaled medication.

Patients with moderate, persistent disease that is only partially responsive to ICS will require second-line prophylactic therapy. There are a number of options but a lack of hard evidence on which to base clinical decisions. The options include doubling the current ICS, switching to a more potent steroid (fluticasone or mometasone), adding a long-acting β-2 agonist (LABA e.g. formoterol, salmeterol), using an LTRA (montelukast, zafirlukast) or adding theophyllines. Expert clinical practice currently would be to use either a LABA or LTRA as additional therapy in a two-month clinical trial and re-evaluate. Patients with severe disease may well require therapy with ICS + LTRA + LABA + oral steroids.

The management of asthma has long been an example of disease management that is directed by the availability of guidelines. There are a number of international versions and those followed in the UK are firmly evidence based and a joint venture of the Scottish Intercollegiate Guidelines Network (SIGN) and the British Thoracic Society (BTS). The SIGN/BTS guideline (2003 with 2004 updates available from the websites of SIGN and BTS, see references) not only recommend drug therapy but also other aspects of disease monitoring and management.

There can be many reasons for apparent poor response to asthma therapy and these are listed below. One of the commonest failings in the management of asthma is that of poor choice and use of inhaler devices. The commonest failing is the use of a pressurized metered dose inhaler (pMDI) without a spacer. There are many devices available but only a few should be in a regular formulary.

Reasons for poor response to asthma therapy

- Poor inhaler technique/inappropriate device
- Poor understanding of disease management
- Poor adherence to treatment regimen
- New allergens or irritants
- Psychological factors
- Life events
- Rarely true non-response to drug

CASE STUDY (continued)

Our boy, now 6 years old, is no longer responding as well to his therapy. He has chronic cough and exercise limitation and variable PEF. His inhaler technique remains good, and he seems to be taking his therapy. The family have acquired a cat. A skin test to cat allergen is carried out and shows a 15-mm reaction. Advice is given that the cat either has to be washed weekly or given away.

Devices for inhaled therapy

Infants (0–2 years)

- pMDI with small volume spacer (AeroChamber, BabyHaler, NebuChamber)
- If all else fails a nebulizer

Pre-school children (2–6 years)

- pMDI with large volume spacer (Volumatic, NebuHaler)
- If all else fails a nebulizer

School age children (7–15 years)

- pMDI with spacer
- Breath-activated dry powder device (Turbuhaler, Accuhaler)
- Breath actuated pMDI

Complications of asthma and its treatment

Most asthma is thankfully relatively benign and of little consequence but can still have large effects on family function and parental wellbeing. There is a lot of concern about drug side effects but again, thankfully, serious problems are rare. Inhaled corticosteroids can cause oral thrush and temporary slowing of growth velocity but long-term studies of those on ICS suggest normal final height although perhaps some delay in puberty. There is enormous controversy about the potential of ICS for effects on bone health and mineralization. It is likely that the doses of ICS and intermittent use of oral steroids necessary in most asthmatic children are of no long-term consequence.

However, high-dose steroids by inhalation or by the oral route are highly toxic with potential for growth delay, adrenal suppression and cushingoid effects. Patients apparently requiring large amounts of therapy must be under expert supervision. There is always a balance to be struck between the severe and potentially fatal effects of uncontrolled asthma and the use of powerful drugs.

Psychological problems are common in severe asthma and may cloud the clinical picture. There can be problems of overlap with psychogenic or habit cough and with vocal cord dysfunction. These may require input from a clinical psychologist or speech therapist.

Prognosis of asthma

Many patients have transient disease in mid-childhood but there is evidence that many of these individuals may have return of disease in adult life. In general, those with the mildest disease have the most benign course. Those with early severe disease are very unlikely to remit and may develop relatively less reversibility of airflow obstruction over time leading to chronic airflow obstruction and severe adult disease. Whether this relates to pre-existing abnormality of lung function and airway development or is purely the result of a disease process is unclear.

There are 15–20 deaths from asthma in childhood and adolescence in the UK each year. Sadly, many of these are thought to be, at least theoretically, preventable.

Management of the acute asthma attack

The mainstay of management of the acute asthma attack is the prompt use of generous doses of inhaled bronchodilator. This can be initially in the form of a dry powder device but is better from multiple doses (8–10 over five minutes) of short-acting β-2 agonist (salbutamol, terbutaline) via a large volume spacer. Where the patient is having difficulties with this method or when hypoxia is present nebulized bronchodilator is required. Moderate episodes responding incompletely or poorly to bronchodilator or severe acute exacerbations should be treated with oral prednisolone 1–2 mg/kg per day for three to five days.

Measurement of oxygen saturation is vital in any child presenting to medical care. Oxygen should be given to produce $SaO_2 > 94$ per cent. This can be by nasal prongs or mask with humidification.

Severe attacks responding poorly to regular one to two hourly salbutamol or terbutaline should have additional four to six hourly nebulized ipratropium. Consideration should then be given to an infusion of aminophylline. A loading dose of 3–5 mg/kg over 20 minutes should be given to those not already on theophylline, followed by an infusion of 1 mg/kg per hour. Tremor is common and hypokalaemia is possible in those given large amounts of salbutamol. Blood gas analysis should show hypoxia but depressed carbon dioxide. If type two respiratory failure ensues, artificial ventilation may be required.

Any patient admitted to hospital with acute asthma presents an opportunity to assess overall asthma control and plan future therapy and review. Most should leave hospital with inhaled steroids. All must be discharged with a clear plan for routine therapy and for acute attacks, an appropriate inhaled form of bronchodilator that they use well and clear plans for follow-up in primary and/or secondary care.

Management of chronic asthma

The child with asthma can be regularly reviewed either in primary or in secondary care by an interested and informed clinician – this may well be an expert nurse. Current and recent symptoms should be reviewed, as should any exacerbations and their management. Particular note should be made of night disturbance and exercise restriction. The current therapy and inhaler technique should be checked and peak expiratory flow can be measured in those old enough to do it well.

Paediatric asthma is a good example of the concept of concordance – working with the patient/parent on an agreed plan of action that involves discussion and joint decisions on any changes in management. A patient doing well can have therapy reduced in a stepwise manner within agreed criteria and any need for increased therapy can be discussed.

KEY POINTS

- Asthma prevalence has peaked in western countries.
- Genetic factors play a part in its expression.
- Most patients have mild disease.
- Many patients' symptoms settle through childhood.
- No therapy has been shown to alter natural history.

CYSTIC FIBROSIS

CASE STUDY

A 2-week-old baby boy is admitted for further assessment after being found to have an elevated serum immunoreactive trypsin (IRT) level on Guthrie card screen taken at 6 days of age. He had one older sibling who is well and has no significant family history.

Genetics and screening

Cystic fibrosis is the commonest lethal genetic disease with a carrier rate of 1 in 25 in caucasian populations and an incidence of 1 in 2200 births. The disease is largely one of white populations and is very unusual in certain races such as Chinese and Australian aboriginal peoples. The defect is in a gene on the long arm of chromosome 7 that codes for a chloride channel named cystic fibrosis transmembrane regulator (CFTR). Varying mutations result in different degrees of failure of production or function of CFTR. The commonest is δ-F508, which is found on 70 per cent of the chromosomes of those affected by cystic fibrosis. No other mutation accounts for more than 4 per cent of mutations. It is becoming clear that there are genotype–phenotype links but other factors, including social circumstances, adherence to therapy and the medical care provided could all influence the outcome. There is believed to be a heterozygote advantage to explain the very high carrier rate and this is thought to be a relative resistance to the worst effects of severe diarrhoeal disease due to altered electrolyte secretion in the gut.

Screening can be carried out antenatally by chorionic villus sampling or amniocentesis of fetuses if both parents are established carriers. Termination of the pregnancy is the only feasible therapy if the fetus is affected. This type of screening is highly controversial in a disease with very variable expression and widely varying prognosis. Postnatal screening is done along with the metabolic and endocrine conditions tested for on the Guthrie blood spot taken at 6 days and on the detection of high levels of IRT with subsequent testing for the commonest cystic fibrosis mutations. Either screening process will result in the failure to detect those with rare mutations. Postnatal screening has been controversial due to the lack of strong evidence of benefit in screened populations. The benefits shown in short-term follow-up studies have been in nutritional parameters and in microbiological colonization. Despite this low level of evidence of benefit, the UK government approved universal postnatal screening in 2003.

Pathophysiology

The defect in CFTR results in abnormal movements of chloride and sodium and hence water across the cell membrane resulting in abnormal consistency of extracellular fluids giving rise to abnormal 'sticky' secretions in the airway lining and abnormal pancreatic exocrine function. There are also physical changes in the fluids and mucus in the respiratory tract which favour the attachment of certain organisms and, in particular, pseudomonads. Most patients have lung disease of varying severity and around 90 per cent of patients require enzyme supplements in childhood.

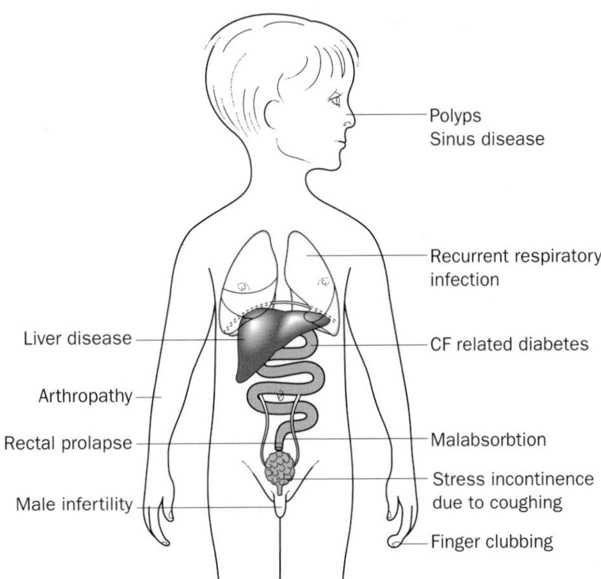

Figure 8.2 Common manifestations of cystic fibrosis

Clinical presentation of cystic fibrosis

The classic picture has been of an infant with recurrent respiratory infection or chronic cough with true failure to thrive, i.e. poor weight gain despite adequate intake. There is associated steatorrhoea. Chronic respiratory problems, rectal prolapse or 'atypical asthma' may be the pattern for later presentation. Rarely, liver disease can be the presenting feature.

Mild disease with unusual genotype may not present until adulthood with mild bronchiectasis or male infertility. The move to universal neonatal screening must result in increased vigilance for these unusual presentations, as they are commonest with rarer mutations that are not covered by the screen for common mutations included in most screening programmes.

Figure 8.2 shows some of the common manifestations of cystic fibrosis.

Treatment of cystic fibrosis

Modern care is delivered by multidisciplinary teams with medical, nursing, dietetic, physiotherapy, psychological and social work support. The average life expectancy is reputed to be over 40 years at the beginning of the twenty-first century. Experience shows that prognosis in childhood has improved dramatically in the past 15 years with death in childhood becoming a rare event, whereas before it was commonplace. However, the prognosis for those reaching adult life with cystic fibrosis has changed much less. Patients and their families must live with inevitable deterioration and the knowledge that although better application of treatment continues there is no real prospect of curative therapy.

Respiratory complications

Recurrent infection with bacterial colonization is a core feature. Early in the disease common pathogens such as viruses, *H. influenzae* subspp. and streptococci are common. *Staphylococcus aureus* is a relatively early colonizer of the cystic fibrosis lung. Prophylactic flucloxacillin has been shown to delay this. Most patients eventually run into clinical problems due to pseudomonal species with progressive lung involvement. The environment of the cystic fibrosis lung is particularly conducive to *Pseudomonas*, which seems to adhere particularly well to cystic fibrosis airway epithelium. Initially this organism may be cultured intermittently in a non-mucoid form and most units will adopt a strategy of courses of IV or combined oral and nebulized therapy to attempt to eradicate *Pseudomonas*. In many patients, it eventually becomes a colonizing organism and develops a mucoid nature. It is thought that much of the damage caused by *Pseudomonas* colonization is as a result of the harmful effects of the host response in terms of the release of proteases and cytokines.

Non-tubercular mycobacteria are fairly frequent colonizers of the cystic fibrosis lung but seldom cause overt clinical disease. Similarly, fungal species such as *Aspergillus* are often found in samples of sputum but may not cause overt clinical problems. However, allergic bronchopulmonary aspergillosis is said to affect 5–10 per cent of cystic fibrosis patients and invasive disease with aspergillosis, especially in damaged and bronchiectatic lung, can be a nasty complication.

Management aims to prevent infection and to treat aggressively when it occurs. Daily physiotherapy with percussion and drainage is used in younger children with a move to more active breathing and expectoration techniques in more mature subjects. It has been shown that regular exercise can augment the positive effects of physiotherapy. Routine immunization is advocated along with annual influenza cover. There is an interest in pneumococcal immunization but no good evidence of its worth, as yet. Similarly, there is interest in antipseudomonal immunization but clinical trials are awaited.

Some clinicians, especially in Denmark, advocate the use of regular courses of intravenous antibiotics every few months to treat and suppress organisms. In the UK, this approach is normally used on a selective basis. Most patients are on regular 'prophylactic' antistaphylococcal antibiotics since diagnosis. These can be doubled in minor infections or augmented with other oral antibiotics as clinically indicated. Intravenous courses are reserved for exacerbations that are more serious or regularly as described above.

There has been a significant increase in the provision of antipseudomonal antibiotics in the past 10–20 years and the development of antibiotic preparations suitable for nebulized administration. Most units use combinations of drugs, such as a fourth-generation cephalosporin and an aminoglycoside. A new therapy gradually finding a place is the long-term administration of azithromycin to reduce respiratory exacerbations in those with pseudomonal colonization.

The concept of mucolytic therapy has always been attractive for obvious reasons. However, this form of therapy has been universally disappointing. The latest compound, dornase alfa (recombinant human DNase) aims to split strands of DNA, which contribute 40 per cent of the viscosity of the cystic fibrosis sputum. Although stunning *in vitro*, this substance given as once daily by nebulizer has been of limited value to relatively few patients. It tends to be used selectively in those shown to benefit.

Nutritional problems

Most patients have pancreatic insufficiency and will have malabsorption, especially of fat, including the fat-soluble vitamins. The presence of malabsorption is indicated by poor weight gain despite an apparently adequate intake and the presence of abnormally bulky offensive greasy stools. There may be rectal prolapse. Laboratory analysis will confirm very low levels of chymotrypsin and excess fat globules in the stool.

The mainstay of nutritional management is a high-energy diet which has plenty of fat. Enzyme replacement capsules are given just prior to each meal or snack with the dose titrated against clinical response. The enzyme capsules have microspheres encased in an acid-resistant capsule to prevent degradation in the stomach. Extra vitamins are also required with preparations high in vitamins A, D, E and K. Particular problems can occur in infancy when 'food battles' are common. In cystic fibrosis, the normal policy of letting the child undernourish at times is detrimental and considerable dietetic and psychology input may help the parents greatly.

Patients with poor nutrition often also have poor respiratory disease and may find it difficult to eat enough to satisfy their increased energy requirements. High-calorie food supplements can be given after and in addition to normal meals. If this is insufficient then enteral feeding with a prepared feed can be administered by nasogastric tube or a gastrostomy. This can normally be given overnight by a feed pump, allowing some remaining appetite for daytime meals.

Gastrointestinal complications

Distal intestinal obstruction syndrome (DIOS) is a common problem with partial or total gut obstruction due to stasis of abnormal bowel contents. Patients prone to this may use simple laxatives in the early stages to prevent escalation of this problem. Established DIOS can be treated with oral gastrografin once complete gut obstruction and perforation are ruled out by clinical and radiological assessment. Further therapy with a bowel preparation solution containing polyethylene glycol is normally very effective. Gut obstruction secondary to strictures consequent to neonatal surgery for meconium ileus is important to bear in mind and can complicate the picture in apparent DIOS.

Gallstones are increasingly recognized and are due to the relative stasis of biliary flow. They are seldom symptomatic in childhood. Cystic fibrosis liver disease is due to biliary disease and often begins to show in mid-childhood. Overt liver dysfunction is unusual in childhood but clinical hepatomegaly, ultrasonographic changes and mild liver function abnormalities are increasingly common with advancing age. Complications such as variceal bleeding require expert clinical management. It has become common practice to commence ursodeoxycholic acid to promote bile flow in those with evidence of significant liver involvement.

Complications in adolescence and adulthood

For the first time in 2001 there were more adults with cystic fibrosis in the UK than children due to the huge improvement in prognosis in childhood. This has led to the development of specialist adult cystic fibrosis units and most paediatric centres will have transition arrangements.

Psychologically, adolescence is greatly complicated by a chronic disease that is progressing. Cystic-fibrosis-related diabetes due to pancreatic destruction starts to increase in incidence in teenage life and is best treated by insulin therapy. Liver disease, progressive lung disease, arthropathy and declining general health can start to feature. However, increasingly people with cystic fibrosis are entering adulthood in relatively good health and able to undertake tertiary education courses, paid employment, etc.

Males with cystic fibrosis are infertile except with use of assisted conception techniques. Females have slightly reduced fertility and may experience decline in disease parameters following pregnancy but produce a healthy child. Very careful liaison between the cystic fibrosis physician and the obstetrician is required.

Terminal respiratory disease can be treated with double lung transplant. Sadly, most patients on the waiting list die, as the organ supply remains low. Patients with cystic fibrosis have a worse survival rate following technically successful transplantation. Transplantation can be complicated by coexisting liver or gut disease or cystic-fibrosis-related diabetes.

Psychosocial factors

Families with a child with any health problem tend to manifest difficulties and cystic fibrosis is no exception. The physical burden of care is particularly heavy and administering treatment may take one to two hours per day every day. Extra treatment such as home administered IV antibiotic therapy for a respiratory exacerbation places further considerable strains. A clinical psychologist and a social worker are vital members of the multidisciplinary team.

Team-based care

There is some evidence that care within a specialized multidisciplinary team caring for a critical mass of patients can lead to better clinical outcomes. However, smaller units with dedicated teams can deliver just as good care. One of the major problems with larger clinics is the problem of cross-infection. There is good evidence that *Burkholderia cepacia* and certain *Pseudomonas aeruginosa* subspp. may be capable of patient-to-patient spread. These organisms have greater potential for bad clinical outcomes and as such are better restricted in their extent. Most large clinics now segregate patients according to microbiological status.

RECURRENT RESPIRATORY INFECTION

A number of children will present with repeated or chronic signs and symptoms of lower respiratory infection with moist cough, intermittent fever and the presence of crackles on auscultation. This is accompanied by chest radiograph changes of opacification, often in one particular lobe. Investigation of these children (see box) is likely to uncover an underlying diagnosis in many.

> Investigations in recurrent respiratory infection
>
> Flexible bronchoscopy
>
> Bronchioalveolar lavage for microbiology and cytology
>
> Computed tomography (CT) scan of chest
>
> PH study and/or barium swallow with TOF study
>
> Videofluoroscopy if primary aspiration suspected
>
> Sweat test ± cystic fibrosis mutation screen
>
> Immunoglobulins and functional antibody testing
>
> Cilia beat frequency and ultrastructure

PRIMARY CILIARY DYSKINESIA

Primary ciliary dyskinesia (PCD) is a condition that probably frequently goes undiagnosed. The cilia are small structures on the surface epithelium of the airways, reproductive tract and cerebral ventricles. They beat synchronously and propel debris and bacteria along and out of the respiratory tract. They therefore form part of the host defence from infection. Cilia have a very complex internal structure which allows them to beat together rather like corn in a field in the wind. Various abnormalities cause absent or dyskinetic movement, resulting in poor mucociliary clearance. This predisposes the subject to respiratory infection with symptoms often starting in neonatal life or in infancy. Correct placement of major organs is dependent on ciliary function and therefore 50 per cent of those with PCD have situs inversus or isolated dextrocardia. Kartagener syndrome with situs inversus, infertility and immotile cilia is part of the spectrum of PCD.

Ciliary function used to be assessed by measuring the time taken to taste a saccharin granule placed at the nares and beaten posteriorly by the nasal cilia. This test was poorly reproducible and inaccurate. Modern assessment of function makes use of very fast video capture of beating cilia. This investigation, along with ultrastructural examination, is an important investigation in those with recurrent respiratory infection. A nasal brush biopsy sample can be rapidly examined to assess the beat frequency and synchronicity of the ciliary motion. Electron microscopy is also useful to assess the presence of any abnormalities of the structure. It is likely that there are many potential individual genetic defects in these complex structures, some of which give rise to aplasia and total absence of function and some that give rise only to abnormal function leading to poor mucociliary clearance.

BRONCHIECTASIS

Bronchiectasis is a diagnosis only really arrived at after HRCT scanning as a plain chest radiograph is poor at picking up early signs. It is a virtually inevitable development in cystic fibrosis but occurs in others particularly following lobar damage from recurrent infection, following foreign body aspiration, in immunodeficiency states and in ciliary dyskinesia disorders. Localized bronchiectasis secondary to pertussis or tuberculosis is now very rare indeed. This form of lung damage is one of the patterns recognized following severe infection in infancy with certain subtypes of adenovirus, influenza and parainfluenza viruses and occasionally following RSV infection.

The mainstays of treatment are chest physiotherapy and aggressive use of antibiotics at the first signs of respiratory infection. Some patients may benefit from 'prophylactic' antibiotics, perhaps a rotation of two to three agents, each given for a month at a time. In addition, this group of patients should be encouraged to have annual influenza immunization. The use of polyvalent pneumococcal immunization is as yet unproved. The development of accompanying rhinosinusitis should always prompt a rigorous search for a systemic cause as it suggests a pan-airway problem.

Few of these patients will go on to develop progressive respiratory disease, as in many the symptoms slowly remit over childhood. Presumably, this is due to resolution of the causative lung damage and the positive effects of lung growth and development. Progressive disease with the development of finger clubbing, chest deformity and chronic suppuration is only likely in those with underlying immunodeficiency or ciliary disorders.

OBSTRUCTIVE SLEEP APNOEA HYPOPNOEA SYNDROME

> **CASE STUDY**
>
> A 9-year-old boy is referred by his general practitioner to the medical clinic because of an increasingly

disturbed sleeping pattern associated with snoring. On closer questioning his parents describe snoring of variable intensity and an irregular breathing pattern during sleep, particularly when he has an intercurrent upper respiratory tract infection. In school, his performance has gone down in the past few months and his teacher has noticed deterioration in his attention span.

Ten per cent of young children snore and 1–2 per cent of pre-school children will have obstructive sleep apnoea hypopnoea syndrome (OSAHS). It is becoming increasingly recognized that this is not a benign problem but that it is associated with significant neurocognitive effects, poor weight gain and behavioural problems including a complex association with attention deficit hyperactivity disorder.

The history in snoring children is poorly discriminant between those with benign primary snoring and those with OSAHS. Children may present with snoring that is loud and often heard outside the bedroom. Parents may further describe pauses in airflow with continued efforts or struggling to breathe preceded by a crescendo of snoring intensity and accompanied by silence due to cessation of airflow consequent on total obstruction. The children are often described as restless and may adopt unusual sleeping positions with the head extended at the neck and the legs folded under the trunk.

Older textbooks state that children with OSAHS do not have daytime somnolence, in contrast to adults with the same syndrome. Recent work on neurocognitive function and behavioural measures suggest that children with OSAHS manifest their sleepiness by being cranky, inattentive and producing poor school performance rather than by falling asleep at work and crashing cars as do adults with OSAHS.

Predisposing factors for obstructive sleep apnoea hypopnoea syndrome

- Craniofacial disorders especially with small jaw
- Down syndrome (one-third have OSAHS)
- Muscle hypotonia
- Obesity
- Large tonsils and adenoids
- Positive family history

Experienced observation along with pulse oximetry can confirm the diagnosis when there is witnessed apnoea and oxygen desaturation. If this is not clear in a child with a compatible history, polysomnography is necessary to confirm the diagnosis. Polysomnography involves the gathering of multiple channels of physiological information to record sleep stage, cardiorespiratory parameters, airflow at the nose and mouth, chest and abdominal movement and respiratory gas exchange. A combination of clinical history and absolute values from polysomnography will allow the diagnosis to be made. Many children have incomplete obstruction and will have multiple hypopnoeas rather than complete apnoea. They also have increased upper airway resistance. It has been postulated that there is a separate disorder (upper airway resistance syndrome) with many of the symptoms of OSAHS but not the same polysomnographic features. Most authorities now consider there is a continuum as demonstrated in Figure 8.3.

Treatment is most often adenotonsillectomy, which in non-syndromic, non-obese children will normally be curative. In adult practice, other forms of upper airway and palatal surgery can be successful, as can dental devices to alter the geometry of the upper airway. Paediatric experience and success with these approaches has been disappointing. There is an intriguing possibility that there may be significant links between childhood OSAHS and adult OSAHS. This is particularly important to investigate because of the clear evidence that OSAHS in adulthood is an independent risk factor for stroke, hypertension and myocardial infarction.

Children in whom some significant degree of obstruction persists will require bi-level positive airway pressure (BiPAP) support at night. This is delivered by a ventilator with the patient wearing a nasal or full face mask during sleep. Bi-level positive airway pressure effectively provides a pressure splint that alters the critical closing pressure of the upper airway, supporting airway tissues and therefore overcoming obstruction.

A combination of ENT surgery and weight loss can also be very effective in those with mixed aetiology.

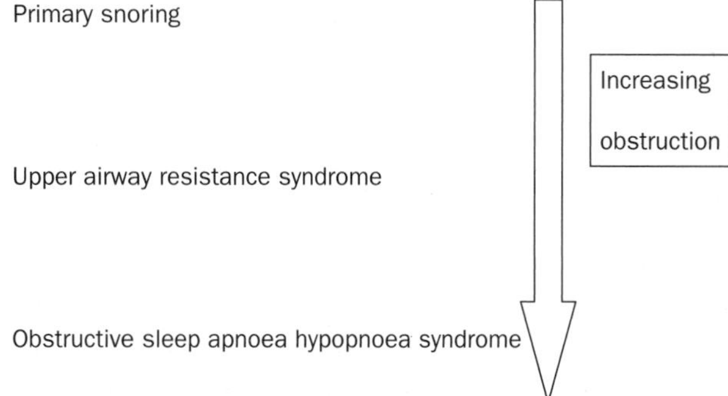

Figure 8.3 Obstructive sleep apnoea hypopnoea syndrome continuum

The so called pickwickian syndrome or obesity hypoventilation syndrome due to severe obesity (body mass index > +3 SD) is becoming commoner in children due to the epidemic in childhood obesity. These children are at very high risk of adverse cardiac outcomes such as systemic hypertension and ultimately cardiac failure. It is postulated that the previously unexplained pulmonary hypertension seen in adults with Down syndrome and structurally normal heart may be due to unrecognized and untreated OSAHS.

RESPIRATORY PROBLEMS IN NEURODISABILITY

With attitudes towards children with neurodisabilities changing, the level of intervention has changed and respiratory difficulties are a significant issue. Children with muscle weakness from Duchenne muscular dystrophy (DMD), congenital myopathies, spinal muscular atrophy (SMA) and other rarer conditions have two main respiratory difficulties. First, they are prone to lower respiratory infection due to ineffective cough and consequent poor clearance of respiratory secretions and the coexistence of gastro-oesophageal reflux or direct aspiration due to poor chewing and swallowing. Second, they may develop respiratory failure, initially at night only, due to decline in muscle power in progressive disorders such as DMD and/or secondary to alteration in their power/weight ratio with growth, maturity or puberty in those with relatively non-progressive disorders such as SMA. The presence of kyphoscoliosis will exacerbate this due to mechanical limitation of chest wall movement.

This group of children is increasingly being offered ventilatory support, normally with non-invasive ventilation and BiPAP. The option exists to provide tracheostomy ventilation at night or full-time ventilation via a tracheostomy. However, when this degree of intervention is necessary careful discussion needs to be undertaken to assess the real benefits and ascertain the quality of life that can be achieved. In DMD it is now accepted that at least 5–10 years of extra life of a quality appreciated by the patients and their carers can be achieved.

Children with neurodisability due to cerebral palsy and progressive neurological disorders can have respiratory infections due to all the factors above but in particular may have direct aspiration associated with chewing and swallowing difficulties and poor protection of the lower airways due to pharyngeal incoordination. There may also be upper airway obstruction due to poor maintenance of airway patency. These children may have particular problems with coexisting asthma as consistent drug delivery can be challenging.

INTERSTITIAL LUNG DISEASE

This term encompasses a collection of clinical pathologies characterized by restrictive lung disease with inflammatory infiltration of the interstitial spaces or alveoli. Most children present in early childhood with dry cough, tachypnoea and clinical signs of hypoxia such as poor growth. The child may have clinical chest deformity and fine crackles may be heard on auscultation. The lungs are stiff (poorly compliant).

Interstitial diseases are rare and not well understood. They can accompany autoimmune disease, other systemic diseases or follow early viral insult, particularly by certain subtypes of adenovirus. Treatment is difficult with no good randomized trials. Hypoxia should be corrected. Most clinicians will institute a trial of steroid therapy in moderate doses. This may well need to be continued in the long term. It is difficult to find convincing evidence that any other drug therapy is effective. A proportion of these patients experience progressive respiratory failure and die. A much larger proportion will have slow remission and be left with a degree of chronic restriction of lung function. It appears that the largest group are those with stable but chronic disease with chest deformity, exercise restriction, poor weight gain and oxygen dependency.

SARCOIDOSIS

This is an unusual condition in childhood but can be found in adolescents. The presentations are similar to those seen in adults with bilateral hilar lymphadenopathy and interstitial changes. Children may present with cough, breathlessness, lethargy and anorexia. Diagnostic tests include measurement of angiotensin converting enzyme or lung biopsy.

REFERENCES

Scottish Intercollegiate Guidelines Network and the British Thoracic Society (2004) *British Guideline on the Management of Asthma*. Guideline no. 63. SIGN/BTS. Available at www.sign.ac.uk/guidelines/fulltext/63/index.html and http://www.brit-thoracic.org.uk/docs/asthmafull.pdf (accessed 26 October 2004).

FURTHER READING

Chernick V, Boat T (eds) (1998). *Kendig's Disorders of the Respiratory Tract in Children*, 6th edn. Philadelphia: WB Saunders.

Ferber R, Kryger M (eds) (1995). *Principles and Practice of Sleep Medicine in the Child.* Philadelphia: WB Saunders.

Silverman M (2002). *Childhood Asthma and Other Wheezing Disorders.* London: Arnold.

Taussig LM, Landau LI (eds) (1997). *Textbook of Paediatric Respiratory Medicine.* St Louis: Mosby.

Chapter 9

Cardiovascular disease

Alan Houston and Trevor Richens

The management of the infant or child with significant heart disease has largely become the remit of the specialist paediatric cardiologist. The general paediatrician must be able to recognize that a cardiac defect is present and understand its possible consequences in order to make an appropriate and timely referral to the specialist cardiologist. To do this it is necessary to have knowledge of common defects and understand their haemodynamic effects. These will determine the presenting features and the urgency of treatment or referral, which is of particular importance in the neonatal period where rapid deterioration can occur and the initiation of appropriate therapy and transfer to a cardiac centre can be life saving.

In the MRCPCH examination, it is likely that the candidate will have to examine a child with a cardiac defect but not an ill neonate. However, knowledge of the diagnosis and management of the neonate is essential and can be tested in other parts of the examination. Thus, general knowledge of all aspects of heart disease is necessary.

THE FETAL CIRCULATION

Anatomy and physiology

The fetal and maternal circulations are connected to the placenta, which provides the fetus with nutrition and oxygen and removes waste metabolites and carbon dioxide. Two umbilical arteries transport fetal blood at lower oxygen level from the distal aorta and a single umbilical vein returns better oxygenated blood (pO_2 30–35 mmHg) through the ductus venosus to the upper inferior vena cava (IVC) and thence the right atrium (Figure 9.1). The umbilical arteries are a continuation of the hypogastric arteries arising from the femoral arteries and become obliterated after birth (persisting as fibrous cords, the lateral umbilical ligaments), and the ductus venosus persists as the ligamentum teres and ligamentum venosum of the liver. The blood returning to the right atrium from the IVC has a higher oxygen content (pO_2 26–28 mmHg) than that from the superior vena cava (SVC), as it is a mixture of blood from the umbilical vein and that from the lower body. It is directed preferentially by the Eustachian valve (a groove in the low right atrium) to the foramen ovale (a flap valve in the atrial septum) and thence through the left atrium and ventricle to the aorta and head and neck vessels. The blood in the SVC has a lower oxygen content (pO_2 12–14 mmHg) and is preferentially directed to the right ventricle and pulmonary artery. Since the pulmonary vessels are collapsed with a high resistance, little goes through the lungs (about 10 per cent) and most passes through the ductus arteriosus to the thoracic and abdominal aorta to supply the lower body, with some going through the umbilical arteries to the placenta and returning at higher oxygenation to the fetal right atrium.

Circulatory changes at birth

When the newborn baby breathes, the alveoli inflate, the pulmonary vascular resistance falls, the pulmonary flow

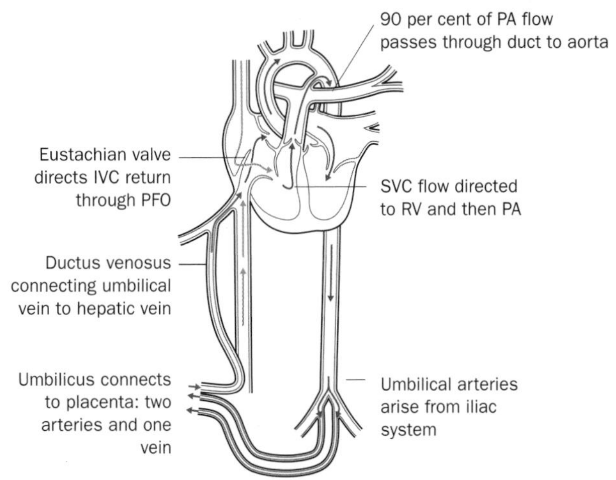

Figure 9.1 The fetal circulation. IVC, inferior vena cava; PA, pulmonary artery; PFO, patent foramen ovale; RV, right ventricle; SVC, superior vena cava

passes through the lungs and the venous return of blood at high oxygen content is established to the left side of the heart and aorta. The placental circulation is cut off and the umbilical cord cut. The ductus arteriosus begins to contract, generally being completely closed by the third to sixth day, and degenerates into an impervious cord, the ligamentum arteriosum, connecting the left pulmonary artery to the arch of the aorta. The practical significance of this structure is that it may form part of a vascular ring causing stridor in infancy or swallowing difficulties in later life. The left atrial pressure rises with the increased venous return, pushing the flap of the foramen ovale against the atrial septum with physiological closure, although a tiny left-to-right flow can often be demonstrated with colour Doppler for some months. In some normal babies, a potential communication can persist into later life, when subsequent right-to-left flow may be the mechanism for a paradoxical embolus.

The clinical importance of understanding the fetal circulation is related to the effect of the patency or closure of the communications in early postnatal life. An umbilical arterial or venous catheter can be inserted through the umbilical vessels in the first hours of life. If a baby is likely to need an atrial septostomy, it is worthwhile keeping the cord moist to facilitate umbilical vein access. The presence or absence of flow through the ductus arteriosus or foramen ovale is important in determining the presentation and management of some forms of significant congenital heart disease in the first days of life, as discussed later (The neonate with suspected congenital heart disease, page 297).

INCIDENCE, ASSOCIATION AND AETIOLOGY

Heart disease is the commonest significant congenital defect with an incidence between 6 and 8 per 1000 live births. A specific aetiological factor is rarely identified as the cause of congenital heart disease but a number of associations have been identified with chromosomal abnormalities, single gene defects, teratogens, maternal drugs, and syndromes (Table 9.1). Perceived wisdom suggests that congenital heart disease is due to polygenic or multifactorial inheritance in which as yet unknown inherited and environmental factors combine to cause the malformation. But the relatively high incidence in the offspring of those with a significant lesion may indicate a greater importance for a single gene defect. The recurrence risk for a cardiac defect depends on the relationship of the affected person, and to a lesser extent the nature of the lesion (Table 9.2).

KEY LEARNING POINTS

- In a child with heart disease consider an associated syndrome or maternal cause.
- If a couple have one child with heart disease the risk of another being affected rises from approximately 0.8 to 3.5 per cent.

Basic classification of cardiac lesions

Acquired

- Rheumatic valve disease
- Kawasaki disease
- Dilated cardiomyopathy
- Infective endocarditis

Congenital

Acyanotic

- Shunt: atrial septal defect (ASD); ventricular septal defect (VSD); persistent ductus arteriosus (PDA)
- Obstruction: pulmonary stenosis; aortic stenosis; coarctation of the aorta

Cyanotic

- Marked hypoxia: simple transposition of the great arteries (TGA); severe tetralogy of Fallot; pulmonary atresia; severe stenosis (including tetralogy of Fallot, single ventricle)
- Mixing situation: single ventricle and no pulmonary stenosis; total anomalous pulmonary venous drainage (TAPVD); hypoplastic left heart syndrome; truncus arteriosus

CLASSIFICATION OF HEART DEFECTS

To understand heart disease in the child it is convenient to consider it under different subgroupings, the most basic being congenital or acquired. Acquired defects are relatively uncommon but should be borne in mind, particularly in the older child. For congenital heart disease the major distinction is between a cyanotic or acyanotic defect. Cyanotic lesions usually present in the first days or weeks of life, are always significant and require urgent referral for a cardiac opinion. Acyanotic lesions may present early (usually needing early referral) or later (often not

Table 9.1 Common associations and heart defects

Association	Defect
Karyotype abnormalities	
Trisomy 21 (Down syndrome)	AVSD or VSD
Trisomy 18 (Edward syndrome)	VSD
Trisomy 13 (Patau syndrome)	VSD
45XO (Turner syndrome)	Coarctation of the aorta, bicuspid aortic valve
Maternal illness	
Congenital rubella	Peripheral pulmonary stenosis, PDA
Diabetes	VSD, transient septal thickening
Phenylketonuria	VSD
Systemic lupus erythematosus	Complete heart block
Maternal drugs/alcohol	
Sodium valproate	Coarctation of aorta, left heart hypoplasia
Lithium	Ebstein anomaly
Phenytoin	VSD, coarctation, semilunar valve stenosis
Isoretinoin	Conotruncal abnormalities
Fetal alcohol syndrome	VSD
Syndromes	
de Lange	VSD
Noonan	Pulmonary valve or artery stenosis
Williams	Supravalve aortic stenosis
Friedreich ataxia	Hypertrophic cardiomyopathy
Jervell and Lange-Nielsen	Prolonged QT
Holt-Oram	Atrial septal defect
VATERL	VSD, tetralogy of Fallot
DiGeorge	Aortic arch and conotruncal abnormalities
CHARGE	VSD, tetralogy of Fallot

ASVD, *a*trio*v*entricular *s*eptal *d*efect; VSD, *v*entricular *s*eptal *d*efect.

CHARGE, *c*oloboma, *h*eart, *a*tresia (choanal), *r*etardation, *g*enital and *e*ar abnormalities.

VATERL, *v*ertebral, *a*nal, *t*racheo*e*sophageal, *r*adial and renal anomalies.

Table 9.2 Risk of an infant having a congenital heart defect

Factor	Risk (per cent)
Pregnancy risk	0.6–0.8
One previous affected child	3–4
Two previous affected children	6–8
Father has congenital heart disease	6–8
Mother is affected	5–15

needing urgent treatment). For routine clinical purposes, acyanotic defects can be considered as those with a shunt or an obstructive lesion. Since the child is acyanotic, the shunt must be left to right and can be at the atrial, ventricular or great artery level, commonly, ASD, VSD and PDA, respectively. In the infant with Down syndrome, an atrioventricular septal defect (AVSD) has to be considered. The common obstructive lesions are pulmonary stenosis, aortic stenosis and coarctation of the aorta. Cyanotic lesions cannot be subdivided so simply. It is necessary to be aware of the common lesions and make the general distinction between those with severe cyanosis/hypoxia and those in whom this is less severe. The former will have TGA or severe obstruction to pulmonary flow. The latter will generally have a situation where the systemic and pulmonary venous returns mix in the heart and there is no obstruction to aortic or pulmonary artery flow so the mixed systemic and pulmonary venous return passes to both the aorta and pulmonary artery. The relative incidences of the common lesions are shown in Table 9.3.

Table 9.3 Approximate incidence of different congenital heart defects

Congenital heart defect	Incidence (per cent)
Acyanotic defects	
Ventricular septal defect	32
Persistent ductus arteriosus	12
Pulmonary stenosis	8
Coarctation of the aorta	6
Atrial septal defect	6
Aortic stenosis	5
Atrioventricular septal defect	2
Total	**71**
Cyanotic defects	
Tetralogy of Fallot	6
Transposition of the great arteries	5
Single ventricle including tricuspid atresia	4
Hypoplastic left heart syndrome	3
Total anomalous pulmonary venous drainage	1
Truncus arteriosus	1
Total	**20**

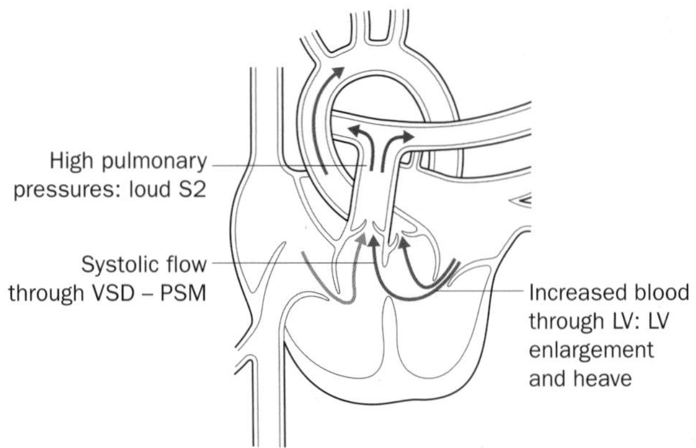

Figure 9.2 Ventricular septal defect (VSD). LV, left ventricle; PSM, pansystolic murmur

KEY LEARNING POINTS

- There are six common acyanotic lesions.
- Of children with Down syndrome, 40 per cent have a cardiac defect (usually VSD or AVSD).
- There is a greater spectrum of cyanotic lesions.

CLINICAL AND HAEMODYNAMIC FEATURES AND MANAGEMENT OF COMMON CONGENITAL ACYANOTIC LESIONS

In many cases, the murmur is the important factor in reaching a diagnosis in an asymptomatic child. However, other features can be important, particularly when there is a significant defect. In addition, an understanding of the haemodynamic factors in each condition helps explain the presence or absence of clinical findings and is included in the following section although it is not mandatory for the MRCPCH examination.

Ventricular septal defect

A defect can be positioned at virtually any site in the ventricular septum. This makes little difference to the clinical effect and signs. Normally the vascular resistance is higher in the systemic than pulmonary circulation, so in systole, blood will flow through the VSD to the pulmonary artery. This produces an increase in pulmonary flow and venous return to the left atrium and ventricle with resultant volume overload and dilatation. The left ventricle dilates to accommodate the increasing venous return and maintain the cardiac output so the pulse volume is usually normal, unless there is severe failure. With a large shunt the ventricular dilation may produce a displaced thrusting apex beat. Blood passes directly from the left ventricle through the right ventricle to the pulmonary artery, so the right ventricle does not dilate. With high pulmonary flow the pulmonary pressure rises and a loud second heart sound and right ventricular heave may be found (Figure 9.2).

In the neonate, there is high pulmonary vascular resistance and little VSD flow thus there may be no murmur in the first day or two of life. Thereafter, the murmur of flow through a VSD is classically harsh and pansystolic but it can be abbreviated and mid-systolic in small defects, particularly muscular ones. The loudness of the murmur is affected by pressure difference between the ventricles and cannot allow an assessment of the size or significance of the defect. With a large shunt and high venous return to the left atrium, a mitral mid-diastolic murmur may result from the high volume flow through the mitral ring, which is of fixed size. This is a similar mechanism to that of mitral stenosis where the flow volume is normal but the orifice reduced. The mitral diastolic murmur is best heard with the bell of the stethoscope.

On rare occasions in an older child with pulmonary vascular disease and Eisenmenger syndrome there is a right-to-left shunt through the VSD and the patient will be cyanosed. This occurs when the pulmonary vascular resistance exceeds the systemic vascular resistance.

The second sound will be accentuated and there may be no systolic murmur, but an early diastolic one due to pulmonary regurgitation is common.

Management

The treatment of a large VSD is generally surgical. However, the infant with a large defect will frequently have problems in the first months from cardiac failure.

Surgical closure, when necessary, is usually undertaken within the first six months of life. The main indications for VSD closure are persistent heart failure (often with feeding difficulty and failure to gain weight) or pulmonary hypertension. If neither of these is present, an expectant policy is usually adopted. Some will close spontaneously, and most of the others do not require closure, even if they are still present into adult life. Although closure is safe in the modern era, the theoretical risk of surgery is greater that that of leaving it alone and giving prophylaxis against infective endocarditis. In a few children there is a large shunt and normal pulmonary artery pressure, and closure is considered prudent after infancy because of the problem of long-term volume overload of the left ventricle. An increasing number of these children are suitable for transcatheter closure.

KEY LEARNING POINTS

- A VSD murmur is usually not heard in the first or second day of life.
- A VSD murmur is not always pansystolic.
- The loudness of the murmur of a VSD is not related to its significance.
- A large shunt is suggested by a displaced apex and mid-diastolic murmur.
- Pulmonary hypertension is suggested by a loud second sound or heave.
- If closure is necessary this is usually before six months of age.

Persistent ductus arteriosus (or arterial duct)

Beyond the neonatal period, an isolated PDA is usually asymptomatic and rarely causes pulmonary hypertension or cardiac failure. Unlike a VSD there is a pressure difference between the aorta and pulmonary artery throughout the cardiac cycle so blood shunts from left-to-right in both systole and diastole (Figure 9.3). There is increased pulmonary artery flow, increased venous return to the left atrium and ventricle and increased output to the aorta, so a large shunt will result in dilatation of the left atrium and ventricle. The increased ventricular output to the aorta and diastolic run off from it to the pulmonary artery can potentially result in high volume or collapsing pulses, similar to the situation in significant aortic regurgitation. However, ductal flow is related to the diameter of the duct and the pressure difference between the aorta and pulmonary artery. With a small duct or pulmonary artery hypertension there may be relatively little flow and the pulses will be normal. In the UK, most ducts are recognized early and it is now unusual to find collapsing pulses in older patients. The murmur is heard under the left clavicle and radiates down the left sternal edge. Since there is a pressure difference across the duct throughout the cardiac cycle, the murmur is continuous, classically crescendo in late systole and falling in volume through diastole.

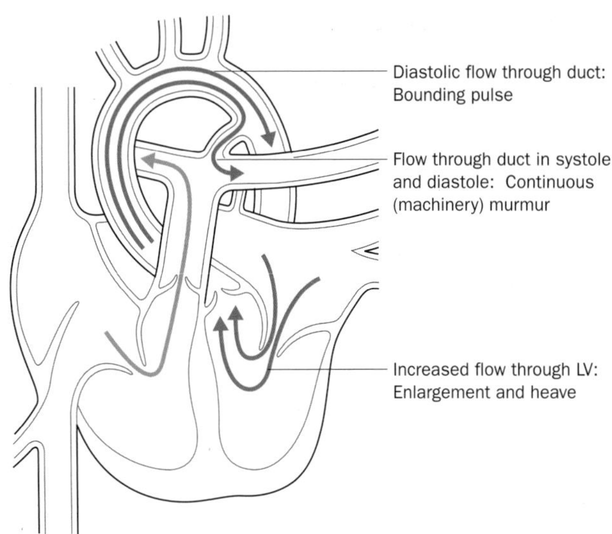

Figure 9.3 Persistent ductus arteriosus. LV, left ventricle

In the preterm baby the question may arise as to whether the increased pulmonary flow through the duct is contributing to the requirement for ventilator support and if its closure would improve the situation. Signs of a classic duct such as high-volume pulse, left ventricular heave and continuous murmur suggest high flow. However, in many there is pulmonary hypertension and the signs can be less marked and the murmur abbreviated, so it is not easy to determine the significance of the duct clinically. Echocardiographic assessment can assist and the main criteria for high flow would be enlargement of the left atrium, generally measured as a ratio compared to the aorta rather than as an absolute value. A ratio of the left atrium to aortic root greater than 1.5:1 has been suggested as indicating high ductal flow. Medical treatment of this takes the form of general supportive measures, fluid restriction and diuretics. Medical closure is successful in some infants using indometacin, given intravenously as three to six doses of 0.1–0.2 mg 12–24 hours apart, or ibuprofen. Relative contraindications to this include raised urea or creatinine, thrombocytopenia, bleeding disorder and necrotizing enterocolitis. When this is not successful and closure is required, this is routinely undertaken by surgical clipping or ligation.

In the older infant or child, closure is routinely recommended when the duct flow is audible on auscultation. In those with a small shunt, volume overload is not a likely problem and the rationale is based on the possible problem of contracting infective endocarditis. The logic of this may be questioned as small VSDs are left alone and not closed. One argument is that ducts do not close spontaneously and closure carries a very low risk, but a VSD may close spontaneously and the risk associated with closure is greater that that of leaving it alone and giving prophylaxis against infective endocarditis. Indometacin is not effective after term and interventional catheterization closure with an occlusion device is successful in most older children.

KEY LEARNING POINTS

- Full volume pulses are not always found with a PDA.
- Indometacin or ibuprofen may effect closure in the preterm baby.
- Transcatheter closure is usually effective in the older child.

Atrial septal defect

The commonest type of ASD (Figure 9.4) is the secundum defect, approximately in the centre of the atrial septum. Less commonly, it is situated high in the atrium (sinus venosus) or low in relation to the atrioventricular valves. The latter, sometimes referred to as a primum defect, is part of the spectrum of the AVSD and now generally called a partial AVSD. The clinical signs of an isolated defect will be the same. However, the partial AVSD can be associated with atrioventricular valve regurgitation due to a cleft in one of the mitral valve leaflets so this may alter the clinical findings.

There is minimal pressure difference between the atria but the impedance to ventricular filling is less in the right than left ventricle with resultant flow from the left to the right atrium and through the tricuspid valve. Left ventricular filling and function are normal and pulses are of normal volume. With a large shunt the right ventricle has to dilate in diastole to accommodate the systemic venous return and the atrial shunt. Significant dilation will produce a right ventricular heave, palpable at the mid to low left sternal edge. The higher flow volume through the pulmonary as compared to the aortic valve with free flow through the

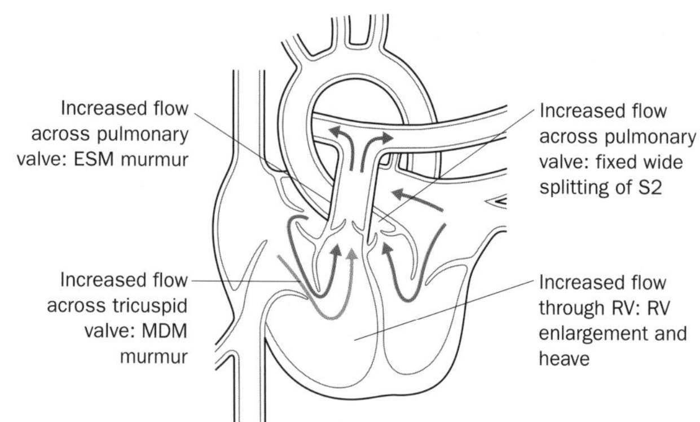

Figure 9.4 Atrial septal defect. ESM, ejection systolic murmur; MDM, mid-diastolic murmur; RV, right ventricle

atrial septum results in wide and fixed splitting of the second heart sound. Since there is little pressure difference with a large ASD, there is little turbulence and a murmur is not heard from the direct left-to-right shunt. Increased volume flow from the right ventricle through the pulmonary valve produces an ejection systolic murmur at the pulmonary area, but with limited radiation to the clavicle. The murmur of an ASD can often be quiet in the early years. With a large atrial shunt the increased volume of flow through the fixed size tricuspid valve in an ASD can produce a mid-diastolic murmur at the lower left sternal edge, the mechanism being similar to the mitral one in a VSD.

Management

Most children with an ASD are asymptomatic but in the long term (from teens to even late adult life) problems may develop with right ventricle failure (from right ventricular volume overload), arrhythmias (from right atrial dilation) and occasionally pulmonary hypertension. Closure is undertaken if there is any more than a small shunt, generally determined by enlargement of the right ventricle on an echocardiogram. A high percentage of secundum defects are amenable to transcatheter closure but the other types require a standard surgical procedure.

KEY LEARNING POINTS

- The signs of an ASD may be minimal in childhood.
- Delay in closure does not usually result in long-term sequelae.
- Fixed splitting of the second sound can be difficult to recognize.
- A large shunt may be manifest by a parasternal heave and diastolic murmur.
- Transcatheter closure is effective in most secundum ASDs.

Aortic stenosis

Obstruction to left ventricle outflow produces a rise in left ventricle pressure, a pressure gradient across the valve (with turbulent systolic flow) and, with increasing severity, left ventricle pressure overload and muscle hypertrophy but not dilation. With severe obstruction, aortic flow will be affected and manifest as a low-volume pulse – however, this is only demonstrable with severe obstruction and is rarely found in the UK or other countries where routine surveillance for a possible cardiac defect is undertaken. The pressure drop and turbulent flow across the valve may be manifest by a thrill palpable in the suprasternal notch or aortic area. An ejection systolic murmur will be audible in the aortic area with radiation up into the neck in valve stenosis. The loudness of the murmur gives little information on the severity of stenosis. In addition, with a pliable stenosed valve, usually bicuspid, an ejection click will be heard, usually best at the low or mid-sternal edge. With subaortic stenosis, the murmur is often better heard at the mid to upper left sternal edge with radiation to the aortic area and there will not be a click.

Aortic stenosis is usually recognized in early life (from a loud murmur) and severe obstruction dealt with before symptoms can occur. Rarely, there may be anginal type chest pain, drop attacks on exertion or exertional dyspnoea. Neonates with critical stenosis can present with circulatory collapse or heart failure.

Indications for intervention would include any symptoms attributable to the defect, a significant gradient on Doppler or catheterization or marked ventricular hypertrophy, particularly if there were ST changes on the electrocardiogram (ECG). The procedure for valve stenosis (surgery or catheter balloon) is generally deferred as long as possible because of the possibility of subsequent significant regurgitation and need for surgical valve replacement. This is not the case for subaortic stenosis and surgery may be undertaken earlier.

KEY LEARNING POINTS

- Clinical assessment of the severity of stenosis is difficult.
- Subaortic stenosis may be misdiagnosed as a VSD.
- A suprasternal thrill is found with both valve and subvalve stenosis.
- Transcatheter balloon dilation is effective in some cases of valve stenosis.

Pulmonary stenosis

Pulmonary stenosis is usually recognized from a loud murmur, and severe obstruction dealt with before symptoms can occur. The neonate with critical pulmonary stenosis can present with cyanosis. Obstruction to right ventricle outflow produces a rise in right ventricular pressure, a pressure gradient across the valve (with turbulent flow) and, with increasing severity, right ventricular pressure overload and muscle hypertrophy but not dilation. Left ventricular filling and function are not affected, and the pulses are normal. There is usually no heave. The pressure drop and turbulent flow across the valve may produce a thrill palpable at the upper left sternal edge. An ejection click may be heard if the valve is pliable. An ejection systolic murmur is maximal in the pulmonary area (upper left sternal edge) with radiation to the left clavicle. Its volume bears little relation to the severity of obstruction.

The indication for intervention generally would be a significant gradient on Doppler. Catheter balloon dilation is usually successful but some cases, where there is a thick and dysplastic valve, require a surgical valvotomy.

KEY LEARNING POINTS

- Clinical assessment of severity is not reliable.
- If in doubt refer to a cardiologist for a Doppler study.
- Transcatheter balloon dilation is usually effective.

Coarctation of the aorta

Coarctation of the aorta (Figure 9.5) is usually situated just beyond the left subclavian artery in the region of the arterial duct. The obstruction results in a pressure gradient between the ascending and descending aorta with reduced volume pulse in the latter. This can be recognized clinically by lower volume pulse in the femorals than arms. Left without treatment, collateral arteries bypass the obstruction with flow through them to the descending aorta. In older patients, a delay in the femoral pulsation compared with the arms may be more apparent than the pulse volume difference.

The presentation of coarctation of the aorta is determined by the severity of the obstruction and ductal patency. The neonate with severe obstruction usually becomes unwell at three to seven days, usually upon

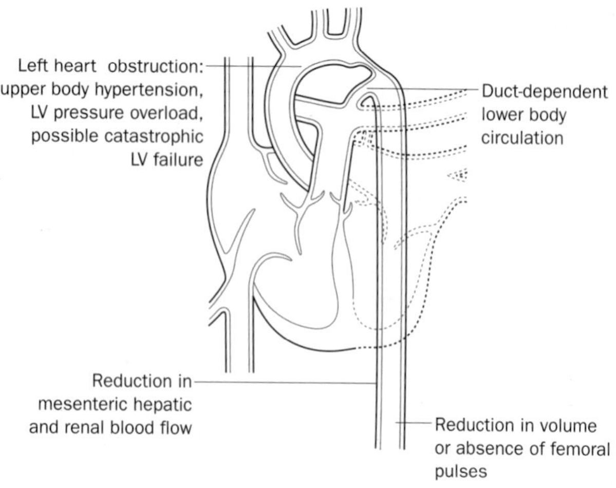

Figure 9.5 Infant coarctation of the aorta. LV, left ventricle

duct closure, and presents with cardiac failure or even circulatory collapse. In some cases, administration of prostaglandin to open the duct can improve the situation and assist in stabilizing the baby before surgery is undertaken. The older asymptomatic patient will be recognized by decreased or delayed femoral pulses, as above. *If the femorals are not examined the diagnosis is missed.* A significant proportion of cases are diagnosed after referral for a cardiac opinion because of a heart murmur, the diagnosis of coarctation having been missed by the referring doctor. Occasionally in older children or adults the diagnosis will be recognized because of systemic hypertension.

Relief of the obstruction is required to reduce the risk and effects of systemic hypertension. It is necessary as an emergency in the ill neonate and as soon as practical in the older patient to minimize the risk of persisting systemic hypertension. In the infant, this is usually undertaken by a surgical procedure. The procedure may use the left subclavian artery to augment the aortic diameter and the left arm pulse is subsequently impalpable. Alternatively, the coarctation segment is excised and the free ends of the aorta reanastomosed. Surgery is required in some older children but in others the obstruction can be dealt with by balloon dilation and/or stenting.

KEY LEARNING POINTS

- The neonate with coarctation presents with heart failure at about three to ten days.
- Do not miss coarctation as systemic hypertension/circulatory collapse may result.
- Feel the femorals as part of any clinical examination.
- Delay in the femorals is only found in older subjects – compare the volume.
- Infants require surgical repair, but older children may be treated by balloon dilation.

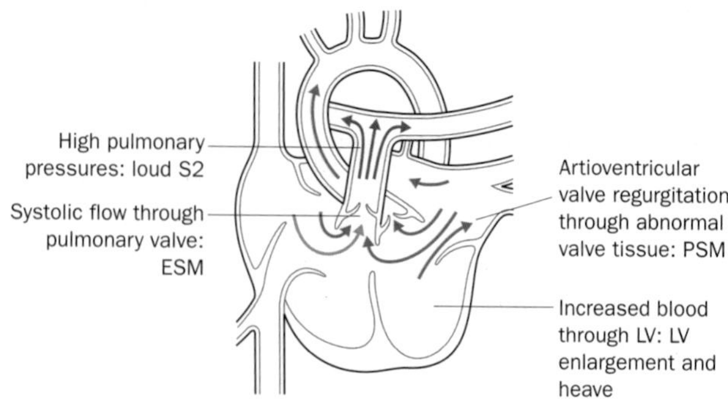

Figure 9.6 Atrioventricular septal defect. ESM, ejection systolic murmur; LV, left ventricle; PSM, pansystolic murmur

Atrioventricular septal defect

An AVSD (Figure 9.6) can present in a similar manner to a VSD or ASD. The basic anatomical defect is that there is a confluent defect with part of both the atrial and ventricular septae being deficient. If the atrioventricular valves are inserted directly into the ventricular septum there is no VSD and the signs are of an ASD. If not, there is both an ASD and VSD and the signs are usually of a large VSD. In addition, there are abnormalities of the inlet valves and regurgitation of variable severity will occur.

Management

Where there is a large ventricular component general medical care is similar to the infant with heart failure and a VSD. In the infant with a large shunt, surgery is necessary before six months of age to minimize the risk of pulmonary hypertension persisting. After surgery, there is still the possibility of problems related to valve regurgitation. If there is only an atrial shunt, surgical intervention can be delayed until the child is older.

KEY LEARNING POINTS

- An AVSD is common in Down syndrome.
- Signs are similar to a VSD but there may be a murmur of mitral regurgitation.

CASE STUDY

At routine clinical assessment at the 39-month screening examination a girl is found to have a murmur but to be otherwise well. On examination, the pulses are normal, there is no heave, there is a systolic thrill in the suprasternal notch, the second sound is normal with an ejection click at the mid left sternal edge and a moderately loud mid-systolic murmur at the base, maximal at the right upper sternal edge and radiating into the neck.

Q. What is the likely diagnosis?

A. Aortic valve stenosis – a murmur at the upper right sternal edge in an acyanotic child is likely to be aortic stenosis but can be an innocent carotid bruit. The suprasternal thrill would not be found in the carotid bruit. The ejection click indicates that the stenosis is at valve level.

Q. What other investigation could you readily undertake and interpret to assess the severity of the lesion.

A. An ECG will be normal with mild-to-moderate obstruction – if this was severe there are likely to be changes of left ventricular hypertrophy or ST changes suggesting ventricular strain.

HEART FAILURE

Heart failure has various definitions. In essence, it implies that the heart cannot meet requirements placed on it by the body. This might occur because a particular cardiac defect requires an increased cardiac output (e.g. VSD, AVSD, PDA), because the myocardium is impaired (e.g. dilated cardiomyopathy, myocarditis), or because the haemodynamic demands of the systemic circulation are too great (e.g. severe anaemia, atriovenous malformation, thyrotoxicosis). In an infant, this usually presents with dyspnoea, sweating, poor feeding and/or failure to thrive. In an older child, the symptoms are more in common with adult heart failure, where exertional dyspnoea, fatigue, orthopnoea and paroxysmal nocturnal dyspnoea predominate. The classic signs in a child are tachypnoea, tachycardia, hepatomegaly and sweating (diaphoresis). Often a heave and gallop will be present. The signs of the underlying condition will also be present, although notably a murmur may be absent in a large VSD or AVSD.

Management

Management of heart failure in a child must tackle both the underlying cause and the effect. The **medical treatment of cardiac failure** takes the form of supporting nutrition and weight gain and specific drug therapy. The infant usually requires nutritional supplements although even with these they may not gain weight and tube feeding may then become necessary. Drug therapy is undertaken with diuretics and afterload reduction. A suitable regimen for the neonate is with diuretics using a loop diuretic such as furosemide (0.5–1.0 mg/kg per dose two to three times daily) and an aldosterone antagonist such as spironolactone (0.5–1.0 mg/kg per dose two to three times daily). Afterload reduction is provided by use of an angiotensin converting enzyme (ACE) inhibitor, most frequently captopril, 0.1–1.0 mg/kg per dose two or three times daily. Prior to starting captopril the serum urea and potassium levels should be checked to ensure they are not raised, in which case introduction should be delayed. Rarely, captopril can produce severe hypotension so it should be introduced in a low dose (0.1 mg/kg) with blood pressure monitoring. The dose is then increased in a graded fashion with blood pressure monitoring after each rise. This generally requires admission to hospital for a few days. In recent years, the addition of a β-blocker has become established therapy and there is now some evidence that it may be more beneficial than ACE inhibitors. Carvedilol is currently the drug of choice, but it is likely that all β-blocking agents are of similar benefit. If the child has a dilated, poorly functioning ventricle, some form of anticoagulation should be considered. An antiplatelet dose of aspirin (2–5 mg/kg daily) is normally sufficient in the absence of identified thrombus within the heart.

Oxygen is often used in infants with heart failure in hospital. If a left-to-right shunt is responsible for this, oxygen will serve as a pulmonary vasodilator and may increase pulmonary blood flow and subsequent volume load. In these situations, it is generally best avoided.

CASE STUDY

A baby girl is referred at 3 weeks of age for assessment. She had a normal, uncomplicated delivery and had been thriving until one week previously. Since then she had been feeding poorly, sweating and her respiratory rate had increased. Examination shows a tachypnoeic infant with normal pulses, marked heave, loud second heart sound and a soft mid-systolic murmur at the lower left sternal edge.

Q. Name two likely diagnoses.

A. Ventricular septal defect and AVSD commonly present with symptoms and signs of heart failure a few weeks after birth – this coincides with a fall in the pulmonary vascular resistance, allowing blood to cross the ventricular septal defect, overloading both the pulmonary circulation and the left ventricle. If the defect is unrestrictive, a murmur may be soft or absent.

Q. What easy investigation will usually distinguish the two?

A. A 12-lead ECG will show left axis deviation in a child with AVSD whereas the axis will normally be to the right in VSD.

INVESTIGATION OF HEART DISEASE

Before considering the investigation of a child with a possible cardiac lesion, it has to be strongly emphasized that an initial clinical assessment is essential. Subsequent tests should then be interpreted in the light of the possible clinical diagnosis.

The chest radiograph and ECG are the only specific cardiac investigations readily available to the general paediatrician. These can give helpful information but echocardiography is often necessary for definitive anatomical and haemodynamic diagnosis, although in some children full elucidation of the lesion requires cardiac catheterization, computed tomography (CT) or magnetic resonance imaging (MRI) studies.

The chest radiograph

The relation between specific radiographic appearances and lesions has long been recognized and reported. However, in the modern age, most patients with cardiac lesions are recognized at an early age and in many there is not enough time for the changes that produce the classic appearances to develop fully. Thus, the chest radiograph may only have a limited part to play in reaching the diagnosis of the child with a suspected cardiac defect. It does have an important place in follow-up and when there may be associated lung disease.

The chest radiograph should be examined for the heart (size and configuration), pulmonary vascularity (normal, increased or decreased) and associated abnormalities. A semiquantitative assessment of the cardiac size can be calculated from the cardiothoracic ratio, the ratio of the cardiac diameter (the sum of the distance from the midline to the most right and left margins of the cardiac shadow) to the maximal internal thoracic one. In normal children, the ratio is less than 0.5 although it can be up to 0.55 in the first two years of life. This is not an absolute value and will be increased if the film is not taken in full inspiration or if it is taken anteroposteriorly, as in infants. The apex tends to be displaced downwards with left ventricular enlargement and directly to the left with right ventricular hypertrophy. In infants, the superior aspect of the cardiac shadow will vary with thymic size and shape. Increased pulmonary blood flow from a large left-to-right shunt is manifest as large vessels passing outwards from the hilum. With pulmonary oedema, the hilar vessels are less easily identified but the bronchi become more easily visible and, if severe, linear septal shadows appear in the lower lateral aspects of the lung fields. Narrow pulmonary vessels with increased lucency of the peripheral fields occur with significant obstruction to pulmonary blood flow.

In the **cyanotic neonate**, the main value of the chest radiograph is to assess the lung fields for abnormal increased markings typical of a lung problem such as respiratory distress syndrome (RDS) or transient tachypnoea of the newborn (TTN). Increased vascular lung markings are usually found in total anomalous pulmonary venous drainage (TAPVD), particularly when it is obstructed, and may be apparent in TGA or hypoplastic left heart syndrome. With a cardiac lesion causing reduced pulmonary flow (any with significant pulmonary obstruction) the lung fields may appear to be oligaemic. In some there is a characteristic appearance (Table 9.4).

Cardiomegaly is almost always found with cardiac failure or a significant cardiac defect resulting in volume overload. It is often caused by enlargement or dilatation of one or both ventricles from a shunt or valve

Table 9.4 Classic radiographic appearances of some cyanotic lesions

Lesion	Appearance
Tetralogy of Fallot	Small boot-shaped heart (absent pulmonary artery segment, apex up and to left); decreased lung markings
Transposition of the great arteries	Egg-on-its-side (when thymus shrinks giving narrow superior mediastinum)
Total anomalous pulmonary venous drainage	Small heart and marked increased lung markings/oedema if obstructed in neonate; snowman appearance of increased superior mediastinum in supracardiac lesions; does not occur in the neonatal period and will not be apparent until after 6 months of age
Ebstein anomaly	Very large/wall-to-wall heart of severe cardiomegaly

regurgitation, or left ventricular dysfunction (cardiomyopathy). In Ebstein anomaly, regurgitation through the tricuspid valve can produce marked right atrial dilatation and severe cardiomegaly (the wall-to-wall heart).

In the older child with a murmur the presence of a significant defect is likely to be apparent on clinical examination. The radiograph is of little practical value in trivial defects and is of virtually no value in deciding if a patient with a possibly innocent murmur has a minor defect.

The appearances in coarctation of the aorta ('figure of 3' at left aortic border), pulmonary stenosis (dilated pulmonary artery segment) and ASD (globular heart and increased lung flow) are not usually apparent in the early years of life and occur only in those in whom a significant defect has been overlooked and treatment delayed.

Barium swallow

In infants with stridor in whom a vascular ring is suspected, a barium swallow is the investigation of choice. A discrete posterior indentation in the oesophagus is indicative either of a ligamentous connection completing the ring or of a double aortic arch. A more diffuse, anterior and inferior indentation has previously been used as a marker of left atrial enlargement although this is now largely obsolete.

KEY LEARNING POINTS

- In the cyanotic neonate increased lung field markings may indicate lung, not cardiac, disease.
- Cardiomegaly is usually found with cardiac failure.
- The characteristic appearance of a specific lesion is not always apparent.

Electrocardiography

With the acceptance of echocardiography, there has become a tendency for paediatricians not to undertake ECG examinations. ECG does, however, have the advantage that it is readily available, carries no risk, can be interpreted with limited cardiology experience or even using the computer program interpretation usually provided by the ECG recording machine. The latter should not be accepted without review of the recording to confirm its accuracy and relevance to paediatric practice. A more detailed but still concise review of paediatric electrocardiography can readily be found in the *BMJ* (Goodacre and McLeod, 2002).

The ECG should be examined in a systematic way, looking in turn at the rate, rhythm, QRS axis and evidence of atrial or ventricular hypertrophy. The PR and QT intervals should be assessed if there are symptoms of fainting or loss of consciousness, particularly if this occurs on exercise.

Rate and rhythm

The standard ECG is recorded at 25 mm/s and standardized at 10 mm to 1 mV. Thus, each small box represents 0.04 s and 0.1 mV, or each larger box 0.2 s and 0.5 mV. The **rate** can be calculated many ways. A simple one is to take 10 large boxes (2 s), count the number of beats in this and multiply by 30 to give the rate in beats per minute. The **rhythm** is usually regular, but with normal sinus arrhythmia, there is a regular minor increase and decrease in R to R interval corresponding to slowing in inspiration and increasing rate in expiration. Where there is irregularity, the relationship of the P wave to QRS complex is examined. The PR interval (onset of P to onset of QRS complex) is usually 70–170 ms in children, increasing to 120–210 ms in adults. In first-degree atrioventricular (AV) block each P wave is followed by a QRS but the PR is prolonged. In 2:1 AV block the PR seems normal but there are two P waves for each QRS, the extra being exactly midway between the P waves preceding the QRS. Wenckebach phenomenon is uncommon in children – the PR interval progressively increases until a P wave is not followed by a QRS. Atrial flutter is most often observed in patients who have undergone previous surgery. It is manifest by regular P waves, usually peaked with a sawtooth appearance, with a QRS after every 2, 3 or 4. In complete heart block or A-V dissociation, the QRS complexes are regular but slow and the P waves are faster with no relation between them and the QRS complexes.

Frontal QRS axis

Full explanation and understanding of calculation of the QRS electrical axis is beyond the remit of this chapter. The electrical or **QRS axis** of the heart is the direction of the maximum electrical force during depolarization. It is assessed from the voltages in the limb leads as from 0° (directly left) in a clockwise direction to 90° (directly inferior) to 180° (right) then 270° (superior) and back to 359° and 0°. To calculate the QRS axis it is necessary to examine the limb leads and calculate the mean voltage from the sum of the R wave minus the S wave in each. If the R is greater than the S in each lead the sum will be positive, if the R is less than the S the sum will be negative.

There are two simple methods of deriving the **approximate** mean frontal QRS axis. The first is to find in which of the leads (I, II, III, aVR, aVL and aVF) the deflections above and below the line are most nearly equal. The mean frontal QRS axis is at right angles to this lead. If aVF is positive, it is between 1 and 179°, if negative between 181° and 359°. Alternatively, as a rule of thumb, the following can be used:

- I positive and aVF positive: 1–89°
- I negative and aVF positive: 91–179°
- I negative and aVF negative: 181–269°, extreme right axis deviation
- I positive and aVF negative: 271–359°, left axis deviation

The normal QRS axis at birth averages 135° (60–160°) and changes gradually to a mean of about 60° (10–100°) at 1 year. Right axis deviation is usually due to right ventricular hypertrophy, but left axis deviation is usually the result of a conduction abnormality of the left ventricle and is characteristically demonstrated with an AVSD tricuspid atresia.

Chamber/ventricular hypertrophy

Criteria for ventricular hypertrophy vary with age. In the early weeks or months of life, right ventricular dominance is normally present, with the left ventricle becoming dominant by the age of 6 months. Right ventricular forces are reflected in the voltage of the R waves in the right (V4R, V1 and V2) and the S waves over the left (V5 and V6) precordial leads. Left ventricular forces are reflected by R waves in the left (V5 and V6) and S waves in the right (V1) precordial leads. An rSR′ pattern (small r initially and larger one subsequently) is commonly associated with an ASD while an RSr′ is often not significant.

Simplified (not comprehensive) criteria suggesting chamber hypertrophy

Right ventricle
- T waves positive in V4R and V1 after 72 hours if R/S more than 1.0
- R in V1 more than 20 mV (0–4 years) or 15 mV for older
- S in V6 more than 10 mV (0–6 months) or 5 mV over 1 year

Left ventricle
- R in V6 more than 12 mV (neonate), 22 mV (6 months to 5 years), 25 mV for older
- S in V1 more than 20 mV at any age
- Sum of S in V1 and R in V5 or V6 >30 mV if under 1 year or >40 mV over 1 year
- Q wave 4 mV or more in V5 or V6
- T wave inversion in V5 or V6 (suggesting strain or ischaemia)

Right atrium
- P waves greater than 3 mV

Left atrium
- Bifid P in any lead with P of more than 0.09 s duration
- Late inversion of P wave in V1 >1.5 mV

QT interval

The QT interval is measured from the beginning of the QRS complex to the end of the T wave. Its duration varies with heart rate but can be corrected for this (QTc) using the RR interval in seconds and the formula:

$$\text{QTc} = \frac{\text{QT}}{\sqrt{\text{RR}}\ \text{(in seconds)}}$$

It is generally less than 0.42–0.44 s and a value of over 0.45 s should be considered abnormal. Its main relevance is in the prolonged QT syndrome where it is associated with the ventricular dysrhythmia torsades de pointes. This can degenerate to ventricular fibrillation and may present as episodes of sudden loss of consciousness with a risk of sudden death. It may also be lengthened in hypocalcaemia, myocardial disease and by certain drugs such as antihistamines, amiodarone and sotalol.

KEY LEARNING POINTS

- Left axis deviation in the cyanotic neonate suggests tricuspid atresia.
- Left axis deviation in an acyanotic child with a shunt suggests AVSD.
- An rSR′ pattern is often found with a significant ASD.
- T wave inversion in V5 or V6 indicates severe left ventricular hypertrophy or strain.
- Measure the QTc in a child with collapse, particularly if precipitated by exercise.

Ultrasound

Detailed knowledge of echocardiography is not expected in the MRCPCH examination but it is useful to understand the basic uses of this technique. The combination of imaging ultrasound with spectral and colour Doppler provides a good assessment of cardiac anatomy, haemodynamics and function. Two-dimensional echocardiography provides cross-sectional images of cardiac and vascular structures, and the M-mode (motion-mode) study a one-dimensional line through a chosen structure, this being of value in making exact measurements. Doppler echocardiography measures blood flow velocity, which can be used to measure pressure differences. Colour Doppler cannot accurately measure high velocities but does superimpose velocity information as a colour-coded signal on the cross-sectional image. Spectral Doppler measures flow velocity relatively accurately.

Imaging (cross-sectional) echocardiography can provide detailed images of intracardiac structures and abnormalities, allowing assessment of chamber sizes and cardiac function. The resolution of cross-sectional echocardiography may not show small defects such as a small VSD or duct; however, these can be demonstrated by colour Doppler flow mapping, which will show the flow velocity signal through the defect. The blood flow velocity is measured, colour coded and then superimposed upon the cross-sectional image. The relatively high velocity through a defect allows it to be picked out even if the defect cannot be imaged. It is important to realize that this is so sensitive that it can demonstrates physiological and normal valve regurgitation and defects such as a small VSD or PDA in which no murmur is audible. Spectral Doppler can measure the maximum velocity of flow from which a pressure drop across an obstruction or between different chambers or vessels can be calculated – the greater the gradient the higher the maximum flow velocity. From this, it is possible to calculate valve gradients and pulmonary artery pressure. Doppler also has some application in the measurement of volumetric flow and thus cardiac output, but the technique has many potential problems and is more of a research than a clinical tool.

KEY LEARNING POINTS

- Cross-sectional imaging shows intracardiac anatomy well.
- Demonstration of small defects requires colour Doppler study.
- Colour Doppler is so sensitive it shows normal physiological appearances which must not be interpreted as abnormal.
- Spectral Doppler allows pressure gradients and pulmonary pressure to be assessed.

Cardiac catheterization

The indications for catheterization in different centres will depend on the availability of equipment and individual expertise with the non-invasive techniques and acceptance of them by the surgeons. Diagnostic cardiac catheterization is undertaken to obtain detailed information on the haemodynamics such as shunt size, pressure gradients, pulmonary artery pressure and pulmonary vascular resistance. Angiocardiography is now less important for the elucidation of intracardiac defects, but it remains necessary for abnormalities of the great arteries or veins, in particular the anatomy of the pulmonary artery and its branches in situations where they are reduced in size.

Assessment of saturation and pressure data

First check if the aorta is fully saturated. A normal high aortic saturation indicates an **acyanotic lesion**. With a left-to-right shunt, there will be a rise in the oxygen level in the chamber at which the shunt occurs: from SVC to right atrium in ASD; at right ventricle in VSD; and pulmonary artery in PDA. If all right-sided oxygen levels are similar and low, and left ones high and similar there is no shunt, then look for evidence of stenosis: a high right ventricular pressure with a fall to pulmonary artery indicates pulmonary stenosis and a fall from left ventricle to aorta indicates aortic stenosis. A low aortic saturation indicates a **cyanotic lesion**. If the right-sided saturations are similar and low but there is a fall from left ventricle to aorta, there is a right-to-left shunt from right ventricle to aorta. There will be equal pressures in the ventricles and the likely diagnoses are tetralogy of Fallot (low pulmonary artery pressure) or Eisenmenger syndrome (high pulmonary artery pressures). In TGA, the saturations will be low in the right atrium, right ventricle and aorta with right ventricle and aortic pressures equal and high. The left atrium, left ventricle and pulmonary artery will have high saturations with low pressure in the left ventricle and pulmonary artery.

Catheterization is increasingly undertaken not for diagnostic purposes but for treatment. Balloon atrial septostomy for TGA and some other condition has long been undertaken and can be performed through the umbilical vein in the first days of life. Balloon dilation is the accepted technique for most cases of pulmonary valve stenosis and some with aortic stenosis and coarctation of the aorta. It may be beneficial in some with arterial stenosis but more frequently this is not of long-term value and insertion of a stent is required. Occlusive procedures are well developed for closure of the arterial duct (except in the preterm baby) and most cases of a secundum ASD. It is also used in selected cases of VSD.

Although cardiac catheterization is a relatively safe procedure, death can occur, most commonly in those with severe pulmonary hypertension. Complications of catheterization include femoral artery occlusion, dysrhythmias, intramyocardial injection with pericardial effusion and cerebral embolus or thrombosis. With interventional procedures there are risks of vessel rupture or device embolization and these should only be undertaken in centres where immediate cardiac surgical support is available.

Magnetic resonance imaging and computed tomography

Magnetic resonance imaging and CT are being used with increased frequency as an adjunct to echocardiography in the diagnosis of congenital heart disease. The non-invasive nature of the investigations gives them clear advantages over catheterization, although as yet catheter intervention is still performed almost exclusively under fluoroscopic control. Almost all aspects of intracardiac anatomy are seen well using MRI, although it is in the detailed assessment of the spatial arrangements of the intracardiac structures that it is of most use. This is particularly true with the widespread availability of three-dimensional and layering reconstruction software. Both MRI and high-speed CT image arteries and veins with great clarity. They are now the investigations of choice for assessment of aortic arch or branch pulmonary artery abnormalities, in addition to the monitoring of repaired coarctation. Magnetic resonance imaging has the advantage that it does not use ionizing radiation, but the slower acquisition times may necessitate a general anaesthetic, which is not required with CT. The prospect of MRI-guided catheter intervention is now being explored in a number of centres. As yet this is a research interest, but the ability to image in three dimensions during catheter intervention may revolutionize the specialty.

CLINICAL SKILLS

Recognition of abnormal findings

Clinical examination of the cardiovascular system is very important, and in most older children with a suspected defect, allows a fairly accurate clinical diagnosis to be reached. It can be less easy in the neonate and a clinical diagnosis may be difficult. Clinical examination of the cardiovascular system will almost always be required in the Part 2 examination. However, a full cardiovascular examination will not always be required, perhaps only palpation and auscultation of the praecordium will be asked for. It is important that you listen to what the examiner is saying and do what they have asked, not just what you want to do! For clinical purposes, a full clinical examination is mandatory. Clinical examination should be undertaken in a systematic manner to ensure all aspects are fully evaluated.

Steps in the systematic examination of the cardiovascular system

All should be recorded as positive or negative findings

General examination

Syndromes/dysmorphism
Cyanosis and clubbing

Evidence of cardiac failure

- Infant: tachypnoea, tachycardia, hepatomegaly
- Older child: breathlessness, oedema, hepatomegaly

Nutrition and growth

Pulses

Rate
Rhythm: regular or not, ectopics, sinus arrhythmia
Volume: normal, increased or decreased
Femorals compared to arm pulses: equal volume, any delay

Praecordium

Inspection

- Deformity: pectus, Harrison sulci
- Scars: median or lateral sternotomy, drain sites

Palpation

- Apex beat: palpable, displaced, interspace and relation to nipple line
- Heave: parasternal, epigastric
- Thrill: timing (almost all systolic), site

Auscultation

- Heart sounds: normal, loud P2, splitting of P2
- Murmur: loudness, quality, timing, maximal site and radiation

Clear presentation of the findings, both positive and negative is appropriate. If an aspect is normal, say so. Otherwise, the examiner may think you have not looked for this. Some indications of how to present the findings are given later (see below). It should be modified as necessary for abnormal findings.

General examination

A general impression of the child's condition is the starting point of the examination.

Nutrition and growth

Failure to gain weight is a common problem in the infant with heart failure. This results from a combination of difficulty in feeding due to breathlessness and increased metabolic requirements. It is not commonly due to cyanotic heart disease alone. However, a number of infants with congenital heart disease tend to be small, not just because of poor intake, and will remain so later in life.

Cyanosis

Cyanosis due to congenital heart disease is central and apparent on the lips or tongue, present at all times and more marked on crying. If there is doubt, oxygen saturation can be measured and this should be done in the right arm. In an examination situation, the infant may be connected to a saturation monitor, so look for this in your general examination. This central cyanosis is distinct from the toddler and young child in whom episodes of facial blueness occur for no apparent reason, presumably related to a change in vascular tone. There is no significant murmur and the child is well during an episode, which lasts for up to about 20 minutes. Characteristically this is noted round the mouth rather than on the lips and the mother will make a circle round the mouth when asked to indicate the site of this. If the child is fully oxygenated and has no physical signs, further investigation is not necessary but the parents must be reassured.

Clubbing

Clubbing is initially recognized as loss of the angle of the nails. It does not occur in early life and will not become apparent until towards the end of the first year.

Heart failure

Heart failure in the infant presents differently from later in life and is usually a mixture of left and right heart failure. The main signs are respiratory (tachypnoea, dyspnoea or indrawing due to increased pulmonary flow or raised left atrial pressure), tachycardia and hepatomegaly (due to raised right atrial and central venous pressure). Other reported signs such as excessive sweating, failure to gain weight and fluid retention are later ones and not commonly found on presentation in the modern era. In the older child, the presentation is similar to the adult with breathlessness and oedema, and signs will include tachypnoea, crepitations or hepatomegaly depending on the cause. Treatment of heart failure has been considered earlier in the chapter (see above).

Presentation of above if normal: A healthy looking, well nourished child; no cyanosis or clubbing; no tachypnoea or hepatomegaly.

Pulse rate and volume and femoral pulses

Pulse rate should be recorded. In the neonate it is usually 120–150 beats per minute, for an infant 85–125, for a 3–5-year-old 75–115, and after 6 years falls progressively to 60–100. Rate will be increased in heart failure or sinus tachycardia due to other factors such as fever or shock. In supraventricular tachycardia (SVT) it will usually not be possible to count the rate by palpation or auscultation as it is over 200 beats per minute. In children the rhythm will usually be regular or, in the older ones, exhibit sinus arrhythmia with the rate increasing on inspiration and decreasing on expiration. Occasional atrial or ventricular ectopics can occur but do not usually indicate a problem. Atrial fibrillation will cause pulse irregularity but is very uncommon in children. Atrial flutter is usually associated with older children with ongoing cardiac problems but the rate will normally be regular.

Pulse volume can theoretically be useful, being decreased with left ventricular outflow obstruction (aortic stenosis) and increased with increased left ventricle output and diastolic run-off (aortic regurgitation and PDA). However, this only occurs with severe lesions that are commonly recognized and treated early in developed countries so pulse volume is usually of limited value. In the infant, these may be apparent at early diagnosis but there will be other more marked signs and the presence of congenital heart disease will not normally be in doubt.

Careful examination of the femoral pulses is mandatory in children. Ideally, the femoral should be palpated with one hand and the right arm pulse with the other. If there is difficult in feeling the radial pulse, try the brachial or axillary. The main abnormality in coarctation is in the volume of the pulses, with femorals being lower. In older children, femoral delay may be apparent. *If the femorals are not examined the diagnosis will be missed.* In active infants, the femorals can be difficult to feel and simultaneous assessment is not possible. However, if they are easily felt or the foot pulses are of good volume there is not likely to be coarctation.

Presentation of above if normal: The pulse was regular, rate xx beats per minute and of normal volume (xx is the measured rate). Comparing the right arm with the femoral, they were of equal volume with no delay.

Blood pressure

Blood pressure should be measured as part of any clinical examination. In the examination situation there may not be time for this so state words to the effect that 'I would normally measure the blood pressure but have not had time to do so'. If coarctation is suspected arm and leg blood pressure measurements are theoretically useful, but this is difficult in younger patients and of limited value.

Praecordial examination

Praecordial examination takes the form of inspection, palpation and auscultation. Percussion of the heart is not normally undertaken.

INSPECTION

Inspection for chest deformities should be undertaken but those related to a cardiac lesion are only apparent with longstanding disease and other signs will normally be apparent.

A median sternotomy scar (centrally down the sternum) usually indicates previous bypass or open heart surgery, and a lateral thoracotomy (in the back approximately along the lower margin of the scapula) indicates previous great artery surgery. A Blalock–Tausig shunt is undertaken for cyanotic lesions with reduced pulmonary artery flow and usually performed on the right, but occasionally on the left. A left thoracotomy is undertaken for surgery for PDA closure, coarctation repair or pulmonary artery banding.

PALPATION

Palpation should encompass three aspects: apex beat, right ventricle heave and presence of a thrill. A displaced apex usually means left ventricle dilation, which in congenital heart disease is due to volume overload. However, it can be difficult to palpate the apex in children – if it cannot be felt it is likely that it is not displaced. A right ventricle heave is felt in the left parasternal area and in the older child indicates right ventricle volume overload, the commonest cause of which is an ASD. It is important to recognize that in the infant with a significant lesion an impulse can commonly be palpated in the subxiphoid area rather than the left sternal edge. This is not simply due to right ventricle overload but can be felt with any hyperdynamic lesion. This sign can be useful in deciding whether an infant has a cardiac or respiratory problem as it is rarely found in the latter.

THRILL

A thrill can be felt where there is a loud (at least 4/6) murmur. It is important to realize that the maximum thrill and volume of the murmur should be found at the same site. If not, reassess the clinical findings. The exception to this is a suprasternal thrill, which is almost always related to aortic stenosis but may occasionally be found with other lesions. This sign can be particularly useful in the patient with subaortic stenosis when the murmur can be loudest at the left sternal edge, suggesting the diagnosis of a VSD.

AUSCULTATION

Auscultation should start with the **heart sounds.** Although much has been written about variations, the only important ones are related to the second sound at the pulmonary area. This can be accentuated in the acyanotic patient with pulmonary hypertension. In cyanotic patients the aorta is often relatively anterior causing the second sound to be accentuated – it rarely indicates pulmonary artery hypertension in this situation. It will be loud in the Eisenmenger syndrome. The second sound can be recognized to be split – the first component being closure of the aortic valve and the second the pulmonary valve. Normally this is wider in inspiration (due to the increased venous return to the right side and thence to the lungs) and narrower in expiration. In the older child with a large ASD, the splitting is wide and does not vary. However, recognition of this is difficult and really beyond the standard required for the trainee paediatrician, albeit a desirable skill. For this, listen to the heart sounds, recognize the first and second and concentrate only on the second. Do not attempt to recognize the breathing pattern but try to distinguish the two components and assess whether they are wider at some time and closer or single at another. In describing the heart sounds it is inappropriate to say 'On auscultation "heart sounds one and two" or "the first and second heart sounds were heard"'. This is the equivalent of saying 'On examination of the abdomen "I palpated the abdomen"'. State that the heart sounds were normal! A third heart sound (just after the second) can be heard in some with heart failure but can also be normal in children and adolescents. Gallop rhythm due to fast heart rate and presence of a summated third and fourth (just before the first) heart sound occurs with heart failure. An ejection click, a sound occurring shortly after the first sound, is associated with a stenotic or bicuspid aortic or pulmonary valve. It occurs when the valve is pliable but does not open fully and its opening is abruptly stopped.

A **murmur** is the main feature that allows an accurate clinical diagnosis of an acyanotic congenital heart defect to be reached. However, it should not be taken in isolation and it is important to assess the features above. The first objective is to find the site of maximal intensity. For this the four classical sites (apex, lower left sternal edge, upper left sternal edge, upper right sternal edge) should be auscultated and the maximal determined. Start at the site of maximal intensity and then move the stethoscope a centimetre or so after listening only for a few seconds. If the intensity is greater, the stethoscope should be moved on for a short time, and so on until it becomes quieter and then back to the loudest site. This will also allow the radiation of the murmur to be assessed. The intensity should then be determined. For a systolic murmur you can use the classification of 1/6 to 6/6, 1/6 being soft, 4/6 associated with a precordial thrill and 6/6 audible with the stethoscope off the chest. Alternatively, at least state whether it is soft, moderately loud or very loud. Diastolic murmurs are rarely loud, and the numerical classification from 1/4 to 4/4 is used. The quality can be difficult to judge with limited experience, particularly for those who are not musical. Timing of a murmur should be assessed not simply as systolic or diastolic but by duration, such as pansystolic (from first to beyond the second heart sound) or ejection/mid-systolic or early or mid-diastolic. A murmur is produced by turbulent blood flow, and it will be apparent over the part of the heart where the turbulence occurs. These are illustrated for the common acyanotic defects in Figure 9.7 and summarized in Table 9.5. Similarly, its timing will be when the flow is occurring, as discussed under specific lesions. When listening for a murmur it is appropriate to use both the diaphragm and bell of the stethoscope – if the bell is not used low pitched mid-diastolic mitral or tricuspid murmurs may not be heard.

Although a murmur is audible with many lesions, it is important to remember that a significant defect can be present with no murmur. For this, the other aspects of examination described above are essential.

PRESENTATION OF ABOVE IF NORMAL

Examination of the praecordium:

- on inspection, there were no deformities and no scars
- on palpation, the apex beat was not displaced being in the xx interspace within the mid-clavicular line, there was no right ventricular heave and there was no thrill (xx is the measured interspace)
- on auscultation, the heart sounds were normal. There was no murmur.

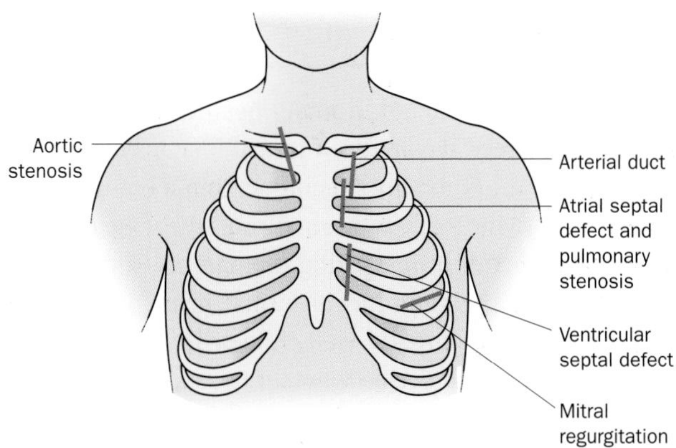

Figure 9.7 Usual sites where murmurs are heard maximally

Table 9.5 Common clinical findings related to anatomical and haemodynamic effects of lesion

	Ventricular septal defect	Atrial septal defect	Persistent ductus arteriosus	Pulmonary stenosis	Aortic stenosis	Coarctation of the aorta
Pulses	Normal	Normal	Collapsing or normal	Normal	Normal or reduced	Femorals reduced or delayed
Ventricular activity	Left (volume) if large shunt. Right if PAH	Right (volume) if large shunt	Left (volume) if large shunt	Right pressure	Left pressure	Left pressure outwith neonatal period
Heart sounds	Loud II if PAH	Wide split II	Normal	Click if pliable valve	Click if pliable valve	Click if bicuspid aortic valve
Murmur						
Systole	Pan/mid-LLSE	Ejection ULSE	Continuous ULSE	Ejection ULSE – clavicle	Ejection URSE – neck	Variable/absent At back
Diastole	Mid apex if large shunt	Mid-LLSE if large shunt		None	None	Unusual

LLSE, lower left sternal edge; PAH, pulmonary arterial hypertension; ULSE, upper left sternal edge; URSE, upper right sternal edge.

KEY LEARNING POINTS

- You are likely to have to examine the cardiovascular system in the clinical exam.
- If so, listen to what the examiner is saying and do what has been asked.
- Palpation of the femoral pulses is mandatory in a full cardiovascular examination.
- In the infant the presence of a subxiphoid heave strongly suggests a cardiac lesion.
- Determination of the site of maximum volume of a murmur is vital for making a diagnosis.

The main clinical findings of acyanotic lesions are given in Table 9.5.

Asymptomatic and possibly innocent murmur

A murmur may be heard in many healthy children with no cardiac defect. A variety of terms have been used for this finding, the commonest being an 'innocent murmur'. Alternatively, the term a 'normal murmur' can be used and may be better in reassuring the parents that there is no defect and the child has a normal heart. When presented with an apparently well child with a murmur the paediatrician has to decide whether the murmur is innocent or not. If it is considered to be due to a cardiac lesion a further decision is required as to whether it is of clinical importance and needs referral to a cardiologist. It is difficult to explain in words how to recognize an innocent murmur and experience is needed before being confident in determining this. However, there are specific features that can assist in making such a judgement.

The child will be healthy and asymptomatic (no cardiac symptoms). There will be no other cardiovascular finding, in particular, there will be normal femoral pulses, no heaves and the second heart sound will be normal. The murmur will generally be soft and systolic (with the exception of the venous hum, which is continuous). It may alter with position, time and the child's condition (tachycardia or fever). In making the assessment it is useful to consider what lesion could produce a murmur at the same site. Since coarctation is diagnosed from the femoral pulses, the distinction is from the common acyanotic lesions, a shunt (ASD, VSD or PDA) or ventricular outlet (pulmonary or aortic) stenosis. Figure 9.7 indicates the common sites of the murmur of an acyanotic lesion. Innocent murmurs can, to some extent, be classified as in Table 9.6, which shows the other likely diagnoses. The commonest is the Still's murmur, which is heard maximally at the mid to low left sternal edge and must be distinguished from a VSD. It may (but not necessarily) decrease in volume if the child is examined sitting up. A similar murmur may be louder toward the apex and radiate towards the left sternal edge. The cause of these murmurs is not known. The carotid bruit is due to flow in the great vessels in the neck, is loudest in the neck and softer in the aortic area, as distinct from aortic stenosis when it will be louder at the upper right sternal edge and softer in the neck. A mid-systolic murmur in the upper left sternal edge is probably from flow across the pulmonary valve, but there is no stenosis. The differentiation would then be from mild pulmonary stenosis or a small ASD. A variation in this is a flow murmur from the pulmonary artery branches, which is more common in preterm babies. This is heard at the base, often on both sides, and radiates to the axillae and to the back. In many cases this disappears as the child grows. The venous hum results from flow in the great neck veins and is louder when sitting up and thus most often recognized in the toddler who has to be examined sitting on the mother's knee. It is usually heard under the right clavicle, but may be audible on the left. It is continuous in timing and has to be distinguished from a PDA. It is best recognized by the fact that it can be made to disappear if the head is rotated, the neck is gently compressed to stop venous flow, or the child lies down.

Table 9.6 Common innocent murmurs and lesions from which they should be distinguished

Type	Site	Distinguish from
Still's	Mid-systolic mid or low LSE	VSD
Apical systolic	Musical, mid-systolic	VSD, mitral regurgitation
Pulmonary	Soft, mid-systolic	Pulmonary stenosis, ASD
Carotid bruit	Mid-systolic, louder in neck than aortic area	Aortic stenosis
Venous hum	Continuous under right clavicle; usually in toddler sitting up; decreases supine, neck movement or pressure	PDA

ASD, atrial septal defect; LSE, left sternal edge; PDA, persistent ductus arteriosus; VSD, ventricular septal defect.

The question often asked is: What investigations should be undertaken in a child with an innocent murmur? If the murmur is clearly innocent, there is no need for any investigation. Investigation may be appropriate if the question is: Is this an innocent murmur or a minor abnormality, e.g. VSD, mild pulmonary stenosis? An ECG may be useful. If it shows the rSR′ pattern of an ASD, or hypertrophy it is possible that the lesion has been wrongly assessed as being of minor clinical significance. However, in distinguishing an innocent murmur from a minor lesion there is virtually no value in undertaking a chest radiograph – it simply exposes the child to radiation.

There is an increasing tendency for paediatricians to refer children for echocardiographic assessment by technical staff with limited training in paediatric echocardiography. The authors have seen incorrect diagnoses on this basis but accept that more and more people are undertaking this. If requesting an echocardiographic examination in a patient with a murmur it is essential that the technician be asked to answer the question: What lesion is considered possible? A blanket request for echocardiography for 'a murmur' is inappropriate. If there is any doubt as to the significance of a murmur and the correct management, the child should be referred for a cardiac assessment. If the cardiologist has any doubt an ultrasound examination can be performed, particularly Doppler to ensure there is no minor defect.

CASE STUDY

At routine clinical assessment at the 39-month screening examination a girl is found to have a soft mid-systolic murmur at the mid to low left sternal edge. This had not previously been commented on. She had previously attended routine examinations and had been admitted to hospital at the age of 30 months with a respiratory illness. She is well with no other cardiovascular findings, in particular, there is no heave and the femoral pulses are normal.

Q. What is the likely diagnosis?

A. Innocent/normal murmur – likely diagnosis for a murmur at the lower left sternal edge is either a VSD or an innocent murmur. A VSD would likely have been heard at the hospital admission.

Q. You examine the child and confirm this diagnosis. What action would you take next?

A. Explain and reassure the parents and discharge from follow-up – an ECG might be a reasonable test that might show an rSR′ if there were an ASD. This is more likely with a murmur at the upper left sternal edge. If there was doubt, a referral to a more experienced colleague would be correct.

THE NEONATE WITH SUSPECTED CONGENITAL HEART DISEASE

Duct-dependent cyanotic lesions

Most of the lesions presenting with significant heart disease in the neonatal period are duct dependent, the neonate appearing well at birth but subsequently becoming ill when the ductus arteriosus closes.

Obstruction to pulmonary flow (oligaemia on chest radiograph)

All cyanotic lesions with obstruction to pulmonary flow have either pulmonary atresia or severe pulmonary stenosis. This can be in the context of a number of different lesions, including severe tetralogy of Fallot, single ventricle or pulmonary atresia with or without a VSD. There is little effect on the fetus since oxygenation is undertaken by the placenta. At birth, cyanosis may not be recognized as the duct will be patent allowing flow from the aorta to the lungs, and thence oxygenated blood back to the heart and onwards to the aorta. As the duct closes, pulmonary flow and return of oxygenated blood to the heart will reduce and cyanosis will become apparent. The severity of cyanosis depends on the degree of pulmonary obstruction and becomes severe for those with pulmonary atresia or severe stenosis.

Emergency treatment with intravenous (IV) prostaglandin to open the duct can be life saving and can be given through the umbilical or systemic veins. Dinoprostone (prostaglandin E2 (PGE2)) is given in the recommended dose of 5–50 ng/kg per minute. The only potential serious side effect of this is apnoea. If this occurs the infusion should be stopped, respiration supported by bag and mask and when breathing recovers the infusion restarted at a lower dose. Alternatively, the infant can be intubated and ventilated. If transfer on PGE2 therapy is necessary it is essential that full facilities for respiratory support are available or the infant is intubated and ventilated. Other side effects include tachypnoea, fever, diarrhoea and jitteriness. In most cases, subsequent surgical intervention initially takes the form of the construction of a modified Blalock–Taussig shunt, which is the insertion of a prosthetic 'tube' between the subclavian and pulmonary artery (usually on the right). This is undertaken through a lateral thoracotomy

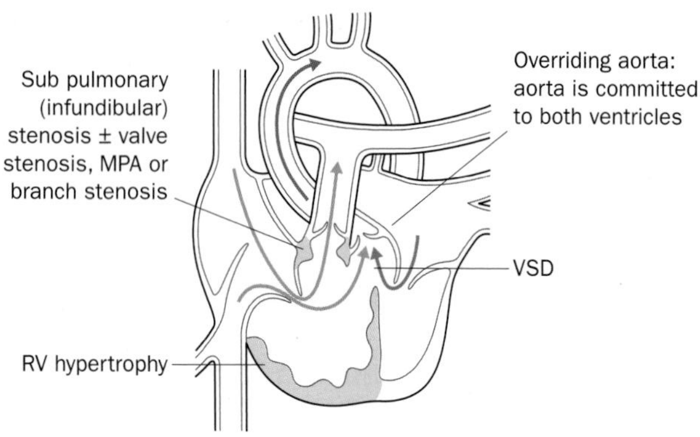

Figure 9.8 Tetralogy of Fallot. MPA, main pulmonary artery; RV, right ventricle; VSD, ventricular septal defect

incision. Subsequent corrective or palliative surgery will depend on the nature of the abnormality.

Tetralogy of Fallot

The main defects in tetralogy of Fallot (Figure 9.8) are a VSD and pulmonary stenosis. The VSD is such that it is overridden by the aorta. The pulmonary stenosis can be at variable sites with narrowing at the level of the pulmonary artery, valve ring or subpulmonary area. This obstruction causes the right ventricular pressure to rise and the development of muscular hypertrophy, as in the original description of the four features of tetralogy.

The clinical presentation will depend on the severity of the outflow obstruction. If very severe, cyanosis will be apparent from birth (as in the preceding discussion). If the obstruction is less severe there may be limited cyanosis, but in most cases, this will become more apparent with time as muscular hypertrophy in the outflow tract becomes more severe and less of the right ventricular output goes to the pulmonary artery and more goes to the aorta.

Clinically, there is variable cyanosis and an ejection murmur due to the pulmonary obstruction – this is often at the mid-sternal edge since the obstruction is below the pulmonary valve. Some patients may experience 'blue spells', probably related to increased subpulmonary obstruction, in which they can become exceptionally cyanosed. Immediate treatment of these is by the use of IV morphine or propranolol and longer-term propranolol until surgery is undertaken.

Surgical repair is by VSD closure and appropriate procedures to relieve any obstruction. In some with significant cyanosis or spells, a Blalock–Taussig shunt is appropriate before this to improve oxygenation and allow the child to grow prior to corrective surgery.

Transposition of the great arteries

In TGA, the pulmonary and systemic circulations function in parallel, not in series (Figure 9.9). The systemic venous (low oxygen) return passes via right atrium to the right ventricle and thence aorta and recirculates round the body. The pulmonary venous (high oxygen) return passes via the left atrium to the left ventricle and back to the pulmonary artery. To survive there must be mixing between the two circulations, largely deoxygenated to the lungs through the duct and oxygenated to the body through the foramen ovale. When the duct closes, survival depends on bidirectional flow through the atrial septum. This can be facilitated by a balloon atrial septostomy to create a tear in the flap valve of the foramen ovale and increase the size of the atrial septal communication. Prior to this, it is appropriate to administer IV prostaglandin to open the duct and improve the oxygenation. The atrial septostomy is usually performed under ultrasound control, using either the umbilical (first days of life) or femoral vein.

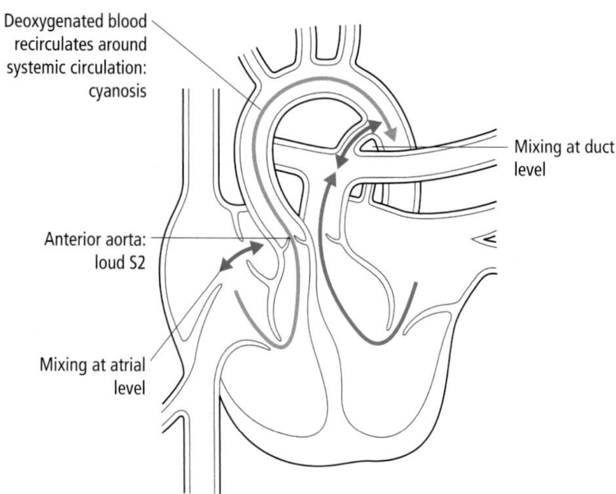

Figure 9.9 Transposition of the great arteries

Subsequent treatment is usually undertaken by an arterial switch operation with attachment of the aorta to the previous pulmonary valve, pulmonary artery to the aortic valve, and transfer of the coronary orifices to the neo-aorta. This has to be undertaken within the first weeks or life. If it is delayed, the normal fall in the pulmonary artery pressure will result in the left ventricle pumping at low pressure and 'de-training' and becoming unable to support the high-pressure systemic circulation after a switch operation.

Duct-dependent lesions with obstruction to systemic flow

Heart failure in the first days of life is a recognized feature of lesions with severe obstruction to aortic flow. This can be at the level of the aortic valve (critical aortic stenosis or left heart hypoplasia) or arch (interrupted aortic arch or coarctation of the aorta). In the fetus, the duct allows flow to the area distal to the obstruction and fetal wellbeing is ensured, but when the duct closes the distal blood supply is reduced. The classic example of this is left heart hypoplasia. The pulmonary venous return to the left atrium cannot continue through the left ventricle to the aorta. The left atrial pressure rises and the blood passes from left to right through the foramen ovale. The mixed systemic and pulmonary venous return flows to the right ventricle, pulmonary artery and, when the duct is open, through the duct to the descending aorta with retrograde flow supplying the arch, ascending aorta and coronary arteries. When the duct closes, the systemic flow is reduced, severe heart failure develops and perfusion of the systemic organs is inadequate. This produces severe collapse and heart failure at about 2 or 3 days of life.

In severe coarctation of the aorta, the head and neck are perfused normally from the left ventricle. Flow to the descending aorta is duct dependent, either through the duct or round the narrowed area if it impinges on the mouth of an open duct. Duct closure limits abdominal perfusion and in severe cases produces severe heart failure and metabolic derangement, usually at 3–7 days of life.

As in the cyanotic lesions, the administration of prostaglandin to open the duct can be life saving.

Clinical features and assessment

The neonate with a cardiac lesion usually presents with cyanosis, tachypnoea or collapse. Where there is respiratory distress or cyanosis there may be difficulty in distinguishing between a cardiac and pulmonary cause of the problem. The following section provides guidance for the paediatrician, but if there is any doubt a paediatric cardiologist should be contacted and the situation discussed.

Severe cyanosis (low pO_2)

In duct-dependent lesions, cyanosis may not be apparent at birth but becomes so as the duct closes. Clinical examination is important but this can be of limited value in the ill neonate. Respiratory signs, particularly tachypnoea or dyspnoea, are likely to be present if there is lung disease but may also be present in some cardiac conditions, particularly if a metabolic acidosis is present. Signs of cardiovascular disease should then be sought. A subxiphoid heave is usually associated with a heart problem but on occasions may be the result of a pulmonary problem causing pulmonary hypertension. It is important to know that significant heart disease can be present in the absence of a murmur or heave, e.g. in uncomplicated TGA. An ejection murmur would suggest outflow obstruction as a possibility.

The chest radiograph is important (see below) to assess the lung fields for any evidence of a neonatal lung condition. Lung fields are relatively clear in most cyanotic cardiac lesions, the major exception being obstructed TAPVD where the lung markings are significantly increased due to pulmonary venous obstruction and the cardiac shadow is classically small. Clear lung fields strongly suggest a cardiac lesion, particularly with heart failure. The heart size, which may be increased in a number of cardiac lesions. It is important to know that the chest radiograph can be interpreted as normal in the neonate with most significant cyanotic cardiac lesions.

A hyperoxic test has been used as a means to try to differentiate heart from lung causes of cyanosis. The basis of this is that if cyanosis is due to a cardiac lesion with reduced pulmonary blood flow or TGA, there will be little rise in blood pO_2 on increasing the inspired gas from air to 100 per cent oxygen. If there is a lung problem, there should be a rise in the oxygen saturation. This is not definitive but failure of the saturation to rise is suggestive of a cardiac cause of cyanosis. Since most of these lesions are duct dependent, it may be more appropriate to assess the effect of IV prostaglandin. This is unlikely to cause a significant deterioration in lung disease, but if the saturation rises, a cardiac cause is almost certainly present. This will also have a therapeutic benefit and can then be continued.

An ECG recorded correctly is difficult to obtain in the acute situation in the neonatal intensive care unit. It is of limited value in identifying a cardiac defect. The exception is in tricuspid atresia (usually with significant pulmonary obstruction) where there is classically left axis deviation and left ventricular hypertrophy.

Respiratory distress with or without moderate cyanosis

In respiratory distress with or without moderate cyanosis, the important decision is between lung disease or a cardiac problem causing heart failure. Both cardiac and respiratory causes can result in decreased pulse volume, although a cardiac lesion with left ventricular outflow obstruction is more likely. The finding of lower-volume femorals than the right arm indicates coarctation of the aorta but this does not usually present in the first day or two of life although interruption of the arch may. Reduced volume arm pulses compared to the femorals may occasionally be found in left heart hypoplasia and an open arterial duct. A murmur may be heard with severe aortic stenosis, but in other conditions may be unimpressive. A subxiphoid heave strongly suggests a cardiac cause.

A chest radiograph is essential. An increase in the lung markings is almost always seen with heart failure and specific findings are likely with neonatal respiratory problems. An increase in the cardiothoracic ratio strongly suggests a cardiac problem. The ECG is of little value. Prostaglandin infusion may improve the situation in left heart outflow problems (left heart hypoplasia, critical aortic stenosis, aortic arch obstruction) but is not a reliable diagnostic test.

KEY LEARNING POINTS

- The differentiation between cardiac and lung disease can be difficult in the neonate.
- If there is any doubt discuss the situation with the paediatric cardiologist.
- The clinical finding of a subxiphoid heave suggests a cardiac lesion.
- Severe cyanosis without respiratory signs suggest a cardiac defect.
- Oxygen rise with prostaglandin make a cardiac defect likely.
- Assess the chest radiograph for the lung fields and heart size.
- ECG is of limited value – do not delay, contact the cardiologist.

CASE STUDY

A baby boy is born at 39 weeks' gestation weighing 3.8 kg. He appears well at birth but at 6 hours is thought to be cyanosed. There are no other abnormal clinical findings. Capillary gases show pH 7.38, pO_2 28 torr, pCO_2 39 torr, base excess 0.

Q. What is the likely diagnosis?

A. Transposition of the great arteries or complex heart disease with pulmonary atresia – low oxygen saturation can be the result of heart or lung disease. Since there is no tachypnoea or other lung findings and a normal pCO_2 this is not likely to be respiratory in origin. The likely cardiac conditions are duct-dependent cyanotic lesions, either TGA or a complex abnormality with severe obstruction to pulmonary flow. The absence of a murmur means that if it were in the latter group it is not likely that there is pulmonary stenosis, but rather pulmonary atresia.

Q. What action could you readily undertake to try to confirm the diagnosis?

A. Give IV infusion of PGE – a chest radiograph would be useful in identifying a lung problem but this is not likely in this case. The hyperoxic test with no significant rise in pO_2 would be in favour of a cardiac cause and thus an appropriate answer. The PGE infusion with a rise in the pO_2 would clearly demonstrate the effect of ductal opening and confirm the diagnosis of duct-dependent cyanotic heart disease.

CASE STUDY

A baby boy is born at 39 weeks' gestation weighing 3.8 kg. He appears well at birth. He feeds poorly, and at 30 hours, he is noted to be unwell with poor colour and breathlessness. On examination he appears unwell with a cyanotic tinge, and respiratory rate is 60 per minute with indrawing. On palpation the liver edge is 2 cm below the costal margin, there is a subxiphoid heave and all pulses are difficult to palpate. No murmur is heard. Saturation is 65 per cent.

Q. What is the likely diagnosis?

A. Hypoplastic left heart syndrome – the infant has heart failure and poor cardiac output, suggesting left ventricular outflow obstruction. It is unlikely to be a lung problem. Since all the pulses are poor arch interruption or coarctation are less likely, and the absence of a murmur would be against critical aortic stenosis.

Q. What investigation could *you readily* undertake to try to confirm the diagnosis (i.e. not echocardiography)?

A. Chest radiograph – this is likely to show cardiomegaly and a generalized increase in lung markings. The cardiomegaly would fit with a significant cardiac lesion. The lung appearances are not those of pulmonary conditions presenting at this age. This will only indicate a cardiac lesion and not the specific diagnosis. Prostaglandin infusion may improve the neonate's condition but is relatively slow to take effect in this case. It should be given but for its therapeutic effect rather than diagnosis.

ACQUIRED HEART DISEASE

Infective endocarditis

Transient bacteraemia is common after many surgical procedures and can result in bacterial endocarditis, usually superimposed on an underlying congenital or rheumatic heart defect. The diagnosis should be considered in any child with a cardiac lesion who is unwell with a febrile illness and antibiotic therapy should not be started until a number of blood samples (ideally six but at least three) have been taken for culture. *Streptococcus viridans* (α-haemolytic streptococcus) and *Staphylococcus aureus* are the main causes of infection in unoperated children, whereas Gram-negative and fungal endocarditis are more often a cause in children with previous cardiac surgery, particularly where there is an intracardiac prosthesis. Failure to grow an organism from blood cultures may result from previous antibiotic therapy or indicate an unusual infecting organism. Haematuria may be present but other 'classic' manifestations of infective endocarditis now are rare. Specific investigations are generally unhelpful though inflammatory markers and white cell count are usually raised and a vegetation may be shown with echocardiography, particularly transoesophageal. Usually the organism isolated should guide antibiotic therapy, however, if none is grown from blood cultures, broad-spectrum cover including that for atypical agents can be used. All antibiotics should be given intravenously and generally for at least six weeks.

Prophylaxis against infective endocarditis is generally recommended for a patient at risk who is undergoing any surgical procedure likely to cause bacteraemia. Infection is more likely with left-sided lesions. Recent recommendations suggest antibiotic cover should be given for any cardiac lesion generating turbulent blood flow or a high-velocity jet. Indications for prophylaxis include surgery to the abdomen, upper respiratory or genitourinary tract, following burns and while receiving IV alimentation. It is required for dental treatment causing bleeding of the gums, particularly extractions, but not for simple fillings or when deciduous teeth are shedding. It is not considered necessary for gastrointestinal endoscopy without biopsy except in those with intracardiac prostheses.

The appropriate prophylactic regimen is determined by the nature of the procedure. Details of a simple suitable antibiotic prophylaxis regimen, taken largely from the recommendations of the British Society for Antimicrobial Chemotherapy, are given in the box below.

Simplified antibiotic prophylaxis regimen against infective endocarditis

Dental extractions, upper respiratory tract surgery

Under local anaesthesia: single oral dose one hour before procedure.

- Over 10 years of age, amoxicillin 3 g or if allergic to penicillin clindamycin 600 mg
- 5–10 years half the dose
- Below 5 years one quarter of dose

Under general anaesthesia: amoxicillin orally four hours before and as soon as possible on waking.

- Over 10 years 3 g each dose
- 5–10 years half the dose
- Below 5 years one quarter the dose

OR

intravenous just before induction and orally six hours later

- Over 10 years: amoxicillin 1 g then 500 mg orally or if allergic clindamycin 300 mg (over 10 minutes) then 150 mg orally
- 5–10 years half the dose
- Below 5 years one quarter of dose

Genitourinary or gastrointestinal surgery or high risk patients (prosthetic material)

- Intravenous amoxicillin and gentamicin
- If allergic to penicillin: IV gentamicin and vancomycin
- Check doses if required to prescribe

For dental treatment a single oral dose of amoxicillin (or clindamycin if allergic to penicillin) 30–60 minutes before the extraction is adequate for most patients. Particular care is required in the patient with an intracardiac prosthesis and parenteral antimicrobial prophylaxis is essential in this situation. Following closure of a PDA, ASD or VSD surgically or with a prosthesis, cover is necessary for the six months after closure but can then be discontinued if closure is complete.

KEY LEARNING POINTS

- Think of infective endocarditis in a child with fever and heart disease.
- Send at least three blood cultures before starting any antibiotic therapy.

- Cover surgical procedures which may produce bacteraemia with antibiotics.
- Single oral dose of amoxicillin or clindamycin for oral procedures.
- Intravenous cover required for those with intracardiac prosthesis.

CASE STUDY

A 5-year-old boy is referred to the general paediatrician with weight loss, fatigue, and a week's history of night sweats. Apart from a history of infective eczema, he has been fit and well, and had a normal 39-month surveillance check. Examination reveals a pale boy, comfortable at rest with a baseline tachycardia and normal blood pressure. He has normal volume pulses, the tip of his spleen is palpable, a mild praecordial heave, normal heart sounds, and a soft 2/6 pansystolic murmur at the apex.

Q. What bedside investigation would you like to do? What signs are you looking for?

A. Urinalysis – the presence of haematuria and absence of white cells would raise the possibility of endocarditis secondary to infected eczema. The absence of the clinical findings seen in subacute bacterial endocarditis (clubbing, splinter haemorrhages, Osler nodes, Janeway lesions) does not mitigate against acute bacterial endocarditis. In the modern era of early detection and treatment, such signs are rarely seen, although splinter haemorrhages are still seen.

Q. Name four other routine investigations to confirm the diagnosis.

A. Blood cultures, echocardiogram, C-reactive protein (CRP), full blood count (FBC). The diagnosis and optimal treatment of endocarditis depends on finding the organism responsible in the blood cultures. Transthoracic echocardiogram may show evidence of vegetation(s), however their absence does not exclude the diagnosis. Transoesophageal echo may be required in children with poor echo images. The CRP shows the normal non-specific rise seen in inflammatory/infective conditions, and the FBC reveals leucocytosis and anaemia.

Mucocutaneous lymph node syndrome

It is important to consider a diagnosis of mucocutaneous lymph node syndrome (Kawasaki) disease to identify the rare but serious complication of coronary artery involvement. Coronary aneurysms and stenoses can develop and result in thrombosis and myocardial infarction, with sudden death in about 1 per cent of children with cardiac manifestations, usually within the first two months of the illness. In most, there are no clinical signs of cardiac disease. Aneurysms usually affect the proximal right or left coronary artery and can be visualized on ultrasound in most children. Stenotic lesions are difficult to demonstrate on echocardiography, and coronary angiography is necessary to demonstrate these. In cases where the aneurysm is less than 8 mm in diameter, complete recovery may take place with regression of the aneurysms and stenotic lesions. The coronary arteries, however, retain abnormal vasomotor properties into adulthood. There is some evidence that high-dose aspirin therapy and high-dose purified human γ-globulin within 10 days of the onset of fever can reduce the incidence of coronary arterial lesions. The difficulty is making the diagnosis early, before the classic peeling of the palms occurs. In the long term low-dose aspirin therapy (3–5 mg/kg per day as a single dose), by reducing platelet aggregation, may decrease the incidence of coronary thrombosis and sudden death in those with coronary lesions. This is generally recommended at diagnosis until it is clear there are no coronary lesions on follow-up.

KEY LEARNING POINTS

- Think of Kawasaki disease, particularly if palmar peeling.
- Give low-dose aspirin initially and continue long term if aneurysms demonstrated.

Rheumatic heart disease

The pathogenesis and non-cardiac manifestations of rheumatic fever are discussed in Chapter 16 (see page 497).

Acute rheumatic fever is now a rare and relatively mild disease in most developed countries but is still common in the developing world. The classic symptoms and signs of acute rheumatic fever are rarely found in the UK and the classic Duckett Jones criteria for making the diagnosis are less apparent. It is important to remember that acute rheumatic fever is rare under 5 years of age. Carditis can cause permanent sequelae, most commonly mitral but also aortic valve disease. In the acute stage, carditis is suggested clinically by the appearance of or change in a significant murmur, pericarditis, arrhythmia or cardiac failure. It must be remembered that innocent murmurs are common in children, particularly associated with a febrile illness, and that an organic murmur may be due to pre-existing congenital heart disease. The commonest organic murmur in rheumatic carditis is an apical systolic one of mitral regurgitation, and if this is severe, an apical mid-diastolic flow murmur may result from high flow. Less commonly, there is aortic regurgitation with a high-pitched, decrescendo early diastolic murmur at the base and left sternal edge. Studies from the 1950s indicated that 10 years after the initial attack the prevalence of chronic heart disease depended on the situation at start of treatment. It increased from approximately 5 per cent in those with no carditis at the start of treatment to 25 per cent in those with an apical systolic murmur, 40 per cent in those with both an apical murmur and a basal diastolic murmur and 70 per cent in those with cardiac failure or pericarditis initially. It is not certain if these figures are valid in the modern era.

There are no specific ECG changes in acute rheumatic fever and although prolongation of the PR interval is frequently found this does not necessarily indicate clinical carditis. Doppler ultrasound can demonstrate valve regurgitation but minimal mitral regurgitation is a physiological condition and can be shown in up to 40 per cent of normal subjects so its significance must be interpreted with caution. The antistreptolysin O (ASO) titre is usually elevated above 200 U/mL and may be much higher for a long period. DNase B is a more sensitive test of previous streptococcal infection but does not start to rise until one to two weeks after infection and peaks at six to eight weeks. The erythrocyte sedimentation rate (ESR) is increased unless heart failure occurs.

The first line of treatment of acute rheumatic fever is penicillin therapy to eradicate any ongoing streptococcal infection. High-dose salicylate therapy provides symptomatic relief but has no long-term effect on the rheumatic process. Glucocorticosteroid therapy is of uncertain value in preventing chronic rheumatic heart disease but is recommended when there is severe involvement. Rheumatic fever is a recurring disease, the risk of recurrence being highest in younger children and decreasing progressively with time after an attack. Each attack carries an increasing risk of a permanent valve defect and antimicrobial prophylaxis against further streptococcal infection should be given throughout childhood and adolescence. This is now usually given orally, though monthly administration of intramuscular benzathine penicillin was previously recommended for those with a severe lesion or possible poor compliance.

KEY LEARNING POINTS

- The presenting features of acute rheumatic fever are less obvious than in the past.
- The ASO titre will be elevated.
- Anti-DNase will rise.
- Penicillin to eradicate any infection is the first line of treatment.
- After an attack, penicillin prophylaxis is necessary until adult life.

CASE STUDY

An 8-year-old boy presented to the neurology department with involuntary movements of his limbs. A systolic murmur was noted and he was referred for a cardiology opinion. In the interim, he had started to become breathless on exertion and was having disturbed sleep. Examination revealed a pale, afebrile, breathless child with normal pulses, a marked praecordial heave and displaced apex. There was a loud gallop, and a 3/6 systolic murmur at the apex radiating to the axilla.

Q. What is the diagnosis?

A. Acute rheumatic fever – the child presented with chorea and a murmur. He then developed symptomatic heart failure due to worsening mitral valve regurgitation, which is evident on the subsequent examination.

Q. What four investigations would you undertake to confirm the diagnosis?

A. A diagnosis of rheumatic fever still requires evidence of preceding streptococcal infection. ASO titre remains the main investigation although some centres are switching to anti-DNase B, which is more sensitive but rises later. Raised inflammatory markers are also a prerequisite for rheumatic fever so analysis of ESR and/or CRP will be required. The diagnosis of carditis would entail an ECG looking for evidence of conduction delay; PR interval prolongation, myocarditis (small complexes) or pericarditis (saddle-shaped ST elevation). An echocardiogram will demonstrate any valve involvement and assess ventricular function.

Dilated cardiomyopathy

Dilated cardiomyopathy is characterized by impaired contraction of the left ventricle causing congestive cardiac failure. The majority are thought to be idiopathic but some are inherited and others are the result of 'burnt-out' myocarditis. The ventricle enlarges and subsequent dilatation of the mitral valve ring may cause mitral regurgitation. Presentation is with cardiac failure and its symptoms: dyspnoea, fatigue and decreased exercise tolerance and signs of tachypnoea, hepatomegaly, oedema and poor volume pulses. There may be a displaced apical impulse, a parasternal or subxiphoid heave, gallop rhythm and a murmur of mitral regurgitation. A chest radiograph will show cardiomegaly and allow distinction from a respiratory cause for dyspnoea. An ECG may show left ventricular hypertrophy and ST changes, or occasionally generalized small QRS complexes. The diagnosis is confirmed by echocardiography demonstrating a dilated, poorly contracting left ventricle with possible mitral regurgitation.

The clinical and echocardiographic features of dilated cardiomyopathy are non-specific and in most cases no cause is identified, though a number of possible causes have to be considered and appropriate investigations undertaken (see box below). It is not common to identify a viral agent. It is not possible to give a clear prognosis at the time of presentation – some deteriorate and die without transplantation, some show little change and others recover. In most cases the aetiology is unknown and treatment is with established heart failure therapy: initially diuretics, ACE inhibitors such as captopril, and aspirin to prevent thrombus formation. Some use digoxin and β-blockers (often carvedilol) are now used regularly in adult heart failure and may be beneficial. Cardiac transplantation should be considered in the most severe cases.

Conditions commonly associated with or causing dilated cardiomyopathy

Infection
- Viral: Coxsackie B usually, but adenovirus and a variety of others
- Some bacterial, parasitic and fungal infections

Neuromuscular disorders
- Muscular dystrophies: Duchenne usually but others
- Congenital myopathies and myotonic dystrophy

Metabolic
- Carnitine deficiency, aminoacidaemias, mucopolysaccharidoses

Drug therapy
- Anthracyclines (adriamycin)

Cardiac lesions
- Anomalous left coronary artery, Kawasaki disease, chronic supraventricular tachycardia

KEY LEARNING POINTS

- Cardiomyopathy is a likely cause of heart failure in a child who was previously well.
- Chest radiograph will show cardiomegaly.

Hypertrophic cardiomyopathy

Hypertrophic cardiomyopathy is usually inherited by an autosomal dominant gene with incomplete penetrance. It is characterized by a non-dilated hypertrophied left ventricle. The hypertrophy often involves the septum more than the free wall, this being known as asymmetrical septal hypertrophy. The morphological features are visualized well using two-dimensional echocardiography. Patients are often asymptomatic, the echocardiogram having been undertaken because of family history or other reasons. Where there is a left ventricular outflow tract gradient, dyspnoea, fatigue on exertion, chest pain, dizziness, syncope and palpitations may occur. The course of the disease is variable. The importance of the condition is that sudden death can occur from a ventricular arrhythmia. Patients with significant abnormalities should avoid intense exercise. A number of different drug therapies (most commonly a β-blocker) have been used in an attempt to delay its progress and prevent sudden death, but none is universally accepted with only amiodarone showing a survival benefit. Implantable defibrillators can be life saving in those with proved episodes of severe ventricular arrhythmias.

KEY LEARNING POINTS

- Most patients are asymptomatic at the time of diagnosis.
- Intense exercise should be avoided.
- The prognosis is difficult to predict.

DISTURBANCES OF RATE, RHYTHM AND CONDUCTION

The usual heart rate for a neonate is 110–150 beats per minute, for an infant 85–125, for a 3–5-year-old 75–115 and after 6 years, the range is 60–100. In sinus tachycardia with fever the rate may rise as high as 200–220 beats per minute in infants and less in older children. Sinus arrhythmia is normal and a common cause of an irregular heartbeat, the rate increasing on inspiration and slowing on expiration. Atrial and junctional ectopic beats are common and seldom give rise to symptoms. Ventricular ectopic beats occur in healthy, asymptomatic children but on occasion result from myocardial disease, electrolyte disturbance or drug ingestion. Ventricular ectopics that disappear on exercise do not require further investigation or treatment.

Supraventricular tachycardia

The clinical picture of supraventricular tachycardia is different in infants and older children. The infant cannot indicate that there is something wrong and an attack may be undetected unless it lasts for more than 24 hours when heart failure may ensue. Poor feeding is the usual initial sign with cardiorespiratory distress subsequently occurring. The older child will usually report feeling a fast heart action or occasionally faintness or chest pain. If the child comes to the attention of the medical services during an episode the fast heart rate can be documented. Many attacks are relatively short lived and infrequent and though the child will present with a history suggesting possible tachycardia, this is rarely diagnostic. Continuous ambulatory electrocardiographic monitoring with an event recorder is then necessary to establish the rhythm during an attack. The event recorder is activated by the child or parent when symptoms occur, the record stored digitally, and then transferred for analysis.

The prognosis for attacks occurring in the first month of life is good. In older children there may be recurrent episodes. There is usually no anatomical cardiac lesion and clinical examination between paroxysms is normal. In an attack, the ECG shows a regular rate of 220–300 beats per minute, the QRS is usually narrow but there may be slurring and widening due to aberrant intraventricular conduction. In a number of older children where the history suggests supraventricular tachycardia, the event monitor will show an increased rate, but less than 200 beats per minute and normal sinus rhythm. They clearly do not have supraventricular tachycardia and often anxiety plays a significant role in their symptoms. Between attacks of supraventricular tachycardia, most children have a normal ECG. In others, the electrocardiographic features of Wolff–Parkinson–White syndrome may be apparent with a short PR interval, broad QRS complex and Δ wave (slurring of the upstroke of R wave) (Figure 9.10). This results from an accessory pathway bypassing the AV node and the electrical impulse passing down this to initiate ventricular contraction distant to the AV node. In an episode of tachycardia, the impulse can pass down this pathway and in a retrograde manner back to the atrium via the AV node to initiate another complex. This complex can then immediately pass back down the accessory pathway to the ventricle and back again to the atrium, thus setting up a re-entry circuit that is self-sustaining.

An episode of acute supraventricular tachycardia initially may be treated with vagal manoeuvres, either the diving reflex, carotid sinus massage or performance of the Valsalva manoeuvre. In the infant, the diving reflex is undertaken by immersing the infant's face in ice cold water or covering the face with a plastic bag filled with ice. All these manoeuvres slow AV node conduction. Intravenous adenosine is now the first-line drug treatment. It blocks passage of the electrical impulse through the AV node terminating the arrhythmia if it is involved. Alternatively, adenosine may slow the ventricular response rate to reveal the underlying atrial rhythm in other situations with an increased atrial rate (e.g. atrial flutter). It is administered in increasing doses (if ineffective) from 0.05 mg/kg, increasing by 0.05 mg/kg (maximum 3 mg) every two minutes to a maximum of 0.25 mg/kg per dose (maximum 12 mg). If this is unsuccessful and the patient is unwell with the tachycardia, cardioversion (usually under general anaesthesia) should be undertaken using a synchronized defibrillator with 0.5–1.0 joule/kg usually being adequate. For less acutely ill infants oral digoxin therapy will usually result in reversion to sinus rhythm within the next 24 hours. A suitable dosage for the infant is 40 μg/kg in three divided doses over the first 24 hours, then 5 μg/kg twice daily for maintenance. For the prophylactic treatment of recurrent episodes, a variety of drugs can be used.

If the ECG shows pre-excitation between attacks many cardiologists would consider digoxin to be contraindicated as it may shorten the antegrade refractory period, making the patient more susceptible to ventricular fibrillation. β-Blockers, disopyramide and flecainide may have a place, and in some children amiodarone is required.

Less commonly SVT can be caused by an ectopic atrial site depolarizing at a rapid rate. This 'automatic' type of SVT can be incidious and incessant sometimes after some weeks. A full description of this is outside the scope of this book.

If the episodes of tachycardia are frequent and troublesome, consideration may be given to transcatheter

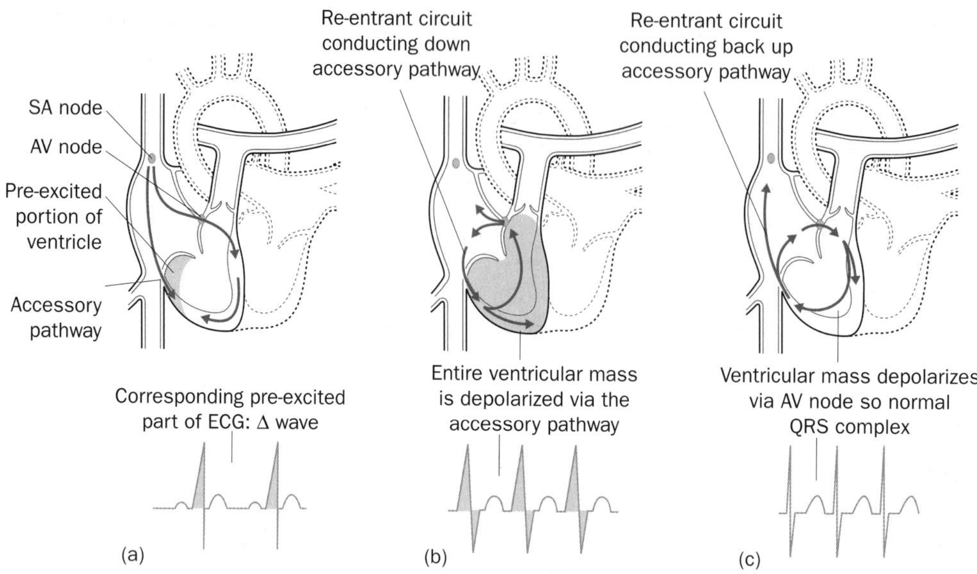

Figure 9.10 Wolff-Parkinson-White syndrome. (a) Mechanism of pre-excitation and Δ wave formation. (b) Mechanism of broad complex SVT. (c) Mechanism of narrow complex SVT. AV, atrioventricular; ECG, electrocardiogram; SA, sinoatrial

radiofrequency ablation of an accessory connection or abnormal focus.

KEY LEARNING POINTS

- In supraventricular tachycardia the rate will be over 200 beats per minute.
- This rate is not possible to count with palpation or auscultation.
- Intravenous adenosine should be given if vagal manoeuvres are ineffective.
- Recurrent attacks of supraventricular tachycardia may be treated by radiofrequency ablation.

Ventricular tachycardia/fibrillation

Ventricular tachycardia or fibrillation is a relatively rare arrhythmia in childhood. Its main importance is in relation to the congenital long QT syndrome that may present with recurrent episodes of syncope as the result of low output polymorphic ventricular tachycardia (torsades de pointes). It often occurs during maximal exercise and can result in sudden death, so syncopal episodes during exercise warrant careful consideration of the possibility of the long QT syndrome (LQTS). A number of different variations are now recognized, including the Jervell and Lange-Nielsen syndrome, which is associated with congenital deafness and an autosomal recessive inheritance. Other forms have an autosomal dominant inheritance. Measurement of the QT interval is detailed under ECG assessment (see above). Treatment of the LQTS takes the form of prophylactic β-blocker therapy often with the insertion of a pacemaker. If there is a family history of unexplained sudden death, or if the child has had a documented cardiac arrest a implantable defibrillator is indicated.

KEY LEARNING POINT

- Think of the LQTS if there are syncopal episodes on exercise.

Congenital complete heart block

In complete heart block (third-degree block), the atria and ventricles beat independently with the atrial rate higher than the ventricular rate. Congenital complete heart block has a recognized association with a maternal systemic lupus erythematosus. Passive transfer from the mother of anti-Ro and anti-La antibodies results in immune damage to the fetal conduction system. The condition is increasingly recognized in the prenatal period by the presence of fetal bradycardia and monitoring for the development of cardiac failure is prudent. In congenital complete heart block without associated heart disease the prognosis is good if there are no symptoms or heart failure in early infancy and the rate is above 55 beats per minute. In others, pacemaker insertion is necessary in the neonatal period or later in life.

KEY LEARNING POINTS

- Complete heart block is associated with maternal systemic lupus erythematosus (anti-Ro antibodies).
- Pacemaker insertion may not be required if the rate is greater than 55 beats per minute.

REFERENCE

Goodacre S and McLeod K (2002) Paediatric electrocardiography. *BMJ* **324**:1382–5.

FURTHER READING

Archer N and Burch M (1999) *Pediatric Cardiology: An Introduction*. London: Arnold.

Gewitz MH (1995) *Primary Pediatric Cardiology*. Armonk, NY: Futura Publishing.

Chapter 10

Gastrointestinal system, hepatic and biliary problems

Peter Gillett

EMBRYOLOGY OF THE GASTROINTESTINAL TRACT

The gastrointestinal tract comprises all components from mouth to anus. In the fourth week of gestation the primitive yolk sac divides into the primitive gut and yolk sac. These are in continuity until the seventh week when the vitelline duct is obliterated. The gut comes from the dorsal aspect of the yolk sac. The primitive gut has three parts: foregut, midgut and hindgut.

The **mouth** is derived from stomodeum, which is lined with ectoderm, and the proximal portion of the foregut, which is endodermal in origin. The **foregut** gives rise to the pharynx, oesophagus, stomach and duodenum down to the ampulla of Vater and the liver and pancreaticobiliary system. The duodenum is composed of distal foregut and proximal midgut. The duodenal loop forms by way of rightward rotation and the classic C-loop forms with the ligament of Treitz fixing the terminal duodenum (fourth part). The liver buds off the distal foregut (second part of the duodenum). The pancreas develops from two buds: a dorsal and a ventral bud of endodermal cells from the foregut. Gut rotation causes the buds and ducts to fuse, forming the main pancreatic duct that joins the common bile duct and enters the second part of the duodenum.

The **midgut** comprises the distal duodenum, small bowel and colon to the proximal third of the transverse colon. The growing abdominal organs squeeze the gut out of the abdominal cavity at 6 weeks' gestation, and it herniates into the extraembryonic cavity (or coelom). At the end closest to the head (cranial) the gut will become small bowel. The caudal limb forms the caecum and colon. A diverticulum forms, which will become the caecum and appendix. The cephalic limb of the midgut forms the jejunum and ileum. The caudal part becomes the distal ileum, caecum, ascending colon and proximal two-thirds of the transverse colon. When outside the embryonic cavity, the gut rotates counterclockwise through 90° (viewed from the anterior aspect of the embryo). In the third month, the cavity is able to accommodate the bowel again and the gut returns to the abdomen. The head end returns with the jejunum first, ending high on the left of the embryo, followed by the ileum which lies in the left side of the cavity. The caudal limb then returns and lies above and in front of the future jejunum and ileum. During this return, the gut loop rotates another 180° counterclockwise, again looking from the anterior position. Rotation is a total of 270°, leaving the caecum and appendix in initial close proximity to the liver, but later descending into the right iliac fossa.

The **hindgut** structures are the distal transverse colon, descending, sigmoid colon rectum and the upper half of the anal canal. The hindgut terminates as a blind-ending sac, in contact with the proctodeum, an ectodermal depression. These apposed layers comprise the cloacal membrane. The bladder forms anteriorly and the urogenital sinus and posterior cloaca form the anorectal canal. The anorectal canal forms the rectum and upper aspect of the anal canal. The lower canal is formed from the ectodermal tissue of the proctodeum and this posterior part of the cloacal membrane breaks down to form the anal opening. Many congenital anatomical abnormalities are explained by the failure of proper development (particularly malrotation).

INVESTIGATIVE PROCEDURES FOR GASTROINTESTINAL DISEASE

Relevant blood and stool investigations for specific conditions are discussed in the appropriate sections.

Percutaneous liver biopsy

Children who have acute or chronic liver disease may need to undergo a biopsy. Platelets should be over 60 000, prothrombin time should be no more than 3 seconds above control and a group and save performed. Fresh frozen plasma (FFP) and/or platelet cover may be required. Ultrasound examination is carried out to exclude grossly dilated ducts, vascular malformations, cysts or abscesses, which are contraindications and many use real-time ultrasound guidance. Complications include bleeding, perforation, pneumothorax, haemopneumothorax and local infection. The children may be kept overnight for observation, nursed on their right side for the first four hours, but after four to six hours, the risk of bleeding is very small. The biopsy is usually taken with the patient on their back, right arm above the head at the point of maximal dullness on percussion, usually at the seventh to tenth intercostal space, mid-axillary line, but it can also be done from an anterior approach. This can be performed under sedation and local anaesthesia or under a quick general anaesthetic depending on local preferences. The present author uses a disposable Hepafix® needle, which is a variation of the Menghini (a hollow coring needle). The Trucut® needle is also used. The breath is held in end-expiration and the needle quickly advanced to a predetermined depth and withdrawn. The core is flushed out of the needle into a container containing formalin.

Transjugular liver biopsy

Where percutaneous biopsy is contraindicated because of uncorrectable coagulopathy, the transjugular route (internal jugular) is employed, usually by radiologists, using a catheter with needle to biopsy the liver from within (hepatic vein). It is not dependent on coagulation results as bleeding occurs into the vascular system. Transjugular liver biopsy is taken in children with prothrombin time prolonged over 5 seconds despite vitamin K, FFP or cryoprecipitate support.

Jejunal biopsy

The original Crosby–Kugler capsule in adults was modified for children, but this technique has been superseded by endoscopy. It involved a metal capsule with a suction port and tubing being passed down to the jejunum and suction applied thus firing an internal cutting device and the sample retained within the port.

Rectal suction biopsy

This is used in suspected Hirschsprung disease or neuronal intestinal dysplasia. A suction-aided device (a biopsy gun with a trigger) with a port is closely applied to the rectal mucosa allowing deep biopsies, including muscularis, to be taken. Histological examination including acetylcholinesterase is done.

Biopsies for disaccharidases

These can be taken endoscopically for measurement of maltase, sucrase, lactase (and trehalase). The levels are expressed as level/g of protein or wet weight of mucosa. Lactase is more sensitive to intestinal inflammatory states than the other enzymes and seems to be the last to recover. Measurement is usually useful in primary disorders such as congenital lactase deficiency or sucrase-isomaltase deficiency.

Breath testing

Malabsorption of carbohydrates results in liberation of hydrogen from bacterial fermentation within the intestine. The hydrogen is excreted in the breath. Usually a baseline hydrogen measurement is taken and then 2 g/kg (maximum 50 g) of the sugar to be tested is ingested in solution. **Lactose** and **sucrose** are the two commonest investigations. The test is dependent on the fermentation (or not) of sugar by bacteria in the colon. Children blow into a plastic bag with a three-way tap for sampling and a read-out (in parts per million, PPM) is given. Baseline elevations in hydrogen can be seen in small bowel bacterial overgrowth. A rise of 10–20 PPM from baseline is indicative of intolerance. **Glucose** and **lactulose** breath testing has been used to look for bacterial overgrowth based on the principle that fermentation and a rise in hydrogen is indicative of proliferation of fermenting bacteria.

Sugar loading tests

Lactose is the most commonly utilized test. Blood is taken for glucose estimation at half-hour intervals for two hours. An increase of 1.7 mmol/L above the pretest glucose level is considered normal. Of value is the clinical response to the load of sugar (symptoms of gassiness, pain, diarrhoea).

Small intestinal permeability tests

Two inert sugars, usually xylose or lactulose (larger sugar) and rhamnose or cellobiose (smaller sugar) are given orally, and the ratio of these sugars is measured in a timed urine collection. The differential absorption gives a measure of increased intestinal leakiness (increased absorption of larger sugars) and loss of surface area (reduced absorption of smaller sugars).

Stool pH, reducing substances, chromatography

Use the fluid part of a stool (the nappy should be inverted or cling film placed inside the nappy so that the whole stool can be collected and the liquid element is not wicked away). A Clinitest tablet is added to a diluted mix with water and a colour change indicates reducing substances from 0 to 2 per cent. One per cent or more is significant. A delay in getting the stool to the lab allows continued fermentation by bacteria and a false positive test. **Stool chromatography** is used if there are significant reducing substances present and can identify patterns of sugar malabsorption which may be helpful, again dependent on which sugars are ingested. However, this should be interpreted carefully. Stool pH values below 5.5 are thought to be indicative of sugar intolerance.

Calprotectin

This white cell protein, measured in stool by enzyme-linked immunosorbent assay (ELISA) can be useful in differentiating causes of diarrhoea (normal in functional diarrhoea such as irritable bowel syndrome (IBS), elevated in inflammatory bowel disease (IBD) and polyps as well as colonic cancer but also in infections). It is gaining popularity in paediatric practice and may be a useful non-invasive marker of disease activity in IBD.

Pancreatic function tests

These are used in investigating **pancreatic insufficiency**, such as in cystic fibrosis or Shwachman–Diamond syndrome or recurrent or chronic pancreatitis. There are indirect and direct tests of pancreatic function. Direct tests measure the production of exocrine secretions under controlled conditions, with the duodenum intubated. Enzyme and fluid production is assessed after stimulation with secretin/cholecystokinin. Indirect tests measure the consequences of poor exocrine function, utilizing stool markers such as trypsin, chymotrypsin, elastase, lipase and faecal fat.

For **faecal fat**, a three to five day quantitative fat estimation of all excreted stools is used in conjunction with a dietary fat intake over the same time when fat malabsorption is suspected. Alternatively, qualitative fat is measured either as a 'spot' microscopy or a steatocrit (a haematocrit tube is centrifuged and the lipid and liquid elements estimated).

Breath tests are available for assessing utilization of triglycerides and starch digestion. Urinary markers are also used: bentiromide is a non-absorbable peptide that is broken down in the small intestine by chymotrypsin and liberates para-aminobenzoic acid, which is measured in the urine. The pancreolauryl test is similar where a fluorescein label is liberated by the breakdown of the parent compound by cholesterol esterase and the fluorescein is absorbed and excreted in the urine where it can be measured.

Blood tests (amylase, lipase) are useful in acute pancreatitis but are not helpful in chronic insufficiency as they are extremely non-specific. Amylase derives from salivary glands as well as the pancreas. Serum immunoreactive trypsin (IRT) using dried blood spots is employed in the detection of pancreatic insufficiency (cystic fibrosis screening). The levels are grossly elevated in the first year of life in children with cystic fibrosis with a quick decline in the second year and sub-normalization by the age of 6 years. There is wide variability in results and it is not of value in discriminating the degree of impairment.

Helicobacter pylori

Breath testing is now commonplace for *H. pylori*. C-14-labelled urea (or the stable isotope C-13) is used and relies on *H. pylori*'s ability to split urea into ammonia and bicarbonate, becoming C-14 or C-13-labelled carbon dioxide, excreted in the breath. False positives occur in younger children due to urea-splitting organisms in the mouth. Rapid *H. pylori* blood testing kits are available for outpatient use and serology is available, often used in the outpatient setting in adult practice (the results are not as accurate in children). It is not useful for evaluating eradication as the antibodies take over a year to disappear.

Motility and pH probe investigation

Manometry is used in investigation of motility disorders such as achalasia, oesophageal spasm and nutcracker oesophagus. Colonic (mostly anorectal) manometry is helpful in the diagnosis of constipation due to motility disorders and disorders of defaecation (Hirschsprung disease, in particular, and other disorders of anorectal function). Biliary (or sphincter of Oddi) manometry, increasingly used in adult practice, is gaining interest in specialist centres. **Electrogastrography** is also used in upper intestinal motility evaluation. A series of electrodes is used over the upper abdomen to evaluate gastroduodenal peristalsis. **pH probe** testing is a means of evaluating acid reflux in children of all ages. Symptom evaluation should select out patients in whom it will be useful. The probe is calibrated and placed transnasally using a standard calculation (Strobel formula). Software analyses the data stored on a recorder and gives a breakdown of important parameters such as percentage time below pH 4 (shown to correlate with development of oesophagitis), long reflux episodes (over five minutes exposure is more significant), patient position (upright, sitting, lying, sleeping), mealtimes and any episodes of heartburn or other symptoms (such as colour change, coughing, choking) marked using an event marker. A diary card is used to document symptoms and activities undertaken over the 24-hour recording period. Most studies are done off medications, but pH probing can help with tailoring requirements of medications as 'on-treatment studies'. Correlation of symptoms and recording is most helpful.

Gastrointestinal endoscopy

Over the past 30 years technology has allowed us to perform diagnostic and therapeutic procedures in the same way as for our colleagues who treat adult patients and has dramatically improved management. Clearly, we approach procedures in a different way. Preparation and age-appropriate explanation are important. Procedures are usually day cases and in most centres in the UK are carried out under general anaesthesia; other units use sedation. For procedures carried out under sedation, combinations of benzodiazepines (midazolam, diazepam) and opiates (pethidine, fentanyl) are used and agents for reversal – flumazenil and naloxone – should always be available. Details of the levels of procedural skills and training competency in paediatric gastroenterology have been detailed by working groups of the British and North American Societies of Paediatric Gastroenterology, Hepatology and Nutrition and numbers and ability need to be 'signed off' by trainers before competency is acknowledged. Antibiotic prophylaxis is used as per standard guidelines (British Society of Gastroenterology, American Society of Gastrointestinal Endoscopy, American Heart Association). Upper endoscopy is the most frequently performed examination before colonoscopy. Endoscopy is possible on all but the smallest neonates. Interventional procedures such as dilatation, variceal banding and sclerotherapy, injection and heater probe treatment of ulcers and cautery/laser therapy of vascular malformations, snare polypectomy and percutaneous gastrostomy (PEG) insertion and newer techniques such as endoscopic fundoplication are performed by paediatric gastroenterologists. Endoscopic retrograde cholangiopancreatography (ERCP), enteroscopy and endoscopic ultrasound are imaging and investigational modalities still used mainly for adults. In the author's centre, these are performed in conjunction with colleagues who treat adult patients. Capsule endoscopy, imaging the small bowel, is also available for children.

Radiology of the gastrointestinal tract

Plain films are used to assess masses and abnormal gas and stool patterns. **Perforation** and **pneumoperitoneum** can be identified, **toxic dilatation** seen in acute colitis, and **pneumatosis intestinalis** and other features of necrotizing enterocolitis. Constipation can be assessed if there are doubts despite history and clinical examination. In addition, **stool marker studies** use different swallowed radiopaque shapes and are used to determine the transit time of the colon (may help differentiate generalized slow transit through the colon from so-called outlet obstruction, seen in megarectum). The **mucosa** can be assessed: thickening of the bowel wall is seen in oedema arising from enteropathy, in vasculitides such as Henoch–Schönlein purpura or in ulcerative colitis. **Foreign bodies** (pins, coins, toys, etc.) and abnormal **calcification** (gallstones, renal stones, etc.) are also detected.

Contrast studies

Contrast studies are used widely to assess the upper intestine, small bowel and rarely (in paediatrics), the large bowel. **Barium swallow** assesses the swallowing mechanism with thin and thicker liquids, frequently in association with speech and language therapists, as a videofluoroscopy, often with more textured larger items as necessary. Aspiration and high-risk reflux can be documented but contrasts are neither sensitive nor specific enough to recommend as a standard test for reflux. Extrinsic compression from rings and tumour masses, hiatus hernia, varices, webs and other abnormalities such as achalasia, and dysmotility disorders can also be seen. The prone pullback study, where a nasogastric tube is passed and contrast trickled as the tube is withdrawn is used to assess the presence of an H-type tracheo-oesophageal fistula. **Barium meal** may detect ulcers in stomach or duodenum and filling defects from masses as well as assessing gastric outlet obstruction and emptying. Duodenal obstruction, malrotation (the duodenal C-loop usually sits to the right of the spine) and volvulus can be assessed by an upper gastrointestinal contrast. Contrast studies are used to look at the small bowel, either as a follow through (SBFT) or enteroclysis (also called a small bowel enema, where the patient has a transpyloric tube passed to get contrast directly into the small bowel). **Barium enema** is seldom used. It can be useful to determine anatomical abnormalities in neonates, to assess malrotation and to assess suspected Hirschsprung disease, often with a delayed or 'post evac' film done 24 hours later. Polyps can be seen on lower contrast studies but would not be first choice in their investigation (colonoscopy is the preferred method, as therapeutic removal can be performed by snare diathermy).

There is little place for enema in the assessment of IBD, again, colonoscopy being the procedure of choice. **Therapeutic contrast studies**: the main role for enema in childhood is for reduction of intussusception. Air enema is the preferred choice, but carbon dioxide systems are increasingly utilized, with barium or water-soluble contrast also used in some instances.

Ultrasound, computed tomography and magnetic resonance imaging

These imaging modalities have revolutionized paediatric gastrointestinal imaging. Ultrasound allows diagnosis and follow-up of tumours, inflammatory masses, abscesses and cysts, to confirm pyloric stenosis and some cases of malrotation, to assess bowel wall thickening in inflammatory bowel disease, liver and splenic parenchymal disease and trauma. It is also helpful in detection of varices and measurement of portal blood flow and the assessment of pancreatic disease. Computed tomography (CT) and magnetic resonance imaging have advanced, particularly in adult practice, for the detection of polyps and other bowel cancers (so-called 'virtual colonoscopy') and MR studies in IBD (assessing bowel involvement and lesions in the perianal area) are increasingly used. MR cholangiopancreatography has revolutionized liver and biliary imaging, reducing the need for ERCP. More recently, the use of **endoscopic ultrasound** (with a variety of different instruments and probes) has revolutionized the detection and staging of gastrointestinal (and respiratory) cancer, allowing fine needle aspiration and biopsy of intrinsic and extraluminal tumours (lung, pancreas).

Radionuclide studies

Studies using ^{99m}technetium-labelled milk in babies are commonly used for detection of **gastro-oesophageal reflux** and to assess aspiration and gastric emptying. Delayed images up to 24 hours may be obtained and can be useful in assessing such complications. Studies with milk or solids such as egg are often combined with reflux studies as **gastric emptying** is easily measured. **Hepatobiliary** scintigraphy is used in babies for investigation of primarily cholestatic liver disease. The baby is given phenobarbital 5 mg/kg per day for five days to prime the liver and then one of the iminodiacetic acid (IDA) compounds (e.g. HIDA, DISIDA or TEBIDA) injected. Images are taken at intervals and excretion into the bowel for up to 24 hours is assessed. Neonatal hepatitis causes diminished uptake into the liver but excretion occurs into bowel, as opposed to good uptake and non-excretion in biliary atresia (and in the hypoplastic diseases).

Meckel diverticulum is also detectable with ^{99m}technetium-labelled pertechnetate, with priming with an H_2-antagonist, traditionally cimetidine. This blocks acid production in the gastric tissue, which is frequently present in Meckel diverticula. Uptake is detected after scanning soon after intravenous (IV) administration of the label, but false negatives do occur. **White cell scanning** is also used in some centres to detect active inflammatory bowel disease in small and large bowel, or to differentiate between active or inactive lesions, for example, a mass due to a narrowed, diseased terminal ileum. **Red cell scanning** can detect gastrointestinal blood loss in situations where there is occult bleeding. It may help localize an area for the surgeon or endoscopist to assess.

VOMITING

Vomiting is a symptom of conditions affecting many organ systems, not just the gastrointestinal tract. Vomiting itself may produce complications requiring investigation and treatment (biochemical derangements, dehydration and upper gastrointestinal bleeding). Nausea (a subjective sensation) is often followed by retching and vomiting (caused by coordinated muscle activity of pharynx, respiratory and gastric muscles that allows contents to be expelled freely without danger to the upper airway). Regurgitation is the effortless reflux of contents into the oesophagus. Motor activity of the vomiting reflex is mediated via the vagus. It may be acute or chronic or cyclic (episodic, recurrent) in nature. Acute vomiting is usually seen in infectious gastroenteritis (along with diarrhoea and abdominal pain) or ingestion of toxic substances and is seen as a discrete episode.

Causes of vomiting

Acute
- Infection (urinary tract infection)
- Ingestions
- Obstruction: congenital abnormalities: malrotation, webs, pyloric stenosis, volvulus
- Raised intracranial pressure (ICP)

Chronic recurrent
- Acid reflux
- Peptic inflammation
- Infection (*H. pylori*, *Giardia*)
- Ménétrier disease (*H. pylori*, cytomegalovirus (CMV) infection)

- Other gastritis from allergy, bile reflux
- Enteropathy from coeliac disease, cows' milk or soy protein
- Dietary intolerances (wheat)
- Crohn disease
- Anatomical
- Achalasia
- Obstruction
- Superior mesenteric artery (SMA) syndrome: immobility, debility from surgery or weight loss
- Malignancies: both gastrointestinal and extraintestinal (raised ICP from brain tumours such as medulloblastoma)

Cyclical/episodic

- Cardiovascular
- Abdominal migraine
- Neurological
- Endocrine: phaeochromocytoma
- Metabolic: medium chain acyl CoA dehydrogenase deficiency (MCAD), porphyria

KEY LEARNING POINTS

- Vomiting is a symptom, often from an acute, self-limiting infection.
- Chronic patterns require careful assessment and relevant investigation.
- Many extraintestinal conditions present with acute or chronic vomiting.

ACUTE AND CHRONIC DIARRHOEA

The definition of acute versus chronic diarrhoea is a continuum, usually with over **three weeks** duration defining chronic. Diarrhoea is an increase in stool water, the overall balance between secretion and absorption of fluid. It also involves an increase in stool frequency and decrease in consistency. Stool volume in excess of 10 g/kg per day in babies and over 200 g per day in children over the age of 3 years is taken to be diarrhoea.

The proximal small bowel is responsible for a huge amount of electrolyte and water shifts, which rapidly reduces the osmolality of the luminal contents to iso-osmolar. The distal small bowel and colon are responsible for most water absorption. Sodium and potassium absorption and chloride and bicarbonate exchange occur by active processes, but water is absorbed passively along a gradient. This fluid regulation is complex and influenced by hormones as well as bacterial toxins, enteric nervous factors, diet, disease states and bowel motility. Nine litres of fluid a day passes the proximal jejunum in older children and adults. This includes the secretions from stomach, duodenum, pancreas and biliary tract. This reduces to 1 L at the distal ileum. The adult colon can absorb 3–4 L/day. In disease states, this process is hindered and diarrhoea results.

Diarrhoea is broadly split into **osmotic** and **secretory**. Often there is overlap in disease states but it is useful to define these.

CASE STUDY: Osmotic diarrhoea

A 4-year-old is referred from their general practitioner (GP) with chronic diarrhoea. Over the last year he has been stooling five times a day, passing a loose watery stool every time. It is associated with crampy central abdominal pain, usually after eating. A full history suggests that he drinks in excess of 2 L per day of apple juice, with a glass taken with each meal and snack. Discontinuation of this for a week resulted in complete resolution of his symptoms.

Watery diarrhoea with abdominal pain in older children strongly suggests a dietary driven problem. A careful history may uncover common dietary causes of loose stools. Common causes are fruit juice, diluting squashes, diet drinks, fizzy beverages, sugar-free gum and boiled sweets. Milk products are also a major factor. Careful elimination of any offending items may well resolve the problem. Included in the differential diagnosis are infections causing mucosal injury, enteropathies, congenital sucrase/isomaltase or acquired lactase deficiency, but also laxatives such as lactulose or milk of magnesia, some vehicles for medicines, such as lactose and sorbitol, high sugar content juices (apple juice), or 'sugar-free' products (sugar-free gum, sweets, fizzy beverages or squash). Bile salt malabsorption can also cause osmotic diarrhoea. Withdrawing the substance results in clinical improvement.

OSMOTIC DIARRHOEA

Malabsorption of a dietary component (solute) produces an osmotic load causing increased fluid losses in the distal small bowel and colon. This causes a large osmotic gap, usually over 50 mmol, i.e. (sodium + potassium) × 2 = faecal osmolality (measured) or 290 mmol/L. Normally the calculation equals 290 mmol/L. Lower total electrolyte values suggest **an osmotically active substance is present.**

Usually **carbohydrate malabsorption** is responsible, resulting in stool pH of <5.5 due to fermentation of the carbohydrate lower down the tract by bacteria, producing lactic acid. Osmotic diarrhoea stops quickly in fasted children.

SECRETORY DIARRHOEA

In contrast to osmotic diarrhoea, secretory diarrhoea continues despite fasting. The fluid balance is the difference between secretion and absorption. Fasting has no influence on stool output in secretory diarrhoea. The equation (sodium + potassium) × 2 = faecal osmolality (measured) is balanced. Faecal sodium is generally above 50 mmol/L. Most diseases do not have a purely secretory component and this must be taken into account when assessing children in the context of diarrhoea. Diarrhoea is associated with excess secretion of neuropeptides (VIPomas, Zollinger–Ellison syndrome, neuro- or ganglioneuroblastomas) in addition to congenital diarrhoeas (chloride, sodium).

Acute diarrhoea

Usually lasting **less than two weeks**, acute diarrhoea is usually caused by infection. Over 4 million deaths occur worldwide each year due to diarrhoea. **Viruses** are the major cause (30–40 per cent) of gastroenteritic infection: rotavirus, enteric adenovirus, astrovirus and calicivirus infection (including Norwalk virus) are commonest.

Bacteria cause diarrhoeal disease via a number of mechanisms:

- **Invasive disease**: by invading the mucosa and multiplying within the surface of the mucosa (*Salmonella*, *Shigella*, *Yersinia*, *Campylobacter*, *Vibrio*).
- **Cytotoxin production**: which alters cell function through direct cell damage (*Shigella*, enteropathogenic *Escherichia coli*, enterohaemorrhagic *E. coli* and *Clostridium difficile*).
- **Enterotoxins**: which cause altered cell salt and water balance without damaging the structure of the cell (*Shigella*, enterotoxic *E. coli*, *Yersinia*, *Aeromonas*, *V. cholerae*).
- **Adherence**: like many of the *E. coli*'s, enterotoxins adhere to the cell membrane and cause flattening of the microvilli. Enterotoxins affect small and large bowel, whereas cytotoxins and enteroinvasive organisms affect primarily large bowel.

Protozoal infection is also common, with *Giardia lamblia* and *Cryptosporidium*, *Entamoeba histolytica* as well as rarer entities (such as *Dientamoeba fragilis*, *Blastocystis hominis* and *Balantidium coli*, *Cyclospora* and *Isospora*).

Nematode infections are described in Chapter 21.

Management

The initial step is to assess the degree of dehydration. A number of similar classification systems are in use, which assess the degree of dehydration as mild (3–4 per cent), moderate (5 per cent) or severe (10 per cent). Laboratory studies are usually unnecessary in mild-to-moderate disease. Blood count, electrolytes, glucose and renal function are important to check in those with severe dehydration or in those who have more complicated problems, such as bloody diarrhoea. Withdrawal of feeds is unnecessary and may delay recovery. Lactose restriction is usually unnecessary and breastfeeding should be continued. Oral rehydration solution (ORS) in mild-to-moderate dehydration should be used in the first four hours with resumption of normal feeding thereafter, followed by an ORS feed of 10 ml/kg per liquid stool as ongoing supplementation, even in children who continue to vomit. A variety of different ORS brands are available. Those most in use in the UK have between 60 and 75 mmol/L of sodium, as opposed to the World Health Organization (WHO) ORS solution which has a higher sodium content of 90 mmol/L. Small frequent feedings using a teaspoon or syringe are effective in rehydrating infants but are labour intensive. Nasogastric tubes feeds are as effective as IV rehydration. Intravenous boluses and rehydration may be necessary in those with severe dehydration (with abnormal vital signs, depressed level of consciousness) or in those who persistently vomit. Chronic consequences of acute infection are lactose intolerance and chronic diarrhoea from enteropathy.

Chronic diarrhoea

Neonatal diarrhoea

Congenital diarrhoeas are rare. Severe diarrhoea usually starts in the first few hours or days of life. Life-threatening dehydration can ensue from conditions including congenital lactase deficiency (see below), glucose-galactose malabsorption, enterokinase deficiency, congenital chloride and sodium diarrhoea, tufting enteropathy and microvillus inclusion disease.

LACTOSE INTOLERANCE

Congenital lactase deficiency is a rare neonatal disorder, though many babies who have diarrhoea are often suspected of having lactose intolerance. It usually presents with very acidic diarrhoea and has been documented in families in Finland. Late-onset deficiency is seen after infections and enteropathic processes, such as coeliac disease. Adult type hypolactasia is described in white, Asian and black populations. It is genetically determined and results in phenotypes typically labelled 'lactose digesters' and 'non-digesters'. Lactose non-digesters develop problems after the toddler years, when lactase levels seem to decline and typical symptoms of diarrhoea, gassiness, recurrent abdominal pain occur, with improvement on a trial of lactose-free diet.

Sucrase-isomaltase deficiency

CASE STUDY

A 5-month-old baby boy presents with acute onset diarrhoea after starting on solids. Discontinuing the feed stops the diarrhoea and investigation, including endoscopy and biopsies for disaccharidases, shows sucrase-isomaltase deficiency. He is managed on a sucrose-free diet initially, with transfer to enzyme replacement.

Watery acidic diarrhoea occurs after introduction of starchy foods at weaning. Diagnosis is made on a sucrose breath test or on intestinal disaccharidase activity on biopsy and treatment is with avoidance of sucrose, glucose polymers and starch in the first year, with toleration of starch intake improving after the age of 3 years. Invertase, a product available to aid digestion of sucrose, can be prescribed.

Coeliac disease

CASE STUDY

A 5-year-old Indian boy complains of increasing lethargy, diffuse crampy abdominal pain, loose stools and a change in mood for six months. The parents have eliminated milk from the diet with some improvement. Examination reveals a pale boy with mild abdominal distension and blood tests reveal iron-deficiency anaemia with a positive coeliac antibody screen. The diagnosis of coeliac disease is confirmed on endoscopic biopsy of the distal duodenum.

Coeliac disease is a 'reversible gluten-sensitive enteropathy in a genetically susceptible individual'. It is commoner in western European populations (where screening will identify 1 in 100–200 individuals), but is also seen in east Indian and South American populations, but rarely in those of African or East Asian descent. **Gluten** from wheat, barley and rye is the toxic element. A trigger infection, typically gastroenteritis, allows the exposure of the mucosa to gliadin, starting a cascade of inflammation mediated by specific restricted T-lymphocytes (DQ2). Human leucocyte antigen (HLA)-DQ2 is the characteristic haplotype found in 90-plus per cent of patients with coeliac disease, with the remainder being HLA-DQ8 positive. Coeliac disease remains a biopsy-proven diagnosis, although serological tests are available with high sensitivity and specificity. Historically, IgA and IgG antigliadin antibodies were used, but these have been superseded by antiendomysial (EMA) and antitissue transglutaminase (tTG). **Selective IgA deficiency** is associated with coeliac disease. With deficiency, coeliac disease is 10 times more likely to occur, but the standard screen will be falsely negative. In this case, IgG antibodies are tested. Histological examination of the duodenum (Marsh grading system) classically shows infiltration of intra-epithelial lymphocytes (IEL) and varying degrees of villous atrophy, from little or no change, to virtually flat (subtotal). The crypts lengthen and the lamina propria is heavily infiltrated with chronic inflammatory cells. Coeliac disease is also responsible for a lymphocytic gastritis and is associated with lymphocytic colitis and collagenous colitis. The mucosal changes improve over the course of a year, with near normalization of histology, but subtle alterations in mucosal T-lymphocyte make-up persist. Antibodies disappear after a year or so, with some taking a while longer. This may allow clinicians to monitor adherence to some extent (i.e. a patient who is persistently positive despite a gluten-free diet is usually non-adherent). Nowadays, a second (or even third) biopsy is not required: the return to negative serology is taken as a proxy for resolution of the mucosal changes. Children who present under the age of 2 years are often re-challenged later ('transient' gluten sensitive enteropathy). The challenge is given before or after the pubertal growth spurt. Such cases are rare if the diagnosis is firmly made with positive serology and confirmatory biopsy before a gluten-free diet is commenced.

Coeliac disease is associated with Down, Turner and Williams syndromes (incidence is typically 5 per cent), type 1 diabetes (5 per cent), autoimmune liver, adrenal, thyroid and connective tissue disease and is linked to infertility, preterm delivery and low birth weight babies. Dermatitis herpetiformis, a blistering skin rash, is also strongly linked. Screening on 'at-risk' groups including family members (10–20 per cent lifetime risk) and even the general population is a matter of much debate. Osteopenia can be seen and diagnosed on a DEXA scan but will normalize after a year on a gluten-free diet. Adequate calcium intake and weight bearing exercises are recommended. Elevation of liver transaminases is reported and resolves on a gluten-free diet. Iron, folate, and less commonly vitamin B_{12}, K (and vitamin A, D and E) deficiency are seen. The risk of intestinal malignancy (upper gastrointestinal cancers and classically enteropathy associated T-cell lymphoma) is increased, but returns to that of the normal population after adherence to a gluten-free diet for about five years. Neurological problems have been described (behavioural changes, unexplained epilepsy, peripheral neuropathies) and have been seen in children with cerebral calcification. These associations are poorly understood. Treatment is adherence to a strict gluten-free diet for life, and patients should be followed regularly with dietetic support.

KEY LEARNING POINTS

- Coeliac disease is common and may present mono- or asymptomatically in at-risk patients.
- Have a low threshold to consider the diagnosis in such patients.

OTHER CAUSES OF ENTEROPATHY

All that is flat is not always coeliac! Other causes of enteropathy include starvation states, post-enteric infection, cows' milk protein enteropathy (CMPE), chronic *Giardia* infection, cryptosporidiosis and human immunodeficiency virus (HIV) infection.

Inflammatory bowel disease (Crohn disease and ulcerative colitis)

CASE STUDY

A 12-year-old girl presents with an eight-month history of diarrhoea, often stooling six or more times a day including night time, with central crampy abdominal pain, reduced appetite, lethargy, early satiety and weight loss. She is pale, has a palpable mass in the right iliac fossa and has chronic anaemia with raised erythrocyte sedimentation rate (ESR) and C-reactive protein (CRP) and low albumin. Further evaluation with small bowel follow through, upper endoscopy and colonoscopy confirms the diagnosis of ileocolonic Crohn disease.

'Regional ileitis' was reported by Crohn *et al.* in 1932 though had been previously described. A quarter of cases present under the age of 18 years and incidence in the Scottish population is high. Smoking is a risk factor but breastfeeding in childhood may be protective. An affected first-degree relative conveys a 10–20 per cent lifetime risk to a family member. Genetic studies have shown a number of candidate genes (e.g. chromosome 16: NOD2/CARD15) which may help identify individuals at risk of future disease and establish their susceptibility to specific disease patterns and distributions. This is a complex disease with an abnormal inflammatory cascade driven by antigens (bacteria, potentially dietary) via the mucosal immune system. Crohn disease presents from mouth to anus. Seventy-five per cent have ileocolonic disease but also present with isolated mouth or perianal changes, small bowel disease or colitis. Mouth ulcers, fever, weight loss, early satiety, anorexia, abdominal pain associated with eating and relieved by stooling and frequent loose stools (day or night time) with or without blood are common. Anaemia, poor growth and delayed puberty may be the only presenting problems. In IBD, other systems may be affected and there is considerable overlap between Crohn disease and ulcerative colitis. Eyes (episcleritis, iritis), joints (swelling, arthritis, arthropathy), skin (erythema nodosum, pyoderma gangrenosum), renal tracts (stones, fistulae) and hepatobiliary system (stones, ascending and sclerosing cholangitis, pancreatitis, autoimmune hepatitis) may be involved. Deep vein thrombosis and other thrombotic/vasculitic complications have been reported. Osteopenia/porosis is common.

Diagnosis is often delayed. Full evaluation at presentation with upper endoscopy and ileocolonoscopy is indicated (Table 10.1). Endoscopic changes typically are of erythema, mucosal thickening, loss of the normal vascular pattern and aphthous ulceration (often linear), patchy in nature (so called 'skip lesions') with fissuring and cobblestoning. Changes of colitis are often seen (rectal sparing is classically described) and distinguishing Crohn colitis from ulcerative colitis is often difficult. Transmural oedema and inflammation may result in stricture and obstruction as well as fistula formation. Adjacent loops of bowel, bladder, vagina, urethra, abdominal wall and the perineum can all be affected. Perianal disease presents with skin tagging, fissures and abscesses. Histologically, Crohn disease causes chronic inflammation with deep layers affected, through to the serosa, ulceration, architectural disruption with branching and destruction of the colonic mucosal glands, crypt abscesses and the presence of non-caseating granulomas.

Ulcerative colitis typically presents with bloody diarrhoea and again may be insidious in onset and initially indistinguishable from an infectious colitis but persistence of symptoms should raise suspicion and prompt further evaluation. It may present with fever, abdominal pain and urgency of stooling, tenesmus and diarrhoea, with or without blood, and, like Crohn disease, investigations

Table 10.1 Investigations for Inflammatory bowel disease (IBD)

Blood tests	Electrolytes, creatinine, glucose, liver function tests, amylase (gallstones, pancreatitis rare), albumin (often low, protein-losing enteropathy), bone chemistry, C-reactive protein, blood count (white blood cells and platelets), erythrocyte sedimentation rate (inflammatory markers raised), prothrombin time (vitamin K), ferritin, vitamin B_{12}, folate, vitamins A, D and E, trace metals (malabsorption), cross-match (transfusion)
Stools	Exclude enteric infection: *Salmonella, Escherichia coli, Shigella, Campylobacter*, amoebic, parasites, *Clostridium difficile* toxin Calprotectin (raised in active IBD, normalizes with clinical improvement)
Imaging	Plain abdominal film (if toxic megacolon or perforation suspected), upper gastrointestinal barium and small-bowel follow through, barium enema rarely in children (endoscopy), ultrasound of abdomen (gall bladder, renal tracts, bowel thickening), magnetic resonance imaging (bowel thickening, complications: perianal disease), bone age (often delayed), DEXA scanning (bone density), white cell scanning
Endoscopic evaluation	Upper endoscopy, colonoscopy and biopsies (up to 30 per cent of children with Crohn disease will have upper gastrointestinal histological changes even in absence of symptoms), surveillance endoscopy is indicated beginning 10 years after diagnosis of ulcerative colitis (and Crohn disease) as increased risk of malignancy

show raised inflammatory markers and anaemia. Endoscopy may show limited distal acute inflammation in milder cases, but extensive confluent pancolitis with erythema, loss of the normal vascular pattern, mucosal thickening, ulceration and friability are often seen with no mucosal sparing (as might be seen in Crohn disease). Acute presentation may progress to fulminant colitis with toxic megacolon and require aggressive treatment with intravenous steroids and immunosuppression, but may inevitably lead to colectomy and ileostomy. Even after thorough evaluation, up to 20 per cent of children fall within an 'indeterminate' category. Most children will enter remission with steroids (or nutritional therapy in Crohn disease), but IBD is a chronic relapsing and remitting condition and may require step-up therapy as indicated in Table 10.2. It is important to remember that IBD also affects the family. A multidisciplinary input from specialist nurses, dietitians, pharmacists, psychologists, surgeons, social workers and schoolteachers is important for patients to manage their condition the best they can.

Table 10.2 Treatment for Inflammatory bowel disease (IBD)

Attaining remission	Steroids: intravenous, oral, topical (suppository, enema) Enteral nutritional therapy: in Crohn disease – elemental E028, polymeric feeds; Modulen-IBD Ciclosporin (acute colitis, usually ulcerative colitis), biological agents Total parenteral nutrition (may be required in debilitated patients)
Maintenance of remission	Aminosalicylic acid (ASA) compounds, sulfasalazine, mesalazine (Asacol, Pentasa, Salofalk) orally or topically (suppository, enema) Antibiotics: metronidazole, ciprofloxacin (in Crohn disease) Probiotics: lactobacillus, bifidobacteria Immunomodulators: azathioprine (6-MP), methotrexate, thalidomide Biological agents: antitumour necrosis factor α (anti-TNF-α)

KEY LEARNING POINTS

- Inflammatory bowel disease is increasing in incidence and is common in children.
- Crohn disease and ulcerative colitis are multisystem diseases and may present atypically.
- Children with chronic diarrhoea and growth issues need IBD actively excluded.
- A multidisciplinary approach, a thorough explanation of the condition and treatment options to the parents and child are paramount to successful care.

GASTROINTESTINAL BLEEDING

CASE STUDY: Mallory–Weiss tear

A 6-year-old girl presents in the early hours of the morning with haematemesis of a large amount of fresh red blood with clots having been vomiting and retching frequently for two days. She is haemodynamically stable when seen in Accident and Emergency. A good history reveals previous episodes of epistaxis but there is no blood on ENT examination. Later that day, endoscopy reveals a 5 mm tear in the fundal area consistent with a traumatic tear.

Table 10.3 Causes of gastrointestinal bleeding

Haematemesis/melaena	Fresh rectal bleeding
Infants Oesophagitis Gastritis, duodenitis and peptic ulcer disease Mallory-Weiss tear, traumatic gastropathy Varices (rarely)	Infants Anal fissure Infectious colitis, cows' milk protein intolerance (colitis/proctitis) Intussusception, Meckel diverticulum, Duplication cyst Vascular malformations (rarely)
Older children and adolescents Oesophagitis Gastritis, duodenitis and peptic ulcer disease Varices Mallory-Weiss tear, traumatic gastropathy Pill-related ulcers	Older children and adolescents Anal fissure Infectious colitis Polyps Lymphoid nodular change Inflammatory bowel disease Henoch-Schönlein purpura Intussusception Meckel diverticulum Haemolytic uraemic syndrome

Bleeding is a worrying symptom for parents and children alike, but significant bleeding is rare. It needs accurate assessment with initiation of appropriate investigations and management.

1 **Has there actually been bleeding and if so, from where?**
   a Upper versus lower?
   b From where, i.e. nose/pharynx/tooth or gum lesion?
   c Is it blood or was what was seen due to food colourings, or medications?
2 **Is the child still bleeding?**
   If yes, ongoing losses need to be taken into account.
3 **How much compromise** has taken place?

Assessment should include pulse, blood pressure, capillary refill, a search for any stigmata of chronic liver disease (varices). Effective triage and supportive treatment is established, with good venous access and regular monitoring of pulse, blood pressure, conscious level and oxygen saturations.

Investigations should include urea and electrolytes, creatinine, liver function tests, glucose, full blood count, CRP, ESR, coagulation and Group and Save (may need cross-match). If the child is vomiting, consider the use of a nasogastric tube. Once the patient is resuscitated and haemodynamically stable, any premorbid conditions or suggestive family history can be ascertained (Table 10.3) and appropriate investigation performed. Upper gastrointestinal bleeding (haematemesis, melaena) should prompt acid blockade with a proton-pump inhibitor (PPI), such as omeprazole, commenced at 1 mg/kg per day. If there is a doubt as to the source of upper bleeding, combined examination with the ENT surgeons may be helpful. Further evaluation with endoscopy is indicated when the patient has stabilized or if the patient continues to have bleeding and endoscopic therapy is indicated. Mallory–Weiss tears, duodenitis and clean-based ulcers usually need no specific intervention. Ulcers are injected with adrenaline (1 in 100 000) around their periphery if at risk of further bleeding. Bleeding ulcers can be coagulated (heater probed) after injection, especially when there is a vessel or overlying clot associated. Upper and lower intestinal polyps are injected at their bases with dilute adrenaline to help stop subsequent bleeding, prior to snare diathermy and removal. Varices are now treated with rubber band ligation – the varix is sucked into a banding device attached to the scope-tip. This has revolutionized management of variceal bleeding. Thrombin glue is also used, particularly for gastric varices.

Polyps

CASE STUDY: Juvenile polyp

A 3-year-old boy presents with the intermittent brisk passage of bright red blood per rectum. He is not in pain. Colonoscopy reveals a large, stalked, ulcerated 3-cm polyp in the sigmoid colon with nil else more proximally. It is injected at its base with adrenaline, then snared and cut off with diathermy. Histological examination confirms that this is a benign or juvenile polyp.

Intestinal polyps are tumours that protrude into the bowel lumen. They are described by their appearance, size and distribution and behaviour. Polyps may be found in asymptomatic patients at screening or because of rectal bleeding and diarrhoea, pain or complications such as intussusception. **Juvenile (or inflammatory) polyps** account for 90 per cent of all polyps in children, usually causing painless, intermittent rectal bleeding between the ages of 2 and 10 years (Table 10.4). They may be multiple rather than solitary and up to a third of cases will present with anaemia secondary to chronic blood loss. Diarrhoea, incomplete evacuation and rectal prolapse are also documented. They rarely recur.

Table 10.4 Polyposis syndromes

Juvenile polyposis	Fifty per cent family history, presents before the age of 10 years with multiple colonic polyps, associations include hydrocephalus, malrotation, Meckel diverticulum and undescended testes
Peutz–Jeghers syndrome	Fifty per cent family history, presents under the age of 10 years with cutaneous freckling pigmentation, usually perioral, buccal, hands and feet; suggested autosomal dominant (AD) inheritance with variable penetrance; may present with abdominal pain and intussusception; intestinal cancer reported and gonadal cancer also associated
Familial adenomatous polyposis (FAP)	AD condition in first to second decade with insidious development of hundreds of sessile colonic, stomach and small bowel lesions with progression to cancer; caused by mutation of the APC gene on chromosome 5; screening before development of lesions is possible – eye exam for retinal hyperpigmentary changes and screening endoscopy is recommended to start at around 12 years of age; colectomy is inevitable in most cases
Cowden syndrome	Multiple hamartomas, papillomas of the lips, tongue and nares, and polyps throughout the gut, particularly stomach and colon, presenting in the second to third decade of life; breast lesions in women can occur, usually fibroadenomas, ductal cancer also reported; thyroid disease
Turcot syndrome	FAP plus neurological problems and tumours – glioblastoma, medulloblastoma; presents in adolescence
Gardner syndrome	Triad of small gastrointestinal polyps affecting stomach, duodenum and colon, soft-tissue tumours and osteomas, appearing in the second decade; tumours are usually epidermoid cysts on the head, neck and trunk, and desmoid tumours which may occur intra-abdominally. Screening endoscopy is indicated and colectomy may be required when the risk of malignancy is raised
Ruvalcaba–Mehyre–Smith syndrome	Rare combination of macrocephaly, pigmented penile lesions and café-au-lait spots, lipomas, colonic polyps, psychomotor retardation and a lipid storage disorder
Cronkhite–Canada syndrome	Pigmented macular lesions, intestinal polyps, onychodystrophy, alopecia usually outwith childhood

KEY LEARNING POINTS

- Acute life-threatening gastrointestinal bleeding in children is uncommon.
- Most lower gastrointestinal bleeding is from fissures, benign polyps or IBD.

GASTRO-OESOPHAGEAL REFLUX AND ITS CONSEQUENCES

CASE STUDY: GOR

A 7-month-old baby girl is referred to you for evaluation of recurrent vomiting, usually after feeds, without blood or bile. The baby is thriving. The parents are both very anxious about the cause and are not reassured by their GP's explanation. You explain that this is very common in infants and that the natural progression is for this to settle and that no investigations are currently required. Positioning is recommended and a feed thickener is commenced with good effect.

CASE STUDY: GORD

An 11-year-old boy complains of postprandial epigastric discomfort, unrelieved by his father's antacid preparation. There is retrosternal discomfort especially after eating spicy or fatty foods and you find that he drinks a lot of caffeinated and fizzy beverages. Advice about reducing triggers (lifestyle changes) is given. You give him a course of ranitidine, which does not help after six weeks, but on switching to omeprazole excellent relief is obtained after only one week.

Gastro-oesophageal reflux (GOR) is common in infants and reduces in frequency into childhood. It ranges from simple 'spitting up', or posseting with no consequences to a major cause of morbidity and mortality with major vomiting and its consequences. Gastro-oesophageal reflux is normal or physiological, whereas GORD is a pathological disease. Infants reflux around 11 per cent of the time (proven on pH probe studies), this figure reducing to less than 6 per cent in the second and subsequent years of life. Reflux occurs after meals, in response to relaxation of the (normally) tonically contracted lower oesophageal sphincter (LOS). Gastro-oesophageal reflux in the first couple of years of life usually resolves, whereas in older children and adults it tends to relapse frequently in around 50 per cent. Gastro-oesophageal reflux disease is very common in children after oesophageal surgery, in chronic chest disease and in neurological conditions and may present atypically or with complications of GORD (peptic stricture or Barrett oesophagus, very rarely cancer) without significant preceding symptoms.

Symptoms of reflux

Typical
- Heartburn
- Postprandial (also bending over, lying flat)
- Acid regurgitation
- Epigastric pain

Atypical
- Vomiting
- Dental enamel erosion
- ENT symptoms
- Respiratory problems (apnoeas, acute life-threatening episodes (ALTE), aspiration pneumonia, asthma, cough)
- Atypical chest pain
- Dystonic movements (Sandifer complex)

Investigations are usually not required, as reflux symptoms are very obvious from the history. Investigations include barium swallow (best utilized to detect complications and anatomical abnormalities rather than reflux for which it is neither sensitive nor specific). pH-metry is the current 'gold standard' investigation but does not indicate non-acid reflux – an important limitation of its use. Endoscopy and biopsy may also be helpful, though many patients are endoscopy negative. Scintigraphy is also used as is manometry and electrogastrography but their role is limited. A newer modality is oesophageal impedance manometry where the movement of fluids past an array of sensors (not pH dependent) is detected and is gaining increasing popularity.

Often no treatment is required, other than simple explanation and reassurance, with the natural history being of resolution within the first two years of life. Treatment is with positioning, feed thickening agents, compound alginate preparations such as Gaviscon®, acid-blocking medications (H_2-receptor antagonists and PPI) and prokinetic agents (domperidone, metoclopramide, cisapride, erythromycin). Reflux (and vomiting) may be due to feed intolerance and a therapeutic change of formula to soy, hydrolysed or elemental feed (or milk-free diet in breastfeeding mothers) may improve symptoms. Older children often follow a relapsing course. Children failing to respond to maximal medical treatment (usually a PPI and prokinetic) or who frequently relapse when coming off medication may be considered for fundoplication (nowadays performed laparoscopically, avoiding an open procedure), but the risks of dumping syndrome, retching and gagging need to be weighed against the benefits of surgery.

KEY LEARNING POINTS

- Often no investigation is required unless complicated reflux is suspected.
- Paradoxically there should be a low threshold to investigate high-risk patients.

ACHALASIA AND OESOPHAGEAL MOTILITY DISORDERS

Achalasia is a primary motor disorder due to absent or decreased relaxation of the LOS, with increased LOS pressure and absent or reduced peristalsis presenting with dysphagia, vomiting (classically at night), weight loss, retrosternal pain and chest infections. Diagnosis is by radiography (air/fluid level, widened mediastinum), barium swallow (breaking at the distal end of a dilated proximal oesophagus) and manometry shows increased LOS pressure, absence of peristalsis and incomplete or abnormal LOS relaxation. Pneumatic dilatation is often performed but definitive laparoscopic Heller myotomy is increasingly used as primary therapy. Other motility problems of smooth muscle include **nutcracker oesophagus** and **diffuse oesophageal spasm.** Secondary disorders occur usually due to reflux, anatomical problems (oesophageal atresia, tracheo-oesophageal fistula), ingestion of caustic substances, connective tissue diseases, neuromuscular disorders and depression.

ACID PEPTIC DISEASE, GASTRITIS, *HELICOBACTER PYLORI*

CASE STUDY: Duodenal ulcer

An 11-year-old girl recently taking naproxen for juvenile idiopathic arthritis is admitted with a three-day history of sudden-onset epigastric pain, which began in the early hours of the morning. She also complains of back pain and passes a number of melaena stools over the next 12 hours. Her haemoglobin drops by 2 g/dL. She is tachycardic but blood pressure is well maintained. Urea and potassium are elevated, suggestive of a recent bleed. After appropriate resuscitation with fluids, she undergoes endoscopy and is found to have gastric antral nodularity (and positive CLOtest®, diagnostic of *H. pylori*) and duodenitis, with a posterior duodenal ulcer with a clean base (i.e. no clot adherent or any sign of a bleeding vessel). She is started on a PPI and has appropriate eradication therapy (PPI, amoxicillin and clarithromycin for one week). Two months later a breath test confirms successful eradication and she remains symptom free.

Acid-related disease is uncommon in children and is seen in less than 5 per cent of children presenting with abdominal pain. Duodenal ulceration is more common than gastric ulceration. *H. pylori* is a Gram-negative organism which infects populations in a cohort fashion. In subsequent generations of children, infection is less common. Developing nations and disadvantaged social groups in the West are more likely to carry *H. pylori*. An approximate 10 per cent lifetime risk of ulcer disease exists when infected. Transmission is faecal–oral and oral–oral. Colonization of the gastric antrum is aided by factors including urease allowing the organism to create an alkaline microenvironment. An initial hypochlohydric state is followed by chronic superficial gastritis and duodenal gastric metaplasia, hypergastrinaemia and reduced duodenal bicarbonate secretion with subsequent ulceration. Some develop an atrophic gastritis, which may lead to gastric cancer, and B-cell lymphomas of the mucosa-associated lymphoid tissue (MALTomas) have been reported in childhood, though rarely. The WHO has determined *H. pylori* to be a grade 1 carcinogen. Patients with a family history of gastric cancer and *H. pylori* should be counselled and offered eradication. In adults on non-steroidal anti-inflammatory drugs (NSAIDs), eradication is recommended. Ten to 20 per cent of duodenal ulcers are *H. pylori*-negative and a history of aspirin or NSAID ingestion should be sought. Coeliac disease, Crohn disease and eosinophilic gastroenteropathy should also be considered as a cause of gastric or duodenal ulceration. Hypersecretory states such as Zollinger–Ellison syndrome, hyperparathyroidism and short bowel syndrome are causes of recurrent and multiple ulcers.

Gastritis is inflammation of the stomach itself, manifesting as nausea, acute or chronic vomiting with or without abdominal pain. In addition to *H. pylori*, other aetiologies include infections (viral such as CMV), allergic, chemical gastritis from bile reflux and iatrogenic (drug therapy, e.g. NSAIDs or aspirin, steroids, chemotherapy).

Debate continues about who should be investigated and treated. Most children with acid-related problems have reflux and oesophagitis and a trial of appropriate therapy is indicated. However for non-responders, investigation may include upper endoscopy and biopsy (with a rapid urease, or CLOtest or specific requests for *H. pylori* histological examination), serological tests (though these are not as accurate in children) and C-14 or C-13 breath testing, although again less reliable than in adults (false positives may be seen in children due to oral urea-splitting organisms). Controversy exists as to whether children with *H. pylori* and recurrent abdominal pain should be treated as eradication may not improve symptoms and *H. pylori* may be an innocent bystander. An infected individual, even if asymptomatic, particularly those with a family history of gastric cancer, should be offered eradication after proper counselling. Eradication can be achieved in over 80 per cent of patients with a seven-day course of a combination of PPI, clarithromycin and amoxicillin or metronidazole. The *British National Formulary* outlines various regimens and local guidelines usually exist due to differences in resistance patterns.

KEY LEARNING POINTS

- In uncomplicated reflux, careful consideration should be given to the need for any investigations.
- Most acid-related abdominal pain is due to reflux, not ulcers.
- Peptic ulcer disease (and *H. pylori*) in children is uncommon.

SHORT BOWEL SYNDROME

This is defined as malabsorption, fluid loss and electrolyte loss following major small bowel resection. It is an extremely challenging problem. The small bowel in term babies is 200–300 cm long, which increases in length to 600–800 cm by adulthood. It has been estimated that as much as 75 per cent of the small bowel can be resected as long as the ileocaecal valve is present, though in preterm babies, this may not apply as the length of bowel is considerably shorter than in full term babies. Resection including the ileocaecal valve contributes to poorer adaptation and complications. Necrotizing enterocolitis is the commonest cause.

Management of small bowel syndrome involves **optimizing nutrition**, the use of hydrolysed, high medium chain triglyceride (MCT) content feeds such as Pregestemil® and Caprilon® or more usually elemental formulas such as Neocate®, with or without the use of total parenteral nutrition (TPN). Small volume trophic feeds allow the mucosa to adapt (as non-feeding causes atrophy of the intestine). Careful measurement of fluid balance is required. **Malabsorption** of fat and carbohydrate, fluid, electrolytes, specific vitamins and nutrients can occur. Specific **deficiencies** of calcium, iron, magnesium and zinc, vitamins A, D, E and K, folate and vitamin B_{12} occur and supplementation may be required. **Bacterial overgrowth** occurs and is promoted by loss of the ileocaecal valve and promotes **D-lactic acidosis** from fermentation of carbohydrates: slurring and diminished mentation and elevated anion gap metabolic acidosis. **Cycled antibiotics** to selectively decontaminate the bowel, such as metronidazole and/or gentamicin given orally, and **probiotics** such as lactobacilli and bifidobacteria are used. High gastrin levels cause **elevated acid secretion** and predispose infants to acid peptic disease. Ranitidine or PPIs, such as omeprazole, are commenced early. Malabsorbed fat binds unabsorbed fatty acids to make soaps and allows oxalate to be reabsorbed in the colon, increasing the risk of **gall stones and renal stones. Cholestatic liver disease** is common, due to sepsis, inspissated bile, gall stones and direct toxic effects to the liver from TPN and antibiotics. **Ursodeoxycholic acid (UDCA)** promotes choleresis and has a protective effect on the liver. **Electrolyte imbalances** occur with chronic diarrhoea (hyponatraemia, hypokalaemia and acidosis) and total body sodium balance, particularly, can be assessed by measurement of urinary sodium (low urinary sodium indicates the need for supplementation). Short chain fatty acid (SCFA) and bile salt malabsorption leads to diarrhoea if the colon is still in continuity. Motility disturbances are common, with fast transit through the jejunum. **Diarrhoea** can be managed with the use of loperamide, codeine and bile salt binding resins such as cholestyramine. Central line infections (skin or colonic bacteria which are translocated across the relatively leaky gut) occur commonly. Long-term TPN has improved survival and quality of life, but death may occur due to infection, liver failure or its complications (bleeding) and lack of venous access. Survival without transplantation correlates with length of residual small bowel, with over 90 per cent surviving with 40–80 cm and 66 per cent survival in those with less than 40 cm. **Small intestinal transplantation** (or isolated liver transplant for chronic liver disease in a child who may eventually adapt) has gained prominence over the last decade due to better immunosuppression and improved techniques, but requires careful assessment and counselling of families about complications including infection (fungal, bacterial, viral such as Epstein–Barr virus (EBV) and CMV), graft rejection and post-transplant lymphoproliferative disease (PTLD).

Causes of short bowel syndrome

- Necrotizing enterocolitis
- Gastroschisis
- Jejunal and ileal atresias
- Neonatal volvulus
- Intussusception
- Congenital short gut syndrome
- Hirschsprung disease (long segment)
- Small bowel Crohn
- SMA thrombosis (severe dehydration)
- Trauma

KEY LEARNING POINTS

- Short bowel syndrome is complex and requires expert multidisciplinary input.
- Total parenteral nutrition has revolutionized management of infants with short bowel syndrome.
- Intestinal failure and liver disease related to short bowel syndrome may require transplantation.

ALLERGIC BOWEL DISEASE AND FOOD INTOLERANCE

CASE STUDY: Cows' milk protein intolerance (CMPI)

A 3-month-old baby girl is seen with bloodstained loose stools with mucus. The child is colicky, irritable and windy and diagnosis is CMPI manifesting as colitis. She is placed on a hydrolysed formula and milk- and soy-free diet and symptoms settle after a few weeks.

Food allergy/intolerance (or hypersensitivity) is a reproducible reaction to a food protein antigen that is immune mediated. Elimination of the offending food will result in resolution and rechallenge will cause the return of the symptoms. Blinded food challenges show, however, that patients and parents overestimate their allergic tendency. Cows' milk protein intolerance may manifest as oesophagitis, gastritis, enteropathy or colitis. Allergic responses types I and IV (immediate and delayed) are both seen to contribute to gastrointestinal allergy (Table 10.5). More than one subtype may be present (see below). Food reactions are either IgE mediated, IgE associated or not. Investigation may include skin prick testing or specific IgE testing on blood, patch testing (to look for delayed or type IV hypersensitivity). In practice, we find such testing generally unhelpful and prefer to take a thorough history and with the help of an experienced dietitian eliminate either specific items which have been highlighted by parents or the patient, or the commonest culprits (cows' milk, soy or wheat) and reintroduce at an interval period after symptom control is established. IgE and non-IgE mediated allergic disease tends to improve with time. Cows' milk protein intolerance prevalence is around 3 per cent based on population studies. Rechallenge is the only way to assess attainment of tolerance, with gradual reintroduction at 12 months of age, and subsequent withdrawal and rechallenge as tolerated. Most children (approx 85 per cent) lose their sensitivity to food allergens (milk, soya, wheat, egg) by the age of 3–5 years.

Table 10.5 Mechanisms of gut-mediated food allergy

IgE associated/ cell mediated, delayed onset/chronic	Includes atopic dermatitis and the eosinophilic gastroenteropathies, which are site specific and dependent on the degree of inflammation present (see below)
Cell-mediated, delayed onset/chronic	Includes protein-mediated oesophagitis, enteropathy, enterocolitis, proctitis, often affecting infants and resolving between the ages of 1 and 3 years and classic 'allergic' bowel disease, coeliac and dermatitis herpetiformis

KEY LEARNING POINTS

- Diet-related symptoms should always be considered.
- Intolerance or allergic symptoms are common in infants.
- Breastfed children may have CMPI through transmission of peptides from maternal diet.

CONSTIPATION

CASE STUDY: Chronic functional constipation

A 2-year-old boy presents with a history of difficulty passing stools from 8 months. The GP is worried about the possibility of Hirschsprung disease and suggested to the parents that he needs a rectal biopsy. You take a careful history and find that stooling was normal until solids were introduced at 6 months.

The diagnosis here is functional constipation. Constipation is the passage of a stool that is difficult or painful and is often associated with soiling. Often, less than three stools per week is considered abnormal. Encopresis is a term used for the involuntary leakage of stool. Soiling is an intrinsic problem in constipation. There are physical, social and psychological issues to take into account. Child protection issues need to be excluded. **Functional constipation** accounts for over 90 per cent of cases.

Constipation is often left too long before it is seen as a problem, or even considered. Inadequate treatment is started, inadequate doses given and before long a pathological pattern emerges. Aggressive medical management and regular support and encouragement are required. Infrequent follow-up and no specific contact person at the GP surgery or hospital (health visitor, practice nurse, paediatric community nurse or nurse specialist, doctor, etc.) will lead to failure. Families benefit from thorough explanation of why this has happened and the reasoning for the treatment plan. Parents often assume that constipation and soiling will settle with a brief period of medication with little or no effort on their part, whereas in reality it may require intermittent disimpaction and long-term medications (months to years) such as softeners and active participation in a toileting programme by them. In the pathological state, constipation may arise from hard stooling which causes the child to withhold and a vicious cycle may ensue. During illness and holidays to hotter climates, reduced fluid intake, lack of activity, lack of privacy or poor toilet facilities, such as at school, all add up to stools getting harder and being more difficult to pass and before long, a pattern of retentive behaviour emerges.

Important questions to ask include: Was there delayed passage of meconium (Hirschsprung disease) and was constipation from the first few weeks? Usually these patients would present with bilious vomiting or generally unwell in the first week or two of life. Were there any other precipitants (illness, a holiday, starting nursery, etc.). Often, no obvious reasons are forthcoming. Constipation frequently reduces appetite, promotes poor weight gain and children may be fractious and unhappy, they may misbehave or may posture to avoid stooling. Dribbling and urinary incontinence or urinary tract infections can occur as a consequence of obstruction. Examination may reveal a faecal mass in the midline, extending up into the left iliac fossa and beyond. Stool is indentable and gentle bimanual palpation may define the problem. The back should be examined for obvious abnormalities of the spine. The lower limbs including the reflexes should be examined. Perianal inspection is important to assess the position of the anus and to exclude local causes of discomfort or reluctance to stool, as well as for evidence of soiling. Rectal exam is helpful in defining anal tone, the size of the ampulla and the presence of stool in children where there is doubt, but only in children likely to cooperate and it is often not necessary.

A plain abdominal film or **transit studies** can define the extent of the problem (see above) when there is doubt. If Hirschsprung's is suspected, **anorectal manometry** or an **unprepped barium enema** may be performed, looking for the classic transition zone of Hirschsprung disease. In poor responders to treatment or those in whom the history or exam has flagged up other underlying potential diagnoses, investigate for electrolyte imbalance, calcium levels, thyroid function and a coeliac screen.

Treatment varies widely – so if a regimen works stick to it. Advice on good **fluid and fibre** intake is essential. The author encourages the use of **star charts and rewards** for successful visits to the toilet, also for days free from soiling. Regular toiletting and positive reinforcement by parents, carers and professionals is vital for success. We have a low threshold for **disimpaction** with sodium picosulphate twice daily until clear then liquid paraffin for **maintenance**. Often, failure is because inadequate amounts of medications are used and disimpaction is not considered or there is refusal to take medications. The child has to be 'on-board' or management will fail. Other medications for disimpaction include bowel cleansing solutions such as Citramag® and Klean Prep®. Stimulant laxatives such as sodium picosulphate or senna may be required as an adjunct to softeners in the long term. Newer preparations such as Movicol® are gaining popularity for disimpaction and maintenance treatment of children. Whatever regimen is used, it should be tailored to the child's needs (and ability to take).

Causes of constipation

Non-organic

- Developmental (cognitive problems, attention deficit hyperactivity disorder)
- Depression
- Constitutional (genetic predisposition, colonic inertia)
- Situational (coercive toilet training, toilet phobia, school toilet avoidance, excessive parental intervention, sexual abuse)
- Reduced stool volume/dry stool (low-fibre diet, dehydration, underfeeding/malnutrition)

Organic

- Anatomic (muscle problems, imperforate anus, anal stenosis, anterior anus, mass, gastroschisis, prune belly, Down syndrome, other neurodevelopmental conditions, Hirschsprung disease, neuronal dysplasia, visceral myopathy)
- Neuropathic problems (spinal cord problems, visceral neuropathy)
- Gastrointestinal (cystic fibrosis, coeliac disease, CMPI)
- Metabolic (hypothyroidism, hypokalaemia, hypocalcaemia, diabetes mellitus, multiple endocrine neoplasia (MEN) type 2B)
- Connective tissue abnormalities
- Drugs

FUNCTIONAL GASTROINTESTINAL DISORDERS IN CHILDHOOD

CASE STUDY: Irritable bowel syndrome

An 8-year-old girl presents with a three-year history of central colicky abdominal pain lasting 15–30 minutes. It occurs before breakfast and sometimes at school, where it will generally pass when she busies herself with activities. She has a tendency to constipation. Her pains worsen when faced with tests at school or other stressors. Exam is normal. You explain that the girl has IBS with constipation predominance. The formulation of visceral hyperalgesia is explained and they are referred to a psychologist for pain management techniques. Working with the family, the psychologist found how to tackle the stressful triggers the girl found brought the pain on and she is now pain free.

Irritable bowel syndrome

Traditionally, the Apley criteria have been applied to children with 'recurrent abdominal pain', recurrent episodes over at least a three-month period affecting normal activity. These have now been superseded by the Rome II criteria, according to which most childhood abdominal pain fits similar adult categories. At least 10 per cent of schoolchildren experience pain regularly. A history fitting these criteria along with normal physical exam and growth pattern is consistent with IBS. Specific dietary precipitants may include lactose, sorbitol, carbonated diet beverages and other natural sugars such as fruit juices (e.g. apple). It is prudent to consider limited investigations such as inflammatory markers, blood count, liver function tests, coeliac screen and stool studies to exclude infection and malabsorption/inflammation in cases where there is doubt or the family need more than verbal reassurance. In some cases, imaging of the abdomen with ultrasound or small bowel follow-through, and in others endoscopy, may be necessary to be definitive in ruling out organic disease. A confident diagnosis and explanation of the condition is important from the outset. It is important for the child and parents to recognize that they must try to maintain their responsibilities of attending school and other commitments as much as possible. It is important to look into the family dynamics and to find out whether there may be an underlying problem which may be amenable to intervention. Often problems are denied or even not appreciated by the family themselves. The psychology team is integral to further assessment and ongoing management of such cases. It is important to discuss the formulation of visceral hyperalgesia (nerve hypersensitivity due to visceral distension in susceptible individuals) and explain the benign nature of the condition. Atypical symptoms should be viewed with caution. Drug treatment may be a helpful adjunct. Concurrent constipation should be treated effectively. Antispasmodics (mebeverine etc.) and tricyclic antidepressants (amitriptyline etc.) have been used with effect in pain management.

Important factors in assessment for IBS

- Child's personality: conscientious, obsessional, insecure, anxious, social difficulties
- Family factors: health problems, preoccupation with illness, high expectations (health, performance), life events

Warning signs

- Young age (under 5)
- Other associated symptoms (vomiting, diarrhoea)
- Nocturnal waking with pain
- Well-localized pain or tenderness
- Weight loss, clubbing, perianal disease
- Poor growth and/or pubertal progression
- Family history of coeliac disease, IBD

Functional abdominal pain

Sometimes symptoms do not meet the criteria for IBS (a common criticism of the original Apley and newer Rome II criteria). Children may have continuous pain; it may have no relation to eating or stooling etc. and may prevent them from sleeping. There may be other symptoms such as headache, tiredness, dizziness or nausea and underlying features of school phobia, anxiety or depression may be evident. Secondary pain may be experienced. Again, adequate explanation and limited but helpful exclusion of other conditions with psychological assessment are helpful.

Abdominal migraine

This is characterized by acute abdominal pain that may last for hours, with acute, debilitating pain in the midline, accompanied by pallor, anorexia, nausea and vomiting. A history of migraine in the child or family may be discovered. Obviously if the child had headaches in addition, the diagnosis is easy. Again, other causes of acute pain need to be considered and ruled out. Response to antimigraine therapy is highly supportive of the diagnosis. Serotonin receptor antagonists such as pizotifen are used frequently to treat abdominal migraine. Cyproheptadine is an alternative.

Cyclical vomiting syndrome

CASE STUDY

A 6-year-old girl presents with a two-year history of vomiting lasting three days, in a very typical pattern each time, starting in the early hours of the morning and vomiting over 20 times an hour at its peak. She is admitted dehydrated to hospital each time, five times a year, and is said to have gastroenteritis, although there are usually no contacts who are unwell. All investigations have been negative, with stools, blood tests and an abdominal ultrasound proving normal.

Cyclical vomiting syndrome consists of recurrent episodes of nausea and vomiting which may last hours or days, usually of similar duration each time and intervals of complete wellbeing in between. Frequency is variable, from a single episode a year to over 50 per year. Symptoms start at a similar time each episode, often at night or early morning. There may be prodromal symptoms but vomiting may start suddenly, worsening over the next few hours. Children are typically 2–7 years old at onset. Family members may have migraine, travel sickness or other functional bowel problems. Pallor, abdominal pain, headache, intolerance to smells, light or sound may be apparent in addition to diarrhoea, blotching and hypertension. There may be a trigger factor in up to 80 per cent of cases such as emotional upsets or infections. Treatment is often difficult, but the early use of ondansetron, ibuprofen or erythromycin may abate symptoms. Frequent episodes may be treated with a variety of different prophylactic medications (none works for all) including erythromycin (as prokinetic), cyproheptadine, amitriptyline, phenobarbital, pizotifen, propranolol or more recently, sumatriptan.

KEY LEARNING POINTS

- A positive diagnosis and explanation is paramount to patient understanding.
- Limited investigations 'up-front' may reassure the family.
- Engage the help of your psychology team and promote them as a major management option.

Table 10.6 Causes of hyperbilirubinaemia in the neonate

Combined factors	Sepsis, congenital infections
Increased production	Blood group incompatibility (ABO, Rhesus), polycythaemia, haemoglobin defects (elliptocytosis, spherocytosis, glucose 6-phosphate dehydrogenase deficiency), bleeding (intra-abdominal, intracranial, traumatic bruising to skin)
Decreased excretion	Increased reabsorption/prematurity (decreased stooling), breastfeeding, drugs, ischaemic hepatic problems, cholestasis and obstruction

LIVER DISEASE IN THE NEONATAL PERIOD AND CHILDHOOD

Jaundice

Bile pigment deposition in the skin causes jaundice, visible when the level reaches 50 μmol/L in the blood. Jaundice is described as **conjugated** (direct hyperbilirubinaemia) and **unconjugated** (indirect hyperbilirubinaemia) (Table 10.6). Bilirubin results from degradation of haemoglobin, or haem, to biliverdin by enzymes in the reticuloendothelial system after the red cells reach the end of their lifespan (90 days in neonates, 120 days in adults). Biliverdin is transported to the liver bound to albumin and taken up into the hepatocytes where it is conjugated with glucuronic acid by glucuronyl transferase and excreted in a water-soluble form into the bile canaliculi as bilirubin diglucuronides (70–90 per cent) and monoglucuronides (up to 30 per cent). Secretion is increased by choleretic agents (phenobarbital) and reduced by hormones (oestrogens) and in pathologic jaundice. Bilirubin is excreted into the small bowel and converted by bacteria in the distal bowel and excreted in the faeces. This section deals with inherited causes of unconjugated jaundice (neonatal unconjugated jaundice and its treatment is covered more fully in Chapter 5) and the major causes of cholestatic jaundice as well as important causes of liver disease in older children.

Unconjugated jaundice (beyond physiological)

CASE STUDY

A 3-day-old breastfed term neonate develops unconjugated hyperbilirubinaemia requiring phototherapy, which drops to a normal level after 1 month.

Liver function tests are normal. He presents again at 10 years with recurrent episodes of short-lived mild jaundice. Again, liver function tests are normal but the total bilirubin is elevated at times, up to 90 mmol/L and falls to within normal.

Breast milk jaundice is the initial diagnosis, but the resolution after one month and subsequent recurrence with normal liver function tests and levels of unconjugated bilirubin under 100 μmol/L are highly consistent with the **Gilbert syndrome.** During breastfeeding, levels can go quite high and advising discontinuation for up to 48 hours with switch to formula feeding may be considered.

Gilbert syndrome

This is one of the hereditary unconjugated hyperbilirubinaemias due to a decrease in hepatic bilirubin UDP-glucuronyltransferase activity of around 50 per cent or more. Levels increase during stress, ill health, in response to menstruation in women and prolonged fasting. It can present with exaggerated early neonatal jaundice and has been linked with pyloric stenosis. It usually re-presents at puberty. Long-term ill health is unusual though patients often complain of non-specific symptoms such as fatigue, nausea, diarrhoea and headache.

Crigler–Najjar types 1 and 2

These two syndromes cause significant unconjugated neonatal jaundice and also arise from mutations of the UGT gene. There is very low activity of glucuronyl transferase in liver. They present with marked unconjugated jaundice in the neonatal period and should be considered in the differential diagnosis when levels exceed 350 μmol/L and are persistent. They can be differentiated clinically by difference in response to phenobarbital (type 2 responds within 48 hours). Type 1 requires prolonged phototherapy (12 hours daily in the long term) to avoid kernicterus and exchange transfusion may be necessary in the acute stages. Treatment is with enzyme inducers in type 2 and auxiliary liver transplantation in type 1.

Conjugated jaundice (Rotor syndrome and Dubin–Johnson)

These deserve a brief mention. **Rotor syndrome** presents with a mixed picture in childhood with over half the bilirubin conjugated and occasionally levels up to 200 μmol/L or more with normal liver function tests. There is no liver abnormality histologically and essentially there is no treatment. **Dubin–Johnson** is commoner and also involves an elevation of both fractions. Again, over half the total level is conjugated but the liver function tests are again normal. It presents in the pubertal period, and may worsen during pregnancy and in women on the oral contraceptive pill. The classic appearance of the liver is black with increased pigmentation but otherwise normal histology. No specific treatment is available.

Neonatal hepatitis syndrome and prolonged jaundice

Children with **jaundice beyond two weeks** need investigation (however limited). Investigation is aimed at establishing if **conjugated** jaundice is present and subsequently **extrahepatic** (surgical causes such as biliary atresia or a choledochal cyst) or **intrahepatic.**

Cholestatic jaundice in the neonate requires a common-sense approach with certain essential investigations and the important surgical causes (as above) excluded and supportive care given as required. Neonates are 'physiologically cholestatic', which does not require much to push them into clinical cholestasis. These underdeveloped mechanisms include reduced secretion and reduced bile acid pool, poor enterohepatic circulation (with the terminal ileum), and qualitative and quantitative differences in bile acids. Bile is toxic to the liver and stimulates inflammation and the fibrosis/cirrhosis sequence. Idiopathic neonatal cholestasis (no specific cause) and biliary atresia are the 'big two', accounting for up to 70 per cent of the total cases. A conjugated level of over 20 μmol/L and over 20 per cent conjugated fraction in an elevated total bilirubin is considered abnormal, however, many babies have a mildly elevated level, eventually settling with time and no specific cause is discovered. It is important to assess liver function tests including γ-glutamyl transferase and alkaline phosphatase (both markers of biliary inflammation), whereas alanine aminotransferase and aspartate aminotransferase suggest hepatocyte damage. Albumin and prothrombin time assess liver synthetic function.

Causes of neonatal cholestasis and liver dysfunction

- Biliary atresia
- Choledochal cyst
- Idiopathic neonatal hepatitis
- α-1-Antitrypsin deficiency
- Alagille and related syndromes
- Bacterial infection
- Infectious hepatitis (TORCH, including CMV, herpes simplex virus (HSV), rubella)
- Bile acid synthetic disorders (progressive familial intrahepatic cholestasis (PFIC))
- Hypothyroidism/pituitarism
- Galactosaemia and other metabolic causes (tyrosinaemia, urea cycle defects)

CASE STUDY: Extrahepatic biliary atresia

A 6-week-old white baby girl presents with jaundice since two weeks. She is deeply jaundiced and has a 3-cm liver. She is feeding well and gaining weight, continuing along the 50th centile. The stools are pale. An ultrasound scan shows no gall bladder. Alanine aminotransferase (ALT) is 300 U/L, γ-glutamyl transferase (GGT) 290 U/L, alkaline phosphatase (ALP) is 600 U/L and conjugated bilirubin is 280 μmol/L. A liver biopsy shows proliferation of the intrahepatic bile ducts, confirming the diagnosis of biliary atresia.

Any jaundiced infant with a conjugated picture like this should raise suspicion. **Biliary atresia** is the main consideration. It results from an idiopathic process destroying the extrahepatic biliary system and causes cholestatic jaundice with acholic stools. Looking at the stools is the single best initial test. There are two types, **embryonic** and **perinatal**. The **embryonic** form is associated with multiple malformations (splenic, cardiac, malrotation), comprises up to a third of cases and presents with no jaundice-free interval, the physiological jaundice of the neonate merging with pathological hyperbilirubinaemia. The **perinatal** form is commoner, with the majority presenting around a month or more with persistent and progressive jaundice after a short jaundice-free period where stools were normal. It is thought to be an acquired lesion and there is experimental evidence in mice that reovirus 3 and rotavirus can cause biliary inflammation and obstruction. Incidence is 1 in 15 000 births. Ultrasound of the liver and biliary system is essential, looking for the calibre and presence of the external system, including the gall bladder and to exclude a **choledochal cyst**. The gall bladder may not be seen if the baby has been fed. Absence does not always mean biliary atresia, but should raise suspicions. Radionuclide scanning with HIDA, DISIDA or TEBIDA (see page 313) should proceed if there is doubt. Classically, there is uptake in the liver but no drainage even after 24 hours. If there is an urgency to obtain definitive diagnosis, as in this baby at 6 weeks of age, the baby should proceed without delay to percutaneous liver biopsy after any coagulation problems are corrected (either with vitamin K or fresh frozen plasma).

Management of biliary atresia has been revolutionized by the introduction of the Kasai portoenterostomy procedure where the extrahepatic portion of the biliary tree is excised and a remnant of the ductal system at the porta hepatis big enough to allow drainage into a Roux-en-Y loop of bowel is identified. Drainage is not successful in up to a half of patients (depending on the operator and the experience of the centre), but generally, the earlier the operation (usually before 8 weeks of age in most series) the better. Drainage, however, is no guarantee of continued success and even operation within the first 60 days may not clear the jaundice. Many infants also develop ascending cholangitis in the postoperative period and need intensive support. Failure of drainage results in progressive cirrhosis and a need for liver transplant within the first two years of life. Many children and teenagers owe their continued good health to the initial drainage procedure they had in the neonatal period.

KEY LEARNING POINTS

- Enquiry about and observing stool colour is important in jaundiced babies.
- Biliary atresia is main 'rule out' diagnosis in neonatal cholestasis.
- Prolonged jaundice after 2 weeks of age should always be investigated.
- Surgery for extrahepatic biliary atresia within 60 days of birth requires prompt investigation, diagnosis and referral.

Work-up for conjugated jaundice (see text)

- Full blood count, ESR
- Coagulation (prothrombin time)
- Electrolytes, creatinine, liver function tests (ALP, ALT, aspartate aminotransferase (AST), GGT, albumin, total protein), CRP
- Total and conjugated bilirubin, α-1-antitrypsin level and phenotype, thyroid function, galactose 1-phosphate uridyl transferase (galactosaemia)
- Urine for reducing substances (galactosaemia), culture (infection), succinylacetone (tyrosinaemia)
- Virology/TORCH infection (hepatitis A, B, C viruses, EBV, HSV, CMV, parvo B19)
- Metabolic disease
- Liver and biliary tree ultrasound (fasting)
- Biliary excretion scan
- Liver biopsy

Other causes

α-1-Antitrypsin deficiency

In this condition, **α-1-antitrypsin** cannot be transported out of the liver and accumulates within the hepatocytes remaining within the endoplasmic reticulum. Infants may be asymptomatic but usually present with hepatomegaly, conjugated jaundice and elevated liver function tests and are found to have a reduced serum α-1-antitrypsin (10–15 per cent of normal values) but there is overlap with the normal range, so protease inhibitor typing is performed (Pi type). Normal phenotype is PiMM. Accumulation is seen in patients homozygous for phenotype PiZZ (protease inhibitor) and causes accumulation of periodic acid Schiff (PAS) positive diastase resistant material in hepatocytes. Only 25 per cent with PiZZ will develop chronic liver disease. It is associated with pulmonary emphysema in the third to fourth decade of life and smoking and significant alcohol intake should be strongly discouraged in childhood. There is an increased risk of liver adenocarcinoma.

Alagille syndrome

Bile duct paucity is divided into syndromic or non-syndromic. **Alagille syndrome** or syndromic paucity is a familial disorder of the human Jagged 1 gene, on chromosome 20. There is a marked reduction or paucity of the intrahepatic bile ducts. Abnormalities are often present in family members and are underrecognized. An autosomal dominant pattern of inheritance is suggested with low penetrance and expressional variability. Facial features include bossed forehead, hypertelorism and small pointed chin and may be more apparent after a few months of age. Presentation is usually within the first 3 months of life, with cholestatic jaundice and pruritus and fat-soluble vitamin deficiency. Around 25 per cent progress to chronic liver disease. Pruritus is particularly severe and often worse than expected for the degree of jaundice but tends to settle after a few years. Elevated cholesterol and triglycerides result in xanthomas and atheromas. Pulmonary stenosis and tetralogy of Fallot are seen. Eye exam reveals evidence of posterior embryotoxon seen in around 90 per cent. Other abnormalities, including butterfly vertebrae (on chest radiograph) and cysts, stones or echogenic kidneys are seen (tubulointerstitial disease is common). Growth is poor, commonly below the 3rd centile and development is commonly delayed.

Endocrine causes

Congenital hypothyroidism and **primary hypopituitarism** may present with conjugated jaundice. Up to 20 per cent of hypothyroid babies are jaundiced. Resolution occurs with specific treatment of the underlying condition.

Tyrosinaemia

Tyrosinaemia is uncommon. Progressive liver dysfunction, renal Fanconi syndrome and hypophosphataemic rickets develop. Infants have enlarged kidneys and liver on examination. Liver function tests are mildly elevated but coagulation is severely deranged. The enzyme fumaryl-acetoacetate hydrolase (FAH) which catalyses the last step of the tyrosine pathway is absent and causes accumulation of succinylacetone, detectable in high quantity in the urine and α-fetoprotein is also elevated. There is a greatly increased risk of hepatocellular carcinoma. A compound (NTBC) has been used with marked improvement in liver function in many patients but they still carry the risk of cancer and despite this, transplantation may be required.

Congenital hepatic fibrosis

This involves abnormalities of the liver with portal hypertension, cystic kidney abnormalities and a risk of ascending cholangitis. It is associated with autosomal recessive polycystic kidney disease. The liver abnormality is because of an arrest in the development of the normal portal and bile duct structures, resulting in plates of ductal elements and fibrosis, resulting in hepatosplenomegaly and portal hypertension and its consequences. The lesions in liver and kidney become very similar as time goes on. Portal hypertensive complications occur and the first presentation is bleeding in up to two-thirds of cases, often between the age 5 years and the early teens. Examination reveals firm hepatosplenomegaly with signs of hypersplenism and varices are prominent. Jaundice is usually not present. Ultrasound helps document portal flows and the extent of liver and kidney disease. Liver biopsy is helpful in assessing fibrosis/cirrhosis. Treatment is with portosystemic shunting, either by radiological means or surgical shunts. Transplantation is indicated in isolated chronic failure or combined with renal transplant.

Progressive familial intrahepatic cholestasis

These disorders are rare and are due to defects in bile transport out of the canalicular cell. **Byler disease** or progressive familial intrahepatic cholestasis (PFIC) **type 1** is the best characterized. It was originally described amongst the Amish community in Pennsylvania, USA. Patients present within the first 3 months of life with cholestatic jaundice, pruritus and enlarged liver and spleen along with diarrhoea. Bilirubin, alkaline phosphatase and aminotransferases are usually elevated but cholesterol and GGT are usually normal. Progressive familial intrahepatic cholestasis **type 2** is **bile salt exporter protein deficiency (BSEP)**, which usually presents with elevated bilirubin, pruritus and may rapidly progress requiring liver transplant. Progressive familial intrahepatic cholestasis **type 3** is due to an abnormality of the multidrug-resistance gene MDR3 and presents in a similar way but patients have elevated cholesterol and GGT. Again, transplant may be required.

Congenital infections

TORCH infections can all affect the liver. **Cytomegalovirus** is the commonest the author has seen in practice, but herpes simplex, syphilis and parvovirus B19 infection should all be borne in mind as causes.

Other metabolic problems

Galactosaemia, mitochondrial and fatty acid oxidation defects, Reye syndrome and peroxisomal defects, Gaucher disease, Niemann–Pick type C, neonatal sclerosing cholangitis and haemochromatosis can all affect the liver but are rare.

Managing patients with cholestasis

There are many aspects to this but there is a commonality to all aetiologies. **Nutrition** is very important. Malabsorption and the subsequent steatorrhoea, **growth issues** and fat-soluble vitamin and trace metal deficiencies need regular monitoring with height and weight measurement, anthropometry and regular blood tests along with close liaison with the dietitian. Adequate calories to maintain growth may mean that up to 150 per cent or more of the recommended daily allowance is required. **Medium chain triglyceride** (easier absorbed in cholestasis) formulas such as Caprilon® or modular feeds (favoured by some centres) may be required. **Fat-soluble vitamins** A, D, E and K need to be supplemented and other deficiencies monitored with regular blood tests. Cholestasis results in retention of toxic bile acids and of cholesterol, resulting in jaundice, pruritus and xanthomas. Medications such as **UDCA (ursodeoxycholic acid)** are used to improve choleresis (bile flow), **rifampicin** and **phenobarbital** are used to improve bile flow through the hepatocytes and **cholestyramine** is used to block the recirculation of bile acids. **Opiate antagonists** (naltrexone), **antihistamines** and **ranitidine** have also been used in attempts to reverse the pruritic effects of bile acids. Lipid lowering agents are sometimes used.

PORTAL HYPERTENSION AND VARICES

CASE STUDY: Portal venous thrombosis

A 7-year-old boy, previously well, presents with a massive haematemesis, requiring resuscitation with fluids and blood transfusion. He is noted to have prominent splenomegaly. He had required hospitalization at birth and had an umbilical venous catheter to administer fluids and antibiotics at that time. Mother remembered that the catheter had been taken out when the surrounding skin had become infected (omphalitis). The diagnosis was confirmed when an ultrasound showed collateral vessels around a portal vein that was obstructed.

Portal hypertension occurs as a consequence of increased pressure within the liver – **intrahepatic portal hypertension** (as we see in chronic liver disease and cirrhosis from many conditions), as a consequence of problems with the **extrahepatic** portal venous system, either **prehepatic** (as in portal vein thrombosis) or **posthepatic**, as in the Budd–Chiari syndrome. Normal portal venous pressure is 5 mmHg. When this pressure (the hepatic venous pressure gradient) exceeds 6 mmHg, portal hypertension exists. At this level, **oesophageal varices** and **splenomegaly** develop. Above 12 mmHg the risk of variceal haemorrhage increases. Haemorrhage, either haematemesis or melaena, development of ascites, a protein-losing enteropathy from portal hypertensive congestion of the small or large bowel wall, or the development of prominent abdominal veins or haemorrhoids may herald the onset of portal hypertension. In contrast to diseases such as biliary atresia, extrahepatic causes such as portal vein thrombosis *do not* have parenchymal liver disease and may recanalize the obstructed vein or develop collateral circulation with time.

Portal hypertensive bleeding from varices may require stabilization with an **octreotide** infusion to reduce splanchnic blood flow, or **terlipressin**, a vasopressin analogue, mostly used in adult practice. **Propranolol**, again used in adult practice, and in some smaller children's studies, has been used to reduce portal venous pressure. **Eradication** programmes reduce the risk of longer-term complications, formerly with **sclerotherapy** but nowadays endoscopic **band ligation** and newer treatment such as **transjugular intrahepatic portosystemic shunting (TIPSS)** has been used to reduce portal pressure and bleeding risk.

Prospective management includes the **avoidance** of **aspirin** and **NSAIDs**, which increase the risk of mucosal ulceration and bleeding. Bleeding that cannot be controlled in this way requires a **Sengstaken** tube inflated to compress the varices and control bleeding while arrangements are made to perform **TIPSS** and **coil** ablation of varices. This has revolutionized the management of bleeding, often used as a bridge to definitive treatment by liver transplant. **Surgical treatment**, shunting of the portal to systemic venous systems (portosystemic shunt), is another option (splenorenal, portacaval, distal splenorenal or the so-called Rex shunt: meso-portal bypass, connecting portal vein and superior mesenteric vein).

Ascites

Ascites is a consequence of chronic liver disease. Ascites associated with chronic liver disease occurs secondary to portal hypertension where the pressure within the liver sinusoids increases the hydrostatic pressure gradient across the cell membrane, resulting in increased lymph production. Leakage through the capsule into the abdominal cavity results in increasing abdominal girth and body weight. Dullness to percussion in the flanks and a fluid thrill are elicited. Ultrasound will confirm ascites (it may help demonstrate fibrinous strands, loculation or a chylous appearance to the fluid) and to mark a suitable position for a diagnostic tap. Some perform this with ultrasound guidance in real time. Paracentesis is primarily used to look for the protein content of the fluid, send culture specimens and to alleviate the tense, uncomfortable build-up of large volumes, tapped with the drain left in place and albumin infused intravenously to compensate for the volume of proteinaceous fluid drained. Volumes of many litres can be drained at one session.

The **serum ascites albumin gradient** can be helpful to categorize ascites: **high gradient ascites**, when the gradient is **over 11 g/L** is seen in portal hypertension, heart failure and Budd–Chiari syndrome, veno-occlusive disease, liver metastases and portal vein thrombosis and **low gradient** ascites (seen in tuberculous peritonitis, pancreatic or biliary ascites) where the difference in albumin is **under 11 g/L**. Ascites in liver disease is high risk for **spontaneous bacterial peritonitis**, usually caused by *Streptococcus pneumoniae*, *Klebsiella pneumoniae* or *Haemophilus influenzae*, with abdominal distension, pain and fever, and is treated with broad-spectrum antibiotics. Prophylactic antibiotics are then given.

LIVER AND RELATED PROBLEMS IN THE OLDER CHILD

Infection

CASE STUDY: Hepatitis A

A 4-year-old girl presents with a seven-day history of malaise and fever followed by diarrhoea and jaundice. Serology confirms that the child has elevated transaminases and acute hepatitis A and after a short period of in-patient support with IV fluids, she is able to go home with no long-term consequences.

Acute and chronic hepatitis and liver failure

Many viral infections cause hepatitis. Hepatitis A is the commonest and is often subclinical in the nursery school age group, spread by the faecal–oral route. Other causes would include hepatitis B (±delta infection), hepatitis C, E and G, CMV, EBV, varicella, HSV, HIV, parvovirus B19, adenovirus, echovirus, measles and cryptogenic non A-G infection. Non-viral causes are implicated, such as amoebic and parasitic infection, bacterial and fungal sepsis. Most viral infections are self-limited and immunity is then conferred, but others are important causes of acute and long-term morbidity. Vertical and acquired infection of HBV and HCV (with or without HIV co-infection) are healthcare issues in developed and developing countries. Persistent infection with HBV and HCV confers increased risk of cirrhosis and hepatocellular carcinoma. Chronic carrier status is common in HBV (with the surface antigen, HBsAg persisting).

Acute infectious hepatitis can lead to **fulminant hepatic failure** (defined as the onset of encephalopathy within eight weeks of the onset of illness) and can be further defined as hyperacute, acute or subacute (depending on duration of onset), with the presence of hepatocellular dysfunction (deranged liver function tests, prolonged prothrombin time and jaundice) and encephalopathy in the absence of evidence of prior liver disease. This will need intensive supportive care and liver transplantation. Other causes in childhood would be drug related (e.g. antibiotics, paracetamol), metabolic (usually in infancy, but Wilson disease usually presents later), autoimmune hepatitis, infiltrative disease and ischaemic insults.

Gall stones

Compared with adult practice, paediatricians rarely see gall stone disease, but with the recent increase in obesity in the West, it may become more prevalent. Gall stone disease is divided into **cholesterol** and **black and brown pigment stones**. Cholesterol stones (non-radiolucent) are commonest in older children, the incidence increasing markedly in girls after menarche. Pigment stones (radiolucent) are commoner in pre-pubertal children, calcium bilirubinate being the major constituent of both. Black stones are associated with conditions causing haemolysis such as sickle cell disease, hereditary spherocytosis and the thalassaemias. Infection predominantly precipitates brown stones, classically in Asian countries where parasites such as *Clonorchis sinensis* (liver fluke) and *Ascaris lumbricoides* (roundworm) are prevalent. The use of drugs (antibiotics like ceftriaxone) increases the risk of stones. Asymptomatic stones can resolve spontaneously, but in older children they should be removed. Treatment is usually with removal at ERCP or surgical: laparoscopic techniques reducing the previous morbidity associated with the procedure. Dissolution therapy with UDCA is of limited benefit and lithotripsy has been tried but is of limited value, usually in solitary radiolucent stones.

Pancreatitis

This is relatively rare in paediatrics. The commonest causes trauma, viral infections and from congenital anatomical abnormalities of the pancreatic duct system. Gall stones are an unusual cause in children. Recent adult studies in those with recurrent episodes suggest a high incidence of cystic fibrosis mutations in affected individuals. Usually, episodes are single and self-limited and often no cause is actually identified. Treatment is supportive.

Non-alcoholic steatohepatitis

This is otherwise known as **non-alcoholic fatty liver disease (NAFLD)**. Obese children are at risk of fatty liver and inflammation, which may lead to cirrhosis. Proposed mechanisms include increased free radical damage by hepatic stellate cells, which produce a cascade of liver inflammation and subsequent fibrotic change. Diagnosis is made on finding moderately elevated aminotransferases or increased liver echogenicity on abdominal ultrasound examination in an obese child. It may be found coincidentally on investigation for other conditions. It is associated with insulin resistance syndromes (acanthosis nigricans), in adolescents increasingly with alcohol abuse and with certain other liver disease (as in cystic fibrosis liver disease and in Wilson disease). It is associated with type 2 diabetes, Turner syndrome, Prader–Willi, Bardet– Biedl and polycystic ovary syndrome. Treatments include vitamin E and UDCA. Recent adult work has looked at the use of steroids. Weight reduction (with sustained programmes including regular exercise) is obviously the most important aspect in tackling NAFLD but prevention must be addressed urgently.

Autoimmune hepatitis

CASE STUDY

A 12-year-old girl is seen by the school doctor. She is well and the parents have not expressed any concerns but she is noted to be jaundiced and has spider naevi on the face and upper chest and other signs of chronic liver disease. Bilirubin and ALT are elevated with positive antinuclear and antismooth muscle antibodies.

This is commonest in young women (75 per cent of cases). There are two main types, type I being commonest, with elevated ALT and positive antinuclear and antismooth muscle antibodies and the second type II with positivity for anti-liver kidney microsomal antibody. Liver histology demonstrates infiltration of mononuclear cells within the portal tracts. Patients may present asymptomatically with coincidental discovery on routine biochemistry. Treatment is with oral steroids until the liver function tests normalize. Azathioprine is often added in but many units continue patients on a long-term small dose of prednisolone as relapse is common. Ciclosporin has been used successfully in the acute stages of autoimmune hepatitis (AIH), but liver transplantation is indicated for those in acute liver failure who do not respond to early therapy. There is an overlap between AIH and **primary sclerosing cholangitis**, which causes chronic inflammation of the intrahepatic and extrahepatic bile ducts. This can be seen on its own or as part of systemic condition like cystic fibrosis, Langerhans cell histiocytosis, inflammatory bowel disease and immunodeficiency syndromes. Sclerosing cholangitis is diagnosed primarily by ERCP or MRCP (showing characteristic beading and stenosis of the intrahepatic bile ducts). Liver biopsy may show non-specific changes of cholangitis and fibrosis.

Wilson disease

CASE STUDY

A 13-year-old boy presents with deteriorating school performance, lethargy, joint pains and tic-like behaviour. He appears jaundiced at presentation to his GP and has hepatosplenomegaly. Further investigations reveal Kayser–Fleischer rings on slit lamp examination as part of his work-up, and a diagnosis of Wilson disease is made.

This is a rare autosomal recessive disorder of membrane-bound copper transport within the endoplasmic reticulum, found on chromosome 13 and presents at different ages, usually beginning in the teenage years. The defect results in reduced copper excretion into bile due to inefficient copper binding to caeruloplasmin and other copper-binding proteins. Liver and neuro-psychiatric symptoms account each for a third of presentations. Hepatic, neurological, neuropsychiatric, haematological and renal problems develop secondary to the high copper levels in plasma and the tissues where it accumulates.

Copper levels in the plasma are elevated and caeruloplasmin level reduced (though some may have levels within the normal range). Liver function tests are usually elevated, but classically the alkaline phosphatase is lower than normal. Glycosuria, aminoaciduria and phosphaturia consistent with renal Fanconi syndrome and renal tract stones have also been documented. Slit lamp exam usually reveals brownish Kayser–Fleischer rings. A 24-hour urine collection pre- and post-penicillamine challenge establishes a baseline elevation of copper in the urine, but a marked rise after challenge. Liver biopsy confirms the diagnosis (assessment of dry liver copper weight and histological examination). Fat accumulation, with ballooning and glycogenation of the hepatocyte nuclei, develops into cirrhosis and necrosis as the disease worsens. Copper deposits in the lenticular nuclei and basal ganglia and can be detected on head MRI, which can also be useful in the work-up if liver biopsy is contraindicated. When a patient is identified, all other family members, particularly siblings, should be screened. Chelation treatment with oral D-penicillamine is commenced. Trientene and zinc have also been used as an adjunct to treatment. Liver transplantation may be required when presentation is with acute liver failure or when chelation fails to halt progression of disease.

LIVER FAILURE AND ORTHOTOPIC LIVER TRANSPLANTATION

Hepatic failure is the end-stage of chronic liver disease. Glucose requirements are high due to liver dysfunction, fluid balance needs to be carefully addressed to avoid overload and ascites and renal impairment are common. Diuretics (spironolactone and furosemide) are often required. Good nutrition is essential and vitamin and trace metal supplementation and coagulopathy and infections are managed proactively. Encephalopathy due to high ammonia levels is treated with laxatives (lactulose) and antibiotics (neomycin) have been used to decontaminate the intestine. Extrahepatic biliary atresia is the major childhood indication for **liver transplantation**. Survival, now at greater than 90 per cent at 1 year in most series, has dramatically improved owing to improved surgical techniques in even the smallest infants and with better immunosuppression regimens (steroids, azathioprine, ciclosporin, tacrolimus, sirolimus, mycophenolate mofetil and monoclonal antibody therapy) and improved intensive care. Graft rejection, bleeding (anastomotic, gastrointestinal ulceration, PTLD), infection, hepatic arterial thrombosis and biliary leakage remain the major post-op complications in addition to drug side effects. Acute rejection occurs in up to 80 per cent of orthotopic liver transplantations in the first few months. Immunosuppression-related problems include infection (bacterial, viral, fungal and opportunistic) and PTLD, a B cell lymphoma driven primarily by EBV infection (present pre-transplant or from an EBV-positive graft). Treatment is by reducing immunosuppression. Split liver grafting and living related donation is being used to address the lack of donor organ availability worldwide.

FURTHER READING AND USEFUL WEBSITES

Baker SS, Liptak GS, Colletti RB, *et al.* (1999) A Medical Position Statement of the North American Society for Pediatric Gastroenterology and Nutrition. Constipation in infants and children: evaluation and treatment. *J Pediatr Gastroenterol Nutr* 29:612–26.

British Society of Gastroenterology. www.bsg.org.uk (accessed 14 November 2004).

British Society of Paediatric Gastroenterology, Hepatology and Nutrition. www.bspghan.org.uk (accessed 14 November 2004).

Children's Digestive Health and Nutrition Foundation. www.cdhnf.org (accessed 14 November 2004).

Coeliac UK. www.coeliac.co.uk (accessed 14 November 2004).

Fasano A, Catassi C (2001) Current approaches to diagnosis and treatment of celiac disease: an evolving spectrum. *Gastroenterology* 120:636–51.

Feldman M, Scharschmidt BF, Sleisinger MH (eds) (1998) *Sleisinger and Fordtran's Gastrointestinal and Liver Disease: Pathophysiology/Diagnosis/Management*, 6th edn. Philadephia: WB Saunders.

GastroHep.com. The global online source for gastroenterology, hepatology and endoscopy. www.gastrohep.com (accessed 14 November 2004).

Hassall E (2001) Peptic ulcer disease and current approaches to *Helicobacter pylori*. *J Pediatr* 138:462–8.

Journal of Pediatric Gastroenterology and Nutrition. www.jpgn.org (accessed 14 November 2004).

Kelly D (ed) (2004) *Diseases of the Liver and Biliary System in Children*, 2nd edn. Oxford: Blackwell.

North American Society for Pediatric Gastroenterology and Nutrition. www.naspghan.org (accessed 14 November 2004).

Rasquin-Weber PE, Hyman S, Cucchiara DR, *et al.* (1999) Childhood functional gastrointestinal disorders. *Gut* **45**(suppl 2):ii60–ii68

Rudolph CD, Mazur LJ, Liptak GS, *et al.*; North American Society for Pediatric Gastroenterology and Nutrition (NASPGHAN) (2002) Guidelines for evaluation and treatment of gastroesophageal reflux in infants and children: recommendations of the North American Society for Pediatric Gastroenterology and Nutrition. *J Pediatr Gastroenterol Nutr* **32**(suppl 2):S1–S31.

Snell RS (1983). *Clinical Embryology for Medical Students*, 3rd edn. New York: Little, Brown and Company.

Walker WA, Goulet O, Kleinman R, Sherman P, Schneider B, Sanderson I (2004) *Pediatric Gastrointestinal Disease, Pathophysiology, Diagnosis, Management*, 4th edn. Hamilton, Ontario: BC Decker.

Wyllie R, Hyams J (1999) *Pediatric Gastrointestinal Disease, Pathophysiology, Diagnosis, Management*, 2nd edn. Philadelphia: WB Saunders.

Chapter 11

Nutrition

Alison M Kelly, Diane M Snowdon and Lawrence T Weaver

Nutrition is concerned with how food is used by the body, interfaces with gastroenterology, metabolism and endocrinology, and is inseparable from growth and development. Diets deficient in particular nutrients may cause specific diseases or syndromes (such as anaemia and scurvy). Overeating causes obesity. Chronic diseases are frequently associated with undernutrition and nutrient deficits. Nutrient deficiencies lead to depletion of tissue stores, derangement of normal biochemistry and disordered tissue function before they are manifest as anatomical changes and may easily go unrecognized. Awareness of poor nutrition is critical to the effective management of many childhood diseases, particularly those that are chronic, and there is evidence that poor nutrition in early life plays a part in the genesis of adult degenerative diseases. Nutrition services should be provided by a team that works together in the clinic, ward and community to provide nutritional support for children.

NUTRITIONAL PHYSIOLOGY AND DIGESTIVE SYSTEM

Ingestion and passage of food into the stomach and then small intestine allows its breakdown by digestive enzymes, including hepatobiliary and pancreatic secretions. Specific transport processes regulate absorption of nutrients, salts and water across the mucosa of the small intestine, followed by fermentation and further salt and water absorption in the colon prior to excretion of waste. The integrity of the gastrointestinal tract relies on the integration of motility, digestion and absorption with immunological and non-immunological mechanisms that defend against harmful substances, while allowing tolerance to certain foreign proteins.

Carbohydrates

Carbohydrates in food consist mainly of starches, sucrose, lactose and non-metabolizable carbohydrates (Table 11.1). Starches require initial digestion by salivary and pancreatic amylases. Hydrolysis of disaccharides and oligosaccharides to their monosaccharide components occurs at the brush border of the enterocyte. Uptake of glucose and galactose by enterocytes occurs via a sodium-dependent co-transporter that facilitates the entry of sodium and monosaccharide down their electrochemical gradients, maintained by Na-K-ATPase at the basolateral membrane. Some oligosaccharides (such as fructo-oligosaccharides, stachyose and raftilose in beans) are not fully digested in the human small intestine. These pass to the colon where they are rapidly fermented to short chain fatty acids. Some starches are less digestible than others (e.g. unripe bananas or raw potato) and resist human enzymes and pass into the colon undigested.

Table 11.1 Dietary sources of macronutrients

Nutrient	Main dietary sources
Carbohydrate	
Starch	Cereals, potatoes, pasta, rice, bread
Sugars	Sucrose, milk products, sweet drinks, confectionery
Fibre	Wholegrain cereals, vegetables, fruit, nuts, pulses
Protein	Meat, milk products, pulses, fish, eggs, vegetables
Fat	
Saturated	Dairy products, meat, confectionery
PUFA $n = 3$	Fish, meat, nuts
PUFA $n = 6$	Vegetable oils, fat spreads

PUFA, polyunsaturated fatty acids.

Carbohydrates provide approximately 4 kcal/g of energy. Glucose is oxidized to produce energy for tissues via an anaerobic pathway (glycolysis) producing pyruvic acid, and an aerobic pathway whereby pyruvic acid is metabolized to carbon dioxide and water. Sugar that is not oxidized is converted to glycogen in the liver or to fat for storage in adipose tissue. Carbohydrates are also an important component of structural and functional glycoproteins and glycolipids.

Proteins

The main sources of protein in foods are meat, dairy products and cereals. Adequate protein supply is particularly important in childhood when rapid growth requires amino acids to provide the building blocks for new muscle and other structural proteins. Ingested proteins are denatured by gastric acid and pepsinogens are converted to pepsins, which act with pancreatic proteases. Following activation by enterokinase, trypsinogen is converted into trypsin and other proteases are activated. Peptides enter the enterocyte either as amino acids, after preliminary digestion at the brush border or as di- or tripeptides, which are then split inside the cell by cytoplasmic peptidases. Amino acids enter and leave enterocytes via numerous sodium-dependent transport systems and di- and tripeptides via a peptide transport system. Amino acids reach the liver via the portal circulation where they are reconstituted into functional proteins such as enzymes, glycoproteins and lipoproteins and distributed to other tissues for growth and repair. Dietary protein is essential to maintain nitrogen balance. All amino acids provide nitrogen for synthesis of human proteins but some dietary amino acids are 'essential' (cannot be synthesized *de novo*). Excess amino acids cannot be stored and are deaminated; the nitrogenous portions are converted to urea in the liver and excreted via the kidneys.

Fats

Dietary sources of fat include meat, milk products, fish and fried foods (see Table 11.1). The majority of ingested fat is in the form of triglycerides. Digestion of fats begins in the stomach under the action of preduodenal lipases. However, pancreatic lipases are most important in the digestion of fats. In the presence of bile salts, they emulsify the ingested lipid droplets in the duodenum. Lipids, including diglycerides, cholesterol esters and fat-soluble vitamins, are solubilized in bile salt micelles. Following diffusion of the micelle into the enterocyte, the products of lipolysis are liberated. Free fatty acids bind to small carrier proteins and approximately 70 per cent of long chain fatty acids are involved in triglyceride resynthesis. Microsomal triglyceride transfer protein transfers resynthesize triglycerides in the rough endoplasmic reticulum where, with phospholipids and cholesterol, they combine with apolipoproteins to form chylomicrons in the Golgi apparatus. Chylomicrons are excreted into the intercellular spaces from which they are taken up into the lymphatics and systemic circulation.

Fats are a major source of energy with a density of about 9 kcal/g, and they are also the main constituent of cell membranes and neural tissue. Linoleic acid and α-linolenic acid are precursors of phospholipids, prostaglandins, leukotrienes, arachidonic acid and docosahexaenoic acid; the latter two are essential constituents of the developing nervous system.

Micronutrients

Vitamins form a group of naturally occurring organic nutrients that have little in common other than their necessity in the diet (Table 11.2). Water-soluble vitamins (B and C) are easily absorbed and are not stored in the body in any great quantity. Fat-soluble vitamins (A, D, E and K) are absorbed with fat, therefore disturbance of fat absorption will reduce their absorption. Fat-soluble vitamins are stored in the body and thus deficiencies in the diet may take longer to affect nutritional status.

Minerals are inorganic elements that are an essential constituent of the diet (Table 11.3). They serve many different biological functions, including structural (calcium in bone), transport (iron in haemoglobin), energy metabolism (phosphate in ATP), endocrine (iodine in thyroid) and enzyme action (molybdenum).

KEY LEARNING POINTS

- The gastrointestinal tract relies on the integration of motility, digestion, absorption and immunological mechanisms for normal functioning.
- Food consists of a combination of macronutrients (carbohydrate, protein and fat) and micronutrients (vitamins and minerals).
- Energy provided by carbohydrate is 4 kcal/g; that provided by fat is 9 kcal/g.
- Fat and carbohydrate are the principal dietary sources of energy; protein provides nitrogen for synthesis of tissues.
- Clinical signs of micronutrient deficiencies occur late and may go unrecognized.

Table 11.2 Dietary sources and functions of vitamins

Vitamin	Dietary source	Function
Thiamine	Wholegrain cereals, nuts, pulses, vegetables, pork meat, milk products, yeast	Co-enzyme in carbohydrate metabolism
Vitamin B_{12}	Milk products, meat, fish, eggs	Co-factor to methionine synthetase
Folic acid	Cereals, green leafy vegetables, milk products, liver	Co-enzyme, essential to metabolism of several amino acids
Vitamin B_6	Vegetables, cereals, milk products, meat, potatoes	Co-enzyme related to protein metabolism, amine synthesis, haem synthesis, glycogen metabolism
Niacin	Cereals, meat, milk products, vegetables	NAD, NADP for oxidoreductases
Riboflavin	Milk products, cereals, meat	Metabolic pathway, cellular respiration
Biotin	Liver, egg, cereals, yeast, milk, meat	Co-factor in fatty acid synthesis, amino acid metabolism
Pantothenic acid	Meat, cereals, green vegetables, yeast, peanuts	Constituent of Co-A esters, essential for lipid and carbohydrate metabolism
Vitamin C	Citrus fruit (juice), potatoes	Collagen synthesis, carnitine and noradrenaline synthesis
Vitamin A	Liver, kidney meat, eggs, milk products, fat spreads, carrots, red peppers, tomatoes	Cell differentiation, fetal development, vision, hearing, growth, immune system
Vitamin D	Cereals, fat spreads, oily fish	Calcium absorption and metabolism, immune system
Vitamin E	Fat spreads, meat, fish, eggs	Antioxidant
Vitamin K	Green leafy vegetables, margarine, soya bean oil	Synthesis of clotting factors II, VII, IX and X

NAD, nicotinamide adenine dinucleotide.

Table 11.3 Dietary sources of minerals

Mineral	Dietary source
Iron	Lean meat, cereals, pulses, fish, eggs
Calcium	Milk, dairy products, fish, dried fruit
Phosphorus	Fish, milk, cereals, meat, poultry, eggs
Potassium	Vegetables, milk products, fruit
Copper	Nuts, cereals, meat, potatoes, legumes
Iodine	Seafoods, milk, dairy products
Zinc	Red meat, milk, cereals, eggs, sea foods
Selenium	Fish, lean meat, wholegrain cereals, eggs, vegetables
Magnesium	Milk products, vegetables, meat, wholegrain cereals
Chromium	Yeast, meat, wholegrain cereals, legumes, nuts

MATERNAL NUTRITION IN PREGNANCY AND LACTATION: EFFECTS ON FETUS

The nutritional status of a mother affects her ability to conceive, feed and rear a healthy baby. Women are most fertile when they are well nourished, and those with low fat mass, because of either poor dietary intake (e.g. anorexia) or excessive physical activity (e.g. athletes) may have delayed puberty and amenorrhoea. Even in women of normal body weight, a short-term reduction in energy intake can cause menstrual disturbance. Obese women have lower fertility rates as well as higher rates of miscarriage and complications of pregnancy, and more babies with congenital malformations.

The body undergoes significant physiological changes after conception, which increase nutritional requirements. The energy cost of normal pregnancy is estimated at around 70 000 kcal (energy content of the fetus, placenta, extra maternal tissues synthesized, basal metabolism of mother and fetus). Energy requirements for pregnant women are around 200 kcal per day above normal requirements. During pregnancy, the average woman gains approximately 12.5 kg. During lactation, the mother loses weight, but her fluid requirements remain high to balance that lost as milk. She continues to require about 500 kcal/day above non-pregnant energy requirements. There is a positive correlation between inadequate maternal weight gain and perinatal mortality. The rate of gain in maternal weight is a significant determinant of infant birth weight, which has been shown to influence infant as well as long-term health.

Requirement for vitamins and minerals also increases during pregnancy but adequate intakes can be achieved by normal diet, although iron is commonly supplemented. Folic acid is an essential co-factor for DNA and protein synthesis, and periconceptional supplementation reduces the incidence of neural tube defects.

Growth and nutrient accretion of fetus and infant

During a normal pregnancy, the fetus grows to an average birth weight of 3500 g and length of 50 cm, and at term should be equipped with sufficient stores of energy (in adipose tissue and liver) and nutrients to enable it to cope with the transition from the intrauterine environment, with its constant nutrient supply, to the extrauterine situation of intermittent enteral feeds.

The placenta transports macro- and micronutrients from the maternal to the fetal circulation by both passive and active mechanisms, and is highly metabolically active. It also has an exocrine function and produces hormones such as growth hormone, insulin-like growth factor and leptin, which play roles in fetal growth. If the placenta is small or dysfunctional, there may be intrauterine growth restriction (IUGR), whereas a large placenta is generally associated with a large fetus.

The body shape, proportions, composition and metabolic rate of the fetus and infant differ from those of the fully grown adult, and this has implications in terms of fluid and nutrient requirements, particularly in preterm babies. The fetus in early life has a high water content with predominance of extracellular sodium and chloride. As it grows, it gains cell mass and intracellular ions, primarily potassium. The fetus accretes calcium, phosphorus and iron in the last trimester although ossification of the fetal skeleton begins at a weight of 700–900 g. Fat is laid down in the fetus at weights over 2600 g and from birth the neonate continues to increase its fat stores until late infancy. This is a vital period for brain growth, which requires a supply of long chain polyunsaturated fatty acids.

Preterm babies

Babies born prematurely are deprived of the opportunity in the third trimester to accrete many minerals such as iron, calcium and phosphate, and these babies have low fat, protein and glycogen stores. It is hard for preterm babies to achieve fetal accretion rates of all nutrients in the postnatal period. However, the fetal growth curve seems a reasonable standard to follow, aiming for a growth rate of 15–20 g/kg per day. Nutritional requirements of preterm babies are shown in Table 11.4. When mother or donor's milk is available, this is the feed of choice and is usually supplemented with sodium, calcium, phosphate, iron and vitamins. Preterm formulas are available which mimic the composition of human milk, but contain the higher recommended amounts of protein, energy, minerals and vitamins.

Table 11.4 Nutritional requirements of the preterm baby

Nutrient	Daily requirement
Calories	110-130 kcal/kg
Carbohydrate	16 g/kg
Protein	3-3.8 g/kg
Fat	7 g/kg
Calcium	3-5 mmol/kg
Phosphorus	2-4.5 mmol/kg
Magnesium	0.5 mmol/kg
Iron	2 mg/kg
Sodium	2.5-6 mmol/kg
Potassium	2-3.5 mmol/kg
Vitamin A	1000 IU (450-850 μg)
Vitamin B_{12}	0.3 μg
Vitamin C	20-30 mg
Vitamin D	400-800 IU
Vitamin E	4-8 mg
Folate	25-50 μg

Intrauterine growth restriction

Intrauterine growth restriction may be symmetrical, caused by poor fetal growth throughout pregnancy, or asymmetrical, usually from poor fetal growth in the last trimester as a result of maternal factors such as placental failure or pre-eclampsia. The asymmetrically IUGR infant, deprived of nutrients in the last trimester, will fail to gain weight, but growth in length and head circumference is usually preserved. If supplied with sufficient nutrients after birth, these infants have catch-up growth and weight gain in the first 6–12 months. Symmetrically IUGR infants have low birth weight with reduced length and head circumference. The cause is fetal (e.g. chromosomal abnormalities, congenital infections or may be multifactorial). These infants catch up growth slowly in spite of good nutritional support, taking three years or more, or never catching up.

KEY LEARNING POINTS

- The nutritional status of the mother affects her ability to conceive, fetal growth and wellbeing during pregnancy, and lactation.
- During normal pregnancy the fetus acquires sufficient stores of energy and nutrients to prepare for extrauterine life.
- The fetus accretes many nutrients during the last trimester of pregnancy – babies born prematurely are deprived of this opportunity.
- Intrauterine growth restriction may be symmetrical, due to poor fetal growth throughout pregnancy, and is usually of fetal origin.

- Asymmetrical IUGR is due to poor growth in the last trimester of pregnancy and is more likely to be maternal in origin, e.g. secondary to pre-eclampsia.

NUTRITIONAL REQUIREMENTS IN HEALTH

Pace of growth changes through childhood and nutritional requirements change to reflect this. Activity levels increase from the relatively immobile infant to the active toddler and young child. Infants grow rapidly and have high energy and nutrient requirements, which demand adequate milk intake and timely introduction of complementary foods to maintain normal growth. Through childhood, growth slows and less energy-dense foods are needed. In adolescence, the pubertal growth spurt is a time of higher requirements for energy and nutrients (Figure 11.1).

Nutrient requirements for children of different ages are defined as dietary reference values (DRVs) (Figure 11.2). The requirement in a group of individuals for a nutrient is assumed to be normally distributed and the mean value is termed the estimated average requirement (EAR). Two standard deviations above is termed the reference nutrient intake (RNI) and intakes above it will almost always be adequate. Two standard deviations below the EAR is known as the lower reference nutrient intake (LRNI) and intakes below it will usually be inadequate for many. Dietary reference values can be used to assess the diet of individuals or groups, to prescribe diets or for labelling foods.

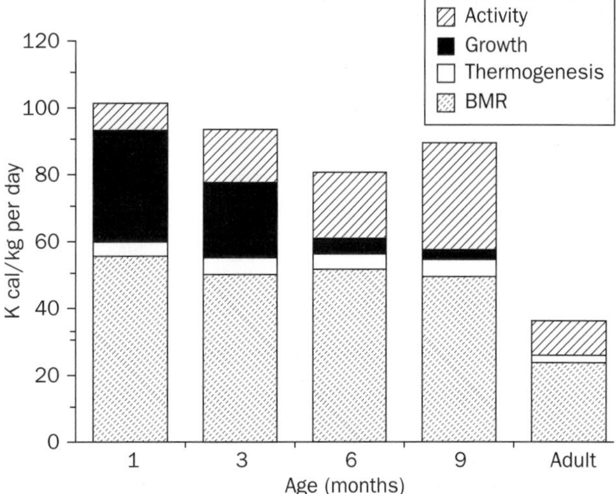

Figure 11.1 Energy requirements during infancy and adulthood. The greatest proportion of energy is used for growth in the neonatal period. BMR, basal metabolic rate (Reproduced with permission from Michaelsen KF, Weaver LT, Branca F, Robertson A (2000) *Feeding and Nutrition of Infants and Young Children*. WHO: Copenhagen)

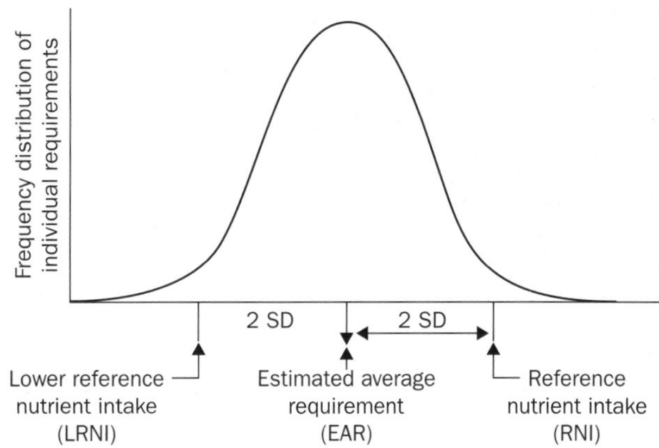

Figure 11.2 Dietary reference values (Reproduced with permission from Michaelsen KF, Weaver LT, Branca F, Robertson A (2000) *Feeding and Nutrition of Infants and Young Children*. WHO: Copenhagen)

Infancy

Human breast milk is the best food for babies and contains all the energy and nutrients needed for the first 6 months of life. It also contains many non-nutritional components, which help adaptation to oral feeding and confer protection against many infections (Table 11.5). Breast milk is a complex fluid of multiple constituents including nutrients, non-nutrients and cells such as lymphocytes and macrophages. Its composition varies between individuals and from day to day and feed to feed. Following parturition small volumes of colostrum are produced containing high concentrations of secretory IgA and lactoferrin. From day 2 to day 5 transitional milk 'comes in', this has higher concentrations of lactose and fat with proportionately less protein. Mature milk is produced from 14 days and milk production is related to infant demand. Foremilk is more watery and contains higher lactose concentrations whereas hindmilk is more energy dense with higher fat content. Over time, concentrations of micronutrients such as iron fall with more rapid decline in zinc levels and at weaning lactose concentration falls with increase in protein and fat content.

Proper feeding is a cornerstone of the care for infants and young children. Appropriate feeding practices encourage mother–infant bonding and psychosocial development. From birth, encouraging breastfeeding is the most important factor in optimal early nutrition. The World Health Organization (WHO) recommends that 'All mothers should have access to skilled support to initiate and sustain exclusive breastfeeding for six months and ensure the timely introduction of adequate and safe complementary foods with continued breastfeeding up to

Table 11.5 Benefits of breastfeeding

Infant		Mother	
Protection against infection	Gastroenteritis Respiratory tract Otitis media	Reduced risk of	Postpartum haemorrhage Anaemia from blood loss Premenopausal breast cancer
Reduced risk of	Sudden infant death Cows' milk allergy	Possible reduced risk of	Ovarian cancer Osteoporosis
	Asthma	Contraceptive effect of lactational amenorrhoea	
Possible reduced risk of	Obesity Autoimmune disease (e.g. diabetes mellitus)	Aids weight loss and return to pre-pregnant weight	
Developmental benefits	Higher IQ scores Improved visual acuity and psychomotor development		

two years or beyond.' Recognizing the unique benefits of breastfeeding, all women should be enabled to practise exclusive breastfeeding as a global goal for optimal maternal and child health and nutrition, and recognizing the need for the reinforcement of a 'breastfeeding culture', the UNICEF and WHO have developed a Baby Friendly Hospital Initiative, which gives accreditation to hospitals that encourage the initiation and support of breastfeeding. This has been taken up in many countries worldwide.

Ten steps to successful breastfeeding

1. Have a written breastfeeding policy that is routinely communicated to all healthcare staff.
2. Train all healthcare staff in the skills necessary to implement the breastfeeding policy.
3. Inform all pregnant women about the benefits and management of breastfeeding.
4. Help mothers initiate breastfeeding soon after birth.
5. Show mothers how to breastfeed and how to maintain lactation even if they are separated from their babies.
6. Give neonates no food or drink other than breast milk, unless medically indicated.
7. Practise rooming-in, allowing mothers and babies to remain together 24 hours a day.
8. Encourage breastfeeding on demand.
9. Give no artificial teats or dummies to breastfeeding infants.
10. Foster the establishment of breastfeeding support groups and refer mothers to them on discharge from the hospital or clinic.

Contraindications to breastfeeding are few, and include galactosaemia, some maternal drugs (listed in the *British National Formulary*) and untreated maternal human immunodeficiency virus infection. Hepatitis B and C or tuberculosis does not preclude breastfeeding although immunization and prophylaxis should be given where appropriate.

Infant milk formulas supply complete nutritional requirements for infants in the first 4–6 months of life (Table 11.6). They are mostly based on cows' milk and resemble human milk but lack many of the components of human milk. Soy-based formulas are suitable for use in galactosaemia and for babies of vegan mothers who do not wish to breastfeed. Unmodified cows' milk is not suitable for babies because of the high renal solute load and low levels of certain nutrients such as iron and vitamins. Full-fat pasteurized cows' milk should be introduced around 12 months.

Complementary feeding or 'weaning' describes the gradual introduction of solid foods along with continued breast or formula feeding. From around 6 months the infant's iron stores become depleted, chewing needs to be developed and milk alone is insufficient to meet the growing nutritional requirements (Figure 11.3). Complementary feeds increase the energy, nutrient and mineral density of the diet although milk continues to supply up to half of energy requirements. Acquisition of feeding skills is a developmental and social progression from coordination of tongue and jaw movements for pureed food to chewing of lumpy textures and finger feeding. Non-wheat cereals, fruit, vegetables and potatoes are suitable first complementary foods. They should be single ingredients and energy dense (>1 kcal/g). Between 6 and 9 months of age, meat, fish, all cereals, pulses, fish and eggs can

Table 11.6 Composition of mature human milk, cows' milk formula, soya milk and follow-on formulas

	Human milk	Formula	Soya milk	Follow-on formula
Energy (kcal/100 mL)	65-75	65-68	67-68	65-74
Protein (g/100 mL)	1.1-1.3	1.4-1.9	1.8-2.2	1.8-2.5
Fat (g/100 mL)	3.7-4.8	2.9-3.8	3.6-3.8	3.1-3.8
Carbohydrate (g/100 mL)	7.0-7.5	7.0-8.3	6.7-6.8	7.2-9.0
Sodium (mmol/100 mL)	0.5-0.9	0.7-1.5	1.0-1.1	1.0-1.4
Chloride (mmol/100 mL)	1.0-1.5	1.1-1.6	1.0-1.4	1.4-1.9
Calcium (mmol/100 mL)	0.8-0.9	1.0-2.2	1.4-1.6	1.8-2.5
Phosphate (mmol/100 mL)	0.45-0.5	0.9-1.8	0.9-1.4	1.6-2.0
Iron (μmol/100 mL)	1.1-1.5	11.6-12.5	11.6-12.5	20-21.5
Vitamin A (μg/100 mL)	44-80	61-100	85	60-80
Vitamin C (mg/100 mL)	3.1-4.5	5.5-5.9	6.8	8-10
Vitamin D (μg/100 mL)	0.6-0.7	1.0-1.1	1.2	1.0-1.8

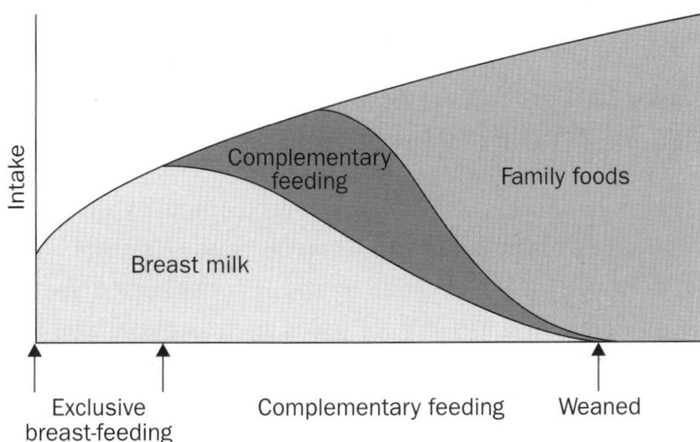

Figure 11.3 Contribution of different food sources to energy intake in infants (Reproduced with permission from Michaelsen KF, Weaver LT, Branca F, Robertson A (2000) *Feeding and Nutrition of Infants and Young Children*. WHO: Copenhagen)

CASE STUDY: Iron deficiency

An 18-month-old infant is referred by her general practitioner (GP) with fussy eating. She was formula fed from birth and solids were introduced at 3 months. She has been drinking cows' milk since 6 months of age, taking 800–1000 mL daily. She eats very little solid food, taking only a few spoonfuls of yoghurt and crisps. Her weight is 12.7 kg (91st centile) and height 80 cm (50th centile). She is pale but examination is otherwise normal. Is the diet likely to be nutritionally adequate? What assessment or investigations should be performed? What advice should be given?

be introduced. Salt should not be added and additional sugars should be given only to improve the palatability of sour fruits. By the time an infant is 1 year old, the diet should be mixed and they can eat chopped family foods.

Vitamin supplements (A and D) are recommended for breastfed babies from 6 months, and for formula-fed infants when formula is replaced by cows' milk. These should ideally continue until 5 years of age and vitamin D supplementation is particularly important for some ethnic groups where there may be risk of rickets. Iron deficiency is a particular risk.

Toddlers and young children

Toddlers and young children continue to develop feeding skills with continued oral and fine motor development and progress from finger feeding at around 12 months to spoon feeding by 2 years and using knife and fork unaided by around 5 years. Toddlers should ideally consume a variety of foods usually given as three main meals with two snacks. With increasing age the energy intake from fat declines and the toddler diet reflects the change from infant feeding, where 50 per cent of energy comes from fat, to the adult diet where not more than 35 per cent of energy should be obtained from fat.

Sufficient iron-containing foods should prevent iron deficiency anaemia, which is not uncommon at this age, and is associated with excessive milk intake. Daily milk consumption of around 500 mL full-fat milk is recommended. Provided growth is normal, semiskimmed milk and lower-fat dairy products should be used from 2 years of age. Foods containing fibre are an essential part of a varied diet. To prevent dental caries all liquids should be given in a cup from 1 year, as sweetened juices taken frequently from bottles with teats cause tooth decay. Fussy eating is common and reflects the growing independence of the toddler. Offering small, energy-dense meals and snacks and restricting juice intake is often effective.

During childhood, the importance of healthy eating patterns should be emphasized and the diet should be similar to that recommended for adults. Habits develop in childhood and it is important to encourage healthy eating at this stage. Diet should be varied and each meal should contain a substantial portion of high-fibre bread, pasta, cereal or potatoes, with a protein source such as meat, fish or pulses as well as vegetables and fruit. Saturated fat intake should be limited by the use of low-fat products and polyunsaturated fatty acids should be used in preference to saturated fats. Sugar intake should also be minimized with avoidance of sweetened beverages, which should be replaced by water.

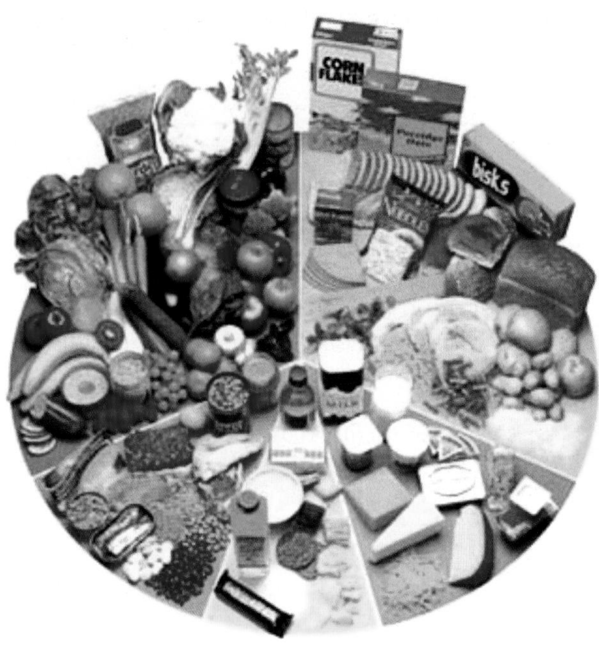

Figure 11.4 Food plate showing categories of different foods that make up a healthy diet (From www.healthyliving.gov.uk)

Adolescents

Adolescence is a time of intense physical and psychological development and period of rapid growth. During this period, the adolescent gains up to 50 per cent of the adult weight, 20 per cent of adult height and 50 per cent of the skeletal mass. This pubertal growth spurt is sensitive to nutrient deprivation. In adolescence peer pressure, concerns over appearance and body image can affect eating, and in extreme cases, anorexia nervosa and bulimia can occur. Obesity is a far greater problem in adolescence. The principles for healthy eating for adolescents are the same as for adults but the adolescent diet can often be based on snacking and high-fat 'fast foods'. A significant number of individuals do not meet the RNI for nutrients such as iron, calcium, zinc and vitamin A.

Healthy eating and public health

Healthy eating and optimal nutrition play a role in growth, development and health both in childhood and adulthood and should have benefits for prevention of many adult diseases linked to premature death, such as coronary heart disease and cancer. Worldwide, malnutrition is a major problem and is a significant cause of infant and child mortality. The WHO estimates that about 30 per cent of children under 5 years are stunted as a consequence of poor feeding and repeated infections. On the other hand, obesity in developed countries is reaching epidemic proportions with its related problems of heart disease, hypertension and diabetes mellitus.

To meet healthy eating recommendations, families should aim to develop a 'healthy eating pattern', which involves eating well-balanced meals. In general, the recommendations are to eat greater amounts of fruits, vegetables, breads, grains, cereals and legumes. The amount of lean meat, poultry and fish consumed should be moderate and use of fatty foods such as butter and oils should be sparing. Polyunsaturated fatty acids should be used in preference to products high in saturated fats. The concept of the healthy eating plate has been used to illustrate this advice and food labelling can be used to help consumers choose appropriate products (Figure 11.4).

KEY LEARNING POINTS

- Nutrient requirements change throughout childhood, reflecting the change in rates of growth and activity at different ages.
- Breast milk is the feed of choice for infants and is recommended exclusively for the first 6 months of life.
- Complementary feeding or 'weaning' is the gradual introduction of solid food along with continued breast or formula milk, starting by 6 months.
- With increasing age the change in diet should result in a fall in the energy supplied by fat, from around 50 per cent in the infant to 30–35 per cent in children.
- Healthy eating habits should be established in childhood and can reduce the adult risk of cardiovascular disease, cancer and obesity.

NUTRITION AND DISEASE

Nutritional requirements are often increased in disease owing to losses (vomiting or diarrhoea), failure of digestion and absorption of nutrients (e.g. coeliac disease, food allergy, cystic fibrosis) and increased energy requirements (e.g. cystic fibrosis). Malabsorption may result from failure of intraluminal digestion or a defect of mucosal function. Clinical signs and symptoms may include diarrhoea, vomiting, abdominal distension and weight loss. Some children present with nutritional or other deficiency states, such as growth failure, iron deficiency or rickets. Specific foods, which cause vomiting, diarrhoea and malabsorption (e.g. cows' milk), may need to be identified. Nutritional support in infants with gastrointestinal disease may involve specific dietary restrictions or support with enteral feeds or parenteral nutrition. Specific nutrient deficiencies are associated with disease (e.g. iron-deficiency anaemia and rickets in vitamin D deficiency). Excess intake of some nutrients (e.g. saturated fat) is associated with high cholesterol levels and an increased risk of atherosclerosis.

Causes of malabsorption

Disorders of intraluminal digestion
Congenital

- Pancreatic: cystic fibrosis; Shwachman syndrome
- Hepatic: hepatitis; hepatocellular failure; cholestasis
- Intestinal: enterokinase deficiency

Acquired

- Pancreatic: chronic pancreatitis
- Hepatic: hepatitis; hepatocellular failure; cholestasis
- Intestinal: bacterial overgrowth

Disorders of intestinal mucosal function
Congenital

- Carbohydrate absorption: glucose-galactose malabsorption; sucrase-isomaltase deficiency; alactasia
- Amino acid absorption: cystinuria; Hartnup disease
- Fat absorption: abetalipoproteinemia; lymphangiectasia
- Electrolyte absorption: chloride-losing diarrhoea; primary hypomagnesaemia; acrodermatitis enteropathica
- Enteropathies: microvillus atrophy; idiopathic

Acquired

- Enteropathies: coeliac disease; food allergy; autoimmune; post-gastroenteritis
- Infections: tuberculosis; giardiasis; hookworm
- Infiltrations: Crohn disease: reticuloses
- Anatomical: intestinal fistulae; short-gut syndrome
- Drugs: chemotherapeutic

There is a vicious cycle between chronic disease and malnutrition. Chronic disease often results in a negative energy and protein balance as a result of anorexia and poor intake, with increased requirements or chronic losses. Undernutrition is associated with an increased risk of infection, poor muscle function, reduced mobility, retarded growth and prolonged admission to hospital. Nutrition support should be provided by a team (see Principles and practice of nutritional support, page 347).

Inflammatory bowel disease

The goal of therapy is to induce and maintain remission of active disease and to correct malnutrition and promote growth. Patients may need iron, folate, vitamin B_{12} and zinc supplements in addition to ensuring adequate energy intake via oral, nasogastric or intravenous (IV) routes. In Crohn disease there has been increasing use of nutritional therapy, with elemental or polymeric feeds, to induce remission and to treat relapse. Five randomized clinical trials comprising 147 children showed that exclusive enteral nutrition was as effective as corticosteroids in inducing remission. It is not clear how enteral therapy works, whether a polymeric (whole protein) feed is as effective as an elemental (amino acid) feed, if large intestinal disease responds as effectively as small intestinal disease, and the role of ongoing maintenance supplementation with enteral feeds. Exclusive enteral nutrition is not effective in the treatment of ulcerative colitis.

Cystic fibrosis

Malabsorption due to pancreatic insufficiency occurs in around 85 per cent of children with cystic fibrosis. Affected infants often have a voracious appetite but are slow to gain weight. Elevated resting and total energy expenditure in children with cystic fibrosis and excessive faecal losses require that total energy intake should be above normal. Malabsorption is exacerbated by abnormal duodenal acidity, intestinal mucosal dysfunction and impaired bile salt excretion. Inadequate absorption of fat-soluble vitamins can cause symptoms, including bleeding (vitamin K deficiency), benign intracranial hypertension (vitamin A deficiency) and haemolytic anaemia or neurological symptoms (vitamin E deficiency), and salt deficiency can result in severe hypochloraemic metabolic alkalosis.

The aim of nutritional management in cystic fibrosis is to prevent malnutrition and support growth by anticipating and treating nutrient deficiencies. To ensure adequate energy intake 150 per cent of the EAR should be supplied, often with supplements such as Maxijul, Polycal or enteral support via nasogastric tube or gastrostomy. Vitamins A, D (150 per cent RNI) and E are also necessary. Pancreatic enzyme replacement is indicated and in older children is 'titrated' against growth, nutritional status and stool fat content. In infants, enzyme supplements can be mixed with a little expressed breast milk or fruit purée.

Coeliac disease

The treatment of coeliac disease with lifelong exclusion of gluten from the diet means avoiding all foods with wheat, barley and rye. Tolerance of oats is variable and some patients also need to exclude these. The education of the children and their parents in this diet needs the help of a paediatric dietitian. Many gluten-free products are freely available, making a restrictive diet easier to tolerate. Some newly diagnosed children, particularly those with a classic presentation, may be malnourished or anaemic. Supplementation with iron, folate, calcium and other nutrients may be required.

CASE STUDY: Coeliac disease

A 2-year-old girl presents with a six-month history of poor growth, abdominal distension and loose stools. Her appetite is poor but she eats a varied diet, which appears adequate for her age. Previously she was well, growing along the 25th centile but her current weight of 9.5 kg is below the 2nd centile. Investigations show normocytic anaemia with low iron stores and negative stool cultures. What is the differential diagnosis and what investigations would be useful? What is the management strategy?

Phenylketonuria

Treatment of phenylketonuria (PKU) is by dietary restriction of phenylalanine as soon as the diagnosis is made, often by the Guthrie test in the neonatal period. Excess production of metabolites, phenylpyruvic acid and phenylethylamine, with high levels of phenylalanine, damages the developing brain. Infant formulas low in phenylalanine are available. Close nutritional supervision and frequent monitoring of serum concentrations of phenylalanine are required. Optimal serum phenylalanine level is 3–15–mg/dL and care must be taken not to overrestrict, as phenylalanine cannot be synthesized by the body and is essential for the rapidly growing infant. Tyrosine also becomes an essential amino acid in this disorder and adequate intake in diet is required. A diet low in phenylalanine is lifelong and strict restriction is particularly important in pregnant women and during brain development in the first 6 years of life.

Diabetes mellitus

Children with type 1 diabetes should eat as 'normal' a diet as possible. Energy intake is calculated on the size of the child, and should be provided as around 55 per cent carbohydrate, 30 per cent fat and 15 per cent protein. In general approximately 70 per cent of the carbohydrate should be taken as complex carbohydrate such as starch, as digestion and absorption are slow, resulting in slow rise in plasma glucose. Refined sugars such as sucrose should be avoided, as they are rapidly absorbed and may cause swings in blood glucose. Diets high in fibre, such as vegetables, wholemeal bread, bran and fruits also help to improve control of blood glucose. The total daily energy intake is divided between breakfast, lunch and dinner, with mid-morning, mid-afternoon and evening snacks. Meal plans are often based on groups of food 'exchanges', but for practical purposes there are few restrictions, so each child can continue a diet based on preference.

Type 2 (maturity-onset) diabetes is becoming more prevalent in children. Many are obese and have abnormal glucose tolerance tests secondary to insulin resistance rather than inadequate secretion. Weight reduction is indicated in children who are obese. Otherwise, nutritional management is similar to that for type 1 diabetes, although insulin therapy is not usually required.

Neurodisability

Nutritional problems are common in children with disabilities, particularly those with severe motor impairment. There may be difficulty chewing and swallowing and spillage of food can compromise food intake. Chronic undernutrition is associated with muscle weakness and poor immune function. Energy requirements are often reduced in non-ambulant children. Assessment of nutritional status can be difficult because of limb contractures or scoliosis. Assessment of oral skills by speech and language therapist can guide management, which may involve changing the consistency of food and giving energy-dense foods or supplements. Gastrostomy feeding is used for children who cannot feed safely orally. Ongoing review should take place to monitor growth and avoid overfeeding. Energy requirement may be lower than the EAR and the amount of feed required to provide sufficient energy might not contain adequate micronutrients. Additional vitamins, minerals and fibre may be required.

CASE STUDY: Neurodisability

A school nurse refers a 6-year-old girl with quadriplegic cerebral palsy for assessment. Her weight has been static for the last 18 months at around 12 kg (below the 0.4th centile). Her height is 102 cm although she has some limb contractures. She feeds orally on mashed foods and drinks juice from a beaker but drools and coughs frequently during feeds. What further assessment is required? What would the management options be and how can the effect of interventions be monitored?

KEY LEARNING POINTS

- Children with chronic disease are susceptible to malnutrition, with poor energy intake secondary to anorexia and increased requirements or losses due to disease.
- The aims of nutritional management are to prevent and reverse malnutrition, anticipate specific nutrient deficiencies and maximize growth potential.
- Enteral therapy is accepted as a primary treatment to induce remission and treat relapse in Crohn disease.
- Children with cystic fibrosis need up to 150 per cent of the EAR for energy and RNI for vitamins A, D and E due to increased energy expenditure and malabsorption.
- Children with diabetes mellitus should eat as normal a diet as possible, following healthy eating recommendations.
- Children with neurodisability are prone to undernutrition due to motor difficulties and may need support with enteral nutrition.

UNDERNUTRITION AND OVERNUTRITION

Failure to thrive or growth faltering are terms used to describe infants and young children who do not achieve expected height and weight gain for age. This can be detected when serial measurements plotted on growth charts show downwards crossing of centiles. Failure to thrive may be due to insufficient intake, excessive requirements or excessive losses of nutrients. Inadequate intake is the commonest cause and is associated with low socioeconomic status. Sometimes hospitalization is required to observe the feeding pattern, particularly in the young infant, but usually the problem is effectively managed by the health visitor in the home. Other causes of failure to thrive, such as cystic fibrosis, coeliac disease or chronic infection, may need to be ruled out. Management of failure to thrive will depend on the underlying cause, but the aim in all patients is the improvement of nutritional status. This will require dietetic advice to look at calorie density of feeds and possible supplementation of macro- and micronutrients.

CASE STUDY: Failure to thrive

A 9-month-old infant is admitted with herpes stomatitis and refusal to feed. Her admission weight is 7 kg (2nd centile) and length 69 cm (9th centile). Her birth weight was on the 50th centile and was maintained until 5 months but had then fallen gradually through the centiles. She normally finger feeds and takes small portions of a variety of solids. She drinks around 200 mL formula milk and several cups of juice per day. Two weeks later the mouth lesions have healed but she still refuses to take a bottle in her mouth and manages only small amounts of pureed foods from a spoon. Her weight has dropped to 6.5 kg (0.4th centile). How should she be managed and which professionals should be involved?

Malnutrition in the developing world and poor communities

Protein–energy malnutrition is a result of dietary deficiency, infective and environmental factors. Milder degrees result in failure to thrive with growth retardation, whereas severe deficiencies cause protein–energy malnutrition (marasmus and kwashiorkor). Worldwide, malnutrition is one of the principal causes of childhood morbidity and mortality.

Marasmus occurs as a result of eating very little of an otherwise balanced diet and is often associated with enteropathy. Clinical features include low weight (<60 per cent median weight-for-age) and wasting of muscles and subcutaneous fat. There may also be associated vitamin deficiencies or diarrhoea. Kwashiorkor occurs at the time of weaning, as a result of a disproportionate reduction in protein intake as total energy intake also falls. With cessation of breastfeeding, the infant loses a ready supply of protein, often replaced with low protein foods such as banana or rice. Growth retardation is associated with oedema, muscle wasting, poor appetite, listlessness and irritability. Other features include sparse hair, anaemia, dermatitis, hepatomegaly, skin changes and micronutrient deficiencies. Atrophy of the pancreas and small intestinal enteropathy lead to malabsorption, steatorrhoea, and deficiencies of fat-soluble vitamins. Small intestinal disaccharidase activities are depressed, leading to carbohydrate intolerance. Plasma protein levels are reduced, and as a consequence, the availability of substances carried on them. The extracellular fluid is hypotonic and circulating cortisol concentrations are high, contributing to fluid retention and hyponatraemia.

Children with protein–energy malnutrition often also have gastroenteritis, Gram-negative septicaemia, respiratory infections or measles. Some children are extremely ill and need admission to hospital with hypothermia, hypoglycemia, drowsiness and stupor, severe diarrhoea and cardiac failure. Mortality can reach 15 per cent for those patients admitted to hospital.

Treatment of marasmus is provision of sufficient food, providing energy intake of around 190 kcal/kg or more. Children are usually hungry and will take this amount orally. Cows' milk is effective and economic in the treatment of kwashiorkor and sugar and vegetable oils are often added to increase the energy content. This diet will provide 96–155 kcal (400–650 kJ), 2–4 g milk protein, 4–6 mmol potassium, 1–3 mmol magnesium and less than 2 mmol Na/kg per day as ideal. Some children can take this by mouth but for those who are unable nasogastric feeding is necessary. Daily supplements of vitamin A and folic acid are recommended and zinc may also be required.

If all goes well the child begins to lose weight, from loss of oedema, within the first three days after admission and continues to do so until the end of the first week. After this there should be a steady weight gain.

Prevention of protein–energy malnutrition requires provision of a good supply of food and prompt treatment of gastroenteritis with oral rehydration therapy. Prolonged breastfeeding up to 2 years should be supported with the use of locally available protein foods. Early re-feeding after episodes of diarrhoea is encouraged.

Obesity

Obesity is caused by a disturbance in the energy balance equation with mismatch of energy intake and expenditure. It can be caused by excess energy intake (consumption of high fat and calorie foods), reduced expenditure (reduction in physical activity levels and increases in sedentary lifestyles) or combination of both. There has been an increase in consumption of high-fat foods and a decline in the intake of fruit, vegetables and cereals in the developed world. Body mass index (BMI) reference centile charts should be used to establish whether a child is obese: BMI >95th centile for age and sex on the UK 1990 BMI reference chart. Numerous studies have documented an increasing trend of childhood obesity, one reporting prevalence rates of 11 per cent in 6-year-olds and 17 per cent in 15-year-olds.

Rarely, obesity is caused by underlying endocrine disorders or associated syndromes (e.g. Prader–Willi syndrome), in which associated dysmorphic features or short stature help identify this very small group (Table 11.7). Obesity in children, as in adults, is linked with

Table 11.7 Causes of obesity

Functional	
Simple obesity	Excessive dietary intake Lack of exercise/mobility (spina bifida, muscular dystrophy)
Organic	
Hypothalamic disturbance	Pituitary tumours
Hyperphagic syndromes	Prader-Willi syndrome Lawrence-Moon-Biedl syndrome
Corticosteroid excess	Cushing's (iatrogenic, pituitary, adrenal)
Hypothyroidism	Thyroid failure
Chromosomal	Down syndrome Klinefelter syndrome
Cerebral disease	Tumours, infection, hydrocephalus

hypertension, altered blood lipids and increased incidence of type 2 diabetes, as well as sleep problems related to airway obstruction. Obesity is also linked to psychological problems in children such as depression and low self-esteem. Preventive strategies promote healthy eating and active lifestyles (e.g. free fruit in schools). Treatment is most effective if the family is willing to make the necessary lifestyle changes and is based on a weight maintenance or modest weight reduction programme achieved by healthier eating, increasing physical activity levels and restricting times of inactivity.

CASE STUDY: Childhood obesity

A 12-year-old boy is referred with nocturnal enuresis. This previously had been infrequent but has recently worsened. Physical examination is normal but his weight is 68 kg (99.6th centile) and height 152 cm (75th centile) giving a BMI of 29, which is obese. On discussion about his weight he becomes upset and reveals that he has been bullied at school about being overweight. Are any investigations necessary and what management should be followed?

KEY LEARNING POINTS

- Failure to thrive or growth faltering describes the infant or young child who fails to achieve expected height and weight gain for age.
- Inadequate food intake is the commonest cause of failure to thrive and is associated with low socioeconomic status.
- Worldwide, malnutrition is one of the principal causes of childhood morbidity and mortality.
- In the developed world, childhood obesity has become increasingly common due to changes in lifestyle, with reduced physical activity and increased consumption of high-calorie foods.

PRINCIPLES AND PRACTICE OF NUTRITIONAL SUPPORT

Nutrition team

Poor nutrition is not only a consequence of specific diseases, but also a feature of most chronic illnesses, follows major surgery and occurs when patients are unable to eat or make proper use of their diet. Children can also become malnourished for non-medical reasons, such as inappropriate or missed hospital meals. Nutrition support has developed as an integral part of the care of sick children both in hospital and in the community.

Nutrition support should be provided by a team led by a paediatrician, trained in clinical nutrition, and comprising dietitians, nutrition nurse specialists, a pharmacist in charge of the preparation and prescription of parenteral solutions, a biochemist responsible for monitoring biochemical outcome and a surgeon with experience of gastrostomies and insertion of IV long lines for parenteral nutrition. Nutrition support may be provided either enterally or parenterally. The enteral route should be used if the gastrointestinal tract is intact, accessible and functional (Figure 11.5). Parenteral nutrition should be reserved for conditions where enteral nutrition is not possible or nutrient requirements cannot be maintained via the gut alone.

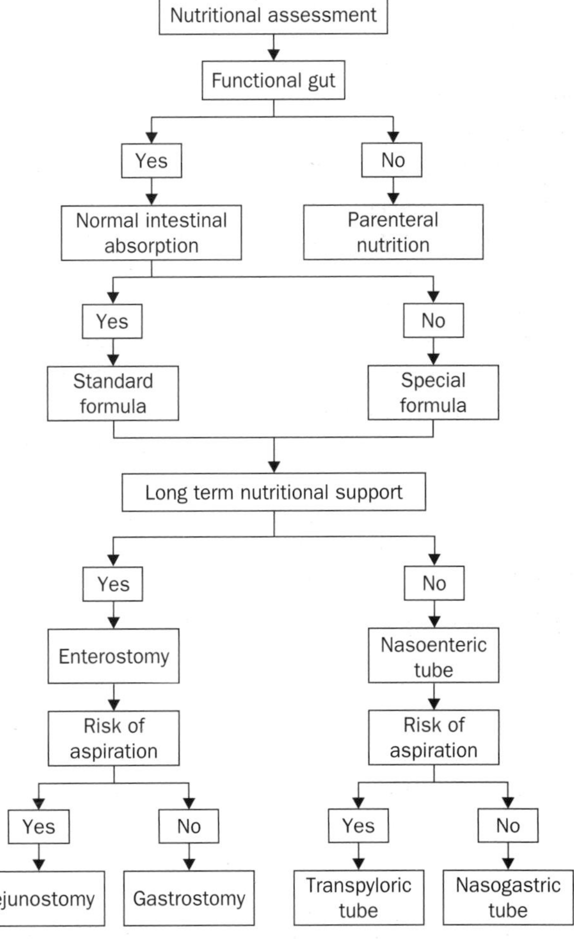

Figure 11.5 Decision making pathways to choice of method of delivery of enteral feeds (Reproduced with permission from Weaver LT, Edwards CA, Golden B, Reilly JJ (2003) Nutrition. In: Mackintosh N, Helms P, Smyth R (eds) *Forfar and Arneil's Textbook of Paediatrics*, 6th edn. Edinburgh: Churchill Livingstone, pp. 561–82)

Enteral nutrition

Enteral feeding is a means by which nutrients are delivered to the gastrointestinal tract by tube or enterostomy. This can be done continuously, as bolus feeds, or intermittently. With continuous feeding, the enteral feed is infused over hours (usually between 8 and 24 hours) using a feeding pump. It is contained within a sterile reservoir feeding bag or bottle. Continuous feeds allow a reasonably high fluid intake with little gastric distension and aspiration. Bolus feeding simulates the usual pattern of feeding, generating a gut hormone response that is greater than that when continuous feeds are given. Feeds can be given at various intervals from hourly to four hourly. Delayed gastric emptying and vomiting are contraindications to bolus feeding and occasionally the dumping syndrome occurs. Intermittent continuous feeding combines the feeding techniques of bolus and continuous feeds. Feeds are usually given via nasogastric tubes, which are easier to introduce and maintain than nasojejunal tubes. Nasogastric tube feeding is also physiological but gastroesophageal reflux and aspiration are more likely to occur.

Enterostomies are a means of delivering enteral feeds directly into the stomach or jejunum when long-term enteral support is required. They are preferred when pharyngeal discomfort is intolerable or risk of aspiration is high. Percutaneous endoscopic gastrostomy (PEG) is an increasingly popular technique of tube placement. Many children who require long-term enteral nutrition have gastrostomies, including many who receive home enteral feeding. There are a range of enteral feeds available for children (Table 11.8), most based on cows' milk, for children with an intact and functional gastrointestinal tract and specialized formulas designed to meet the altered nutrient needs of children with specific clinical disorders.

Parenteral nutrition

Parenteral nutrition is a means by which nutrients are delivered via the vein. It may provide complete nutritional support – total parenteral nutrition (TPN) – or be combined with enteral feeding. Whereas gastrointestinal failure is an absolute indication for parenteral nutrition, complete exclusion of luminal nutrients is frequently neither essential nor desirable. Even if only minimal volumes of enteral feed can be given in addition to parenteral nutrition, this helps to reduce cholestasis by stimulating bile flow and pancreatic secretions, maintaining splanchnic blood flow and providing nutrition to enterocytes. Infants need around 470 kJ/kg per day (112 kcal/kg per day) and this decreases to about 40 per cent of this value in adult life. When attempting to reverse long-term growth failure energy supply should be related to expected rather than actual weight.

Table 11.8 A selection of commercially available enteral feeds and specialized infant formulas

Feed	Protein	Composition per 100 ml				Uses	Manufacturer
		Protein (g)	Energy (kcal)	Fat (g)	Carbohydrate (g)		
Nutrini	Caseinates	2.75	100	4.4	12.3	1–6 years old	Cow & Gate
Nutrini energy	Caseinates	4.1	150	6.7	18.5	1–6 years old	Cow & Gate
Paediasure	Whey and caseinates	3.0	100	5.0	11.0		Abbott Laboratories
Elemental 028	Essential and non-essential amino acids	2.0	78	1.3	14.4	Severe gastro-intestinal tract impairment	Scientific Hospital Supplies (SHS)
Nutramigen	Casein hydrosylate	1.9	68	3.4	7.5	Cows' milk protein intolerance	Mead Johnson
Neocate	L-amino acids	1.95	71	3.5	8.1	Food allergy or intolerance	SHS
Caprilon	Whey protein	1.5	66	3.6 25% LCT:75% MCT	7.0	Hepatic disease	SHS
Kindergen	Whey and essential amino acids	1.5	101	5.2	12.1	Chronic renal failure	SHS
Pepdite 1+	Soya and pork hydrolysate	2.8	88	3.5	11.4	Gastrointestinal tract impairment	SHS

L/MCT, long/medium chain triglyceride.

Nitrogen (protein) is supplied as a solution of synthetic crystalline essential and non-essential L-amino acids. In children, histidine, proline, tyrosine, taurine, alanine and cystine/cysteine are required during infancy in addition to the eight amino acids regarded as essential in adults. Glucose is the carbohydrate of choice for parenteral nutrition because it is metabolized by all cells. High infusion rates may lead to hyperglycaemia, glycosuria and osmotic diuresis. Tolerance can usually be achieved by increasing intake over a number of days. Lipid emulsions are non-irritant to veins, calorie dense and provide essential fatty acids. A dual-energy system comprising both fat and glucose leads to improved protein synthesis, less water retention and less fatty infiltration of the liver.

Bone mineralization is dependent upon adequate supply of calcium and phosphate. The limited solubilities of calcium and phosphate need to be taken into account. There is no ideal vitamin or trace element solution for children over 10 kg. Selenium is now given routinely. Zinc requirements may be high particularly in children with gastrointestinal fluid losses. Chromium added to long-term parenteral nutrition regimens has been associated with hepatic and renal impairment. The prescription of parenteral nutrition is covered below.

Short-term parenteral nutrition can be given using a standard peripheral venous cannula so long as dextrose concentration is <12.5 per cent. Maintaining peripheral venous access becomes increasingly difficult with duration of parenteral nutrition and interruptions to infusion can lead to suboptimal nutritional intake. Central venous catheterization (CVC) provides reliable venous access and should be considered when parenteral nutrition is required for more than a week. Sepsis is a serious complication. Major unexpected biochemical disturbances are rare. One common problem is cholestasis, from lack of enteral feeding. Other complications of parenteral nutrition include thromboembolic events, granulomatous pulmonary arteritis and pulmonary hypertension.

A volumetric pump should be used to deliver parenteral nutrition fluids. For children receiving prolonged parenteral nutrition, cyclical nutrition (given over less than 24 hours) should be considered. This allows time off and helps to protect against cholestasis and hepatic dysfunction. Home parenteral nutrition is now an option, facilitated by the development of the nutritional support industry and hospital outreach services. It offers children who would otherwise become institutionalized the possibility of realizing growth and developmental potential, a good quality of life and a reduced risk of complications such as CVC sepsis. Suitable patients are those with long-term gastrointestinal failure who are medically stable and have adequate home circumstances. The carers must be motivated and capable of becoming expert in home therapy.

CASE STUDY: Parenteral nutrition

A 4-month-old baby boy is transferred from the neonatal surgical unit following extensive small bowel resection (including terminal ileum) for neonatal volvulus. He cannot tolerate enteral feeds and has short-bowel syndrome requiring long-term parenteral nutrition. His birth weight was on the 50th centile but his weight is currently on the 0.4th centile. Skinfold thickness measurements are on the 2nd centile. Outline the strategy for providing adequate nutrition for this infant. What nutrient deficiencies is he at risk of?

KEY LEARNING POINTS

- Nutrition support should be provided by a multidisciplinary team.
- Enteral nutrition is a means by which a nutritionally complete feed can be delivered to the gastrointestinal tract via a tube or enterostomy.
- The enteral route should always be used if the gastrointestinal tract is intact and functional.
- Parenteral nutrition can be used to deliver nutrients via a vein in those patients in whom enteral feeding is not possible or in combination with enteral feeding.
- For patients stable on parenteral nutrition, home parenteral nutrition can be used with motivated parents and trained professional support.

ASSESSMENT

Nutritional assessment is the evaluation of a patient's nutritional status and requirements. It is a means by which the undernourished or overnourished child can be identified and the nutritional effects of therapy and interventions monitored.

Dietary assessment

Dietary assessment should be carried out by a paediatric dietitian with the skills to ensure that all aspects of intake are considered, including assessment of the quantities of food eaten. Retrospective, three, five or seven-day food record diaries are sometimes used. Dietary assessment of an infant who is less than 6 months of age should include assessment of the mother's nutritional status while pregnant and her lactation if she is breast-feeding.

Anthropometry

Anthropometry is the measurement of physical dimensions, such as weight, height and skinfold thickness. These measurements are carried out at different ages and compared with reference standards. Anthropometry is a reasonable guide to energy and protein status. Low height-for-age, 'stunting', is an index of chronic undernutrition and low weight-for-height, 'wasting', is an index of more acute undernutrition. The BMI – weight (kg)/height $(m)^2$ – is also a simple and useful tool for assessing or monitoring overweight and underweight and reference charts are now available. Growth reference charts are vital tools for nutritional assessment. Without accurate and up-to-date body weights and heights, rational calculation of nutritional assessment cannot be made. Chapter 14 covers anthropometry in more detail.

Biochemical and haematological assessment

Biochemical and haematological assessment can be made by measurement of nutrient concentrations or biochemical markers of nutritional status in the blood or urine. However, circulating concentrations of nutrients are not always an accurate measurement of tissue stores. Commonly measured nutrients are blood urea, a measure of protein intake, plasma amino acids (to look for specific amino acid deficiencies in children taking a diet low in protein), alkaline phosphatase as a marker for rickets and ferritin and total iron binding capacity as a measure of iron status.

Clinical assessment

Clinical assessment is used in association with anthropometry and to detect signs of specific nutritional deficiencies. Isolated nutrient deficiencies rarely occur alone but physical signs, such as glossitis or angular stomatitis, may be detected. Physical signs of protein–energy malnutrition, specific vitamin and mineral deficiencies, including rickets and scurvy may be seen, but it should be remembered that physical signs are a late manifestation of nutrient deficiency.

Functional and physiological assessment

Functional and physiological assessment may reveal evidence of delayed walking (e.g. vitamin D deficiency and rickets) or delay in general development with broader nutritional deficiency.

PRESCRIPTION OF PARENTERAL NUTRITION

Parenteral nutrition may be the sole source of nutrients as TPN or may contribute in part if some enteral feed is tolerated. This should be taken into account when prescribing parenteral nutrition. Parenteral nutrition is prescribed in terms of carbohydrate (per cent solution), protein (g/kg), fat (g/kg) and electrolyte (mmol/kg) content. Vitamins and minerals are usually added as a standard additive solution. It is normal practice to build up the parenteral nutrition content over a number of days as tolerated (Figure 11.6).

ANSWERS TO QUESTIONS POSED IN THE CASE STUDIES

Case study – Iron deficiency (page 343)
The main energy source is cows' milk and this diet is likely to be deficient in iron. Full blood count showed hypochromic, microcytic anaemia and serum ferritin was low. Management is with iron supplements and dietary advice to reduce the intake of cows' milk and promote intake of solids.

Case study – Coeliac disease (page 346)
If assessment of the diet suggests that it is adequate then there must be either malabsorption or increased energy requirements. The differential diagnosis therefore includes causes of malabsorption (see box page 343) and chronic diseases (e.g. cystic fibrosis). Management of coeliac disease involves lifelong exclusion of gluten from the diet and the assistance of a paediatric dietitian is required to advise the family and ensure an adequate diet.

Case study – Neurodisability (page 347)
Dietary assessment should determine if intake is adequate for this child's requirements, and anthropometry, including skinfold thickness measurements, can help to assess nutritional status. Speech and language assessment of oromotor skills should be carried out and videofluoroscopy examination will help assessment of swallowing.

PARENTERAL NUTRITION PRESCRIPTION FORM
Pharmacy Department:

Please complete all the information requested below when ordering Parenteral Nutrition

- ☺ A separate form must be completed for each patient each day (PN bags will be prepared for Saturday and Sunday from Friday's prescription)
- ☺ All requests must be received and confirmed by **11 am at the latest**
- ☺ Please phone_ _ _ _ _ if you require advice on prescribing PN
- ☺ Please ensure all blood is taken before 9.30 am. If blood results are not reported by 11 am the previous days results will be used. See over for recommended minimum monitoring.

Patient name ______________________ **Ward** __________

Hospital number* ______________________ **Consultant*** __________

Weight ______________________ **D of B*** __________

Indication for TPN* ______________________

Central/peripheral line *must be completed on day 1 of parenteral nutrition only

Aqueous rate	
Lipid rate	
Lipid (g/kg)	
Protein (g/kg)	
Glucose (%) (max 10% for peripheral admin)	
Standard electrolytes (see reverse for details)	Based on NN Bag/standard electrolytes/kg

Modified electrolytes:

Sodium (mmol/kg)	
Potassium (mmol/kg)	
Calcium (mmol/kg)	
Phosphate (mmol/kg)	
Magnesium (mmol/kg)	
Acetate formula	Yes/no

Additional comments:

Prescriber's signature ______________________ **Date** __________

Name (please print) ______________________ **Page no** __________

Figure 11.6 Prescription sheet for parenteral nutrition

If the child can swallow safely then energy supplements may be helpful, but if not then an alternative route of feeding such as nasogastric or gastrostomy feeding should be considered, taking into account its risks and benefits. If intragastric feeding is commenced careful nutritional follow-up is required to ensure provision of adequate nutrients and avoid overfeeding.

Case study – Failure to thrive (page 347)

This child is failing to thrive and has aversion to foods secondary to the oral lesions. Involvement of a speech and language therapist will help manage the feeding problem and a dietitian will help to assess the dietary intake and advise on increasing energy intake. Feeding from a beaker cup and finger feeding was established and high-energy formula milk given to replace the low calorie juice.

Case study – Childhood obesity (page 349)

Management should aim to maintain weight by encouraging healthy eating in all members of the family (controlling excess intake of saturated fat, fizzy drinks, and snacks; encouraging five portions each day of fruit and vegetables), increasing physical exercise and reducing periods of inactivity. Psychological support may also be required to help self-esteem. If there is no evidence of short stature or dysmorphic features investigations are unlikely to be helpful.

Case study – Parenteral nutrition (page 351)

A multidisciplinary nutrition team best provides long-term parenteral nutrition management. Central venous line insertion will facilitate parenteral nutrition delivery. Adequate calories should be provided for normal growth and to allow for catch-up. Parenteral nutrition should deliver sufficient amounts of all nutrients but small amounts of enteral feeds should also be given to facilitate intestinal adaptation. Monitoring growth and micronutrient status should guide ongoing management. Owing to the loss of the terminal ileum, fat malabsorption and deficiencies of fat-soluble vitamins and vitamin B_{12} should be considered but these nutrients should be provided in parenteral nutrition.

FURTHER READING

Doherty CP, Reilly JJ, Paterson WF, Donaldson MDC, Weaver LT (2000) Growth failure and malnutrition. In: Walker WA *et al.* (eds) *Pediatric Gastrointestinal Disease.* Toronto: Dekker, 12–27.

Michaelsen KF, Weaver LT, Branca F, Robertson A (2000) *Feeding and Nutrition of Infants and Young Children.* Copenhagen: WHO.

Weaver LT (2003) Feeding the normal infant, child and adolescent. *Medicine* 31:39–42.

Weaver LT, Prentice A (2003) Nutrition in infancy. In: Morgan JB, Dickerson WT (eds) *Nutrition in Early Life.* London: Wiley, 205–32.

Weaver LT, Edwards CA, Golden B, Reilly JJ (2003) Nutrition. In: Mackintosh N, Helms P, Smyth R (eds) *Forfar and Arneil's Textbook of Paediatrics*, 6th edn. Edinburgh: Churchill Livingstone, 561–82.

Chapter 12

Urinary tract problems

Jim Beattie and Amir F Azmy

URINARY TRACT: EMBRYOLOGY, PHYSIOLOGY AND IMAGING

EMBRYOLOGY/PRENATAL DEVELOPMENT

The urinary tract develops from the cloaca and the intermediate mesoderm. The definitive functional kidney in the human, the metanephros, results from the sequential development and involution of two more primitive sets of tubules, the pronephros and the mesonephros (Figure 12.1).

The pronephros, which is non-functional in humans, develops during the third and regresses by the fifth post-conceptual week. When the pronephros degenerates, its duct becomes the mesonephric duct – which in some species is the mature kidney but there is no proof of function in the human embryo. The mesonephric duct in turn eventually becomes the ureteric bud, which is essential for formation of the metanephros.

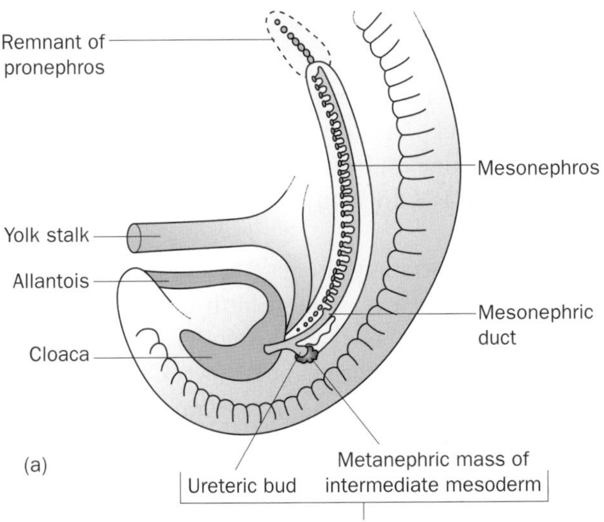

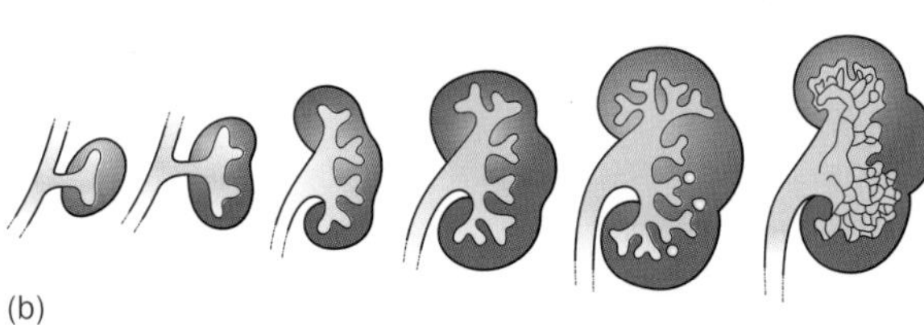

Figure 12.1 (a, b) Embryonic/fetal renal development (redrawn from Gray DL, Crane JP (1988) Prenatal diagnosis of urinary tract malformation. *Pediatr Nephrol* **2**:326–33)

The metanephros is the final stage in human renal development. The ureteric bud appears by the fifth post-conceptual week as a branch of the mesonephric duct but as the ureteric bud extends in a superior direction, the metanephric mass of mesoderm (metanephric blastema) condenses into the metanephros. The ureteric bud branches in succession to form the ureter, pelvis, calyces and collecting tubules. The metanephric blastema forms the glomeruli and upper part of the nephrons. The first nephron development occurs around the eighth post-conceptual week and nephron development continues until 34 weeks' post conception.

The upper portion of the bladder is derived from the allantois and the lower portion from the cloaca. The fibrous cord known as the urachus is formed from the remainder of the allantois and connects the bladder to the umbilicus.

Fetal renal function

In fetal life, excretory function is accomplished by the placenta that receives approximately 50 per cent of the fetal cardiac output. The fetal renal blood flow accounts for only 2–4 per cent of the cardiac output at term compared to 15 per cent in the neonate. Fetal renal blood flow is maintained at a low rate by a combination of low mean arterial blood pressure and the influence of such factors as the renin–angiotensin system, the renal sympathetic nervous system, renal and systemic prostaglandins, the kallikrein–kinin system and atrial natriuretic peptide. Glomerular filtration rate (GFR) is low in fetal life and increases towards term but remains constant in relation to kidney weight. After birth (see below) the GFR rises rapidly via recruitment of superficial cortical nephrons and an increase in the individual nephron filtered load.

In fetal life, there is a high rate of renal tubular sodium excretion that decreases with increasing gestational age. Fetal urine is hypo-osmotic but can be concentrated and diluted by alterations in maternal hydration and varies from 230 to 660 mL per day. The fetal urinary sodium and phosphate levels decrease while the creatinine increases with increasing gestation, whereas the fetal urinary urea, calcium and potassium levels generally remain unchanged. The fall in fetal urinary sodium and phosphate and accompanying increase in creatinine levels with gestational age is consistent with increasing GFR and tubular maturation.

KEY LEARNING POINTS

- The urinary tract results from the sequential development and involution of primitive sets of tubules. The first nephron appears around the eighth post-conceptual week and nephron development continues until 34 weeks' post conception.
- Fetal urinary sodium and phosphate levels fall progressively with increasing gestation and are a sensitive indicator of increasing fetal GFR and tubular maturation.

POSTNATAL RENAL DEVELOPMENT

Perinatal and postnatal renal function

Most known renal homoeostatic mechanisms are operative in the fetus although fluid and electrolyte regulation is accomplished almost entirely by the placenta. At birth, the regulatory and excretory demands are placed entirely on the kidney whose performance will largely be dependent on the gestational age of the neonate.

It is conventional to correct renal function to a standard body size of 1.73 m^2, which represents the average body surface area of a standard man. There are, however, theoretical and physiological limitations with the use of this correction, and in a research setting it is probably more appropriate to use absolute values of GFR.

In the term baby the GFR at birth is approximately 25 mL/minute per 1.73 m^2 and that of the 31-week gestational baby is 10–15 mL/minute per 1.73 m^2 (Table 12.1). In the term baby the GFR increases by 50–100 per cent during the first two weeks of life with a more gradual increase thereafter, reaching adult levels (80–120 mL/minute per 1.73 m^2) by 12–18 months of age. For the baby born before 34 weeks' gestational age, GFR rises slowly until the baby reaches a post-conceptual age of 34 weeks after which a rapid rise is observed following completion of nephrogenesis.

Table 12.1 Changes in perinatal and postnatal renal function

	Preterm	Term		
	0–3 days	0–3 days	14 days	8 weeks
Urine volume (mL/kg per day)	15–75	20–75	25–120	80–130
Urine osmolality (mOsm/kg)				
Max:	400–500	600–800	800–900	1000–1200
Min:	30–50	50	50	50
Glomerular filtration rate (mL/minute per 1.73 m^2)	10–15	15–20	35–45	75–80

Measurement of glomerular filtration rate

Inulin as a reference solute for GFR estimation is mainly used as a research tool. In clinical practice, particularly in infants, accurate measure of GFR may be obtained by the use of radiopharmaceuticals, e.g. ^{99m}Tc-DTPA, ^{125}I-iothalamate and ^{51}Cr-EDTA. The main advantage of the isotopic methods is the lack of a requirement for a timed urine collection.

In the older child, a creatinine clearance involving a timed (preferably 24-hour) urine collection as well as a plasma creatinine estimation carried out during the collection period is sufficiently accurate for use in clinical practice.

Glomerular filtration rate may be estimated from the plasma creatinine level, and at birth this approximates the mother's value (average 75 μmol/L). In term babies the level falls rapidly during the first week and thereafter there is a slow increase as a reflection of increasing muscle mass with age and adult values are reached by the age of 12 years (see Appendix A). Glomerular filtration rate may be estimated using the formula $k \times$ length (cm) divided by plasma creatinine (μmol/L). The value of the constant k varies with age and gender:

- Low birth weight infants (<2.5 kg) – 30
- Normal infant 0–2 years – 40
- Girls 2–16 years – 49
- Boys 2–13 years – 49
- Boys 13–16 years – 60

The sequential estimation of GFR by this formula in an individual patient with renal disease gives the clinician useful information but it is important that occasional formal clearance estimations are performed for comparison.

POSTNATAL CHANGES IN RENAL TUBULAR FUNCTION

Sodium homoeostasis

The relationship of tubular function to gestational age is relatively complex. The infant of low gestational age at birth behaves as a salt loser and may develop negative sodium balance that may result in hyponatraemia. This apparent glomerulotubular imbalance is probably due to a combination of proximal renal tubular immaturity and partial resistance of the distal tubule to aldosterone. However, it is also consistent with the progressive decrease in extracellular fluid volume with increasing gestation that necessitates a reduction in body sodium content from 120 mmol/kg at 8 weeks to 80 mmol/kg at 40 weeks' gestational age.

In the term neonate, renal tubular excretion of sodium is increased at birth but by the third day of life a term neonate is able to maximally conserve sodium in a similar way to the adult. In contrast, the ability to excrete a sodium load is blunted, probably because of the high circulating plasma aldosterone level and the relatively low GFR.

Water homoeostasis

A reduction in total body water, as well as extracellular fluid volume, is also part of normal gestational development and correlates with increasing fetal urine production during the third trimester. During the first several hours of life, urine volume of a 28 weeks' gestation neonate averages 4 mL/kg per hour whereas that of a term baby is 1 mL/kg per hour. Diluting capacity of babies of >30 weeks' gestation is at least the equivalent to that of the adult in that the urine osmolality may be lowered to 30–50 mOsm/kg. However, despite this capability excessive rates of fluid administration to premature babies are associated with expanded extracellular fluid volume and increased incidence of patent ductus arteriosus, bronchopulmonary dysplasia and necrotizing enterocolitis.

In contrast to diluting capacity, the maximum urinary concentrating capacity of the neonate is significantly lower than that of the older child or adult. Normal adult values are generally achieved by the age of 1 year.

Acid–base homoeostasis

At birth, control of acid–base balance is removed from the placenta and taken over by the neonate's kidney and lungs. Whereas the arterial pH of the premature and term neonate is similar to that of adults, the plasma bicarbonate level is normally lower, varying from 14–16 mmol/L in premature to 21 mmol/L in the term baby. The normal adult range of 24–26 mmol/L is achieved by 2 years of age. These differences reflect the reduced net acid excretion (i.e. the sum of the hydrogen ion excreted as ammonia and titratable acidity minus bicarbonate) and the low renal bicarbonate threshold.

At a practical level, it is important to recognize these differences since attempts to increase the plasma bicarbonate level above the renal threshold by the administration of bicarbonate will be unsuccessful and may run the risk of sodium overload.

In summary, the neonatal kidney is capable of rapid adaptation to extrauterine life but it is important to recognize the significant physiological differences in renal function compared with the adult who has quite a different body composition. If the infant is subjected to stress, disease or over judicious fluid and electrolyte administration, renal adaptation may be inadequate.

KEY LEARNING POINTS

- Glomerular filtration rate is low in both preterm and term babies and babies of <34 weeks' gestation have a delayed physiological increase in GFR.
- Preterm neonates have high urinary salt loss but also have a limited ability to excrete a sodium and water load because of a low GFR.
- Bicarbonate reabsorptive capacity is low, particularly in the preterm baby, and neonates and infants have lower plasma bicarbonate concentrations than adults.
- Maximum urinary concentrating capacity of the neonate is significantly lower than the older child and adult and this level is achieved by 12 months of age.
- Despite incomplete maturation, the neonatal kidney is functional and glomerulotubular imbalance is more apparent than real. The presence of 'immature' kidneys should not be used to explain disturbances in fluid and electrolyte balance or increase in plasma urea and creatinine.
- Sequential estimation of GFR using height/plasma creatinine ratio is useful and more convenient than formal clearance methods.

URINARY TRACT IMAGING

Whenever imaging of the urinary tract is required, the least invasive technique should always be chosen. In addition, algorithms are particularly useful since they require agreement between clinicians and radiologists as well as ensuring rational use of imaging resources.

Ultrasound

Ultrasound is a non-invasive technique with no radiation burden and should be available on all units responsible for the care of children. Ultrasound provides anatomical detail of the urinary tract as well as the retroperitoneal intra-abdominal structures. Accurate measurements of renal length are possible, allowing the development of normal renal growth charts (Figure 12.2). In the presence of an abdominal mass, ultrasound can define the origin and nature of the mass and determine whether it is cystic or solid. The neonatal renal ultrasound is different from that of the older child in that there is a less clear distinction between the renal cortex and medulla and occasionally in the neonate the medulla may appear hyperechoic to the unskilled observer and may suggest the diagnosis of multiple cysts when in fact it is normal.

The colour Doppler ultrasound as a non-invasive method of assessing blood flow is very useful in the context of renal transplantation, in the diagnosis of renal venous/inferior vena cava thrombosis in the neonate and in the assessment of patients with possible renal artery stenosis.

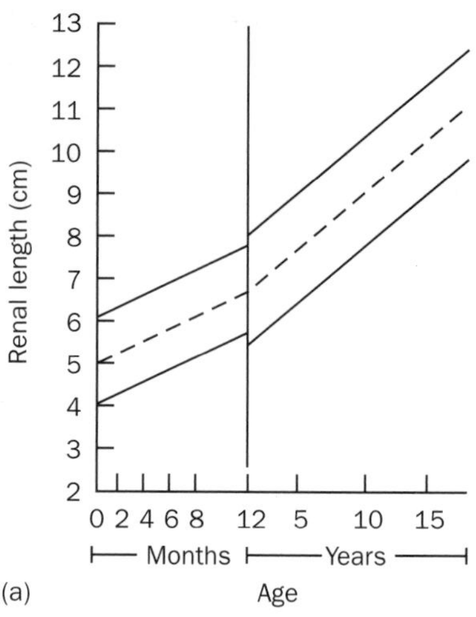

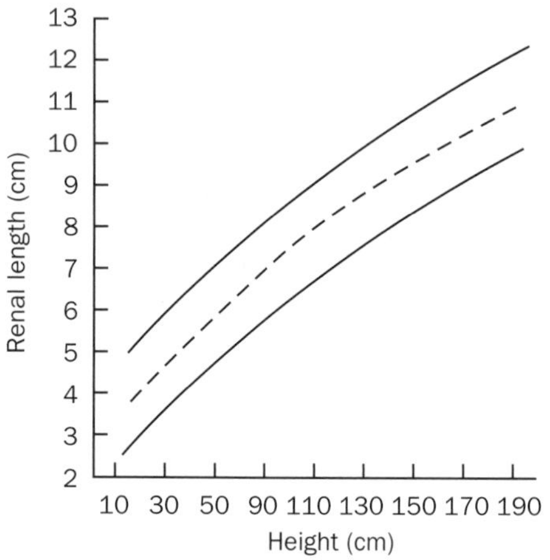

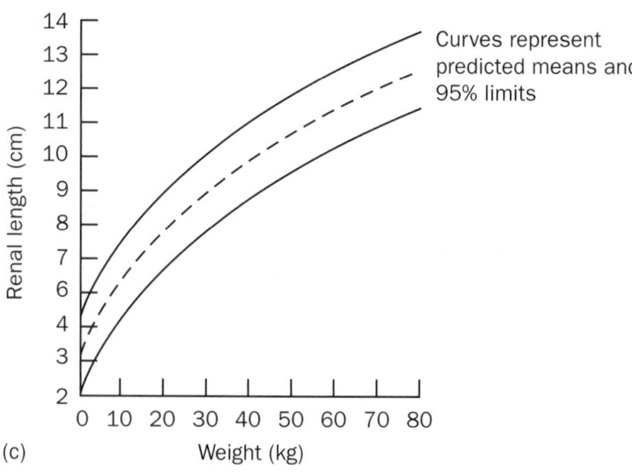

Figure 12.2 (a–c) Renal ultrasound length centiles (redrawn from Han BK and Babcock JS (1985) Sonographic measurements and appearance of normal kidneys in children. *AJR Am J Roentgenol* **145**:611–16)

Radioisotopes

Dynamic scanning (^{99m}Tc-DTPA/MAG3 or ^{123}I-Hippuran)

Dynamic scanning using ^{99m}Tc-DTPA/MAG3 or ^{123}I-Hippuran is indicated for the establishment of differential renal function, in the presence of dilatation of the collecting system on ultrasound, following surgery on the pelvis or ureter, following renal transplantation and for indirect cystography. Indirect cystography using either ^{99m}Tc-DTPA or ^{99m}Tc-MAG3 is a non-invasive technique for the follow-up of vesicoureteric reflux (VUR) previously documented by micturition cystourethrography (MCUG) or direct radionuclide cystography (see below) and in girls presenting with urinary tract infection (UTI) for the first time.

The technique however requires a significant degree of cooperation, is not possible in the child who is not consistently continent and is less sensitive than both contrast and direct radionuclide cystography.

Static scanning (^{99m}Tc-DMSA)

^{99m}Tc-DMSA carries a higher radiation dose than the isotopes used in dynamic scanning but is the most sensitive technique for the detection of renal parenchymal damage associated with UTI/VUR. It also allows a more accurate evaluation of differential function and is the method of choice in the investigation of potential renovascular hypertension and when a non-functioning moiety of a duplex system or an ectopic kidney is suspected.

Radioisotope cystogram (^{99m}Tc-pertechnetate)

The direct radioisotopic cystogram is similar to the MCUG in that it requires bladder catheterization but instead of contrast being instilled into the bladder a small dose of radioisotope mixed with normal saline is instilled. The advantages are the high sensitivity and the very low radiation dose. The main disadvantage is that no comment on the urethral or bladder anatomy is possible.

Plain radiograph and intravenous urogram

The advantage of the plain abdominal radiograph is in the detection of nephrolithiasis, which may be overlooked by ultrasound examination, and visualization of the lumbosacral spine in the evaluation of possible neuropathic bladder dysfunction.

Requests for an intravenous urogram (IVU) should be tailored to specific situations and this should result in a fewer number of radiographs and a lower radiation dose. One of the main indications is the finding of a small kidney(s) on ultrasound and/or isotope examinations in the absence of VUR. The advantage of the IVU in this context is mainly to establish calyceal anatomy. Further indications are in suspected renal dysplasia, medullary necrosis, medullary sponge kidney, pelviureteric junction (PUJ) obstruction, complicated duplex system and vesicoureteric junction (VUJ) obstruction.

Micturating cystourethrography

Micturating cystourethrography is still the definitive method for assessing the bladder and urethral anatomy. The most frequent indication for MCUG is in infants under the age of 1 year presenting with UTI but other indications are the presence of ureteric dilatation and the suspicion of neuropathic bladder on ultrasound.

Antegrade and retrograde pyelography

Antegrade pyelography requires the presence of an experienced operator and is usually carried out under general anaesthesia in order to provide some anatomical detail of the pelvis and ureter in the presence of a dilated upper urinary tract.

Retrograde pyelography is carried out at the same time as cystoscopy. The indications for retrograde pyelography are mainly in the evaluation of suspected VUJ obstruction or as a substitute for antegrade pyelography in the evaluation of possible PUJ obstruction.

Arteriography

This is an invasive investigation that has a high radiation dose and should be reserved for special situations. Generally indications are suspected renal vascular disease, post-traumatic haematuria or prior to intervention procedures, e.g. embolization of arteriovenous malformation or balloon dilatation.

Computed tomography scanning

The main indication for abdominal/renal computed tomography (CT) scanning is the finding of a mass lesion on ultrasound. Generally speaking, CT is not a helpful investigation of suspected polycystic kidney disease in childhood.

Magnetic resonance imaging

There are two main indications for magnetic resonance imaging (MRI). First, in the child with neuropathic bladder with no obvious cause, where full imaging of the spine is necessary in order to detect both intrinsic and extrinsic spinal cord pathology. Secondly, MRI may also be useful in suspected renal artery stenosis although the sensitivity is highest in osteal rather than peripheral arterial stenosis and may not preclude angiography.

KEY LEARNING POINTS

- Ultrasound is the most useful and least invasive form of urinary tract imaging available.
- Radioisotope imaging has replaced IVU as second-line imaging of the urinary tract, particularly in the assessment of patients with UTI.
- Computed tomography and MRI imaging have very restricted indications.

CORE SYSTEM PROBLEMS

FETAL UROPATHY

Malformation of the urinary tract is among the commonest of all congenital malformations and within the heading of fetal uropathy there is a very diverse group of disorders (see box below). Prior to the introduction of routine antenatal ultrasonography these anomalies remained undetected until later presentation prompted investigation. The frequency of fetal uropathy detected on antenatal ultrasonography varies from 0.2 to 0.7 per cent. However, the incidence is much higher in women with a family history of urinary tract disease such as renal agenesis, multicystic dysplastic kidney (MCDK), obstructive uropathy, polycystic kidney disease (PKD) or reflux nephropathy.

Ninety-five per cent of fetal kidneys can be identified on ultrasound by 22 weeks' gestation and this is early enough to consider termination if the anomaly is severe. Interpretation of fetal ultrasound may be difficult however, since transient dilatation of the urinary tract occurs in up to 10–20 per cent of fetuses in the third trimester and up to 50 per cent fetuses with 'abnormal' antenatal scans are normal on postnatal follow-up.

Spectrum of fetal uropathy

Dysplasia

- Multicystic dysplasia
- Obstructive, e.g. posterior urethral valves
- Isolated
- Prune belly syndrome

Cystic kidney disease

- Autosomal recessive polycystic kidney disease
- Autosomal dominant polycystic kidney disease
- Familial juvenile nephronophthisis
- Medullary sponge kidney

Obstructive uropathy without dysplasia

- PUJ obstruction
- VUJ obstruction

Others

- VUR
- Duplication anomalies
- Ureterocele
- Agenesis
- Ectopia/fusion anomalies

Oligohydramnios remains the most reliable clinical marker of disordered fetal renal function since the amniotic fluid is largely fetal urine but a normal amniotic fluid volume does not indicate the presence of normal fetal renal function. Analysis of fetal urine may be used to determine whether intervention is appropriate. Increased fetal urinary levels of sodium and to a lesser extent calcium are more likely to be seen with urinary tract obstruction or renal dysplasia.

Dysplasia

CASE STUDY: Renal dysplasia

An otherwise well term neonate is noted to have an enlarged left kidney on abdominal palpation. Serial antenatal ultrasound scans from 20 weeks' gestation had revealed a 'cystic' left kidney and a normal right kidney and bladder. Postnatal ultrasound showed a large left kidney with multiple cysts consistent with multicystic dysplastic kidney (MCDK).

Dysplasia is caused by an abnormality in renal development at the stage of the metanephros. Histologically, dysplasia is characterized by the presence of primitive tubules, metaplastic cartilage and sometimes bone. The commonest manifestation of renal dysplasia is MCDK, which occurs in around 1 in 4000 live births and is the most frequently diagnosed prenatal renal abnormality after hydronephrosis. It is unilateral in 90 per cent of cases. The affected kidney contains multiple non-communicating cysts of varying sizes and is non-functional. Associated abnormalities of the contralateral kidney occur in 25 per cent of cases, e.g. VUR, PUJ obstruction. The great majority of cases are managed conservatively in view of the very low risk of hypertension and malignancy.

Renal dysplasia may also occur with urinary tract obstruction and as an isolated phenomenon. Although obstructive cystic dysplasia, e.g. in posterior urethral valves (PUV), may be similar histologically to MCDK the two conditions are easily differentiated by ultrasound and by radionuclide scan, which tends to show some functioning parenchyma. The pattern of dysplasia and outcome is dependent on the time of onset of the obstruction and location of the lesion.

Isolated dysplasia presents with early onset renal failure and the diagnosis is usually based on the ultrasound findings of small echogenic kidneys.

Bladder outlet obstruction

This may be caused by urethral agenesis, persistence of the cloaca, urethral stricture or posterior urethral valves (PUV). PUV occurs only in males and is the commonest cause of bladder outlet obstruction with an incidence of 1 in 5000 to 1 in 8000. Of the babies not diagnosed prenatally, approximately 50 per cent will present with symptoms in the first year of life, 25 per cent of these in the neonatal period. The prenatal ultrasound findings of hydronephrosis, mega ureter, thick trabeculated bladder and oligohydramnios are characteristic. Prenatal diagnosis of PUV may allow early intervention and thereby salvage renal function although this is yet unproved. After birth, if the renal function is good, cystoscopy and diathermy of the valves may be carried out but in the presence of poor renal function and marked hydronephrosis, vesicostomy is preferred. The long-term prognosis is dependent upon both the severity and duration of obstruction. Of boys presenting in infancy, 25–30 per cent are at risk of renal insufficiency in childhood and the risk of renal failure is directly proportional to the degree of renal dysplasia present at birth. Later in life, however, bladder dysfunction becomes a significant factor in the progression of renal failure.

Prune belly syndrome

This (or triad syndrome) is characterized by deficiency of abdominal musculature, bilateral cryptorchidism and a dilated non-obstructive urinary tract. Ninety-five per cent of cases occur in boys and approximately 20 per cent of cases die perinatally from severe pulmonary hypoplasia. More than 70 per cent have VUR and the majority will develop endstage renal failure by late childhood.

Cystic kidney disease

CASE STUDY

A baby girl of 36 weeks' gestation developed increasing respiratory distress requiring intubation and ventilation within 30 minutes of delivery. This was the mother's first pregnancy and an ultrasound one week before delivery confirmed the clinical suspicion of oligohydramnios and showed the fetal kidneys to be enlarged. Postnatal ultrasound showed large diffusely echogenic kidneys, consistent with autosomal recessive polycystic disease (ARPKD).

Autosomal recessive polycystic disease

The incidence of ARPKD varies from 1 to 6000 to 1 to 40 000 but within a given family the severity and presentation is relatively constant and falls into a typical autosomal recessive pattern of inheritance. The liver lesion is different from that in autosomal dominant polycystic kidney disease (ADPKD) and consists of biliary duct hyperplasia and hepatic fibrosis and is uniformly present. When diagnosed prenatally, the ultrasound findings in ARPKD are of large echogenic kidneys. When oligohydramnios is present prenatally the baby is likely to have severe renal failure and to be at risk of dying with pulmonary hypoplasia. Advances in neonatology have improved the survival for all but those with the most severe pulmonary hypoplasia and the current 10-year survival is around 50 per cent. Some older children and adolescents present with portal hypertension secondary to hepatic fibrosis.

Autosomal dominant polycystic disease is by far the commonest inherited renal disease with an incidence of 1 in 200 to 1 in 1000. Linkage analysis and positional cloning have led to advances in isolation of genes and gene products responsible for ADPKD and two genes have been identified (PKD1 and PKD2). Large echogenic kidneys may be seen on antenatal ultrasound and parental ultrasound examination is vital in the absence of a family history.

The familial juvenile nephrolithiasis/medullary cystic disease (FJN/MCD) complex

This refers to a series of diseases that histologically have a similar finding of chronic tubulointerstitial fibrosis. Familial juvenile nephrolithiasis is inherited as an autosomal recessive and MCD as autosomal dominant. In both conditions the renal size on ultrasound is generally normal. Familial juvenile nephrolithiasis (FJN) tends to present with an early history of significant polyuria and polydipsia and progressive renal insufficiency, often with inappropriate degree of anaemia but minimal abnormal urinalysis or hypertension. The commonest extrarenal manifestation of FJN is a pigmentary retinopathy but congenital hepatic fibrosis and skeletal abnormalities may also be present. The diagnosis may be confirmed by renal biopsy or more recently by mutational analysis.

Medullary cystic disease typically presents in adulthood although when presenting in children hypertension, haematuria and proteinuria are more likely.

Medullary sponge kidney (MSK)

This is usually diagnosed in adulthood following presentation with renal stones, haematuria or UTI. The diagnosis of MSK is made on IVU and MSK is either inherited as autosomal dominant or occurs sporadically with the incidence of 1 in 5000 to 1 in 20 000.

Congenital urinary tract obstruction without renal dysplasia

CASE STUDY

A baby boy, 4 weeks of age, is referred for investigation because of the finding of an abnormal prenatal ultrasound scan. At 18 weeks' gestation, pelvicalyceal dilatation (PCD) was noted in the left fetal kidney. This appearance persisted and at 36 weeks' gestation, the fetal pelvic diameter was 15 mm. Postnatal ultrasound showed isolated left PCD 17 mm in diameter, consistent with PUJ obstruction.

Most PUJ obstruction occurs early in the first trimester and this is the commonest site of upper urinary obstruction. There is a slight male predominance and a left-sided predilection and the condition is bilateral in approximately 5 per cent of cases. If not detected prenatally, presentation may be throughout childhood with an abdominal mass, intermittent vomiting and abdominal pain usually lateralized, haematuria and UTI. The diagnosis can be suspected on ultrasound but MCUG and ^{99m}Tc-MAG3/DTPA are necessary to confirm the diagnosis.

The main indications for corrective surgery (pyeloplasty) are marked pelvic dilatation (>30 mm), calyceal dilatation or a decrease in differential function of 10–15 per cent. If the initial differential function of the affected kidney is 15 per cent or less, uninephrectomy should be carried out.

Vesicoureteric junction obstruction

This is less common and is due to a congenital obstruction of the distal ureter. The diagnosis should be suspected in the presence of hydronephrosis and hydroureter in the absence of VUR and confirmed by IVU or occasionally retrograde pyelography. Management is by surgical ureteric reimplantation.

Other urinary tract malformations

CASE STUDY

A 3-year-old girl presents for the first time with a febrile UTI. Urinary tract ultrasound and ^{99m}Tc-DMSA scans show a relatively enlarged right kidney and a normal left kidney consistent with a duplex right kidney.

Duplication of the urinary collecting system

This may be incomplete, involving a bifid renal pelvis or it may be complete with two ureters and two ureteric orifices. These are the commonest anomalies of the urinary tract. In complete duplication, the higher and more laterally placed ureteric orifice that drains the lower moiety of the duplex kidney is more likely to reflux. The ectopic upper moiety ureter that enters the bladder in a lower and more medial position is more likely to be obstructed but may also reflux. In general, the further the ureteric orifices are from the normal position the more dysplastic is the associated renal tissue.

Ureterocele

This is a cystic dilatation of the intravesicular ureter. It is often related to the ureter of the upper moiety of a duplex system but can also occur in a normally located single ureter. It is increasingly being diagnosed on prenatal ultrasound. Postnatally, the majority of cases will present with UTI in infancy. Once the lesion is suspected on ultrasound, MCUG is very important because of the high likelihood of VUR to the ipsilateral lower pole as well as the contralateral side. A ^{99m}Tc-DMSA scan helps determine the relative function of the related renal segment and this will influence the management decision, i.e. either a conservative approach or partial nephrectomy

Bilateral renal agenesis

This is associated with virtual absence of amniotic fluid after 13–14 weeks' gestation and has an incidence of approximately 1 in 3000 births whereas **unilateral renal agenesis** affects 1 in every 600 individuals. Parents and siblings of children with bilateral renal agenesis have 5 per cent incidence of unilateral agenesis. Up to 15 per cent of patients with unilateral agenesis have abnormalities of the contralateral kidney such as ectopia or malrotation. There is no increased risk of renal insufficiency in unilateral renal agenesis.

Ectopic kidneys

These are most often pelvic and occasionally thoracic and the majority of ectopic kidneys have VUR, and as many as 50 per cent of the contralateral kidneys are also abnormal. Crossed renal ectopia and horseshoe kidneys are examples of fusion abnormalities. The latter are characterized by an isthmus of fibrous tissue joining the lower poles of the kidneys. The condition is usually diagnosed in childhood when associated with other congenital anomalies and in syndromes such as trisomy 18, Turner syndrome and neural tube defects.

Vesicoureteric reflux

This may be found following investigation of fetal renal pelvis dilatation (RPD), or as a coincidental finding in the contralateral ureter following investigation of suspected PUJ obstruction or MCDK. There is no clear consensus on the investigation of fetal RPD, but the algorithm given in Figure 12.3 reflects the majority view.

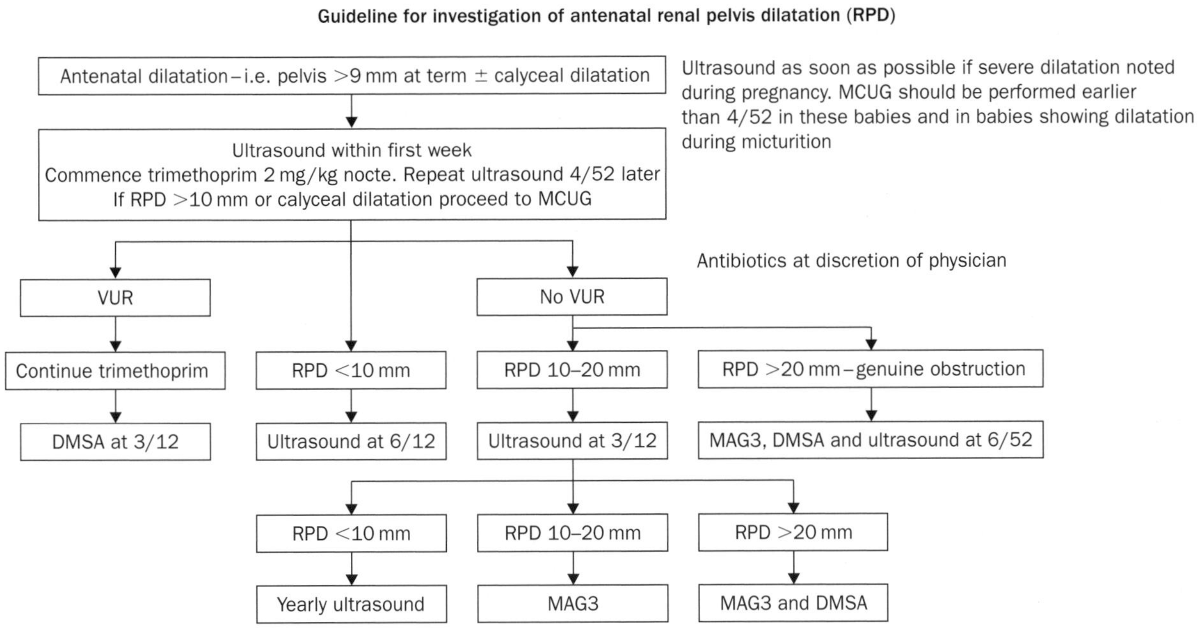

Guideline for investigation of antenatal renal pelvis dilatation (RPD)

Antenatal dilatation – i.e. pelvis >9 mm at term ± calyceal dilatation

Ultrasound as soon as possible if severe dilatation noted during pregnancy. MCUG should be performed earlier than 4/52 in these babies and in babies showing dilatation during micturition

Ultrasound within first week
Commence trimethoprim 2 mg/kg nocte. Repeat ultrasound 4/52 later
If RPD >10 mm or calyceal dilatation proceed to MCUG

Antibiotics at discretion of physician

VUR → Continue trimethoprim → DMSA at 3/12

RPD <10 mm → Ultrasound at 6/12

No VUR → RPD 10–20 mm → Ultrasound at 3/12

No VUR → RPD >20 mm – genuine obstruction → MAG3, DMSA and ultrasound at 6/52

Ultrasound at 3/12 → RPD <10 mm → Yearly ultrasound

Ultrasound at 3/12 → RPD 10–20 mm → MAG3

Ultrasound at 3/12 → RPD >20 mm → MAG3 and DMSA

Figure 12.3 Evaluation of pelvicalyceal dilatation. VUR, vesicoureteric reflux; MCUG, micturition cystourethrography

KEY LEARNING POINTS

- Severe oligohydramnios detected before 24 weeks' gestation is a poor prognostic indicator for survival in the neonatal period.
- Unilateral hydronephrosis is the most commonly diagnosed fetal urinary tract abnormality and may be caused by VUR, PUJ or VUJ obstruction.
- Bilateral hydronephrosis may be caused by VUR but should raise the suspicion of bladder outlet obstruction.
- Where large echogenic kidneys are detected on antenatal ultrasound, in the absence of a positive family history, parental ultrasound should be offered.

URINARY TRACT INFECTION AND RELATED PROBLEMS

Urinary tract infection is one of the commonest bacterial diseases in childhood, affecting 8 per cent of all girls and 1 per cent of all boys within the first 10 years of life and associated with fever in 50 per cent. There is a significant female predominance except within the first six months of life and the recurrence rate is 50 per cent in girls and 15 per cent in boys. The diagnosis is based on urine microbiology. Mid-stream urine sample (MSSU) or clean-catch urine (CCU) ($\geq 10^5$ colony-forming units (CFU)/mL) is the preferred sampling method unless, in view of clinical urgency, suprapubic aspiration (any Gram-negative or $>10^3$ Gram-positive organisms) or urethral catheterization ($>10^3$ CFU/mL) is required since urine collected in sterile adhesive bags and urinary pads are associated with a high rate of contamination.

The finding of pyuria on urine microscopy (>10 white blood cells (WBC)/mm^3 in boys and $>50/mm^3$ in girls) is a helpful rapid investigation in a child suspected of UTI since pyuria is present in practically all episodes of first symptomatic UTI. In recurrent UTI, however, significant pyuria may be absent in 25 per cent of cases. In addition, pyuria does not always indicate the presence of significant bacteriuria.

Combination dipstick urinalysis measuring leucocyte esterase activity and urinary nitrite is faster and less expensive than urine microscopy. Urine culture may be avoidable if leucocyte esterase and nitrite are absent in children over the age of 2 years, since urinary tract symptoms are more reliable evidence of infection but the technique has a lower sensitivity in infants.

The main offending organism in community-acquired UTI is *Escherichia coli*, which accounts for up to 75 per cent of cases in childhood. The remaining 25 per cent are caused by a combination of enterococci, *Klebsiella*, *Proteus*, *Serratia* and others.

It is generally assumed that almost all bacterial UTI occur via the ascending route. Urinary stasis is therefore of importance, be it as a result of anatomical obstruction, VUR, incomplete or inefficient voiding habits, low fluid intake or constipation. However, a number of patients have none of the foregoing risk factors and other mechanisms are likely to be involved such as periurethral colonization by uropathogenic bacteria as well as impairment of lower urinary tract defence mechanisms.

CASE STUDY

An infant of 5 weeks of age was admitted with a short history of fever and reluctance to feed. Clinical examination was normal apart from the finding of irritability. Dipstick urinalysis showed haematuria, proteinuria, nitrites and leucocyte esterase. Peripheral white cell count was 17.4×10^9/L (9.9×10^9/L neutrophils), C-reactive protein (CRP) 352 mg/L (normal: 0–10), cerebrospinal fluid (CSF) protein 0.5 g/L, CSF glucose 3.7 mmol/L. He was treated with intravenous cefotaxime and showed a good clinical response. Subsequent venous blood culture showed no growth but a CCU prior to antibiotics showed $>10^5$ CFU/mL of lactose-fermenting coliforms. Urinary tract ultrasound revealed an enlarged left kidney that was moderately hyperechoic and showed some upper pole swelling. The right kidney appeared normal. Subsequent MCUG showed unilateral dilated (grade III) VUR on the left and ^{99m}Tc-DMSA scan showed diminished uptake in the left upper pole but normal uptake by the right kidney.

Early diagnosis and prompt treatment of UTI is especially important during the first years of life and all infants and children with a temperature >38°C with no definite cause found should have a urine sample examined. Other indications for examining urine are unexplained vomiting or abdominal pain, failure to thrive, prolonged jaundice in the neonate, haematuria, hypertension and suspected child sexual abuse.

When considering urinary tract imaging, it is useful to distinguish those symptoms that are likely to be consistent with acute pyelonephritis ('upper tract') from those more consistent with acute cysto-urethritis ('lower tract').

Upper tract
- Fever
- Lethargy
- General malaise
- Vomiting
- Loin pain

Lower tract
- Dysuria
- Urgency, frequency
- Wetting
- Frank haematuria
- Non-specific abdominal pain

Those patients with 'upper tract' symptoms particularly if recurrent, have a higher likelihood of urinary tract abnormalities and this should be reflected in the imaging protocol (see box below). The same criteria should apply to those patients who are found on screening or coincidentally to have asymptomatic bacteriuria.

Imaging guidelines for UTI

0–1 year
- Ultrasound, ^{99m}Tc-DMSA and MCUG

>1 year
- Ultrasound, ^{99m}Tc-DMSA (if 'upper tract' symptoms)
- ^{99m}Tc-DMSA (if 'upper tract' symptoms, recurrence or family history of VUR/renal scarring)
- MCUG or isotope reflux study if abnormality on initial imaging

Management

The choice of antibiotics should be based on a 'best guess' policy until the sensitivity of the organism is available. However, if there is no clinical response within 24–48 hours the antibiotic should be changed. The following antibiotics are suitable for oral administration:

- Trimethoprim
- Co-amoxiclav
- Nitrofurantoin
- Cephradine

Intravenous therapy should be considered in the infant and young child and in all patients who are sufficiently ill to warrant hospital admission. Third generation cephalosporins, e.g. cefotaxime, ceftazidime or ceftriaxone or a combination of aminoglycoside and amoxicillin would be appropriate. The current evidence suggests that a 2–4 day course is sufficient for 'lower tract' infections. For 'upper tract' infections a 7–10 day course of oral therapy is as effective as intravenous therapy but the use of oral therapy in this context is dependent on the child being able to tolerate oral medication. Despite the fact that there is little evidence base, prophylaxis should be considered at least until investigation of the urinary tract has been completed. The agents commonly used for prophylaxis include:

- Trimethoprim 1–2 mg/kg per day
- Nitrofurantoin 1 mg/kg per day

- Co-amoxiclav 0–1 125/31 2.5 mL per day, 1–6 125/31 5 mL per day, 6–12 250/62 5–10 mL per day.

The long-term management of infants and children with a history of recurrent UTI, imaging abnormalities, e.g. VUR or renal scarring should be individualized. However, it would seem appropriate to maintain patients with documented risk factors on prophylaxis until the age of 5 years.

Vesicoureteric reflux

This is defined as a retrograde flow of urine from the bladder to the ureters and is a common finding (30 per cent) in patients with UTI. Early data suggested that primary VUR occurs in approximately 1 per cent of healthy neonates; however, investigation of patients with MCKD or antenatally diagnosed RPD suggests the prevalence is higher (up to 17 per cent). VUR may also occur as a secondary phenomenon in the context of urethral obstruction, neuropathic bladder dysfunction or severe dysfunctional voiding. The association of VUR with UTI and renal scarring or **reflux nephropathy** led to the concept that VUR plays a role in the pathogenesis of both. The prevalence of VUR is typically higher in younger patients with UTI and decreases with age and there is a significant spontaneous resolution rate particularly in those with lower grades.

It is likely that the inheritance of VUR is autosomal dominant with variable penetrance. Approximately one third of siblings of index patients with VUR/RN also have VUR, usually of a mild degree although most (75 per cent) do not have a history of UTI. There is no consensus on screening, but if the index case has significant VUR/RN, selective imaging of siblings or offspring should be discussed and a low threshold for investigation of febrile illness highlighted.

Within the last 15–20 years both single centre and multinational studies have demonstrated that the incidence of UTI, renal growth, and the development of new renal scars or progression of existing scarring was similar in patients who underwent continuous antibiotic prophylaxis compared to those who underwent surgical reimplantation. The main indications however for antireflux surgery, either formal reimplantation or endoscopic (subureteric Teflon injection (STING)), are failure of medical therapy or non-compliance. Other indications are poor renal growth or progression of renal scarring.

Coarse renal cortical scarring

This is found in about 10 per cent of children with UTI. Recognized risk factors are early (within the first 3 years of life), repeated and inadequately treated infection and anatomical obstruction. The pathogenesis of renal scarring in patients with VUR, particularly high grade, is sex dependent. In boys, prenatal dysplasia is more likely whereas in girls, acquired post-infective scarring is more likely. Other relevant factors particularly in patients who have no demonstrable VUR, are dysfunctional voiding, bacterial virulence factors and the host inflammatory response.

Outcome

Although most children with UTI have excellent prognosis, there may be long-term implications in a small group especially those with obstructive malformations and high-grade VUR with scarring. Long-term follow-up of women who presented in childhood with symptomatic or covert bacteriuria have a three times greater incidence of acute pyelonephritis compared with controls. In addition, there is an increased incidence of pre-eclampsia in those women who have renal scarring.

Although hypertension and chronic renal insufficiency are recognized long-term risk factors in patients with bilateral renal scarring, fortunately recent prospective data suggest the risk is small and probably restricted to those with renal dysplasia.

KEY LEARNING POINTS

- Clinical features of UTI are often non-specific and every young child with an unexplained fever should have a urine culture.
- A negative combination dipstick urinalysis result does not exclude UTI particularly in infants.
- All children should have a urinary tract ultrasound after a first proved UTI. Subsequent investigation should be dictated by age, presenting symptoms and family history.
- VUR is found in up to 30 per cent of children with a history of UTI but renal scarring may occur in the absence of VUR.
- The pathogenesis of renal scarring in association with VUR is sex-specific with prenatal dysplasia being prominent in boys and post-infective scarring in girls.
- The long-term risk of hypertension in patients with unilateral renal scarring is very small but patients with bilateral renal scarring require lifelong review.

DAY AND NIGHT WETTING

Prior to considering the definition of day and night wetting, it is useful briefly to consider normal voiding milestones. Bladder emptying is frequent and uninhibited from birth to 6 months, but by the age of 6–12 months voiding is less frequent due to central nervous inhibition. In the second year of life there is a progressive development of conscious perception of bladder fullness and from 3 to 5 years of age the child develops the ability to inhibit voiding both unconsciously and voluntarily. The majority of children achieve daytime continence by the age of 3 years and night time continence by the age of 5 years.

A useful operational definition of nocturnal enuresis therefore is a child of 5 years or older who wets at least once per week. The definition of day wetting is less precise but a useful operational definition is the presence of wetting episodes occurring on a daily or alternate day basis in a child over the age of 5 years. Day and night wetting may be primary or secondary, the latter is defined on the basis of a period of more than six months reliable continence.

Nocturnal enuresis

CASE STUDY

A 10-year-old boy was referred to the outpatient clinic because of primary nocturnal enuresis. Serial urinalysis and culture carried out by his general practitioner (GP) was negative. On closer questioning, he had an increased daytime urinary frequency but had no history of day wetting. He had an older sibling who was enuretic until the age of 12 years and his father also admitted to being enuretic until the age of 13 years. Physical examination and blood pressure were normal as was urinalysis; urine culture was sterile.

This affects 10–15 per cent of 5-year-olds, but there is a spontaneous remission rate of around 15 per cent per annum with a resultant prevalence rate in adolescents and adults of <1 per cent. There is a male predominance and a higher likelihood of primary enuresis in early childhood but both become less marked in later childhood and adolescence.

Nocturnal enuresis is said to be more likely in the first-born child, in children from a lower socioeconomic background, emotionally and developmentally delayed children, and institutionalized children whether they be of normal or subnormal intelligence. The current understanding of the pathophysiology of nocturnal enuresis remains rather confused. Perhaps the most important factor is a genetic predisposition to delayed maturation of nocturnal continence. If both parents have a history of nocturnal enuresis the offspring have up to a 75 per cent risk but in the absence of family history the risk is 15 per cent. In support of maturational delay is the fact that nocturnal continence is an acquired skill, the strong genetic background, the very high natural remission rate and finally the response to conditioning therapy.

The majority of children with nocturnal enuresis have no organic disease and in practice the only two conditions which should be considered are those presenting with polyuria and UTI. It is, however, very uncommon for enuresis to be the only symptom/sign in patients presenting with polyuria. Nocturnal enuresis, however, may be the presenting symptom in up to 15 per cent of children with UTI and there is also a higher incidence than expected in patients who are found to have covert bacteriuria. Successful treatment of UTI cures or improves enuresis in up to 30 per cent.

Initial evaluation

This should include a detailed history of the nocturnal episodes as well as daytime micturition pattern since a history of increased daytime urinary frequency is common. Clinical assessment should include examination of the abdomen, lumbosacral spine, perineum and lower limb reflexes. If clinical examination, routine urinalysis and culture are normal there is no indication for urinary tract imaging.

Management

This may best be considered under general measures and specific therapies, i.e. pharmacological and conditioning. An important aspect of general management is the development of a positive and supportive attitude. These patients are best seen in a nurse-led clinic since a prolonged period of treatment is likely. A simple form of record keeping is important for both the therapist and the patient to assess improvement and this type of recording will vary according to the maturity of the patient. There is no evidence that fluid restriction helps but there is some value in avoiding excessive drinking. In view of the fact that the wetting episode generally happens within the first three hours after going to bed, trying to pre-empt this by waking the child may result in a dry night or at least a less wet night.

Only imipramine and desmopressin (DDAVP) (Desmospray/Desmotabs) have been evaluated in properly conducted clinical trials. The response rate during treatment varies from 50 to 80 per cent but there is high relapse rate when these agents are discontinued. Both medications are useful for short-term treatment on particular occasions such as school camps or holidays or as a morale boosting exercise. If therapy with these agents are successful they may be continued for prolonged periods but it is advisable to discontinue therapy every three months to establish whether a spontaneous remission has developed.

Two main types of conditioning therapy are available. Firstly, the dry bed training regimen, which involves an intensive waking schedule. There is no doubt that this method can be effective but it needs considerable skill from the therapist and maximum compliance from the family and is therefore generally not applicable for domestic use.

The more frequent form of conditioning therapy used is the enuretic alarm. Wetness results in the alarm sounding and waking the child. However, alarms are awkward to use and the child must be well motivated and compliant. Children of 7 years or older tend to cooperate readily but treatment below the age of 7 requires patience and determination by the family. Initial response to the alarm may be as high as 80 per cent with a relapse rate as low as 20 per cent. In addition the cost of an enuretic alarm is relatively small and it therefore makes economic as well as clinical sense to consider this mode of therapy.

Day wetting

CASE STUDY

A 6-year-old girl was referred for evaluation of primary day and night wetting. Serial urinalysis was normal and urine cultures showed no significant bacteriuria. There was no significant family history and she had two younger siblings. On closer questioning she also had associated significant urge, and produced a firm stool every three to four days. Her day wetting frequency was around two to three times per day of a moderate degree requiring regular change of underwear. General physical examination including examination of her spine and lower limbs was normal. Her urinalysis was also normal and urine culture sterile. She underwent a urinary tract ultrasound that apart from showing mild thickness of the bladder wall was completely normal.

Accurate estimates of day wetting are difficult to obtain because of lack of clarity of definition. With these provisos the prevalence of isolated day wetting is around 1 per cent and combined day and night wetting 1.5 per cent in 5–10-year-old children. There is a female preponderance particularly in patients with primary day wetting and a spontaneous remission rate similar to that of nocturnal enuresis of 15 per cent per year.

Table 12.2 Causes of day wetting

Urge incontinence	Transient wetting
Stress incontinence	Negligible wetting
Giggle micturition	Careless wetting

Table 12.2 lists the common causes of day wetting but by far the commonest is **urge incontinence** secondary to primary detrusor instability. **Stress incontinence** in childhood is rare but occasionally the child with urge incontinence dampens their pants when coughing or straining. **Giggle micturition** is a relatively rare but troublesome condition in which the child has a complete and involuntary void associated with an episode of laughing or giggling. **Transient wetting** may happen in association with the increased frequency associated with UTI. **Careless wetting** is seen in the child who does not take enough time to void but may also be seen in emotionally disturbed children. Although a congenital abnormality of the urinary tract such as ectopic ureter is frequently considered as a cause of day wetting, this is very rare and is characterized by constant wetting.

Urge incontinence is associated with significant bacteriuria in 50 per cent of girls but only a minority lose their symptoms when the bacteriuria is eradicated. There is commonly a history of chronic constipation.

In some patients, ultrasound will reveal thickening of the bladder wall but the majority will have no other abnormality. A small minority of patients with significant dysfunctional voiding may develop progressive renal parenchymal damage. This is as a result of the combination of strong uninhibited detrusor contractions counteracted by pelvic floor contraction and holding on manoeuvres such as squatting, sitting or pressing the heel into the perineum. The resultant high bladder pressures are transmitted to the upper urinary tract.

Evaluation

The evaluation of a child with day wetting is similar to that of night wetting in that an accurate history should be taken and, in addition frequency/volume data should be recorded. Examination of the abdomen, lumbosacral spine and perineum and lower limb reflexes should be done as a routine. In view of the high incidence of bacteriuria, routine urinalysis and urine culture is important and ultrasound imaging should be arranged particularly to assess bladder emptying.

It is relatively easy to consider the diagnosis of **neuropathic bladder dysfunction** (NBD) in a child with an overt spinal problem such as spina bifida, spinal cord tumour or trauma. It should also be considered in patients at higher risk, e.g. those with anorectal anomalies, cerebral palsy and transverse myelitis. The presentation of covert NBD in patients with sacral agenesis or spinal cord tethering is generally delayed but should always be considered in a child with delayed continence, particularly when associated with UTI, constipation, poor urinary stream, continual dribbling and impaired bladder emptying clinically or on ultrasound scanning. Subsequent detailed upper and lower urinary tract evaluation including urodynamic assessment is necessary in patients with suspected NBD.

Management

As with nocturnal enuresis, general measurements are important and the therapist should be confident of cure and as supportive as possible. The simplest measures are to encourage good fluid intake, regular/timed voiding, either by the clock or by the use of mobile alarm system and to aggressively manage any associated constipation. If urinary infection has been detected it is logical both to eradicate bacteriuria and prevent recurrence with the use of prophylaxis. Although there are few data on the efficacy of anticholinergic therapy in day wetting, most clinicians would give a trial of these agents, e.g. oxybutynin, if the above measures are unsuccessful.

More complex behavioural training regimens including the use of biofeedback may be used and are particularly appropriate for the child who has failed to respond to simple methods and may be vital for the child whose incoordinated voiding leads to progressive upper urinary tract damage. Patients with NBD or suspected NBD are best managed within a multidisciplinary nephro-urology service since they may be at high risk of renal scarring and renal functional impairment. The main aims of management are to ensure satisfactory bladder and upper urinary tract drainage in the short term and the achievement of continence in the long term ideally by intermittent clean urethral catheterization or by the Mitrofanoff (continent urinary diversion) procedure.

KEY LEARNING POINTS

- A genetic predisposition is the most important aetiological factor in nocturnal enuresis.
- Desmopressin and imipramine are the only drugs shown to be of benefit in nocturnal enuresis but enuresis alarms are the most effective therapy in accelerating remission.
- Primary detrusor instability is the commonest cause of day wetting and is strongly associated with UTI and constipation.
- Covert NBD should be suspected in a child with delayed continence, particularly when associated with UTI, constipation, poor urinary stream, continual dribbling and impaired bladder emptying.

HAEMATURIA AND PROTEINURIA

Haematuria and to a lesser extent proteinuria are common manifestations of a wide variety of urinary tract diseases and as such are best dealt with together. Haematuria may be frank, i.e. obvious to the naked eye, or microscopic. The widespread availability of urinary dipstick analysis allows rapid confirmation of frank haematuria as well as an increased diagnostic rate of microscopic haematuria and proteinuria. It is important to appreciate the causes of red urine other than haematuria, e.g. certain foodstuffs and drugs and urates in the young infant, as well as circumstances in which the dipstick records the presence of blood but no red cells are visible on microscopy, i.e. haemoglobinuria and myoglobinuria.

False positive dipstick for proteinuria may be found if the urine is very alkaline or highly concentrated, with the use of certain drugs and for both haematuria and proteinuria, if the testing instructions are not adhered to. In view of the sensitivity of dipstick testing persistent abnormalities, i.e. + or more should be confirmed, in the case of haematuria by urine microscopy particularly requesting the laboratory to look for casts and to comment on red cell morphology. With proteinuria a single voided, preferably early morning urine sample should be sent for protein/creatinine ratio. This correlates closely with 24-hour excretion and the normal range is <20 mg/mmol, with values of 20–200 defined as mild to moderate and >200 as 'nephrotic range' proteinuria.

In conditions in which the glomerular filter is disturbed, there will be a relatively larger concentration of higher molecular weight proteins, e.g. globulin, compared with disease in which there is minimal or no disruption to the filtration mechanism. This led to the development of the urine protein selectivity index, with a high index indicating predominant albuminuria. However, this is no longer used as a substitute for further investigation, particularly renal biopsy.

The prevalence of microscopic haematuria in schoolchildren is 0.5–1 per cent; isolated proteinuria 0.03 per cent and microscopic haematuria and proteinuria 0.06 per cent. The causes of haematuria and proteinuria are given below. The differential diagnosis of haematuria includes a substantial number of non-glomerular causes whereas the vast majority of cases of persistent proteinuria are of glomerular origin. Figures 12.4 and 12.5 show

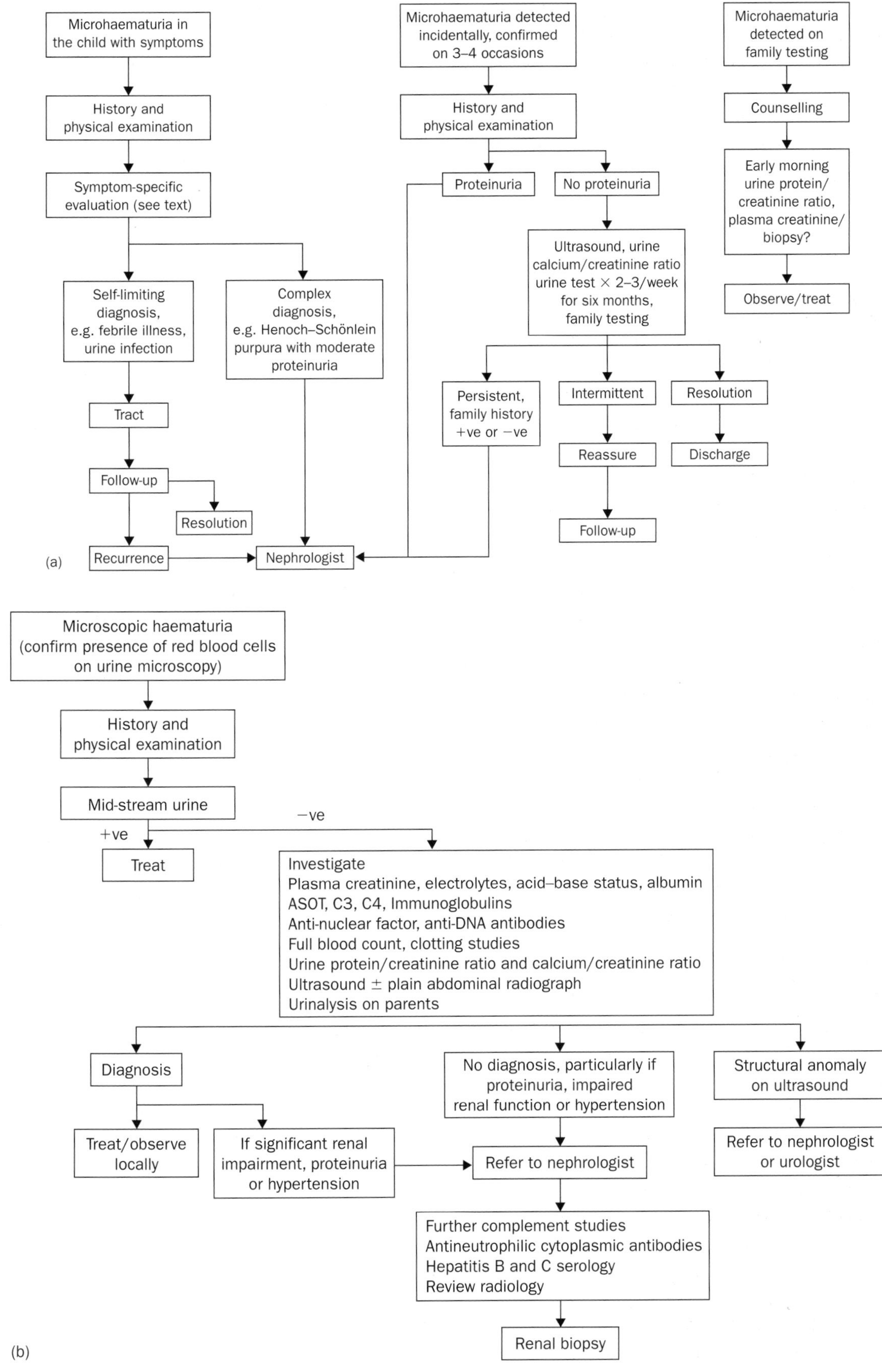

Figure 12.4 (a, b) Evaluation of haematuria (redrawn from Webb NJA, Postlewaithe RJ (eds) (2003) *Clinical Paediatric Nephrology*, 3rd edn. Oxford: Oxford Medical Publications)

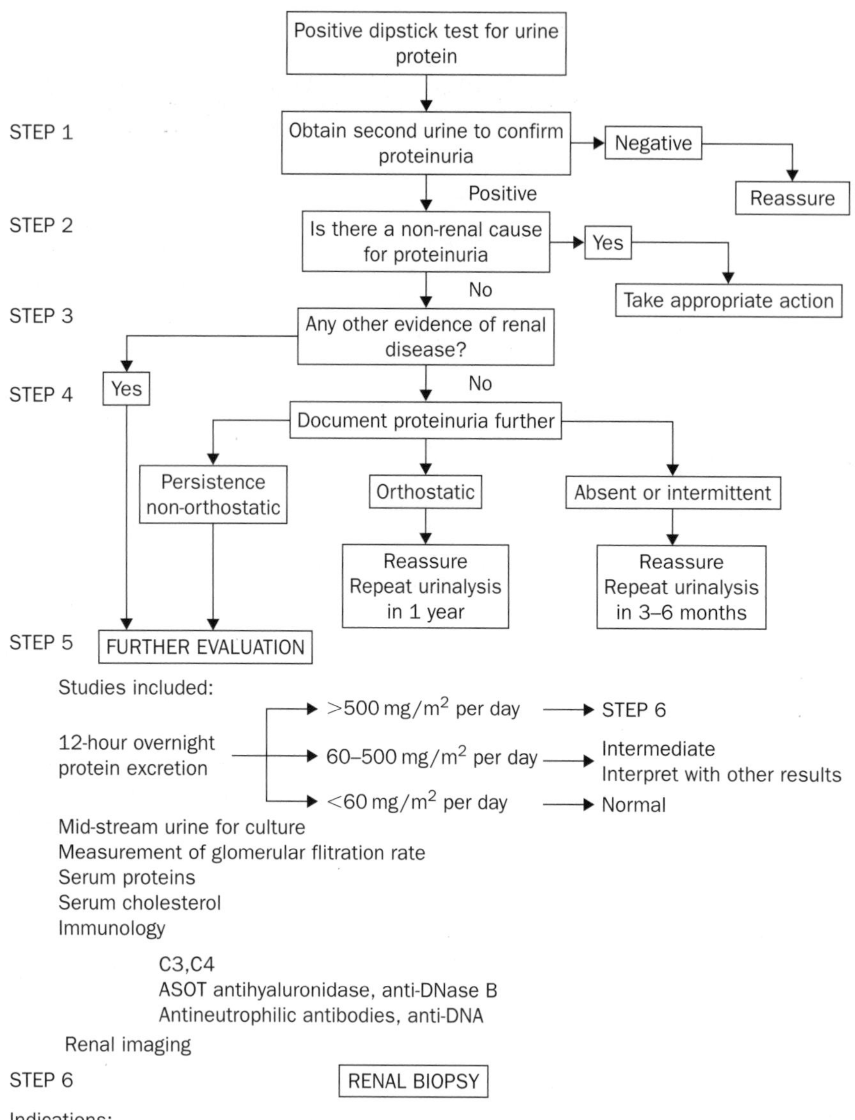

Figure 12.5 Evaluation of proteinuria (redrawn from Webb NJA, Postlewaithe RJ (eds) (2003) *Clinical Paediatric Nephrology*, 3rd edn. Oxford: Oxford Medical Publications)

suggested algorithms for the investigation of haematuria and proteinuria, respectively.

> Causes of haematuria
>
> **Glomerular**
> - Primary (including post-infectious) glomerulonephritis
> - Glomerulonephritis secondary to systemic disease
> - Hereditary/familial nephropathies
>
> **Non-glomerular**
> - UTI (bacterial, viral, schistosomal, etc.)
> - Tumour
> - Calculi and/or hypercalciuria
> - Trauma
> - Structural disease, e.g. obstructive uropathy, cystic disease
> - Drugs, e.g. cyclophosphamide
> - Factitious

> Causes of proteinuria
>
> **Variable**
>
> Orthostatic/postural
>
> Transient, e.g. fever, UTI, congestive cardiac failure

Fixed
Glomerular
- Primary (including post-infectious) glomerulonephritis
- Glomerulonephritis secondary to systemic disease
- Hereditary/familial nephropathies
- Drug-induced, e.g. gold, penicillamine
- Others, e.g. reflux nephropathy, sickle cell disease

Non-glomerular
- Fanconi syndrome
- Acute tubular necrosis
- Structural disease, e.g. obstructive uropathy, cystic disease
- Heavy metal poisoning

Non-glomerular haematuria

CASE STUDY

A 3-year-old previously well boy was referred following an episode of frank haematuria associated with lower abdominal pain but no dysuria or fever lasting for 48 hours. Urine culture showed a significant growth of *Proteus* and he received appropriate antibiotic therapy. Physical examination was normal and urine dipstick showed microscopic +++ haematuria and ++ proteinuria. Abdominal radiograph and ultrasound showed a staghorn calculus in the left kidney. Subsequent plasma biochemical profile, urine calcium, urate and oxalate/creatinine ratios and amino acid chromatography were normal.

Renal calculi or nephrolithiasis are important although relatively uncommon non-glomerular causes of haematuria. In the Middle East, North Africa and the Indian subcontinent, urate bladder stones still predominate, whereas in Western Europe and in North America renal calculi are equally likely to be associated either with UTI or an underlying metabolic problem (Table 12.3).

Calcium oxalate or phosphate is the main constituent of one third of all stones and 80–90 per cent of non-infection related calculi. Idiopathic hypercalciuria, defined as hypercalciuria in the presence of a normal plasma calcium and the absence of any identifiable factors increasing urinary calcium excretion, is the commonest underlying

Table 12.3 Causes of renal calculi

Radio-opaque	Radiolucent
Struvite (magnesium ammonium calcium phosphate)	Urate
	Primary
Calcium (with or without hypercalciuria)	HGPRT deficiency
Idiopathic	APRT deficiency
Loop diuretic therapy	G6-P deficiency
Total parenteral nutrition	*Secondary*
Distal renal tubular acidosis	Tumour lysis
Hypocitraturia	Short gut syndrome
Hyperparathyroidism	Xanthine
Hypothyroidism	Xanthinuria
Excess vitamin D administration	
Dent disease	
Oxalate	
Primary hyperoxaluria	
Enteric hyperoxaluria	
Cystine	
Cystinuria	

HGPRT, hypoxanthine-guanine phosphoribosyltransferase; APRT, adenine phosphoribosyltransferase; G6-P, glucose 6-phosphate.

'metabolic' problem and may present with haematuria alone. Medullary nephrocalcinosis may be associated with metabolic causes of renal calculi, but cortical nephrocalcinosis is only seen following renal cortical necrosis. A scheme for the investigation of renal calculi and/or nephrocalcinosis is given below.

Evaluation of nephrolithiasis and/or nephrocalcinosis

- Ultrasound and abdominal X-ray.
- Biochemical stone analysis when possible. If the biochemical stone analysis suggests a cystine stone, the key investigation is urinary amino acid chromatography. If analysis suggests a uric acid stone the key investigations are urinary urate creatinine ratio, plasma urate, plasma HGPRT and APRT. If analysis suggests a struvite stone, metabolic evaluation is unnecessary.
- If the biochemical stone analysis suggests calcium oxalate/calcium phosphate or if there is no stone recovered, the following investigations should be carried out:
  - Urinalysis and pH
  - Urine culture

- Urinary calcium, oxalate and urate creatinine ratios
- Urinary citrate creatinine ratio
- Urinary amino acid and organic acid screen
- **If spot urines are abnormal, a second voided early morning urine sample should be taken and subsequently a 12–24 hour collection.**
- Plasma urea and electrolytes calcium, phosphate, magnesium, parathyroid hormone, urate, 25 and 1,25 $(OH)_2$ D_3

The general management of renal calculi is to prevent or relieve obstruction and infection whether primary or secondary to stone formation. Ultrasound and abdominal radiographs are both important and IVU may be necessary to establish calyceal anatomy prior to lithotripsy or percutaneous nephrolithotomy. Ureteric stones may be removed by a Dormia basket. The risk of recurrence will depend on the likely aetiology but is generally <10 per cent and a high non-milk fluid intake should be encouraged in all forms of renal stone disease.

Glomerular haematuria

CASE STUDY

A 9-year-old boy was referred with a 2-year history of isolated microscopic haematuria initially detected following an episode of suspected appendicitis. His father had undergone cystoscopy and IVU after having had dipstick positive haematuria documented on an insurance medical examination, but there was no family history of renal disease or deafness. General physical examination, blood pressure, plasma and urine biochemistry, urine culture, ultrasound and abdominal radiograph were normal. Urine dipstick analysis of the patient, his father and one of his two siblings showed +++ haematuria but no proteinuria. Percutaneous renal biopsy revealed normal light and immunofluorescent microscopy but on electron microscopy, the glomerular basement membrane (GBM) was uniformly thin with no splitting.

Thin basement membrane nephropathy

This is a form of benign familial nephropathy usually presenting with microscopic but occasionally frank haematuria with an autosomal dominant inheritance. The main differential diagnosis is that of **Alport disease**, an X-linked dominant condition that may present in a similar fashion and with or without a family history of renal disease or deafness. In boys with Alport syndrome coexistent proteinuria is likely on presentation although renal function is usually preserved until adolescence. Light and immunofluorescent microscopy may be normal in the early stages but attenuation and splitting of the GBM is diagnostic.

CASE STUDY

A 12-year-old boy was referred with an 18-month history of recurrent episodes of painless frank haematuria associated with upper respiratory tract infection but occasionally following swimming, occurring every six to eight weeks. He was otherwise well and there was no notable family history. General physical examination, blood pressure, plasma creatinine, albumin and C3/4, urine calcium/creatinine ratio and culture and ultrasound and abdominal radiograph were normal. Urine dipstick showed ++++ haematuria and ++ proteinuria and protein/creatinine ratio was 125 mg/mmol. Urine microscopy showed abundant red cells but no casts. Percutaneous renal biopsy revealed diffuse mesangial hypercellularity of a moderate degree. Immunofluorescence showed mesangial deposition of IgA and IgG. Electron microscopy was normal apart from showing mesangial deposits.

Primary mesangial IgA nephropathy

This was previously known as Berger disease and is a primary glomerulonephritis classically presenting with recurrent frank haematuria in late childhood or adolescence. The prognosis is generally better in childhood compared with adulthood but the presence of interim abnormal urinalysis and particularly the presence of significant proteinuria is of concern.

A very similar mesangial IgA nephropathy is seen as part of the syndrome of Henoch-Schönlein purpura (HSP). Up to 25 per cent of patients with HSP will have abnormal urinalysis, most commonly isolated microhaematuria although a small number may develop nephrotic syndrome or a rapidly progressive glomerulonephritis. Fortunately, only 1 per cent of patients with HSP have significant renal disease.

Acute post-infectious glomerulonephritis

Usually post-streptococcal, this is relatively uncommon in developed countries and presents with frank haematuria, proteinuria, red cell casts on urine microscopy and varying degrees of oliguria, fluid retention and hypertension. The presence of significant renal insufficiency is atypical and full recovery takes place in the great majority although microscopic haematuria may persist for up to 12–24 months.

Asymptomatic proteinuria

> **CASE STUDY**
>
> A 12-year-old girl was referred because of the finding of proteinuria. She had been investigated at the age of 8 years following a history of recurrent UTI and found to have a unilateral scarred kidney but no evidence of VUR and had been asymptomatic in the interim. Dipstick urinalysis of a random specimen showed ++++ proteinuria and the protein/creatinine ratio was 265 mg/mmol. Physical examination, blood pressure, plasma albumin, creatinine, and complement and autoantibody screen were normal. Three first morning urine samples (EMU) were submitted for protein/creatinine ratio and all showed a value of <20 mg/mmol. Review 12 months later continued to show proteinuria on a random specimen but analysis of EMU samples remained normal.

The mechanisms underlying postural or orthostatic proteinuria remain unclear but all the available evidence indicates that postural proteinuria as an isolated finding is benign. The prognosis of fixed proteinuria (see box above) which is mainly of glomerular origin is, however, variable.

> **KEY LEARNING POINTS**
>
> - Urinalysis and microscopy should be done to confirm that red urine is due to haematuria.
> - UTI is the commonest cause of frank haematuria.
> - The finding of isolated microscopic haematuria in the majority of children is short lived and does not require extensive assessment.
> - The finding of haematuria either frank or microscopic, in association with significant proteinuria, hypertension or impaired renal function warrants further specialist investigation.

OEDEMA

Oedema denotes an abnormal increase in the interstitial fluid compartment and may be localized or generalized. Oedema of an extremity should suggest a localized venous or lymphatic obstruction, either congenital, e.g. Turner syndrome and primary lymphoedema, or acquired, e.g. sickle cell disease or HSP. The causes of generalized oedema are given below, and rarely does the differential diagnosis present a clinical problem. Initial assessment should include urinalysis and measurement of the plasma albumin.

> Causes of generalized oedema
>
> Renal: nephrotic syndrome; acute glomerulonephritis; acute renal failure; chronic renal failure
>
> Cardiac: congestive cardiac failure
>
> Hepatic: chronic liver disease; hepatic venous outflow obstruction
>
> Neonatal: extreme prematurity; perinatal asphyxia; hyaline membrane disease; haemolytic disease; congenital lymphoedema; Turner syndrome; cystic fibrosis

Nephrotic syndrome

This is the commonest renal disorder leading to generalized oedema. The two mechanisms underlying oedema formation in nephrotic syndrome, are firstly the 'underfill model' and secondly the 'overfill model'. The main clinical correlate of the former model is steroid sensitive nephrotic syndrome (SSNS) where a reduction in plasma colloid oncotic pressure consequent on the fall in plasma albumin (usually to <20 g/L), results in a net movement of plasma water into the interstitial fluid and a reduction in plasma volume. The latter mechanism is more likely to apply in steroid resistant nephrotic syndrome and is due to a primary impairment of urinary sodium excretion leading to salt and water retention resulting in an expansion in the plasma and interstitial fluid compartments.

Childhood nephrotic syndrome is a heterogeneous disorder due to a variety of primary glomerular diseases in 90 per cent and in the remainder a feature of multisystem disease. The classic features of hypoproteinaemia (plasma albumin <25 g/L), 'nephrotic range' proteinuria and oedema may be associated with haematuria, either microscopic or frank, hypertension or a reduction in GFR.

Causes of nephrotic syndrome

Infancy

- Primary glomerular disease: (0–6 months): congenital nephrotic syndrome (Finnish and Non-Finnish types); MCD; focal and segmental glomerulosclerosis (FSGS)
- Secondary: congenital infection, e.g. syphilis, toxoplasmosis, cytomegalovirus (CMV); Denys–Drash syndrome (XY pseudohermaphroditism); systemic lupus erythematosus (SLE)

Childhood

- Primary glomerular disease: MCD; FSGS; membranoproliferative glomerulonephritis (MPGN); membranous nephropathy
- Secondary: HSP; SLE

The spectrum of underlying histological abnormalities varies with age, and outwith the first year of life until mid-childhood the commonest is MCD. With increasing age the spectrum changes and alternative histologies, particularly FSGS and MPGN become commoner. In contrast, MCD only accounts for approximately 25 per cent of adults with nephrotic syndrome. The spectrum within the first year of life is also different in view of the influence of congenital nephrotic syndrome, the onset of which is within the first three months of life.

The incidence of nephrotic syndrome is around 5 per 100 000 children per year with a prevalence of 1 per 6000 children. There is a significant racial variation in susceptibility with an incidence of 16 per 100 000 in Asian children in the UK.

Although the advent of percutaneous renal biopsy has helped enormously, it should be appreciated that histological classification still remains rather crude and non-specific, in that different histological appearances may have a similar therapeutic response and similar histological appearances may have quite different natural histories.

The therapeutic response to corticosteroid therapy plays a dominant role in the assessment of nephrotic syndrome in childhood in contrast to adult practice. The child with no adverse features such as onset within the first six months of life, macroscopic haematuria in the absence of UTI, significant hypertension, hypocomplementaemia and a low GFR, who has a consistently good response to corticosteroids may never undergo biopsy and is assumed to have MCD.

The natural history of SSNS/MCD is good with all patients eventually achieving a spontaneous remission and none developing renal insufficiency or hypertension. The great majority (60–90 per cent) will experience at least one relapse and 20 per cent will continue to relapse 10 years following presentation. Unfortunately despite the good long-term prognosis, there is a 3–4 per cent fatality rate from potentially avoidable complications of the nephrotic state and/or treatment, the main ones being infection and thrombosis. The specific management principles of SSNS/MCD are outlined in Table 12.4.

Although some children with FSGS respond to corticosteroids albeit partially, the non-MCD group are generally steroid resistant and as a group have a poorer prognosis and tend to be under the care of a paediatric nephrologist.

Table 12.4 Levels of management of steroid sensitive nephrotic syndrome

1	Initial episode	Prednisolone 60 mg/m^2 per day (max. 80 mg) for one month Prednisolone 40 mg/m^2 on alternate days (max. 40 mg) for one month Progressive withdrawal by 10 mg/m^2 each week over the next month
2	First two relapses	Prednisolone 60 mg/m^2 per day (max. 80 mg) until remission followed by 40 mg/m^2 on alternate days (max. 40 mg) for one month
3	Frequent relapser	Prednisolone 0.1–0.5 mg/kg on alternate days for 3–6 months
4	Relapse on prednisolone >0.5 mg/kg alternate days	Levamisole 2.5 mg/kg alternate days for 4–12 months
5	Continuing relapsing course on prednisolone >0.5 mg/kg alternate days	Cyclophosphamide 2 mg/kg per day for 12 weeks or chlorambucil 0.2 mg/kg per day for 8 weeks
6	Post-alkylating therapy relapse	As 2–3 above
7	Continuing relapsing course on prednisolone >0.5 mg/kg alternate days	Ciclosporin 5 mg/kg per day for 12–24 months

KEY LEARNING POINTS

- Nephrotic syndrome is commoner in boys, in the 2–5 year age group and minimal change disease is the commonest histological lesion.

- The child with nephrotic syndrome is at risk of hypovolaemia and primary peritonitis, both of which present with abdominal pain.
- Intravenous albumin is *not* a routine treatment for all patients with relapse of nephrotic syndrome and may be dangerous in the patient who is not hypovolaemic.
- Adverse factors on presentation, e.g. hypertension, macroscopic haematuria, impaired GFR and/or hypocomplementaemia warrant specialist referral.

POLYURIA AND POLYDIPSIA

The definition of polyuria is somewhat arbitrary since normal urine volumes in childhood are ill defined and the factors influencing urine volume vary with maturity. However, a working definition is a daily urine volume >1 L in the pre-school child, >2 L in the school-age child and >3 L in adolescents and adults.

Increased frequency of micturition is sometimes confused with polyuria. In the former small volumes of urine are passed repeatedly but the total daily volume is normal. If there is difficulty in distinguishing the two, a frequency/volume chart should be completed.

Nocturia, defined as the passage of urine at night in the absence of nocturnal enuresis and/or nocturnal enuresis, is a common finding in patients with polyuria although both may be present in patients with increased urinary frequency associated with UTI. Polydipsia is defined as an abnormally increased oral fluid intake and may be primary or secondary.

Causes of polyuria and polydipsia

Increased fluid intake: primary polydipsia; psychogenic polydipsia

Urinary concentration defect:

- Increased osmotic load, e.g. diabetes mellitus, total parenteral nutrition, chronic renal failure (CRF)
- Central diabetes insipidus, e.g. post-trauma/surgery, cerebral malformation, idiopathic, inherited
- Nephrogenic diabetes insipidus, e.g. inherited or secondary to CRF, obstructive uropathy, acute tubular necrosis (ATN), Fanconi syndrome, hypokalaemia, hypercalcaemia

CASE STUDY: Polyuria and polydipsia

A 3-year-old boy was referred with a history of several months of excessive drinking and relatively poor appetite although his weight gain was satisfactory and dipstick urinalysis was normal. He tended to wake at least once at night for a drink and took predominantly milk or diluted fruit juice. He was otherwise asymptomatic and general physical examination was normal. Routine plasma biochemical assessment was normal and following overnight fluid deprivation the urine osmolality was 850 mOsm/kg.

In practice it is useful to establish if the child is non-selective in their choice of fluids, whether they wake from sleep to drink or require a large drink first thing in the morning and whether they drink from inappropriate sources, e.g. toilet pans, bath water. If some or all of these factors are present, it is strongly suggestive of an organic cause for the polydipsia.

Primary polydipsia is a relatively common problem in the young child beyond infancy. The polydipsia is always selective and nocturnal drinking is variable. If the physical examination and urinalysis are normal, a trial of substituting water for all or part of the daily fluid intake will resolve the polydipsia. **Compulsive water drinking** or **psychogenic polydipsia** is a rare disorder in older children and adolescents and is associated with emotional or psychiatric disorders.

Assessment of a patient with a suspected urine concentration defect should include simple baseline plasma electrolytes, glucose, calcium and urinary tract ultrasound. Assuming these are normal, controlled water deprivation with or without DDAVP is warranted. However, this is a potentially hazardous procedure and should *not* be undertaken if the plasma sodium (PNa) is elevated. In this circumstance, DDAVP (0.5 μg/m^2 parenterally or 5 μg/m^2 intranasally) should be given and a urine osmolality (Uosm) estimated four hours later (adequate response >800 mOsm/kg).

If the patient is adequately hydrated and the PNa is normal, fluid deprivation should be undertaken over six to eight hours or until 3 per cent of the body weight is lost should this occur first. If at any time during the test the Uosm exceeds 800 mOsm/kg, deprivation can be stopped. At the end of the six- to eight-hour period, the PNa and Uosm should be checked and if the Uosm is <800 mOsm/kg, DDAVP should be given as above and a further Uosm and PNa checked four hours later.

CASE STUDY: Polyuria and polydipsia

A 9-week-old infant was seen for review at the infant follow-up clinic. He was one of triplets born at 34 weeks' gestation, had an uneventful neonatal period and was discharged home at the age of 3 weeks. He was formula-fed but compared with his two siblings, his weight gain was poor and he was described as being frequently unsettled and despite being apparently 'hungry', took his milk feeds slowly but fed avidly when offered water. On examination he was irritable, but was not clinically dehydrated and developmentally appropriate. Investigations included normal dipstick urinalysis, urine microscopy and urinary tract ultrasound; plasma sodium was 161 mmol/L, urea 11 mmol/L and creatinine 60 μmol/L. Following admission, he was given DDAVP 0.5 μg intramuscularly and Uosm four hours later was 151 mOsm/kg.

Diabetes insipidus

This is a generic term applied to a number of disorders with similar clinical features with the hallmark being polyuria and polydipsia in the absence of osmotic diuresis (see box above). These features may not be obvious in the infant who demonstrates irritability, frequent feed requirements, unexplained fever, constipation, failure to thrive and delayed development. Infants, in contrast with older children who are able to regulate their fluid intake, are at significant risk of hypernatraemic dehydration.

In central diabetes insipidus (CDI) secondary to a complete defect in antidiuretic hormone (ADH) secretion and in nephrogenic diabetes insipidus (NDI), there will be no significant change in the Uosm during fluid deprivation but the Posm often exceeds 300 mOsm/kg. Following DDAVP, the Uosm should be >800 mOsm/kg in CDI but will remain unchanged in NDI. In partial CDI the Uosm will be 300–800 mOsm/kg but will show an adequate response to DDAVP.

Almost all patients with congenital NDI are males but female siblings may have a mild form of the disorder only demonstrable by fluid deprivation. Acquired NDI occurs more frequently and usually in the context of some form of intrinsic renal disease. Adolescents with psychogenic polydipsia may demonstrate a suboptimal response to water deprivation and DDAVP (Uosm 500–800 mOsm/kg), but the Posm remains normal.

CASE STUDY: Polyuria and polydipsia

A 13-month-old infant was referred with chronic constipation and failure to thrive. He was a single child of elderly but healthy parents who felt he had been unwell for over a year. On examination he was pale, irritable and hypotonic and his weight was significantly below the 3rd centile. Urine dipstick showed + glycosuria and proteinuria. Further investigations were as follows: plasma Na 164 mmol/L, bicarbonate 12 mmol/L, phosphate 0.6 mmol/L, glucose 5 mmol/L, urea 15 mmol/L and creatinine 61 μmol/L and urine amino acid chromatography showed gross generalized amino aciduria.

Fanconi syndrome

This is characterized by a generalized disturbance in renal tubular function with at least initially, well preserved glomerular function. The cardinal clinical features are growth retardation, polyuria and rickets in association with a normal plasma anion gap metabolic acidosis, hypophosphataemia, hypokalaemia and generalized aminoaciduria.

There are multiple causes, but nephropathic cystinosis is the commonest cause in Europe and North America. This is a disorder of lysosomal cystine transport of autosomal recessive inheritance that leads to excessive intracellular accumulation of free cystine in many organs including the kidney.

Causes of renal Fanconi syndrome

Primary

- Cystinosis
- Tyrosinaemia
- Galactosaemia
- Fructosaemia
- Lowe syndrome
- Wilson disease
- Dent disease
- Glycogen storage disease
- Idiopathic
- Mitochondrial cytopathy

Secondary

- Chemotherapy, e.g. cisplatin, ifosfamide
- Drugs, e.g. outdated tetracycline
- Heavy metal poisoning
- Post renal transplantation
- Amyloidosis

In contrast to the early onset and severity of the infantile or nephropathic form, the intermediate or adolescent form does not present until the second decade and in the adult type there is no renal involvement despite cystine deposition elsewhere, e.g. cornea.

The therapy of Fanconi syndrome is either specific and/or supportive. Examples of specific therapy are the elimination of the underlying metabolic defect in galactosaemia or fructose intolerance, removal of the offending drug and the use in cystinosis of an agent designed to prevent further intracellular accumulation of cystine, e.g. cysteamine.

Supportive therapy should include adequate salt, water and nutritional supplementation and bicarbonate, electrolyte and phosphate replacement. In addition, calcium supplements as well as 1-α or 1,25[OH]2 vitamin D therapy are needed to control the metabolic bone disease.

Other conditions exist where there is a selective defect in tubular function, e.g. proximal (bicarbonaturia) and distal renal tubular acidosis (reduced H^+ ion excretion), isolated renal glycosuria and isolated phosphaturia in X-linked hypophosphataemic rickets. In addition, selective defects in amino acid reabsorption exist, e.g. dibasic aminoaciduria in cystinuria and neutral aminoaciduria in Hartnup disease.

KEY LEARNING POINTS

- The majority of children with polydipsia do not have impaired urinary concentrating ability.
- Children with renal tubular disease present with non-specific symptoms in early life and may experience significant clinical dehydration associated with relatively trivial intercurrent illness.
- Chronic constipation, growth retardation and rickets are classic features of a renal Fanconi syndrome

OLIGURIA AND ACUTE RENAL FAILURE

Acute renal failure may be defined as a sudden decrease in renal function over a period of hours or days accompanied by retention of nitrogenous waste and disturbance of fluid and electrolyte balance. Accurate estimates of the incidence of ARF in infancy and childhood are lacking although the general impression is that both the incidence and mortality is less than adults, perhaps with the exception of ARF in the neonate. As a result of improved techniques in the care of the seriously ill neonate, ARF has assumed greater importance in infants who would previously have succumbed to immaturity, overwhelming sepsis or complex cardiac malformations. **Oliguria** is defined as a urine volume of <1 mL/kg per hour (infant) and <0.5 mL/kg per hour (child), and although not a prerequisite for diagnosis, since it is absent in up to 50 per cent of cases, is of considerable prognostic importance. Other helpful parameters for the definition of ARF include a 50 per cent increase in plasma creatinine over baseline or a rise of >50 μmol/L per day. In the neonate ARF is present if the plasma creatinine is >130 μmol/L after the first 24 hours of life in association with a daily increase of >20 μmol/L.

Although the spectrum of ARF in infants and children (see box below) may be considered under prerenal, i.e. perfusion failure, renal parenchymal and obstructive causes, in practice a number of factors may operate in the individual case. In developing countries, the main cause is acute tubular necrosis (ATN) following salt and water depletion secondary to acute gastroenteritis. In developed countries, haemolytic uraemic syndrome (HUS), postcardiac surgical ARF and ARF as part of multiorgan failure are commoner.

Causes of acute renal failure in infancy and childhood

Hypovolaemia, e.g. acute gastroenteritis, septicaemia, cardiac surgery, burns, nephrotic syndrome, salt wasting CRF

Parenchymal disease, e.g. HUS, neonatal renal vein thrombosis, acute glomerulonephritis, acute pyelonephritis, nephrotoxins

Urinary tract obstruction, e.g. posterior urethral valves, calculus obstruction

The value of plasma urea measurement is limited in view of the effects of intravascular volume depletion, dietary protein intake, drug therapy and any cause of increased catabolic rate such as sepsis. The value of the urinary indices (Table 12.5) is in distinguishing prerenal, i.e. volume/diuretic responsive ARF, from that of established renal failure but they have limitations in the very preterm infant (gestational age <32 weeks). Ultrasound Doppler imaging is extremely useful in determining renal size and structure, the presence of urinary tract obstruction and renal venous and arterial flow.

Table 12.5 Urinary indices in acute renal failure

	Prerenal	Established
Urinary sodium (mmol/L)	<30	>30
Fractional excretion of sodium	<1 per cent	>1 per cent
U/P urea (child and adult)	>10	<10
U/P urea (infancy)	>5	<5
U/P osmolality	>1.15	<1.15

CASE STUDY: Acute renal failure

An 18-month-old previously well girl presented with a three-day history of diarrhoea which was described as bloody 24 hours prior to admission. Shortly before admission, she developed a generalized clonic convulsion. She had not been reported to pass urine on a previous 24-hour period. On examination she had mild generalized oedema, and her blood pressure was recorded at 120/90 mmHg. Investigations on admission revealed a plasma sodium of 128 mmol/L, potassium 6.2 mmol/L, urea 40 mmol/L, bicarbonate 12 mmol/L, osmolality 296 mOsm/kg, haemoglobin 8.5 g/dL, platelets 40×10^9/L and her blood film revealed a microangiopathic haemolytic uraemia. She remained oliguric and within 12 hours, she was started on peritoneal dialysis.

CASE STUDY: Acute renal failure

A 3-year-old boy presented with a history of anuria and abdominal pain of 24 hours duration. He had been seen by his GP on one occasion previously because of apparent dysuria and frank haematuria which had settled with oral antibiotic therapy. On examination he was pale but well perfused and in no significant distress. His blood pressure was recorded at 110/80 mmHg and abdominal examination revealed no tenderness, rebound or guarding and no abdominal organomegaly. No urine was available for analysis and his plasma sodium was recorded at 139 mmol/L, potassium 6 mmol/L, chloride 100 mmol/L, bicarbonate 18 mmol/L, urea 24 mmol/L and creatinine 250 μmol/L.

Abdominal radiograph revealed calcification in the region of the left kidney and overlying the pelvic brim. Abdominal ultrasound showed left-sided hydronephrosis and hydroureter but no evidence of a right kidney. A diagnosis of calculus obstruction was made and he underwent percutaneous nephrostomy under ultrasound guidance. Subsequent nephrostogram revealed a staghorn calculus of the left kidney and ureteric obstruction. He had a retrograde removal of the ureteric calculus and subsequently underwent extracorporeal shock wave lithotripsy.

Wherever possible, preventive strategies should be encouraged in clinical circumstances known to be associated with a risk of ARF, e.g. cardiac surgery and chemotherapy for acute lymphoproliferative disorders. The level of monitoring should be appropriate to the degree of clinical illness and this will vary from a minimum of careful fluid balance, daily weight and regular blood pressure recording to a level generally associated with intensive care management. Intravascular volume depletion should be corrected by rapid infusion of plasma or normal saline (20–60 mL/kg). If oliguria persists in the presence of an adequate blood pressure, central venous pressure (CVP) monitoring and inotropic support is indicated. Despite the widespread use of low-dose dopamine (1–5 μg/kg per minute) there is little evidence of efficacy and there are also important questions about potential complications, e.g. intestinal ischaemia leading to possible bacterial translocation.

If the blood pressure and CVP are adequate and when low urinary tract obstruction has been ruled out, a diuretic challenge should be considered (furosemide 1–5 mg/kg by slow intravenous injection). The value of both high-dose loop diuretics and mannitol in oliguric ARF remains unproved but the response to diuretic therapy suggests prerenal ARF. In some patients, oliguria may be reversed with no accompanying improvement in plasma biochemistry. However, this conversion is of clinical benefit since not only is the patient easier to manage but there also appears to be less morbidity and mortality associated with non-oliguric ARF. If hypertension develops, oral hydralazine or nifedipine is preferable to the use of β-blockers. In hypertensive encephalopathy intravenous hydralazine or intravenous labetalol should be used.

Fluid and nutritional requirements are related to metabolic rate and energy expenditure and energy

Table 12.6 Management of hyperkalaemia

	Dosage	Onset	Duration
10 per cent calcium gluconate	0.5 mL/kg	1-5 minutes	1 hour
Salbutamol	2.5-5 mg (neb) 4 mg/kg (IV)	30 minutes	2 hours
8.4 per cent sodium bicarbonate	2 mL/kg	30 minutes	2 hours
50 per cent dextrose and	0.5 g/kg per hour		
Insulin	0.15 U/kg per hour	30 minutes	6 hours
Furosemide	2 mg/kg	Variable	Variable
Calcium/sodium resonium	1 g/kg	1-2 hours	6 hours
Renal replacement	-	Variable	Variable

neb, nebulizer; IV, intravenous.

requirements should be approximated. The fluid prescription in ARF is based on the predicted insensible water losses plus losses. This regimen should allow a daily weight loss of 1–2 per cent and the enteral route for fluids and nutrition is preferred. A high calorie (75–100 calories/kg per day) and low protein (1 g/kg per day) formula should be used although the protein prescription can be liberalized if renal replacement therapy (RRT) is instituted. Sodium and potassium should be restricted to less than 1 mmol/kg per day of enteral feeds and avoided in parenteral fluids.

When ARF develops the drug prescription chart should be scrutinized since many schedules require modification and unfortunately this important consideration is frequently omitted. The priority in the treatment of hyperkalaemia (Table 12.6) is dictated by the presence of major electrocardiogram (ECG) abnormalities that tend to occur at a potassium level of 8 mmol/L. The risk of major dysrhythmias is enhanced by the presence of acidosis and hypoxia and may therefore occur at lower levels. Correction of an uncompensated metabolic acidosis with 8.4 per cent sodium bicarbonate (1–2 ml/kg) will also transiently reduce the plasma potassium but may precipitate symptomatic hypocalcaemia/hypomagnesaemia, particularly in infants. In most circumstances the above therapy is used to stabilize the clinical situation prior to the introduction of RRT. The decision to initiate RRT in ARF is relatively easy in the presence of resistant hyperkalaemia, severe metabolic acidosis, fluid overload or symptomatic uraemia. More often however, the decision is based on the predicted course and fluid/nutritional/blood product requirements rather than on arbitrary biochemical values.

Despite the technical feasibility of haemodialysis and increasing popularity of continuous haemofiltration, peritoneal dialysis remains a popular mode of therapy for ARF, particular in infants and young children with uncomplicated ARF. Conventional haemodialysis is dependent on available expertise and is generally restricted to the patient in whom peritoneal dialysis is contraindicated or has failed or to the potentially ambulant patient in whom a prolonged course is likely. In the patient with multiorgan failure, conventional haemodialysis has effectively been replaced by continuous haemofiltration and this technique has gained wide acceptance as safe and effective therapy in the critically ill infant and child. The main disadvantage of both haemodialysis and haemofiltration relate to the need to maintain dependable vascular access and continuous anticoagulation and despite the widespread use of haemofiltration, there is no evidence of a reduction in the high mortality (60 per cent) associated with ARF in the critically ill child.

KEY LEARNING POINTS

- The early detection of hypovolaemia and obstructive aetiology in a child presenting with ARF is important.
- Early management includes a fluid challenge if hypovolaemia is suspected and the use of an intravenous loop diuretic when circulatory status is secured.
- Children with anuria or persistent oliguria are likely to need RRT.
- Always examine the drug kardex in a child with ARF.

CHRONIC RENAL FAILURE

Although the lower limit of GFR is 80 mL/minute per 1.73 m^2, chronic renal failure is defined by a GFR of <50 mL/minute per 1.73 m^2 since it is only below this level that a rise in plasma creatinine occurs and clinical and metabolic abnormalities become progressively more apparent. In contrast to the rapidity of onset of ARF however, the loss of renal function occurs over a period of months and years. Endstage renal failure, defined by a GFR of <10 mL/minute per 1.73 m^2 indicates the stage when RRT, either dialysis or transplantation is necessary.

In Europe and the USA, the reported incidence of CRF and endstage renal failure in the 0–15 year age group is 23 and 5 per million child population, respectively. Of those with endstage renal failure, the majority are in the 6–14 year age group, but the proportion <6 years of age and in particular those <2 years of age has been increasing in recent years.

The distribution of primary renal disease in the child with endstage renal failure differs markedly from an equivalent adult population in that structural renal disease and hereditary/familial nephropathies predominate with acquired disease, e.g. glomerulonephritis becoming prevalent only in the adolescent age group (Table 12.7).

Table 12.7 Causes of chronic renal failure in childhood

Primary renal disease	0–2 years (%)	0–15 years (%)
Glomerulonephritis	14	29
Pyelonephritis/interstitial nephritis	15	24
Hereditary/familial nephropathy	14	16
Congenital hypoplasia/dysplasia	24	14
Haemolytic uraemic syndrome	17	5
Others	16	11

The child with CRF may present in a variety of ways and since the course maybe insidious, symptoms may not develop until an advanced stage. In this situation, distinction between ARF and CRF maybe difficult but features suggestive of CRF are short stature/failure to thrive, history of longstanding polyuria/polydipsia, signs of longstanding hypertension, a normochromic normocytic anaemia, small or structurally abnormal kidneys on ultrasound and radiological evidence of rickets or hyperparathyroidism.

CASE STUDY: Chronic renal failure

A baby boy was born by elective LUSCS at 36 weeks' gestation because of fetal uropathy. Antenatal ultrasound scanning at 32 weeks' gestation undertaken because of reported diminished fetal movements, had shown a reduced liquor volume and marked bilateral pelvicalyceal dilatation (PCD) and a poorly emptying bladder. His birth weight was 2.1 kg and he required no resuscitation and was admitted to the special care baby unit (SCBU). General examination was normal apart from the finding of a palpable bladder and mild tachypnoea. Plasma creatinine at 6 hours of age was 85 μmol/L and was associated with a mild metabolic acidosis. Urinary tract ultrasound showed gross bilateral PCD (pelvic diameters 20–25 mm), bilateral hydroureter and small echogenic kidneys with numerous small cortical cysts and a thick walled bladder. MCUG confirmed the provisional diagnosis of posterior urethral valves and showed severe bilateral VUR into dilated and tortuous ureters. A urethral catheter was inserted but the plasma creatinine climbed to 230 μmol/L by day 21 and the ultrasound appearances remained unchanged. On day 28 he underwent surgical excision of the posterior urethral valves and creation of a vesicostomy. He was discharged on a low protein, phosphate and potassium milk formula with sodium chloride and bicarbonate supplements given via a nasogastric tube. Additional medication included calcium carbonate, 1-α(OH)2 vitamin D_3 and prophylactic trimethoprim. Subcutaneous human erythropoietin (HUEPO) was introduced at the age of 3 months. His weight remained below but parallel to the 3rd centile and his length remained between the 3rd and 10th centiles. At the age of 11 months the plasma creatinine was 400 μmol/L and he was started on automated peritoneal dialysis and the vesicostomy was closed. His subsequent progress was satisfactory, although because of poor statural growth, human growth hormone (HGH) was introduced at the age of 2 years and at the age of 3 years (weight 14 kg) he underwent a successful living related donor transplantation from his mother.

CASE STUDY: Chronic renal failure

A 7-year-old girl was referred by her GP because of the finding of an elevated plasma creatinine (190 μmol/L) and a low haemoglobin (8.1 g/dL). She had been increasingly lethargic over the previous 3 months and had longstanding polydipsia and primary nocturnal enuresis. She was the youngest of three children to healthy parents and there was no extended family history of renal disease. Apart from pallor, physical examination including blood pressure was normal and urinalysis showed a trace of proteinuria only. Renal ultrasound showed normal-sized kidneys with poor corticomedullary differentiation and wrist radiograph showed a bone age of 5.5 years and features of rickets. In view of the clinical suspicion of familial juvenile nephronophthisis, blood was submitted for DNA analysis and a mutation in the FPHP1 gene was found, confirming the above diagnosis. She was treated with dietary protein restriction, alkali therapy, activated vitamin D and both HUEPO and HGH. The plasma creatinine rose progressively over the following two years and was associated with progressively worsening symptoms. By the age of 9 years, the plasma creatinine level was 600 μmol/L and automated peritoneal dialysis was instituted, but within 3 months she underwent a successful cadaveric transplantation.

The management of the child with CRF is best coordinated by a multidisciplinary team in the setting of a dedicated clinic. **Growth pattern** abnormalities are common when the GFR falls below 25 mL/minute per 1.73 m^2 and the infantile (up to 2 years) and the pubertal components are most vulnerable. Malnutrition secondary to the almost universal anorexia of CRF is a major growth retarding factor. **Nutritional support**, particularly to enhance energy intake in order to reduce catabolism and control phosphate, protein and potassium intake, and attention to sodium and water balance is vital at all ages, especially in the polyuric infant with congenital renal disease. In addition to dietary phosphate restriction, control of **secondary hyperparathyroidism** generally requires activated vitamin D therapy as well as control of metabolic acidosis with alkali therapy, which has the additional benefit of growth enhancement and control of hyperkalaemia. However, there remains a cohort of children with CRF whose growth velocity remains poor despite optimal control of nutrition, osteodystrophy and acidosis and in this group, recombinant HGH is recommended.

Another common complication of CRF is a **normochromic normocytic anaemia**, which although multifactorial, is predominantly secondary to a reduced renal production of erythropoietin deficiency. In the past, this complication led to a regular blood transfusion requirement for patients with endstage renal failure with the accompanying risk of sensitization. However, with the introduction of recombinant erythropoietin that is given intravenously or subcutaneously once to three times weekly, the need for transfusion has been abolished.

Since the majority of patients with CRF will experience a progressive decline in renal function, irrespective of the primary renal disease, attempts should be made to slow the decline. The most important interventions are adequate control of blood pressure, osteodystrophy and nutritional status and to a lesser extent, angiotensin-converting enzyme (ACE) inhibitor therapy in patients with high-grade proteinuria. However, whatever time is available before the development of endstage renal failure should be used to prepare the child and their family for the challenges of RRT.

Renal transplantation is the preferred form of RRT for children with endstage renal failure and currently, 20 per cent of children undergo 'pre-emptive' transplantation when the GFR falls <10 mL/minute per 1.73 m^2 and before dialysis is required. If pre-emptive transplantation is not available or does not occur, uraemic symptoms such as lethargy and vomiting, significant and resistant hyperkalaemia and diuretic resistant salt and water retention generally indicate the need for dialysis. The type of dialysis, i.e. haemodialysis or peritoneal dialysis, should be tailored to the individual and their family, the aim being to ensure as normal an existence as possible.

Haemodialysis, which should be undertaken in specialist centres, is used as first line therapy in 25 per cent of children but may also be used as back up therapy in patients on peritoneal dialysis, following abdominal surgery or during periods of catheter malfunction/removal. The main challenge in haemodialysis is the maintenance of adequate long-term vascular access which is best provided by the surgical creation of a forearm arteriovenous fistula. In the young child, however, this is technically difficult and for this reason, and to avoid the trauma of repeated needling of a fistula, the use of long-term double lumen central venous catheters have become popular. The main disadvantages of central vascular access are recurrent sepsis and stenosis or occlusion of large central veins. This latter complication in a child who may have many years of RRT in store may have significant long-term consequences.

The majority of children with endstage renal failure on chronic dialysis are managed by peritoneal dialysis, either by four daytime exchanges and an overnight dwell (CAPD) or more frequently, several overnight automated exchanges by a portable machine and a long daytime dwell (CCPD). Both techniques are simple, effective, home based and enable more consistent school attendance and travel. The main disadvantage is peritonitis, however, the risk of this complication may be minimized by stringent antiseptic measures.

The ultimate goal for children with endstage renal failure should be transplantation since this offers the potential for normal health and full rehabilitation, neither of which can be achieved on chronic dialysis. There has been a progressive improvement in renal allograft and patient survival over the recent years due to improvements in pre-, peri- and postoperative care and advances in immunosuppressive therapy, particularly calcineurin inhibitors, e.g. ciclosporin and tacrolimus. There is a wide variation in the use of living related donors from >80 per cent in Scandinavia to <20 per cent in the UK. The current allograft survival from national registry data at one year and five years is 91 per cent and 80 per cent for living related donors grafts and 83 per cent and 65 per cent for cadaveric donor grafts, indicating that changing practice has narrowed the short-term survival gap between living related donor and cadaveric donor grafts. In addition to more effective immunosuppression, cadaveric donor graft survival is enhanced by close human leucocyte antigen (HLA) matching and avoidance of young child donors, because of the increased risk of graft vascular thrombosis.

The continuing challenges in this field are to optimize patient and graft survival, decrease acute and chronic graft rejection and minimize both the short- and long-term side effects of immunosuppressive agents and the risk of recurrent disease in the graft.

KEY LEARNING POINTS

- The symptoms of CRF are very non-specific but growth failure, unexplained anaemia and polyuria are common.
- Hypertensive encephalopathy and congestive cardiac failure may be the first presentation of advanced renal failure.

- Management of the child with chronic and endstage renal failure is multidisciplinary.
- Successful renal transplantation is the treatment of choice for children with endstage renal failure.
- Living related renal transplant donation is commoner in childhood endstage renal failure.

HYPERTENSION

Systolic blood pressure rises and diastolic blood pressure falls during the first few weeks of life, they then stabilize until the age of 5 years and rise subsequently. Before puberty, blood pressure levels are similar in boys and girls, but during adolescence the rise in systolic blood pressure is greater in boys than in girls. The increase in blood pressure with age is largely due to increases in height and weight, thus the blood pressure of tall heavy children will be greater than that of short thin children of the same age. In addition, for any given height, an overweight child will have a higher blood pressure than a child whose weight is appropriate for their height. A number of large population studies have resulted in the establishment of normal values for blood pressure in relation to age, sex and height (see Appendix C). Hypertension in childhood and adolescence is therefore defined as blood pressure measurements repeatedly exceeding the 95th percentile, rather than on absolute values. In the neonate in contrast, threshold values of 90/60 mmHg (term) and 80/50 mmHg (preterm) are widely used.

The most accurate **method of blood pressure measurement** is direct intra-arterial measurement. Of the two popular non-invasive methods, mercury sphygmomanometry and oscillometry, the former is still regarded as the gold standard and should be used as calibration for the latter. For each of the non-invasive methods every attempt should be made to settle the infant or child who should be in a sitting or supine position. In addition, it is important to use the largest cuff that will fit as too small a cuff will overestimate blood pressure.

Ambulatory blood pressure monitoring (ABPM), is useful as a diagnostic tool in children with borderline casual recordings and in the assessment of anti-hypertensive control and can be successfully applied to the pre-school age group. It should be appreciated that ABPM data in normal children are limited but that those available suggest that daytime ABP is significantly higher than casual recordings at rest.

The **prevalence of hypertension** in children and adolescents is estimated to be between 1 and 3 per cent.

Table 12.8 Causes of hypertension

	Infancy	Childhood
Vascular	Renal artery/aortic thrombosis Coarctation	Coarctation
Renal	Renal parenchymal disease Renal failure	Renal parenchymal disease Renal failure
Drugs	Corticosteroid therapy Cocaine intoxication	Corticosteroid therapy
Catecholamine excess	Phaeochromocytoma Neuroblastoma	Phaeochromocytoma Neuroblastoma
Others	Bronchopulmonary dysplasia Extracorporeal membrane oxygenation	Renal tumours Conn and Cushing syndromes Congenital adrenal hyperplasia

The great majority have a minor increase in blood pressure, are asymptomatic and are presumed to have essential hypertension. However, 1 per 1000 have severe and symptomatic hypertension usually secondary to renal disease. The reported prevalence of hypertension in high-risk neonates varies from 0.7 to 2.5 per cent, compared with that of 0.2 per cent in healthy neonates. The age-related common causes of hypertension are given in Table 12.8.

CASE STUDY: Hypertension

A term baby boy presented with frank haematuria at the age of 36 hours. He was born by SVD to a 21-year-old mother with insulin-dependent diabetes mellitus. He had mild perinatal asphyxia, with an Apgar score of 4 and 7 at 1 and 5 minutes, respectively and was admitted to the SCBU for observation and, apart from transient hypoglycaemia, appeared well. Laboratory investigations showed: haemoglobin 15.2 g/dL, platelet count 55 $\times 10^9$/L, plasma creatinine 69 μmol/L. Abdominal ultrasound showed a swollen left kidney with absent intrarenal venous flow. No specific therapy was started and he was fit for discharge at the age of 10 days. Blood pressure on discharge was 85/60 mmHg.

He was reviewed at the age of 1 month when the blood pressure was 100/65 mmHg and 110/72 mmHg by the age of 3 months. ^{99m}Tc-DMSA was undertaken at this point and showed a normal right kidney but a small scarred left kidney contributing 25 per cent of differential function. At the age of 6 months, the blood pressure is currently 90/60 mmHg on atenolol 20 mg/day and nifedepine 10 mg twice daily.

CASE STUDY: Hypertension

A 10-year-old girl was admitted with a three-day history of increasing cough, exertional dyspnoea and orthopnoea. She had been generally unwell for the previous three months with anorexia, lethargy and pallor. On examination, she was centrally cyanosed and in significant respiratory distress (SAO_2 85 per cent). Auscultation revealed a praecordial triple rhythm and diffuse bilateral basal crackles. Blood pressure was 180/120 mmHg and funduscopy showed grade IV hypertensive retinopathy. Shortly after admission, she had a respiratory arrest and underwent endotracheal intubation and following intubation abundant pink secretions were aspirated. Chest radiograph showed cardiomegaly and bilateral interstitial pulmonary oedema. Laboratory investigations showed: haemoglobin 7.5 g/dL, plasma creatinine 965 μmol/L, urea 45 mmol/L and potassium 6.3 mmol/L. She was given intravenous furosemide 5 mg/kg over 30 minutes and an infusion of nitroglycerin was given as an antihypertensive. Subsequent abdominal ultrasound showed small dysplastic kidneys and a wrist radiograph showed changes of hyperparathyroidism. Echocardiography showed a thickened left ventricular wall but otherwise normal intracardiac and aortic arch anatomy. There was no significant response to intravenous furosemide but following haemodialysis she was successfully extubated although she remains dependent on dialysis. Current oral antihypertensive therapy includes enalapril, nifedipine and doxazosin.

The extent to which hypertension is investigated depends on the severity and persistence, since transient hypertension maybe seen in a number of circumstances, e.g. ARF, acute glomerulonephritis, HSP, drug-related, CNS disease/injury, etc. If persistent, patients with **borderline** hypertension (systolic and/or diastolic blood pressure around 95th percentile) require little more than a careful history including a family history of hypertension and medication use, e.g. oral contraceptive and clinical examination. Subsequent evaluation may be limited to urinalysis, ECG, plasma creatinine and abdominal ultrasound. More detailed evaluation is necessary in patients with **moderate** hypertension (blood pressure >95th percentile with no end organ damage) and **severe** hypertension (blood pressure >10–20 mmHg above the 95th percentile with end organ damage).

Evaluation of sustained hypertension

Initial investigations

Urinalysis

Urine culture

Urea and electrolytes, liver function tests, C-reactive protein and full blood count

±Peripheral plasma renin and aldosterone (following 30 minutes of recumbency and preferably off treatment)

Spot urine for catecholamines

Chest radiograph

Electrocardiogram and echocardiograph

Renal ultrasound with Doppler

Secondary investigations

Are guided by the findings from the above preliminary investigations along with the clinical findings and include:

1 Renal aetiology suspected:
- DMSA scan
- Direct or indirect cystogram
- Intravenous urography
- Renal angiography
- Renal venous renin sampling
- Renal biopsy

2 Catecholamine excess suspected
- ^{123}I MIBG scan
- Computed tomography (CT)/magnetic resonance imaging (MRI)
- Abdominal angiography with selective venous sampling

3 Corticosteroid excess suspected
- Urinary steroid profile
- Steroid suppression tests
- Adrenal CT/MRI
- Selective adrenal venous steroid sampling

Table 12.9 Antihypertensive drugs commonly used in children

Drug	Route	Normal starting dose	Normal dose range	Divided doses/day
Amiloride*	Oral	0.1 mg/kg per dose	0.4 mg/kg per day; 20 mg/day (maximum)	1–2
Atenolol	Oral	1 mg/kg per dose	1–2 mg/kg per day	1
Captopril	Oral	0.05 mg/kg per dose	0.5–3 mg/kg per day	3
Clonidine	IV	0.002 mg/kg per dose	0.002–0.006 mg/kg per day	2
	Oral	0.005 mg/kg	0.01–0.08 mg/kg per day	2
Diazoxide*	IV	0.5–1 mg/kg	1–10 mg/kg per day	By rapid infusion
Enalapril	Oral	0.2 mg/kg	0.2–1 mg/kg per day (max. 40 mg/day)	1
Esmolol	IV	50 μg/kg per minute	100–300 μg/kg per minute	Infusion only
Furosemide	IV	0.5 mg/kg per dose	0.5–4 mg/kg per day	1–4
	Oral	0.5 mg/kg per dose	1–4 mg/kg per day	1–4
Hydralazine	IV stat followed by infusion	0.1 mg/kg per dose stat (max. 10 mg)	Infusion 10–50 μg/kg per hour	As an infusion
	Oral	0.2 mg/kg per dose	1–8 mg/kg per day	3–4
Hydrochlorothiazide	Oral	1 mg/kg per dose	1–4 mg/kg per day	2
Labetalol	IV	0.5 mg/kg per h	1–3 mg/kg per h	Infusion only
Metolazone	Oral	0.1 mg/kg per dose	0.1–3 mg/kg per day	1
Minoxidil	Oral	0.1 mg/kg per dose	1–2 mg/kg per day	2
Nifedepine	Oral/sublingual	0.25 mg/kg per dose (capsular contents drawn by syringe to make correct dose)	1–2 mg/kg per day	4
	Slow release tablets	0.5 mg/kg per dose	1–2 mg/kg per day	2–3 (used in older children)
Phenoxybenzamine*	Oral	0.2 mg/kg per dose	1–4 mg/kg per day	2
	IV	0.5 mg/kg over 1 hour (stat dose)	1–2 mg/kg per day	2–4 (need intensive care facilities)
Phentolamine*	IV	0.1–0.2 mg/kg per dose	Titrated to response	Infusion only (used for control of hypertensive episodes during pheochromocytoma surgery)
Prazosin	Oral	0.005 mg/kg per dose; max. 0.25 mg	0.05–0.4 mg/kg per day	4
Propranolol	Oral	1 mg/kg per dose	1–10 mg/kg per day	3
Sodium nitroprusside*	IV	0.5 μg/kg per minute	0.5–8.0 μg/kg per minute	Infusion only (protect from light and monitor blood cyanide levels)
Spironolactone	Oral	0.5 mg/kg per dose	1–3 mg/kg per day	2
Triamterene*	Oral	1 mg/kg per dose	1–6 mg/kg per day	1–3

*Drugs used under special circumstances for specific indications.
Source: Webb NJA, Postlethwaite RJ (eds) (2003) *Clinical Paediatric Nephrology*, 3rd edn. Oxford: Oxford Medical Publication.

All patients with hypertension irrespective of the aetiology and specific therapy require general advice on diet, exercise and lifestyle and this may be the only measure necessary in patients with borderline hypertension. Moderate dietary sodium restriction with particular emphasis on the avoidance of popular junk foods and effective weight control in obese individuals is wise. Table 12.9 gives a list of commonly used antihypertensive drugs in children.

KEY LEARNING POINTS

- The diagnosis of hypertension should be made on several recordings using appropriate equipment and using published normative data.
- Hypertension may present with unusual features such as facial palsy, congestive cardiac failure, failure to thrive.
- The primary aims of investigation are to establish the presence and extent of end organ damage and aetiology.
- Control of hypertension is important irrespective of the aetiology and precipitous falls in blood pressure should be avoided.

COMMON FLUID AND ELECTROLYTE ABNORMALITIES

Disturbances in fluid, electrolyte and acid–base abnormalities are a frequent occurrence in practice and occur in a variety of clinical circumstances varying from the previously well infant with acute gastroenteritis to the critically ill infant and child in the paediatric intensive care unit (PICU).

Clinical evaluation, particularly **assessment of extracellular and intravascular volume,** is of paramount importance in patients with fluid and electrolyte disturbance and laboratory measures should always be regarded as complementary.

Random urinary sodium (Na) and chloride concentration, fractional excretion of Na: {FENa(per cent) = (UNa × plasma creatinine)/PNa × urine creatinine) × 100}, calculated plasma osmolality {2 × plasma Na + glucose + urea (in mmol/L)}, plasma osmolal gap {measured − calculated osmolalities}, and urine osmolality are very useful adjuncts to clinical assessment, particularly when faced with abnormalities in plasma sodium.

CASE STUDY: Fluid and electrolyte disorders

A 6-year-old boy being treated for acute lymphocytic leukaemia in relapse and intracerebral abscess developed increasing somnolence followed by a grand mal convulsion. Plasma sodium and osmolality taken shortly after the convulsion was 115 mmol/L and 241 mOsm/kg and urinary sodium and osmolality 55 mmol/L and 251 mOsm/kg, respectively. On examination, he was drowsy but localizing to painful stimuli (Glasgow Coma Score 10) and had no focal neurological deficit. Syndrome of inappropriate ADH secretion (SIADH) was diagnosed and in view of the severity of the neurological symptoms, intravenous 3 per cent NaCl was infused at 4 mL/kg per hour until the plasma sodium reached 125 mmol/L.

There are many causes of hyponatraemia (plasma Na < 130 mmol/L), but only two underlying mechanisms, firstly, a loss of sodium in excess of water, and secondly, a gain of water in excess of sodium. Pure sodium deficiency is very rarely observed, the association with fluid deficit being the norm and in practice hyponatraemia in hospitalized patients of all ages is more likely to be due to water retention. The key factors in the evaluation of a patient with hyponatraemia are accurate assessment of the status of extracellular fluid volume, plasma osmolality and urinary sodium concentration (Figure 12.6).

Differential diagnosis of hyponatraemia

Factitious (Posm high): e.g. hyperglycaemia; mannitol

Pseudo (Posm normal): e.g. hyperlipidaemia; hyperproteinaemia

True (Posm low):

1 Loss of sodium in excess of water
  - Extrarenal (UNa < 20 mmol/L): gastrointestinal, e.g diarrhoea, vomiting, fistula, etc.; skin, e.g. heat stress, cystic fibrosis, adrenal insufficiency; third space, e.g. burns, pancreatitis, ascites, intestinal obstruction
  - Renal (UNa > 20 mmol/L): diabetic ketoacidosis; diuretic therapy; Fanconi syndrome; mineralocorticoid deficiency/resistance; salt-wasting CRF

2 Gain of water in excess of sodium
- Non-oedematous states (UNa > 20 mmol/L): SIADH; psychogenic polydipsia; adrenal insufficiency; hypothyroidism; antidiuretic drugs
- Oedematous states (UNa > 20 mmol/L): nephrotic syndrome; cardiac failure; hepatic failure; renal failure (UNa > 20 mmol/L)

CASE STUDY

A 21-day-old breastfed infant was admitted with a history of irritability. His weight on admission was 3.2 kg (birth weight 3.5 kg) and he was felt to be mildly jaundiced and dehydrated, but there was no history of vomiting or diarrhoea and he was keen to feed. Plasma sodium and osmolality was 165 mmol/L and 337 mOsm/kg and a random urine sodium and osmolality 11 mmol/L and 812 mOsm/kg, respectively. Hypernatraemic dehydration secondary to failure of breastfeeding was diagnosed and he was given intravenous N/5 saline in 5 per cent dextrose at a rate to replace the calculated fluid deficit over a 48-hour period. Formula feeds were introduced and the plasma sodium was normal on discharge five days later.

The two mechanisms that result in hypernatraemia are loss of water in excess of sodium and gain of sodium in excess of water. The commonest presentation of hypernatraemia in clinical practice is in association with a fluid deficit. The key factors in the evaluation of a patient with hypernatraemia are an accurate assessment of the status of extracellular fluid volume and urine osmolality (Figure 12.7).

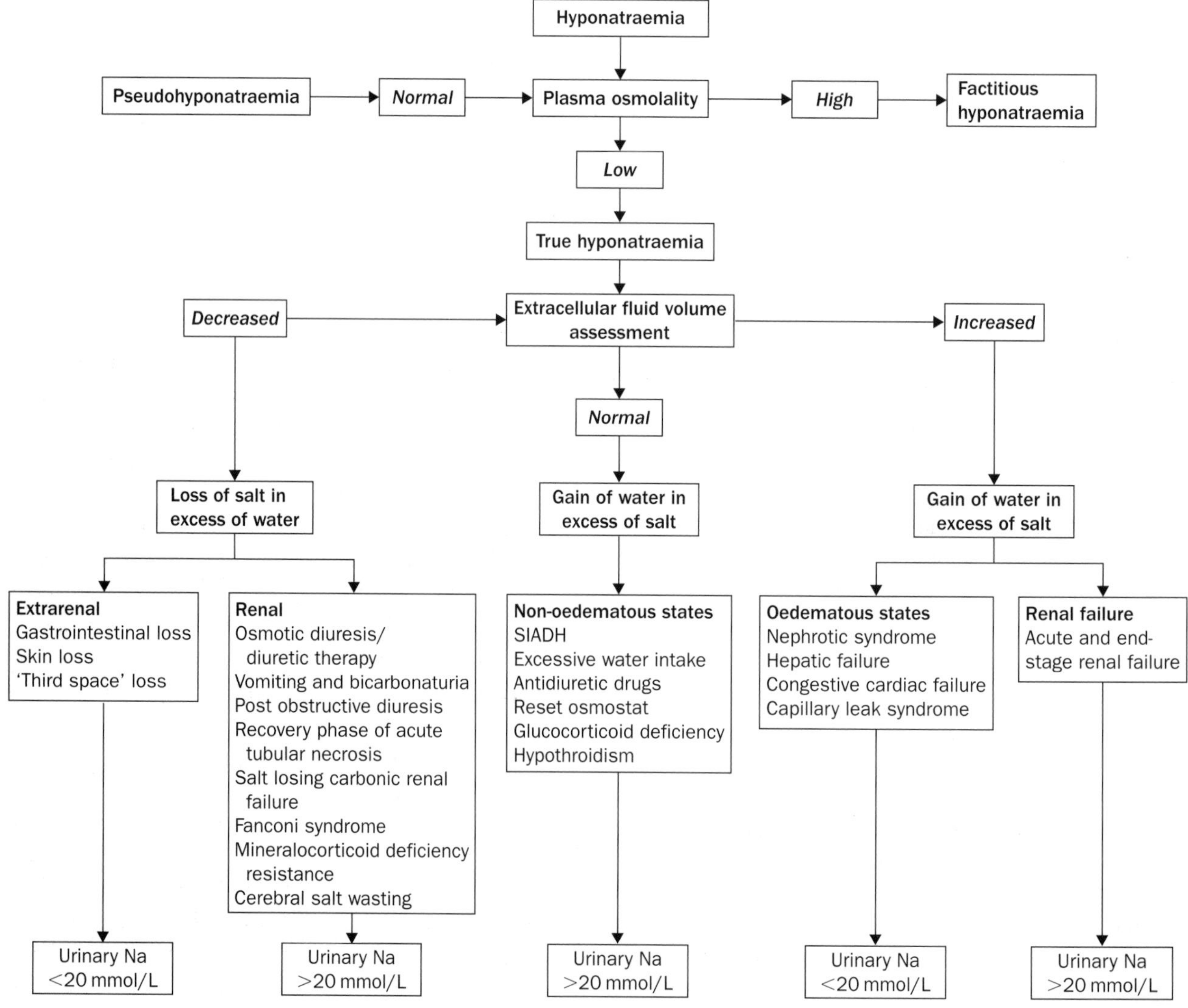

Figure 12.6 Evaluation of hyponatraemia

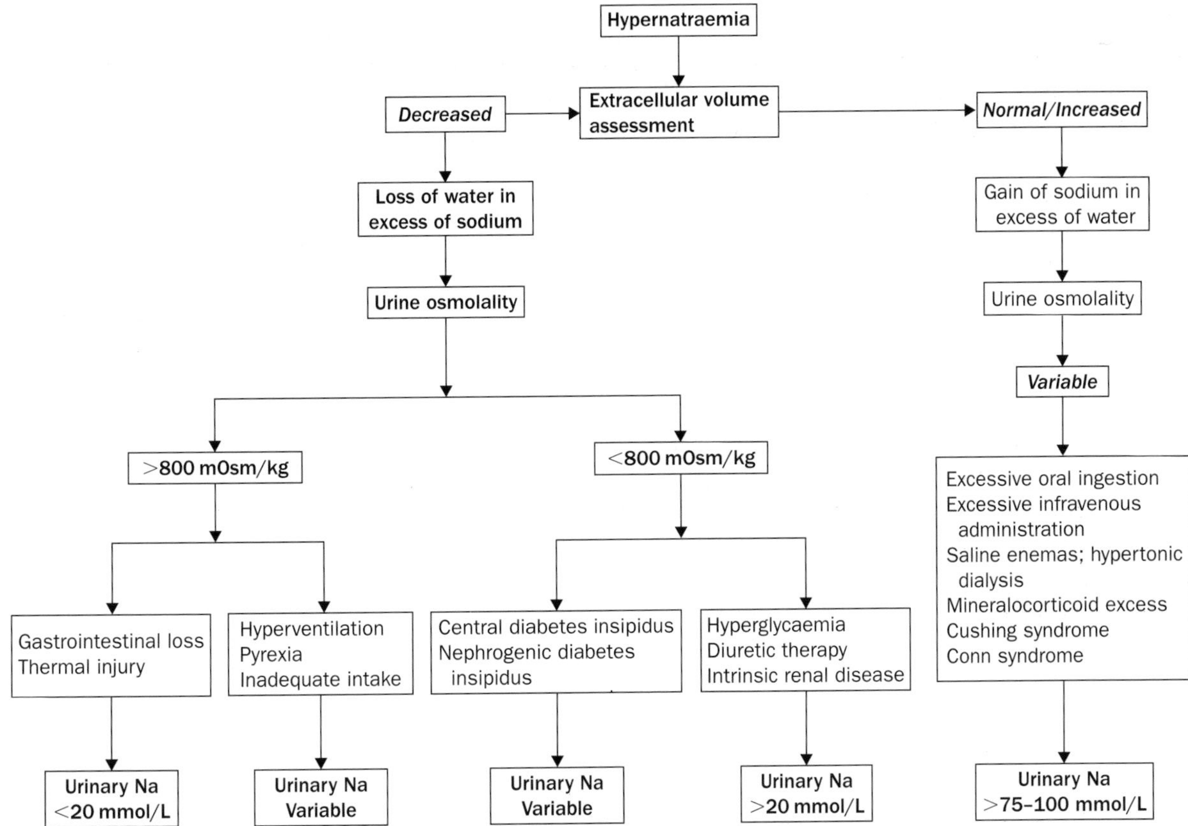

Figure 12.7 Evaluation of hypernatraemia

Differential diagnosis of hypernatraemia

Loss of water in excess of sodium

- Extrarenal (Uosm > 800 mOsm/kg; UNa < 20 mmol/L): gastrointestinal loss; burns; hyperventilation; pyrexia; inadequate water intake
- Renal (Uosm < 800 mOsm/kg; UNa variable): Central and nephrogenic diabetes insipidus; diabetic ketoacidosis; diuretic therapy; intrinsic renal disease

Gain of sodium in excess of water (Uosm variable; UNa > 75–100 mmol/L)

- Excess oral ingestion, e.g. in milk/nasogastric feeds, sea water
- Excess intravenous administration, e.g. 8.4 per cent sodium bicarbonate, hypertonic sodium chloride
- Saline enema
- Mineralocorticoid excess, e.g. Cushing and Conn syndromes

CASE STUDY

A 15-week-old breastfed baby girl was admitted for further investigation of failure to thrive and recurrent effortless vomiting (birth weight 3.9 kg and admission weight 4.9 kg). She was shown to have mild gastro-oesophageal reflux on barium swallow 5 weeks previously but the vomiting continued despite the introduction of Gaviscon®. Investigations revealed a plasma Na of 131 mmol/L, Cl 80 mmol/L, K 2.2 mmol/L and HCO_3 31 mmol/L with a normal urea and creatinine. Urinary Na and Cl were 15 and 12 mmol/L, respectively, and sweat Cl was 103 mmol/L.

Hypokalaemia may result from total body potassium deficiency or as a result of re-distribution between the extracellular and intracellular fluid compartments. The commonest cause of hypokalaemia is either acute or chronic gastrointestinal loss but another non-renal cause is excessive loss through the skin and patients with cystic fibrosis may present with a pseudo-Bartter syndrome.

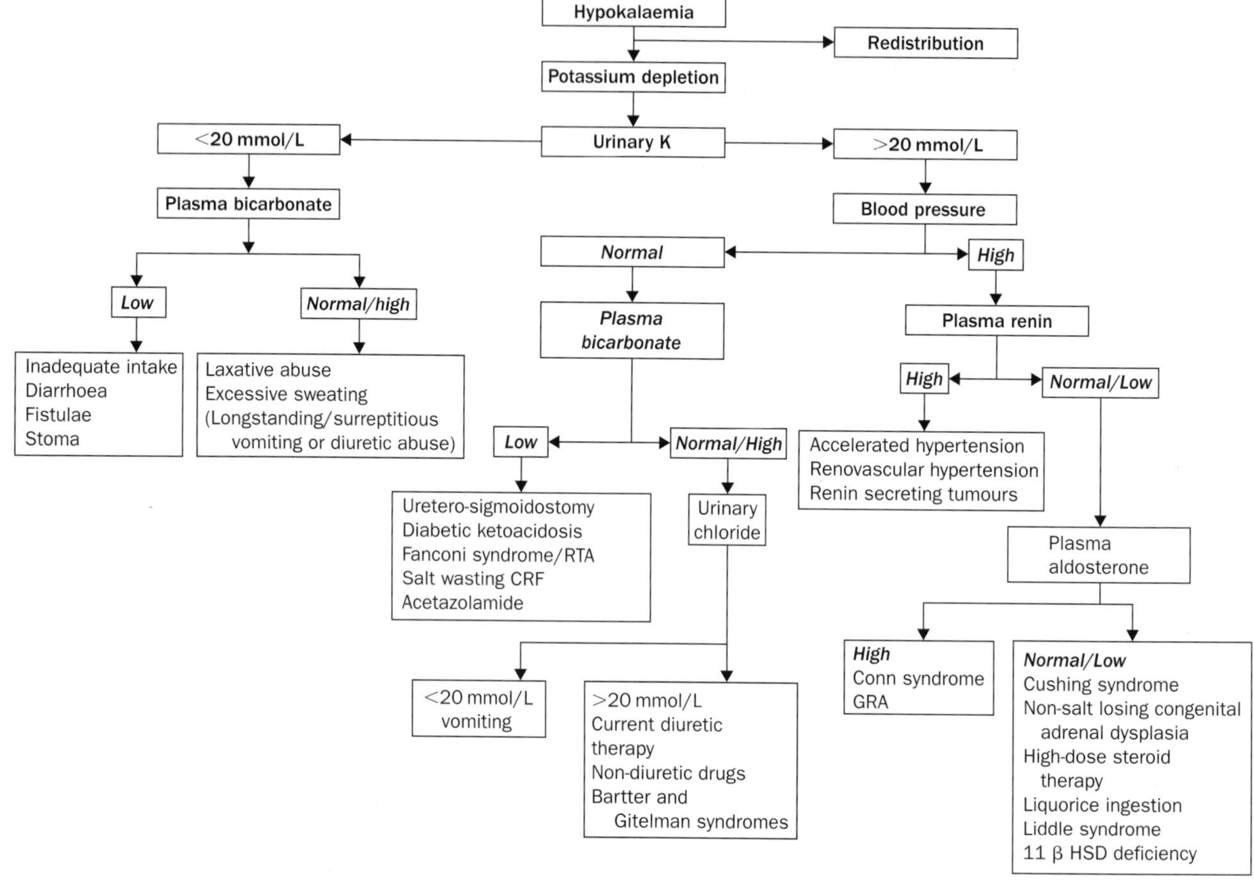

Figure 12.8 Evaluation of hypokalaemia

The key factors in the evaluation of hypokalaemia are blood pressure, urinary potassium concentration, and plasma bicarbonate and renin levels (Figure 12.8).

Differential diagnosis of hypokalaemia

Associated with total body deficiency

Inadequate intake (UK $<$ 20 mmol/L)

Extrarenal loss (UK $<$ 20 mmol/L)

- *Low plasma HCO_3*: Diarrhoea, gastrointestinal fistulae and stomas
- *Normal/high plasma HCO_3*: Laxative abuse, excessive sweating in cystic fibrosis

Renal loss (UK $>$ 20 mmol/L)

- *BP normal*

Low plasma HCO_3: Urinary/gastrointestinal diversion; Fanconi syndrome, renal tubular acidosis (RTA); salt-wasting CRF; diabetic ketoacidosis

Normal/high plasma HCO_3: recurrent vomiting; diuretic therapy; Bartter syndrome

- *BP high*

Low plasma renin: corticosteroid therapy; Cushing and Conn syndromes; liquorice ingestion

Elevated plasma renin: accelerated hypertension; renovascular hypertension; renin-secreting tumours

Redistribution hypokalaemia

Metabolic/respiratory alkalosis

Insulin administration

CASE STUDY

A 9-month-old boy with complex cyanotic congenital heart disease was admitted with worsening heart failure associated with acute bronchiolitis. His baseline medications were furosemide, spironolactone and captopril. Initial investigations revealed a plasma Na of 130 mmol/L, Cl 80 mmol/L, K 7.2 mmol/L, HCO_3 26 mmol/L, urea 15 mmol/L and creatinine 105 μmol/L.

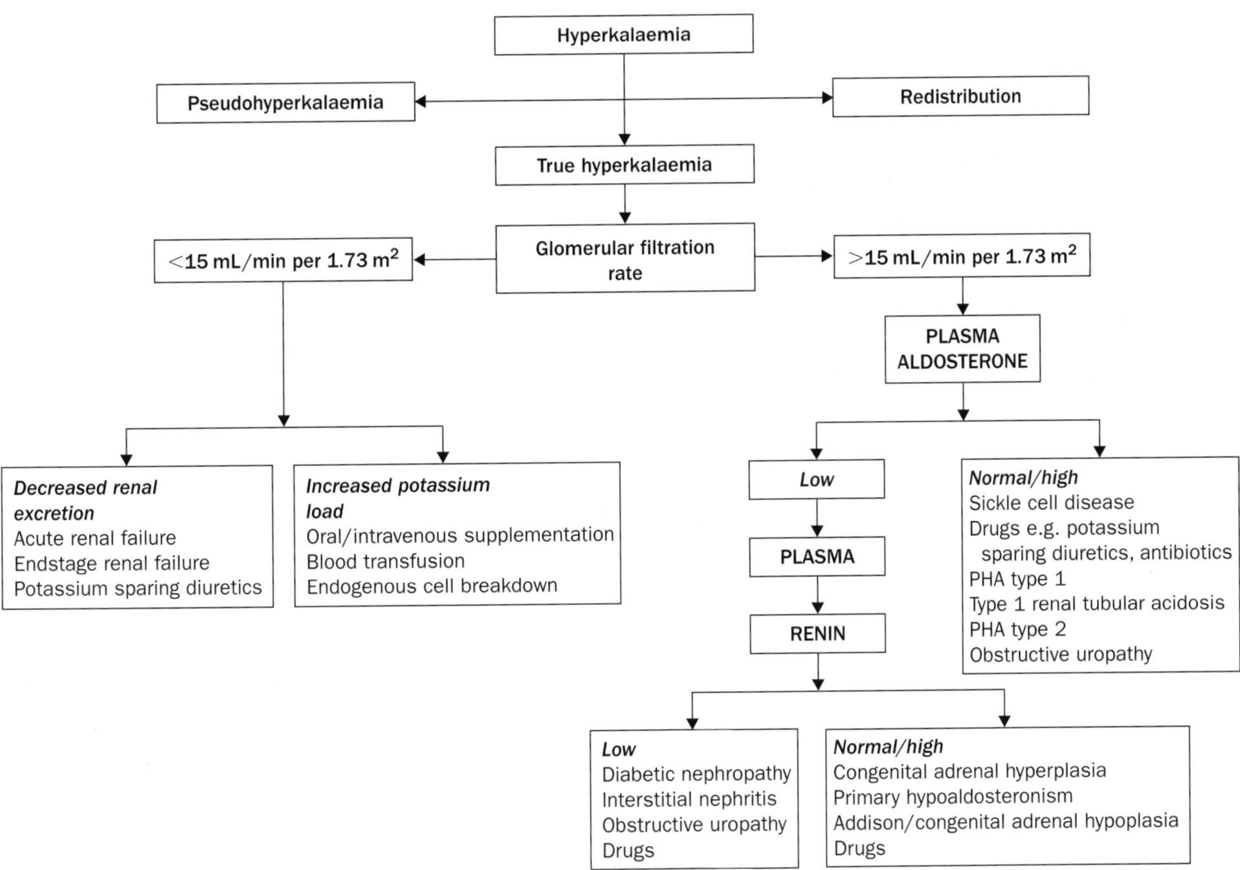

Figure 12.9 Evaluation of hyperkalaemia

> Differential diagnosis of hyperkalaemia
>
> Pseudohyperkalaemia: e.g. *in vitro* haemolysis, extreme leucocytosis or thrombocytosis
>
> True hyperkalaemia
>
> - *Normal renal function*
>
> Low plasma aldosterone: congenital adrenal hyperplasia, Addison disease; primary hypoaldosteronism; ACE-inhibitors, non-steroidal anti-inflammatory drugs, ciclosporin therapy
>
> Normal/high plasma aldosterone: pseudohypoaldosteronism; RTA; obstructive uropathy; sickle cell nephropathy; potassium-sparing diuretics
>
> - *Impaired renal function*: ARF, CRF; potassium-sparing diuretics; oral supplementation; blood transfusion
>
> Redistribution hyperkalaemia
>
> - Metabolic and respiratory acidosis
> - Mineralocorticoid/insulin deficiency
> - β-Blockers

True hyperkalaemia may result from excess administration, decreased renal excretion or as a result of re-distribution between the extracellular and intracellular fluid compartments. The commonest cause of hyperkalaemia is renal failure, both acute and chronic. The combination of salt wasting and hyperkalaemia should suggest adrenal insufficiency, primary hypoaldosteronism or pseudohypoaldosteronism. Hyperkalaemia is also a recognized complication of the use of ACE-inhibitors, particularly if there is coexisting reduction in effective circulating volume and consequent low GFR. In addition, potassium-sparing diuretics are likely to induce hyperkalaemia if the GFR is low for any reason. The key factors in the evaluation of hyperkalaemia are the GFR and plasma aldosterone levels (Figure 12.9).

KEY LEARNING POINTS

- Clinical assessment of extracellular fluid volume is essential in the evaluation of hyponatraemia and hypernatraemia, since the total body sodium may be normal, increased or decreased.

- Oral rehydration therapy in diarrhoeal-induced hyponatraemia and hypernatraemia is safe in children who are not shocked.
- The commonest cause of hypokalaemia in children is extrarenal loss in acute or chronic gastrointestinal disease.
- Hyperkalaemia may result from an increase in total body potassium or from maldistribution between the extracellular and intracellular fluid compartments.

COMMON ACID–BASE ABNORMALITIES

Cellular, tissue and organ systems function best with an extracellular pH of 7.35–7.45. pH is a mathematical expression of H^+ ion concentration *viz.* pH = $-\log[H^+]$. The concentration of H^+ ion at pH 7.00 is 100 nmol/L and 40 nmol/L at pH 7.40. Within the range of pH of 7.26 and 7.45, H^+ concentration can be estimated as [80 − the decimal of the pH].

Physiological pH is maintained by several buffer systems designed to maintain a stable H^+ ion concentration. The most important of these buffer systems and the one that enables identification of the major acid base abnormalities is the bicarbonate (HCO_3)/carbonic acid (H_2CO_3) system. HCO_3 represents the metabolic component of the buffer pair and PCO_2 (as the major component of H_2CO_3), represents the respiratory component. The HCO_3 can be estimated by measuring the total carbon dioxide content (T_{CO_2}) in venous serum or plasma and it is also possible to derive the HCO_3 from arterial blood, using the Henderson–Hasselbalch equation: $HCO_3 = 24 \times PCO_2/[H^+]$. It should be remembered that the estimated value is 1–3 mmol/L higher than the derived value. When an underlying disease process generates an acid–base disorder by increasing or decreasing HCO_3 or PCO_2, the other is adjusted in the same direction by physiological compensation in order to reduce the magnitude of change in pH. Compensation is defined as *absent* if the opposing variable is unchanged, *partial* if the opposing variable has changed but the pH remains abnormal and *full* if the pH is normal.

The first step in the assessment of acidaemia (low pH) and alkalaemia (high pH) is to establish the directional change (up or down) in HCO_3 and PCO_2 and to make a judgement as to whether this explains the change in pH. In a simple disorder (Table 12.10) alteration in only one of these variables will account for the change in pH.

Table 12.10 Simple acid–base disorders

	Metabolic acidosis	Metabolic alkalosis	Respiratory acidosis	Respiratory alkalosis
Primary change	$\downarrow HCO_3$	$\uparrow HCO_3$	$\uparrow PCO_2$	$\downarrow PCO_2$
Compensation	$\downarrow PCO_2$	$\uparrow PCO_2$	$\uparrow HCO_3$	$\downarrow HCO_3$
Effect on pH	↓pH	↑pH	↓pH	↑pH

CASE STUDY: Acid–base disorders

A 6-week-old infant who had been admitted 24 hours previously with acute bronchiolitis is noted to have had a progressive rise in respiratory and heart rate and increasing oxygen requirement. On examination, he was in significant respiratory distress with widespread crepitations audible on auscultation and had an O_2 saturation of 92 per cent in 2 L/minute of oxygen. A sample of capillary blood revealed the following results: pH 7.26 ($[H^+]$ 54 nmol/L), PCO_2 60 mmHg and PO_2 45 mmHg. A simultaneous venous sample revealed a plasma HCO_3 of 26 mmol/L.

The primary event in **respiratory acidosis** is a rise in PCO_2 and, during the acute phase, i.e. up to 24 hours, only buffering takes place but after this period, renal compensation takes place with the generation of additional HCO_3.

CASE STUDY: Acid–base disorders

A 4-year-old girl presents with a two-day history of fever and general malaise and a one-day history of headache. On admission she was drowsy and had evidence of meningism. She was also noted to be tachypnoeic but chest auscultation, oxygen saturation and chest radiograph were normal. Lumbar puncture revealed elevated CSF protein and reduced glucose and microscopy showed 250 polymorphs/mm^3 and Gram-positive cocci. In view of the tachypnoea, capillary blood gas was analysed. The pH was 7.52, PCO_2 25 mmHg, and the HCO_3 on a venous sample was 21 mmol/L.

The initial event in **primary respiratory alkalosis** is a fall in PCO_2. Buffering occurs as a result of release of $[H^+]$ from the cells and within several hours there is a compensatory increase in renal HCO_3 excretion. Disorders that drive ventilation independent of CO_2 resulting in a

Table 12.11 Differential diagnosis of metabolic acidosis

High plasma anion gap	Normal plasma anion gap
Ketoacidosis e.g. diabetic, starvation	Gastrointestinal HCO_3 loss **(+ve UAG)** e.g. diarrhoea, bowel augmentation, cystoplasty
Renal failure	Renal HCO_3 loss **(−ve UAG)** e.g. renal tubular acidosis, acetazolamide, Fanconi syndrome
Other e.g. intoxication with ethylene glycol, methanol, salicylate, lactic acidosis either primary or secondary to circulatory failure	Other e.g. total parenteral nutrition, cholestyramine, adrenal insufficiency

respiratory alkalosis, include inflammatory and mass lesions of the CNS, psychiatric disorders and centrally acting drugs and chemicals, e.g. salicylates. Other causes are hypoxaemia secondary to pneumonia, pulmonary oedema, and thromboembolism and hypovolaemia.

CASE STUDY: Acid–base disorders

A breastfed term neonate born by SVD presented in the postnatal ward at the age of 30 hours with reluctance to feed and abdominal distension. On examination, she was generally unwell looking with poor peripheral perfusion and tachypnoea. A venous blood culture was taken and she was given 20 mL/kg of 4.5 per cent human albumin solution and intravenous cefotaxime and metronidazole. An arterial sample showed a pH of 7.15, PCO_2 33 mmHg and base deficit 12. Plasma HCO_3 was 12 mmol/L and lactate was 6 mmol/L. At laparotomy four hours later, several centimetres of ischaemic small bowel were removed.

The primary event in **metabolic acidosis** is a fall in the HCO_3 and the compensatory fall in PCO_2 is due to stimulation of CNS receptors by the low pH. The **plasma anion gap** [(Na + K) − (Cl + HCO_3)] is the key assessment in the differentiation of the causes of metabolic acidosis into those with an excess of circulating acid, e.g. ketoacidosis, lactic acidosis and those with a loss of HCO_3 (Table 12.11). In distinguishing an extrarenal from a renal cause of a normal anion gap metabolic acidosis, estimation of the **urinary anion gap [(UNa + UK) − UCl]** is more useful than estimation of the urinary pH. Urinary ammonium is a much more sensitive indicator of the renal response to acidosis and since it is excreted in the urine as ammonium chloride, the urinary chloride is used as a proxy for ammonium. In renal hyperchloraemic acidosis, urinary acidification is deficient, i.e. (UNa − UK) > UCl.

Table 12.12 Differential diagnosis of metabolic alkalosis

Volume deplete/ Chloride sensitive	Volume replete/ Chloride unresponsive
Upper gastrointestinal losses e.g. vomiting, nasogastric suction Chronic diuretic therapy Cystic fibrosis Chronic respiratory failure	Cushing syndrome Non-salt-losing congenital adrenal hyperplasia Bartter syndrome Hypoaldosteronism, primary, secondary, pseudo Severe potassium deficiency Liquorice ingestion

CASE STUDY: Acid–base disorders

A 6-week-old formula fed boy presented with a five-day history of increasingly forceful vomiting with no associated diarrhoea or reluctance to feed. On examination he was restless but alert, and mildly dehydrated. A test feed revealed a pyloric tumour that was later confirmed on abdominal ultrasound scan. Capillary blood revealed a pH of 7.54, PCO_2 48 mmHg and base excess 11. Plasma HCO_3 was recorded as 33 mmol/L and plasma sodium 129 mmol/L.

The primary event in **metabolic alkalosis** is a rise in plasma HCO_3. The resultant increase in pH leads to compensatory hypoventilation and a rise in PCO_2. The key assessment in the differentiation of the causes of metabolic alkalosis is the urinary Cl concentration as this is a better indicator of the status of extracellular fluid volume than urinary Na and a value of <20 mmol/L indicates depletion (Table 12.12).

CASE STUDY: Acid–base disorders

A 12-year-old boy with advanced chronic respiratory failure secondary to cystic fibrosis was admitted with cor pulmonale and was started on regular diuretic therapy. Capillary blood on admission revealed a pH of 7.32, PCO_2 80 mmhg and base excess 6. Plasma HCO_3 was recorded as 41 mmol/L. The pH was 7.41 48 hours later and the plasma HCO_3 49 mmol/L with no change in PCO_2. His condition stabilized after one week and the diuretic therapy was stopped. Unfortunately he then developed acute gastroenteritis secondary to rotavirus and repeat investigation showed a pH of 7.1, PCO_2 80 mmHg and plasma HCO_3 of 24 mmol/L.

The above case demonstrates an example of a **mixed acid–base disorder**, i.e. respiratory acidosis/metabolic alkalosis and respiratory acidosis/metabolic acidosis. In contrast to simple disorders, the change in **both HCO_3** and PCO_2 can explain the observed change in pH, however the variable with the bigger percentage change indicates the major component of the mixed disorder.

KEY LEARNING POINTS

- The first step in the evaluation of acidaemia and alkalaemia is to establish the directional change in PCO_2 and HCO_3 and to make a judgement as to whether this explains the change in pH.
- The plasma anion gap is essential for the differentiation of metabolic acidosis.
- The urinary anion gap is important for the differentiation of a normal plasma anion gap metabolic acidosis.
- The urinary chloride is important in the evaluation of metabolic alkalosis.
- In contrast to a simple acid–base disorder in which a change in PCO_2 *or* HCO_3 explains the change in pH, in a mixed disorder change in both measures can explain the change in pH.

COMMON UROLOGICAL PROBLEMS

Undescended testis

There are several reasons for failure to palpate the testis. Perhaps the commonest is where the testis descends normally but is difficult to palpate as in the obese child, if masked by the external oblique muscle or if retractile. Less commonly, a testis maybe congenitally absent, one or both maybe cryptorchid (intra-abdominal, groin, suprascrotal or gliding) or ectopic (perineal or inguinal).

If the testis cannot be palpated in the scrotum by 12 weeks of age surgical referral is indicated. In the patient with bilateral undescended testes, abdominal ultrasound and karyotyping should be carried out and human chorionic gonadotrophin (hCG) stimulation considered in order to establish the presence of testicular tissue. The examination of choice to detect intra-abdominal testes is laparoscopy and orchidopexy should be undertaken around 12 months of age in order to maximize long-term fertility. There is an increased risk of malignancy in children with cryptorchid testes that is not altered by orchidopexy, however, fixing the testis in the scrotum allows early detection of tumour development. Intra-abdominal testes that cannot be brought down into the scrotum and small unilateral atrophic testes should be removed.

Hypospadias

This is due to a failure of the urethral folds to unite over and cover the urethral groove. As a result, the urethral meatus is situated proximal to the glans, the foreskin is hooded and in severe forms, there is chordee that causes abnormal curvature of the penis. The incidence is 1 in 300 boys and the classification is based on the position of the urethral meatus, i.e. anterior (65 per cent), middle (15 per cent) and posterior (20 per cent).

In mild forms urinary tract imaging is unnecessary, as the incidence of associated abnormality is very low. In severe forms, particularly if associated with undescended testis, abdominal ultrasound, MCUG and karyotyping should be performed. Surgical repair, both single-stage for minor degrees and two-stage for more significant deformities, is carried out between 6 and 18 months of age.

Indications for circumcision

Balanitis obliterans xerotica or lichen sclerosis et atrophicus causes severe phimosis and is the only absolute indication for circumcision. Other relative indications are recurrent balanitis, paraphimosis and for religious and cultural reasons.

Wilms tumour

This is one of the commonest paediatric solid tumours and usually presents with an abdominal mass before the age of 2 years. Hypertension may be present in 25 per cent and haematuria in 15 per cent. Wilms tumour may occur in isolation or in association with a syndromic diagnosis such as WAGR and Denys–Drash. Three genetic loci have been linked with Wilms tumour, two on chromosome 11 (p13 and 15) and one on chromosome 17 (q12–21), however the mode of operation of these loci remains unclear.

The main differential diagnosis of an abdominal mass in a child <2 years is that of neuroblastoma. The presence of calcification on abdominal radiograph supports the diagnosis of neuroblastoma. Abdominal ultrasound and CT will define whether the mass is solid or cystic, the relationship to the kidney, enlargement of para-aortic lymph nodes and assessment of invasion of tumour thrombus in the renal vein or inferior vena cava. Computed tomography is the preferred imaging for staging, that also includes laparotomy and histology, which is favourable in 90 per cent:

1 Tumour localized to the kidney and completely excised
2 Tumour extends beyond the kidney but completely excised
3 Residual intra-abdominal tumour due to incomplete excision or peritoneal spill due to tumour rupture
4 Haematological spread to liver, lung, bone and brain
5 Bilateral Wilms tumour (occurs in 5 per cent).

Chemotherapy is indicated in tumours considered inoperable, in very large tumours where the risk of rupture is significant, in bilateral disease, in the presence of intracaval extension of tumour thrombus and for stage 4 disease.

The acute scrotum

The presence of an acutely tender and swollen scrotum should alert one to the possibility of **testicular torsion,** the commonest cause of an acute scrotum in childhood with an incidence of 1 in 4000 and a surgical emergency. The testis on the affected side is high in the scrotum due to shortening of the spermatic cord secondary to the twist and the presence of a transverse lie of the contralateral testis supports the diagnosis. Doppler ultrasound will show diminished testicular blood supply but urgent surgical exploration should not be deferred.

Differential diagnosis of the acute scrotum

Testicular torsion
Torsion of the appendix testis
Acute epididymitis
Idiopathic oedema of the scrotum
Trauma
HSP

The clinical presentation of **torsion of the appendix testis** is similar but palpation early in the clinical course may reveal a tender nodule in relation to the testis or epididymis. Doppler ultrasound shows a normal testicular blood supply and conservative management is appropriate. **Acute epididymitis** is suggested by a preceding history of dysuria or increased urinary frequency or the presence of a urethral discharge. At an early stage, palpation will reveal localized epididymal tenderness and Doppler ultrasound will show increased blood supply. Management is with a combination of broad-spectrum antibiotics and analgesia. The finding of oedema of the scrotum with no testicular or epididymal tenderness, associated with erythema either limited to the scrotum or extending into the perineum or upper thigh is suggestive of **acute idiopathic oedema of the scrotum.** The aetiology is unknown but is thought to have an allergic basis and the condition resolves rapidly without treatment. Finally, an **incarcerated inguinal hernia** may present for the first time with an acute tender swelling of the upper scrotum and groin associated with vomiting and abdominal pain. Urgent surgical exploration is necessary.

FURTHER READING

Belman B, King LR, Kramer SA (eds) (2002) *Clinical Pediatric Urology*, 4th edn. London: Martin Dunitz.

Webb NJA, Postlewaithe RJ (eds) (2003) *Clinical Paediatric Nephrology*, 3rd edn. Oxford: Oxford Medical Publications.

Chapter 13

Diabetes

Kenneth J Robertson

BASIC KNOWLEDGE

ANATOMY

The endocrine pancreas comprises 1–2 million islets of Langerhans – these are nests of cells, ~70 per cent of which are insulin-producing β-cells. The rest produce glucagon (α-cells), somatostatin (δ-cells) and pancreatic polypeptide (PP-cells).

EPIDEMIOLOGY

Type 1 diabetes mellitus is mainly a disease of white populations with marked geographical variation in incidence. The incidence is highest in Finland (50/100 000 per year under 15 years) and other northern European countries, but there are anomalies. Sardinia has an incidence of more than 30/100 000 per year. Japan, on the other hand, has an incidence of only around 2/100 000 per year. However, in almost all areas studied, the annual incidence is rising at a rate (often around 2–3 per cent per annum) hugely greater than that which could be explained by genetics. Careful study (e.g. via the EuroDiab programme) has established that these are true secular trends and not simply a result of improving registration systems.

AETIOLOGY

The vast majority of children with diabetes have type 1 disease of autoimmune aetiology. However, this is a heterogeneous condition with numerous potential triggering factors on a background of genetic susceptibility. At least 20 genes have been implicated in the latter including the human leucocyte antigen (HLA) and insulin genes, but the genetic contribution to disease has been calculated to be around 40 per cent so environmental factors are obviously important. Although none have yet been conclusively identified, several possible triggers have been proposed. Of these, viral infections (particularly with enteroviruses) have been extensively studied and associations found with the onset of autoimmunity, which often begins in the first year or two of life. Other potential aetiological agents are early introduction of cow's milk protein and dietary nitrates, but neither has been demonstrated to be causal in humans. A process of T-cell mediated progressive destruction of the pancreatic β-cells culminates in the presentation of diabetes with a peak age of onset of 10–14 years. It is possible that the process of decline in β-cell function is non-linear and that second or third environmental insults are involved.

DIAGNOSIS AND INITIAL MANAGEMENT

'Walking wounded'

When β-cell function has reached around 10–20 per cent, insulin production is barely sufficient and any additional stress renders it inadequate. This explains why pyrexial illness or even a stressful event may be associated with the onset of symptoms. In regions with a high incidence of type 1 diabetes, the majority of children present in the 'walking wounded' category with no metabolic decompensation. The key symptoms are polyuria, polydipsia and weight loss. Hyperglycaemia is a direct result of insulin deficiency, which causes reduced peripheral uptake of glucose but also counterregulatory hormone (glucagon, growth hormone, cortisol)-induced glucose production via gluconeogenesis and glycogenolysis of stores in liver and muscle. The renal threshold for glucose is around 10 mmol/L so glycosuria precipitates polyuria with thirst, which then triggers polydipsia. The thirst in diabetes is obviously pathological – it is extreme and distressing if not slaked. Children will often drink many litres, frequently even of things they did not previously like, and the thirst continues through the night which is, in any case, usually interrupted by the repeated need to urinate. Diabetes must always be considered immediately in cases of secondary nocturnal enuresis.

Diagnosis is confirmed by the history, usually of several weeks duration, and the finding of glycosuria (with or without ketonuria, see below) and hyperglycaemia. Occasionally a child presents with a suggestive history but with no supporting laboratory evidence. It is then necessary to conduct a glucose tolerance test. Haemoglobin A1c (Hb A1c) should not be used alone for diagnostic purposes but elevation may be taken as supportive evidence. The differential diagnosis includes psychogenic polydipsia (unassociated with weight loss and rarely nocturnal) and diabetes insipidus (very rare and easily distinguished by lack of glycosuria). Compulsive juice drinking by toddlers is common and easily distinguished by degree from pathology.

Autoantibodies to islet cells, insulin, glutamic acid decarboxylase (GAD) and others are found in 85–98 per cent of children with type 1 disease at presentation. It is rarely necessary to measure these but in cases of doubt about the type of diabetes, testing can be helpful if not diagnostic.

KEY LEARNING POINTS

- Transient hyperglycaemia may be associated with stress or pain.
- Be very reluctant to diagnose type 1 diabetes without a supportive history.

Ketoacidosis

Delay in the diagnosis of type 1 diabetes inevitably leads to the development of ketoacidosis. Prolonged hyperglycaemia temporarily 'paralyses' the remaining β-cells so that a state of complete insulin deficiency ensues. Counterregulatory hormones then provoke lipolyis with a consequent increase in plasma non-esterified fatty acids which are converted to ketone bodies by β-oxidation (Figure 13.1). Ketosis often causes abdominal pain and vomiting with abdominal muscle rigidity – occasionally mistaken for a surgical problem – and further dehydration. The reduction in pH in ketoacidosis is a consequence of both ketone production and peripheral lactic acidosis secondary to decreased peripheral perfusion.

The combination of continuing polyuria despite shock and deep sighing respiration should prompt the diagnosis of diabetes when combined with the prodromal history of polyuria, polydipsia and weight loss.

Kussmaul breathing is an attempt to blow off acid and, although regularly mistaken as a sign of respiratory illness, once witnessed is never forgotten. The lung fields are clear, there is no stridor, and chest expansion and air entry are increased.

The management of ketoacidosis should involve the use of a predefined protocol tailored for local circumstances (see the website www.diabetes-scotland.org for examples). The following principles must be adopted:

- correction of shock
- steady replacement of fluid deficit
- commencement of intravenous (IV) insulin.

Diabetic ketoacidosis carries significant morbidity and mortality that can be minimized by meticulous attention to details of treatment with scrupulous monitoring of

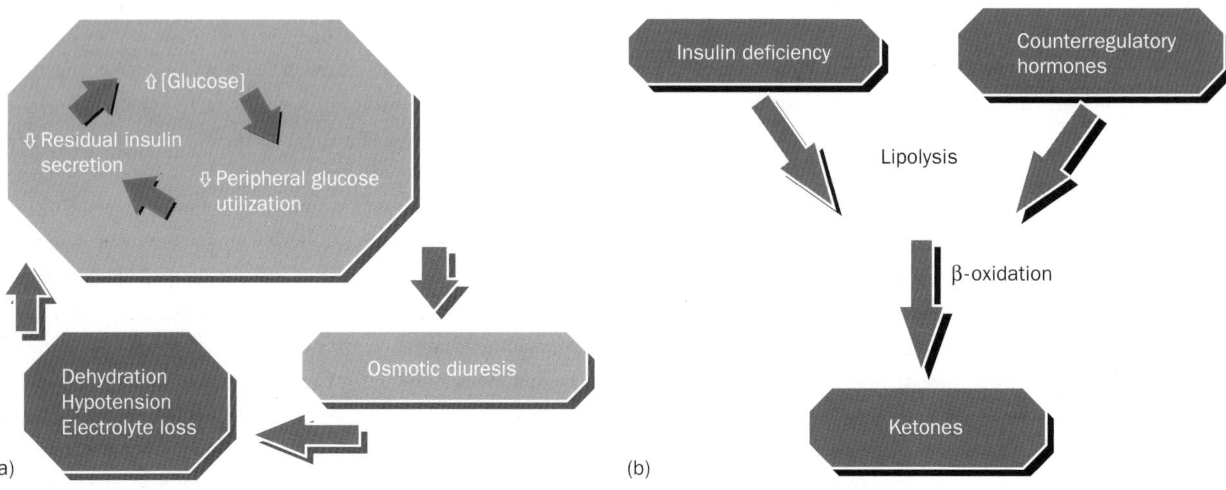

Figure 13.1 Type 1 diabetes: (a) disordered carbohydrate metabolism and (b) disordered lipid metabolism.

response. Cerebral oedema is the commonest cause of death, its onset usually 6 to 18 hours after beginning treatment heralded by reduction in consciousness and headache. Contrary to popular belief, the cause is not understood, and is not solely due to overhydration, but hypotonic fluids should be avoided.

KEY LEARNING POINTS

- Even very dehydrated patients may still be polyuric because of osmotic diuresis.
- Fluid replacement in diabetic ketoacidosis (DKA) should always be according to the local protocol.
- Hourly neurological observation and attention to detail is essential.
- Bicarbonate should not be used in the treatment of DKA.

Commencing insulin and the honeymoon period

Subcutaneous insulin should be commenced as soon as rehydration and restoration of acid–base status have been achieved. There is no justification for continuing IV insulin on a sliding scale until 'blood sugars have stabilized'. Choice of insulin regimen is discussed below but it is usually possible to move straight to this from IV insulin without the need for a period on four to six hourly subcutaneous soluble insulin. A 30-minute gap should be left between the first subcutaneous injection and the discontinuation of IV insulin to allow time for absorption and to prevent rebound ketosis.

Initial insulin resistance usually wanes after 7 to 10 days of treatment. The temporary return of endogenous insulin production results in a fall in the dose required. This 'honeymoon period' may last weeks or months, during which time blood glucose control is often extremely good. Controversy exists over whether aggressive initial therapy (IV or subcutaneous insulin) affects duration.

THE DIABETES TEAM

The patient (and their family) is the most important member of the diabetes care team. Self-management is crucial and the major contributor to the success of care, measured in terms of short-, medium- and long-term outcomes. Diabetes is unlike most chronic diseases in that it cannot be ignored even for a single day. Accordingly, the emphasis should be upon providing the family with the tools to look after it on a day-to-day basis. This is the role of the multidisciplinary diabetes team.

Insulin is an essential mainstay but it has to be balanced by a carefully regulated intake of food. The paediatric dietitian is skilled in helping children (and their families) adjust to the regular eating required and to understand the elements of diet – carbohydrate, protein and fat. Traditionally, the advice has concentrated upon carbohydrates but the 'diabetic diet' now pays attention to the requirement to restrict the intake of saturated fat because of its associations with obesity and macrovascular morbidity. The major issue for most children is regulation of sweet intake and they have to be taught to limit these to pre-exercise and occasionally at the end of starchy meals when the simple carbohydrate absorption from the gut will be delayed. In the UK, exhortation to increase the intake of fruit and vegetables is frequently necessary.

A diabetes nurse specialist usually provides much of the teaching and they will get to know the family well. This familiarity is essential because the context of care must be understood before change can be implemented. For example, knowledge of housing or marital circumstances can alter profoundly the interventions that are appropriate. A vital early task is to teach the family about blood glucose monitoring which must be undertaken regularly. Interpretation and action upon the results is the cornerstone of self-management. Except in environments without access to blood glucose monitoring equipment, urine glucose monitoring has no role in the care of type 1 disease.

The diabetes team should have ready access to support from psychology because psychological problems are common in any chronic disease. In diabetes, frequent issues are needle phobia, fear of hypoglycaemia and low self-esteem. The effect of anxiety upon blood sugar control can be dramatic – presumably mediated via adrenaline – and so intervention is urgent. Social problems such as housing issues and the effect of poverty upon dietary choices are common so close liaison with social services is essential.

Most diabetes teams have a predefined programme of teaching for new families. They will also provide continuing support both in the community and via the clinic. The degree of support lessens as families become accustomed to managing diabetes but needs also change with the age of the child. A point of particular importance is the recognition that when a child develops diabetes at a young age, the parents are solely responsible for care. As the child grows, the transfer of knowledge and understanding of the condition has to be managed otherwise wrong assumptions may be made about an adolescent's skills just because 'she has had diabetes for 10 years'.

UNUSUAL DIABETES

Paediatric diabetes has not traditionally been a diagnostic speciality, but this is beginning to change because of increased understanding of the genetics of the condition and also because of secular changes in society. In the USA, some states are now reporting as many as 50 per cent of new adolescents with diabetes are type 2. This is predominantly because of a dramatic increase in obesity and sedentary behaviour. Native Americans and those of Hispanic origin are genetically at higher risk and account for most such patients but type 2 diabetes is also appearing in white children and adolescents with the incidence expected to rise. Diabetes in cystic fibrosis is usually due to involvement of the pancreatic islets in the general destruction of the exocrine pancreas. The incidence is increasing because of longer survival in cystic fibrosis. At least five types of mature-onset diabetes of the young (MODY) have now been identified, each due to a single gene defect. Accordingly, the term 'monogenic diabetes' is now preferred. These conditions are all rare and associated with a family history of early-onset diabetes. Unless genetic diagnostic facilities are available, they are mainly treated like type 1. A variety of syndromes are associated with glucose intolerance and diabetes, e.g. Bardet-Biedl, Prader–Willi and Pearson syndromes as well as congenital muscular dystrophies.

Neonatal diabetes is rare and usually transient. It is associated with low birth weight and is thought to be due to late switching-on of insulin production. It is often related to unipaternal isodisomy of the short arm of chromosome 6.

Aetiological classification of diabetes (World Health Organization, 2001)

1 Type 1 diabetes (β-cell destruction, usually leading to absolute insulin deficiency)
   - Immune-mediated
   - Idiopathic
2 Type 2 diabetes (may range from predominantly insulin resistance with relative insulin deficiency to a predominantly secretory defect with insulin resistance)
3 Other specific types
   - Genetic defects of insulin action (e.g. lipoatrophic diabetes)
   - Genetic defects of β-cell function (e.g. MODY)
   - Diseases of the exocrine pancreas (e.g. cystic fibrosis)
   - Endocrinopathies (e.g. Cushing syndrome)
   - Drug- or chemical-induced (e.g. glucocorticoids)
   - Infections (e.g. congenital rubella)
   - Uncommon forms of immune-mediated diabetes
   - Other genetic syndromes sometimes associated with diabetes (e.g. Prader–Willi syndrome)
4 Gestational diabetes mellitus

TECHNOLOGY

The daily grind of managing diabetes has been eased and the outcomes improved by the application of technology to the processes of delivering insulin. For the economically privileged, these advances are likely to offer independence from insulin injection within a few years but many more will benefit from advances in injection systems and blood glucose monitoring equipment. Insulin technology itself continues to make important contributions to care. Many children now deliver their insulin with pen systems. These make the 'drawing-up' of doses simpler, speed the injection process and some models even record details of the last dose, which is invaluable to parents, e.g. at the end of a school day.

Insulin pump therapy is popular in the USA and northern Europe but uptake in the UK has been minimal, largely due to differences in funding arrangements. There is little evidence that these devices improve overall blood glucose control but they probably reduce the incidence of severe hypoglycaemia and can markedly improve quality of life for some patients because of the greater flexibility around eating. Pump use demands particularly careful self-monitoring.

Inhaled insulin will soon become a commercial reality. It will be for use around meal times and will require to be used with a basal (long-acting) insulin which will still need to be injected, albeit less frequently. Concerns remain around the safety of long-term use.

Blood testing is the bane of most patients' lives. New systems allow collection of tiny aliquots of blood from sites other than sensitive fingertips and these are proving popular. A variety of bloodless glucose monitoring systems are appearing on the market. All are expensive and rather limited in application but advances in this sector are expected to be rapid.

Much exciting work is being done in the field of biotechnology, with recent publicity for the Edmonton protocol of steroid-sparing immunosuppression allied to intrahepatic injection of cadaveric pancreatic islets. Such work is fascinating but many obstacles (not least the availability of suitable β-cells) have to be overcome before such procedures become routine.

PREVENTION

Although type 2 diabetes associated with obesity and sedentary lifestyle has been shown to be preventable with behaviour modification, this is not true of type 1 diabetes. Several immune interventions have been tried and have failed, and two large studies have recently reported negative results: the European Nicotinamide Diabetes Intervention Trial (ENDIT) and the Diabetes Prevention Trial Type-1 (DPT-1) in the USA, which intervened with low-dose subcutaneous insulin or oral insulin in those at high risk of developing the disease. ENDIT was an attempt to reduce chromosomal damage in the T-cell-mediated autoimmune attack and DPT-1 to alter the immune response to a putative autoantigen. Since no intervention is known to work, it is unethical to test the autoantibody status of any child outwith the structure of an intervention trial.

CORE SYSTEM PROBLEMS

INSULIN REGIMEN

The choice of insulin regimen should be based upon knowledge of the patient's lifestyle, activity levels and eating plan. Necessarily this may change and flexibility by the diabetes team is important. Choice is often also influenced by cultural norms. In most of northern Europe, a multiple injection, basal bolus system is usual, but in the UK, most children are still on twice daily premixed insulin. In Scotland, a recent shift towards a three injection per day regimen with premix before breakfast, soluble before the evening meal and isophane insulin in the late evening has failed to improve the average Hb A1c. However, there is some evidence that this is less likely to be associated with nocturnal hypoglycaemia and that it is also beneficial in combating the dawn phenomenon of blood glucose rising in the early hours of the morning because of release of growth hormone and sex hormones during puberty. In many instances, the incorporation of a lunchtime injection of insulin is made more difficult by issues around assistance at school and reluctance of children to be seen injecting by their friends.

Rapid-acting insulin analogues have proved popular partly because their rapid onset of action obviates the requirement with soluble insulin of leaving a 30-minute gap between injection and food. The new ultra-long-acting analogues may offer a good platform of basal insulin on which to apply boluses of rapid-acting insulin but their best use in children has yet to be clarified. Insulin pump programmes now routinely use rapid-acting insulin analogues. Currently, there is a push towards using basal bolus regimens with long- and short-acting analogues in children and adolescents. It is vital to realize that such changes will only help if accompanied by intensive dietetic and nursing support as the insulin must be tailored to food intake.

Whatever regimen a patient uses, it is important for them and their family to understand what the components do and how to adjust them. Most centres now provide written guidance. An example is shown in Figure 13.2.

HYPOGLYCAEMIA

Fear of hypoglycaemia underpins many of the difficulties associated with managing diabetes. Children fear ostracism at school if they collapse or do something embarrassing while 'hypo' and parents worry about unnoticed nocturnal hypoglycaemia and sudden death. Although it is a key aim of treatment to avoid debilitating hypoglycaemia, it is an inevitable consequence of good glucose control that there will be occasional mild hypoglycaemic symptoms. Most well-controlled patients will report symptomatic hypoglycaemia once or twice per week. Of course, this usually occurs for a known reason – late for a meal or snack or extra exercise without extra carbohydrate. Learning to recognize risk situations and to take avoiding action (usually an extra snack) receives major emphasis in early teaching. Similarly, ability to recognize early symptoms and knowing how to deal with them effectively, but not over-enthusiastically, is vital.

KEY POINTS

- Hypoglycaemia is always due to hyperinsulinaemia – either absolute or relative to ambient blood glucose.
- Follow treatment with rapid-acting carbohydrate with a starchy carbohydrate, e.g. a biscuit, to prevent recurrence.
- Families of children with diabetes should all have glucagon and know when and how to use it.

What to do if your blood glucose results are too low or too high?

Aim for most blood glucose results to be in the 'target range' of 4–10 mmol/L.
If three consecutive results, at the same time of day, are *not* in the 'target range', consider:

1 Diet : time of day, amount and type of food eaten
2 Exercise : time of day, amount of activity and food taken before activity
3 Injections : time of day, time before meals and if injection sites healthy
4 Illness : see 'Sick Day' guidelines (Figure 13.3)

Once these factors have been considered, adjustment of insulin dosage is required

How to adjust insulin doses?

The following questions need to be answered in order to appropriately adjust insulin dosage:

1 Whether to increase or decrease the insulin dose
2 When to adjust the insulin dose
3 How much to adjust the insulin

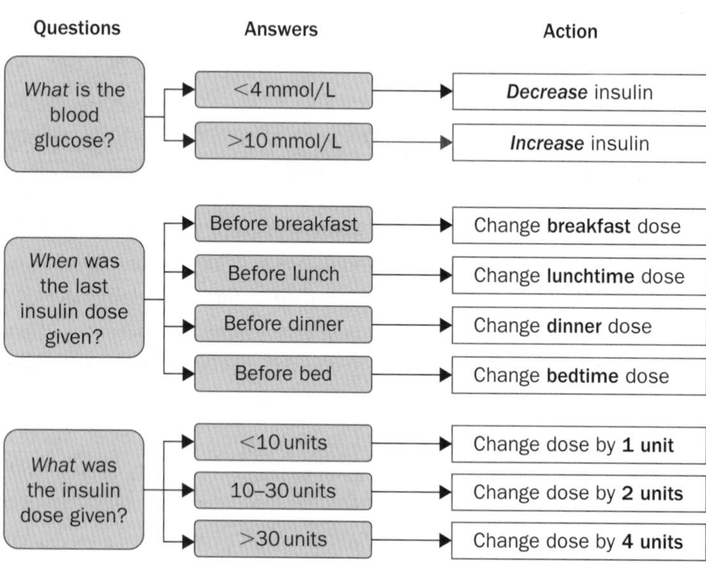

Figure 13.2 What to do if your blood glucose results are too low or too high: an example of written guidance (courtesy of Dr I Craigie)

Hypoglycaemic unawareness

CASE STUDY

A well-controlled 10-year-old girl with diabetes complains that she has had three episodes of hypoglycaemia at school in the last week with no warning.

In some ways, all toddlers are hypoglycaemia unaware and this is a major reason why it is dangerous to strive too officiously for tight control in this group. However, the term is normally reserved for those who have previously recognized 'hypo' symptoms but lose the ability to do so. Characteristically, this occurs in two situations:

- when blood glucose control has been very tight for some time, perhaps with frequent mild 'hypos'
- following one or more severe hypoglycaemic episodes.

The dangers of this situation are obvious with the risk of severe neuroglycopenia leading to sudden collapse and loss of consciousness before any autonomic warnings. Fortunately, it is usually possible to reverse this unawareness by allowing control to be less tight and studiously avoiding all hypoglycaemia for a few months. There is no good evidence that hypoglycaemic unawareness is more prevalent in those using human as opposed to porcine or bovine insulins.

Surreptitious insulin administration

> **CASE STUDY**
>
> A 9-year-old boy, who previously had poor control, has recently dropped his Hb A1c by 2 per cent to 8 per cent. His insulin requirement has fallen from 1 U/kg per day to 0.75 U/kg per day, but he continues to have hypoglycaemic attacks, two of which required glucagon administration by his mother. These episodes have all been in the late evening despite him eating his evening meal and bedtime snack. He has not been particularly active and his weight has risen slightly on the centile chart.

This is not an uncommon scenario. A move from hypertrophied injection sites to a fresh area can be responsible for a fall in insulin requirement and more 'hypos'. Weight gain in conjunction with hypoglycaemia should trigger a check of thyroid function and antithyroid antibodies. However, the timing of episodes has to be taken into account. This boy gave his own insulin injections and resented not being able to eat sweets in the evenings like his friends. Since he knew that his blood sugar results before bed would betray sweet eating, he had taken to giving himself extra insulin in the evenings. Management of such a situation is not usually too difficult although outright confrontation is rarely helpful. It is frequently only necessary to have a general discussion around the possible causes and to indicate that taking extra insulin is potentially very dangerous. Recognition of the motivation is also important and allowing some sweets after a starchy evening meal may remove the problem. In a few instances, it may be necessary to seek help from a psychologist with experience of diabetes.

SICK DAYS

> **CASE STUDY**
>
> A 5-year-old girl, who has had diabetes for two years, develops a viral infection with pyrexia and vomiting. Her parents are concerned and telephone for advice.

Understanding how to manage 'sick days' is a core competency in diabetes care. Many centres provide families with written guidance (Figure 13.3) on what to do but ready and informed telephone advice is also a vital element in minimizing hospital admission and reducing secondary ketoacidosis.

As with any problem, having accurate information is essential so the first step is to perform more blood glucose estimations than normal – hourly tests may be necessary. Without this information, it is hazardous to predict the correct treatment. In most pyrexial illnesses blood glucose would be expected to rise because of the increase in metabolic rate and increased insulin demand. However, young children often have gastroenteritic symptoms which reduce (or halt) intake/absorption of carbohydrate with likelihood of hypoglycaemia. Persistently low glucose readings may be an indication to reduce slightly the normal insulin doses but there is never a case for withholding insulin completely even if the child is taking nil-by-mouth, although hospital admission is likely to be necessary for the provision of fluids. High blood glucose readings should be a stimulus to check urinary ketones. 'Moderate' or 'large' ketonuria coupled with high glucose is a strong warning that ketoacidosis is imminent without urgent action. Extra insulin will be required and should be delivered as soluble or rapid-acting analogue. Doses may be repeated every two to three hours until the blood glucose responds. Throughout, the state of hydration is critical and fluids should be administered frequently and in small volumes. These should be both sugar-free and sugar-containing because it is important to try to maintain carbohydrate intake, e.g. in the form of high-energy drinks.

Parents need to know when admission is prudent and this should be before dehydration is established. Essentially, failure to control elevated blood glucose and ketone production and/or continued severe vomiting are absolute criteria for hospitalization. Other criteria include lack of parental confidence, exhaustion or geographical considerations.

> **KEY LEARNING POINTS**
>
> - Insulin should never be stopped during 'sick days'.
> - Extra blood testing is essential.
> - Extra insulin may be required.
> - Carbohydrate must still be given – usually in liquid form.

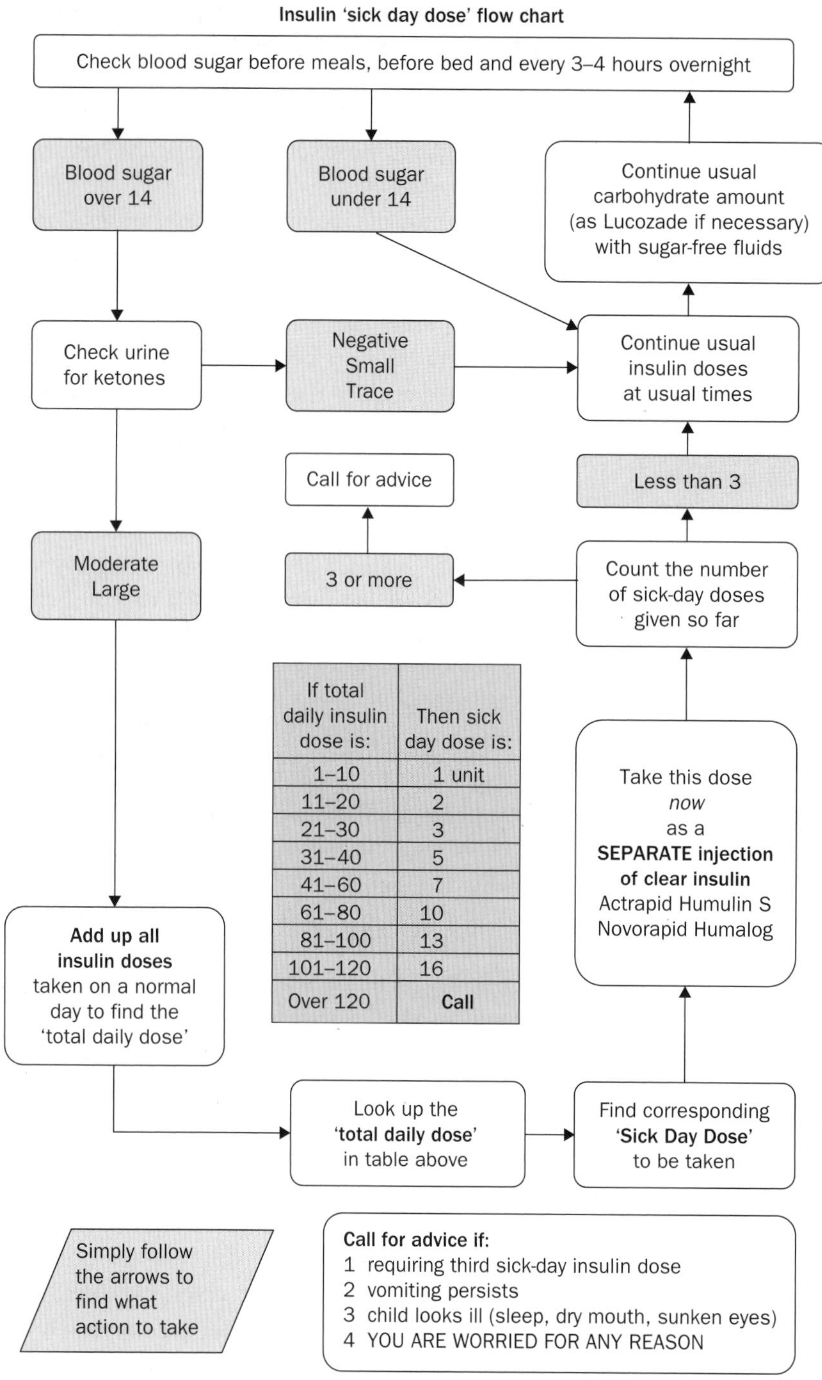

If total daily insulin dose is:	Then sick day dose is:
1–10	1 unit
11–20	2
21–30	3
31–40	5
41–60	7
61–80	10
81–100	13
101–120	16
Over 120	**Call**

Figure 13.3 An example flow chart for insulin 'sick day dose' (courtesy of Dr I Craigie)

ADOLESCENCE

CASE STUDY

A 14-year-old boy has a Hb A1c level of 12.5 per cent, although from diagnosis until recently it was running around 8 per cent. He is not interested in his diabetes.

Adolescence is traditionally a very difficult time in the management of diabetes. It is not surprising since the last thing individuals struggling to establish their own identity need is a health problem of such proportions that ignoring it, even for a short while, can be fatal. Many, if not most, teenagers regularly miss insulin injections and routinely eat outwith recommendations. The latter is, of course, entirely normal adolescent behaviour and, with the power of peer group pressure especially great in this age group, not surprising. Knowledge of this should shape the consultation when patients have very poor control. There is likely to be very little mileage in long discussions around subtle adjustment of insulin dose or addition or subtraction of small portions of carbohydrate from the diet. When control is very poor it is important to concentrate on the absolute basic requirement to take insulin. Often, compromising on the requirement to do blood tests relieves the pressure felt by the teenager. A non-judgemental approach to their poor adherence to the routine of diabetes can also help. The prime concerns when managing teenagers should be to keep them out of ketoacidosis and to keep them coming to clinic. Most adolescents will go through a period of rebellion against their diabetes and usually this is accompanied by a period of poor control. The evidence suggests that most will settle down but it can be a very traumatic time for both patient and carers waiting for this turnaround. Access to a psychologist is essential. It is important not to forget the increased physiological requirement for insulin during puberty and to ensure that sick days are managed tightly because deterioration to ketoacidosis is especially rapid when underlying metabolic control is poor.

TODDLERS

CASE STUDY

A mother is struggling to cope with a wilful 2-year-old with newly diagnosed diabetes who regularly refuses food.

Most toddlers are faddy eaters but are consistent enough for a standard insulin injection regimen to be sustainable. However, mealtimes can become a battleground and some children seem to relish the distress that refusal to eat causes their parents who fear consequent hypoglycaemia. This is, of course, in the context of a patient too young to recognize or articulate the sensations provoked by the autonomic signals engendered by hypoglycaemia. Paediatric dietetic advice may help with suggestions to leave finger-foods around so that falling blood glucose might provoke the child to eat. Failure should trigger a rethink of insulin strategy and one approach that lessens anxiety dramatically is to use fast-acting insulin analogues post prandially. These new insulins begin to act within 10 minutes of subcutaneous administration so a dose can be pegged to actual food consumed with minimization of the post-prandial glucose peak.

CO-MORBIDITY

Since diabetes is the commonest metabolic/endocrine disorder, it frequently occurs in individuals who have other diseases. However, other autoimmune diseases are more likely in someone who already has one. The conditions most frequently associated with diabetes are autoimmune hypothyroidism, coeliac disease and Addison disease, in that order. The majority of paediatric clinics in the UK now screen regularly for these although controversy remains around screening for antiendomysial antibodies in asymptomatic children. The imposition of a gluten-free diet is dependent upon a positive diagnosis by jejunal biopsy, but is still a difficult additional burden to bear when there has been no preceding bowel upset or disruption of growth. Clearly, there is no such dilemma when symptoms have provoked testing. Hypothyroidism should be suspected when insulin requirement falls and frequent 'hypos' occur, often accompanied by weight gain. It is unusual for this to progress to the classic signs of hypothyroidism before diagnosis. Addison disease is rare but lethargy, weakness, falling insulin requirement, 'hypos' and appearance of pigmentation are all characteristic.

COMPLICATIONS

The Diabetes Control and Complications Trial (DCCT) proved the strong association between long-term blood glucose control (as measured by Hb A1c) and the microvascular complications of retinopathy, nephropathy and neuropathy. Dramatic reductions in risk accompany tight control achieved by a combination of intensive insulin therapy and robust support from a dedicated diabetes team. In the DCCT, the intensively managed group also experienced a threefold increase in severe hypoglycaemia but no obvious, associated morbidity. Unfortunately, the youngest patient in the study was 13 years old and relatively few adolescents were included so recommendations tend to be extrapolations. Nonetheless, other evidence shows that the prepubertal period is not risk free so the aim should still be to achieve as good control of glucose as possible without debilitating hypoglycaemia.

Overt diabetic complications are rare in childhood but screening for microalbuminuria (a proved forerunner of proteinuria) and background retinopathy should begin early (see the guidelines of the International Society for Pediatric and Adolescent Diabetes (ISPAD), 2000) because effective interventions are available – angiotensin-converting enzyme (ACE)-inhibitor therapy and laser treatment, respectively.

The major killer in diabetes is macrovascular disease manifested as myocardial infarction and stroke. These are strongly correlated with hypertension and hyperlipidaemia. The evidence for monitoring and intervention for these problems in children is currently lacking but it is clear from other work that early dietary habits have a profound impact upon morbidity so emphasis upon getting it right from the outset is crucial.

KEY LEARNING POINTS

- Hb A1c should be measured every three to four months.
- Levels should be as low as possible without frequent or severe hypoglycaemia.
- Control should be slightly less tight in the under-5s.

FURTHER READING AND USEFUL WEBSITES

Children with diabetes. The on-line community for kids, families and adults with diabetes.
www.childrenwithdiabetes.com (accessed 1 November 2004).

Court S, Lamb W (eds) (1997) *Childhood and Adolescent Diabetes.* Chichester: Wiley.

Diabetes Control and Complications Trial Research Group (1993) The effect of intensive treatment of diabetes on the development and progression of long term complications in insulin dependent diabetes mellitus. *N Engl J Med* 329:977–86.

Diabetes Scotland Homepage. www.diabetes-scotland.org (accessed 1 November 2004).

Hanas R (2004) *Type 1 Diabetes in Children, Adolescents and Young Adults*, 2nd edn. London: Class Publishing.

International Society of Pediatric and Adolescent Diabetes. *Consensus Guidelines 2000.* Zeist, the Netherlands: Medical Forum International. Available at www.ispad.org (accessed 1 November 2004).

Kelnar CJ (ed) (1994) *Childhood and Adolescent Diabetes.* London: Arnold.

The National Institute for Clinical Excellence guidelines on diabetes (2004) are available from its website (www.nice.org.uk).

Chapter 14

Endocrinology

Malcolm DC Donaldson and Wendy F Paterson

BASIC HORMONE PHYSIOLOGY, GROWTH AND PUBERTY

BASIC HORMONE PHYSIOLOGY

An organism consisting of millions of cells cannot function without sophisticated communication between the cells – extracellular communication. The nervous system communicates by electrochemical signals, the immune system by chemical signals, and the endocrine system by chemical mediators known as hormones.

Hormones

- Hormones are needed for growth and development, reproduction, homoeostasis (e.g. blood pressure and blood glucose), and organization of energy (production, utilization and storage). Classically hormones act in an endocrine fashion, carried in the circulation to distant tissues. However, a hormone may also exert its effect on adjacent cells (paracrine action) or on its own cell (autocrine action).
- Endocrine systems characteristically show biorhythms. Examples include the daily (circadian) rhythm of cortisol secretion, the monthly menstrual cycle and the seasonal variation in growth hormone secretion.
- A single hormone may have multiple functions, for example testosterone (nitrogen retention, increase in body hair, penile growth, etc.). In contrast, a single function, such as glucose homoeostasis, may require multiple hormones (insulin, glucagon, growth hormone, cortisol and catecholamines).

Types of hormone

Hormones fall into two main groups: **peptides** and **steroids**.

Peptides range in size from the complex peptides (e.g. luteinizing hormone), intermediate size peptides (e.g. insulin), small peptides (e.g. adrenocorticotropic hormone (ACTH)) and dipeptides (e.g. thyroxine) to single amino acid derivatives (e.g. serotonin). Peptides are synthesized by protein biosynthesis and then undergo cleavage and modification.

Steroid hormones are synthesized from cholesterol and modified by hydroxylation and cleavage of the molecule. They can be subdivided into hormones with an intact steroid B ring (e.g. cortisol) and a broken B ring (vitamin D metabolites). Steroids are not water soluble and require carrier proteins, including non-specific proteins such as albumin and specific carriers such as sex hormone and thyroid-binding globulins. It is important to distinguish between free (active) and bound (inactive) hormone when interpreting laboratory data.

Hormone receptors

The water-soluble peptide hormones bind to cell surface receptors comprising extracellular, transmembrane and intracellular domains. Activation of these receptors results in signal transduction through a second messenger system. The three classes of cell surface receptor are those with intrinsic tyrosine kinase activity (e.g. the insulin receptor), receptors which recruit tyrosine kinase activity (e.g. the growth hormone receptor), and the G-protein coupled receptors (e.g. the ACTH receptor) (Figure 14.1a). Activation of the G-protein coupled receptor results in cleavage of the α-subunit from the G-protein. The α-subunit becomes activated and in turn activates the adenylate cyclase system resulting in an increase in intracellular cyclic adenosine monophosphate (AMP).

The steroid hormone receptors are located in the cytoplasm of the cell and consist of a variable region, a DNA-binding domain, a hinge region, and a ligand-binding domain (Figure 14.1b). The steroid molecule binds to the ligand domain of the receptor and the receptor–steroid complex enters the nucleus of the cell where mRNA transcription occurs.

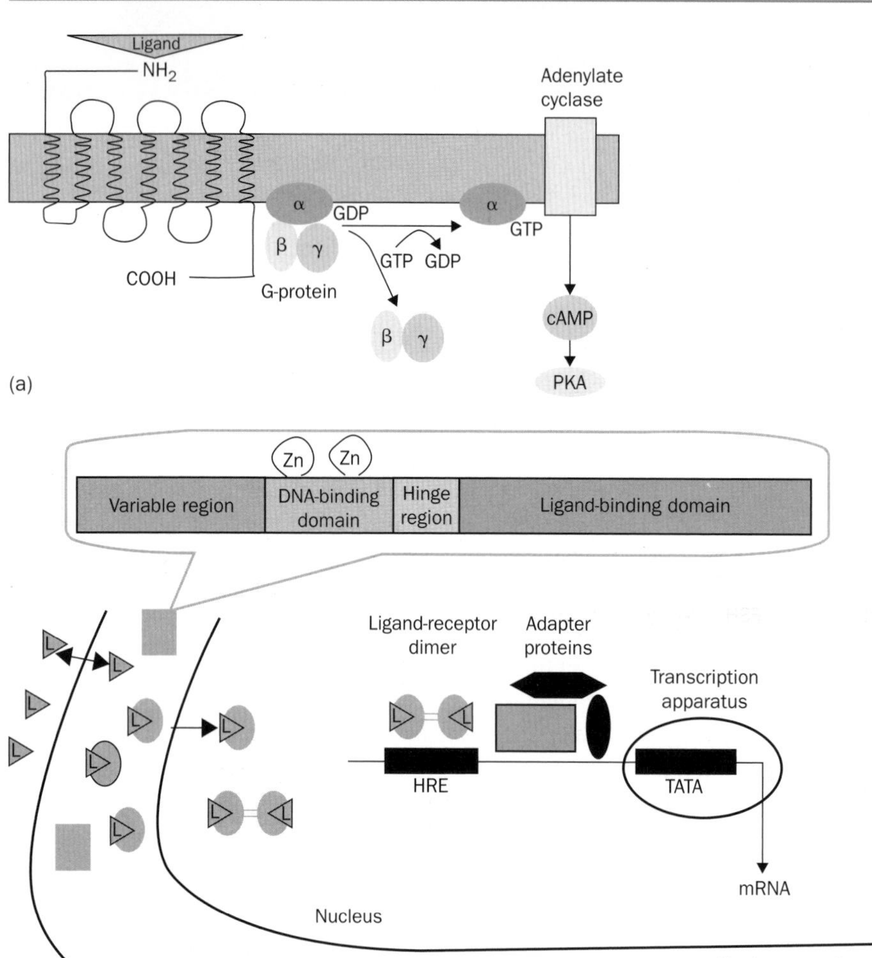

Figure 14.1 (a) Signal transduction in a G-protein coupled class of peptide receptor. Ligand binds to extracellular domain of cell surface receptor, activating the G-protein with dissociation of the alpha subunit and generation of GTP. This in turn activates the adenylate cyclase system, resulting in increased production of intracellular cyclic AMP and protein kinase activity. (b) Signal transduction in nuclear receptors. Ligand (e.g. steroid molecule) binds to receptor which undergoes conformational change (symbolized by change from square to oval). The ligand-receptor complex then enters nucleus, dimerizes and binds to hormone responsive element (HRE) of nuclear DNA, activating the TATA promoter box, leading to transcription and new protein synthesis

Endocrine feedback systems

Many hormone systems, notably those of the hypothalamo–pituitary axis, operate by negative feedback (Figure 14.2). For example, the secretion of thyroxine (T4) following pituitary stimulation results in inhibition of further hypothalamo-pituitary stimulation, whereas insufficient circulating T4 prompts release of hypothalamic thyrotropin-releasing hormone (TRH) and thyroid-stimulating hormone (TSH). The secretion of releasing hormones by the hypothalamus is also influenced by the higher centres (e.g. the ACTH response to danger/stress).

In disorders involving the hypothalamo–pituitary axis it is helpful to think in terms of the site of the defect – primary (target gland), secondary (pituitary) and tertiary (hypothalamic) deficiency. In primary deficiency the pituitary hormones will be abnormally elevated, whereas in secondary and tertiary deficiency they will be low.

Molecular genetic considerations

One or more genes encode each hormone, receptor and enzyme involved with hormone synthesis. Mutations, alterations in the nucleotide sequence of genes due either to changes in DNA length (insertions and deletions) or to substitution of bases (point mutations) may result in altered structure and function of the protein concerned, the nature depending on the site and size of the mutation. Mutations in the genes encoding hormone synthesis will naturally result in loss of function, but mutations in hormone receptor genes may cause either loss of function (**inactivating**) or gain of function (**activating**) alterations.

KEY LEARNING POINTS

- Hormones may have endocrine, paracrine or autocrine action.
- Endocrine systems show biorhythms; many operate by negative feedback.

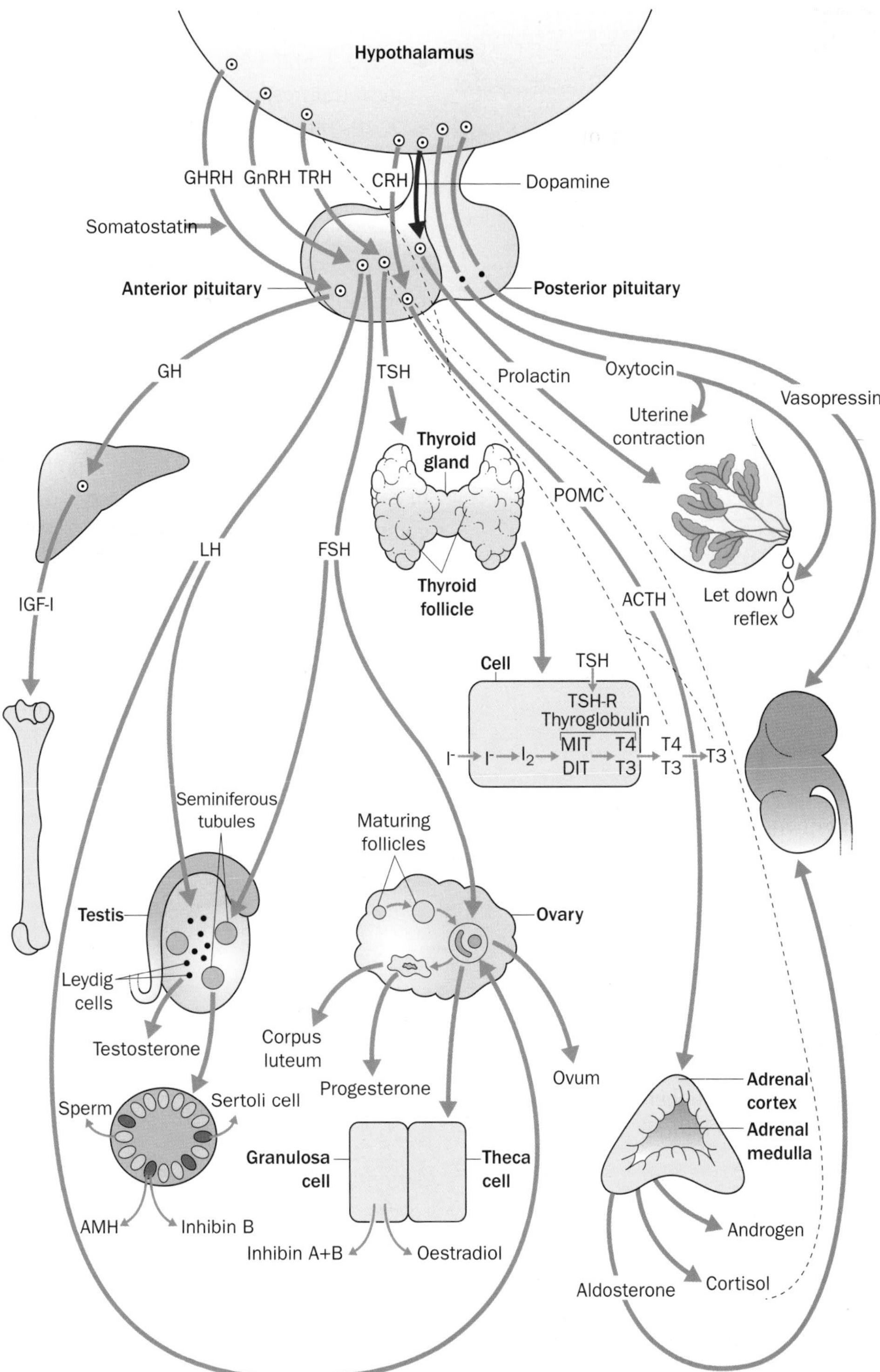

Figure 14.2 Schematic diagram of pathways under hypothalamo-pituitary control

- Most hormones are either peptides or steroids; peptides are water soluble, whereas steroids are not and require carrier proteins.
- Hormones act through receptors; peptide hormone receptors are situated on the cell membrane whereas steroid receptors are located within the cell.
- Gene mutations result in loss of function of hormones and either loss or gain of function of receptors.

PHYSIOLOGY OF GROWTH AND PUBERTY

The term childhood refers to the period of life during which the dominant features are:

- growth – increase in size, and
- development – increase in skills.

It follows, therefore, that childhood begins at conception rather than birth. In practical terms childhood can be considered to end at 16–18 years, by which time sexual maturation and final height are usually achieved, and the individual is adult in terms of social and legal status.

Types of growth and development

- Somatic growth
  - Head circumference
  - Supine length/standing height
  - Weight
- Secondary sexual development
- Neurodevelopment
- Educational development
- Social development and integration

These indices of growth and development are useful in:

- measuring mass health (e.g. height status of child population)
- supporting the diagnosis of normality (normal somatic growth and development)
- detection of disease (e.g. delayed talking in deafness, poor linear growth in Crohn disease)
- monitoring the health of children with known disease (e.g. somatic growth, pubertal development and school performance in children with diabetes mellitus or cystic fibrosis).

Somatic growth

Head circumference

The occipitofrontal circumference (OFC) is a measure of brain growth. Occipitofrontal circumference should be routinely measured as an index of somatic growth from birth to 2 years, by which time head growth is largely complete.

Weight

Weight is a measure of all the body's tissues and fluctuates from day to day depending on food intake and activity. Weight gain is extraordinarily rapid but decelerating *in utero* and during the first 2 years of life. It is useful to remember that weight is (very roughly):

- 1.1, 2.2, and 3.3 kg at 28, 34 and 40 weeks' gestation respectively
- 7, 10, and 12 kg at 6, 12 and 24 months of age.

The rapid growth during infancy demands a high energy intake (roughly 100 kcal/kg). This high calorie requirement, together with the helplessness of infants and their tendency to frequent infections, explains why weight faltering (failure to thrive) is such a common problem.

Length/height – the infantile–childhood–pubertal model (Figure 14.3)

Until approximately 2 years of age supine length is measured, after which standing height is preferred. Examination of a standard height chart shows that there are three main components to the growth curve.

- Infantile phase (rapid growth from 0–2 years):
  - a continuation of the rapid but decelerating intrauterine growth phase
  - largely growth hormone and thyroxine independent
  - dependent on factors such as nutrition, placental function and insulin-like growth factors IGF-I and IGF-II.

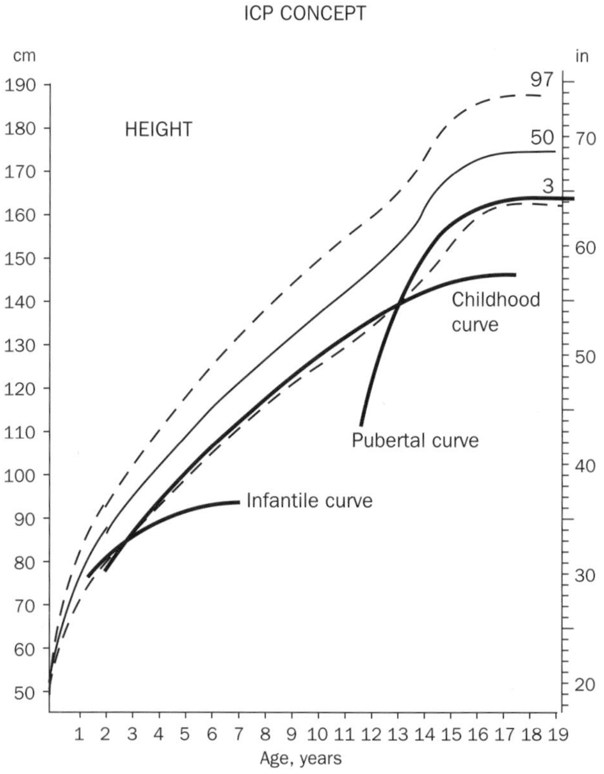

Figure 14.3 The ICP (infantile-childhood-pubertal) model of linear growth from birth to achievement of adult height. In the absence of growth hormone and/or thyroxine secretion, the child will follow the infantile growth trajectory; in the absence of sex steroid secretion, the childhood trajectory will persist

- Childhood phase (2–12 years):
  - slower and slightly decelerating curve
  - growth hormone and thyroxine dependent.
- Pubertal phase (approximately 12 years to final height):
  - caused by an increase in growth hormone secretion, stimulated by the sex steroids
  - acceleration in growth is limited by fusion of the epiphyses, caused by oestrogen in both boys and girls.

The ICP concept is useful in understanding growth patterns. For example, prolonged intrauterine growth retardation (IUGR) will result in impaired growth during the infantile phase, the child following a programmed trajectory of reduced growth after birth. Failure to maintain the height centile during the childhood phase of growth should, in the absence of obvious environmental factors or ill health, prompt a search for growth hormone and/or thyroxine deficiency. Delayed puberty will be associated with prolongation of the childhood growth trajectory.

Growth charts, centile lines and standard deviations

Height is normally distributed. Therefore, a group of children at any given age will show a bell-shaped or Gaussian distribution of height, with most subjects falling around the mean. Traditionally the growth chart has been divided up into the 50th, 25th and 75th, 10th and 90th, and 3rd and 97th centiles. In terms of standard deviations, the 50th centile equates to 0 SD, and the 25th and 75th centiles approximate to −1 and +1 SD respectively. The 3rd and 97th centiles are almost the same as the 95 per cent confidence limits, +2 and −2 SD.

In recent years, the 9-centile charts of Freeman and Cole have been developed (Freeman *et al.*, 1995), comprising the 0.4th, 2nd, 9th, 25th, 50th, 75th, 91st, 98th and 99.6th centiles (Child Growth Foundation (CGF), London, 1996). The 0.4th and 99.6th centiles equate to −3 and +3 SD, respectively and are useful for community screening. The other advantage of the CGF charts is that they reflect current UK height and weight data. However, the cross-sectional nature of the charts results in smoothing of the pubertal growth curve, making it less representative of growth in the individual child than the traditional style Buckler–Tanner charts (Tanner and Buckler, 1997) that are based on both cross-sectional and longitudinal data.

Linear growth in childhood

Size at birth is weakly correlated with childhood stature, the former being related more to intrauterine environment and nutrition than to genetic factors. Between birth and the age of 2 years the individual 'tracks' onto his/her genetic centile, determined by the parental heights (see below). Therefore, by the age of 2 years the height status of the individual will have been declared. The time-honoured observation that a 2-year-old child is half his/her adult final height reflects this phenomenon of 'tracking'.

Thereafter, **the healthy child stays on his/her centile until puberty**. At this point there is considerable variability, related to the age of onset, duration and intensity of the pubertal growth spurt.

Factors affecting height

- Age.
- Sex – boys are slightly taller than girls during the prepubertal years.
- Race – e.g. Scandinavians are tall, Mediterranean races tend to be short.
- Nutrition – an environmental factor that contributes to height differences between races.
- Birth weight – little effect on childhood height unless small for gestational age.
- Pubertal status – early developers are taller for age than late developers.
- Parental heights – the underlying genetic influence on height.
- General health – growth may be affected adversely by any chronic illness, e.g. Crohn disease, chronic renal failure.
- Specific growth disorders – e.g. growth hormone and thyroxine deficiency.
- Socioeconomic status – children from privileged areas are taller on average than children from poor areas.
- Severe psychosocial deprivation.

Normal puberty

Puberty occurs when the hypothalamus secretes gonadotrophin-releasing hormone (GnRH), resulting in luteinizing hormone (LH) and follicle-stimulating hormone (FSH) release from the pituitary (see Figure 14.2). The gonadotrophins act on the gonads, stimulating sex steroid production, which in turn brings about secondary sexual development.

Pubertal staging

Secondary sexual development is assessed according to the method of James Tanner.

GENITAL STAGING

- G1 – pre-pubertal penis, testes and scrotum; testes <4 mL in volume

- G2 – laxity, rugosity and reddening of the scrotum with testes enlarged to 4 mL or greater, but the penis remaining pre-pubertal
- G3 – enlargement of the penis with further development of the scrotum and testes
- G4 – further penile development with broadening as well as lengthening, further development of scrotum and testes, testicular volume usually 12 mL or greater
- G5 – adult development, testes 15–25 mL.

NB: Testicular volume is not necessarily correlated with the genital stage. For example, a boy with genital enlargement due to adrenal androgen excess could be G3 or G4 but with 2 mL testes (pre-pubertal). Moreover, with normal puberty there is considerable variation in testicular volume at a given stage so that although it is usual to have testes of 10–15 mL at G4, some boys at G2 have 10 mL testes and other boys at G4 have 8 mL testes.

BREAST STAGING

- B1 – no breast tissue present
- B2 – breast budding, often felt as a hard wedge of tissue underneath the areola
- B3 – definite breast mound but not adult size
- B4 – projection of the areola from the breast mound at a different angle
- B5 – adult

PUBIC HAIR STAGING

- P1 – no pubic hair
- P2 – the beginnings of pubic hair which is fine, wispy and not readily visible from a distance
- P3 – adult-type pubic hair (coarse, dark, curly) with distribution limited to the symphysis pubis and labia majora
- P4 – near-adult in type and distribution
- P5 – adult, with extension to the thighs and lower abdomen

AXILLARY HAIR STAGING

- A1 – no axillary hair
- A2 – some axillary hair but not yet adult
- A3 – adult amount of axillary hair

Milestones of puberty in relation to peak height velocity

Age at entering into puberty depends on ethnicity, environmental factors such as nutritional status and genetic factors. The first sign of puberty in girls is usually breast development occurring at a mean age of about 11.0 years. Breast budding is associated with enhanced height velocity, girls achieving their peak height velocity (PHV) at a mean age of 12 years, coinciding with B2–3 (Figure 14.4). By the time the girl has mature breast development (B4) the height velocity is decreasing and once menarche has occurred (mean age 13.0 years) she is usually near to her adult final height.

Boys enter puberty only a little later than girls (mean age 11.1 years), the first sign being enlargement of the testes and laxity of the scrotum (G2). At this stage the boy is still in the childhood phase of growth, with height velocity the same or slower than in G1. It is only when the penis starts to enlarge (G3) that height velocity increases, with boys achieving PHV at the age of 14 years coinciding with G4 and the voice breaking. Even when boys reach G5 they are still growing significantly. Mean PHV in boys is slightly higher than in girls (9.4 versus 8.5 cm/year).

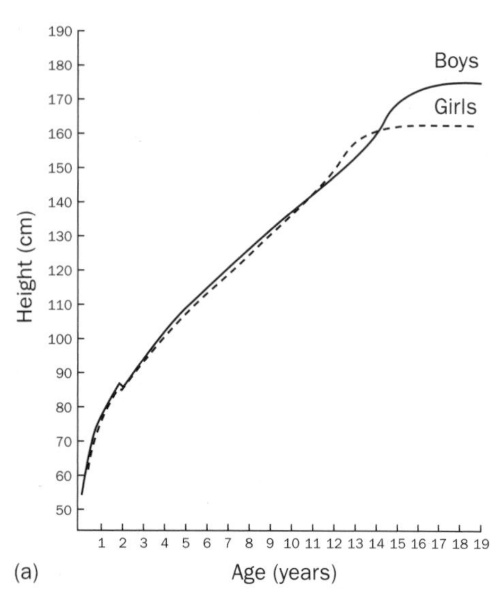

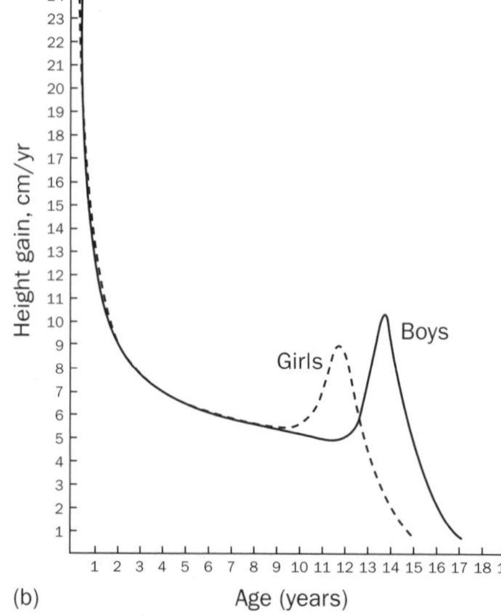

Figure 14.4 Distance and height velocity growth curves for boys (solid line) and girls (dotted line) illustrating (i) the two-year difference in age at peak height velocity, (ii) the more intense pubertal growth spurt in boys and (iii) the resultant 12.5 cm (5 inches) difference in final height between males and females (Reproduced with permission from Tanner *et al.*, 1983)

In adulthood, therefore, men are taller than women by 12.5–14 cm (5–5.5 inches) due to three factors:

- starting their pubertal growth spurt two years later than girls
- having a more intense pubertal growth spurt than girls
- being slightly taller than girls during childhood.

Growth assessment

Good growth assessment depends on accurate measurement of both the child and the parents; accurate transcription of growth data on to an appropriate growth chart; calculation of mid-parental height and target range; calculation of height velocity; pubertal staging and assessment of bone age.

Accurate measurement

The child is measured standing straight with both feet together and heels pressed back against the wall. The outer canthus of the eye is aligned with the external auditory meatus (Frankfurt plane). The Holtain stadiometer is the gold standard of measuring equipment in the UK, but less expensive devices such as the Leicester Height Measure are accurate, although less robust. Parents should be measured, as reported heights are often inaccurate.

Transcription on to growth charts

Decimal age is calculated by referring to the decimal calculation table on the height chart. Each day is expressed as a fraction of the year, in decimal format. For example, if a boy was born on 25 May 1993, his date of birth in decimals is expressed as 93.395. To calculate his decimal age to any particular date, his date of birth is simply subtracted from the decimalized actual date. If the date was 9 September 2003, this would be written as 103.688 so that the child's decimal age would be 103.688 − 93.395 = 10.293 years.

Measurements should be entered accurately as a neat, small dot. The dots should not be joined up since this assumes regular linear growth.

Calculation of mid-parental height and target range (Figure 14.5)

The 12.5–14 cm sex difference must be corrected for by adding this amount to the maternal height on a boy's growth chart and subtracting from the paternal height on a girl's growth chart. The calculation is as follows:

Girls

- Plot the mother's height
- Plot father's height − 12.5 cm (13 or 14 cm is the correction factor used by some centres)
- Plot the mid-parental height (MPH) by taking the mean of these two measurements
- Plot the target range as 2 standard deviations (8.5 cm) on either side of the mid-parental height

Boys

- Plot father's height
- Plot mother's height + 12.5 cm (13 or 14 cm is the correction factor used by some centres)
- Plot the MPH
- Plot the target range (MPH ± 8.5 cm) (10 cm is the 2SD measurement recommended on some growth charts)

Example: Father = 173 cm
Mother = 152.5 cm (corrected height 152.5 + 12.5 = 165 cm)
MPH = (173 + 165)/2 = 169 cm
Target range for sons = 169 ± 8.5 cm = 160.5–177.5 cm

The MPH and target range can be considered as the growth chart centiles for the family concerned, MPH corresponding to the 50th centile (0 SD). The upper end of the range is the 97.5th centile and at the lower end the target range is the 2.5th centile. Under normal circumstances the child's height centile will fall within the parental target range centiles.

Calculation of height velocity

Height velocity is the distance grown in centimetres, divided by the interval in years. The preferred interval is one year with minimum and maximum intervals of 0.5 and 1.3 years. This is because short time intervals magnify measurement errors and long intervals will mask any variability in growth rate.

Example: Child X – date of birth 5.1.95
Measures 116.2 cm on 23 May 2002 (decimal age 7.378)
Measures 123.0 cm on 12 June 2003 (decimal age 8.433)
Height velocity = (difference in height)/(difference in time)
= (123.0 − 116.2)/(8.433 − 7.378) cm
= 6.8/1.055
= 6.4 cm/year

Bone age assessment and plotting (see Figure 14.5)

The chronological age indicates the duration of growth and development. In contrast, assessment of skeletal maturity gives an indication as to how 'far' the individual has progressed in physical terms. Skeletal maturity or bone age is estimated from the appearance of the epiphyses of the left wrist and hand. The most popular systems are those of Tanner and Whitehouse, Greulich and Pyle, and Bailey-Pinneau. In the UK, most centres use the radius, ulna and small bone method devised by Tanner and Whitehouse (RUS(TW2)) (Tanner *et al.*, 1983). This method has recently been revised to take into account the secular trend in physical maturity, evident throughout the developed world. The resultant TW3 method is valid for European, European-American and Japanese children (Tanner *et al.*, 2001). In both TW2 and TW3 systems, a maturity score is awarded to individual epiphyses the sum of which is then converted to a bone age which is plotted on the growth chart as height for bone age denoted by an open circle and connected to the epiphyses height for chronological age by a dotted line (see Figure 14.5). In a healthy child, the height centile for bone age will be more closely related to the adult centile than height for chronological age. Bone age is useful in evaluating the prognosis for final height in healthy children, and in monitoring children with growth disorders who are receiving treatment. It is of limited diagnostic value.

KEY LEARNING POINTS

- Childhood is defined as a period of growth (increase in size) and development (increase in skills).
- Somatic growth, secondary sexual development, neurodevelopment, educational and social development are helpful indices of child health and can be used both to detect and monitor disease.
- Head circumference, a measure of brain growth, is a valuable index of normal growth from 0 to 2 years.
- The three phases of linear growth are infantile (0–2 years), childhood (2–12 years) and pubertal (12 years to adulthood).
- Between birth and 2 years an individual tracks onto his/her genetic centile and stays on this centile until puberty. Deviation above or below the centile demands an explanation.
- The height of a child will depend on genetic, environmental, nutritional and health factors.
- Skeletal maturity or bone age is an objective assessment of physical maturity and is expressed on the growth chart as height for bone age (see Figure 14.5).
- Onset of puberty in both sexes is around the age of 11 years, but girls differ from boys in having their peak growth spurt some two years earlier (see Figure 14.4), this being the main reason why girls are approximately 12.5 cm (5 inches) shorter than boys at final height.
- Calculation of the MPH and target range gives the 50th, 3rd and 97th centiles for the child's family; in normal children the height usually falls within the parental target range centiles.

GROWTH PROBLEMS

Growth problems can be broadly defined as:

- Short stature
- Weight faltering or failure to thrive
- Growth failure
- Tall stature
- Obesity
- Sexual precocity
- Delayed puberty

SHORT STATURE

CASE STUDY

An 8-year-old girl is referred because she is small compared with her peer group and her younger sister is catching up with her in height. She has a history of middle ear infections. She is doing well in school but finds mathematics difficult. She is hypertensive, with weak femoral pulses and a wide carrying angle at the elbow.

Short stature is defined as height below the 3rd centile, equivalent to two standard deviations below the mean. The causes of short stature can be memorized using the acronym NIDSCED.

*N*ormal variant short stature
*I*ntrauterine growth retardation
*D*ysmorphic syndromes
*S*keletal dysplasias
*C*hronic systemic disease
*E*ndocrine disorders
*D*ire social circumstances

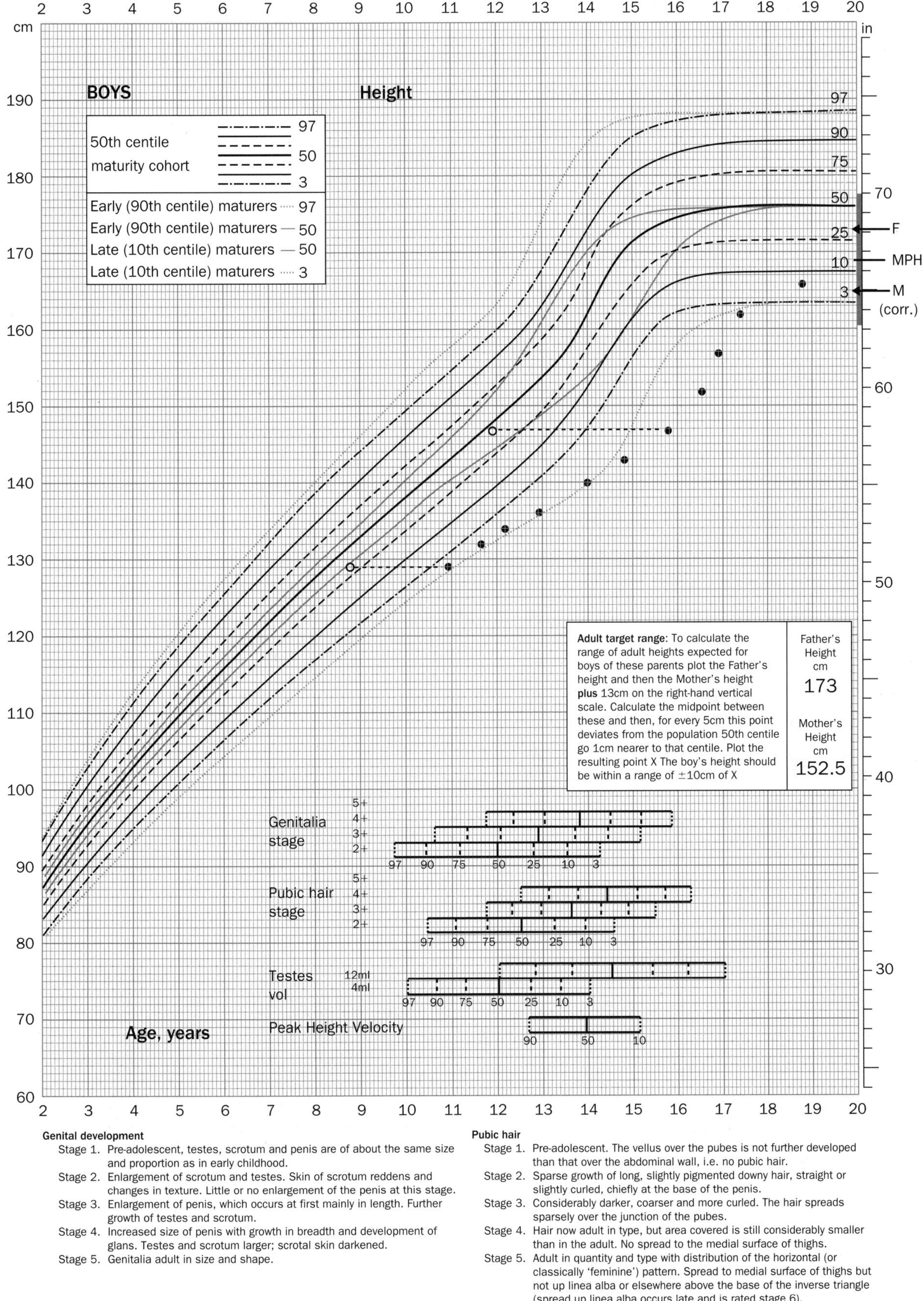

Figure 14.5 Growth chart of a boy with constitutional short stature and delayed puberty, showing paternal height (F for father), corrected maternal height (M corr), midparental height (MPH) and target range (MPH ± 8.5 cm). Height for bone age is represented as an open circle. Note the marked bone age delay, peri-pubertal growth deceleration and eventual catch-up growth resulting in final height within the parental target range

Normal variant short stature

This can be subdivided into genetic short stature and constitutional delay, although in practice there is considerable overlap between the two variants.

Normal genetic short stature

- The child looks short but normal.
- One or both parents are short but normal.
- Child's bone age is not significantly delayed.
- NB: If one parent is particularly short a dominant growth disorder such as a skeletal dysplasia or growth hormone deficiency, rather than normal genetic short stature, could be responsible.

Constitutional delay (see Figure 14.5)

- Child looks short but normal and younger than chronological age.
- Parents are of normal stature but one of them may have been short during childhood and had a late adolescence.
- Bone age is usually delayed.
- Child is destined to have a late puberty with delayed growth spurt and subsequent catch-up growth, final height usually at the lower end of the parental target range.

Intrauterine growth retardation

The term IUGR is used when impairment of fetal growth is sufficient to cause the baby to be small for gestational age (SGA) – birth weight below the 3rd centile for gestational age (equivalent to −2 SD). Intrauterine growth retardation can be subdivided into two types: asymmetrical and symmetrical.

Asymmetrical IUGR is the result of third trimester malnutrition. At birth, the baby is thin, with relative sparing of length and head growth, and there is catch-up growth during infancy. In contrast, symmetrical IUGR results from prolonged intrauterine growth impairment so that the baby is *proportionately* small at birth and remains small during childhood with only partial (if any) catch-up growth.

Intrauterine growth retardation is commonly seen in a variety of dysmorphic syndromes including fetal alcohol syndrome and Russell–Silver (RS) syndrome. Infants with RS show triangular facies often with expanded skull vault giving the impression of hydrocephalus, downturned mouth, and clinodactyly (incurving of the little finger). Asymmetry of the limbs is a characteristic but not invariable feature. A small proportion of children with RS show maternal disomy of chromosome 7, and deletion of a paternal gene (as yet undiscovered) is the presumed cause in most cases.

Dysmorphic syndromes

A dysmorphic syndrome is suggested by a constellation of features, variable both in presence and severity, that may include some of the following:

- unusual phenotype – characteristic facies, unusual hands etc.
- growth problems – usually short, but sometimes tall, stature
- learning difficulties
- congenital anomalies (especially cardiac and renal)
- gonadal problems – e.g. cryptorchidism, hypospadias.

There are a large number of recognized syndromes although many children have unclassified or 'private' syndromes. Down syndrome is by far the commonest disorder, RS has already been mentioned, and a brief account of three other relatively common conditions – Turner, Noonan, and fetal alcohol syndrome – will be given here.

Turner syndrome

Turner syndrome (TS) affects 1 in 2000–2500 girls and is caused by loss or abnormality of the second X chromosome in at least one major cell line. The classic triad consists of (i) short stature, (ii) ovarian dysgenesis and (iii) a variable array of dysmorphic traits. The short stature is partly explained by loss of critical genes (including the SHOX gene) from the short arm of X. About 50 per cent of patients show the 45,XO karyotype, and most of the remaining girls show a mosaic pattern, e.g. 45,X/46,XX or 45,X/46,XisoXq. Clinical features result from:

- lymphoedema – causing coarctation of aorta, neck webbing, puffy hands and feet, and the characteristic hypoplastic often hyperconvex nails with puffy nail folds (Figure 14.6)

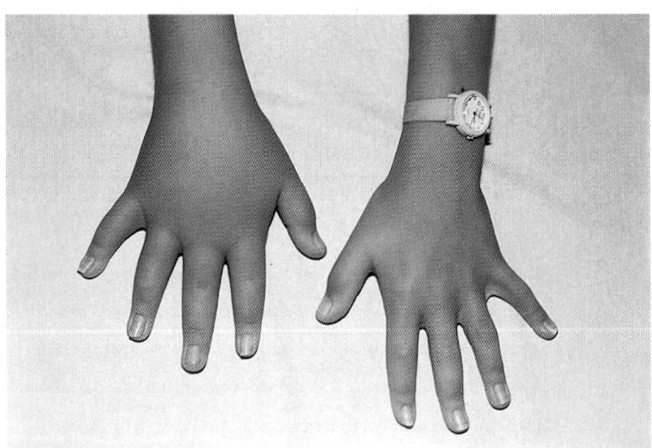

Figure 14.6 Hands of a girl with Turner syndrome. Note lymphoedema, more marked on the right, with characteristic hyperconvex nails and hypoplastic terminal phalanges

- skeletal dysplasia – accounting in part for the short childhood stature, impaired growth at puberty, wide carrying angle at the elbow and shield chest
- ovarian dysgenesis – resulting in pubertal failure and infertility.

Middle ear sepsis with effusion is very common in TS, often requiring surgery. Cardiac problems include coarctation of the aorta, biscuspid aortic valve with or without stenosis, high blood pressure and (in adulthood) aortic root dilatation. Intelligence is usually normal but specific learning difficulties (e.g. with mathematics) often cause educational difficulties particularly if compounded by middle ear problems.

The short stature of TS is treated with growth hormone and the ovarian dysgenesis by induction of puberty with oestrogen.

Noonan syndrome

This condition occurs in both sexes and may be inherited as an autosomal dominant (gene defect unknown) although most cases are sporadic. A mutation in the PTPN11 gene is detectable in roughly a third of clinically diagnosed cases. Clinical features include wide carrying angle, wide spaced eyes, and prominent ears, mild learning difficulties, cryptorchidism, and cardiac defects, commonly pulmonary stenosis. Short or borderline short stature and delayed puberty are the rule. The degree of shortness is often insufficient to persuade the family and clinician to treat with growth hormone.

Fetal alcohol syndrome

Babies are born SGA, may have congenital heart disease, e.g. ventricular septal defect, and remain short during childhood with reduced head circumference, short concentration span and learning difficulties. The characteristic facies – malar hypoplasia, short palpebral fissures and short philtrum – are not always evident, and the diagnosis comes mainly from the history of maternal alcoholism in a short, previously SGA child, with behaviour, concentration and learning problems.

Skeletal dysplasias

Skeletal dysplasias can be broadly divided into:

- those principally affecting the long bones, e.g. achondroplasia, hypochondroplasia and metaphyseal dysplasia.
- those affecting the spine as well as the long bones, e.g. spondylometaphyseal dysplasia.

The spinal dysplasias will result in a short spine whereas the chondrodysplasias result in short limbs. The obvious disproportionate short stature of achondroplasia and severe hypochondroplasia is easy to diagnose but subtle disturbance of body proportions requires careful clinical assessment. The sitting height and leg length (obtained by subtracting sitting height from standing height) should be plotted on the appropriate growth charts.

Chronic systemic diseases

Any chronic condition – gastrointestinal, cardiac, respiratory, renal, neurological, metabolic, rheumatological – can cause short stature and poor growth. Most chronic systemic disease is itself evident, but some gastrointestinal and renal disorders are notoriously silent so that chronic renal failure, Crohn disease and coeliac disease may present to the growth clinic with short stature, growth failure and delayed puberty.

Endocrine disorders

The great majority of short children have no endocrine deficiencies. Growth hormone and thyroxine deficiency, and glucocorticoid excess (Cushing syndrome) will cause not only short stature but also growth failure.

Psychosocial deprivation

Severe psychosocial deprivation and physical/emotional abuse or neglect can cause profound growth impairment sometimes in association with a history of hyperphagia, polydipsia, polyuria and enuresis. Examination may show a short child who may be plump, resembling the hypopituitary state. Growth hormone levels are low in this situation, but response to exogenous growth hormone is poor, and there is dramatic catch-up growth when the child is removed from the home (Albanese *et al.*, 1994).

Investigation of short stature

The majority of short children have normal variant short stature, and a good history and examination will usually render investigation unnecessary. Children with IUGR, dysmorphic syndromes and skeletal dysplasias are investigated as appropriate with involvement of the clinical geneticist and radiologist. When chronic disease is suspected detailed investigation may be needed including a search for malabsorption and inflammatory bowel disease. It is important to identify psychosocial growth failure to avoid inappropriate investigation and treatment with growth hormone.

As a rule it is wise to investigate children whose height falls outside the parental target range centiles, although the majority will turn out to have constitutional delay. In the first instance it is appropriate to carry out short stature screening investigations, followed by endocrine stimulation tests as necessary.

Short stature screening investigations

Blood

- Full blood count (FBC) and film, ferritin, red cell folate (screening for chronic gastrointestinal disease, e.g. malabsorption)
- IgA antiendomysial or tissue transglutaminase (TTG) antibodies (screening for coeliac disease)
- Creatinine, urea and electrolytes, calcium and phosphate (screening for renal disease)
- T4 and TSH, cortisol, (prolactin), and IgF_1 (endocrine screening)
- Chromosomes

Urine

- Ward urinalysis, clean catch sample for culture
- Fasting early morning urine osmolality

Diagnostic imaging

- Bone age
- Abdominal ultrasound
- Skeletal survey if dysplasia suspected (in consultation with radiology department)

Other

- EDTA and heparin sample for molecular genetic studies, and clinical photographs if syndrome suspected

Management of short stature

Management of short stature depends on the underlying cause and by the extent to which the child and family regard the shortness as a problem. Simple reassurance and estimation of ultimate height is usually sufficient in genetic short stature and constitutional delay. Growth hormone is indicated for growth hormone insufficiency (see below) and is also licensed for the treatment of TS and IUGR. The role of growth hormone in other short stature conditions such as normal variant short stature (NVSS) is controversial. Extensive research has been carried out to determine the effect of GH on short- and long-term growth in NVSS. The results suggest an average improvement in final height of 4–6 cm with GH therapy. However, there is considerable debate as to the cost-effectiveness versus benefits of this treatment (Finkelstein *et al.*, 2002).

FAILURE TO THRIVE/WEIGHT FALTERING

Failure to thrive is a term applied to infants and preschool children denoting failure to gain weight at an appropriate rate so that the child appears thin. Most failure to thrive is non-organic, and if a careful history and examination do not suggest a physical cause then investigations will usually be non-contributory. Failure to thrive is discussed further in Chapter 11.

GROWTH FAILURE

CASE STUDY

A girl develops tiredness, weight gain, and slow growth with height on the 10th centile at 7 years (previously on the 50th). Examination shows pallor, hypertrichosis, and squaring of the facies. Thyroid function tests confirm severe hypothyroidism with positive thyroid peroxidase antibodies.

Growth failure is defined as failure to achieve and maintain a height velocity that it is appropriate for both age and maturity. Unlike short stature, which may be normal or abnormal, growth failure is by definition abnormal. However, true growth failure must be distinguished from the decelerating growth trajectory of constitutional delay (see Figure 14.5). It is important to make a distinction between short stature, failure to thrive and growth failure (see the case study above); these three growth problems may occur singly or in combination.

TALL STATURE

CASE STUDY

A boy is referred aged 12 years with tall stature. He is not obviously dysmorphic but his height falls outwith the parental target range. Bone age is one year advanced. Cardiac ultrasound shows a dilated aortic root and mild mitral valve prolapse.

Tall stature is defined as height above the 97th centile, equivalent to two standard deviations above the mean.

The causes can be remembered using the acronym NODSPE:

*N*ormal variant tall stature
*O*besity
*D*ysmorphic syndromes
*S*exual *P*recocity
*E*ndocrine

Normal variant tall stature

This can be subdivided into normal genetic tall stature and constitutional advance groups – the mirror images of normal variant short stature.

- In normal genetic tall stature:
  - the child looks normal but tall
  - there is little or no bone age advance
  - one or both parents are tall.
- In constitutional advance
  - the child is tall but looks normal and older than chronological age
  - there is bone age advance
  - child goes on to display early puberty, achieving final height earlier than usual.

Obesity

This is usually expressed in terms of the body mass index (BMI) calculated according to the formula weight (kilograms) divided by height (metres) squared. The BMI value is plotted onto a centile chart (Child Growth Foundation BMI chart, CGF, 2 Mayfield Avenue, London W4 1PW). Overweight, obesity and severe obesity can be defined as BMI >85th, >95th, and >98th centiles, respectively.

The increased calorie intake associated with simple obesity results in an increase in height velocity. The child will be relatively tall, with height in the upper half of, or above, the parental target range centiles and show an advance in bone age. Obesity is discussed further in Chapter 11.

Dysmorphic syndromes

There are a large number of overgrowth dysmorphic syndromes, which are either classified or unclassified.

Dysmorphic syndromes causing tall stature include the sex chromosome aneuploidy syndromes such as Klinefelter (47,XXY) and its variants, and the 47,XYY syndrome. Marfan syndrome is an important diagnosis to consider in a tall child and, being a dominant disorder, may be present in one of the parents. Sotos syndrome is a relatively common dysmorphic syndrome associated with tall stature, macrocephaly with prominent forehead, large hands and feet, and poor coordination. Bone age is advanced so that adult height is not excessive.

Sexual precocity

Premature sexual maturation, due to oestrogen or androgen excess, will cause increased height velocity with tall stature and bone age advance. Depending on the severity of the sexual precocity, adult final height may be compromised due to premature closure of the epiphyses, resulting in the paradox of tall stature during childhood and short stature in adulthood. Children with overgrowth disorders associated with learning disability are also prone to early puberty, which will compound the tall stature.

Endocrine disorders

Apart from sexual precocity these include thyrotoxicosis and growth hormone excess, causing true gigantism (see next section).

SEXUAL PRECOCITY AND DELAYED PUBERTY

These problems are discussed in the next section.

KEY LEARNING POINTS

- Growth and pubertal problems encompass short and tall stature, thin and fat children, early and late developers, and growth failure.
- The causes of short stature can be memorized according to the acronym NIDSCED.
- The majority of short children have normal variant short stature but care must be taken to identify children with chronic disease, dysmorphic syndromes such as TS, psychosocial deprivation, and growth hormone deficiency.
- Following careful clinical assessment investigation of short stature is often unnecessary. It is wise to investigate children who fall outside the parental target range centiles.
- Causes of tall stature can be remembered according to the acronym NODSPE.
- Clinical evaluation of tall children includes taking a family history, enquiring about learning difficulties, recognizing dysmorphism and carrying out pubertal staging.

ENDOCRINE DISORDERS

These will be considered under the following headings:

- Disorders of systems under hypothalamo-pituitary control. These systems comprise the growth, gonadal, thyroid, and adrenal axes, dopamine and prolactin, the posterior pituitary hormones, and the satiety system
- Diabetes mellitus and hypoglycaemia (covered in Chapter 13)
- Disorders of sexual differentiation
- Calcium and bone disorders
- Late endocrine effects of treatment for childhood cancer
- Miscellaneous endocrine disorders (gut, kidney, adrenal medulla, pineal)

DISORDERS OF SYSTEMS UNDER HYPOTHALAMO-PITUITARY CONTROL

The hypothalamo–pituitary unit (see Figure 14.2)

The hypothalamus develops as a downgrowth from the floor of the third ventricle, extending to form the pituitary stalk or infundibulum and the posterior pituitary or neurohypophysis. An outgrowth from the roof of the primitive mouth containing a lumen (Rathke pouch) meets the neurohypophysis and differentiates into the anterior pituitary, with a thin intermediate lobe, and disappearance of Rathke pouch.

The hypothalamus is situated at the base of the 3rd ventricle with the optic chiasm above and anterior to the pituitary stalk. The pituitary gland is situated in the pituitary fossa, or sella turcica.

The median eminence of the hypothalamus produces the pituitary-releasing hormones. These are secreted into the capillaries of the hypophyseal-portal system in the pituitary stalk (vascular transport). The supraoptic and paraventricular nuclei of the hypothalamus produce oxytocin and vasopressin, which travel along neural channels in the pituitary stalk to the posterior pituitary where they are stored (neural transport).

Growth hormone axis

Growth hormone-releasing hormone (GHRH) is modulated by somatostatin to cause pulsatile release of growth hormone mainly occurring during sleep. Growth hormone stimulates release of IGF-I from the liver and bone which results in promotion of skeletal growth. In addition to its indirect effect on growth, growth hormone promotes protein synthesis, lipolysis, and glucose release so that severe growth hormone deficiency will result not only in short stature but also muscular weakness, adiposity, and a tendency to hypoglycaemia.

TESTS OF GROWTH HORMONE AXIS

Growth hormone is a dynamic hormone and random levels are of limited value in assessment. Overnight sampling to determine pulsatile secretion is the most physiological approach, but too labour intensive to be practical in a clinical setting. Growth hormone reserve can be tested by provocative stimuli such as insulin-induced hypoglycaemia, glucagon, arginine and clonidine. Opinions vary as to the best test. Overnight fasting, a prerequisite of growth hormone provocation tests, can result in hypoglycaemia in a hypopituitary child so that whatever test is used it is important to take safety precautions. Intravenous access must be secure with a good-sized cannula *in situ*, oxygen and suction facilities should be available, and the procedure must be performed by experienced staff. If hypoglycaemia occurs, the symptoms can be quickly and safely relieved with Lucozade, a readily available glucose drink (Galloway *et al*., 2002).

The arbitrary cut-off value for peak growth hormone following stimulation or during an overnight profile is 20 mU/L. Results will vary within the same individual child from day to day and according to the type of assay used. Partial growth hormone insufficiency is defined as peak levels between 10 and 20 mU/L, severe insufficiency between 5 and 10 mU/L and complete insufficiency <5 mU/L. Growth hormone levels cannot be considered in isolation from the clinical picture. Short children and those with constitutional delay may show low growth hormone levels at certain stages, notably in mid-childhood and before puberty. Low growth hormone levels are also seen in psychosocial deprivation. It is therefore useful to use the term **insufficiency** when low levels of growth hormone have been found in an individual who may turn out to have normal pituitary function and to reserve the term **deficiency** for individuals in whom true permanent lack of growth hormone is certain.

When growth hormone excess is suspected a glucose tolerance test can be carried out to determine whether or not growth hormone levels suppress to <5 mU/L in response to the oral glucose load.

Growth hormone insufficiency

CASE STUDY

A 3-year-old boy is admitted with a history of headache and vomiting for the past six weeks. His parents have noticed that his growth has slowed over the past year. On examination, he is below the 3rd centile for height, on the 10th for weight, and has an afferent defect in the right pupil with papilloedema on fundoscopy.

True growth hormone deficiency is rare, the great majority of short children having an anatomically normal hypothalamo-pituitary axis. Growth hormone insufficiency can be classified according to the following:

- cause (congenital or acquired)
- nature (true permanent deficiency or functional/temporary insufficiency)
- severity (complete, severe or partial)
- whether isolated or part of multiple anterior pituitary deficiency.

Classification of growth hormone insufficiency according to cause/nature

Temporary insufficiency – conditions in which growth hormone levels may be low on stimulation testing but normal on retesting at a later date:

- Normal variant short stature – including constitutional delay
- IUGR
- Psychosocial deprivation
- Turner syndrome

Permanent growth hormone deficiency due to abnormality of hypothalamo-pituitary axis:

Congenital

- Idiopathic
- Inherited causes (autosomal recessive, autosomal dominant, X-linked)
- Developmental defects (e.g. septo-optic dysplasia)
- Hypothalamic disorders (e.g. Prader–Willi syndrome)

Acquired

- Tumours adjacent to hypothalamo-pituitary axis (e.g. craniopharyngioma, optic glioma)
- Surgery to the hypothalamo-pituitary axis.
- Cranial radiotherapy (e.g. for medulloblastoma)
- Granulomatous disease (e.g. Langerhans cell histiocytosis)

CAUSES OF GROWTH HORMONE DEFICIENCY

Congenital

Most isolated congenital growth hormone deficiency is idiopathic and sporadic. Traction on the pituitary at breech delivery is a traditional cause of growth hormone deficiency but is rarely seen nowadays. Isolated growth hormone deficiency can be due to gene defects affecting GHRH, its receptor, or growth hormone itself (Figure 14.7). Gene mutations affecting the transcription factor Pit 1 cause growth hormone, prolactin and TSH deficiency, while Prop 1 mutations cause growth hormone, prolactin, TSH and gonadotrophin deficiency. An important developmental cause of growth hormone deficiency is septo-optic dysplasia.

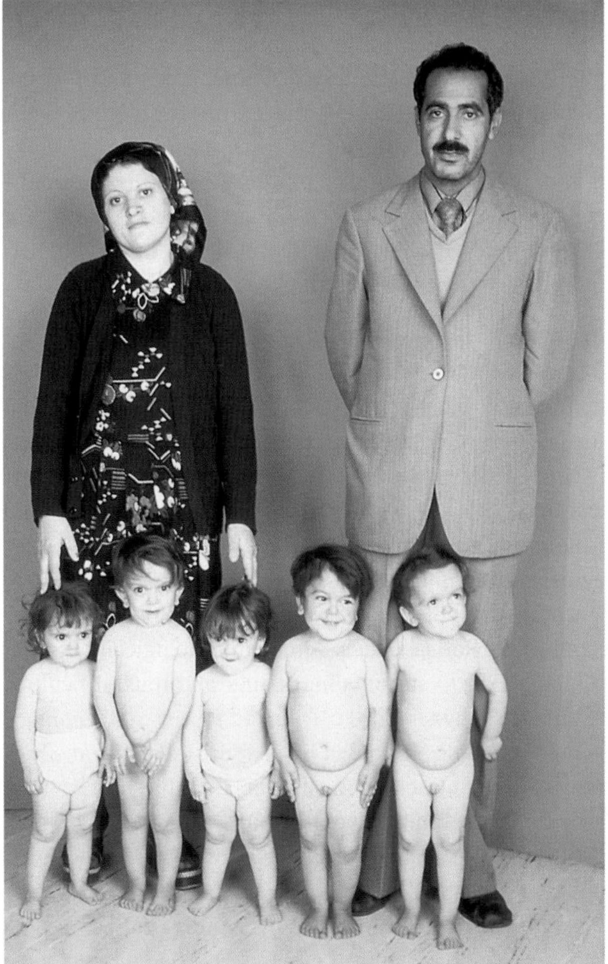

Figure 14.7 Autosomal recessive growth hormone deficiency in two sibships. Two brothers married two sisters, the brothers being first cousins to the sisters. The photograph shows one parent from each family with five of the seven children. Note the growth hormone deficient facies and habitus of the children whose ages range between 2 and 7 years. (Reprinted with permission from *Journal of Medical Genetics*)

Septo-optic dysplasia comprises a triad of hypothalamic hypopituitarism, optic nerve hypoplasia and absent septum pellucidum. The cause of this and more severe midline developmental defects is largely unknown but disordered function of various transcription factors involved in organogenesis, possibly related to teratogens is a possibility. The degree of hypopituitarism and visual impairment are variable. Severely affected children present in the neonatal period with hypoglycaemia and prolonged jaundice (due to ACTH deficiency), micropenis (from gonadotrophin deficiency) and roving nystagmus (indicating visual impairment). Growth hormone deficiency is invariably seen if other pituitary hormones are deficient. Diabetes insipidus is absent in the majority of cases. Some children show learning disability whereas intelligence is normal in others.

Acquired

Causes include tumours in the region of the hypothalamo-pituitary axis such as craniopharyngioma, cranial irradiation either as treatment for a tumour in this region (e.g. optic nerve glioma in neurofibromatosis) or for central nervous system (CNS) prophylaxis (e.g. craniospinal irradiation in medulloblastoma), Langerhans cell histiocytosis and trauma.

Craniopharyngioma is a tumour arising from the remnants of the Rathke pouch. Although histologically benign, it is adherent to surrounding tissues and thus difficult to remove, usually contains calcium and has a cystic component. Symptoms are caused by pressure on adjacent structures so that presentation may be with (i) short stature, growth failure and polydipsia (due to growth hormone deficiency and diabetes insipidus), (ii) visual failure with temporal field loss and (iii) hydrocephalus from third ventricle obstruction. Treatment is by shunting for the hydrocephalus, surgical removal of as much tumour as possible whilst trying to avoid injury to surrounding structures followed by radiotherapy if this is incomplete, pituitary replacement therapy and involvement of the visual impairment team when appropriate.

ASSESSMENT AND TREATMENT OF GROWTH HORMONE DEFICIENCY

Growth hormone deficiency should be anticipated in situations such as postoperative craniopharyngioma and following craniospinal irradiation for medulloblastoma. The axis is assessed by a growth hormone stimulation test and co-administration of GnRH and TRH. Synthetic ACTH (tetracosactide (Synacthen®)) must also be given if the growth hormone stimulus used does not stimulate cortisol secretion. Children should also undergo pituitary magnetic resonance imaging (MRI), not only to exclude the presence of a tumour but also to determine pituitary size, the presence and site of the posterior pituitary bright spot and the pituitary stalk (absent in some congenital anomalies).

The short, slowly growing child with low growth hormone levels but no obvious congenital or acquired cause for hypopituitarism is often labelled as having 'idiopathic growth hormone deficiency'. In practice, most of these children will be found on subsequent evaluation to have normal pituitary function and to have been displaying normal variant short stature. Nevertheless, a course of growth hormone therapy may be helpful in this situation.

GROWTH HORMONE TREATMENT

This is given as a single nightly subcutaneous injection in a dose of 5 mg/m^2 per week for pre-pubertal children and 7 mg/m^2 per week for pubertal children. A variety of devices exist for growth hormone administration, the most popular being the pen injectors. Input from an endocrine specialist nurse is invaluable in training families how to give the growth hormone injections and in overseeing compliance. Response to treatment is assessed by monitoring the height velocity at four monthly clinic visits. Compliance can be gauged by measuring IGF-I levels.

GROWTH HORMONE RESISTANCE

Mutations in the growth hormone receptor will result in the phenotype of growth hormone deficiency with elevated growth hormone levels and low IGF-I levels – Laron dwarfism – the cause of short stature in African pygmies. Functional dislocation of the growth hormone/IGF-I axis is also seen in some chronic conditions such as poorly controlled diabetes mellitus, Crohn disease, and chronic renal failure.

Growth hormone excess

Growth hormone excess due to a growth-hormone-producing adenoma in children causes gigantism, the counterpart of acromegaly in the adult. True gigantism is extremely rare and is suspected in the context of inappropriate tall stature with increased height velocity, failure of growth hormone to suppress to below 5 mU/L following a normal glucose load, and the finding of a pituitary lesion on imaging. Growth hormone excess can also be seen in the McCune–Albright syndrome and in multiple endocrine neoplasia type 1. The treatment of choice is surgery followed by radiotherapy if this is incomplete. The long-acting somatostatin analogue octreotide can be used to reduce pituitary growth hormone secretion.

KEY LEARNING POINTS

- Growth hormone stimulation testing should only be carried out in units with adequate resources and staffing.
- Growth hormone **insufficiency** – stimulated growth hormone levels <20 mU/L – may be seen in individuals without true GH **deficiency**, e.g. normal variant short stature.

- Congenital growth hormone deficiency may be idiopathic, inherited or part of a developmental anomaly (e.g. septo-optic dysplasia).
- Acquired true growth hormone deficiency occurs as a result of cranial tumours and/or radiotherapy in the region of the hypothalamo-pituitary axis and rarely Langerhans cell histiocytosis.
- Growth hormone therapy is given as a subcutaneous nightly injection by the family; input from a specialist nurse is important in overseeing compliance.

Gonadal axis (see Figure 14.2)

Secretion of GnRH from the hypothalamus is minimal during childhood until the age of 7–8 years when the pulsatile release of LH begins. From around 10–11 years the LH pulses are sufficient to stimulate enough sex steroid production to result in the external signs of puberty.

Testicular physiology

The testis is divided into two notional compartments – the seminiferous tubules containing the haploid and diploid germ cells and Sertoli cells, and the interstitial tissue containing Leydig cells. Sertoli cells exert a paracrine 'nursing' effect on the germ cells. Spermatogenesis results from complex interaction of pituitary LH and FSH, intratesticular testosterone secreted by Leydig cells, and inhibin B which is secreted by Sertoli cells and which inhibits pituitary FSH.

Ovarian physiology

Six months after birth the ovary has achieved the maximum number of primordial follicles which then decrease steadily until the menopause. The onset of ovulation completes the first meiotic phase and the second phase develops after ovulation and before fertilization. Gonadotrophin secretion results in the enlargement of 10–20 follicles/month. In the follicular phase, FSH stimulates androstenedione secretion in the theca cells, and induces its conversion to oestradiol in the granulosa cells by the enzyme aromatase. An LH surge in mid-cycle causes ovulation followed by the formation of a corpus luteum and progesterone secretion (luteal phase). The granulosa cells of the ovaries produce inhibin A and B, which inhibit FSH secretion. Stimulation of the stromal cells of the ovary by LH results in androgen production.

Tests of gonadal axis

- Basal LH and FSH measurement is useful in the assessment of primary gonadal failure in which case FSH will be elevated (usually >10 U/L).
- Luteinizing-hormone-releasing hormone (LHRH) test. Administration of the releasing hormone LHRH 100 μg intravenously, measuring LH and FSH at 0, 15, 30 and 60 minutes will demonstrate:
  - a pre-pubertal response: LH peak <5 U/L and LH response < FSH response
  - a pubertal response: LH peak >5 U/L, LH response > FSH response.
- Plasma basal serum testosterone and oestradiol. Standard oestradiol assays are not sufficiently sensitive to detect the low but significant levels found in the early stages of puberty (10–50 μg).
- Human chorionic gonadotrophin (hCG) test, measuring Leydig cell reserve:
  - short hCG test: 1500 units of hCG intramuscularly, taking blood for serum testosterone before and four days later
  - long hCG test: hCG 100 units/kg (maximum 1500 units) intramuscularly twice weekly for three weeks. This test serves not only as an aid to diagnosis, but also as therapy for cryptorchidism and micropenis.
- Pelvic ultrasound. In experienced hands this will identify:
  - uterine length, configuration and presence of endometrial echo (reflecting oestrogen effect)
  - ovarian volumes, number and size of follicles (reflecting gonadotrophin secretion).

In puberty uterine length and fundo-cervical ratio increase giving the characteristic heart-shaped appearance, and a thick endometrial stripe indicates that menses are imminent; ovarian volumes are usually 3 mL or greater in volume with several discernible follicles.

Sexual precocity

This is defined as premature sexual maturation, irrespective of cause, occurring in girls before the age of 10 years and boys before the age of 11 years. The classification and causes of sexual precocity are shown in Table 14.1.

TRUE PRECOCIOUS AND EARLY PUBERTY

CASE STUDY

A girl of 8 years presents with a six-month history of breast development and mood swings. Always tall, she has been growing particularly fast recently. Her mother and older sisters experienced menarche at 11 years. Examination shows a tall girl with stage B2 breast development, no café-au-lait patches, and normal fundoscopy.

Table 14.1 Classification and causes of sexual precocity

True precocious and early puberty	
Idiopathic – common in girls, rare in boys	
Tumours within hypothalamus, e.g. hypothalamic hamartoma	
Tumours adjacent to hypothalamus, e.g. optic glioma, suprasellar germinoma	
Central nervous system disorders, e.g. hydrocephalus, cerebral palsy, learning disability	
Low-dose cranial irradiation, e.g. cranial prophylaxis in childhood leukaemia	
Previous exposure to sex steroids ('priming'), e.g. simple virilizing 21-hydroxylase deficiency, drugs such as oxymethalone	
Precocious pseudopuberty	
Boys	Girls
Virilizing and feminizing adrenal adenomas	Feminizing and virilizing adrenal adenomas
Activating LH receptor mutations	Virilizing ovarian tumours
Germline defects causing Leydig's cell adenoma	Feminizing granulosa cell tumours of ovary
Somatic defects causing testotoxicosis	McCune–Albright syndrome (caused by mosaicism for activating GS-α mutation).
Drugs (e.g. oxymethalone)	
Exaggerated adrenarche	
Incomplete sexual precocity in girls	
Isolated premature thelarche	
Thelarche variant	
Isolated premature menarche	

LH, luteinizing hormone.

Precocious and early puberty is the domain of girls in whom it is usually idiopathic. It is rare in boys in whom an underlying lesion is likely.

History and examination

The key features are breast and genital development in girls and boys, respectively, and in both sexes a variable combination of pubic hair, increase in growth rate, moodiness, body odour, and sometimes acne. The family patterns of puberty (menarche in females, growth spurt and voice breaking in males) should be obtained. Underlying causes of precocious puberty such as learning disability and CNS disorders, cranial irradiation, headache (suggestive of raised intracranial pressure), family history of neurofibromatosis and café-au-lait patches should be sought.

Examination will show a child who is usually tall for age, height above the target range centiles. The exception to this is the child with concomitant growth hormone deficiency. Bone age is advanced by >1 year. In boys palpation of the testes will show bilateral enlargement to 4 mL or greater, with or without penile enlargement and pubic hair. Breast staging in girls will show at least stage B2 development, but assessment can be difficult in obese girls in whom simple adiposity may masquerade as stage B3. It is essential to examine the fundi, looking for optic nerve atrophy due to pressure from a pituitary lesion adjacent to the hypothalamo-pituitary axis (e.g. an optic glioma). The skin should be carefully examined for café-au-lait patches (seen in neurofibromatosis and McCune–Albright syndrome).

Investigations

The cornerstone of diagnosis is the LHRH test which will almost always show a pubertal LH response in true precocious and early puberty. Pelvic ultrasound in girls will usually show the characteristic pubertal uterus and ovaries. The cause of precocious puberty should be sought by cranial MRI, in which resolution is superior to a computed tomography (CT) scan.

Treatment

Treatment of precocious and early puberty is with GnRH analogue which, when given in pharmacological doses, causes downregulation of gonadotrophin secretion. The decision whether or not to medically treat precocious and early puberty must take into account the girl's height status, learning ability, age of onset and intensity of the puberty, and the feelings of the girl and her family. Treatment with GnRH analogue probably improves final height outcome in precocious puberty but probably not in early puberty. The main benefit of treatment is psychological in preventing progression of pubertal signs and menses. This can be particularly valuable in girls with learning disability.

A number of preparations are available including goserelin (Zoladex®) which is given as a depot injection into the subcutaneous fat of the anterior abdominal wall either as 3.6 mg every four weeks or 10.8 mg every 10–12 weeks (Paterson *et al.*, 1998). Treatment is continued until the age of 10 or 11 years, menses starting about one to two years after stopping treatment.

PRECOCIOUS PSEUDOPUBERTY

> **CASE STUDY**
>
> A girl of 3 years is referred with a three-month history of pubic hair development and aggressive behaviour. Examination shows a child of normal stature in relation to parental heights. There is clitoral enlargement, stage P3 pubic hair and a mass in the lower abdomen. Plasma androgens are elevated, LH and FSH completely suppressed.

This term is applied to sexual precocity arising from causes outside hypothalamo-pituitary control. The diagnosis is suggested in boys with sexual precocity when one or both testes are pre-pubertal in volume. Most precocious pseudopuberty in girls is virilizing in nature, therefore readily distinguished clinically from true precocious and early puberty.

Feminizing lesions are exceedingly rare in boys. Diagnosis may be difficult in girls with feminizing lesions due to adrenal adenomas and ovarian tumours. The crucial distinction between true and pseudoprecocious puberty is made by the LHRH test which shows a pubertal response in the former and suppression in the latter. In girls the possibility of **McCune–Albright syndrome** should be considered. This condition is due to an activating mutation of the GS α subunit, affecting some of the cells in specific tissues. This mosaic pattern produces café-au-lait patches on the skin, fibrous dysplasia in the bones, ovarian hypersecretion, and more rarely adrenal steroid and pituitary growth hormone excess.

Treatment of precocious pseudopuberty depends on the underlying cause.

Isolated premature thelarche

This common condition is usually seen in pre-school girls. There is isolated breast development whereas height, growth rate, bone age and pelvic ultrasound are normal for age. Investigation is usually unnecessary but the LHRH test will show FSH dominance, often with peak FSH levels of >20 U/L. The aetiology of the condition is still unknown and may be due to higher FSH levels than usual, or to enhanced sensitivity of the breast tissue. No treatment is required.

Thelarche variant

This descriptive term is applied to girls, usually of school age, who show persistent isolated breast development in the context of a normal or slightly increased height velocity, modest bone age advance, and sometimes vaginal bleeding, but a pre-pubertal LHRH test. Possibilities such as true puberty with an initially negative LHRH test and precocious pseudopuberty (e.g. McCune–Albright syndrome with isolated ovarian involvement) should be considered and the girl kept under surveillance.

Isolated premature menarche

Occasionally pre-pubertal girls show cyclical vaginal bleeding in the absence of any other features of sexual precocity. The condition should be distinguished from non-endocrine causes of vaginal bleeding such as child abuse and vaginal tumours (e.g. rhabdomyosarcoma). The investigation of choice is a pelvic ultrasound scan which, when taken during an episode of bleeding, will show an endometrial echo.

Exaggerated adrenarche

Adrenal puberty or adrenarche occurs in both sexes between the ages of 6 and 8 years. It is usually a subclinical event characterized by increased adrenal androgen secretion with a slight increase in height and weight velocity. Some children, especially girls, exhibit signs of mild androgenicity such as weight gain, greasy skin and hair, mild acne, body odour and the development of pubic and axillary hair, the former being more evident over the labia majora. This condition is called exaggerated or amplified adrenarche and is more likely to occur in children who have shown IUGR. It must be distinguished from serious causes of androgen excess such as adrenal enzyme disorders and adrenal/gonadal tumours but these usually cause severe virilization. Occasionally exaggerated adrenarche is seen before the age of 6 years, in which case the term premature adrenarche is appropriate.

Delayed/incomplete puberty

> **CASE STUDY**
>
> A 14-year-old boy received total body irradiation prior to bone marrow transplant for leukaemia at 9 years. Pubertal staging is G4P4A2 but testicular volumes are smaller than normal at 6 mL, FSH elevated at 20 U/L. The family are asking about his prospects for fertility.

Delayed puberty can be arbitrarily defined as no signs of puberty in a girl aged 13 years or a boy aged 14 years. It is the domain of boys, in whom constitutional delay is much the commonest cause. Delayed puberty is classified as either central (with an intact or impaired axis) or primary gonadal (Table 14.2).

HISTORY AND EXAMINATION

Important aspects to consider are (i) previous growth history, (ii) clues as to the cause of the delayed puberty and (iii) the psychological effect of the problem.

Constitutional delay in growth and adolescence (CDGA) (Figure 14.8) is usually seen in a child with long-standing short, or borderline short, stature compounded by a deceleration in growth rate from the age of 9 or 10 years. General health is good but there is often a history of asthma. Most but not all cases have a family history of pubertal delay. The presence of tiredness and lack of energy should arouse suspicion of an underlying chronic illness, and prompt a careful system review. General health and the psychological impact of the pubertal delay can be gauged by enquiring about school attendance and performance, participation in sporting activities, and leisure pursuits. Kallmann syndrome can be screened for by asking the boy if he can smell toast burning or unpleasant odours, such as rotting eggs. The past medical history may disclose causative factors such as previous treatment for childhood cancer (e.g. chemotherapy and radiotherapy),

Table 14.2 Causes of delayed and abnormal puberty

Central delay		Gonadal impairment	
Intact axis	**Impaired axis**	**Boys**	**Girls**
Constitutional delay in growth and adolescence Chronic illness Eating disorders (e.g. anorexia nervosa)	Congenital hypopituitarism LHRH deficiency - 7isolated - with anosmia (Kallmann syndrome) - Prader-Willi syndrome Tumours adjacent to hypothalamo-pituitary axis (e.g. craniopharyngioma, suprasellar germinoma) Surgery and radiotherapy	Anorchia Bilateral cryptorchidism Klinefelter syndrome Prader-Willi syndrome Noonan syndrome Radiotherapy (e.g. for testicular relapse in leukaemia)	Gonadal dysgenesis (e.g. Turner syndrome) Radiotherapy (e.g. total body irradiation in preconditioning for bone marrow transplant Galactosaemia

LHRH, luteinizing-hormone-releasing hormone.

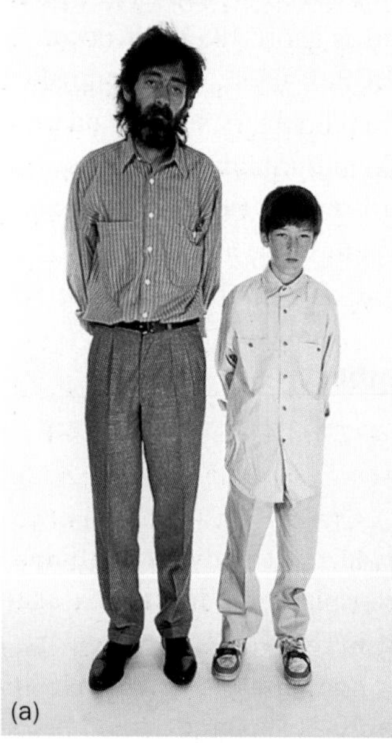

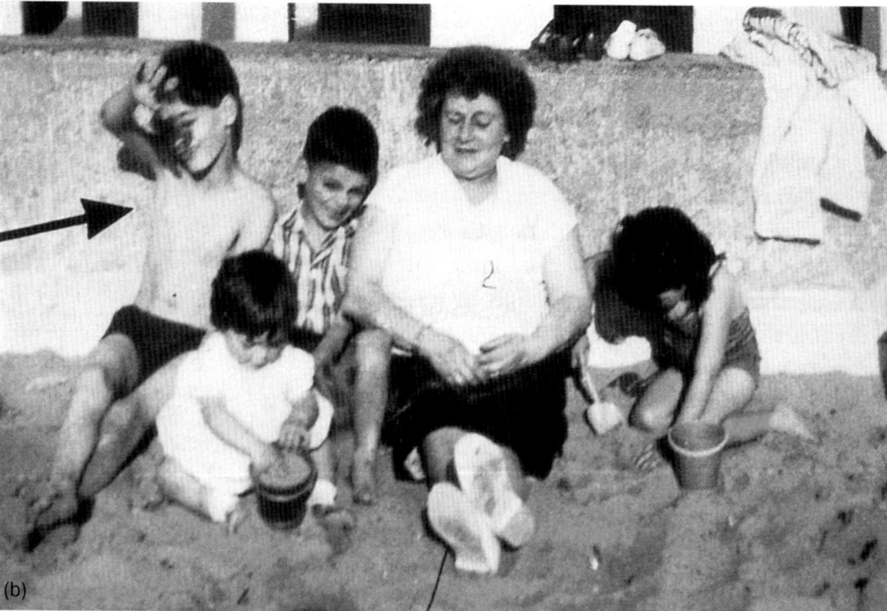

Figure 14.8 Father and son with constitutional delay in growth and puberty. The son is aged 12 years in (a) and the father (arrowed in b) is shown at age 14 years. No investigation was required in the son (reproduced with permission from Harcourt Publishers Ltd)

cryptorchidism, and pituitary disorders. Examination includes accurate measurement of the patient and parents, pubertal staging, nutritional assessment, a search for dysmorphic features (e.g. stigmata of TS), measurement of blood pressure, and examination of fundi for optic disc pallor (indicating a suprasellar lesion).

INVESTIGATIONS

The diagnosis of CDGA can usually made clinically, and most boys do not require investigation (Donaldson and Paterson, 2000). In girls, it is advisable to check the chromosomes for TS. If chronic systemic disease is suspected from the history and examination the patient must be investigated accordingly along similar lines to short stature screening (see previous section). When hypogonadism is suspected assessment includes gonadotrophin and sex hormone measurement before and after stimulation with LHRH and hCG, pelvic ultrasound examination, a formal smelling test, and cranial imaging. Unfortunately, the LHRH test cannot distinguish between the normal prepubertal state and central hypogonadism although a completely flat response suggests the latter.

MANAGEMENT OF DELAYED/INCOMPLETE PUBERTY

Physiological delay

Management of CDGA involves reassurance and counselling. Prediction of adult height, for example using the RUS(TW2) or TW3 systems of Tanner and Whitehouse, is helpful in giving the family a realistic height prognosis. In boys with CDGA aged 11–13 years the anabolic steroid oxandrolone in doses of 1.25–2.5 mg at night for three to six months enhances height velocity. Boys aged 13 years or more can be offered a course of intramuscular testosterone 100 mg monthly for three months to increase height velocity and genital maturation without causing final height impairment (Kelly *et al.*, 2003). Girls with CDGA are difficult to treat because of the tiny doses of oestradiol required to initiate puberty. In selected cases ethinylestradiol 2 μg daily or on alternate days for a one to two year period can be considered provided the patient is under strict endocrine supervision.

Impaired gonadal axis

Testosterone and oestrogen replacement will obviously be necessary in cases such as craniopharyngioma, TS and anorchia where gonadotrophin or sex steroid secretion is absent. Where the gonadal axis impairment is partial, for example following total body irradiation or in Klinefelter syndrome, treatment may be unnecessary or supplementation rather than full replacement may be required. For boys an effective testosterone regimen for induction is Sustanon® 100 mg intramuscularly once every six weeks for one year, 100 mg intramuscularly once every four weeks for a second year, then 250 mg intramuscularly every four weeks for a further year. Thereafter a suitable maintenance treatment – testosterone tablets, patches, intramuscular injections or subcutaneous pellets – should be chosen by the young adult and his doctor. For girls, an effective induction regimen is ethinylestradiol 2 μg daily for one year, 4 μg daily for a further year, then 6, 8 and 10 μg daily for four months followed by norethisterone 5 mg daily for the first five days of each calendar month in order to shed the endometrial lining and cause a period. Thereafter the girl and her doctor/gynaecologist should choose an appropriate maintenance regimen such as the oral contraceptive pill, hormone replacement therapy (HRT) and various patch preparations.

Miscellaneous pubertal problems

> **CASE STUDY**
>
> A 15-year-old girl is referred because her periods, which commenced aged 11 years but have never been regular, have stopped. On examination she is obese and hirsute with darkening of skin in the axillae (acanthosis nigricans). Investigation shows hyperinsulinism, elevated plasma androgens, and a basal LH of 12 U/L. Pelvic ultrasound shows 4 mL ovaries with a normal number of follicles.

Miscellaneous pubertal problems include **gynaecomastia** in boys, which commonly presents around the time of puberty and is presumably due to increased sensitivity of the breast tissue to the small amounts of oestrogen aromatized from testosterone. In most boys, the gynaecomastia settles spontaneously but severe cases cause considerable distress. A history of learning/behaviour difficulties and inappropriately small testes should lead to a search for Klinefelter syndrome, but this condition rarely presents with isolated gynaecomastia. If the gynaecomastia is causing distress with no immediate signs of resolution, it is appropriate to consult a plastic surgeon for consideration of subcutaneous breast reduction/liposuction.

In girls, immaturity of the hypothalamus frequently results in anovulatory cycles causing **menstrual disturbance** with infrequent/irregular periods and prolonged bleeding. Norethisterone 5 mg daily for 5 or 10 days will help shed the endometrial lining and stop the irregular bleeding, and is preferable in the first instance to the oral contraceptive pill, which simply suppresses the axis. The **polycystic ovary syndrome** (PCOS) is suggested by a combination of hyperandrogenism and ovulatory dysfunction, with weight gain, increased body hair, acne and infrequent/irregular periods. Investigations show raised fasting insulin, basal LH and serum androgens. Polycystic ovaries are usually but not always present. Treatment is with either metformin to increase insulin sensitivity or Dianette® (a combination of oestradiol and the antiandrogen cyproterone acetate), or both.

KEY LEARNING POINTS

- Precocious and early puberty is the domain of girls and usually idiopathic. Evaluation is by clinical assessment together with pelvic ultrasound evaluation and LHRH test.
- Boys with precocious and early puberty are more likely to have an intracranial lesion.
- If desired, puberty can be suppressed by downregulating pituitary gonadotrophin secretion using a GnRH analogue, given in depot form.
- Mild androgen excess in girls and boys aged 6–8 years is usually due to exaggerated adrenarche.
- Delayed puberty is the domain of boys in whom it is usually physiological. A short course of testosterone therapy may be helpful in boys with constitutional delay.

Thyroid axis

Embryology and morphology of the thyroid gland

At 4 weeks' gestation a downgrowth from the floor of the pharynx becomes a diverticulum. This descends into the neck, leaving a tract known as the thyroglossal duct which usually disappears during the sixth week. The bilobed diverticulum develops into the thyroid gland with two lateral lobes connected by a narrow, thin band of tissue in front of the trachea called the isthmus. Differentiation of the thyroid gland is controlled by a variety of transcription factors including TTF1, TTF2 and Pax 8. Thyroid dysgenesis may result from deficiency or abnormality of these and other factors. The fetal thyroid is able to form thyroglobulin by about the fourth week *in utero* and to synthesize thyroxine (T4) by week 10, up to 2 weeks before fetal TSH becomes detectable. During this first trimester the fetus is dependent on the small amounts of maternal T4 that pass through the placenta, so that severe iodine or thyroxine deficiency in the mother will have an adverse effect on fetal neurodevelopment. Figure 14.2 shows the interaction between TSH and the thyroid cell, and the synthetic steps involved with thyroxine production. The substrates for thyroxine are dietary iodide, which is oxidized in the thyroid to iodine, and tyrosine. Tyrosine is iodinated to produce mono- and diiodothyronine (MIT and DIT) which are then coupled to form tri- and tetraiodothyronine (T3 and T4). Outer and inner ring deiodination of T4 by the deiodinase enzymes DI, D II and D III result in the production of triiodothyronine (T3), the active metabolite, or reverse T3 (rT3), the inactive form. Both T4 and T3 are inactivated by sulphation. Modulation of the enzyme systems causing deiodination and sulphation of the thyroid hormones produces the appropriate concentration of T3 in specific tissues, such as brain, heart, muscle and pituitary gland. T4 and T3 bind to α- and β-receptors in the target tissues and have a profound influence on cellular metabolism. In children, thyroid hormones are essential for linear growth in childhood and neurodevelopment up until the end of the second year of life, and for metabolism, cardiovascular health and neurological function throughout life.

Thyroid assessment

HORMONE MEASUREMENT (TABLE 14.3)

The levels of total T4 are influenced by thyroid-binding globulin (TBG). Total T4 levels are therefore low in TBG deficiency, giving the spurious impression of hypothyroidism. For this reason most laboratories prefer to measure free T4. Neonates have higher T4 and fT4 than older children, reflecting increased TSH activity around the time of birth. Basal TSH is elevated in primary hypothyroidism, low in secondary hypothyroidism, normal or slightly elevated in tertiary hypothyroidism and suppressed ($<$0.05 mU/L) in hyperthyroidism. The TRH test shows an exaggerated response in primary hypothyroidism, a flat response in secondary hypothyroidism and a sustained rise in tertiary hypothyroidism.

Table 14.3 Measurement of thyroid hormones

Thyroid hormones		TSH (mU/L)	
T4	60–160 nmol/L	Basal	0.55–5.5
Free T4	9–26 pmol/L	30 minutes after TRH (200 μg IV)	5–30
T3	0.8–2.8 nmol/L	60 minutes after TRH	<30-minute value

TRH, thyroid releasing hormone; TSH, thyroid stimulating hormone.

Measurement of T3 is usually unnecessary in hypothyroidism but helpful in the monitoring of hyperthyroidism, since preferential conversion of T4 to T3 in hyperthyroid states causes T3 to be relatively higher.

THYROID ANTIBODY MEASUREMENT

In Graves disease TSH receptor antibody activity is measured as the percentage displacement of TSH binding (normal <10 per cent). In autoimmune or Hashimoto thyroiditis antibodies to thyroid peroxidase (TPO) are present (normal <35 IU/mL). Measurement of TPO antibody has replaced thyroglobulin and thyroid microsomal antibody assays in most laboratories.

THYROID IMAGING

Thyroid ultrasound determines the shape, size and consistency of the thyroid gland. Isotope scanning confirms the presence and site of thyroid tissue, identifies non-functioning and hyper-functioning nodules, and measures increased iodine uptake in conditions such as dyshormonogenesis, thyroiditis, and Graves disease. When malignancy is suspected, fine needle aspiration (FNA) should be done in liaison with an adult pathology service.

Classification of thyroid disorders in childhood

Hypothyroidism

Congenital

Transient

- Neonatal hypothyroxinaemia
- Transient neonatal hypothyroidism
- Hyperthyrotropinaemia

Permanent

- Thyroid dysgenesis: absent thyroid gland (agenesis); ectopic gland; hypoplastic gland *in situ*
- Dyshormonogenesis

Acquired

- Hashimoto disease.
- Antithyroid drugs, e.g. carbimazole
- Radiation, e.g. following radioiodine treatment for Graves disease
- Thyroid surgery, e.g. total thyroidectomy for carcinoma

NB: Congenital hypothyroidism, if not detected by newborn screening, may present later in childhood.

Hyperthyroidism

- Neonatal Graves disease
- Graves disease
- Hashimoto disease
- Drugs, e.g. amiodarone

Goitre

Hypothyroid

- Iodine deficiency
- Dyshormonogenesis
- Hashimoto disease

Hyperthyroid

- Graves disease
- Hashimoto disease

Euthyroid

- Physiological, e.g. puberty
- Hashimoto disease
- Iodine deficiency
- Thyroid carcinoma (usually papillary)

HYPOTHYROIDISM

CASE STUDY

A 10-day-old neonate is referred by the neonatal screening laboratory when the capillary blood sample taken on day 4 of life shows a TSH of 400 mU/L. She was born at term weighing 4000 g. On examination, she is still jaundiced with a large tongue, an umbilical hernia, and cool dry skin. Plasma fT4 is <5 pmol/L, and TSH >150 mU/L. Isotope and ultrasound scanning show no thyroid tissue.

Hypothyroidism can be classified according to:

- duration – transient or permanent
- cause – congenital or acquired
- site – primary (thyroid), secondary (pituitary) and tertiary (hypothalamic)
- severity – compensated (axis is impaired but still able to maintain fT4 levels within the reference range), or decompensated (fT4 is subnormal).

Neonatal thyroid problems

Preterm babies have relatively low T4 levels which may decrease below the reference range during perinatal illness – neonatal hypothyroxinaemia. Mild persistent TSH elevation (hyperthyrotropinaemia) may be due to delay in maturation of the thyroid axis, but needs to be distinguished from mild compensated congenital hypothyroidism. Transient neonatal TSH elevation with or without low T4 is seen in sick babies, e.g. due to prematurity and/or congenital malformations and following exposure to iodine for surgical procedures.

Permanent congenital hypothyroidism

Primary congenital hypothyroidism (CH) is relatively common (1 in 4000 live births) in contrast to secondary and tertiary hypothyroidism (1 in 50 000 births). The features of primary CH include coarse facies with enlarged tongue and hoarse cry, umbilical hernia, dry skin, hypothermia, lethargy and prolonged jaundice. The presence of goitre suggests dyshormonogenesis or iodine deficiency as the cause. Primary CH can be detected in all but the mildest cases by newborn screening. This is carried out by obtaining dried blood spots for TSH measurement by heel prick sampling between days 4 and 7, at which time the neonate should be on milk, thus enabling phenylketonuria screening to be done at the same time. Neonates with TSH values of >10–15 mU/L are referred. Those not on full milk feeds by day 7 should still have TSH sampling at the usual time, with a second sample for phenylketonuria screening at a later date.

Thyroid dysgenesis resulting in an absent, ectopic or hypoplastic gland accounts for 80 per cent of cases in the UK. A variety of recessive enzyme disorders disrupting T4 synthesis – dyshormonogenesis – accounts for the remaining 20 per cent. Dyshormonogenesis is suggested by the presence of goitre, and/or when CH occurs in siblings. The association between dyshormonogenesis and deafness is known as Pendred syndrome.

Thyroid imaging helps to distinguish true from transient CH and is of value in genetic counselling. Isotope scanning must be performed while TSH is still elevated, ideally within a week of starting treatment, and can be complemented by ultrasound imaging.

Screening has transformed the outlook for neonates with primary CH in whom treatment can now be started at 10–14 days of age. Prior to treatment, a good venous sample must be obtained for fT4 and TSH measurement, both to confirm the diagnosis and give a guide to prognosis. Neonates with initial fT4/T4 levels below <5 pmol/L (<40 mmol/L) may show a 10-point reduction in IQ score, with subtle motor, auditory and vestibular problems.

The optimal dose of thyroxine in infancy is controversial. There is some evidence that postnatal treatment with T4 in a relatively high dose (10–16 μg/kg per day) can redress any IQ deficit but there is concern that this might increase behaviour and concentration problems at a later age. Doses of 7–8 μg/kg per day (25 μg daily from birth) are associated with prolonged TSH elevation, implying underreplacement. In recent years, the present authors have started giving 50 μg daily for the first 10 days then 37.5 μg (approximately 10 μg/kg daily), adjusting the dose thereafter according to clinical progress and TSH levels. After the first year, treatment is relatively straightforward, giving 3–5 μg/kg per day of T4. The child is seen 6 to 12 monthly to adjust the dose according to body weight/surface area, using T4 and TSH measurement to monitor compliance.

Acquired hypothyroidism

Autoimmune thyroiditis or **Hashimoto thyroiditis** is by far the commonest cause of acquired hypothyroidism. Children with other autoimmune diseases such as diabetes mellitus, and with chromosomal disorders such as TS and Down syndrome are at increased risk (Figure 14.9) so that screening is indicated (Noble *et al.*, 2000). Common presenting features are goitre, hypothyroid symptoms such as pallor, tiredness, weight gain and cold intolerance, and occasionally features of hyperthyroidism. Examination shows euthyroid, hypothyroid or hyperthyroid features depending on the phase of the illness, goitre present or absent, and occasionally other features of autoimmune disease such as vitiligo and alopecia. In Down syndrome, the clinical features are difficult to differentiate from the syndrome itself so that annual screening, e.g. by measuring capillary TSH, is recommended. TPO antibodies are usually but not always positive at presentation. Treatment is with very low initial doses of thyroxine, increasing in small increments at a slow pace (e.g. by 25 μg every two months), until a target dose of 3–4 μg/kg per day is achieved. More rapid increments may be associated with marked adverse symptoms including poor concentration, behaviour disturbances, fatigue and irritability.

Secondary and tertiary hypothyroidism are seen in the context of hypothalamo-hypopituitary disease and almost never in isolation from other anterior pituitary hormone deficiencies. Thyroxine replacement will be necessary for end-stage or ablated Graves disease, and following removal of the thyroid gland (e.g. for carcinoma).

HYPERTHYROIDISM

> **CASE STUDY**
>
> A 10-year-old girl with a family history of diabetes and pernicious anaemia presents with a four-month history of heat intolerance, weight loss and poor concentration. On examination, she is tall with a smooth symmetrical goitre and tachycardia but no exophthalmos. Investigations show TSH suppression with high fT4 and T3, TSH receptor antibodies are negative but TPO antibodies are >1000 IU/mL.

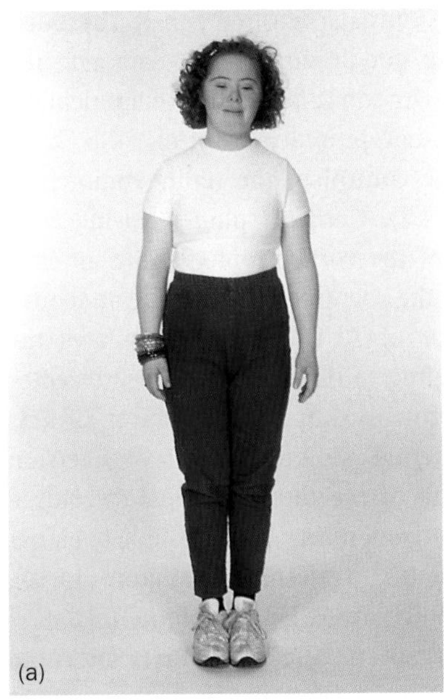

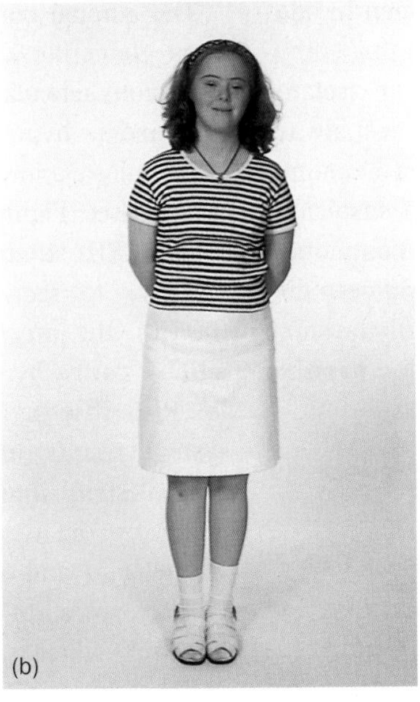

Figure 14.9 Adolescent with Down syndrome before and after detection and treatment of hypothyroidism (due to Hashimoto thyroiditis) on school-based capillary thyroid stimulating hormone (TSH) screening programme

Neonatal Graves disease

This occurs in a small proportion of babies of affected mothers and is due to transplacental transfer of TSH receptor antibodies. The condition can be severe, with tachycardia, failure to thrive, irritability and diarrhoea. The diagnosis is confirmed by measuring neonatal fT4, T3 and TSH, and by demonstrating TSH receptor antibodies in both the mother's and the baby's serum. Treatment, which may be required for several months, is with Lugol iodine solution initially together with carbimazole 0.5–1.0 mg/kg per day.

Paediatric Graves disease

This is much rarer but also more severe in children than in adults. There is a female preponderance. The presenting features include heat intolerance with irritability and hyperactivity, deteriorating school performance, rapid growth, weight loss despite an increased appetite, palpitations and diarrhoea. There is often a family history of thyroid disease. Examination shows a diffuse goitre, exophthalmos that is rarely severe, relative tall stature, choreiform movements, tremor and tachycardia. The diagnosis is confirmed by demonstrating elevated fT4 and T3 levels with complete TSH suppression. Both TSH receptor and TPO antibodies are usually positive. Initial treatment is with propranolol 1 mg/kg per day in three divided doses adjusted according to response, and carbimazole or propylthiouracil given in the doses of 0.5 and 5 mg/kg per day, respectively. Following initial stabilization the fT4 and T3 levels will fall so that the dose of antithyroid drug should either be reduced (titration method) or thyroxine added (block and replace method). Both regimens have their advocates, but the latter is unsuitable in children with particularly severe thyrotoxicosis and/or poor compliance in whom blockade may not be achievable, even with high doses of carbimazole (>1 mg/kg per day).

Paediatric Graves disease does not remit for many years. Alternatives to medical therapy such as surgery and radioiodine should be considered in children with compliance difficulties, and/or those in whom symptom control is poor. The recurrence of thyrotoxicosis following surgery together with the risk of unsightly keloid scarring has led some centres in recent years to prefer ablative treatment with radioiodine followed by thyroxine replacement.

Hashimoto thyroiditis

About 5 per cent of cases with Hashimoto thyroiditis will show a hyperthyroid phase. The condition is distinguished from Graves disease by the absence of exophthalmos and TSH receptor antibodies. Medical treatment is easier to administer in Hashimoto than Graves disease and non-medical strategies such as surgery and radiotherapy are not normally required.

Drug-induced hyperthyroidism

The thyroxine analogue amiodarone is used as an antiarrhythmic drug and can produce a variety of clinical patterns including hypo- and hyperthyroidism. In such cases the minimum necessary dose of amiodarone should be used, and the patient treated either with carbimazole or thyroxine depending on thyroid status.

GOITRE

Throughout the world, iodine deficiency is the main cause of (usually euthyroid) goitre. In the iodine-sufficient UK, euthyroid goitre is usually due to Hashimoto disease, while modest thyroid enlargement may be seen in adolescence and pregnancy. The presence of enlarging euthyroid goitre, especially if the gland shows an isolated nodule, is suspicious of thyroid carcinoma, almost always papillary in children. Isotope and ultrasound examination of the thyroid is indicated, with FNA of suspicious areas followed by surgical exploration. The commonest cause of hypothyroid goitre in the UK is Hashimoto disease, dyshormonogenesis accounting for only a small proportion of cases. Hyperthyroid goitre is due to either Graves or Hashimoto disease.

KEY LEARNING POINTS

- Primary congenital hypothyroidism is detected by neonatal screening for TSH elevation on blood spot samples from the heel prick on days 5–7.
- Hashimoto disease usually presents as hypothyroid or euthyroid goitre and occasionally with hyperthyroidism.
- Graves disease is rare in childhood but the condition is more severe in the paediatric age range and does not remit for many years.
- Thyroid carcinoma, although rare, should be considered in the context of an enlarging euthyroid or nodular goitre in the absence of thyroid autoantibodies.

Adrenal axis

Embryology and morphology of the adrenal gland

The adrenal gland is divided into:

- the inner medulla, derived from the neuroectoderm of the neural crest
- the outer cortex, derived from the mesoderm.

The adrenal cortex consists of three zones: the outer zona glomerulosa, the middle zona fasciculata and the inner zona reticularis. The zonae fasciculata and reticularis are under hypothalamic-pituitary control, the zona glomerulosa under the control of the renin–angiotensin system (see Figure 14.2). Corticotrophin-releasing hormone (CRH) stimulates the corticotrophs of the anterior pituitary to secrete the peptide pro-opiomelanocortin (POMC), the precursor of ACTH, which stimulates the adrenal cortex by binding to the melanocortin-2 receptor (MCR-2) that is G-protein coupled. Activation of this system results in steroid synthesis, with conversion of cholesterol into one of the three principal steroids – glucocorticoid (e.g. cortisol), mineralocorticoid (e.g. aldosterone) and androgen (e.g. testosterone) (Figure 14.10). Cortisol secretion results in ACTH inhibition (negative feedback) whereas cortisol insufficiency causes increased ACTH secretion. The skin pigmentation in ACTH excess is due partly to an increase in the breakdown products of POMC, including melanocyte-stimulating hormone (MSH) and also because the ACTH molecule has affinity for the MCR-1 receptors in the skin.

Assessment of adrenal function

MINERALOCORTICOID FUNCTION

This is reflected by the blood pressure, electrolytes and plasma renin activity. In deficiency states blood pressure and sodium are low, potassium and renin high; in states of excess, blood pressure is elevated, potassium is low and renin suppressed.

GLUCOCORTICOID FUNCTION

Assessment of cortisol excess involves measuring fasting 8 am and sleeping midnight cortisol samples (looking for loss of diurnal rhythm), urine-free cortisol on three consecutive 24-hour urine collections, and carrying out the low-dose dexamethasone suppression test (see below). ACTH is high when cortisol deficiency is due to a primary defect and low with secondary or tertiary insufficiency).

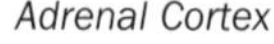

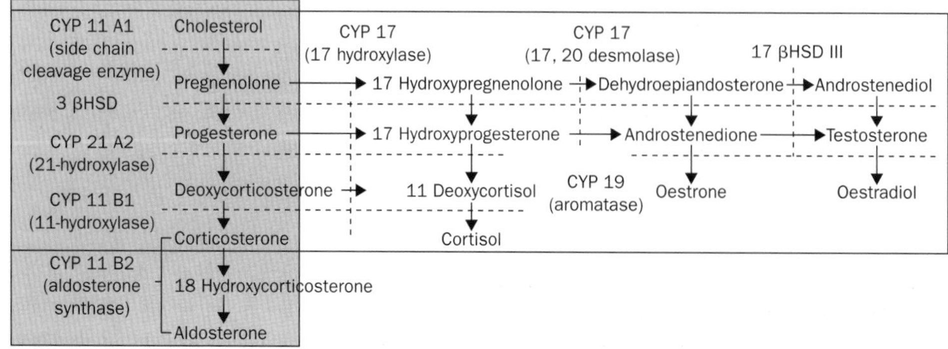

Figure 14.10 Pathways of steroid synthesis in adrenal cortex

Synacthen is given in standard (250 μg) dose to estimate adrenal reserve in primary adrenal insufficiency, and low (500 ng/1.73 m^2) dose when secondary or tertiary deficiency is suspected.

ANDROGEN STATUS

If androgen deficiency or excess is suspected then a standard Synacthen test is done, measuring basal ACTH, and the steroid precursors 17-hydroxyprogesterone (17-OHP), dehydroepiandrosterone sulphate (DHAS) and androstenedione before and 60 minutes after stimulation. Adrenal imaging is simplest using ultrasound but CT and MRI provide better resolution and should always be sought if adrenal pathology (e.g. tumour) is seriously suspected.

Classification of adrenal disorders

Adrenal insufficiency and excess can be classified (Table 14.4) according to:

- cause – congenital and acquired
- site – primary, secondary and tertiary

Table 14.4 Classification of adrenal disorders

Adrenal insufficiency		
Glucocorticoid	**Mineralocorticoid**	**Androgen**
Primary Congenital Congenital adrenal hyperplasia (CAH) Adrenal hypoplasia congenita (AHC) Familial glucocorticoid deficiency Acquired (Addison disease) Autoimmune Tuberculosis Adrenoleucodystrophy Surgery, drugs (e.g. cyproterone)	*Aldosterone deficiency* Congenital AHC CAH (21-hydroxylase, 3β-HSD and StAR protein deficiency) Aldosterone synthetase deficiency Acquired Addison disease *Aldosterone resistance* (pseudohypoaldosteronism) Inactivating defect of epithelial sodium channel (recessive, severe) Dominant/sporadic defect (less severe)	AHC CAH (StAR protein, 3β-HSD, and 17α-hydroxylase deficiency) Other enzyme defects 17, 20 desmolase and 17β-HSD deficiency
Secondary and tertiary Congenital Hypopituitarism, e.g. septo-optic dysplasia Acquired Tumours Pituitary surgery Iatrogenic – withdrawal of exogenous steroids		
Adrenal excess		
Glucocorticoid (Cushing syndrome)	**Mineralocorticoid**	**Androgen**
Primary Adrenal tumour Primary micronodular hyperplasia McCune–Albright syndrome Secondary Pituitary Cushing disease Iatrogenic steroid administration Oral Skin preparation Intranasal steroids Inhaled steroids Ectopic ACTH syndrome	Primary and secondary hyperaldosteronism Fludrocortisone overdosage Liquorice excess CAH (11β- and 17α-hydroxylase deficiency) 11β-HSD 2 deficiency (apparent mineralocorticoid excess) Glucocorticoid suppressible hyperaldosteronism Activating defect of epithelial sodium channel (Liddle syndrome)	Exaggerated adrenarche Virilizing adrenal tumour Cortical adenoma Carcinoma CAH (21- and 11β-hydroxylase deficiency)

ACTH, adrenocorticotropic hormone; HSD, hydroxy steroid dehydrogenase.

- pathway principally affected – mineralocorticoid, glucocorticoid and androgen.

PRIMARY ADRENAL INSUFFICIENCY

CASE STUDY

A baby boy named John presents on day 10 of life with poor weight gain, vomiting, and poor colour during the preceding 24 hours. On examination the baby weighs 3200 g (birth weight 3600 g) and is severely dehydrated with pigmentation of the genitalia which show apparent hypospadias with bifid scrotum. Electrolytes show plasma sodium 110 mmol/L and potassium 7.8 mmol/L.

Congenital causes

Adrenal hypoplasia congenita (AHC) is usually inherited as an X-linked disorder caused by a mutation in the DAX-1 gene. Features include salt wasting with failure to thrive, dehydration, hyponatraemia and hypoglycaemia together with increased pigmentation due to ACTH excess. There may be a history of early infant death in maternal male relatives. The Synacthen test will show low normal or even normal basal cortisol levels but with little or no response to a standard dose.

Familial glucocorticoid deficiency is an autosomal recessive disorder in which the adrenal cortex is unresponsive to ACTH. This results in severe cortisol deficiency with hypoglycaemia and jaundice but no salt wasting since the renin–angiotensin system is unaffected. In about 50 per cent of cases, an inactivating mutation of the ACTH receptor gene can be found.

Congenital adrenal hyperplasia (CAH) is the name given to a group of five enzyme defects causing impaired cortisol synthesis with consequent increase in ACTH secretion and adrenal enlargement (see Figure 14.10). By far the commonest variety is 21-hydroxylase deficiency (21-OHD), caused by deletion of the active 21B gene, its partial or complete replacement by the inactive 21A pseudogene or by a point mutation in the 21B gene. The enzyme deficiency and ACTH drive lead to deficiency of glucocorticoid and mineralocorticoid, and androgen excess, respectively.

The phenotype in 21-OHD relates to the severity of the enzyme defect and the sex of the patient. The clinical forms are as follows:

- Salt wasting (SW-21-OHD) – accounting for 70–80 per cent of childhood cases
- Simple virilizing (SV-21-OHD) – accounting for 20–30 per cent
- Non-classical (NC) – seen in female adolescents and in adulthood.

SW-21-OHD in males causes failure to thrive, vomiting and dehydration, usually presenting between 5 and 10 days after birth – the salt wasting crisis. Untreated, these neonates die quickly. Examination shows wasting and dehydration with pigmentation of the scrotum due to the ACTH excess. Biochemistry shows hyponatraemia (sodium often $<$110 mmol/L), hyperkalaemia, acidosis and hypoglycaemia, and the diagnosis is confirmed by measurement of the precursor steroid 17-α-hydroxyprogesterone, which will be grossly elevated.

SW-21-OHD in females results in prenatal virilization with enlargement of the clitoris, narrowing of the lower vagina to form a urogenital sinus, and fusion of the labia majora (Figure 14.11). In severe cases, the baby appears to be a boy with hypospadias and undescended testes. Appropriate assessment includes analysis of chromosomes to show a 46,XX complement, pelvic ultrasound to show a uterus, and measurement of 17-OHP. If incorrectly diagnosed as males, these babies present in salt wasting crisis.

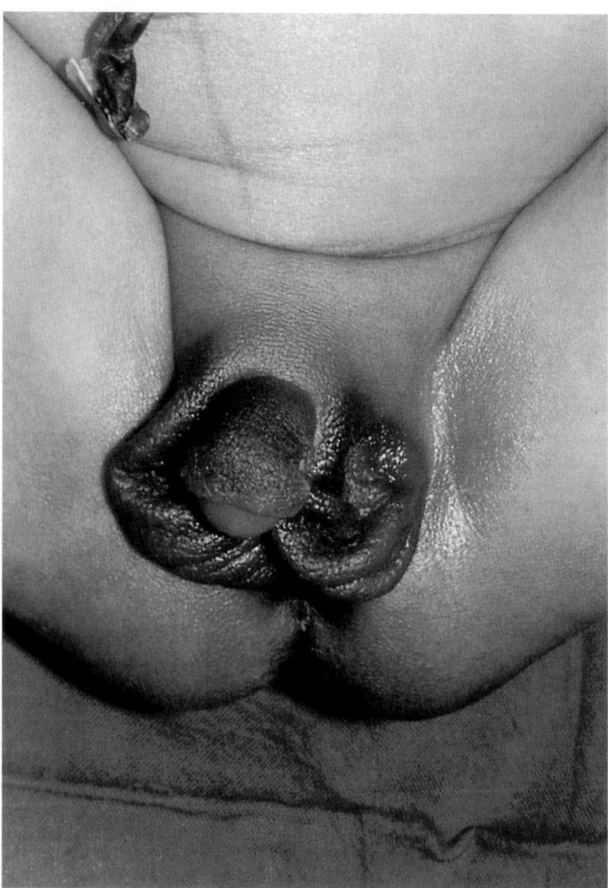

Figure 14.11 Genitalia of neonate with lax, rugose labioscrotal folds, clitoro-phallus with perineal hypospadias and no palpable gonads. Karyotype was 46,XX and serum 17-hydroxyprogesterone (17-OHP) greatly elevated, consistent with 21-hydroxylase deficiency

SV-OHD in girls and boys usually presents between 2 and 5 years of age with the features of androgen excess. Tall stature with bone age advance is a constant feature and there may also be greasy skin and hair with acne, behaviour problems, and pubic hair. The clitoris or phallus is enlarged and in boys the testes are pre-pubertal in volume. Following treatment, almost all children develop true precocious puberty due to the priming effect of the androgens.

Management

21-Hydroxylase deficiency is treated with glucocorticoid to suppress ACTH and thus androgen overproduction under basal conditions, giving increased doses at times of stress (e.g. intercurrent illness and surgery) and mineralocorticoid to replace aldosterone deficiency. Girls require surgery to reduce clitoral size while preserving the neurovascular supply and to open out the lower vagina so as to allow menstruation and intercourse at a later date. The timing of surgery is controversial. In the UK, clitoroplasty and vaginoplasty are usually performed as a one-stage procedure towards the end of infancy, with further vaginal surgery around the age of 10 years.

The key to successful management is for the family to have a good understanding of the condition, sufficient to ensure reasonable compliance and regular clinic attendance. The family must have written instructions concerning management of acute illness, which involves increasing the oral hydrocortisone dose initially, giving it intramuscularly in the event of drowsiness or vomiting. In clinic, the growth rate is monitored closely and the glucocorticoid dose adjusted to keep pace with body surface area. Most patients grow well on hydrocortisone 10–15 mg/m^2 per day and fludrocortisone 100–150 μg/m^2 per day but obesity is a common problem especially in girls. Bone age is measured annually, and biochemistry assessed every 6 to 12 months by measuring either serum or capillary blood spot 17-OHP.

Prenatal treatment and screening

Virilization in an affected female fetus can be prevented or minimized by treating the mother with dexamethasone provided that this is begun no later than 9 weeks' gestation and preferably by 5–6 weeks. At 9–10 weeks chorionic villous sampling enables fetal sexing and mutational analysis to be carried out and treatment is discontinued if the child is a male or an unaffected female. Although effective, prenatal treatment is controversial. Only one in eight fetuses will benefit because of the 1 in 4 chance of the baby having 21-OHD, and the 1 in 2 chance of being female, while the long-term effects of prenatal dexamethasone treatment on the brain and cardiovascular system are unknown.

Neonatal screening for 21-OHD can be carried out on day 2 of life by capillary sampling for 17-OHP. With efficient screening and prompt treatment the salt losing crisis and gender misassignment can be pre-empted and late presentation with sexual precocity eliminated. Unfortunately, neonatal screening, now routine in many parts of mainland Europe and North America, is still not practised in the UK.

ACQUIRED ADRENAL INSUFFICIENCY

> **CASE STUDY**
>
> A boy of 6 years is admitted with tiredness and weight loss. He is found to be pigmented and investigation shows elevated ACTH and renin levels with grossly impaired response to Synacthen (basal and peak cortisol 294 and 183 nmol/L respectively). He is given hydrocortisone and fludrocortisone replacement and is well for a year but then re-presents with loss of vision.

Addison disease

This is usually autoimmune in nature and may be associated with other conditions such as Hashimoto thyroiditis, diabetes mellitus type 1, hypoparathyroidism, vitiligo, alopecia, malabsorption and hepatitis. The triad of mucocutaneous candidiasis, hypoparathyroidism and Addison disease is characteristic of autoimmune polyendocrinopathy with cutaneous ectodermal dysplasia (APECED) caused by a mutation of the autoimmune regulator gene on chromosome 21. Other causes of Addison disease include tuberculosis, previous bilateral adrenalectomy for Cushing syndrome, and drugs including metyrapone and cyproterone. An important cause in males is X-linked adrenoleucodystrophy (ALD) which is associated with progressive neurological symptoms usually preceding but occasionally following the development of adrenal insufficiency.

The symptoms of Addison disease are insidious with initial lethargy (especially in the mornings), increased frequency of and difficulty shaking off intercurrent illness, and pigmentation – all attributable to cortisol deficiency. In the later stages vomiting due to aldosterone deficiency occurs. Astute diagnosis is needed to pre-empt the Addisonian crisis – hypotension and circulatory collapse, impaired conscious level leading to coma, hyponatraemic dehydration with hyperkalaemia and hypoglycaemia.

The clinical diagnosis is confirmed by documenting elevation of ACTH and renin, and performing a standard

Synacthen test under controlled conditions since this investigation may precipitate an adrenal crisis. Very long chain fatty acids (VLCFA) must be measured in boys to exclude ALD. An autoantibody screen (including adrenal antibodies) and measurement of calcium and phosphate, thyroid function, haemoglobin and liver function tests should be performed to detect accompanying autoimmune diseases.

SECONDARY AND TERTIARY ADRENAL INSUFFICIENCY

The symptoms are similar to those seen with primary adrenal insufficiency except that salt wasting does not occur. Congenital ACTH deficiency is seen in the context of idiopathic congenital panhypopituitarism and septooptic dysplasia, and may present with hypoglycaemia and prolonged jaundice in the neonatal period. Acquired secondary adrenal insufficiency is seen in patients with tumours adjacent to the hypothalamo-pituitary axis, e.g. craniopharyngioma, and as a relatively rare late effect of radiotherapy in the treatment of childhood cancer. Adrenal insufficiency also occurs when chronic steroid medication is suddenly discontinued. The inhaled steroids, particularly fluticasone (see below), may cause adrenal suppression with symptoms of chronic steroid insufficiency, complicated by acute decompensation with hypoglycaemia.

TREATMENT OF GLUCOCORTICOID INSUFFICIENCY

In hypopituitary patients, hydrocortisone 8–10 mg/m^2 per day is usually sufficient. In primary adrenal insufficiency, the starting dose is 12 mg/m^2 per day, but considerably higher doses may be required. Aldosterone replacement, where appropriate, is given as fludrocortisone 100 μg daily, increasing to 150–200 μg daily in adolescence.

ADRENAL STEROID EXCESS

> **CASE STUDY**
>
> A 2-year-old boy with Down syndrome is admitted for investigation of gross Cushing syndrome. Morning and midnight cortisol levels, however, are not recordable (<25 nmol/L). Further enquiry reveals that the child has been treated with intranasal betamethasone for six months.

Mineralocorticoid excess (rare)

Mineralocorticoid excess occurs in the 11β- and 17β-hydroxylase deficient varieties of congenital adrenal hyperplasia. A mutation in the gene encoding for the enzyme aldosterone synthetase results in a chimeric enzyme under aldosterone control, causing glucocorticoid suppressible hyperaldosteronism. Deficiency of the enzyme 11 β-hydroxysteroid dehydrogenase type II, which inactivates cortisol to cortisone in the kidney, leads to swamping of the aldosterone-binding sites in the renal tubules by cortisol – so-called apparent mineralocorticoid excess (AME).

Glucocorticoid excess

Glucocorticoid excess gives rise to **Cushing syndrome.** The classic clinical features comprise obesity with the typical fat distribution giving the characteristic moon face, buffalo hump, and truncal obesity with relatively thin arms and legs; hirsutism; striae; acne; hypertension; and short stature with growth failure. Cushing syndrome is readily differentiated from simple obesity on the grounds of height status, although the occasional patient with obesity and normal variant short stature may cause confusion.

The diagnosis is made by demonstrating lack of circadian rhythm, increased urine-free cortisol on three consecutive 24-hour urinary estimations and failure of cortisol to suppress to <50 nmol/L during the low-dose dexamethasone suppression test (0.8 mg of dexamethasone six hourly for 48 hours, followed by measurement of plasma cortisol at 9 am the following day).

Diagnosis of the *cause* of Cushing syndrome involves investigations best carried out in a specialist centre. The high-dose dexamethasone suppression test results in cortisol suppression in pituitary Cushing syndrome (Cushing disease) but not in adrenal Cushing or ectopic ACTH secretion. In selected cases, bilateral inferior petrosal venous sampling of ACTH following CRH administration is required to confirm Cushing disease. High-resolution MRI of the adrenal gland and pituitary gland may show the lesion.

Iatrogenic Cushing syndrome rarely presents a diagnostic problem when oral or dermatological treatment has been given, but the significance of intranasal preparations (e.g. betamethasone) and high-dose inhaled steroids (e.g. fluticasone) can be overlooked. The diagnosis is suggested when there are cushingoid features in the context of steroid administration, low/unrecordable basal cortisol and ACTH and an impaired cortisol response to standard or low-dose Synacthen.

Iatrogenic Cushing syndrome is treated by withdrawal of steroid medication where possible, ensuring that hydrocortisone cover is given during the first year in cases where there is severe adrenal insufficiency. Adrenal tumours are treated surgically. Cushing disease (Figure 14.12) is treated where possible with transsphenoidal hypophysectomy followed if necessary by pituitary irradiation. Cortisol excess due to McCune–Albright syndrome or to inoperable adrenal carcinoma can be treated with agents such as metyrapone and ketoconazole.

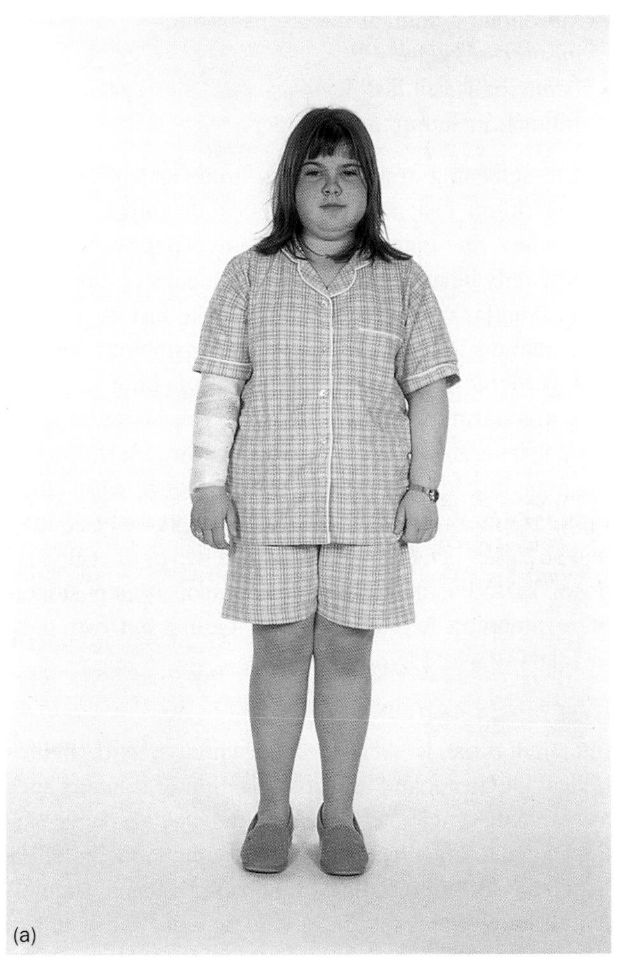

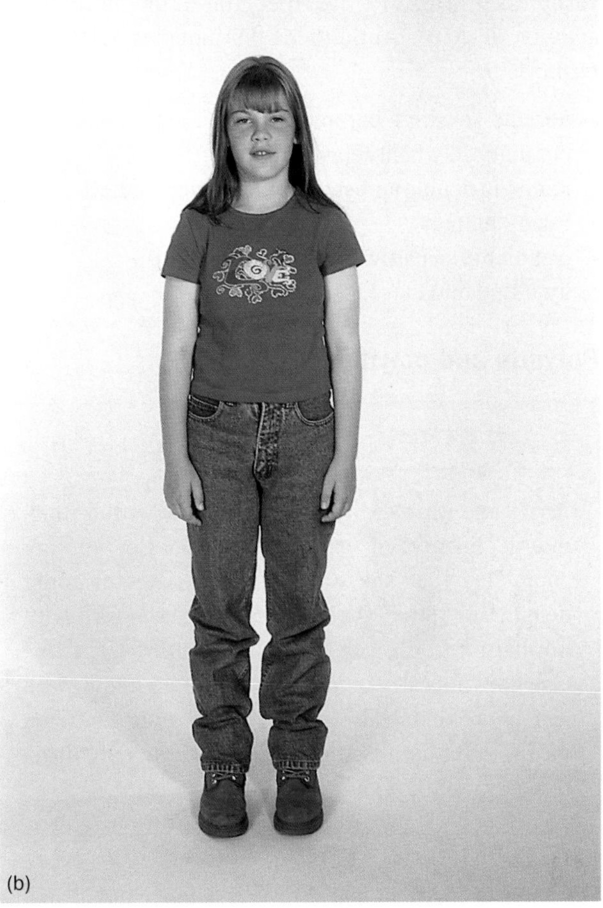

Figure 14.12 (a, b) Cushing disease in a 7-year-old girl. Despite no adenoma being identified during pituitary exploration, cortisol levels were not recordable postoperatively, followed by remission of the clinical features and catch-up growth as shown in (b), taken 15 months after (a)

Adrenal androgen excess

This is seen with adrenal tumours and in the two commonest forms of congital adrenal hyperplasia (see above). Adrenal tumours usually feature a fairly short history (i.e. several months) of virilization sufficient to cause clitoral/phallic enlargement and, in contrast to 21-OHD, tall stature and bone age advance are not present. Investigations include the measurement of serum and urinary steroids, and adrenal imaging. Surgery is the treatment of choice and, in tumours <5 cm diameter, is usually curative. Children with adrenal tumours merit genetic review since some cases are related to the Li–Straumer gene anomaly, linked with familial malignancy.

KEY LEARNING POINTS

- The symptoms of adrenal insufficiency are insidious. Glucocorticoid deficiency causes fatigue, weakness, difficulty in shaking off and susceptibility to infections, hypoglycaemia and ultimately acute collapse; mineralocorticoid deficiency causes vomiting with hyponatraemic dehydration and hyperkalaemia.
- The standard Synacthen test is used for diagnosing primary adrenal insufficiency, and the low-dose Synacthen test is used for secondary and tertiary deficiency.
- The management of the 21-OHD variety of CAH involves patient and family education. Prenatal treatment to prevent virilization in females is effective but controversial.

Posterior pituitary (see Figure 14.2)

Arginine vasopressin (AVP), also called antidiuretic hormone (ADH) and oxytocin are nonapeptides, each with antidiuretic and pressor effects. Antidiuretic hormone acts primarily on the collecting tubule of the nephron to cause water retention and oxytocin acts principally on uterine muscle and on the let-down reflex during lactation. The ADH analogue 1-desamino-8-D-arginine vasopressin (DDAVP) has four times the antidiuretic activity of ADH. Antidiuretic hormone is released in response to:

- volume-sensitive baroreceptors in the systemic circulation, which relay signals to the paraventricular and supraoptic nuclei in the hypothalamus
- osmolality-sensitive osmoreceptors in the hypothalamus.

Polyuria and polydipsia

CASE STUDY

An 18-month-old girl is seen in clinic with a four-month history of excessive thirst. Her mother complains that she wakes several times at night demanding 'juice'. On examination, she is well with normal nutrition, height on 50th centile. The clinician does not carry out any investigations and instead merely recommends giving water only between meals. After an unsettled few weeks, the polydipsia resolves.

Excessive drinking in a healthy pre-school child is almost invariably due to habit drinking and can be cured by banning all fluid except for water between meals. It is unnecessary to subject these children to a water deprivation test, the result of which will often be difficult to interpret due to a functional urine concentration defect secondary to depletion of solute in the renal medulla.

Organic polyuria and polydipsia are caused by:

- osmotic diuresis in diabetes mellitus and chronic renal failure
- renal salt wasting in renal tubular disorders and aldosterone deficiency
- renal tubular impairment caused by chronic hypokalaemia and hypercalcaemia
- antidiuretic hormone deficiency – cranial diabetes insipidus (DI)
- arginine vasopressin resistance – nephrogenic DI.

Cranial DI results in severe polydypsia. Pre-school children may be so desperate for fluids as to drink water from the bath or lavatory, and fluid deprivation results in agitation with rapid development of hypernatraemia and hyperchloraemia. The causes of cranial DI are:

- tumours in the hypothalamo-pituitary area (e.g. craniopharyngioma)
- autosomal dominant mutations in the vasopressin gene
- Langerhans cell histiocytosis
- trauma, including neurosurgery.

The screening test for DI is urine osmolality after an overnight fast, a value of 800 mOsmol/kg or more excluding the diagnosis. The water deprivation test should only be undertaken in exceptional situations by a team familiar with the technique. If the history, clinical examination, and cranial MRI indicate pathology consistent with cranial DI, water deprivation is both unnecessary and hazardous. When no cause can be found serial cranial imaging should be performed in order to detect an evolving lesion. Cranial DI is treated with either intranasal or oral DDAVP starting with doses of about 5 and 50 $\mu g/m^2$ per day, respectively, in two or three divided doses. DDAVP can be given subcutaneously in postoperative situations (e.g. craniopharyngioma) but care must be taken to avoid hyponatraemia.

HYPODIPSIA AND ADIPSIA

Impaired thirst is seen in some children with neurological handicap, and as a complication of tumours such as craniopharyngioma. These children may also have partial DI due to impaired osmoreceptor function with failure to secrete AVP in response to increased plasma osmolality, although the response to volume depletion is intact. Chronic hypernatraemic dehydration may result and rapid fluid replacement may induce fitting. Management is with a combination of DDAVP and a minimum daily target for fluid intake.

DOPAMINE AND PROLACTIN

Dopamine secretion inhibits prolactin, which is therefore elevated in hypothalamic hypopituitarism. Prolactin is low in Pit 1 and Prop 1 deficiency. Prolactin-secreting tumours are exceptionally rare in children.

The satiety system

Leptin, a peptide produced by the adipose cells, binds to receptors in the hypothalamus and inhibits secretion of neuropeptide Y (NPY), causing satiety. Conversely low leptin levels during fasting result in lack of NPY inhibition and increase in appetite. Leptin stimulates POMC production, one of whose cleavage products is MSH. By binding to its receptor MCR-4, MSH inhibits NPY so that the net effect of leptin on POMC is to cause satiety.

Hyperphagia is most commonly seen in the context of simple obesity from overeating. This produces hyperinsulinaemia with acanthosis nigricans (darkening of the skin in the axillae) in some subjects, predisposing to type

2 diabetes in later life. Steroid treatment stimulates the appetite and is one of the factors causing obesity in CAH.

Rarely mutations occur in the gene encoding leptin, its receptor, and the MCR-4, causing impaired satiety with consequent severe obesity. Impaired satiety is seen in various learning disability syndromes, including Bardet- Biedl syndrome and, most notoriously, Prader–Willi syndrome.

Prader–Willi syndrome

Prader–Willi syndrome results from loss of paternally imprinted gene(s) from the 11–13q region of chromosome 15. In over 70 per cent the cause is a deletion in the critical region in the sperm fertilizing the ovum. In about 20 per cent of cases the cause is maternal disomy where the baby inherits both chromosomes 15 from the mother thus losing the paternal contribution to the 11–13q area. Loss of protein(s) critical in neurodevelopment are presumed to cause the classic features of hypothalamic dysfunction with hyperphagia, hypogonadism and temper tantrum, together with hypotonia and learning disability. Mean IQ (70) is within the range of mild learning disability but traits such as rigid thinking, perseveration and impaired verbal memory result in a lower performance IQ.

The clinical presentation of Prader–Willi syndrome is classic with reduced fetal movements and extreme floppiness at birth resulting in little movement, little or no cry and poor feeding so that a nasogastric tube is required. Gross motor milestones are delayed. At 2–3 years the hyperphagic phase of the condition begins so that unless strict dietary surveillance is practised, the child rapidly veers from being thin to becoming obese. There is usually moderate short stature with an impaired growth response to obesity and most subjects show low growth hormone levels on stimulation testing. Bilateral cryptorchidism is the rule in males with absent or incomplete puberty whereas females show delayed but complete puberty with oligomenorrhoea.

Management involves intensive dietetic, physiotherapy, speech and language, and occupational therapy input during the first year. Strict dietary control and early nursery placement will enhance development and pre-empt the hyperphagic phase of the condition. Management of obsessional behaviour, temper tantrums, skin picking and perseveration becomes a challenge during the childhood and adolescent years. Growth hormone treatment may be helpful in improving both linear growth and body composition. Males require testosterone supplementation from late adolescence onwards. Appropriate placement, occupation and dietary control are needed in adulthood to avoid the complications of morbid obesity such as type 2 diabetes, sleep apnoea and respiratory failure.

DISORDERS OF SEXUAL DIFFERENTIATION

Physiology of sex determination and differentiation (Figure 14.13)

- Sex determination is the differentiation of the indifferent gonad into testis or ovary.
- Sex differentiation is the differentiation of the internal and external genitalia into male or female structures.

Sex determination

Presence of the SRY (*S*ex determining *R*egion of the *Y* chromosome) gene, which interacts with other genes on the autosomes and X chromosome, influences migration of primordial germ cells from the dorsal endoderm of the yolk sac to the indifferent gonad at the urogenital ridge in the 4th and 5th weeks of gestation. This results in testicular differentiation and testosterone production by 9 weeks' gestation. In the absence of SRY, ovarian differentiation takes place but little is known concerning the genes involved.

Sex differentiation

Internal genitalia (Figure 14.13a)

From 7 weeks' gestation the fetus possesses a double system – the Wolffian system with potential for male development and the Müllerian system with potential for female development. In the absence of a gonad the Wolffian system involutes while the Müllerian system forms the fallopian tubes, uterus, and upper third of the vagina. If a testis is present, production of anti-Müllerian hormone (AMH) from Sertoli cells results in active suppression of the Müllerian system while testosterone production from Leydig cells develops the Wolffian system into the epididymis, vas deferens, seminal vesicles and ejaculatory ducts.

External genitalia (Figure 14.13b)

In the absence of a testis, the urogenital sinus forms the lower two-thirds of the vagina and the urethra and the common anlage differentiates into the clitoris, labia minora, and labia majora. In the presence of a testis, testosterone is converted to dihydrotestosterone by the tissue enzyme 5α-reductase resulting in narrowing of the urogenital sinus to form the posterior urethra and prostate gland. The genital tubercle of the common anlage develops into the glans penis (homologous with

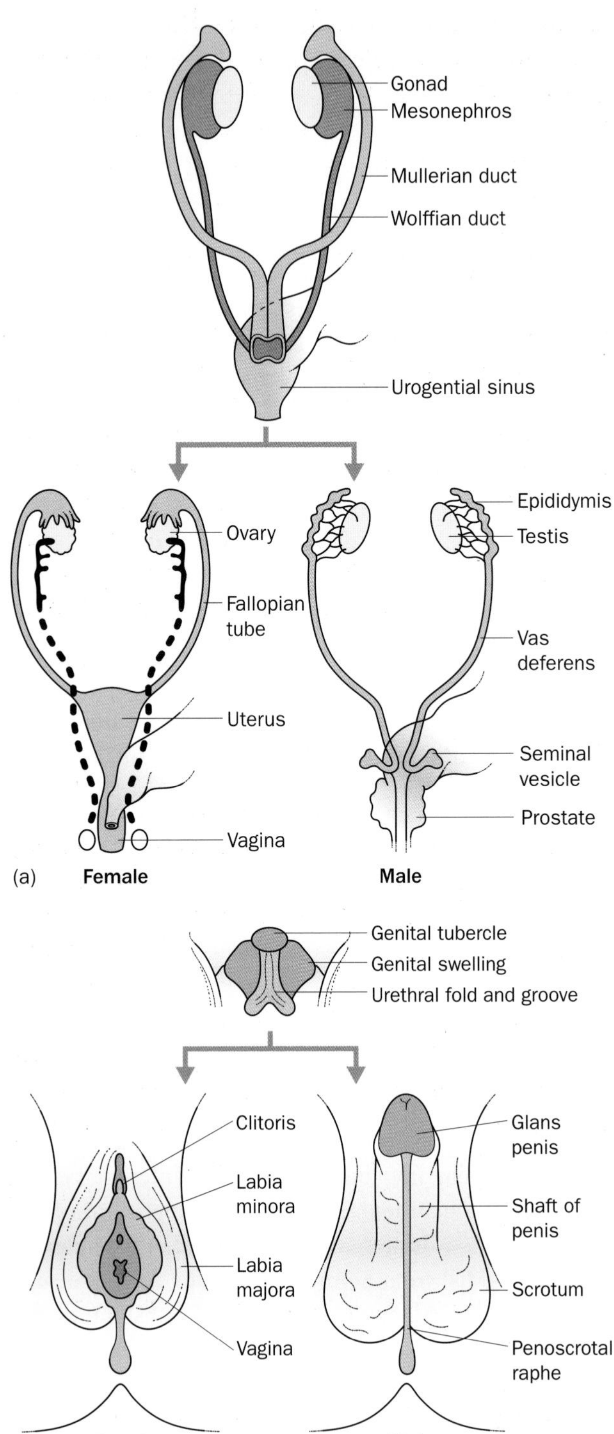

Figure 14.13 Primary sex differentiation. (a) In the presence of a testis the internal genitalia develop from the Wolffian system, with atrophy of the Müllerian system, while the common anlage differentiates into male external genitalia. (b) In the absence of a testis, the Wolffian system atrophies, the Müllerian system develops, and the common anlage differentiates into female external genitalia

the clitoris), the urethral folds into the shaft of the penis (homologous with the labia minora) enclosing the distal urethra and the genital swellings fuse to form the scrotum (homologous with the labia majora).

Definitions and classification of disorders of sexual differentiation

Intersex is when the genotype is at partial or complete variance with the sexual phenotype. The term **ambiguous genitalia** has been used to describe a form of intersex in which the external phenotype is neither definitely male nor female but the term **complex genital anomalies** is more appropriate and has less disturbing connotations for the family.

Intersex can simply be classified as male undermasculinization (previously called male pseudohermaphroditism) in which the karyotype is 46,XY or a variant thereof, female masculinization (previously called female pseudohermaphroditism) in which the karyotype is 46,XX, and true hermaphroditism (very rare) in which karyotype is either 46,XY or 46,XX and both ovarian and testicular tissue are present. Disorders of sexual differentiation can be grouped according to the karyotype.

Disorders in which both X and Y chromosomes are present

- Male undermasculinization
  - Androgen deficiency
    - Pituitary hormone deficiency
    - Biosynthetic testicular defect
    - Gonadal dysgenesis
  - Androgen resistance
    - Complete
    - Partial
- Less severe disorders of penile/testicular and breast development
  - Hypospadias
  - Micropenis
  - Cryptorchidism
  - Gynaecomastia
  - Aneuploidy syndromes e.g. Klinefelter syndrome (47,XXY), 47,XYY syndrome

MALE UNDERMASCULINIZATION

Androgen deficiency

> **CASE STUDY**
>
> An infant born at 39 weeks' gestation weighing 2700 g is noted to have bifid labioscrotal folds with a 3-cm clitoro-phallus, and perineal urethra. A gonad is palpable in the inguinal canal on one side only. Pelvic ultrasound examination shows a vagina and uterus. The karyotype is 45,X/46,XY. Gender assignment is discussed with the family.

Hypopituitarism causes cryptorchidism and micropenis rather than complex genital anomaly. Biosynthetic defects in androgen synthesis (see Figure 14.10) are rare but important because they respond to androgen treatment. Gonadal dysgenesis may occur with: 46,XY karyotype and complete sex reversal (pure gonadal dysgenesis); 45,X/46,XY karyotype with streak gonad on one side and dysgenetic testis on the other with or without stigmata of TS (mixed gonadal dysgenesis); and with autosomal abnormalities (e.g. 10q deletion, 9p deletion, SOX9 mutation causing camptomelic dwarfism).

Complete androgen insensitivity syndrome (CAIS)

Complete insensitivity to testosterone results in normal female external genitalia, absent internal male structures and intra-abdominal testes. Production of AMH is normal, so that uterus and upper third of vagina are absent. Since oestrogen sensitivity is normal, aromatization of testosterone results in normal breast development at the time of puberty. Complete androgen insensitivity syndrome may present in infancy with an inguinal hernia in a phenotypic female or with amenorrhoea and sparse pubic hair in late adolescence. Karyotype is 46,XY and pelvic ultrasound shows no female structures. At puberty, serum testosterone levels are in the normal male range, and the gonadotrophin response to GnRH is enhanced.

An inactivating mutation of the androgen receptor gene on the X chromosome can be demonstrated in 80 per cent of cases. Following discovery of the index case the family should be counselled about the 50 per cent risk of CAIS in future genetically male children, and the 50 per cent chance of genetically female children being carriers. An honest explanation of the condition must also be given to the patient, who needs to understand that the uterus and upper third of the vagina are absent, so that menstruation and childbearing will not be possible. Gonadectomy is required to pre-empt the development of malignant change and can either be carried out before puberty, in which case puberty must be induced with low-dose oestrogen, or after spontaneous puberty is complete, followed by oestrogen replacement.

Partial androgen insensitivity (PAIS)

This causes variable undermasculization, for example micropenis with hypospadias and bifid scrotum, in a 46,XY subject with suppression of Müllerian structures. The diagnosis is suggested by a history of affected relatives, and by demonstrating high/high normal testosterone levels after stimulation with hCG. An inactivating mutation of the AR gene is found in less than half the patients. In contrast to CAIS, gender assignment in severe PAIS is problematic, particularly since the response of the genitalia to androgen at the time of puberty cannot be predicted with certainty during infancy.

Idiopathic male undermasculinization

In the majority of babies with male undermasculization no endocrine abnormality can be demonstrated although, in the absence of an identifiable mutation of the AR gene, it is difficult to exclude a form of PAIS in which the defect is distal to the AR.

LESS SEVERE DISORDERS OF PENILE/TESTICULAR AND BREAST DEVELOPMENT

Isolated penile or glandular hypospadias and unilateral cryptorchidism tend to be referred to the paediatric surgeon. The chance of finding an endocrine abnormality in these situations is small. By contrast, children with bilateral cryptorchidism and/or severe hypospadias should be assessed for a possible endocrine disorder such as partial androgen insensitivity, or an underlying syndrome (e.g. Noonan). Gynaecomastia, commonly seen in pubertal boys, is discussed under miscellaneous pubertal disorders (see page 425).

ANEUPLOIDY SYNDROMES

Klinefelter syndrome (47,XXY) usually presents in adulthood with infertility but may be seen following amniocentesis, or in the course of investigating behaviour and learning difficulties in childhood. At puberty Leydig cell function is relatively spared leading to spontaneous puberty but the testes are small (2–3 mL) in volume, and the boy may show some gynaecomastia with relatively long legs (eunuchoid habitus). Endocrine investigations show high basal gonadotrophins (particularly FSH), with low normal testosterone levels. Testosterone supplementation may be offered during the pubertal years to limit skeletal disproportion. Individuals with a Y chromosome and more than two X chromosomes (e.g. 48,XXXY) show more severe intellectual and gonadal impairment.

Disorders in which only X chromosome(s) are present

- Female masculinization
  - Congenital adrenal hyperplasia (see adrenal axis)
  - Congenital anomalies affecting genitourinary and anorectal systems
  - 46,XX male (due in some cases to transfer of SRY to X chromosome)
  - Rarities (e.g. maternal drugs and androgen secreting tumours, aromatase deficiency)
- Normal female genitalia with little or no virilization
  - Gonadal dysgenesis
    - Turner syndrome (45,X and its variants) (see short stature)
    - Pure gonadal dysgenesis (karyotype 46, XX)
    - Biosynthetic defects (see adrenal axis)

- Aneuploidy syndromes
  - Triple X syndrome (47,XXX)

Pure gonadal dysgenesis (with either 46,XX or 46,XY karyotype) is seen in girls with pubertal failure in the context of normal stature, elevated basal FSH and LH levels, and hypoplastic uterus on pelvic ultrasound. Ultrasound imaging by an inexperienced observer may lead to a diagnosis of uterine absence being made, causing unnecessary distress to the girl and her family. Treatment is with oestrogen and progesterone replacement, as described in the section on puberty.

CALCIUM, VITAMIN D AND BONE DISORDERS

Bone physiology and metabolism

Bone is responsible for forming a rigid structure and also acting as a reservoir for calcium, phosphate and base. The two types of bone are **trabecular**, e.g. the vertebrae and flat bones of the skull, and **cortical**, e.g. the diaphyses of the long bones.

Bone is composed of:

- organic matrix (mainly collagen)
- inorganic mineral phase of hydroxyapatite
- osteoblasts, which promote bone synthesis
- osteoclasts, which promote bone absorption
- osteocytes, which are embedded within mineralized bone.

Bone growth, by bone formation of the periosteal surface and resorption at the endosteal surface, and elongation at the growth plate (metaphysis) occurs in childhood and adolescence, whereas bone remodelling – the balance between bone formation (reflecting osteoblastic activity) and bone resorption (osteoclastic activity) – is a lifelong process. Bone mass increases during childhood and adolescence, the peak bone mass being achieved during the third decade. Longitudinal growth of long bones occurs in the following sequence:

1. proliferation of columns of cartilage cells (chondrocytes)
2. hypertrophic differentiation of chondrocytes within growth plate
3. formation of matrix around hypertophic chondrocytes
4. matrix becomes invaded by blood vessels
5. apoptosis and calcification of surrounding matrix
6. calcified tissue is resorbed and replaced by bone trabeculae.

The process of endochrondral ossification results from a complex interaction of a number of hormones including parathormone-related peptide (PTHRP), growth hormone, and IGF-I. The influence of paracrine factors is important, notably that of fibroblast growth factor (FGF) which interacts with its receptor (FGFR3) to regulate chondrocyte proliferation. Activating mutations in the gene encoding FGFR3 result in achondroplasia and hypochrondroplasia. Chondrocyte hypertrophy is regulated by PTF-related peptide which is inhibited by the signalling molecule Indian Hedgehog protein (IHH).

Calcium metabolism

Ninety-nine per cent of the body's calcium is in the skeleton in the form of hydroxyapatite. The serum calcium concentration ranges between 2.2 and 2.6 mmol/L and is influenced by circulating levels of albumin. Approximately 50 per cent of calcium is in the active ionized form. Calcium is an essential intracellular and extracellular element, particularly in the nervous and muscular systems. The balance of calcium in the body reflects intestinal absorption, urinary excretion and skeletal accretion. The hormones principally involved in calcium and bone metabolism are:

- Vitamin D
- Parathyroid hormone
- Calcitonin.

The gene encoding parathyroid hormone (PTH) is localized to chromosome 11p. Parathyroid hormone is synthesized in the four parathyroid glands situated adjacent to the thyroid gland in the neck. Its release is stimulated by hypocalcaemia and inhibited by hypercalcaemia via a specific calcium-sensing receptor. Physiological PTH secretion increases calcium absorption from bone, increases renal tubular reabsorption of calcium, renal phosphate excretion and intestinal calcium absorption.

The gene encoding calcitonin is also localized to chromosome 11p. Calcitonin is secreted by the chief 'C' cells of the thyroid gland. Calcitonin is known to antagonize the action of PTH and vitamin D but appears to play a relatively minor role in calcium homoeostasis.

Vitamin D is a term referring to a group of compounds known as sterols, whose basic structure is related to cholesterol. Naturally occurring forms are ergocalciferol (D_2) and cholecalciferol (D_3). Cholecalciferol is derived from the diet (e.g. fish, oil) and also by conversion of 7-dehydrocholesterol by ultraviolet light in the skin. Cholecalciferol (D_3) is converted into 25 (OH) D_3 in the liver, and to 1,25 $(OH)_2$ D_3 in the kidney due to 25 and 1 α-hydroxylase activity, respectively. Vitamin D increases serum calcium by increasing intestinal absorption, mobilizing calcium from bone and, in physiological amounts, decreasing renal calcium excretion. In therapeutic situations vitamin D therapy increases calcium excretion, causing problems in the treatment of hypocalcaemic disorders.

Hypocalcaemia

CASE STUDY

A 5-year-old girl with partial complex seizures, which are refractory to anticonvulsant, is admitted with a further seizure. On examination, she is short and obese with rounded facies. Plasma electrolytes show calcium 1.5 mmol/L, phosphate 3 mmol/L. Parathormone is 14 pmol/L (normal <5.5), fT4 normal, TSH 11 mU/L (normal <5.5).

Hypocalcaemia is defined as serum calcium <2.2 mmol/L although symptoms are more likely with values <2 mmol/L. Symptoms include paraesthesias, often felt in the mouth and hands, muscle cramps, carpopedal spasm, mood changes, diarrhoea and convulsions. Physical signs include dry skin, coarse hair, brittle nails and enamel hypoplasia of the teeth. Tapping over the facial nerve in the parotid region results in facial twitching (Chvostek sign) and inflation of the blood pressure cuff to above systolic pressure for a few minutes results in wrist and finger flexion (Trousseau sign).

Causes of hypocalcaemia

Neonatal

Transient
- Prematurity
- Birth asphyxia
- Infant of diabetic mother
- Maternal vitamin D deficiency
- High phosphate load in unsuitable milk
- Parenteral nutrition
- Exchange transfusion
- Hypomagnesaemia

Permanent
- Hypoparathyroidism (22q deletion syndromes including DiGeorge spectrum)
- Isolated congenital
- Other

Childhood

Hypoparathyroidism
- Congenital hypoparathyroidism presenting in childhood
- 22q deletion
- PTH deficiency with renal anomalies and deafness
- Autoimmune disease (isolated or in association with other autoimmune disorders (e.g. Addison disease)
- Post surgery (e.g. total thyroidectomy)

PTH resistance
- Albright hereditary osteodystrophy
- Hypomagnesaemia

Vitamin D deficiency and failure (rickets)

Chronic renal failure

If hypocalcaemia is suspected or confirmed, blood should be taken for calcium, magnesium, phosphate, alkaline phosphatase, parathormone and 25-cholecalciferol. Additional blood should also be taken for 1,25-cholecalciferol and stored for possible measurement at a later date. The initial treatment of hypocalcaemia is with oral calcium 15 mg/kg per day in three to four divided doses. If there is marked symptomatic hypocalcaemia the calcium can be given intravenously as 10 per cent calcium gluconate 0.3 mL/kg over 5–10 minutes, followed by a maintenance infusion of 10 per cent calcium gluconate 0.2 mL/kg per hour but extreme care should be taken as even a small quantity of extravasation into the tissues can cause severe necrosis.

Hypoparathyroidism

This is either congenital or acquired in aetiology. Congenital hypoparathyroidism may be related to 22q deletion, which includes DiGeorge spectrum. Hypoparathyroidism may occur where the parathyroid glands are structurally intact but there is a disorder of the calcium-sensing mechanism. Acquired hypoparathyroidism is usually autoimmune in nature. Parathyroid hormone resistance is seen in Albright hereditary osteodystrophy (AHO), also called pseudohypoparathyroidism. Albright hereditary osteodystrophy is caused by an inactivating mutation of the GS α-subunit, principally in bone and kidney tissue, and the phenotype is characteristic with short stature, rounded facies and short 4th and 5th metacarpals. The management of hypoparathyroidism is with vitamin D therapy, since PTH is not available for therapeutic administration, and would have to be given subcutaneously several times per day. Either 1-α (OH) D_3 or 1,25 $(OH)_2$ D_3 are given as a single daily dose of 25–50 ng/kg per day, aiming to keep the serum calcium at 2.0–2.2 mmol/L, accepting a serum phosphate in the upper half of the reference range, and trying to keep the urine calcium/creatinine ratio

<1. Calcium supplementation with oral calcium salts (e.g. Sandocal) may be required. If hypercalcuria occurs despite a low normal serum calcium the diuretic hydrochlorothiazide or chlorothiazide can be added in the doses of 1.25 or 12.5 mg/kg per day in order to decrease renal calcium excretion and raise serum calcium, allowing a reduction in vitamin D dosage. The child is seen three to four monthly in clinic and the parents should be warned to look out for the key symptoms of hypercalcaemia due to vitamin D excess – anorexia, mood change, polyuria and polydipsia.

Hypercalcaemia

CASE STUDY

A 5-year-old girl is admitted with tiredness, thirst, loss of appetite and secondary enuresis. There are no physical signs. Plasma calcium is elevated at 3 mmol/L, wrist radiograph is suggestive of osteoporosis. Full blood count is unremarkable, but bone marrow aspiration shows acute lymphoblastic leukaemia.

Hypercalcaemia is defined as serum calcium >2.65 mmol/L. The symptoms include anorexia, polyuria and polydipsia, mood change, abdominal pain and constipation. Biochemistry shows a rise in plasma creatinine due to (usually reversible) renal impairment. The calcium to creatinine ratio in the urine will be >1.0 mmol/mmol in all hypercalcaemic states other than hypocalcuric hypercalcaemia.

Causes of hypercalcaemia

Infantile onset

- Neonatal
- Primary
- Hyperparathyroidism (due to a mutation of the calcium sensing receptor gene)
- Idiopathic hypercalcaemia of infancy
- Williams syndrome

Childhood onset

- Vitamin D excess (usually iatrogenic)
- Hyperparathyroidism (rare) due to: isolated adenoma; multiple endocrine neoplasia types 1 and 2a; tertiary hyperparathyroidism
- Familial hypocalcuric hypocalcaemia
- Malignant disease, e.g. leukaemia
- Immobilization
- Sarcoidosis

The hypercalcaemia of infancy and Williams syndrome can be managed by low-calcium diet which will not usually be required in the long term. Neonatal primary hyperparathyroidism is treated surgically. Iatrogenic hypercalcaemia is treated by temporary discontinuation of vitamin D and calcium supplements, restarting at a lower dose once the hypercalcaemia has resolved. Acute hypercalcaemia can be managed with intravenous saline, frusemide and steroids.

Rickets

CASE STUDY

A 3-year-old boy of Pakistani origin is referred with irritability, fatigue and difficulty walking. He is hypotonic with marked lumbar lordosis, swollen wrists and ankles.

Rickets is defined as failure to calcify the matrix of the growth plate together with excessive accumulation of unclassified cartilage and bone matrix – osteoid. The four mechanisms are vitamin D deficiency and failure, calcium deficiency, phosphate deficiency (especially seen in preterm babies), and acidosis.

Causes of rickets

Vitamin D deficiency and failure

- Dietary insufficiency; lack of sunlight; malabsorption, e.g. coeliac disease
- 25-Hydroxylase deficiency in liver disease
- 1α-Hydroxylase deficiency in chronic renal failure
- 1,25 $(OH)_2$ D_3 receptor defect

Calcium deficiency

- Preterm and ill babies
- Severe dietary deficiency

Phosphate deficiency

- Preterm and ill babies
- X-linked dominant hypophosphataemic rickets
- Fanconi syndrome

Distal renal tubular acidosis

The symptoms and signs of rickets include irritability, muscle weakness and hypotonia with swollen wrists and ankles, swollen costochondral junctions, resulting in the 'rickety rosary', increased lumbar lordosis with waddling gait, and (in the 1,25 $(OH)_2$ D_3 receptor defect) alopecia (Figure 14.14). Biochemistry shows calcium usually

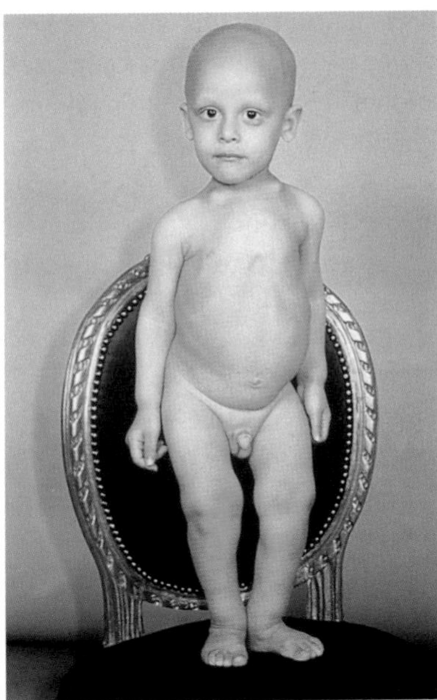

Figure 14.14 Three-year-old boy with vitamin D receptor defect causing severe rickets with alopecia

low-normal or frankly subnormal associated with symptoms of hypocalcaemia, low phosphate (except in renal osteodystrophy) and high alkaline phosphatase. Parathyroid hormone is high except in hypophosphataemic rickets, 25 (OH) D_3 is low in dietary deficiency, normal or low-normal in other causes whereas 1,25 $(OH)_2$ D_3 is normal, or high-normal in dietary rickets and high with a receptor defect.

The treatment of rickets depends on the underlying causes. Dietary deficiency is treated with calcium, phosphate, or vitamin D_3 supplements as appropriate, giving 50–150 μg/day of vitamin D_3 for two weeks, then 10 μg daily. In chronic renal failure, vitamin D can be given as calcitriol 0.25–2 μg daily. Hypophosphataemic rickets is treated with phosphate 50–70 mg/day in four to six divided doses and calcitriol 15–20 ng/kg per day initially. Children with the 1,25 $(OH)_2$ D_3 receptor defect are unresponsive to vitamin D therapy and treated with high doses of intravenous calcium via a central line. Following healing of the rickets, remission is maintained by high-dose oral calcium replacement.

Osteopenia and osteoporosis

Osteoporosis is defined as bone mineral density (BMD) >2 standard deviations below the mean. Bone mineral density is assessed by dual energy X-ray absorptiometry (DXA), a valuable tool in monitoring the bone health of individual patients with chronic disease. Assessment of BMD in childhood and adolescence is rendered difficult by variable size but reference ranges for age and height are now available. Volumetric as opposed to aerial assessment negates the influence of body size.

Causes of osteoporosis and osteopenia include osteogenesis imperfecta (severe autosomal recessive form, often fatal, and milder autosomal dominant form), idiopathic juvenile osteoporosis, chronic inflammatory disease (including chronic juvenile arthritis), Cushing syndrome, sex steroid deficiency and immobilization.

Treatment of osteoporosis in childhood is supportive with analgesia, physiotherapy and splints. Dietary calcium and vitamin D intake should be optimized, and the underlying disease treated where possible. When steroid administration is responsible, the minimal steroid dose should be sought. Osteoporosis due to hypogonadism and growth hormone deficiency should be treated with endocrine replacement therapy. Treatment with bisphosphonates (e.g. pamidronate) has greatly improved the quality of life and prognosis for severe osteogenesis imperfecta, reducing pain, decreasing fracture incidence, and increasing bone mineral density. However, the long-term safety and outcome with bisphosphonate treatment is unknown.

LATE ENDOCRINE EFFECTS OF TREATMENT OF CHILDHOOD CANCER

The endocrine manifestations of childhood cancer relate to effect of:

- the original disease (e.g. suprasellar tumour causing hypopituitarism) – see above
- the treatment for the original disease (e.g. surgery, chemotherapy, and ionizing radiation).

Surgery

Surgery in the hypothalamo-pituitary region for craniopharyngioma, optic glioma, etc. is likely to result in permanent hypopituitarism with diabetes insipidus. Total thyroidectomy for thyroid carcinoma results in lifelong hypothyroidism requiring thyroxine replacement.

Treatment involving ionizing radiation

Low-dose cranial irradiation

This was until relatively recently given routinely for the prophylaxis of CNS relapse in acute lymphoblastic leukaemia (ALL). Doses of 1800 cGy resulted in the combination of early puberty (especially in girls) and mild growth hormone insufficiency causing blunting of the adolescent growth spurt with a consequent reduction in final height, although not usually enough for the family and child to wish for growth hormone treatment. This problem has been largely eliminated by using high-dose intravenous and intrathecal methotrexate in ALL unless there is CNS involvement or a particularly high peripheral white cell count at presentation.

High-dose cranial irradiation

In ALL complicated by CNS relapse cranial irradiation is given in a dose of 2500 cGy, which is sufficient to cause frank growth hormone deficiency. Doses of 3000 cGy and higher are used for tumours in the hypothalamo-pituitary area (e.g. optic glioma, craniopharyngioma) when surgery is not feasible and the lesion is enlarging so that vision is compromised. Patients with malignant germinoma and medulloblastoma are treated with biopsy/surgery followed by craniospinal irradiation, giving 3000 cGy to the axis and a 1000 cGy posterior fossa boost.

With doses of ≥3000 cGy growth hormone deficiency within two years is almost inevitable. Gonadotrophin, TSH and ACTH secretion are usually unaffected although ACTH deficiency may occur as a particularly late feature. Spinal irradiation results in impaired spinal growth with loss of sitting height. Growth hormone therapy following craniospinal irradiation (e.g. for medulloblastoma) improves leg length but not spinal growth, so that target height is not reached and segmental disproportion is increased. Radiation scatter from spinal irradiation may also cause damage to the thyroid gland, with TSH elevation, and to the gonads, with FSH elevation.

Bone marrow transplantation

Autologous bone marrow transplantation for relapsed ALL, acute myeloblastic leukaemia (AML) and some solid tumours, e.g. neuroblastoma, involves conditioning prior to the transplant with total body irradiation (TBI) in a dose of 1000 cGy, and cyclophosphamide or melphalan administration. TBI causes mild-to-moderate growth hormone insufficiency, may cause mild compensated hypothyroidism with TSH elevation and invariably causes germ-cell damage to the gonads with FSH elevation. Gonadal impairment is more pronounced in girls than in boys. Thus whereas most boys progress through puberty spontaneously albeit with reduced testicular volumes and reduced or absent sperm count, girls usually require oestrogen supplementation. Pelvic ultrasound may show a reduction in the uterine size from a direct effect of the irradiation.

Chest and abdominal radiotherapy

Hodgkin disease is rarely managed with radiation but when this is used in the chest and neck region primary hypothyroidism may result. It is considered good practice to give thyroxine treatment to cause complete suppression if TSH elevation is found, in order to minimize the chance of thyroid carcinoma developing. Wilms tumour in the abdomen is rarely treated with radiotherapy nowadays, but when this is carried out ovarian failure may result, together with asymmetric growth of the lumbar spine.

Chemotherapy

Chemotherapy has an additive effect with radiotherapy and may contribute to the hypopituitarism seen in medulloblastoma survivors. Treatment with cyclophosphamide and melphalan will cause germ-cell impairment. The hypothyroidism seen in Hodgkin disease is partly related to chemotherapy.

MISCELLANEOUS DISORDERS: ADRENAL MEDULLA

Phaeochromocytoma may be seen in isolation or as part of multiple endocrine neoplasia type 2a. It presents with intermittent hypertension, sweating and episodic headache. Treatment is surgical. Patient with **neuroblastoma** present to the general paediatrician and oncologist with pallor, sweating and abdominal mass, sometimes with hypertension. Urine catecholamines are elevated. **Gastrointestinal tumours** are suspected in cases with episodic diarrhoea associated with flushing and tachycardia.

ACKNOWLEDGEMENT

I would like to thank Professor Angela Huebner from Dresden, Germany, for supplying Figure 14.1 a and b.

REFERENCES

Albanese A, Hamill G, Jones J, Skuse D, Matthews DR, Stanhope R (1994) Reversibility of physiological growth hormone secretion in children with psychosocial dwarfism. *Clin Endocrinol* 40:687–92.

Donaldson MDC, Paterson WF (2000) Assessment and management of delayed puberty. *Curr Paediatr* 10:275–83.

Finkelstein BS, Imperiale TF, Speroff T, Marrero U, Radcliffe DJ, Cuttler L (2002) Effect of growth hormone therapy on height in children with idiopathic short stature: a meta-analysis. *Arch Pediat Adolesc Med* 156:230–40.

Freeman JV, Cole TJ, Chinn S, Jones PRM, White EM, Preece MA (1995) Cross-sectional stature and weight reference curves for the UK, 1990. *Arch Dis Child* **73**:17–24.

Galloway PJ, McNeill E, Paterson WF, Donaldson MDC (2002) Safety of the insulin tolerance test. *Arch Dis Child* **87**:354–6.

Kelly BP, Paterson WF, Donaldson MDC (2003) Final height outcome and value of height prediction in boys with constitutional delay in growth and adolescence treated with intramuscular testosterone 125 mg per month for 3 months. *Clin Endocrinol* **58**:267–72.

Noble SE, Leyland K, Findlay CA, *et al.* (2000) School based screening for hypothyroidism in Down's syndrome by dried blood spot TSH measurement. *Arch Dis Child* **82**:27–31.

Paterson WF, Hollman AS, Reid S, McNeill E, Donaldson MDC (1998) Efficacy of Zoladex LA (goserelin) in the treatment of girls with central precocious or early puberty. *Arch Dis Child* **79**:323–7.

Tanner JM, Buckler JMH (1997) Revision and update of Tanner-Whitehouse clinical longitudinal charts for height and weight. *Eur J Pediatr* **156**:248–9.

Tanner JM, Whitehouse RH, Cameron N, Marshall WA, Healy MJR, Goldstein H (1983) *Assessment of Skeletal Maturity and Prediction of Adult Height (TW2 method)*, 2nd edn. London: Academic Press.

Tanner JM, Healy MJR, Goldstein H, Cameron N (2001) *Assessment of Skeletal Maturity and Prediction of Adult Height (TW3 method)*, 3rd edn. London: WB Saunders.

FURTHER READING

Raine JE, Donaldson MDC, Gregory JW, Savage MO (2001) *Practical Endocrinology and Diabetes in Children*. Oxford: Blackwell Science Ltd.

Chapter 15

Metabolic disorders

Peter Robinson

CLINICAL FEATURES, PRINCIPLES OF DIAGNOSIS AND BIOCHEMICAL INVESTIGATIONS

CLINICAL FEATURES OF METABOLIC DISORDERS IN THE NEONATE

The ill neonate

Most babies with inherited metabolic disease will be born at term and well at birth (Chakrapani *et al.*, 2001). They become unwell after a clear asymptomatic interval of hours or days. Poor feeding, vomiting, dehydration (with weight loss of 10–15 per cent), encephalopathy or tachypnoea may be early signs. **Encephalopathy** may be characterized by periods of varying hypertonia or hypotonia or abnormal 'cycling' movements. Sustained hypertonia is characteristic of maple syrup urine disease (MSUD). There is hyperventilation in the absence of respiratory or cardiac abnormalities in severe **acidosis** and in **hyperammonaemia**, in which there may be a metabolic **alkalosis. Hypoglycaemia** may present subtly – poor feeding, apathy, pallor and sweating – or may present with convulsions. **Liver failure** may present as vomiting, bruising or bleeding (including intracranial bleeding) and jaundice. Always ask about consanguinity and ask about previous early neonatal deaths or illness, progressive or stepwise developmental delay or other neurological abnormality in other family members. A few disorders cause excretion of chemical intermediates that may impart an unusual smell to skin, urine or vomitus. The clinical features in acute metabolic disorders may be similar to those of sepsis: be prepared to reconsider presumed sepsis in a term baby with no risk factors for infection who does not respond to antibiotic therapy.

> **KEY LEARNING POINTS**
>
> - Babies with inherited metabolic disease generally present after a symptom-free interval of hours or days after birth with non-specific signs often initially thought to be due to infection.
> - Common presentations are with encephalopathy, metabolic acidosis, hypoglycaemia or liver failure.
> - Hyperammonaemia can cause respiratory alkalosis.

The neonate with dysmorphism

A minority of disorders of intermediary biochemistry present at birth with dysmorphism. The chemical substances that accumulate in these disorders affect cell migration and tissue formation. Untreated maternal phenylketonuria causes low birth weight, microcephaly with poor formation of the corpus callosum, minor facial abnormalities, cardiac septal defects, aortic arch abnormalities and cleft palate. Pyruvate dehydrogenase deficiency causes bifrontal narrowing, high forehead and other facial features like those of the fetal alcohol syndrome. These facial features, cardiomyopathy and cystic renal disease occur in the severe form of multiple acyl CoA dehydrogenase deficiency. Typical features of Zellweger syndrome, in which peroxisomes are absent, are high forehead and wide fontanellae, hypotonia and poor feeding, hepatomegaly and liver dysfunction, with epiphyseal stippling at the knee. The features are due to accumulation of long-chain fatty acids, with secondary effects on tissue structure and sterol synthesis. Cholesterol and sterol synthesis is impaired in Smith–Lemli–Opitz syndrome. The dysmorphic features (which may be very mild) are microcephaly, ptosis, upturned nose, hypoplastic genitalia and syndactyly of the second and third toes. Abnormal glycosylation of structural and transport molecules occurs in the congenital disorders of glycosylation. Only type Ia is not rare. It may present in the early neonatal period with low birth weight and failure to thrive, limb and hand contractures, abnormal skin, cardiomyopathy and pericardial effusions.

Where 'storage materials', normally degraded from structural molecules in connective tissues accumulate due to lysosomal enzyme deficiencies, the dysmorphic features will progress relentlessly after birth. There may be generalized abnormalities such as skeletal ossification (dysostosis multiplex), hepatosplenomegaly, thickened skin and subcutaneous tissues, hernias and corneal clouding and hydrops. In I-cell disease (named after the inclusion bodies representing abnormal lysosomes), in which there is functional deficiency of many lysosomal hydrolases and GM1 gangliosidosis in which glycolipids accumulate, abnormalities are already present at birth. The other disorders in this very large group present later.

KEY LEARNING POINTS

- An increasing number of dysmorphic syndromes are due to metabolic disorders that affect tissue differentiation and organogenesis *in utero*. These cause dysmorphism that is present at birth but does not progress.
- In disorders such as the lysosomal enzyme disorders, there is continued accumulation of storage materials after birth. Dysmorphism may be present at birth or appear later and will progress.

CLINICAL FEATURES OF METABOLIC DISORDERS IN THE OLDER CHILD

Recurrent encephalopathy, precipitated by incidental infections, or fasting, may cause episodes of confusion, ataxia, vomiting or prostration in the older child. There may be many minor episodes with spontaneous recovery, or the child may present gravely ill after a first episode. Focal signs do not rule out a metabolic disorder: visual loss or stroke can occur with hyperammonaemia and in mitochondrial encephalopathy with lactic acidosis and stroke-like episodes (MELAS). Moderate developmental delay or isolated speech delay is not likely to have a metabolic cause.

Motor developmental delay is common in organic acidaemias and in some fat oxidation defects. Stepwise **loss of acquired skills** (after intercurrent infection, fasting, fever or immunization), suggests an organic acidaemia. This particularly applies to the catastrophic neurological change which is characteristic of glutaryl CoA dehydrogenase deficiency (glutaric aciduria type I). **Failure to thrive** because of poor feeding or specific aversion to protein foods or vomiting often occurs after weaning, especially in infants who have been breastfed. **Hepatosplenomegaly**, other organomegaly (tongue, kidney, adrenal glands), corneal clouding, skeletal abnormalities and progressively coarse facies suggest storage disorders. Remember that seemingly unrelated symptoms and signs in several organ systems may occur and should prompt the question: What could link these problems?

KEY LEARNING POINTS

- Symptoms and signs in apparently unrelated organ systems may suggest an inherited metabolic disease.
- Severe symptoms after minor infective illnesses or a period of fasting should suggest a metabolic disorder.
- Minor motor developmental delay or isolated speech delay are not likely to be the result of a metabolic disorder.
- Focal neurological signs do not rule out a metabolic cause for encephalopathy or coma.

PRINCIPLES OF PRENATAL DIAGNOSIS

The standard prenatal screening methods (ultrasound, maternal α-fetoprotein, chromosome analysis) do not detect inborn errors of metabolism. For most metabolic disorders, the fetus is structurally normal and imaging by ultrasound, radiography or magnetic resonance is not informative. There must be a previously affected child or a known risk because of family history and an accurately established diagnosis in the index case before attempting prenatal diagnosis. The methods available are:

- mutation analysis of chorionic villus samples
- direct enzyme measurement in chorionic villus samples
- enzyme measurement in cultured cells from chorionic villus or fetal amniocytes
- direct chemical analysis of amniotic fluid (if an abnormal metabolite accumulates).

For enzyme measurement, the enzyme must be expressed in chorionic villus cells or cultured amniocytes. The enzyme activity must be high enough and the assay methods accurate enough to distinguish reliably an affected fetus from a carrier or normal fetus. If diagnosis can only be by enzymology and the enzyme is not expressed in chorionic villus cells or amniocytes and only in fetal blood or liver, fetal cordocentesis or fetal liver biopsy may be performed. These invasive techniques are rarely used. Diagnosis is highly dependent on a very small number of specialized laboratories in different countries and each case must be discussed and planned well in advance.

KEY LEARNING POINTS

- It is necessary to have a secure diagnosis in the index case by the proposed analytical method before attempting a prenatal diagnosis.
- Antenatal diagnosis is sometimes made by chemical analysis of amniotic fluid, but more usually by measuring enzyme activity or by mutation analysis of chorionic villus cells or amniotic fluid cells.
- The appropriate methods are changing very fast as more diseases have identified mutations, so enzymology and metabolite assays are less likely to be used in the future.

CLINICAL AND NUTRITIONAL IMPORTANCE OF THE MAJOR METABOLIC PATHWAYS

The metabolic pathways with the greatest clinical and nutritional importance are those of amino acids and ammonium, fatty acids and glucose. These are involved in synthesis (anabolic processes in growth and tissue repair) and breakdown (catabolic processes during fasting and the stress of infective illnesses and injury). The urea cycle functions to convert highly toxic ammonium produced when nitrogen is removed from amino acids to the far less toxic, water-soluble urea, which is excreted. Fatty acids are oxidized directly as energy-releasing fuel by heart, muscle and kidney. Fatty acids are also oxidized in liver for synthesis of ketones (β-hydroxybutyrate and acetoacetate) for export to other tissues. Glucose is used for energy production in glycolysis and ultimately completely oxidized in the citric acid cycle. Glucose storage as glycogen and its subsequent release are impaired in the glycogen storage diseases. Important intermediates such as pyruvate, alanine, glycerol and acetyl CoA link the glucose, amino acid and fatty acid pathways.

Prevention of catabolism and promotion of anabolism are central in managing the urea cycle and amino acid disorders, the organic acidaemias and the fat oxidation disorders because it is the demand made on poorly functioning catabolic pathways that leads to illness. This is best understood by an understanding of the fast–feed cycle.

Fast–feed cycle

On fasting, there is no dietary carbohydrate to provide glucose. Glycogen stores in the liver are broken down to release glucose. As blood glucose slowly falls, insulin concentration falls and glucagon rises, activating lipolysis. This releases fatty acids and glycerol from fat stores. Glycerol can be converted to glucose. Fatty acids cannot be converted to glucose but are used directly for energy by skeletal and cardiac muscle and renal cortex. Brain and renal medulla remain dependent on glucose. There has to be a net source of carbon skeletons so that glucose can be synthesized by the process of gluconeogenesis. This source is the proteins in skeletal muscle that are hydrolysed to release amino acids. The branched-chain amino acids (leucine, isoleucine and valine) are deaminated in muscle to their corresponding ketoacids, which are released into the circulation and passed to the liver, ultimately producing glucose or ketones. In parallel, pyruvate or lactate produced by glycolysis in peripheral tissues is taken up by muscle and transaminated to alanine. Alanine is released and taken up by the liver, transaminated (the nitrogen metabolized to urea) and the carbon skeleton reconverted into glucose.

Feeding restores a supply of carbohydrate, stops gluconeogenesis and the liver again disposes of glucose by its conversion to glycogen. Insulin levels rise and glucagon falls. The high ratio of insulin to glucagon is a prime effector of the switch from catabolism to anabolism. Ketosis is reversed. Fatty acids, some amino acids and protein are resynthesized.

In acute illness, nutritional management is very important to recovery. This means adequate carbohydrate, with insulin sometimes necessary to allow its proper utilization, and, in the urea cycle disorders and the organic acidaemias, controlled restriction of amino acid or protein intake. Maintenance therapy in these disorders has to include protein or amino acid restriction. Overrestriction may cause the catabolic state of acute illness to continue, and eventually leads to poor growth, vomiting and anorexia. Intake of protein above the requirement for tissue repair and growth is not tolerated in the organic acidaemias or urea cycle disorders because the excess cannot be metabolized to 'safe' substances. The minimum safe amount is determined individually.

KEY LEARNING POINTS

- Illness results from 'energy insufficiency' in the disorders of fatty acid oxidation, glycogen breakdown and gluconeogenesis.
- Disorders affecting catabolic pathways present with 'intoxication' due to ketoacidosis, lactic acidosis and high ammonia. Examples are the organic acidaemias and the urea cycle disorders.
- Fasting stress typically causes metabolic decompensation in the disorders of intermediary metabolism because normal regulation of the fast–feed cycle cannot take place.
- Management in acute illness must include promotion of an anabolic state.
- Maintenance treatment must include a controlled nutritional intake.

INVESTIGATIONS FOR COMMON METABOLIC DISORDERS

In an acute illness, **first-line** investigations, available in most hospital laboratories, can confirm or deny a suspicion of a metabolic disorder. **Second-line** investigations, complex analyses such as amino acids and organic acids, may be available in only specialized, regional laboratories. **Third-line** investigations such as measurement of complex enzymes or DNA analyses may be available only in supraregional reference laboratories or in other countries. It is important to be able to choose tests appropriately (Table 15.1) to avoid expensive and unfruitful unnecessary investigation.

Table 15.1 Investigations for common metabolic disorders

Investigation	Typical example of abnormality
First-line investigations (general investigations)	
Blood	
Full blood count	Neutropenia, thrombocytopenia acutely in some organic acidaemias; macrocytic anaemia in some disorders of vitamin B_{12}, folate and methionine metabolism
Coagulation screen	Mildly abnormal in fat oxidation defects, urea cycle disorder in crisis; very abnormal in tyrosinaemia type I galactosaemia and mitochondrial liver disease
Urea and electrolytes	Severe dehydration; hypokalaemia in organic acidaemias
Glucose	Hypoglycaemia; hyperglycaemia due to insulin resistance in organic acidaemias and other acute disorders
Bicarbonate	Low in metabolic acidosis
Chloride	May be high in acidosis of renal tubular origin or intestinal bicarbonate loss
Blood gas analysis	Metabolic acidosis; respiratory alkalosis early in hyperammonaemia
Cholesterol, triglycerides	High cholesterol in familial hypercholesterolaemia and other hyperlipidaemias; low cholesterol in abetalipoproteinaemia and usually in Smith-Lemli-Opitz syndrome and some other rare lipid disorders
Urate (plasma and urine)	High in Lesch-Nyhan syndrome and some other purine disorders, glycogen storage disease (GSD) type I; acutely high in fat oxidation disorders and organic acidaemias; low in some purine disorders and molybdenum co-factor deficiency (combined sulphite oxidase deficiency and xanthine oxidase deficiency
Transaminases	Liver disease; myopathies; very high in acute hepatic ischaemia or early after liver necrosis
Alkaline phosphatase	High in many forms of bone disease, bile salt synthesis disorders; low in hypophosphatasia
Creatine kinase	Modestly elevated in fat oxidation defects and in GSD type III and some metabolic myopathies; massively elevated in the rhabdomyolysis of some fat oxidation disorders

(Continued)

Table 15.1 *(Continued)*

Investigation	Typical example of abnormality
Urine	
Urine acetoacetate 'ketones'	Very valuable screening test: positive result in a neonate suggests an organic acidaemia; always negative in hypoglycaemia due to hyperinsulinism; positive result does not exclude a fat oxidation defect
Urine-reducing sugars ('Clinitest')	Positive in galactosaemia, but unreliable
Second-line investigations (specific investigations)	
Blood	
Ammonia	See detailed discussion in text: high in a range of metabolic and non-metabolic disorders
Plasma amino acids	Specific patterns: High phenylalanine, low tyrosine in hyperphenylalaninaemia High leucine, isoleucine, valine in maple syrup urine disease (MSUD) High methionine, homocystine and homocysteine, low cystine in classic homocystinuria Detectable argininosuccinic acid (ASA) in ASA lyase (ASAL) deficiency, high citrulline in ASA synthetase (ASAS) deficiency Non-specific patterns: High glutamine, alanine in hyperammonaemia High methionine, tyrosine, phenylalanine in liver disease High alanine in lactic acidosis, low alanine in ketosis with hypoglycaemia High glycine in organic acidaemias and 'non-ketotic hyperglycinaemia'
Lactate	High in shock, tissue hypoperfusion; high (with hypoglycaemia) in GSD I, disorders of glucose synthesis; high in some fat oxidation disorders and organic acidaemias and also in primary lactic acidoses and disorders of oxidative phosphorylation; cerebrospinal fluid (CSF) lactate may be high in respiratory chain disorders or other lactic acidoses affecting brain. Lactate/pyruvate ratio may be useful in determining the cause of high lactate, but is otherwise not relevant
Carnitine	Low in primary and secondary carnitine deficiency (many fat oxidation disorders and organic acidaemias), high in hepatic carnitine-palmitoyl transferase deficiency
β-Hydroxybutyrate	Low in hyperinsulinism, high in all forms of ketoacidosis
Non-esterified fatty acids (NEFA or FFA)	Low in hyperinsulinism, high ratio of NEFA to β-hydroxybutyrate in fat oxidation disorders (normal ratio is <1; ratio >2 very abnormal)
Acylcarnitines	Specific, often diagnostic analytical patterns in fat oxidation disorders and organic acidaemias
Plasma very long chain fatty acids	Elevated in disorders of absence of peroxisomes (Zellweger syndrome), or deficiency of specific peroxisomal enzymes (X-linked adrenoleucodystrophy, Refsum disease)
Plasma transferrin electrophoresis	Highly specialized test: abnormal in disorders of protein glycosylation (see Dysmorphic syndromes)
Pterins (biopterin, neopterin)	Highly specialized test: measured in blood and/or urine or CSF. Blood pterins as secondary screening tests in all cases of persistent hyperphenylalaninaemia to look for disorders of biopterin metabolism (about 1 per cent of cases of hyperphenylalaninaemia)
Copper (plasma, urine, liver)	Elevated urinary and liver copper in Wilson disease; low plasma copper in Menkes disease
Caeruloplasmin	Low in Menkes disease
Porphyrins	Can be measured in blood, urine and faeces; diagnostic in the acute (hepatic) and cutaneous porphyrias
Sterol analysis	Plasma; identifies abnormal cholesterol biosynthesis as in Smith–Lemli–Opitz syndrome
Bile acid analysis	Plasma, urine; highly specialized test: useful in some peroxisomal disorders and disorders of bile salt synthesis
CSF	
Biogenic amine metabolites	Homovanillic acid (HVA; from dopamine), vanillylmandelic (VMA; from adrenaline, noradrenaline), 5-hydroxyindoleacetic acid (5HIAA; from serotonin); abnormal in biopterin defects and other disorders of amine synthesis, with movement disorder or extrapyramidal signs
Urine	
Urine glycosaminoglycans and oligosaccharides	Elevated in mucopolysaccharide disorders and some other syndromes of dysmorphism and developmental delay (see Dysmorphic syndromes)
Urine organic acids	Dicarboxylic aciduria in fat oxidation disorders; specific abnormalities in medium-chain acyl CoA dehydrogenase (MCAD) deficiency (see text) Other organic acids in: methlymalonic aciduria, propionic aciduria, isovaleric aciduria and others

(Continued)

Table 15.1 *(Continued)*

Investigation	Typical example of abnormality
Urine orotic acid	Typically elevated in the urea cycle disorders, lysinuric protein intolerance and also in hereditary orotic aciduria
Urine succinylacetone	Elevated in tyrosinaemia type I
Others	
Light microscopy, electron microscopy	Vacuolation or inclusion bodies or granules of storage material material in peripheral blood lymphocytes or marrow aspirate in lysosomal storage disorders and some other neurodegenerative disorders. Megaloblastic anaemia in some disorders of vitamin B_{12} metabolism and related disorders
Third-line investigations (confirmation)	
Enzymology	Possible for many disorders with a single or multiple enzyme deficiencies; some enzymes expressed in plasma, red blood cells, lymphocytes, platelets, fibroblasts; others may be specific to liver or muscle. May be available only in highly specialized laboratories
Mutation analysis	May be an alternative to, or supplement biochemical analyses; highly specialized and requires up-to-date knowledge of new developments; must be discussed with a reference laboratory

For hypoglycaemia, the test profile outlined is essential at the time of presentation as diagnosis depends on interpreting the complex changes and counterchanges in physiological adaptation to fasting or other stresses.

KEY LEARNING POINTS

- Relatively simple, first-line tests will often suggest or refute a metabolic disorder, particularly in hypoglycaemia, acidosis and in encephalopathy.
- Test results must be interpreted in the light of the physiological state of the patient. High insulin levels are not helpful unless there is hypoglycaemia at the time. Ketosis at the time of hypoglycaemia excludes hyperinsulinism as the cause.
- Blood samples taken at the time of an acute illness may afford an opportunity for diagnosis that is not reproducible and saves a great deal of effort later.

CORE SYSTEM PROBLEMS

HYPOGLYCAEMIA

You must recognize symptoms and signs of hypoglycaemia and measure glucose formally in any child with altered consciousness. In very premature neonates in the first three days of life, glucose may be as low as 1.1 mmol/L without an underlying abnormality. In term neonates it may be as low as 1.7 mmol/L in the first three days and 2.2 mmol/L in the remainder of the first week. Thereafter, glucose of 2.6 mmol/L or lower requires investigation.

Table 15.2 Substances tested for in hypoglycaemia

Intermediary metabolites	Hormones	Others
Glucose Lactate β-Hydroxybutyrate Free fatty acids (NEFA)	Insulin, C-peptide Cortisol Growth hormone	Urea and electrolytes Bicarbonate Transaminases and bilirubin Capillary blood gas analysis Urate Creatine kinase Ammonia Amino acids Carnitine and acylcarnitines (Ethanol)

Collect the first-passed urine, test for 'ketones' (acetoacetate) by test strip and then freeze at −20 °C for organic acid analysis.

A low result found by test strip in a capillary blood sample must be confirmed by a laboratory sample. The best chance to determine the underlying cause is at presentation: correction of hypoglycaemia will rapidly reverse the physiological–biochemical effects and countereffects, which are clues to the underlying causes (Bonham, 1993).

Blood should be taken for the intermediary metabolites and hormones (Table 15.2) immediately before correction of hypoglycaemia. Not all are routine tests and you will need to warn your laboratory to separate and store the samples for later analysis. Priority can be given to the most appropriate test if you have not been able to obtain enough blood for them all. The others provide valuable information and can be carried out after initial correction of hypoglycaemia but should not be delayed beyond an hour.

CASE STUDY: Severe persistent neonatal hypoglycaemia

A 2-hour-old neonate presents with a convulsion. Capillary blood glucose is low and not recordable. He responds initially to an intravenous (IV) bolus of glucose, but has recurrent hypoglycaemia. Insulin is 8 mU/L when glucose is 1.0 mmol/L. β-Hydroxybutyrate and non-esterified fatty acids (NEFAs) are both very low.

In neonates, the most common cause of **severe persistent hypoglycaemia** is hyperinsulinism. This is due to diffuse or focal islet cell hyperplasia of the endocrine pancreas, much less commonly to an adenoma. The rate of glucose infusion required to keep glucose at or just above 3.0 mmol/L is over 12 mg/kg per minute and may be 25 mg/kg per minute or more.

Glucose mg/kg per minute = (per cent glucose infusion × rate of infusion (mL/hour))/(weight (kg) × 6)

Management is complex, requiring a prolonged effort of maximal medical therapy with diazoxide, glucagon, octreotide and nifedipine before radical (more than 95 per cent) pancreatectomy for diffuse hyperplasia, or targeted surgery if normal regions of the pancreas can be identified and preserved (Aynsley-Green *et al.*, 2000).

In infants and young children, the history should include:

- recent infectious illness
- recent fasting interval and the normal dietary habits
- previous episodes suggestive of recurrent hypoglycaemia
- accidental ingestion (e.g. alcohol consumption or oral hypoglycaemic agents) and drug therapy (e.g. β-blockers).

Important features in the clinical examination include:

- presence of acidotic breathing (organic acidaemia or lactic acidosis)
- hepatomegaly (glycogen storage diseases, fat oxidation disorders, some disorders of gluconeogenesis)
- jaundice (liver failure) or splenomegaly (portal hypertension)
- myopathy (fat oxidation disorders)
- short stature and relative obesity for height and micropenis (hypopituitarism and growth hormone deficiency), and pigmentation (adrenal failure).

Ask about symptoms after exercise (glutamate dehydrogenase (G+LDH) regulatory defect with hyperammonaemia) or paradoxical hypoglycaemia two to four hours after meals (hyperinsulinism in older children).

CASE STUDY: Hypoglycaemia, hepatomegaly, ketosis and lactic acidosis

A 9-month-old boy is admitted with bronchiolitis. He is sweaty (and tachypnoeic and wheezy). He is found to have 10 cm hepatomegaly. Random blood glucose is 1.5 mmol/L. Further investigation shows lactate 10.3 mmol/L, β-hydroxybutyrate 2.3 mmol/L, urate 0.58 mmol/L and cholesterol 7.4 mmol/L. Liver biopsy confirms glycogen storage disease type 1 by enzymology.

CASE STUDY: Hypoglycaemia and ketosis

A 16-month-old girl is admitted at 8.30 am with a non-febrile convulsion. Glucose on presentation is 1.8 mmol/L. She ate poorly the day before because of a respiratory tract infection. She is on the tenth centile for weight. Lactate is normal. β-Hydroxybutyrate and NEFA are both elevated, with a normal ratio. Cortisol is high and insulin is low. Urine organic acids show only heavy ketosis.

The history and the pattern of results are typical of **idiopathic ketotic hypoglycaemia**, the commonest cause of childhood hypoglycaemia, but this is a diagnosis of exclusion. It usually presents in toddlers, perhaps with hypoglycaemic seizures.

Treatment of hypoglycaemia

Glucose infusion

- *Give* 2 ml/kg 10 per cent glucose IV over two to three minutes.
- *Follow* with an infusion of 10 per cent glucose at the maintenance rate appropriate to the age of the child.
- *Check* blood glucose after 10 and 30 minutes and afterward if necessary.
- *If* the history suggests hypopituitarism or hypoadrenalism give hydrocortisone IV 2 mg/kg.

See Table 15.3 for rates of infusion.

Table 15.3 Glucose infusion rates

Age	Rate ml/kg per hour	Glucose g/kg per hour	Glucose mg/kg per minute
<1 year	5	0.5	8.3
1-5 years	4	0.4	6.7
>5 years	3	0.3	5.0

Figure 15.1 shows a diagnostic flow chart for diagnosis of metabolic and endocrine disorders causing hypoglycaemia (Table 15.4). Hypoglycaemia can result from hepatocellular failure and some other liver conditions, but is unlikely to be the presenting feature. The causes are shown in Figure 15.2.

JAUNDICE AND HEPATOCELLULAR FAILURE

Most causes of simple prolonged jaundice are not metabolic, and you should consider **haemolysis, blood group incompatibility, infection** (including urinary tract infection and congenital infections) and **hypothyroidism**. It is essential to have considered and to urgently confirm or rule out **biliary atresia**. In the ill preterm neonate, long-term parenteral nutrition and delay in initiating enteral nutrition may contribute. In hypopituitarism, there may be mixed conjugated and unconjugated hyperbilirubinaemia but the presentation is usually dominated by lethargy, perhaps hypothermic episodes and recurrent hypoglycaemia. There may be clinical findings of large head in relation to length, a small mid-face, which may emphasize frontal bossing, and micropenis. Babies with **cystic fibrosis** may have low-grade hyperbilirubinaemia and elevated transaminases. Jaundice (due to unconjugated bilirubin) may return in a minority of babies with **pyloric stenosis**, and these may later turn out to have Gilbert syndrome, mild bilirubin glucuronidase deficiency.

In the metabolic diseases, there is usually hepatomegaly and at least modest elevation of transaminases. Prolonged jaundice may blend imperceptibly with **liver failure.**

CASE STUDY: Early cholestatic jaundice, vomiting and cataract

A 5-day-old baby has been feeding poorly and is vomiting. Liver function tests reveal mixed conjugated and unconjugated hyperbilirubinaemia. Ophthalmoscopic examination shows a central cataract.

Cholestatic jaundice occurs in **galactosaemia** and in some cases of **α-1-antitrypsin deficiency**. You must never forget **galactosaemia** (galactose 1-phosphate uridyl transferase (GALT) deficiency) in any ill jaundiced neonate or infant who has had milk. Most will present with mixed conjugated and unconjugated jaundice in the first week, some later, but never beyond 6 months of age. Vomiting, jaundice, poor feeding and poor weight gain are universal. Cerebral oedema and encephalopathy can occur. 'Oil-drop' cataracts can be seen by an ophthalmoscope within days of birth. *Escherichia coli* sepsis is not uncommon,

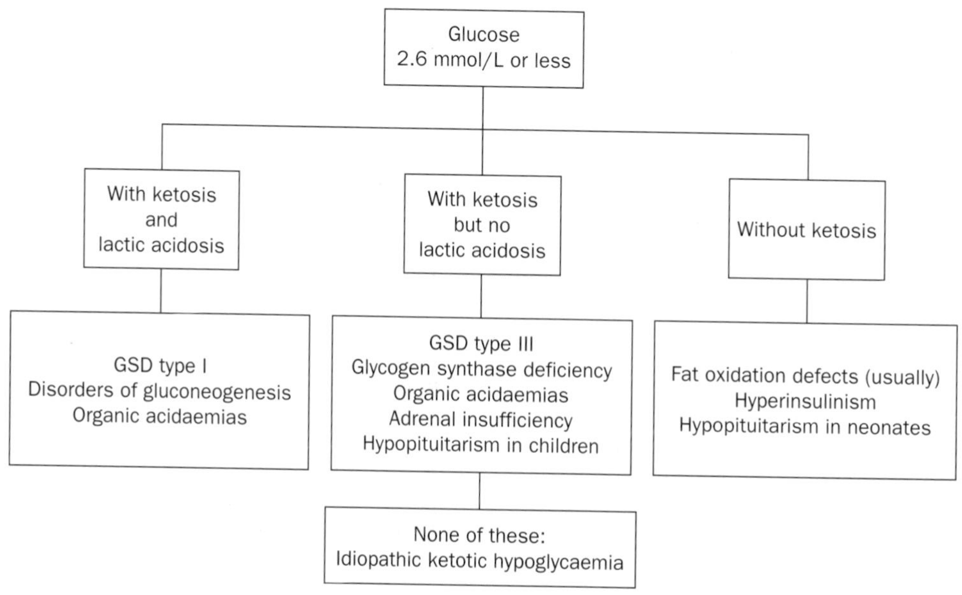

Figure 15.1 Metabolic and endocrine disorders causing hypoglycaemia. GSD, glycogen storage disease

Table 15.4 Disorders causing hypoglycaemia

Types	Clinical features	Key investigations	Management/outcome
Ketosis and severe lactic acidosis			
Glycogen storage disease (GSD) types Ia–d	Hypoglycaemia or hepatomegaly by 3–6 months, fasting tolerance 2–3 hours, 'doll face', short stature, bleeding due to platelet dysfunction. Types Ib and Ic associated with, oral ulceration, immune dysfunction and Crohn-type inflammatory bowel disease	High lactate (up to 12–15 mmol/L) falls with glucose, constant high triglycerides and cholesterol, high urate, high transaminases. With glucagon lactate rises, no glycaemic response. Diagnosis by assay of fresh liver biopsy (or DNA analysis in some cases) Neutropenia in Ib and Ic	2–3 hourly daytime feeds, corn starch; overnight enteral feeds to maintain normoglycaemia and suppress lactic acidosis; allopurinol; restrict lactose and sucrose; check renal function and bone status/calcium excretion. Risk of adenomas of liver
Fructose 1,6-bisphosphatase deficiency	May be lethal in early neonatal period; hepatomegaly	Severe lactic acidosis at time of hypoglycaemia. Occasionally non-ketotic. Diagnosis by enzymology of liver or white cell preparation.	Frequent feeds. Avoid fructose in infancy. Symptoms lessen in early childhood
Pyruvate carboxylase deficiency	Neonatal type	Severe lactic acidosis and hyperammonaemia. Very low PC activity in white cells or fibroblasts	Avoid fasting; glucose and bicarbonate during episodes of decompensation
	Native American type	Severe mental retardation	Neonatal form lethal
	'Benign' type	Recurrent hypoglycaemia and ketosis during intercurrent illnesses, well otherwise. Normal development. Some PC activity	
Ketosis and moderate lactic acidosis			
Organic acidaemias (see Table 15.6)	Hypoglycaemia is rarely the main presenting feature. Vomiting, hyperventilation, dehydration, encephalopathy	Ketoacidosis is severe. Lactate 4–7 mmol/L. Urine organic acids diagnostic	Need fluid replacement, bicarbonate, carnitine. Low protein diet or feed based on specific amino acid restriction. High risk of adverse neurological outcome
Ketosis but no lactic acidosis			
Glycogen synthase deficiency (also called glycogen storage disease type 0)	Short stature; no hepatomegaly	Extremely rare. Lactic acidosis and hyperglycaemia after meals or in glucose tolerance test (GTT). Very low liver glycogen content (<1 per cent, normal 3–5 per cent) Diagnosis requires liver biopsy. Presentation very similar to idiopathic ketotic hypoglycaemia	Avoid fasting
Glycogen storage disease type III	May have lactic acidosis after meals or after overcorrection of hypoglycaemia or after a GTT. Hepatomegaly and myopathy prominent	High red cell glycogen. High CK. Less severe than GSD I. Diagnosis by enzyme assay in white cells	Frequent daytime meals. Corn starch. High protein late evening meal. May require overnight tube feeding as in GSD 1. Milder course. Clinical features improve but cardiomyopathy develops in late childhood and adulthood

(*Continued*)

Table 15.4 *(Continued)*

Types	Clinical features	Key investigations	Management/outcome
Pituitary/adrenal insufficiency	Recurrent vomiting episodes and pigmentation in primary adrenal failure. Short stature, relative macrocephaly and micropenis in early-onset hypopituitarism. Hypoglycaemia does not occur in isolated growth hormone deficiency.	Cortisol should be at least 500–600 nmol/L in the normal response to hypoglycaemia. High ACTH in primary adrenal failure.	Short Synacthen test to exclude adrenal disease is mandatory if normal cortisol response has not been shown at the time of hypoglycaemia.
Without ketosis			
Hyperinsulinism	In 60 per cent onset of hypoglycaemia within 72 hours of birth. Often macrosomic. >12 mg/kg per minute total glucose intake needed to maintain blood glucose at >2.6–3.0 mmol/L; 35 per cent present at 1–12 months; 5 per cent at over 1 year	Insulin is >3 mU/L when glucose is <2.0 mmol/L: that is, lack of the physiological complete suppression of insulin during hypoglycaemia. In neonatal forms insulin may be very high (50–150 mU/L). Very low NEFA and β-hydroxybutyrate (no ketosis). Dramatic rise in blood glucose with IM glucagon. Mutations of SUR 1 gene or Kir6.2 gene on chromosome 11p15.1 are known in some diffuse lesions. In focal lesions loss of maternal alleles of the imprinted 11p15 in affected tissue. Both are autosomal recessive. Mutations of GLDH (glutamate dehydrogenase), or glucokinase cause autosomal dominant forms. Modest hyperammonaemia (50–150 μmol/L) occurs independently of hypoglycaemia in GLDH deficiency	Diazoxide 15 mg/kg per day with chlorothiazide – but most neonates are unresponsive. Intravenous glucagon infusion. Subcutaneous somatostatin analogue (octreotide). Rarely, response to nifedipine. Trial of intensive medical therapy before surgery, or long-term medical therapy. Diffuse β-cell hyperplasia (60 per cent); 95 per cent pancreatactomy; focal adenomatous hyperplasia (35 per cent) local resection. Aim is to achieve normal (not excessive) growth with a safe fasting interval of eight hours
Fatty acid oxidation defects (see Table 15.8)	Illness precipitated by fasting stress. Rarely presents in the neonatal period. Encephalopathy and slow recovery of consciousness after correction of hypoglycaemia. High risk of cerebral oedema. Hepatomegaly only during decompensation	Raised ratio (>2) of NEFA to β-hydroxybutyrate (normal is 0.6–1.0 after a long fast or in hypoglycaemia). Ketosis may occur and does not exclude these disorders. May have raised CK, AST, ALT, urate when symptomatic. Carnitine low except in the hepatic type of carnitine palmitoyl transferase deficiency. Dicarboxylic aciduria and/or acylcarnitine profile may be diagnostic	Treat cerebral oedema, carnitine. Fat-modified diet in some disorders. Some defects dominated by skeletal or cardiac myopathy and rhabdomyolysis

ALT, alanine transaminase; AST, aspartate transaminase; CK, creatine kinase; NEFA, non-esterified fatty acids.

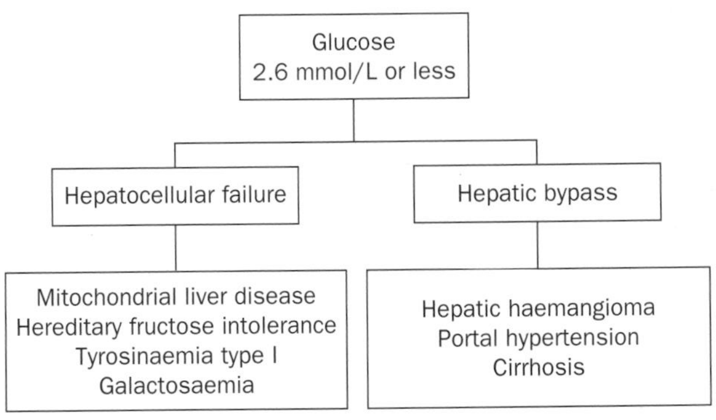

Figure 15.2 Hepatic disorders causing hypoglycaemia

but hypoglycaemia is rare. There is renal tubular dysfunction, which means that glucose, galactose and perhaps lactose may all be present in urine, if there has been recent lactose ingestion. These may not be present if the child has been feeding poorly, vomiting or was given IV fluids. Thus in any ill child, urine testing will not reliably confirm or exclude galactosaemia, and you must request red-cell GALT measurement. This may be invalidated because of recent transfusion; if so, you may make the diagnosis by demonstrating that both parents have enzyme activities in the heterozygote range. Stop all lactose-containing feeds if you suspect galactosaemia.

Rare causes of prolonged cholestatic jaundice in neonates are the disorders of bile salt synthesis and Niemann–Pick disease. It also occurs in the peroxisomal disorders, and in some of the congenital disorders of glycosylation and GM1 gangliosidosis but the other serious structural and neurological abnormalities will dominate the clinical presentation. These are discussed later in the chapter.

CASE STUDY: Prolonged jaundice, hypotonia and eventual liver failure

An infant had mild prolonged conjugated hyperbilirubinaemia, hypotonia and developmental delay. Transaminases were initially normal. He had moderately elevated blood and cerebrospinal fluid (CSF) lactate. Jaundice cleared very slowly over five months. During an intercurrent infectious illness at 10 months of age, he developed recurrence of severe jaundice and fatal hepatocellular failure. He had reduced activity of cytochrome *c* oxidase (complex IV of the respiratory chain) in muscle and liver.

Liver failure may present with rapidly evolving jaundice (or none), vomiting, bruising and with haematesis, pulmonary haemorrhage or intracranial haemorrhage. Liver failure, with very prominent jaundice and lactic acidosis, occurs in mitochondrial liver disease or respiratory chain disorders, where there may be mitochondrial (mt)DNA point mutations, deletions and duplications (normal quantities of abnormal mtDNA) or mitochondrial depletion (reduced quantities of normal mtDNA), or so-called somatic mutations affecting nuclear genes which regulate mitochondrial function or gene expression.

CASE STUDY: Liver failure due to tyrosinaemia type I

A 3-month-old infant presented with vomiting and poor weight gain. 'Routine' electrolytes and liver function tests showed low calcium, very low phosphate, mildly elevated transaminases, and very high alkaline phosphatase, indicating liver disease and metabolic bone disease. Coagulation screen showed an abnormal prolonged prothrombin time, in contrast with the mild transaminitis, characteristic of this disorder. Urine succinylacetone was high.

This is one of the major causes of metabolic liver failure in early childhood (Table 15.5). It can present in the first few weeks of life with liver failure, renal tubulopathy and biochemical rickets or later in milder forms. The earlier the presentation, the more severe and aggressive is the course. Before specific therapy with 2-(2-nitro-4-trifluoromethylbenzoyl)-1,3-cyclohexanedione (NTBC) became available, those who did not die of liver failure were at very high risk of developing fatal hepatocellular carcinoma.

Wilson disease is a disorder of copper metabolism, only rarely presenting in childhood, and invariably at over 5 years of age. Adolescents and young adults may present with the neurological features. The defective gene encodes a copper-transporting ATPase expressed in liver. Menkes disease (see Dysmorphic syndromes, page 469), is also due to a copper-transporting ATPase, but expressed in most tissues except liver.

PERSISTENT OR RECURRENT EPISODES OF METABOLIC ACIDOSIS

In the early neonatal period, you must exclude congenital heart disease such as coarctation of the aorta, hypoplastic

Table 15.5 Metabolic causes of jaundice and hepatocellular failure

Type	Clinical features	Key investigations	Management/outcome
Hepatocellular failure			
Hereditary fructose intolerance	Seizures, collapse after first exposure to fructose on weaning. Tolerance develops with time but with continued exposure liver failure with jaundice, ascites and failure to thrive and renal tubular disease may supervene. Patients self-select a sucrose and fructose free diet. Lack of dental caries	Hypoglycaemia, hypophosphataemia, high urate and lactic acidosis with acute exposure to fructose. Low activity of fructose aldolase B on liver biopsy.	Patients are normal on a fructose-free diet
Mitochondrial liver disease or respiratory chain disorders	Fulminant liver failure with coagulopathy, severe jaundice, bleeding in neonatal period, 'neonatal haemochromatosis'	Loss of respiratory chain complexes by mitochondrial or nuclear gene point mutations, deletions, or mitochondrial DNA depletions. Muscle, liver tissue required for diagnosis.	Some may reverse with supportive therapy. Liver transplantation (but beware multisystem disorders with later myopathy or mitochondrial encephalopathy)
Tyrosinaemia type I	Neonatal and infantile onset: liver failure with prominent coagulopathy, renal tubular disease with phosphate losses. Later onset: renal and bone disease, peripheral neuropathy and porphyria-like neurological crises. Very high risk of fatal hepatocellular carcinoma if untreated	Tyrosine elevated in blood and urine but is not specific. Succinyl acetone present in urine. Fumarylacetoacetase reduced in fibroblasts. Hypoglycaemia may sometimes be caused by reduced hepatic clearance of insulin	May need haem arginate for acute porphyric crises. Ninety per cent respond to NTBC. Liver transplant in non-responders or pre-emptively in hepatocellular carcinoma
Galactosaemia	Vomiting, jaundice, hepatomegaly, encephalopathy at 2–5 days of age. Cataracts are seen within a week	Renal tubular disease in the acute illness means urine may have glucose, lactose and galactose. Only reliable test in a very ill child is red cell galactose 1-phosphate uridyl transferase, but invalidated if recent blood transfusion	*E. coli* sepsis may coexist. Stop lactose containing feeds immediately. Cataracts and liver disease resolve. Reduced IQ, with speech dyspraxia. Most girls have primary ovarian failure. May be late neurological deterioration and tremor in adult life
Wilson disease	Presents at over 5 years with chronic active hepatitis, fulminant kiver failure or cirrhosis. Neurological signs in adolescence or early adulthood: tremor, drooling, dysarthria. Behavioural change, cognitive impairment, psychosis in 10–20 per cent of adults	Low total serum copper. 24-hour urine copper increased after 1 g/day penicillamine. Caeruloplasmin low but may be normal in hepatic failure. Kayser–Fleischer rings (but not present in early disease). Liver copper raised	Zinc prevents copper absorption. Penicillamine and trientine chelate copper and increase copper excretion. Tetrathiomolybdate binds copper in the gut and in blood. Liver transplant for fulminant disease or poor response to drugs
α-1 antitrypsin deficiency	May present as cholestatic jaundice with dark urine and pale stools and hepatomegaly, or later in infancy with a hard cirrhotic liver and portal hypertension.	α-1 antitrypsin level is unreliable, should perform Pi phenotype analysis	Supportive therapy; transplantation
Bile salt synthesis disorders			
5-β-reductase deficiency	Prolonged cholestatic neonatal jaundice, resulting in fat and fat-soluble vitamin malabsorption, rickets	Bile salt analysis in blood and urine (specialized laboratories only)	Bile salt replacement with ursodeoxycholic acid and chenodeoxycholic acid cause dramatic improvement

aortic arch, critical aortic stenosis and hypoplastic left heart. Metabolic acidosis may occur in renal dysplasia. You must exclude an acidosis of renal tubular origin. Later in the neonatal period, sepsis, particularly bowel sepsis and ischaemia as in necrotizing enterocolitis, may initially have only metabolic acidosis as a presenting feature.

CASE STUDY: Neonatal methylmalonic aciduria

A 3-day-old infant presents with vomiting, lethargy and poor feeding. There is weight loss of 15 per cent of body weight. There is metabolic acidosis with low chloride and a high anion gap. The urine tests positive for acetoacetate. Organic acid analysis identifies large amounts of methylmalonic acid.

Persistent acidosis may be due to an organic acidaemia or a primary lactic acidosis (Ozand and Gascon, 1991a,b). Organic acids are derived from chemical intermediates in the breakdown of amino acids (most from leucine). The initial step in the catabolism of amino acids not used directly for protein synthesis is removal of the amino group as ammonium ion: the remaining carbon 'skeleton' is then degraded in a series of steps to eventually form 'ketones' (acetoacetate and β-hydroxybutyrate) or glucose or both. The organic acidaemias are deficiencies of one or more of these steps. Fatty acid oxidation defects may cause abnormal organic aciduria but less commonly cause metabolic acidosis except for the lactic acidosis of long-chain hydroxyacyl-CoA dehydrogenase deficiency (LCHAD) deficiency and very long-chain hydroxyacyl-CoA dehydrogenase deficiency (VLCAD) deficiency, and are considered separately. In the glycogen storage diseases high lactic acid is well buffered and does not cause severe metabolic acidosis. There may, however, be persistent systemic acidosis due to ketoacidosis and lactic acidosis in the disorders of gluconeogenesis when the hypoglycaemia may be intermittent, and therefore less obvious (see Hypoglycaemia, page 452).

CASE STUDY: Isovaleric acidaemia

A 3-year-old boy presents with vomiting. He remains very lethargic for 48 hours despite fluid replacement and has very low plasma bicarbonate but recovers. Mother reports that any infectious illnesses make him unwell and that he becomes ataxic before vomiting starts. Urine organic acid analysis shows the presence of large amounts of isovaleric acid.

The commonest organic acidaemias are methylmalonic acidaemia, propionic acidaemia and isovaleric acidaemia. They may have a catastrophic presentation in the neonatal period with metabolic acidosis, ketoacidosis and encephalopathy, which may lead to deep coma. Isovaleric acidaemia, especially, may present much later. Note that the presence of ketones (acetoacetate) in the urine of a neonate is unusual, even during fasting, and strongly suggests an organic acidaemia. There may be hepatomegaly and hyperammonaemia severe enough to mimic a urea cycle disorder. Hypoglycaemia or hyperglycaemia may occur. Transient anaemia, neutropenia and thrombocytopenia occur and resolve spontaneously. (Note that these may wrongly appear to reinforce an initial diagnosis of sepsis.) Propionic acidaemia may present later with developmental delay, a movement disorder with choreoathetosis and with a T-cell immunodeficiency and rash. Methylmalonic acidaemia may present with recurrent vomiting, failure to thrive and motor developmental delay. Methylmalonic aciduria is most commonly caused by near total absence of methylmalonyl CoA mutase deficiency (mut_0) but there are forms with some residual activity (mut_-) and some due to defects in metabolism of vitamin B_{12}, a cofactor for the mutase enzyme (see the section on Vitamin-responsive disorders, page 471).

Glutaric aciduria type I may present with ketosis and acidosis, but may also present with minimal or no organic aciduria as a devastating encephalopathy. It is considered in the section on acute encephalopathy (page 461). Glutaric aciduria type II results from deficient or unstable electron transfer flavoprotein (ETF) or electron transfer flavoprotein-ubiquinone oxidoreductase (ETF-QO). These proteins are part of the final energy-producing enzymes involved in metabolism of fatty acids and organic acids from many amino acids, hence the alternative name, multiple acyl CoA dehydrogenase deficiency (MADD). A severe form (MADD-S) will present in infancy and is associated with dysmorphic facies. A milder form (MADD-M), has acidosis, little ketosis, hypoglycaemia and skeletal and cardiac myopathy. Table 15.6 summarizes the metabolic acidoses.

Table 15.6 Investigations in suspected organic acidaemias

Type	Clinical features	Key investigations	Treatment/outcome
Methylmalonic aciduria (MMA) Propionic aciduria (PA) (For variant forms of methylmalonic aciduria see Vitamin-responsive disorders, page 471)	May have severe neonatal encephalopathy and ketoacidosis or present later with vomiting, failure to thrive, developmental delay. Often dystonic motor disorder in PA. Hyperammonaemia common in the acute stage. PA may develop late cardiomyopathy	Urinary ketones (acetoacetate); ammonia; plasma amino acids often show high glycine; transient pancytopenia; low free and high or low total carnitine; specific acylcarnitines. Urine organic acids: MMA – methylmalonic acid, methylcitrate, 3-hydroxypropionate. PA – propionylglycine, 3-hydroxypropionate, methylcitrate	Aggressive treatment of neonatal acidosis with hypercaloric fluid replacement, bicarbonate, carnitine. May require dialysis, especially with hyperammonaemia. Initial protein restriction, then minimum protein for normal growth. Some MMA respond to hydroxocobalamin. Carnitine for secondary deficiency and for toxin removal. Outcome varies from severe to mild or no intellectual impairment. Long term renal failure likely in MMA
Isovaleric aciduria	As above, often well after infancy and usually less severe. 'Sweaty feet odour'	Urine organic acids show isovalerylglycine, 3-hydroxyisovaleric acid. Specific acylcarnitines	Often a good outcome. Glycine therapy (250 mg/kg per day or more) allows detoxification by means of high excretion of isovalerylglycine in urine and permits a relaxed protein intake
Maple syrup urine disease (Branched chain ketoaciduria)	Early presentation: ketoacidosis, hypertonus,encephalopathy Late presentation: intermittent ataxia, spasticity, dystonia, failure to thrive. Sweet, 'hot maple syrup' smell	Urine DNPH test detects ketoacids other than β-hydroxybutyrate and acetoacetate. Amino acids show very high leucine, isoleucine and valine (the 'branched-chain amino acids'). Organic acids show the related ketoacids 2-ketoisocaproic acid, 2-ketoisovaleric acid and 2-keto, 3-methylvaleric acid	Early aggressive therapy as for MMA and PA but lowering the high branched-chain amino acids (BCAAs) requires a complex semi-artificial diet with specific restriction of the 3 BCAAs and adequate amounts of the other essential amino acids. Good outcome depends on early recognition. May, rarely, respond to thiamine
Multiple carboxylase deficiency (see also Biotinidase deficiency in the Vitamin responsive disorders)	Ketoacidosis in the neonatal period or very early infancy. Male cats' urine odour	Organic acids reflect the 4 non-functional carboxylases: methylcrotonylglycine, 3-hydroxypropionate, lactate, 3-hydroxyisovalerate	Initial treatment as for PA and MMA, but responds within hours to 20–40 mg biotin which stabilizes the protein–biotin enzyme complex
Glutaric aciduria type II MADD-S MADD-M	 Severe neonatal presentation, overwhelming acidosis and dysmorphism Acidosis, modest ketosis. May have cardiomyopathy and skeletal myopathy	 Organic acids show glutaric acid, and many glycine conjugates of organic acids and fatty acids	 May respond to riboflavin and glycine. Carnitine
Pyruvate dehydrogenase deficiency	Severe persistent lactic acidosis. X-linked E_1 complex deficiency may be lethal to males. Females show facial dysmorphism, microcephaly, seizures, basal ganglia cysts and absent corpus callosum	High lactate, lactate/pyruvate ratio normal (<25:1). Diagnosis very complex: due to genetic deficiencies of molecular subunits of the enzyme complex: E_1, E_2, E_3 and 'protein X'. High BCAAs in E_3 complex deficiency	No treatment effective. High fat, low carbohydrate diet may reduce lactic acidosis
Pyruvate carboxylase deficiency		Lactic acidosis, ketosis, sometimes hypoglycaemia. Hyperammonaemia and high lactate/pyruvate ratio (>35:1) in the severe neonatal form	Fluid replacement, glucose, bicarbonate for intermittent symptoms in the milder forms. Severe form lethal

MADD, multiple acyl CoA dehydrogenase deficiency.

Investigations in suspected organic acidaemias

First line

- Full blood count
- Urea and electrolytes
- Glucose
- Bicarbonate
- Chloride
- Ammonia
- Blood gases and pH
- Urine testing for acetoacetate

Second line

- Blood lactate
- Plasma amino acids
- Plasma β-hydroxybutyrate
- Blood spots for acylcarnitine analysis
- Urine organic acid analysis by gas chromatography mass spectrometry

Anion gap = sodium + potassium − (chloride + bicarbonate). Normal is 10–18 mmol/L. The ion gap (unmeasured ions) is increased in ketoacidosis, including lactic acidosis and the organic acidaemias, and normal (with a compensatory high chloride) in conditions of renal and intestinal bicarbonate loss.

ACUTE ENCEPHALOPATHY INCLUDING INTRACTABLE SEIZURES AND REYE SYNDROME

Acute encephalopathy is a feature of very many metabolic disorders, especially hyperammonaemia, the fat oxidation defects, and organic acidaemias. **Glutaric acidaemia type I** (glutaryl CoA dehydrogenase deficiency) is considered here because it can present without the usual features of the organic acidaemias. **Intractable seizures** in the neonatal period may result from a small number of metabolic disorders. **Reye syndrome** is an acute non-inflammatory encephalopathy with hepatocellular failure, of uncertain aetiology (Table 15.7).

CASE STUDY: Glutaric aciduria type I

An apparently normal 1-year-old boy has a flu-like illness but becomes drowsy, extremely irritable and later is unable to be roused. Two days later in hospital, he has regained consciousness but has dystonic movements. A year later, he has profound motor deficit, with dystonia, feeding difficulties and severe gastro-oesophageal reflux.

Devastating acute illness occurs in two-thirds of cases. Children may be entirely asymptomatic until the first encephalopathic event. Some may present because of macrocephaly, with subdural effusions and arachnoid cysts and variable developmental delay. Peak age of neurological deterioration is under 1 year, with few relapses after 3 years. Identified asymptomatic siblings should be treated aggressively at the first sign of encephalopathy. Glutaric acid and 3-hydroxyglutaric acid are usually but not always found in urine.

CASE STUDY: Glycine cleavage defect

A term neonate, hypotonic at birth, develops apnoea at 4 hours of age requiring ventilatory support, and myoclonic seizures. Hiccups are also prominent and mother recalls these *in utero*. Seizures prove unresponsive to anticonvulsants. The ratio of CSF glycine to plasma glycine is abnormally high.

Glycine cleavage defect, or **non-ketotic hyperglycinaemia** causes neonatal onset epileptic encephalopathy and usually profound early hypotonia and apnoea, which may require respiratory support.

CASE STUDY: Pyridoxine responsive seizures

A neonate has seizures from the first day of life. They do not respond to anticonvulsants but stop clinically and electrically when a test dose of 50 mg pyridoxine is given intravenously with electroencephalographic (EEG) monitoring. The child remains free of seizures on an oral maintenance dose of 10 mg daily.

A trial of pyridoxine (50–100 mg IV), with EEG monitoring of the effect should be given to any child with a difficult seizure disorder to identify **pyridoxine dependency with seizures**. This disorder is associated with increased glutamate and decreased γ-aminobutyric acid (GABA) in CSF, but the precise underlying cause is not clear. (A very small number of infants who have not responded to pyridoxine may respond to pyridoxal phosphate.)

Table 15.7 Acute encephalopathy, epileptic encephalopathy and Reye syndrome

Disorder	Clinical features	Key investigations	Treatment/outcome
Glutaryl CoA dehydrogenase deficiency (Glutaric aciduria type I)	Macrocephaly. Some entirely normal until severe acute encephalopathy. Hyperpyrexia may occur. Dystonia and quadriplegia result from basal ganglia, putamen and caudate nuclei injury, sparing cerebral cortex	Organic acid analysis shows glutaric acid and 3-hydroxyglutarate, but this may be absent, even in severe encephalopathy. Fibroblast enzyme analysis. MRI brain shows subdural effusions and basal ganglia lesions, frontotemporal atrophy	Riboflavin, carnitine and diet restricted in lysine and tryptophan. Aggressive therapy for acute encephalopathy as for the organic acidaemias. Vigabatrin, valproate, benzodiazepines, ketamine dextromethorphan may reduce acute injury. Outlook dismal after encephalopathy
Non-ketotic hyperglycinaemia (glycine cleavage defect)	Neonatal hypotonia, hiccups, apnoea. Severe epileptic encephalopathy with myoclonic seizures. Near-absent post-neonatal neurological development. A few rare mild or transient cases described	EEG shows so-called burst-suppression pattern which is non-specific. High urine and blood glycine. Ratio of CSF glycine to plasma glycine 0.06–0.10 (normal is <0.04). The glycine cleavage system can be assayed in lymphocytes	Benzodiazepines, ketamine, dextromethorphan may block glycine-dependent neuronal receptors. Sodium benzoate (250–500 mg/kg per day) may lower glycine levels. Treatment is largely ineffective for the severe cases
Vitamin B_6-dependent seizures	Seizures of prenatal or neonatal onset, rarely later, resistant to standard anticonvulsants	Increased glutamate, decreased GABA in CSF. Immediate EEG resolution with pyridoxine is diagnostic	Pyridoxine 10–50 mg/day
Isolated sulphite oxidase deficiency Molybdenum co-factor deficiency	Neonatal epileptic encephalopathy, later lens dislocation	Increased urine thiosulphate. Low plasma and urine urate and high urine xanthine and hypoxanthine in molybdenum co-factor deficiency	None
Folinic acid-dependent seizures	Early-onset seizures, cardiomyopathy	Folate metabolites abnormal in CSF	Rapid and complete response to folinic acid 2–5 mg/day
GABA transaminase deficiency	Severe epileptic encephalopathy, tall stature, severe retardation	Increased CSF GABA. High fasting growth hormone	Early childhood death
Glucose transport protein deficiency	Severe epilepsy, retardation, microcephaly	Ratio of CSF glucose to blood glucose less than 0.35	Ketogenic diet: a good outcome depends on early recognition.
Reye syndrome	Biphasic course (see text), vomiting, rapidly evolving encephalopathy and coma. Seizures rare except in deep coma and ominous	Ammonia raised (may be transient). Raised transaminases. Prolonged prothrombin time. Amino acids show elevated lysine and glutamine. Glucose may be low. Liver histology: diffuse pan-lobular fatty change, macrovesicular or mixed microvesicular and macrovesicular fatty change. Abnormal large mitochondria with disrupted cristae on electron microscopy. Post-mortem: 'fatty degeneration of the viscera': fatty change in liver, heart, renal tubules, skeletal muscle and pancreas	Correct hypoglycaemia. Treat cerebral oedema – ventilation, cooling, head-up nursing, thiopental, monitoring of intracranial pressure to maintain cerebral perfusion. Encephalopathy and hepatopathy improve within days but survival or neurological recovery depend on the depth of coma and treatment of cerebral oedema. (Diagnosis is by exclusion, after a search for specific underlying disorders)

CSF, cerebrospinal fluid; EEG, electroencephalography; GABA, γ-aminobutyric acid; MRI, magnetic resonanse imaging.

Sulphite oxidase deficiency causes an infantile epileptic encephalopathy and may later cause lens dislocation. The less rare **molybdenum co-factor deficiency** combines sulphite oxidase deficiency and xanthine oxidase deficiency. **Folinic acid dependent seizures** may respond to folinic acid with immediate cessation of seizures and normal long term development. **GABA transaminase deficiency** causes an epileptic encephalopathy, high growth hormone levels and increased somatic growth. GABA is greatly increased in CSF. **Glucose transport protein deficiency** causes seizures, microcephaly and severe developmental delay. CSF glucose is low. A ketogenic diet provides alternative fuel for brain and allows a good outlook with early recognition and treatment, provided severe brain injury has not already occurred. **Peroxisomal disorders** may cause intractable seizures, due to an associated neuronal migration disorder (see the section on Peroxisomal disorders, page 477).

Reye syndrome is defined as an acute non-inflammatory encephalopathy (less than 8 white cells/mm^3 in CSF), with **elevation of ammonia** to more than three times the measuring laboratory's upper limit of normal, or **elevation of transaminases** (aspartate aminotransferase (AST) and alanine aminotransferase (ALT) or serum glutamate-oxalate transaminase (SGOT) and serum glutamate-pyruvate transaminase (SGPT)) to more than three times the measuring laboratory's upper limit of normal, and, no more reasonable explanation for the condition. Hypoglycaemia, often coexistent, especially in infants, is not one of the diagnostic criteria. The disorder has a biphasic course, with a prodromal virus-type illness, followed by a period of apparent recovery, followed by the onset of intractable ('pernicious') vomiting. There is then a rapid neurological deterioration with early irritability, confusion and aggressiveness ('combativeness') evolving to coma.

The condition has been linked by epidemiological studies, and some experimental studies to the administration of aspirin, and this led, in the UK, to the withdrawal of aspirin for use in children under 16 years of age, except on the advice of a doctor. Other associations are with influenza A and varicella. The rapid rise to prominence of the disorder and a dramatic fall after the restriction of aspirin use suggests that this is a distinct entity, but it must be distinguished from the many conditions that may mimic it and cause 'Reye-like illnesses'. By far the most important are the fat oxidation disorders.

Disorders that cause coma and abnormal liver function tests

- Septicaemia with shock
- Haemorrhagic shock and encephalopathy syndrome
- Near-miss sudden infant death syndrome
- Fulminant hepatitis
- Meningitis
- Severe generalized viral illness: adenovirus, varicella
- Hypoxic brain and liver damage
- Severe dehydration
- Encephalopathies causing convulsions and requiring intramuscular injections
- Salmonellosis and shigellosis
- Wilson disease

Genetic or familial disorders that have mimicked Reye syndrome

- Mitochondrial fatty acid oxidation defects
- Primary (systemic) carnitine deficiency
- Organic acidurias
- Urea cycle defects
- Respiratory chain defects
- Maple syrup urine disease
- Hereditary fructose intolerance
- Fructose 1,6-bisphosphatase deficiency
- α-1 Antitrypsin deficiency
- Glycerol kinase deficiency
- Familial haemophagocytic lymphohistiocytosis
- Cystic fibrosis

Drugs or toxins that have mimicked Reye syndrome

- Aflatoxin
- Margosa oil
- Unripe ackee fruit containing hypoglycins
- Hornet stings
- Insecticide exposure (Budworm spraying)
- Salicylate poisoning
- Paracetamol poisoning
- Valproate toxicity

DISORDERS OF β-OXIDATION OF FATTY ACIDS

Fatty acids are oxidized for energy in some tissues, or to ketones in the liver. β-Oxidation of fatty acids involves their being transported (at first bound to carnitine as palmitoyl carnitine) across the mitochondrial membranes, and then undergoing repeated cycles of reactions that shorten them. A series of enzymes of differing chain-length specificity is involved. Deficiencies of nearly all the steps in this process are known (Rinaldo *et al.*, 2002). Because production of ketones is impaired ketosis is limited but not absent. The ratio of free fatty acids (NEFA) to β-hydroxybutyrate is increased during fasting. (In the well-fed state lipolysis is suppressed and both NEFA and β-hydroxybutyrate are low. The ratio is then uninterpretable.) Impaired fatty acid oxidation in mitochondria leads to peroxisomal β-oxidation of the accumulating monocarboxylic acids and production of dicarboxylic acids, which may appear in the urine.

The main clinical presentation is encephalopathy, thought to be due to the accumulating dicarboxylic acids. There is often hypoglycaemia, but encephalopathy occurs first. Urinary excretion of dicarboxylic acids may be diagnostic in some disorders (e.g. medium-chain acyl CoA dehydrogenase (MCAD) deficiency) or much less specific or absent (as in carnitine cycle defects and in the long-chain disorders). The unoxidized fatty acids accumulate as fatty-acylcarnitine esters, of varying length from 14-carbon length (C_{14}) to 4-carbon length (C_4), and may be detected by acylcarnitine analysis of plasma or dried blood spots, allowing specific diagnosis. Except for carnitine-palmitoyl transferase deficiency type I (hepatic type), in which carnitine is normal or high, there is a secondary carnitine deficiency because of renal losses of acylcarnitine in these disorders.

CASE STUDY: Medium-chain acyl CoA dehydrogenase deficiency

A 2-year-old boy is admitted after rotavirus diarrhoea, with sleepiness and confusion. His glucose level is 2.4 mmol/L. He takes 24 hours to return to full consciousness despite IV glucose replacement and subsequent normal glucose results. Plasma β-hydroxybutyrate is a little elevated but the NEFA to β-hydroxybutyrate ratio is over 3. Urine organic acids show hexanoylglycine and suberylglycine, with little ketosis. DNA analysis confirms homozygosity for the common mutation of MCAD deficiency.

Medium-chain acyl CoA dehydrogenase deficiency is one of the commonest inborn errors of metabolism in white populations. The typical age at presentation is 1–3 years. One child in three suffers irreparable brain injury or death at the time of the first encephalopathic episode. Note that encephalopathy precedes hypoglycaemia, which may not be present.

Cardiomyopathy is common in all the fatty acid oxidation disorders except MCAD deficiency and carnitine-palmitoyl transferase deficiency type I. Long-chain 3-hydroxyacyl CoA dehydrogenase deficiency has particular additional complications of an evolving pigmentary retinopathy with loss of colour vision by early adult life and peripheral neuropathy.

Women pregnant with a fetus affected by this disorder have a high risk of acute fatty liver of pregnancy (AFLP) or haemolysis, elevated liver enzymes and low platelets (the HELLP syndrome).

CASE STUDY: Very-long-chain acyl CoA dehydrogenase deficiency

A boy first presented in the neonatal period with sweating and poor feeding and was found to be hypoglycaemic. Acylcarnitine analysis, enzymology and mutation analysis confirmed VLCAD deficiency. By 3 years, he was having recurrent episodes of mild encephalopathy with muscle pain and weakness and sometimes dark urine. This was despite overnight tube feeding and a diet in which long-chain fats were largely replaced by medium-chain triglycerides.

Intermittent muscle pain, weakness and myoglobinuria (with very high creatine kinase in blood) are characteristic of all the carnitine transport defects and the long-chain fat oxidation disorders. It may occur for the first time in adulthood in type II carnitine-palmitoyl transferase deficiency. Carnitine-palmitoyl transferase deficiency type I presents in childhood with cardiac and skeletal myopathy, hepatomegaly and encephalopathy with hypoglycaemia.

Carnitine transporter deficiency presents very similarly. Cells cannot take up carnitine and there are high urinary carnitine losses. Carnitine levels in blood are extremely low. The disease responds dramatically to carnitine. Carnitine is widely used in all these disorders, though this use has not been subject to controlled clinical trials.

Table 15.8 summarizes the disorders of β-oxidation of fatty acids.

NEAR-MISS COT DEATH

Despite a large number of metabolic diseases individually associated with sudden unexplained death in infancy,

Table 15.8 Disorders of β-oxidation of fatty acids

Deficiency	Clinical features	Key investigations	Management/outcome
Short-chain acyl CoA dehydrogenase	Neonatal onset: vomiting, encephalopathy, liver disease, myopathy Adult onset: myopathy, encephalopathy	Hypoglycaemia; variable organic aciduria – ethylmalonic acid, adipic acid, methylsuccinate, butyrylglycine. Elevated butyryl carnitine. Fibroblasts show reduced oxidation of short-chain (C4) acyl CoA	Normal diet. MCT is contra-indicated. Carnitine
Medium-chain acyl CoA dehydrogenase (common)	Encephalopathy. No cardiomyopathy or skeletal myopathy. The commonest of these disorders (incidence 1:10 000)	Hypoglycaemia, high NEFA/β-hydroxybutyrate, low plasma carnitine. Specific dicarboxylic aciduria (hexanoylglycine, suberylglycine); elevated hexanoyl (C8)- and octanoyl (C8)-carnitine; 80–90 per cent homozygous for the common ΔG985 mutation. Enzymology may be unreliable	Normal diet. MCT is contra-indicated. Avoid long fasting periods. Carnitine
Long-chain 3-hydroxyacyl CoA dehydrogenase and 'Trifunctional protein' deficiency	Encephalopathy, myopathy, cardiomyopathy. Liver disease may evolve to cirrhosis. Later onset peripheral neuropathy and pigmentary retinopathy. High incidence of maternal AFLP and HELLP syndrome	Hypoglycaemia, high NEFA/β-hydroxybutyrate, lactic acidosis, low plasma carnitine, C14 hydroxyacylcarnitine elevated. Confirmed by enzymology or mutation analysis	Low fat, high carbohydrate diet, MCT. Carnitine. Supplements of essential fatty acids and fish oils may prevent progression of retinopathy which typically causes loss of peripheral (night) vision and loss of colour vision by 20s
Very-long-chain acyl CoA dehydrogenase deficiency	Encephalopathy, hepatomegaly, cardiomyopathy, skeletal myopathy. May have vomiting, loose stools due to intestinal dysmotility	Hypoglycaemia, high NEFA/β-hydroxybutyrate low plasma carnitine, non-specific dicarboxylic aciduria; elevated C14 unsaturated acylcarnitine	Low fat, high carbohydrate diet, MCT. Carnitine
Carnitine-palmitoyl transferase I	Encephalopathy, hepatomegaly	Hypoglycaemia, high NEFA/β-hydroxybutyrate, high free and total carnitine, high palmitoyl-carnitine, no organic aciduria. Confirmation by enzymology on cultured fibroblasts.	Low fat, high carbohydrate diet; fat supplemented as MCT. Short fasting periods; may require overnight continuous feeding
Carnitine-acylcarnitine translocase	Encephalopathy, cardiomyopathy, skeletal myopathy	Hypoglycaemia, high NEFA/β-hydroxybutyrate, low plasma carnitine, encephalopathy. Confirmed by enzymology	Low fat, high carbohydrate diet, MCT
Carnitine-palmitoyl transferase II	Infantile: facial dysmorphism, cystic changes in kidney, cardiomyopathy, encephalopathy Adult: fasting or exercise-induced rhabdomyolysis	Hypoglycaemia, high NEFA/β-hydroxybutyrate, low plasma carnitine, variable and non-specific dicarboxylic aciduria: elevated long-chain acylcarnitines. Adult: elevated creatine kinase, myoglobinuria precipitated by fasting or exercise. Confirmed by enzymology	Low fat, high carbohydrate diet, MCT. Carnitine. Myoglobinuria in adults may be massive and cause renal failure
Carnitine transporter deficiency (primary carnitine deficiency)	Like type I carnitine-palmitoyl transferase deficiency	Extremely low plasma and tissue carnitine. Absent carnitine uptake in cultured fibroblasts	Carnitine 100–200 mg/kg per day

MCT, medium-chain triglyceride; NEFA, non-esterified fatty acids.

cot death, collectively they account for no more than 1 per cent of cases. Cases will have had hours or days of symptoms before apparent acute collapse. Most identified causes are due to fatty acid oxidation disorders, particularly medium-chain acyl CoA dehydrogenase deficiency. There may be profound secondary metabolic abnormalities in the absence of a primary metabolic disorder in an infant or young child rescued from acute cardiorespiratory vascular collapse, including hypoglycaemia or hyperglycaemia, metabolic acidosis and lactic acidosis. Severe hyperammonaemia up to 400 μmol/L may occur but is transient, lasting no more than a few hours. Alanine transaminase, AST and creatine kinase (CK) may be high, reflecting extreme tissue hypoxia. Serial measurements of AST and ALT with a rapid rise and fall over a few days may indicate liver cell necrosis. Other secondary clinical problems include cerebral oedema, acute renal tubular necrosis and poor myocardial function. High fever, acidosis, diarrhoea (perhaps blood stained) and hypoglycaemia are not uncommon, and may lead to suspicion of haemorrhagic shock encephalopathy syndrome. For any collapsed child the investigations for acute encephalopathy and acidosis should be undertaken, and the profile for hypoglycaemia, if appropriate. Stored blood spots for acylcarnitine analysis are particularly valuable for the fat oxidation defects and the organic acidaemias. If the child is not going to survive, then blood should be taken, plasma and cells separated, and frozen. Urine should be frozen for organic acid analysis and a record kept of all drugs given, so that drug metabolites can be distinguished. If necropsy is performed, the finding of microvesicular fatty change in liver, cardiac and skeletal muscle and kidney is suggestive of a fat oxidation defect. A fibroblast culture should be set up from skin or pericardium. Analysis of vitreous humour may permit discovery of peri-mortem hypoglycaemia, or hypernatraemia or uraemia.

FAILURE TO THRIVE

Some metabolic disorders will have failure to thrive as the presenting symptom, but there will usually be multisystem disease, with anorexia and vomiting, or malabsorption, and often neurological abnormalities. They are dealt with elsewhere but collated here (Table 15.9). For detailed information, refer to the appropriate section.

DEVELOPMENTAL DELAY AND NEURODEVELOPMENTAL REGRESSION

Special metabolic investigations are not indicated in isolated delay in speech and language development or motor development or autism. Children presenting to secondary level services with global developmental delay merit investigation. The history is important in determining whether there has been loss of acquired skills, the hallmark of developmental regression, or slowing of acquisition of new skills, which may not indicate a progressive disorder. Devastating loss of skills, with the development of motor dysfunction after an encephalopathy is a characteristic of glutaric acidaemia type I, also associated with a large head. Leigh syndrome may also present after an acute illness. Additional clues to a possible metabolic disorder are parental consanguinity, recurrent unexplained illness, hypotonia, cataract,

Table 15.9 Metabolic disorders presenting mainly as failure to thrive

Condition	Clinical features	Refer to
Propionic acidaemia and methylmalonic acidaemia	Vomiting, gastro-oesophageal reflux, delayed motor development	Organic acidaemias
Ornithine carbamoyl transferase deficiency (mild)	Anorexia, recurrent vomiting	Hyperammonaemia
Lysinuric protein intolerance	Vomiting, anorexia, extreme growth retardation, hepatosplenomegaly	Amino acid disorders
Abetalipoproteinaemia	Steatorrhoea	Lipid disorders
Wolman disease (infantile cholesterol ester hydrolase (acid lipase) deficiency	Infant-onset severe steatorrhoea	Lipid disorders
*My*o*N*euro*G*astro*I*ntestinal *E*ncephalopathy (MNGIE)	Diarrhoea, gastrointestinal dysmotility, small head	Mitochondrial disorders
Pearson syndrome	Steatorrhoea, anaemia, lactic acidosis	Mitochondrial disorders
Biotinidase deficiency	Vomiting, rash, immunodeficiency, seizures	Vitamin disorders
Transcobalamin II deficiency	Diarrhoea, stomatitis, anaemia	Vitamin disorders (B_{12})

deafness (conductive or sensorineural or both), and dysmorphism – particularly coarse facial features, bone and skin abnormalities, and hair abnormalities. It is important to identify treatable disorders or disorders that will have a risk of recurrence in other children.

A detailed birth history and a careful clinical examination are paramount. Mucopolysaccharidosis III (Sanfilippo disease) is likely to be overlooked in a delayed and hyperactive child, as the physical features can be very mild (see Lysosomal storage diseases, page 477). Table 15.10 lists the investigations considered in developmental delay.

For severe, early-onset developmental failure consider Tay–Sachs disease, Sandhoff disease, infantile Gaucher disease and, for regression in an older child, metachromatic leucodystrophy or, later, Niemann–Pick disease type C (see Sphingolipidoses in Table 15.18).

CASE STUDY: 'Cerebral palsy' and crystalluria

An 8-month-old boy shows motor developmental delay, and spasticity of all limbs, with dystonia, but seems interested in his surroundings and is very visually aware. Mother recalls red-pink discoloration of nappies. Plasma and urine uric acid are both grossly elevated.

This child has Lesch–Nyhan syndrome, due to hypoxanthine-guanine phosphoribosyl transferase deficiency (HGPRT deficiency). There is X-linked inheritance. Urate crystals may precipitate from urine. This disorder progresses relentlessly, despite treatment to reduce urate synthesis and excretion with allopurinol. Risk of renal stones and ultimate renal failure is high. The diagnosis is confirmed by enzyme assay in red cells. The boy's mother should be tested for carrier status for risk of recurrence.

CASE STUDY: Brain stem signs in an infant

An 18-month-old boy develops rapid breathing and nystagmus after chickenpox. Both disappear after a few days. Over the next few months mother notes occasional choking with drinks and a deterioration in his walking. He stops learning new words and becomes ataxic. Blood lactate after a carbohydrate meal is 4.0 mmol/L and CSF lactate is 5.2 mmol/L. Magnetic resonance imaging (MRI) scan of the head shows bilateral basal ganglia lesions. He has a relapsing, deteriorating course over the next five years.

This boy has Leigh syndrome. It can present earlier, or much later. The pathological lesions are demyelination,

Table 15.10 Investigations in developmental delay

Investigations	Condition
First-line	
Chromosomes, including analysis specifically for fragile sites on X chromosome	Chromosomal abnormalities and fragile X syndrome
Calcium	Hypocalcaemia, hypoparathyroidism
Thyroid function tests	Congenital or acquired hypothyroidism
Creatine kinase	Duchenne muscular dystrophy, some fat oxidation defects
Blood lead	Lead poisoning
Biotinidase	Biotinidase deficiency (see Vitamin disorders, page 471)
Plasma and urine urate	Purine/pyrimidine disorders, especially Lesch-Nyhan syndrome (high) and molybdenum co-factor deficiency (low), but both are very rare
Second-line	
Plasma lactate (post-prandial)	Mitochondrial encephalopathies/oxidative phosphorylation disorders – mitochondrial or nuclear DNA mutations
Plasma amino acids and total homocysteine	Hyperphenylalaninaemia (if no neonatal screening), homocystinurias (see Amino acid disorders), vitamin B_{12} disorders (see Vitamin disorders, page 471)
Ammonia	Urea cycle disorders
Free carnitine	Low in the fat oxidation disorders and some organic acidaemias
Very long chain fatty acids	Abnormal in peroxisomal disorders (see Peroxisomal disorders, page 477)
Urine organic acids and orotic acid	Organic acidaemias, fat oxidation defects, urea cycle disorders
Urine glycosaminoglycans and oligosaccharides	Mucopolysaccharidoses and oligosaccharidoses (see Lysosomal disorders, page 477)

necrosis and gliosis in the basal ganglia, brain stem, cerebellum and cerebral cortex. This condition may be due to the final common pathway of a number of conditions affecting brain energy metabolism (see Mitochondrial diseases, page 477).

> **CASE STUDY: Regression and behaviour problems at school**
>
> A 6-year-old boy has lost skills and become clumsy and dysarthric. There are no dysmorphic features. Deep tendon reflexes are absent. After a recent family holiday, he remains rather tanned. Very long chain fatty acid analysis is abnormal.

This boy has X-linked adrenoleucodystrophy. This disorder is one of the peroxisomal disorders (see Peroxisomal disorders, page 477). It can present from childhood to early adulthood, with neurological features and signs of adrenal failure in varying combinations. The childhood form progresses to decerebration within a few years. Pigmentation is due to primary adrenal failure and elevated adrenocorticotrophic hormone (ACTH).

HYPERAMMONAEMIA

Measure plasma ammonia in any child who presents with altered consciousness or coma where the cause is not injury, epilepsy or other recognized encephalopathy. Presence of focal signs, including hemiplegia and visual loss does not rule out hyperammonaemia. Infants will be drowsy and irritable and may vomit. There may be abnormalities of tone and posture with abnormal 'cycling' movements. Failure to recognize and treat hyperammonaemia may be devastating.

The normal range is less than 40 μmol/L for term babies and older children, up to 65 μmol/L in well preterm babies and up to 180 μmol/L for ill preterm babies. In metabolic disorders, it is over 200 μmol/L and may reach 1500–5000 μmol/L in the urea cycle disorders.

Measuring urine orotic acid can be helpful in diagnosis. This is derived from accumulated carbamoyl phosphate in the disorders of the urea cycle (especially in ornithine carbamoyl transferase deficiency), and in lysinuric protein intolerance (see the section on Amino acid disorders, page 471). It is not found in carbamoyl phosphate synthase (CPS) deficiency and *N*-acetylglutamate synthase (NAGS) deficiency (Table 15.11), or any of the other disorders.

Table 15.11 Causes of hyperammonaemia

In the neonate	
Inherited disorders of the urea cycle	Ornithine carbamoyl transferase deficiency (not uncommon). X-linked inheritance
	Argininosuccinic acid synthase deficiency (citrullinaemia)
	Argininosuccinic acid lyase deficiency (argininosuccinic aciduria)
	N-acetyl glutamate synthase deficiency
	Carbamoyl phosphate synthase deficiency
Organic acidaemias	Propionic acidaemia
	Methylmalonic acidaemia
	Pyruvate carboxylase deficiency (rare)
Others (transient)	Transient neonatal hyperammonaemia
	Perinatal asphyxia
	Intravenous feeding and excessive protein intake
	Ill preterm neonates
	Neonatal herpes simplex infection
In the infant and older child	
Urea cycle disorders	As above
Organic acidaemias	As above
Other disorders of ammonia metabolism	Lysinuric protein intolerance
	Hyperammonaemia, homocitrullinaemia and hyperornithinaemia
Liver disease	Advanced liver disease, including cystic fibrosis
	Reye syndrome
Miscellaneous	Idiosyncrasy to sodium valproate
	Infection with urea-splitting organisms (especially *Proteus* spp.) in an obstructed, dilated urinary tract

Treatment of hyperammonaemia

Associated hypoglycaemia, acidosis, dehydration or sepsis should be treated. For ammonia above 150 μmol/L sodium benzoate and sodium phenylbutyrate therapy is used. These conjugate with glycine and glutamine, forming products that are rapidly excreted in urine. Success depends on adequate urine output. In all cases except arginase deficiency, arginine is given: it is a catalyst for any residual enzyme activity and also becomes an 'essential' amino acid in these disorders, as it cannot be synthesized. Very high ammonia at presentation (>350 μmol/L) should be treated urgently by dialysis. Efficiency is different for different methods: haemodialysis > haemodiafiltration ≫ peritoneal dialysis. Dialysis will also be necessary if renal function is poor or renal tract obstruction cannot be corrected rapidly. The drugs are continued as long-term therapy in the urea cycle disorders (Urea Cycle Disorders Conference Group, 2001).

The outlook for rescue from severe neonatal hyperammonaemia due to urea cycle disorders is grim, but neonates with hyperammonaemia of the newborn (transient, with no underlying biochemical deficiency), vigorously treated, do well.

CASE STUDY: Mild ornithine carbamoyl transferase (OCT) deficiency

A 2-year-old girl has had repeated admissions to hospital because of vomiting, which usually resolves after a brief period of IV fluids. In between she eats poorly. In one admission, she is noted to be ataxic and irritable. Blood ammonia is 240 μmol/L. Amino acids later show high glutamine and alanine, but no other abnormal amino acids are present. Urine contains orotic acid, but no abnormal organic acids.

This child has mild OCT deficiency, hence the presentation well beyond the neonatal period. It can mimic 'cyclical vomiting'. Very mildly affected females with OCT deficiency may have recurrent headaches and intolerance of high-protein meals. Diagnosis may be based on enzymology on liver biopsy tissue but is now more reliably based on mutation analysis of the OCT gene.

In the organic acidaemias and the fatty acid oxidation defects, ammonia probably accumulates because of inhibition of synthesis of carbamoyl phosphate. In classic Reye syndrome, the cause is a generalized impairment of mitochondrial function.

CASE STUDY: Transient hyperammonaemia of the newborn

A baby boy, 34 weeks' gestational age, presents with tachypnoea at 8 hours. A chest radiograph shows no abnormality and, in particular, no sign of respiratory distress syndrome (RDS) or pneumonia, and blood gases in air are normal. At 16 hours he is refusing to feed and is vomiting tube feeds. At 24 hours ammonia is 1000 μmol/L. Ammonia falls extremely quickly in response to IV arginine followed by brief haemodiafiltration. There is no rebound rise in ammonia after dialysis is discontinued and full feeds are tolerated quickly.

This disorder occurs invariably in preterm babies and presents earlier than the true metabolic causes of hyperammonaemia. It may be due blood bypassing the liver because of a persistent ductus venosus that later closes spontaneously. Glutamine is low in relation to the high level of ammonia. A flow chart for the diagnosis of metabolic causes of hyperammonaemia is presented in Figure 15.3.

METABOLIC DISORDERS PRESENTING AS DYSMORPHIC SYNDROMES

Some babies will present with **non-progressive dysmorphism at birth**, due to teratogenic effects of small molecules on intrauterine development. The infant of a mother with untreated (occasionally unrecognized) **severe hyperphenylalaninaemia** may have microcephaly (90 per cent) and congenital heart defects (20 per cent), especially coarctation of the aorta and ventricular septal defect. There are mild mid-face abnormalities such as hypertelorism, epicanthic folds, and perhaps cleft palate and oesophageal atresia. Some **organic acidaemias** and **X-linked pyruvate dehydrogenase** deficiency (a cause of lactic acidosis) cause facial and other abnormalities, similar enough to suggest a common mechanism, with some features of **fetal alcohol syndrome**.

Storage disorders cause progressive changes to initially normal tissues. Some affected babies will be clearly abnormal at birth, the rest presenting insidiously in the first months or years.

Disorders affecting **multiple peroxisomal functions** cause major abnormalities of organ development and differentiation with early dysmorphic features, multisystem disease and severe neurological impairment. Disorders of

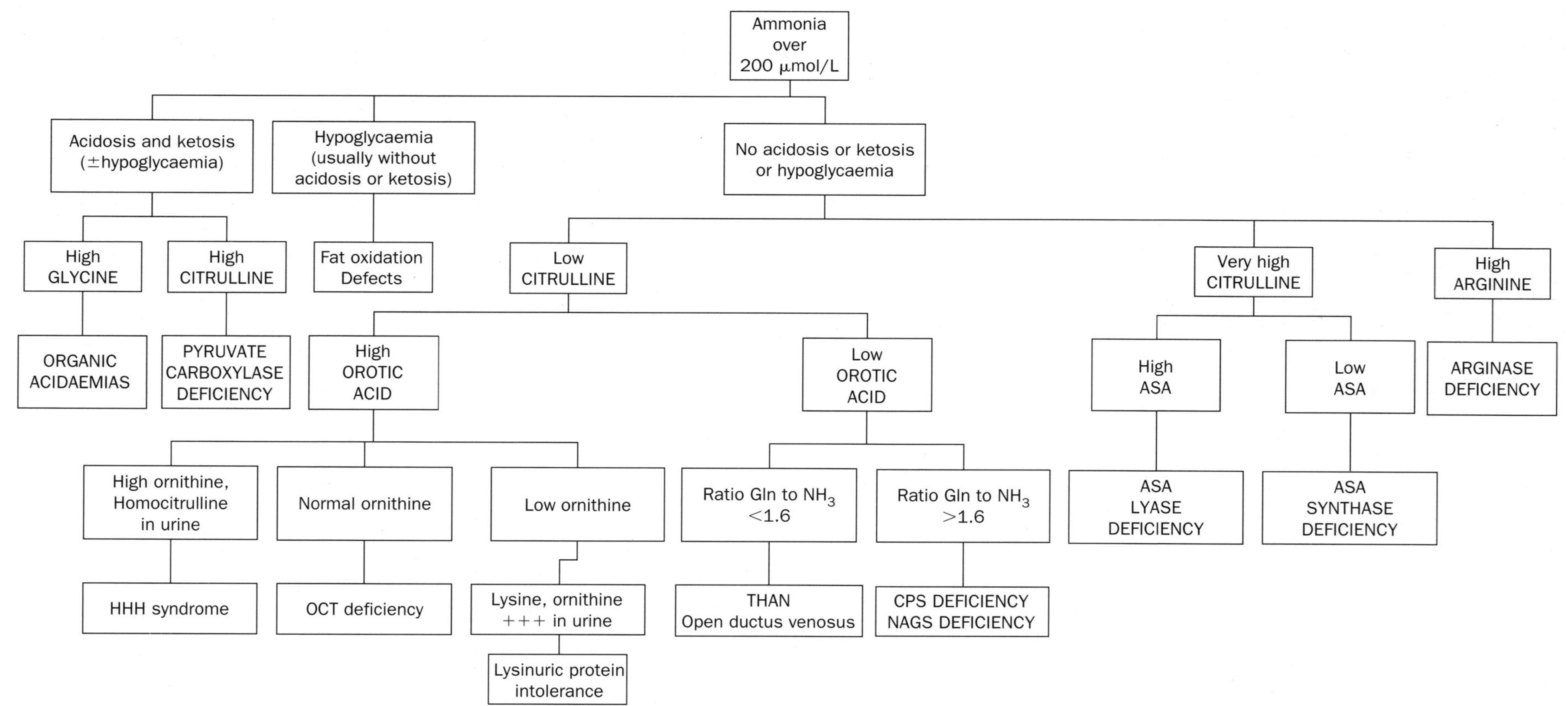

Figure 15.3 Metabolic disorders causing hyperammonaemia. ASA, argininosuccinate acid; CPS, carbamoyl phosphate synthase; Gln, glutamine; HHH, hyperammonaemia-hyperornithinaemia-homocitrullinaemia; NAGS, *N*-acetylglutamate synthase; OCT, ornithine carbamoyl transferase; THAN, transient hyperammonaemia of the newborn

single peroxisomal enzymes do not have dysmorphism. Boys with Menkes disease may look normal at birth but present by 2 months of age (Table 15.12).

DISORDERS OF INTERMEDIARY METABOLISM INCLUDING CARBOHYDRATE, AMINO ACID, AMMONIA, FATTY ACID AND VITAMIN METABOLISM

Carbohydrate disorders

Many of the important disorders of carbohydrate metabolism have been considered in relation to **hypoglycaemia** (the glycogen storage diseases I and III and disorders of gluconeogenesis), and the hepatic effects of **galactosaemia** and **hereditary fructose intolerance**. The other hepatic storage diseases present with hepatomegaly. Pompe disease is a generalized lysosomal storage disease and has multisystem effects: cardiomyopathy and others in infants and myopathy in older, late presenting, adults. Two muscle glycogenoses present with only muscle symptoms.

Amino acid disorders

Hyperphenylalaninaemia due to deficiency of phenylalanine hydroxylase (PAH) is numerically the most important amino acid disorder. Therapy with a specialized low-phenylalanine diet is highly effective in preventing the almost inevitable severe impairment of mental developmental that it causes. **Tyrosinaemia type I** has liver and renal abnormalities as its most immediate consequence and hepatocellular carcinoma as its most lethal and is considered in the section on hepatocellular failure. **Homocystinuria** loosely refers to cystathionine β-synthase deficiency, a disorder of sulphur-containing amino acids, in which methionine, homocysteine, homocyst*ine* (which is a dimer of homocyst*eine*) and other mixed disulphides accumulate. These damage connective tissues, causing abnormalities of the lens, skeleton and intimal layer of blood vessels. Mental and behaviour abnormalities are variable, and unexplained.

Maple syrup urine disease behaves like an organic acidaemia, though it tends not to cause a severe metabolic acidosis and ketosis is variable. It results from deficiency of the branched-chain ketoacid decarboxylase that carries out the first step in the metabolism of the ketoacids of leucine, isoleucine and valine. Leucine accumulation most closely relates to the symptoms. A leucine-derived ketoacid is thought to account for the characteristic smell from body fluids found in acute episodes of illness. **Non-ketotic hyperglycinaemia** is discussed in the section on acute metabolic encephalopathy (page 461). **Cystinuria** is one of the commonest metabolic causes of renal stone disease (but still rare in renal stone disease in general). **Lysinuric protein intolerance** is due to a disorder of transport of dibasic amino acids with losses of lysine, and ornithine and arginine in the intestine and the renal tubules. Secondary effects cause severe failure to thrive and delayed mental development, recurrent vomiting after protein-containing meals (hence the name), osteoporosis, hepatosplenomegaly and anaemia, and interstitial lung disease.

Disorders of vitamin metabolism

Vitamins usually have roles as co-factors for enzymes. Some severe vitamin deficiency states cause disease by impairing these enzymes. Biochemical vitamin-responsive diseases result from conditions that may affect metabolism of the vitamins to active forms, or binding of vitamins to form their vitamin–apoenzyme complexes (Bartlett, 1983). Forms of **cobalamin** (vitamin B_{12}) undergo processing before being chemically active. **Biotin** requirements are much greater than can be sustained from the normal diet and biotin is salvaged from some enzyme-co-factor proteins to be recycled. Deficiency of the enzyme for this activity, biotinidase, causes deficiency of four biotin-dependent enzymes and a progressive, often lethal multisystem disease.

Pyridoxine is a co-factor for cystathionine β-synthase and a proportion (up to 50 per cent in some populations) of patients with classic homocystinuria will respond to pyridoxine in large doses (up to 500 mg per day). Pyridoxine dependency with seizures is considered with the disorders causing refractory epilepsy.

Rarely, mild variants of propionic aciduria and MSUD may respond to **thiamine**. **Riboflavin** is given for congenital methaemoglobinaemia, glutaric aciduria type I and glutaric acidaemia type II (multiple acyl CoA dehydrogenase deficiency): see Organic acidaemias (page 459).

See Table 15.13 for a summary of these disorders.

Disorders of lipoprotein metabolism

Plasma lipoproteins transport cholesterol esters and triglycerides between tissues. Cholesterol and triglycerides form an inner core. This is surrounded by a protein and lipid coat. The proteins (called apolipoproteins or apoproteins) bind to receptors on cells and to enzymes. The lipoproteins differ in properties which allow their physicochemical classification (by centrifugation, electrophoresis) and identifying excess or deficiency of lipoproteins

Table 15.12 Metabolic disorders presenting as dysmorphic syndromes

Condition	Clinical features	Key investigations	Treatment/outcome
Non-progressive teratogenesis			
Maternal hyperphenylalaninaemia	Heart defect, microcephaly	Maternal phenylalanine	
Some rare organic acidaemias, females with X-linked pyruvate dehydrogenase deficiency	Mid-face dysplasia, long philtrum, sloping or prominent forehead, narrow bifrontal diameter agenesis of corpus callosum	Urine organic acids Blood lactate	
From birth, progressive			
Some lysosomal diseases, particularly GM1 gangliosidosis, β-glucuronidase deficiency (MPS VII), I-cell disease, neuraminidase deficiency	Coarse facies, corneal clouding, gum hypertrophy, dysostosis multiplex, hepatomegaly, hernias, some may cause oedema or hydrops	Plasma, white cell lysosomal enzymes	See Lysosomal storage diseases (page 475)
Peroxisomal disorders, Zellweger syndrome	Wide open fontanelle, high forehead, epicanthic folds, ear abnormalities, hypotonia, cataract and pigmentary eye abnormalities, hepatomegaly, renal cysts, chondrodysplasia calcifications, cryptorchidism	Plasma very long chain fatty acids Red cell plasmalogens	See Peroxisomal diseases (page 475)
Menkes disease (X-linked)	'Cherub' facies, sparse, brittle stubby hair. Developmental arrest at a few months, epilepsy, hypothermia, hydroureter and vesicoureteric reflux, intracranial haemorrhages	Very low plasma copper and caeruloplasmin. Hair abnormal on electron microscopy. Skeletal abnormalities. Abnormal copper uptake studies in fibroblasts	Copper histidine injections may alter the course, if started very early, but death often by 3 years
Later, progressive			
Lysosomal storage diseases	Varying with disease type: coarse facial features, corneal clouding, bone abnormalities, organomegaly, regression	Urine glycosaminoglycans and oligosaccharides. Lysosomal enzymes	See Lysosomal storage diseases
Smith–Lemli–Opitz syndrome	Microcephaly, upturned nose, ptosis, syndactyly of 2nd and 3rd toes, cryptorchidism and renal abnormalities, failure to thrive	Low cholesterol (often), high 7-dehydrocholesterol	
Disorders of glycoprotein synthesis: CDG type Ia is the most common	Inverted hypoplastic nipples, cryptorchidism, abnormal fat pads and *peau d'orange*, joint contractures, cardiomyopathy, pleural and pericardial effusions, olivo-ponto-cerebellar hypoplasia	Abnormal transferrin electrophoresis, low hormone binding proteins	See Lysosomal storage diseases

CDG, congenital disorders of glycosylation; MPS, mucopolysaccharidosis.

Table 15.13 Disorders of intermediary metabolism

Type	Clinical features	Key Investigations	Treatment/outcome
Carbohydrate disorders			
Pompe disease (GSD type II)	This is a lysosomal storage disorder. Does not cause hypoglycaemia Infantile form: large tongue, hypotonia, infiltrative cardiomyopathy Adult or late childhood form: slowly progressive skeletal myopathy	In cardiomyopathy, very large QRS complexes on ECG, 'bright' appearance of myocardium on echocardiogram. Very low α-1,4 glucosidase in fibroblasts, plasma (peripheral WBCs unreliable due to isoenzyme forms). Vacuolated peripheral bood lymphocytes	Early cardiomyopathy causes death in infancy. Experimental enzyme replacement therapy has been successful
Andersen disease (GSD type IV)	Does not cause hypoglycaemia. Extremely rare. Usually causes developmental delay, liver cirrhosis, skeletal myopathy and cardiomyopathy in early childhood; some patients have non-progressive chronic liver disease, or only CNS disease	Liver biopsy shows a non-branching plant-type starch accumulation in brain, liver muscle. Low 'branching enzyme' in peripheral blood leucocytes	Measures for liver cirrhosis. Liver transplant is uncertain in this multisystem disease
McArdle disease (GSD V) and Tarui disease (GSD VII)	Do not cause hypoglycaemia. Weakness, fatiguability, muscle pain and stiffness. Symptoms are earlier, and more severe in GSD VII, and in GSD VII there is a mild haemolytic anaemia. Worse with exercise but a 'second wind' phenomenon may occur. (This may be due to using fatty acids, not carbohydrate for energy during sustained exercise)	High blood urate and creatine kinase after exercise. On ischaemic exercise lactate does not rise, but urate and ammonia do. This test is not reliable as subjects have to continue exercise through pain. Muscle phosphorylase activity reduced in GSD V and muscle phosphofructokinase reduced in GSD VII	Encourage graded non-extreme exercise. Carbohydrate supplements during exercise (but may worsen symptoms in GSD VII)
Hers disease (GSD VI) and GSD IX	Present with hepatomegaly and mild, if any, hypoglycaemia. Growth delay in mid-childhood reverses at or before puberty	Clinically similar: differences are in the involved enzymes and inheritance: type VI is autosomal recessive liver phosphorylase deficiency and type IX is autosomal recessive liver phosphorylase b kinase deficiency. Phosphorylase kinase has four subunits encoded on different autosomal chromosomes and the X chromosome, so there are various forms with different tissue specificity variously recessive or X-linked. Mutation analysis available for some	Treatment may not be necessary. Uncooked corn starch is used for smooth fasting glucose control or improved exercise tolerance or endurance if indicated
Fanconi–Bickel syndrome (GSD XI)	Hepatomegaly, large kidneys, failure to thrive, and severe renal tubular defect causing rickets	Fasting hypoglycaemia is mild and variable. Glycogen stored in liver and proximal renal tubules. Galactose intolerance. Mutations in the glucose transporter 2 (GLUT2) gene	No specific therapy available

(*Continued*)

Table 15.13 *(Continued)*

Type	Clinical features	Key investigations	Treatment/outcome
Amino acid disorders			
Hyperphenylalaninaemias including isolated phenylalanine hydroxylase (PAH) deficiency (98 per cent) and defects of biopterins; dihydropteridine reductase (DHPR) deficiency, GTP cyclohydrolase deficiency, 6-pyruvoyl tetrahydrobiopterin synthase deficiency (1–2 per cent)	Sustained hyperphenylalaninaemia impairs normal brain development, with mental retardation and autistic behaviour patterns. Incidence 1 in 6000 to 1 in 50 000 worldwide. 1 per cent of cases are due to disorders of synthesis or recycling of tetrahydrobiopterin (BH_4), a co-factor for PAH and the hydroxylases for the synthesis of L-dopa and 5-hydroxytryptophan. These cause signs of dopamine, serotonin and noradrenaline neurotransmitter deficiencies	Normal phenylalanine (Phe) is 60–90 μmol/L. Neonatal screening identifies all cases where (Phe) is $>$240 μmol/L. Phe $>$400 μmol/L requires therapy. Phe $>$700 μmol/L and often $>$1200 μmol/L at screening is 'classic' phenylketonuria (PKU), with Phe metabolites in urine and high risk of adverse outcome if untreated. Blood biopterins, red cell DHPR activity and sometimes tests of responsiveness to biopterin therapy needed to exclude BH_4 disorders. Over 300 mutations known in PAH deficiency	For PAH deficiency: semi-artificial low-phenylalanine diet needed for life. Good intellectual outcome if adequate Phe control in childhood. Adequate therapy to lower Phe is essential in pregnancy to avoid teratogenic effects (early fetal loss, congenital heart defects, facial malformations, microcephaly and low birth weight). For biopterin defects: BH_4 and neurotransmitter replacement therapy with L-dopa/carbidopa and 5-hydroxytryptophan. Folinic acid for DHPR deficiency. BH_4 alone may lower Phe adequately without the need for specific diet. Variable long-term outcome
Cystathionine β-synthase deficiency, classic homocystinuria	Lens dislocation causing increasing myopia is a common presentation where there is no neonatal screening programme. Developmental delay (not invariable), tall stature and 'marfanoid' habitus and osteopenia. Untreated, very high risk of arterial and venous and pulmonary thromboembolism and stroke	Homocystine in urine can be detected by the nitroprusside test; high homocysteine and methionine in plasma. Other disorders cause 'homocystinuria', but have other features: disorders of vitamin B_{12} absorption or transport or metabolism, methionine synthase deficiency, 5,10-methylene tetrahydrofolate reductase deficiency	Some respond to high doses of pyridoxine alone. For others: low-methionine semi-artificial diet, folic acid, antithrombotic drugs – aspirin, dipyridimole. Outcome best for treatment after neonatal screening
Lysinuric protein intolerance	Varied clinical signs. Vomiting after protein meals; failure to thrive and short stature. Immunodeficiency and a lupus-like syndrome. Hepatosplenomegaly. Lung disease with alveolar proteinosis and interstitial cholesterol crystalline deposits may cause death	Mutations in the SCLA7 gene for amino acid transport in intestine, renal tubule. Arginine, ornithine and lysine low in blood and high in urine. Hyperammonaemia and orotic aciduria after protein meals. Anaemia and thrombocytopenia. Osteopenia. T-cell dysfunction	Low protein diet; oral citrulline to replace arginine
Cystine-lysinuria	Cystine-containing renal stones in a minority – many remain asymptomatic	Cystine-lysinuria (also excreted are ornithine and arginine). At least three allelic genes involved	Stones likely if 24-hour excretion of cystine exceeds 400 mg per day or maximum urine concentration exceeds 1.25 mmol/L (300 mg/L). High fluid intake to encourage urine output of 1.66 L/m^2 body surface area

			per day. Alkalinization of urine for maximum solubility of cystine is of doubtful benefit and may not be achievable
Ornithine aminotransferase deficiency (gyrate atrophy of the retina)	Visual loss (with night blindness) beginning after 10 years of age, cataract. Characteristic retinal appearance	High plasma ornithine, without other evidence of the HHH syndrome (See section on causes of high ammonia). Enzyme assay on fibroblasts, liver	Pyridoxine may lower plasma ornithine in some cases. Low arginine diet may further lower ornithine and oral lysine may increase urinary ornithine excretion: all may help to stabilize retinal function
Disorders of vitamin metabolism			
Vitamin B_{12} disorders: Vitamin B_{12} is absorbed as hydroxocobalamin but active as methylcobalamin and adenosylcobalamin. Methylcobalamin is co-factor for the methionine synthase complex; adenosylcobalamin for	Methylcobalamin deficiency: neurodevelopmental regression, seizures, subacute degeneration of the spinal cord, homocystinuria, megaloblastic anaemia, retinopathy	Homocystinuria and high plasma homocysteine. Low plasma methionine. Megaloblastic marrow. MRI may show abnormal myelination in brain and spinal cord	1000 mg hydroxocobalamin or methylcobalamin or adenosylcobalamin (initially daily, then reduced), folate; betaine to raise methionine may stabilize or reverse neurological decline
methylmalonyl CoA mutase (see Methylmalonic aciduria). Disorders of absorption or protein binding transport of B_{12} will affect both:	Adenosylcobalamin deficiency: vomiting, ketoacidosis (mild)	Urine organic acids analysis shows methylmalonic aciduria	Some forms may respond to hydroxocobalamin or adenosylcobalamin: otherwise treat as mut_{-} or mut_0 methylmalonic aciduria
disorders of subcellular organelle release or conversion will cause loss of one or both functions. Cobalamin disorders with varying features are designated cblA to cblH	Severe failure to thrive, diarrhoea, anaemia with transcobalamin II deficiency which affects B_{12} transport		
Biotin disorders			
Biotinidase deficiency (See also multiple carboxylase deficiency in the organic acidaemias)	Onset at about 6 months old as biotin is depleted. Failure to thrive, perioral, perinasal and blepharal dermatitis, hair loss; T-cell immunodeficiency. Demyelination involving lower brain stem causes stridor, optic atrophy, long tract signs. Seizures	Enzyme can be measured in plasma and dried blood spots (screening is possible). Specific abnormal organic aciduria reflects the four affected carboxylase enzymes (see Organic acidurias)	Biotin 10–20 mg daily reverses all abnormalities except for established CNS signs
Thiamine disorders			
Thiamine responsive megaloblastic anaemia	Includes deafness, diabetes mellitus	Megaloblastic anaemia	Thiamine 25–100 mg/day reverses most findings: deafness responds variably
Thiamine responsive propionic aciduria and maple syrup urine disease	See organic acidaemias		

(Continued)

Table 15.13 *(Continued)*

Type	Clinical features	Key investigations	Treatment/outcome
Pyridoxine disorders			
'Classical homocystinuria' due to cystathionine-β-synthase deficiency	See amino acid disorders		
Pyridoxine dependent seizures	See intractable seizures		
Riboflavin			
Glutaric acidaemia type II (multiple acyl CoA dehydrogenase deficiency; MADD)	See organic acidurias		

CNS, central nervous system; EEG, electroencephalography; GSD, glycogen storage diseases; HHH, hyperammonaemia-hyperornithinaemia-homocitrullinaemia; MRI, magnetic resonance imaging; WBC, white blood cell.

allows a broad classification of disease types. Knowledge of the structures of these molecules is expanding and diseases may eventually be classified by the apoproteins involved, or by mutation analysis. Chylomicrons and very low density lipoprotein (VLDL) are rich in triglycerides. Low density lipoprotein (LDL) and high density lipoprotein (HDL) are rich in cholesterol. **Lipoprotein lipase** binds to chylomicrons and VLDL and cleaves triglycerides to fatty acids and glycerol to be used as energy sources. The chylomicron remnants are taken up by the liver. VLDL is eventually converted to LDL.

Low density lipoprotein is broken down in lysosomes by **acid lipase**, also called **cholesterol ester hydrolase**. The released cholesterol is stored. HDL activates **lecithin-cholesterol acyl transferase** and becomes further enriched with cholesterol. HDL is in turn taken up by the liver and serves to transport cholesterol from the periphery to the liver. It has an antiatherogenic effect. Table 15.14 gives an overview of lipoprotein disorders.

DEFECTS OF CELLULAR ORGANELLES: MITOCHONDRIA, PEROXISOMES AND LYSOSOMES

Mitochondria are the organelles involved in the production of high-energy chemical intermediates from the oxidation of fatty acids, the metabolism of acetyl CoA in Krebs' cycle, pyruvate metabolism and, eventually, storage of energy as ATP following oxidative phosphorylation in the respiratory chain. The respiratory chain is the multienzyme complex intimately bound to the inner and outer mitochondrial membranes. Some of the components of the respiratory chain are encoded by nuclear DNA; abnormalities are inherited as autosomal recessive traits. Others are encoded by the mtDNA genome that is exclusively of maternal origin: abnormalities may be passed from mother to child as dominant traits with variable expression.

Mitochondrial disorders (Table 15.15) affect metabolically active tissues throughout the body and a hallmark is progressive, multisystem disease in which organs are affected in sequence (Nissenkorn *et al.*, 1999). Most are believed to result from nuclear gene defects. Some, including important and distinctive syndromes, are due to point mutations, deletions or duplications in mtDNA, or due to depletion of mtDNA, causing, as time passes, fewer mitochondria and failing enzyme expression. Expression varies within families and the same mutations may cause different constellations of symptoms and signs.

Investigation is highly complex. Careful investigation of organ function will highlight the multisystem disease. Lactate may be raised, with a high lactate to pyruvate ratio. Elevated CSF lactate, if found, is a very important and suggestive abnormality. Even in the mtDNA deletion syndromes expression varies between tissues. Muscle biopsy and analysis including histochemistry or direct assay of respiratory chain enzyme activity, mutation analysis and quantitative measurement of mtDNA are indicated.

Peroxisomal disorders

Peroxisomes have a role in oxidation of fatty acids (most importantly of the long structural molecules of cell membranes, including long branched fatty acids from the diet, pristanic acid and phytanic acid) and in the synthesis of bile acids and ether phospholipids, and in glyoxylate metabolism. The disorders (Table 15.16) can be grouped as:

- those with absence of peroxisomes causing near complete loss of peroxisomal functions
- those with loss of multiple enzymes
- those with loss of single enzymes.

The best recognized conditions are **Zellweger syndrome, adrenoleucodystrophy** and **Refsum disease. Acatalasaemia** is a peroxisomal disorder that impairs neutrophil function and leads to necrotizing gingivitis and other oral infection. **Hyperoxaluria** causes precipitation of calcium oxalate in the kidney, then later in other organs after renal failure develops. **Mevalonate kinase** deficiency affects steroid synthesis and causes minor dysmorphic features. It may present as an immune deficiency disorder, with periodic fever and hyperimmunoglobinaemia (hyper IgD). Mevalonic acid is present in large amounts in plasma and urine.

Lysosomal disorders and congenital disorders of glycosylation

Lysosomes are intracellular organelles containing hydrolases active in acid conditions. These break down complex constituent molecules of cells and intercellular tissues; deficiency of one, or of multiple enzymes, causes them to accumulate. There are effects on connective tissues, nervous tissue and brain, internal organs and the skeleton. Lysosomal disorders are classified by the type of storage material present. They represent a very wide group of disorders, many extremely rare. Their importance is increased because some are common in some racial groups (Tay-Sachs disease and Gaucher disease in Ashkenazi Jews), some relatively treatable by bone-marrow transplantation (Hurler syndrome), and an increasing number will be treatable by recombinant enzyme replacement therapy

Table 15.14 Disorders of lipoprotein metabolism

Type	Clinical features	Key investigations	Treatment/outcome
High cholesterol			
Familial hypercholesterolaemia (FH): autosomal co-dominant, 1:500 incidence, due to abnormalities of hepatic LDL-cholesterol receptors	Premature atherosclerosis (men before 50 and women before 60), xanthomas, xanthelasma. Severe childhood atherosclerosis in homozygotes	Raised LDL-cholesterol and normal triglycerides. Total cholesterol nearly always >7.5 mmol/L in heterozygotes, and >15 mmol/L in homozygotes. Screening of families with early ischaemic heart disease. Analysis of LDL-receptor mutations	Dietary restriction of total fat and cholesterol. Decision to use drug therapy is strongly influenced by male sex and the family history of severity and age of onset of ischaemic heart disease. Resin binding agents colestipol and cholestyramine have limited effectiveness. Fibrates. Statins (simvastatin, atorvastatin and others) inhibit HMG CoA reductase and reduce cholesterol synthesis but have a theoretical risk of impairing sex-sterol synthesis in puberty. For homozygotes: statins, plasmapheresis, liver transplantation
Familial ApoB-100 deficiency: 1:700 incidence	Clinically, as for FH	Analysis of mutations in the ApoB-100 apolipoprotein	As for FH
High cholesterol and triglycerides			
Familial combined hyperlipidaemia: autosomal dominant, up to 1:33 incidence in some communities	Increased obesity, hyperinsulinism and glucose intolerance, coronary heart disease and peripheral vascular disease	High VLDL and LDL and triglycerides	Low fat diet, exercise, avoidance of other risk factors. Statins in adulthood – unlikely to present in childhood, but 20–30 per cent will have abnormal lipids in childhood
Lecithin-cholesterol acyl transferase (LCAT) deficiency: autosomal recessive	Proteinuria at 3–4 years, corneal opacity at puberty. Haemolytic anaemia in adult life, and eventual renal failure. Early atherosclerosis	High total cholesterol and triglycerides. Foamy storage cells in bone marrow.	Reduced dietary fat. Renal replacement therapy.
Cholesterol ester hydrolase (acid lipase) deficiency Severe, infantile: Wolman disease Mild, adult: cholesterol ester storage disease (CESD)	Wolman disease – fatal in infancy, with steatorrhoea, hepatosplenomegaly and enlarged and calcified adrenals. CESD – hepatomegaly, liver fibrosis, premature atherosclerosis	Usually high plasma total cholesterol and triglycerides: sometimes normal in Wolman disease but liver lipids massively high. Foamy storage cells in bone marrow. Enzymology in fibroblasts	Statin drugs in the adult form. Infantile form is invariably fatal.
High triglycerides			
Familial lipoprotein lipase deficiency: autosomal recessive	Childhood presentation with abdominal pain, recurrent pancreatitis, hepatosplenomegaly, eruptive xanthomas, but no premature atherosclerosis	Creamy layer over clear plasma in a blood sample refrigerated overnight. Triglycerides over 20 mmol/L before symptoms occur, may reach very high levels.	Very-low-fat diet (2–4 g/day) is dramatically effective. Medium chain triglyceride may be used as energy supplement.

Apoprotein CII deficiency: autosomal recessive	As lipoprotein lipase deficiency but no xanthomas or hepatosplenomegaly. Haemolytic anaemia and high risk of diabetes	As for LPL deficiency	As for LPL deficiency
Familial hypertriglyceridaemia: autosomal dominant	Mostly asymptomatic, but metabolic syndrome, associated with obesity, glucose intolerance, hyperuricaemia, hypertension	Triglycerides 5–10 mmol/L	Carbohydrate restriction, fibrates or nicotinic acid; fish oils, exercise
Low cholesterol and triglycerides			
Familial abetalipoproteinaemia and hypobetalipoproteinaemia: autosomal recessive	Fat malabsorption, steatorrhoea, vitamin E and vitamin A deficiency	Low cholesterol and triglycerides, low VLDL and LDL. Ancanthocytes. Apoprotein B deficiency	Low fat diet, possibly medium chain triglycerides. Vitamin A and E supplements
Low cholesterol, normal or high triglycerides			
Tangier disease: autosomal recessive	Large orange tonsils. Corneal opacity. Peripheral neuropathy. Haemolytic anaemia and thrombocytopenia	Plasma total cholesterol below 2.6 mmol/L because of almost complete absence of HDL. Low apo AI and AII. High triglycerides	Low-cholesterol diet prevents cholesterol storage in tonsil and intestinal mucosa

HDL, high density lipoprotein; LDL, low density lipoprotein; VLDL, very low density lipoprotein.

Table 15.15 Defects of mitochondrial metabolism

Condition	Clinical features	Investigations	Treatment/outcome
Leigh syndrome	Subacute necrotizing encephalomyelopathy, brain stem dysfunction, respiratory abnormalities, dystonia, ataxia, nystagmus, peripheral neuropathy	NARP and MELAS mutations, complex I (NADH-ubiquinone reductase) and complex IV (cytochrome *c* oxidase) deficiency. Mitochondrial or nuclear (autosomal). Some associated with pyruvate dehydrogenase deficiency. Characteristic abnormalities on brain MRI scan	Outlook poor, but variable. High-fat, low-carbohydrate diet may help in lactic acidosis. Anecdotal reports of benefit from many co-factor therapies: thiamine, riboflavin, vitamin C, biotin, Coenzyme Q (ubiquinone), menadione, lipoic acid. Dichloroacetate may lower high lactate
MELAS	*M*itochondrial *E*ncephalopathy, *L*actic *A*cidosis, *S*troke-like episodes, recurrent vomiting, 'migraine', cortical blindness	3243A > G mutation in mtDNA and others	
Alpers disease	Explosive onset of epilepsy, with characteristic EEG, slow myoclonus, later preterminal liver failure	As MELAS	
MERRF	*M*itochondrial *E*ncephalopathy, *R*agged *R*ed *F*ibres on muscle biopsy	8344G > A mutation in mtDNA and others	

(Continued)

Table 15.15 *(Continued)*

Condition	Clinical features	Investigations	Treatment/outcome
NARP	*N*eurodegeneration, *A*taxia, *R*etinitis *P*igmentosa	8933T > G mutation in mtDNA and others	
LHON	*L*eber *H*ereditary *O*ptic *N*europathy	11778G > A mutation in mtDNA and others;	
MNGIE	*M*yo*N*euro*G*astro*I*ntestinal *E*ncephalopathy, microcephalopathy, spastic diplegia, sparse hair, microvillous atrophy, intestinal dysmotility	mtDNA deletions	
DIDMOAD syndrome	*D*iabetes *I*nsipidus, *D*iabetes *M*ellitus, *O*ptic *A*trophy, *D*eafness	mtDNA mutations (including 11778G > A mutation)	
Kearns–Sayre syndrome	Progressive external ophthalmoplegia, and ptosis, proptosis, cardiac conduction defects, myocardial hypertrophy, pigmentary retinopathy, renal tubular and renal cystic disease, sensorineural deafness	mtDNA deletions and duplications	
Pearson syndrome	Lactic acidosis, pancreatic insufficiency, anaemia with ring sideroblasts, myopathy, liver disease	mtDNA deletions. Neonatal survivors may evolve to Kearns–Sayre syndrome	

EEG, electroencephalography; MRI, magnetic resonance imaging; mtDNA, mitochondrial DNA.

Table 15.16 Peroxisomal disorders

Type	Clinical features	Important investigations	Treatment/outcome
Loss of all peroxisomal functions			
Zellweger syndrome	Typical dysmorphic features (see section on Disorders with dysmorphism), hepatomegaly, liver failure, severe hypotonia, cataract, deafness, neuronal migration disorder, seizures, stippled epiphyses, renal cysts	Elevated very long chain fatty acids (VLCFA), low red cell plasmalogens (derived from ether phospholipids), abnormal bile acids, raised phytanic acid	Dietary restriction of VLCFA, or bile acid replacement unsuccessful. Possible benefit from DHA (docosahexanoic acid) methylester. Generally death in infancy
Neonatal adrenoleucodystrophy	No dysmorphic features, but brain demyelination, adrenal atrophy, neurological regression in early infancy	Elevated VLCFA, low or normal plasmalogens, raised bile acids, phytanic acid and pristanic acid	As Zellweger syndrome
Infantile Refsum disease	Slow neurodevelopmental regression	As adrenoleucodystrophy	Dietary restriction may slow progression

Loss of multiple peroxisomal functions			
Rhizomelic chondrodysplasia punctata	Short upper segments of the limbs, contractures, bone dysplasia, ocular abnormalities, developmental regression	Normal VLCFA, bile acids and pristanic acid, low plasmalogens, high phytanic acid. Deficiency of four peroxisomal enzymes is linked to absence of a receptor common to their expression	Death in mid-childhood
Loss of single peroxisomal functions			
X-linked adrenoleucodystrophy	Variable features, stroke-like episodes, demyelination, absent reflexes, late-onset adrenal failure, with pigmentation. Variable predominance of the neurological or adrenal features.	Elevated VLCFA	Lorenzo's oil (1:4 ratio of the triglycerides of erucic acid and oleic acid) lowers VLCFA but does not alter clinical course. Early bone marrow transplantation *may* be useful. *Adrenal steroid replacement*
Refsum disease	Usually adult onset peripheral neuropathy, ataxia, pigmentary retinopathy, night blindness, ichthyosis, raised CSF protein	Elevated phytanic acid. Absent phytanic acid oxidase activity	Plasmapheresis at induction of treatment, then dietary restriction of phytanic acid
Other very rare disorders DHAPAT deficiency (resembles chondrodysplasia punctata), pseudo-Zellweger syndrome, pseudo-neonatal leucodystrophy	Some features of the related disorders of multiple functions, but with loss of single enzyme functions		

Table 15.17 Classification of lysosomal storage disorders

Disorder	Stored material
Mucopolysaccharidoses	Glycosaminoglycans ('GAGs'): complex polysaccharides with amino sugars
Oligosaccharidoses	Short complex sugars (glycoproteins)
Sphingolipidoses	Complex glycolipids linked to ceramide and called sphingolipids, globosides and gangliosides
Mucolipidoses	GAGs, glycoproteins, glycolipids – a combination of many of the above
Others (see specific sections)	Pompe disease (glycogen storage disease type II): glycogen-linked oligosaccharides
	Cystinosis: intracellular free cystine
	Acid lipase deficiency: cholesteryl esters (see Lipid disorders)

Table 15.18 Lysosomal disorders and congenital disorders of glycosylation (CDG)

Condition	Clinical features	Important investigations	Treatment/outcome
Mucopolysaccharidoses Type I–Hurler and Scheie Type II–Hunter (X-linked) Type III–Sanfillipo Type IV–A Morquio A Type IV–B Morquio B Type VI–Maroteaux-Lamy Type VII–Sly Type VIII–DiFerranti	All except types IS (Scheie), IV and VI are associated with mental retardation. All except type IS (Scheie) and type III have skeletal changes, very severe in type IVA. All except type IS (Scheie) and types III and IV have hepatosplenomegaly and other soft tissue changes. Corneal clouding in all except type III and severe in type IS (Scheie)	Abnormal urine GAGs in all except type IVB. Skeletal survey for bony abnormalities. Precise diagnosis depends on measurement of specific enzymes in plasma, white cells or fibroblasts – see detailed references	Type IS, mild forms of type II and type IVA may have long lifespan. Early hyperactivity is characteristic of type III. Soft tissue changes and effects on internal organs are greatest for Type IH (Hurler) and severe forms of type II – large tongue, upper airway obstruction, deafness, cardiomyopathy, hernias, diarrhoea. Hydrocephalus may occur. Odontoid hypoplasia in type IV may require spinal fusion to prevent cord pressure. BMT lessens mental deterioration in type IH if performed early but enzyme replacement therapy (ERT) is now available for type IH, IS and II
Sphingolipidoses Gaucher disease	Type I presents with anaemia, thrombocytopenia, splenomegaly, bone pain and fractures and episodic fever at any age beyond early childhood. In Type II there is severe neurological deterioration in infancy because of central nervous system involvement and lung infiltrates	'Gaucher cells' in marrow. Deficient glucocerebrosidase enzyme	ERT now available, but ineffective in type II
Niemann–Pick disease	Hepatomegaly, splenomegaly, cholestasis, (see liver disease), feeding difficulties and neurological deterioration in infants – type A. Type B is in older children and adults with hepatosplenomegaly, high cholesterol, lung infiltrates	Sphingomyelinase deficiency in type A and B. Type C has mild splenomegaly, perhaps cholestasis in infancy, loss of upward gaze and cataplexy and is due to a disorder of intracellular cholesterol metabolism, with normal sphingomyelinase. Foamy cells in bone marrow in all. Type D occurs in Nova Scotia, enzyme defect unknown	Symptomatic only
Fabry disease	X-linked inheritance. Effects on autonomic ganglia cause disabling burning pain in hands and feet. Angiokeratomas of abdomen, buttocks. Later, cardiomyopathy and renal failure	α-Galactosidase deficiency	Renal transplantation, but ERT now available
Tay–Sachs disease and Sandhoff disease (GM2 gangliosidosis)	Presentation as infantile, juvenile and adult forms Infantile: hypotonia, large head, extreme startle to sound. Lack of progress, then loss of skills	'Cherry red spot' at the macula Tay–Sachs disease: absent hexosaminidase A Sandhoff disease: absent hexosaminidase B	None. In some populations, screening for Tay–Sachs disease heterozygotes may avoid carrier matings

(*Continued*)

	with visual and hearing loss and epilepsy; eventually decorticate. Hepatomegaly in Sandhoff disease, not Tay–Sachs.		
GM1 gangliosidosis (also galactosialidosis, with combined deficiency of β-galactosidase and neuraminidase as in sialidosis)	Coarse features and bone changes at birth, perhaps neonatal hydrops, hepatosplenomegaly, neurological deterioration in the 'generalized' form. Milder childhood or adult presentation possible	'Cherry red spot' at the macula Absent β-galactosidase (the same enzyme as Morquio B)	None
Metachromatic leucodystrophy (MLD) and Austin disease	Infantile, childhood and adult presentations. Infantile: delayed development, hypotonia, loss of speech, ataxia, optic atrophy, eventual quadriplegia. Juvenile form proceeds more slowly. Adult form: dementia, psychosis, ataxia	Deficient arylsulphatase A. (Austin disease is due to multiple sulphatase deficiencies and combines MLD with features of five of the MPS disorders and X-linked icthyosis)	None. Death before 10 years in the infantile form of MLD
Mucolipidoses Inclusion-cell disease Pseudo-Hurler polydystrophy	I-cell disease is very similar to Hurler's disease, but presents in the neonatal period, and has an even faster progression. Gum hyperplasia is very prominent. Pseudo-Hurler polydystrophy is like a mild variant of Hurler disease	Multiple hydrolases decreased in fibroblasts and leucocytes, but increased in plasma, due to failure to store these enzymes in the lysosomes. Storage material remains as inclusion bodies within lysosomes, visible microscopically. No urinary GAGs are excreted.	Death before 10 years in I-cell disease. Survival to early adult life in pseudo-Hurler polydystrophy. BMT has not been successful
Oligosaccharidoses Sialidosis Mannosidosis Fucosidosis Aspartylglycosaminuria	Mild variable coarse facial features, deafness and mild skeletal changes. Angiokeratomas of the skin of the abdomen, legs and perineum in fucosidosis. High sweat sodium in fucosidosis	Urinary oligosaccharides. Exact diagnosis depends on measurement of specific enzymes in plasma, white cells or fibroblasts – see detailed references	No specific treatment
Congenital disorders of glycosylation (CDG) Type I a-h Type II a-d and x	Large number of disorders, all very rare except type Ia, which causes variable developmental retardation, seizures, stroke-like episodes, cerebellar hypoplasia, cardiomyopathy, hypoplastic nipples, thick *peau d'orange* skin and fat pads over lateral buttocks Type Ib: diarrhoea, failure to thrive, without dysmorphism	Classified by plasma transferrin electrophoresis (abnormal in all type I and most type II), and by specific enzyme defects. Low antithrombin III and factor XI common in all. Should be considered in all delayed children, especially if dysmorphic, and with any evidence of other system disorders: failure to thrive, hepatic fibrosis, ataxia, neuropathy (Westphal *et al.*, 2000)	Only Type Ib has specific therapy: dramatic improvement with oral mannose, which permits normal protein glycosylation

GAG, glycosaminoglycan; BMT, bone marrow transplantation.

(approved by regulatory bodies for Gaucher disease, Fabry disease and Hurler disease, and at present subject to trial, in Hunter disease and Pompe disease but extremely expensive). The clinical presentation overlaps so much that a confident clinical diagnosis is often not possible. Biochemical complexity means that diagnosis is not easy and there are no simple screening tests. Some disorders share enzyme deficiencies, or have multiple deficiencies. Suspected cases must be discussed with the laboratories involved so that results are not misinterpreted or diagnoses missed.

The congenital disorders of glycosylation are disorders of the Golgi body and endoplasmic reticulum. Sugar residues are added to complex molecules variously forming cell surface markers and transport proteins. (These substances are eventually degraded in the lysosomes). There is a very complex family of these disorders, with widespread consequences (Tables 15.17 and 15.18) (Westphal *et al.*, 2000).

REFERENCES

Aynsley-Green A, Hussain K, Hall J, *et al.* (2000) Practical management of hyperinsulism in infancy. *Arch Dis Child Fetal Neonatal Ed* **82**:F98–F107.

Bartlett K (1983) Vitamin-responsive inborn errors of metabolism. *Adv Clin Chem* **23**:141–98.

Bonham JR (1993) The investigation of hypoglycaemia during childhood. *Ann Clin Biochem* **30**:238–47.

Chakrapani A, Cleary MA, Wraith JE (2001) Detection of inborn errors of metabolism in the newborn. *Arch Dis Child Fetal Neonatal Ed* **84**:F205–F210.

Nissenkorn A, Zeharia A, Lev D *et al.* (1999) Multiple presentation of mitochondrial disorders. *Arch Dis Child* **81**:209–14.

Ozand PT, Gascon GG (1991a) Organic acidurias: a review. Part 1. *J Child Neurol* **6**:196–219.

Ozand PT, Gascon GG (1991b) Organic acidurias: a review. Part 2. *J Child Neurol* **6**:288–303.

Rinaldo P, Matern D, Bennet MJ (2002) Fatty acid oxidation disorders. *Annu Rev Physiol* **64**:477–502.

Urea Cycle Disorders Conference Group (2001) Proceedings of a consensus conference for the management of patients with urea cycle disorders. *J Pediatr* **38**(suppl): S1–S80.

Westphal V, Srikrishna G, Freeze HH (2000) Congenital disorders of glycosylation: Have you encountered them? *Genet Med* **2**:329–37.

FURTHER READING AND USEFUL WEBSITES

Blau N, Duran M, Blaskovics M, Gibson KM (eds) (2002) *Physician's Guide to the Laboratory Diagnosis of Metabolic Diseases.* Heidelberg: Springer-Verlag.

Fernandes J, Saudubray J-M, van den Berghe G (eds) (2000) *Inborn Metabolic Diseases: Diagnosis and Treatment*, 3rd edn. Berlin: Springer-Verlag.

Scriver CR, Beaudet AL, Sly WS, Valle D, Vogelstein B, Childs B (eds) (2001) *The Metabolic and Molecular Bases of Inherited Disease*, 8th edn. New York: McGraw-Hill.

Detailed information about clinical features and the genetics of all the inherited metabolic diseases is available from the website of On-line Mendelian Inheritance in Man (OMIM) at www.ncbi.nlm.nih.gov/entrez/query.fcgi?db = OMIM (accessed 4 November 2004).

Links to this and many other sites, including information about laboratories undertaking specialized assays and parents' organizations, are available through the website of the Society for the Study of Inborn Errors of Metabolism at www.ssiem.org.uk (accessed 4 November 2004).

Chapter 16

Musculoskeletal and connective tissue disorders

Janet M Gardner-Medwin, Paul Galea and Roderick Duncan

BASIC KNOWLEDGE

DEVELOPMENT OF WALKING AND GAIT IN CHILDHOOD

Knowledge of the variation in the musculoskeletal system throughout childhood is fundamental to identifying deviations from normal (Figure 16.1). Proportions of the limbs and ranges of movement of the joints change throughout childhood. For example, healthy neonates have increased mobility at the ankles and wrists but more restricted movement at the elbows and knees compared with infants just a few months older. The tibia is normally bowed in neonates and infants compared to older children, giving a bow-legged appearance.

Children under 2 years normally have flat feet, with a broad-based gait and extended arms as walking starts. At age 3–4 years children's joints remain supple but the posture changes, and many will demonstrate flat feet, genu recurvatum, an exaggerated lumbar lordosis, and a knock-kneed appearance. Gait analysis has shown that there are many changes in the pattern of walking throughout the first seven years of life. Thereafter the pattern is broadly similar to that seen in adults. The adult musculature develops with the onset of puberty although adolescents remain more mobile, with greater ranges of movements

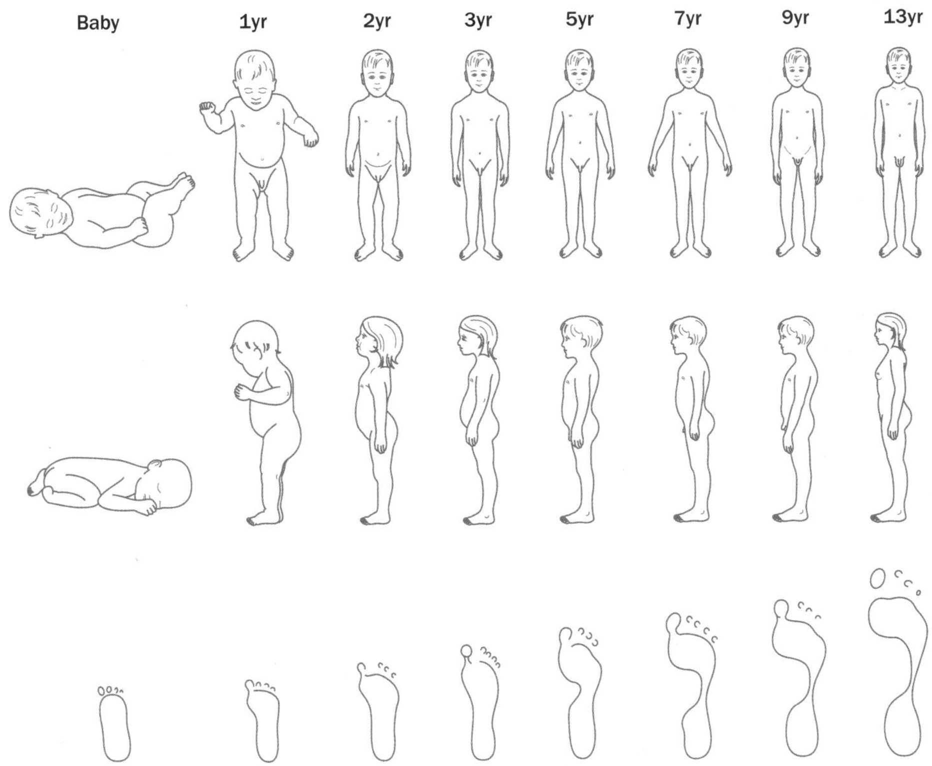

Figure 16.1 Changes in the normal musculoskeletal proportions, posture and footprints throughout childhood

than adults, particularly at the knees and elbows. Ethnic differences are important, with more hypermobility in the black population.

PATHOPHYSIOLOGY OF THE JOINT AND BONE GROWTH

Bones change in size, shape and structure throughout growth developing by ossification of pre-existing cartilage. Long bones consist of a shaft, the **diaphysis** and a proximal and distal **metaphysis**, the flared portion at the end of bone. Each of these is separated from the **epiphysis** by the growth plate or **physis**. Epiphyses start as cartilaginous structures, and gradually ossify, with one or more **secondary ossification centres** until the epiphyses and metaphyses fuse, marking the end of growth. Testosterone stimulates bone growth but eventually results in physeal fusion at the end of puberty. Thyroxine and growth hormone also stimulate bone growth. The local mechanical environment also has an effect on growth of the long bones and is largely responsible for the remodelling seen after fractures in children. Skeletal bone age can be estimated by the radiological stage of ossification of the bones and fusion of the **physes**, usually measured at the wrist.

Joints may be fibrous (sutures of the skull), cartilaginous (symphysis pubis) or synovial (most skeletal joints). In the synovial joint, bone is covered by hyaline cartilage, with synovium attaching to the cartilage enclosing the joint space. The synovium produces small quantities of synovial fluid that lubricates the joint and provides nutrition for the cartilage. Hyaline cartilage promotes frictionless motion and absorbs the shocks of weight bearing. In arthritis, the synovium becomes inflamed with increased synovial fluid production, increased cellularity and alteration of the cytokine milieu. This intra-articular environment is destructive to cartilage, and once the protective layer of cartilage is removed, the underlying bone is eroded.

Enthesitis

The point of insertion of tendon, ligament, fascia or capsule into bone is called the enthesis, and is an active metabolic site in childhood. It is prone to mechanical (plantar fasciitis or Achilles tendonitis), growth-related (e.g. Osgood–Schlatter disease and other osteochondritides) or inflammatory stress (as in human leucocyte antigen (HLA)-B27-related disease such as enthesitis-related arthritis). Point tenderness limited to the site of enthesis is characteristic (Figure 16.2).

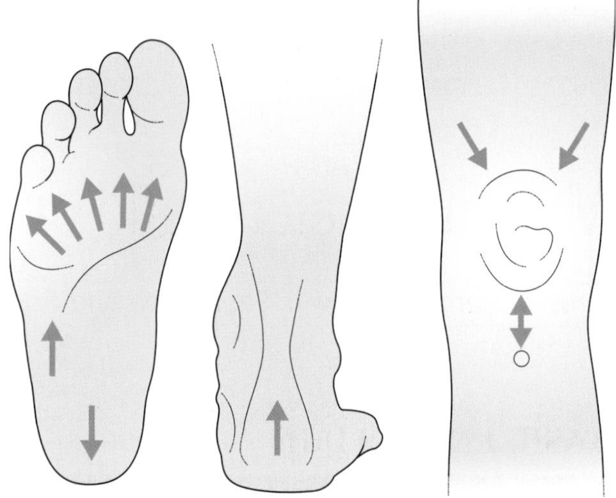

Figure 16.2 The points of insertion of the plantar fascia, the Achilles tendon, and tendons around the knee (enthesis)

INTERPRETATION OF RHEUMATOLOGICAL INVESTIGATIONS

There are no diagnostic tests in rheumatology, and diagnoses such as arthritis or systemic lupus erythematosus (SLE) are made by clinical history and examination supported by thoughtful interpretation of a few judicious investigations.

Autoantibodies

Antinuclear antibodies (ANA) are found in 5 per cent of healthy, normal children, and several autoimmune diseases, and other conditions, particularly infection (Table 16.1). The finding of a positive ANA is not a *specific* test for SLE, or juvenile idiopathic arthritis (JIA). However ANA is very *sensitive* for SLE, making the diagnosis of SLE in the absence of ANA exceedingly unlikely. Higher titres of ANA (>1:640) are more likely to be associated with autoimmune disease. Many laboratories report low titres of ANA as negative to avoid confusion (1:20 up to 1:80) because of their occurrence in the normal population.

Conversely, **antibodies to dsDNA** are very *specific* for SLE, in that they are not associated with other conditions. However, dsDNA is not very *sensitive* for SLE as only 50 per cent of children with SLE are dsDNA positive. They are more likely to be positive in sicker children with renal or cerebral involvement. The antibodies reflect disease activity and may disappear with improved disease management. Therefore, many children with SLE

Table 16.1 Causes of positive antinuclear antibody (ANA)

Rheumatic disease	Systemic lupus erythematosus Dermatomyositis Sjögren syndrome Scleroderma Vasculitis Juvenile idiopathic arthritis
Drug-induced	Carbamazepine Isoniazid Sulfasalazine Chlorpromazine
Hepatic disease	Autoimmune hepatitis Primary biliary cirrhosis
Pulmonary disease	Idiopathic pulmonary fibrosis Primary pulmonary hypertension
Infections	Chronic infections Transiently with acute infections
Malignancy	Lymphoma Leukaemias Solid tumours
Haematological	Idiopathic thrombocytopenic purpura Autoimmune haemolytic anaemia
Others	Endocrine disease, e.g. diabetes mellitus Endstage renal failure After organ transplantation
Normal, healthy individuals	

are dsDNA negative, particularly those in whom the diagnosis of SLE is less obvious.

Rheumatoid factors (RFs) are a group of autoantibodies produced in response to an inflammatory stimulus. They may be transiently positive following infection. They are present in about 5 per cent of children with JIA. These tend to be girls over 10 years of age who have a severe form of the disease similar to adult rheumatoid arthritis, with rheumatoid nodules, an aggressive, erosive, symmetrical small and large joint arthritis. The significance of a positive RF without this supporting clinical picture is less clear.

HLA-B27

Human leucocyte antigen B27 is one of the histocompatibility antigens found in 10 per cent of the population. Its presence does not establish a diagnosis, but is strongly associated with clinical diagnoses of psoriatic arthropathy (20 per cent), enthesitis related arthritis (95 per cent), inflammatory bowel disease (50 per cent), Reiter syndrome (80 per cent), or anterior uveitis (50 per cent).

Full blood count, erythrocyte sedimentation rate and C-reactive protein

Skilful interpretation of the full blood count including the differential count in children can be very valuable. In a child with presumed inflammatory arthritis features such as a raised white cell count and platelet count are expected to be in proportion to the acute phase response. Erythrocyte sedimentation rate (ESR) and C-reactive protein (CRP) may be normal in a child with significant inflammation, for example in a child with an oligoarthritis, and importantly do not rule out bone and joint sepsis. A low or normal platelet count should raise suspicion that marrow infiltration, and a diagnosis such as acute lymphoblastic leukaemia (ALL) is the underlying cause of arthritis, and a bone marrow biopsy should be taken. A persistently low lymphocyte count is also a feature of SLE. The erythrocyte sedimentation rate and C-reactive protein are non-specific markers of inflammation, but can help in supporting diagnoses such as in SLE where the ESR is raised with a normal CRP. A rising CRP in SLE should alert the clinician to possible intercurrent infection.

MUSCULOSKELETAL IMAGING

Plain radiographs

Plain radiographs are the most valuable investigation in children with bone pain, or following trauma. It is essential to interpret the radiographs with knowledge of the clinical history and particularly the examination findings. The presence of secondary ossification centres, growth plates and the wide variation in the appearance of radiographs in the normal child makes an experienced paediatric radiologist invaluable.

Radiographs are not a valuable investigation to diagnose JIA. A child with a short history of joint swelling will have no specific features diagnostic for JIA on a plain radiograph, which will just confirm the clinically apparent effusion and soft tissue swelling. The value of a radiograph in a child with new joint swelling is to exclude diagnoses other than JIA, or as a baseline for monitoring disease progression. Diagnoses such as the metaphyseal fractures of non-accidental injury (Figure 16.3), the metaphyseal lucencies of ALL (Figure 16.4), or bony tumours (Figure 16.5) may be identified. Late in the course of the JIA, radiographic features of disease damage, such as loss of joint space (reflecting cartilage loss) and bony erosions, become apparent.

Technetium-MDP bone scan

This short-acting radioactive isotope is actively taken up by bone and especially around the physes. It highlights areas of increased osteoblastic activity as caused by inflammation, infection and tumours, but is non-specific. In conditions with variable osteoblastic activity such as leukaemia it may be unreliable. One of the problems frequently encountered in children is that the musculoskeletal pathology is often situated around the joint or the metaphyses. The high uptake of radioisotope by the growth plates can obscure subtle abnormalities, and in many situations magnetic resonance imaging (MRI) is the preferred imaging modality.

Magnetic resonance imaging

Magnetic resonance imaging with gadolinium contrast is becoming the standard imaging modality, after plain radiographs, in children with suspected musculoskeletal problems. With modern machines the anatomical detail is vastly superior to computed tomography (CT). The accurate interpretation of images relies on accurate clinical information and they must be read in conjunction with plain films. Certain bone lesions, for example, are more reliably diagnosed on radiographs. MRI with gadolinium contrast gives detailed pictures of the joint, long before radiographic abnormalities appear. It can show articular cartilage, fluid and soft tissue structures of the joint, identifying altered signal, thinning, erosions and deep cartilage loss. Earliest features, such as synovitis, can be directly imaged supporting therapeutic intervention earlier in the disease course. Magnetic resonance imaging is useful in the clinically atypical joint to identify mimics of synovitis such as haemangiomas, inflammatory muscle disease and pigmented villonodular synovitis (PVNS).

KEY LEARNING POINTS

- There are no diagnostic tests in rheumatology, and diagnoses such as arthritis or SLE are made by accurate clinical history and examination

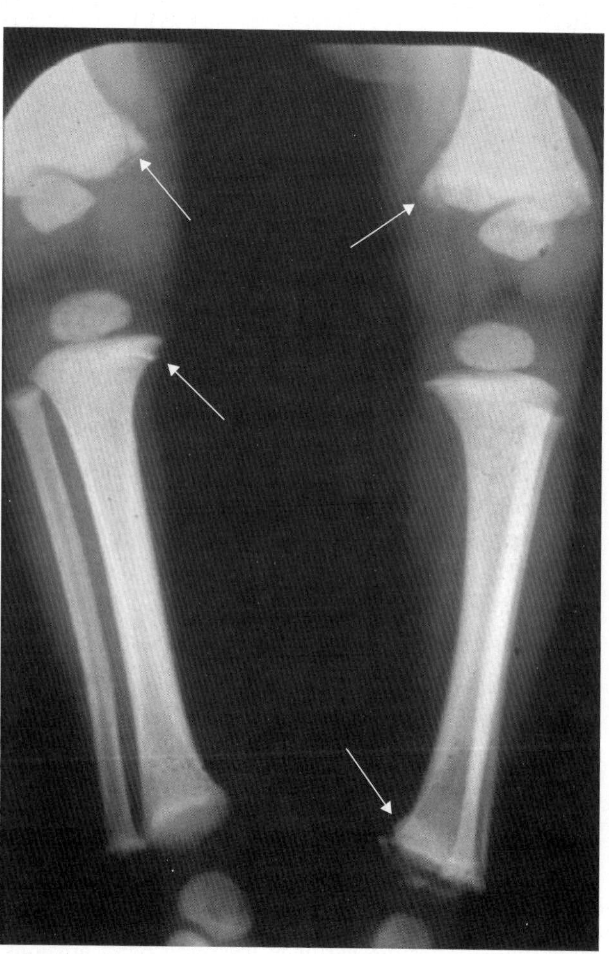

Figure 16.3 Metaphyseal fractures of non-accidental injury

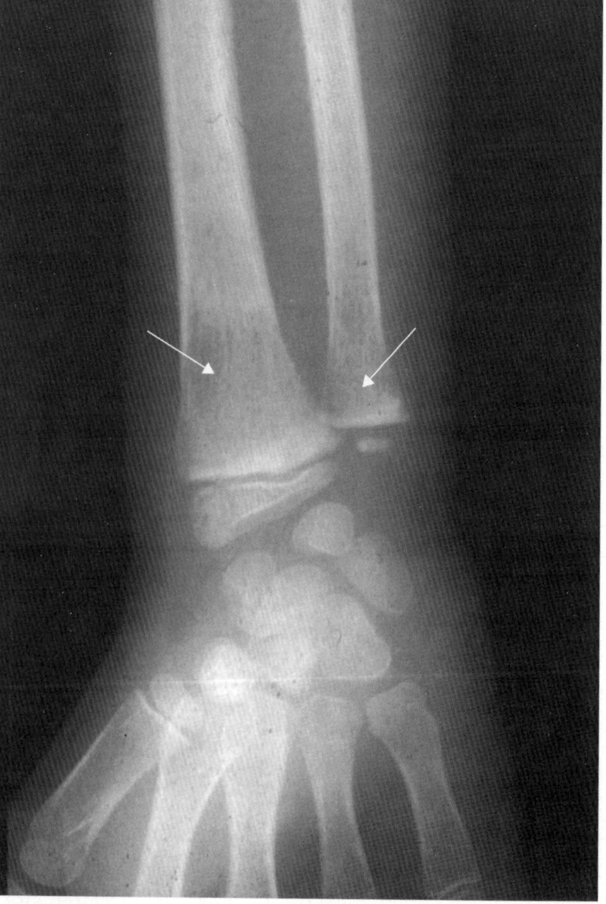

Figure 16.4 Metaphyseal lucency in acute lymphoblastic leukaemia

supported by thoughtful interpretation of a few judicious investigations.

- Enthesitis is common in children, and easily identified by point tenderness at the critical sites.
- The ANA is not specific for SLE or JIA, and is found in lower titres in healthy children.
- Rheumatoid factor is a non-specific test. The clinical features are critical to making the diagnosis.
- A normal full blood count in the face of an unwell child and a significant acute phase response should raise the possibility of marrow infiltration.
- A radiograph is an inappropriate investigation to diagnose arthritis, septic arthritis or osteomyelitis early in the disease process. It is of value in many other musculoskeletal pathologies.
- An MR image interpreted by a paediatric radiologist is valuable in imaging the musculoskeletal system.

CORE SYSTEM PROBLEMS

Musculoskeletal pain and other problems are common during childhood, occurring in 4–30 per cent of children and encompass common benign conditions from hypermobility and nocturnal idiopathic pain, to life-threatening conditions such as non-accidental injury and

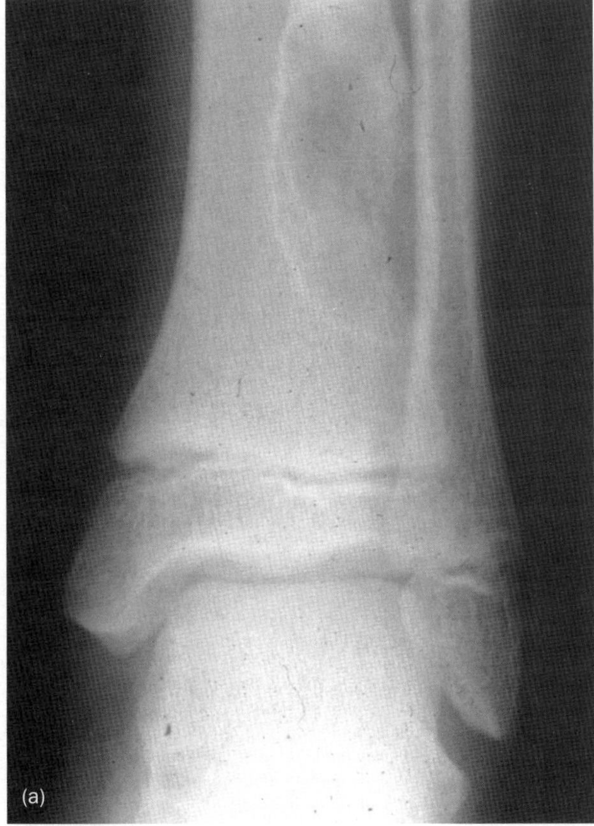

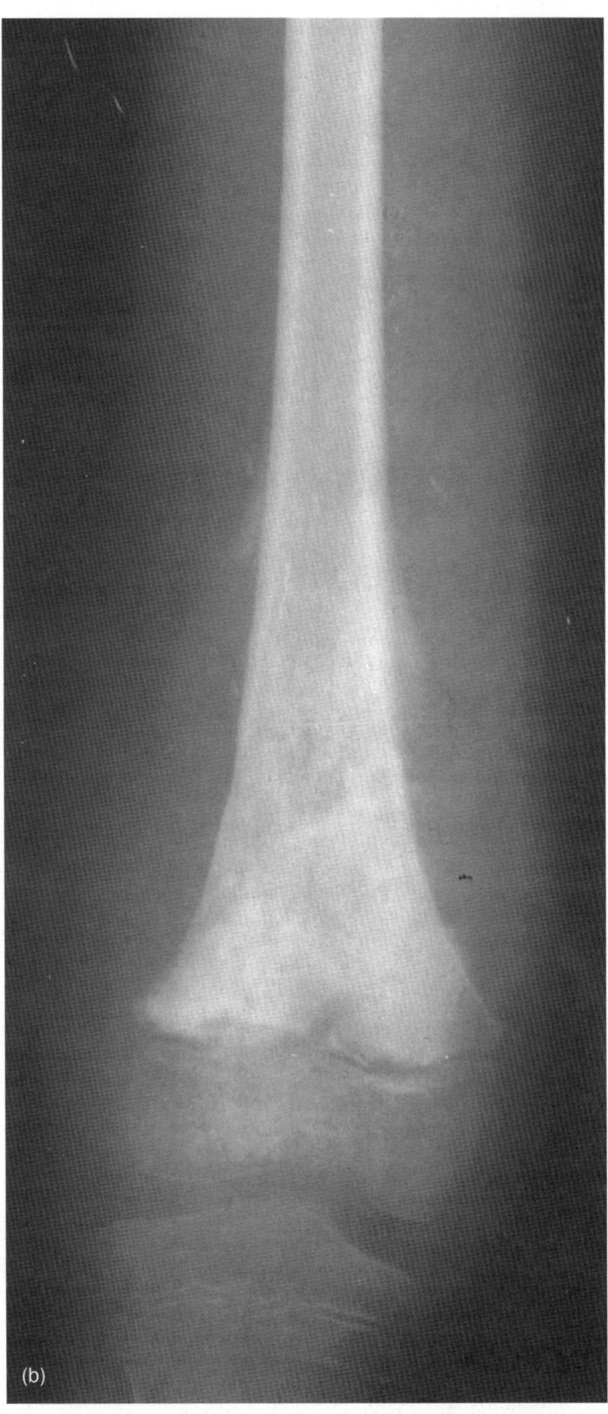

Figure 16.5 Non-ossifying fibroma and osteosarcoma. These figures show the typical radiographic appearances of a benign non-ossifying fibroma (NOF) (a) and a malignant bone tumour (osteosarcoma). (b) The NOF presents as a well-circumscribed area of bone destruction with a sclerotic margin. There is no breach in the cortex, periosteal reaction or a soft tissue mass. The osteosarcoma radiograph shows a poorly defined lesion with a large soft tissue mass and a periosteal reaction

Table 16.2 The new classification of juvenile arthritis, clinical features, and comparison with old classifications and adult disease

Characteristic	JIA	Clinical features*	JRA (USA)	JCA (Europe)	Adult equivalent
Age at onset	<16 years		<16 years	<16 years	
Minimum duration of arthritis	6 weeks		6 weeks	3 months	
Subtypes	Systemic arthritis	Systemic manifestations often precede arthritis: evening spikes of fever dipping to subnormal in the mornings; evanescent salmon-coloured rash on the trunk, axillae and inner thighs most marked at the height of the fever; lymphadenopathy, splenomegaly, serositis and pallor. An aggressive polyarticular arthritis can develop and is associated with a worse prognosis	Systemic onset JRA	Systemic onset JCA	Adult Still disease
	Oligoarthritis	Arthritis in up to four joints. This pattern of arthritis has the strongest association with uveitis, particularly in ANA-positive girls	Pauciarticular JRA	Pauciarticular JCA	-
	Persistent	Continues to involve < 4 joints throughout the disease course			
	Extended	Affects more than four joints after the first six months and is associated with a worse prognosis than persistent oligoarthritis			
	Polyarthritis (RF-negative)	Affects five or more joints in first six months of disease. Tests for RF are repeatedly negative	Polyarticular JRA *(RF does not alter classification)*	Polyarticular JCA	-
	Polyarthritis (RF-positive)	Affects five or more joints in first six months of disease. Tests for RF are positive on two occasions at least two months apart		Juvenile rheumatoid arthritis (JRA)	Rheumatoid arthritis
	Enthesitis-related arthritis	Boys > 8 years old, HLA-B27 positive, or family history of HLA-B27-associated disease. Asymmetrical large joints arthritis of the lower limbs, enthesitis in the feet, knees and pelvic girdle. Lumbosacral spine and sacroiliac involvement rare in childhood, but may develop ankylosing spondylitis as older teenagers/adults	Excluded	Juvenile spondyloarthropathies (including juvenile ankylosing spondylitis, juvenile psoriatic arthritis, Reiter syndrome and arthropathies of inflammatory bowel disease)	Ankylosing spondylitis
	Psoriatic arthritis	Arthritis and psoriasis may occur together. In the absence of psoriasis, a family history or nail features of psoriasis such as nail pitting may be found. The asymmetrical arthritis typical involves large and small joints (e.g. dactylitis)	Excluded		Psoriatic arthritis
	Other	Arthritis that either does not fulfil criteria for any category or fulfils criteria for more than one category. It is hoped new disease groups will emerge from this category	-	-	-

* See Figure 16.5 for pattern of arthritis.
ANA, antinuclear antibody; HLA, human leucocyte antigen; JCA, juvenile chronic arthritis; JIA, juvenile idiopathic arthritis; JRA, juvenile rheumatoid arthritis; RF, rheumatoid factor.

malignancy. Clinical history and examination, supported by a comprehensive knowledge of the normal childhood musculoskeletal system and by the judicious use of a few appropriate investigations, remain the mainstay of diagnosis.

INFLAMMATORY

Juvenile idiopathic arthritis

CASE STUDY

A 3-year-old girl developed a limp several weeks after an upper respiratory infection. This was attributed to an irritable hip, but did not resolve. She had difficulty getting out of bed, and had a wet bed most mornings, but was reported as playing happily in nursery most afternoons although the limp persisted. Her right knee was swollen with an effusion, fixed in 15° of flexion, and despite the flexion the right leg was 1 cm longer than the left when standing. There was marked muscle wasting of the medial quadriceps muscle just above that knee. Slit lamp examination revealed inflammatory cells in the anterior chamber of the eye. Diagnosis: JIA, oligoarthritis.

The classification of juvenile arthritis has been complicated by transatlantic differences in nomenclature, being defined as juvenile chronic arthritis (JCA) (European) or juvenile rheumatoid arthritis (JRA) (America and Canada). A new classification, juvenile idiopathic arthritis, aims to unify these previous classifications, facilitate research, and further understanding of these diseases (Table 16.2).

Aetiology and epidemiology

The aetiology/ies of JIA remain elusive. A genetic predisposition has been suggested through the HLA associations. The prevalence is 30–150 per 100 000 children and incidence of JIA is 5–18 per 100 000, a similar incidence to childhood diabetes.

Clinical manifestations

Arthritis presents with **persistent** joint swelling. There may be associated stiffness typically early morning and after periods of immobility (gelling) which is often more prominent than pain.

The involved joints are swollen. The range of movements may be variably limited, as may the degree of warmth and erythema. Disuse atrophy affecting the surrounding muscles, and in younger children limb length discrepancies, may be apparent. Systemic upset, particularly tiredness and lethargy, may be underestimated. The pattern of joint involvement may help to identify the subgroup of JIA (Figure 16.6).

Differential diagnosis

Juvenile idiopathic arthritis remains a clinical diagnosis. Investigation aims at the exclusion of other diagnoses and establishing baseline measurement for assessing the outcome of JIA. Arthritis in childhood has a wide and important age-dependent differential diagnosis.

Differential diagnosis of arthritis in children

Inflammatory

Juvenile idiopathic arthritis
Inflammatory disease: inflammatory bowel disease, sarcoid, cystic fibrosis, autoimmune hepatitis
Haematological malignancies: leukaemia, lymphoma
Malignancy: neuroblastoma
Reactive: post-streptococcal, rheumatic fever, post-enteric, post-viral
Infection: septic arthritis, osteomyelitis, tuberculosis, Lyme arthritis
Irritable hip, discitis
Systemic disease: SLE, vasculitis (Kawasaki disease, Henoch–Schönlein purpura, rarer systemic vasculitides), juvenile dermatomyositis, scleroderma
Down's arthritis

Mechanical

Osgood–Schlatter disease and other eponymous osteochondritides
Chondromalacia patellae
Scheuermann disease
Hypermobility, pes planus
Growing pains (nocturnal idiopathic pain syndrome)
Inherited: skeletal dysplasias, congenital dislocation of the hip
Collagen disorders: e.g. Ehlers–Danlos, Marfan, Stickler syndromes
Storage disorders e.g. mucopolysaccharidoses/lipidoses
Avascular necrosis and other degenerative disorders: Perthes', slipped upper femoral epiphysis, idiopathic chondrolysis, spondylolysis and listhesis

Trauma: accidental and non-accidental injury
Haematological: haemophilia and haemoglobinopathy (sickle predominantly)
Metabolic: rickets, hypophosphataemic rickets, hypo/hyperthyroidism, diabetes, purine metabolism

Tumours of cartilage bone or muscle

Benign: osteoid osteoma, pigmented villonodular synovitis, haemangioma
Malignant: synovial sarcoma, osteosarcoma, rhabdomyosarcoma, Ewing tumour

Psychological

Idiopathic pain syndromes
Local, e.g. reflex sympathetic dystrophy
Generalized, e.g. fibromyalgia

Management of juvenile idiopathic arthritis

Management of children with JIA requires a multidisciplinary approach, the early introduction of

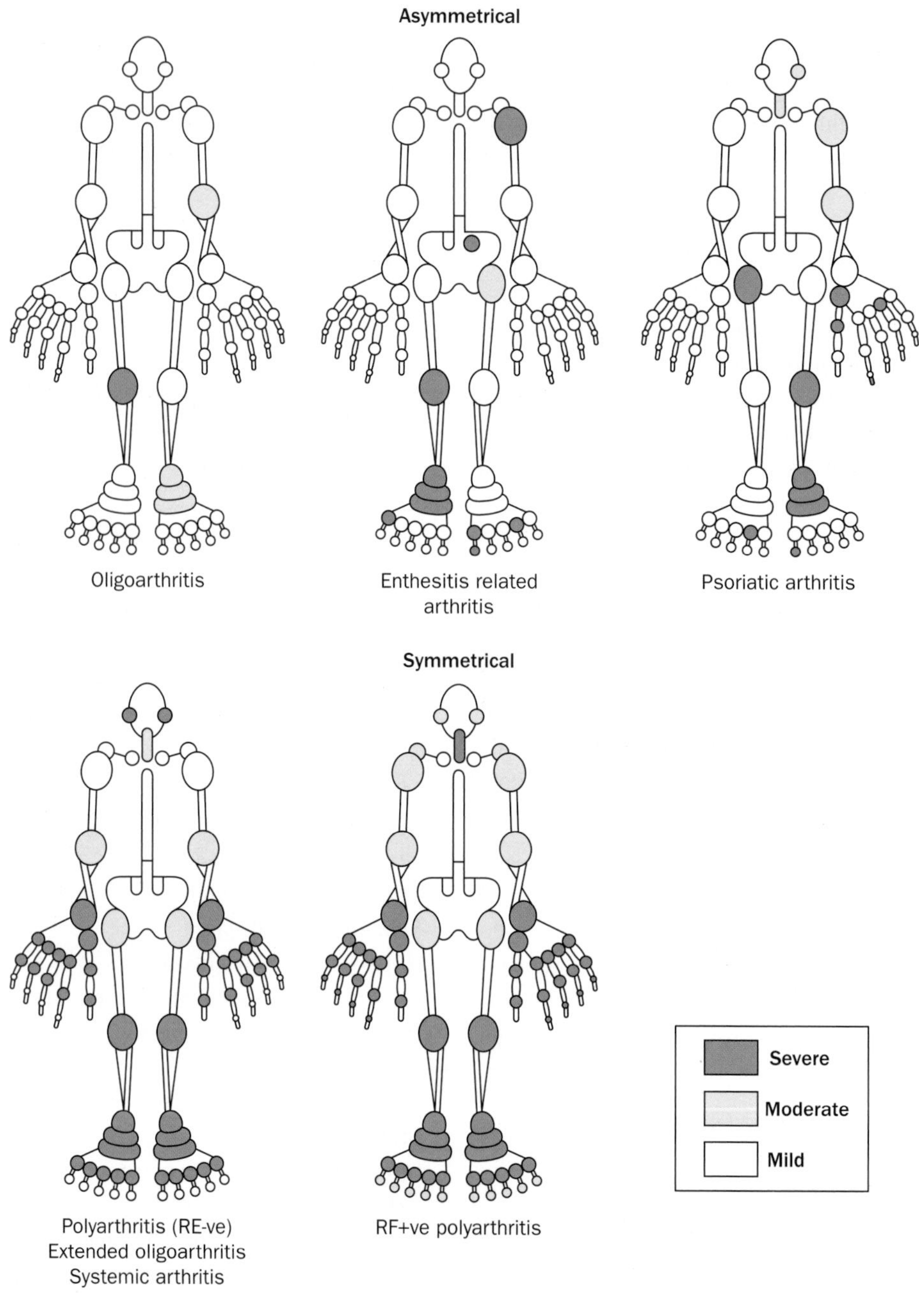

Figure 16.6 Pattern of joint involvement in different types of juvenile idiopathic arthritis

treatment to prevent damage, and meticulous clinical monitoring.

Multidisciplinary management

The primary aim of treatment is the preservation of joint function and vision. Children with arthritis require a multidisciplinary team approach addressing the ongoing school needs, activities of daily living, physical and mental growth, and the transitional needs of adolescence. A central, ongoing programme of disease management and education for the child, parents, school, and involved professionals should support these aims. The impact of chronic disease, pain, and real or perceived abnormalities of body habitus have a major impact on the social and psychological development of children with arthritis. Disease management must address these issues from an early age if these children are to achieve their full potential as individuals with autonomy, adult relationships, independence, and a vocation.

Drug therapy

ARTHRITIS

Non-steroidal anti-inflammatory drugs (NSAIDs) and steroid joint injections are the mainstays of drug treatment in the child with oligoarthritis. Septic arthritis should always be excluded in any child with a monoarthritis. For most children, no further joints become involved, and this pattern of arthritis is associated with a good prognosis, although these children remain at significant risk of uveitis. For polyarthritis of all types early introduction of methotrexate and rapid disease control using steroids (intra-articular, intravenous or occasionally oral) is the treatment of choice. Subcutaneous methotrexate has improved efficacy and is widely used in children. Sulfasalazine is useful in the management of children with enthesitis-related arthritis and arthritis associated with inflammatory bowel disease. The mainstay of treatment for systemic involvement remains steroid therapy, either oral or intravenous, as pulsed methylprednisolone. Biological agents (antitumour necrosis factor (anti-TNF) agents), and autologous bone marrow transplantation are emerging as new therapies for those with the most resistant disease.

GROWTH

Arthritis has a major impact on the growing skeleton. Growth and bone mass are markedly reduced by persistent inflammation, immobility and use of corticosteroids. Growth hormone in these children has had limited success, but may be warranted in the most severe cases. Inflammatory arthritis accelerates bone growth resulting in elongated limb length and bony overgrowth around the joint, and advanced bone age. Radiographic estimation of bone-age is of no value in a child with wrist arthritis. Early fusion of the growth plate resulting from inflammation eventually results in a shortened limb on the affected side. Arthritis causes the temporomandibular joint to fuse early, producing micrognathia and overbite, or asymmetrical jaw opening following unilateral arthritis. The promotion of a balanced diet is important as up to 50 per cent of children with JIA have protein-energy malnutrition because of increased energy expenditure.

UVEITIS

Chronic anterior uveitis is a cause of significant morbidity in JIA, with asymptomatic, progressive loss of vision, most commonly in the youngest children. The prognosis for vision is generally good if it is identified and treated early. Three to six monthly slit-lamp ophthalmoscopy screening is mandatory for all children with JIA until the child is old enough to recognize subtle painless changes in vision (accepted as 12 years old), or until joint disease has been quiescent for at least seven years. Children with a positive ANA and an oligoarticular course are at the greatest risk of uveitis (30 per cent incidence). It must not be forgotten that other groups of JIA carry a 10 per cent risk.

KEY LEARNING POINTS

- Arthritis is characterized by persistent joint swelling.
- Juvenile idiopathic arthritis is a clinical diagnosis, with no diagnostic tests.
- Transient joint swelling in children is likely to be associated with conditions such as hypermobility.
- Juvenile idiopathic arthritis is an umbrella term for a group of diseases. It is not adult rheumatoid arthritis. Only 5 per cent of children are RF-positive and have a disease similar to adult rheumatoid arthritis.
- Treatment aims at the rapid suppression of disease activity, preserving vision and joint structure, and return to full function.
- Multidisciplinary management and patient and parent education are critical to outcome.

Malignancy

CASE STUDY

A 10-year-old boy developed a widespread polyarthritis with effusions in his knees, wrists, and fingers. His joints were exquisitely tender to touch but particularly over the metaphyses. He had lost weight, and had an ESR 120 mm/h, Hb 10.2 g/dL, WCC 2.4×10^9/L, neutrophils 1.5×10^9/L, lymphocytes 0.9×10^9/L, platelet count 300×10^9/L. Diagnosis: Acute lymphoblastic leukaemia, and associated arthritis.

Musculoskeletal features are reported in 11–50 per cent of haematological malignancies, and 15–25 per cent of neuroblastomas at presentation. Bone tumours in children are rare, but are often diagnosed late, significantly affecting the prognosis. Malignancy should be considered in every child with a musculoskeletal presentation.

Haematological malignancies

Lymphomas and particularly leukaemia may present with musculoskeletal features, usually an oligoarthritis, which most commonly affects the knee and may be clinically indistinguishable from JIA. Pain may be localized over the metaphyses or may be non-specific (see Figure 16.4). Bone pain may be confused with that of arthritis. A high index of suspicion is required. An ESR that is raised out of proportion to the arthritis, or a platelet count or white count that are low or normal should raise concern. Blast cells are not necessarily found on the blood film. Where doubt exists, a bone marrow biopsy should be performed.

Neuroblastoma

Neuroblastoma is the commonest tumour causing bony metastases in childhood, presenting with musculoskeletal pain in a third of cases. There may be accompanying fever, misery and occasionally rash and joint swelling which mimic systemic arthritis. A high index of suspicion must be maintained. Bone scintigraphy should be done and bone marrow aspirate and urinary catecholamines tested.

Bone tumours

Bone tumours are uncommon in childhood, but often diagnosed late. Malignant bone tumours seen in childhood are very aggressive and early diagnosis is essential. The vast majority, however are benign. A bone tumour should never be considered benign without seeking an expert opinion.

Bone tumours (Table 16.3) may present with bone pain, a mass, a pathological fracture or as an incidental finding. The pain may be worse when straining or at night, persistent, aching, or boring in nature. However, the pain

Table 16.3 Commonest bone tumours of childhood

Lesion	Presentation	Natural history	Management
Simple bone cyst	Geographic area of bone destruction often an incidental finding in the proximal humerus or femur or as a pathological fracture	Can act as a stress riser which predisposes to pathological fracture	Observation, local steroid injection
Fibrous cortical defect	Incidental finding around the knee or ankle	Resolves with time	Observation
Osteochondroma	Cartilage-capped exostosis presents as a mass, usually around the knee	May remain symptomatic, growth stops at skeletal maturity	Excision if doubt regarding the diagnosis or if symptoms warrant
Langerhans cell histiocytosis	Either as solitary or multiple bone lesions Diabetes insipidus and systemic involvement seen in Letterer-Siwe and Hand-Schüller-Christian diseases	Systemic involvement must be sought	Multidisciplinary, with treatment according to degree of involvement. Bone lesions often heal after biopsy
Fibrous dysplasia	May affect one or more bones and may present as McCune-Albright syndrome	Variable, with progressive deformity in more severely affected cases	Surgical excision or stabilization where necessary
Ewing tumour	May be systemically unwell with bone pain and a mass	A highly malignant tumour which metastasizes to lungs and to bone marrow	Neoadjuvant chemotherapy and surgical resection where feasible
Osteosarcoma	Bone pain, mass or pathological fracture	A highly malignant sarcoma which metastasizes to lungs	Neoadjuvant chemotherapy and surgical resection

is not usually very specific, and therefore its significance may be missed. It is essential to exclude a bone tumour with a radiograph in cases where bone pain attributed to injury does not improve as expected, or is more severe than the history of trauma would suggest (see Figure 16.5). Most young adults presenting with a malignant bone tumour have been found to have a mass at presentation, which emphasizes the need for careful clinical examination. If they are located near a joint they may cause an effusion. Weight loss, fever, anaemia and a raised ESR may be present. Radiographs may be diagnostic, but bone scintigraphy may help identify small tumours, which are difficult to demonstrate on plain radiographs. Bone tumours are best managed by clinicians who specialize in this area. A multidisciplinary team from oncology, orthopaedics, pathology and radiology must manage malignant tumours. They should have access to a full range of support services.

Bone and joint infection

The clinical picture of bone and joint infection has changed dramatically in the past 50 years. In the developing world, however, the situation remains static with bone and joint infection causing considerable impairment and disability. Tuberculosis remains a major health problem in areas where human immunodeficiency virus (HIV) is endemic, and is increasing again in Europe and North America where drug resistance is a new problem. *Haemophilus influenzae* septic arthritis is less common in areas where vaccination programmes are successful.

Septic arthritis

Septic arthritis is a surgical emergency. Changes in articular cartilage composition can be observed within hours of inoculation. The commonest infecting organisms are *Streptococcus aureus* and *S. pyogenes* (see Table 16.4). Children are systemically unwell with fever and headache, and may have other foci of infection (septicaemia, meningitis, pharyngitis). Classically the joint is exquisitely painful, held immobile (pseudoparalysis), hot, swollen, and red. The child resists passive movements and is unwilling to weight bear on the infected joint. There may be associated bone pain from osteomyelitis. Differentiating septic arthritis from transient synovitis of the hip can be problematic. The diagnosis of septic arthritis of the hip will be correct in 99 per cent of cases if the following are present:

- pyrexia above 38.5°C within the past week
- inability to weight bear
- a raised ESR above 40 mm/h
- WBC greater than 12×10^9/L.

Diagnosis is made by urgent aspiration of the joint (under general anaesthetic), immediate Gram stain, and subsequent culture of synovial fluid. The prognosis is improved when an organism is identified (see Table 16.4), and every attempt to get cultures before antibiotics should be made. Blood cultures may less reliably identify the organism. Radiographs are not valuable at acute presentation, confirming only non-specific clinical features such as effusion and soft tissue swelling. They are useful later to document the damage caused by septic arthritis, including loss of joint space, erosions and ankylosis.

Osteomyelitis

The incidence of acute haematogenous osteomyelitis is declining in European populations. The reasons are unclear, but may relate to bacterial, host or environmental factors. Previously the classical presentation was an acutely ill child with a pyrexia, local erythema and tenderness. Now it is much more common for it to present in a subacute manner. Osteomyelitis can occur in association with septic arthritis. Acute osteomyelitis is usually caused by *S. aureus*, or group A streptococcus, but any of the organisms which cause a septic arthritis may be involved (see Table 16.4). A history of recent varicella zoster infection is not unusual. Osteomyelitis in children usually involves the metaphysis, and may be associated with a bland effusion of the adjacent joint (Figure 16.7). There is point tenderness at the site of infection, often night pain, and a limp. Pyrexia is often absent. Radiographs early in the course of the disease are usually normal, and bone scans are more sensitive early in the disease course. Where radiographic change occurs, a geographic or motheaten pattern of bone destruction and a periosteal reaction are typical (see Figure 16.7). Identification of the causative organism tends to be associated with an improved outcome. Management is with blood cultures, bone aspiration, a prolonged course of high-dose intravenous antistaphylococcal antibiotics (e.g. 100 mg/kg per day flucloxacillin intravenous in four divided doses) and cast immobilization.

Tuberculosis

Tuberculosis, once rare outside developing countries, is rising in incidence, and drug resistant strains are increasingly encountered. Bone and joint tuberculosis is usually secondary to infection elsewhere, most commonly pulmonary. It has an insidious onset and can present as a septic arthritis, osteitis or as a vertebral osteitis. Treatment is with antituberculous therapy, and surgery may be required later. Diagnosis can be made quickly with polymerase chain reaction (PCR), while culture results over six weeks are required for drug sensitivities. A reactive arthritis, Poncet disease, is recognized with tuberculosis.

Table 16.4 Organisms associated with septic and reactive arthritis

Organisms/disease	Septic arthritis/Osteomyelitis	Reactive arthritis
Staphylococcus aureus *Haemophilus influenzae* *Streptococcus pneumoniae*	Commonest organisms in all ages (HIB vaccination associated with a falling incidence of haemophilus)	*Streptococcus*: acute rheumatic fever (painful, migratory arthritis) or post-streptococcal arthritis (large joints especially knee with bland persistent effusions)
Enterococcus *Candida* spp. Group B streptococcus *Staphylococcus epidermidis*	Neonates susceptible to different organisms, may present with sepsis, but few systemic features may be observed initially. Tends to be diagnosed late in the neonate, with an associated poorer outcome	
Gonococcus	Sexually active adolescents and in neonates (vertical transmission). Typical vesicopustular rash, systemic features such as fever may occur	
Shigella flexneri *Salmonella spp.* *Yersinia enterocolitica* *Campylobacter jejuni* *Clostridium difficile*	*Salmonella* spp. associated with sickle cell disease	Fever, diarrhoea and abdominal cramps followed by an oligoarthritis starting 1–3 weeks later and lasting weeks to months. Yersinia can be associated with uveitis, conjunctivitis and myocarditis. Reiter syndrome (arthritis, conjunctivitis, oral and genital ulceration and severe dysuria) is associated with enteric or genitourinary infections
Lyme's arthritis	Infection caused by a spirochete (*Borrelia burgdorferi*) which is a tick-borne disease causing a typical rash, erythema chronicum migrans, episodic arthritis, meningitis, encephalitis and uveitis. Late features if untreated include a chronic arthritis and severe neurological involvement (encephalomyelitis, polyradiculopathy)	
Tuberculosis	Increasing frequency. Causes a chronic monoarthritis, indolent presentation, extremely destructive. Pott disease (vertebral osteomyelitis). Synovial fluid should be sent for Ziehl–Neelsen stain, and culture	Poncet disease – a reactive arthritis in response to tuberculosis

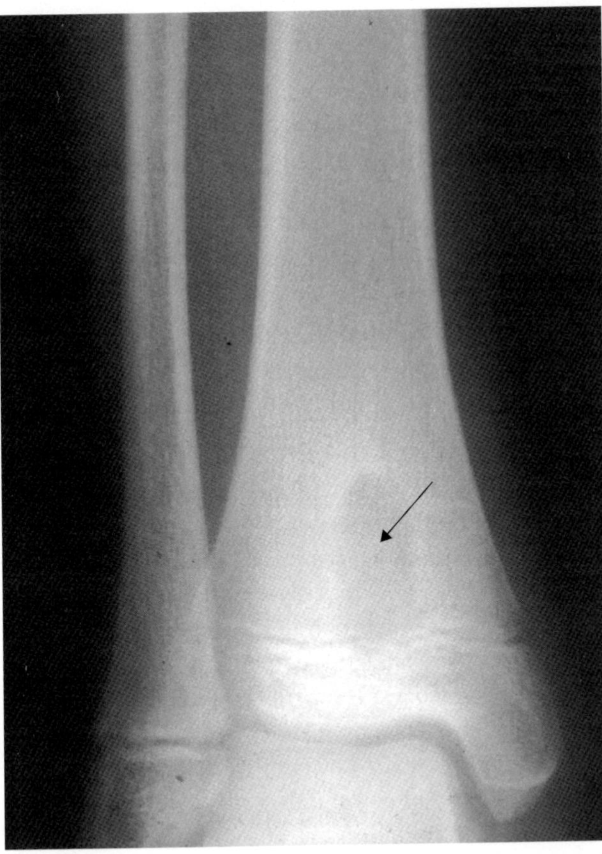

Figure 16.7 Osteomyelitis (Brodie abscess) in a child with unfused growth plates (arrow)

Reactive arthritis/Reiter syndrome/ post-enteric arthritis

Reactive arthritis is triggered by infectious agents outside the joints. Table 16.4 outlines the common organisms. Specific constellations of features such as rheumatic fever (streptococcus) or Reiter syndrome (post-enteric or genitourinary) are recognized. Reactive illness usually settles over a number of weeks but may take up to three months or longer. Full recovery is expected but reinfection may trigger further illness. Treatment with anti-inflammatory drugs reduces inflammation and controls pain. Appropriate therapy to clear residual organisms is required. Early antibiotic therapy for the treatment of enteric bowel infection has not been shown to have any benefit on the duration of manifestations of reactive arthritis. Rheumatic fever requires particular treatment and is discussed in Chapter 9 (page 302).

Reiter syndrome is a post-infectious or reactive condition consisting of the triad of urethritis, arthritis, and conjunctivitis. Most commonly, it is associated with *Shigella*, *Salmonella* or *Yersinia* dysentery, but the possibility of sexually acquired infection, particularly *Chlamydia*, should not be overlooked in older boys. Reiter syndrome is associated with HLA-B27, and the predominance in boys, the pattern of both the arthritis and eye involvement, and the association with enthesitis and keratoderma blennorrhagicum are similar to enthesitis-related arthritis, raising aetiological questions about both conditions. Reiter syndrome is a self-limiting illness in most children.

Post-viral infection

TRANSIENT SYNOVITIS

Transient synovitis of the hip (irritable hip) is an idiopathic disorder often preceded by infection. Children between the ages of 3 and 10 years develop a sudden or gradual onset of pain in the hip associated with limping. The hip is held in a position of maximum comfort: flexed and externally rotated. Internal rotation increases the pressure within the hip joint. It is painful and resisted. The pain may be referred to the knee. Hip ultrasound usually confirms an effusion. Radiographs may be normal, or less often show the effusion. The ESR and white count are normal, or occasionally mildly raised and are not usually helpful in management. Where there is doubt about the diagnosis, and a septic arthritis is suspected, aspiration of the hip joint is mandatory and has the added benefit of relieving the pressure. However, most children can be managed conservatively. Children will naturally hold their hip in the position of most comfort, so minimizing intracapsular pressure. Traction adds nothing, and can be damaging if it forces the hip into a position of raised intracapsular pressure. Analgesics or NSAIDs may be helpful. Children will choose to stay on bed rest until the hip is comfortable enough to allow them to mobilize. The natural history of the condition is for the pain to resolve over a few days and usually no more than a week. Perthes disease is associated with irritable hip in approximately 1 per cent of cases, but the nature of this association is unclear.

Discitis

It is unclear whether discitis is infectious in aetiology or not. Acute discitis, in the absence of associated vertebral osteomyelitis, is a self-limiting illness, not associated with culture of organisms. Peak onset is between 1 and 3 years, presenting with back pain and stiffness. The child refuses to walk, causing diagnostic confusion with irritable hip, and may complain of non-specific features common in this age group, such as abdominal pain. There may be low-grade fever. Examination demonstrates well-localized tenderness, usually in the lumbar spine. Radiographs are normal until late in the disease, and bone scan and MRI are the most useful investigations (Figure 16.8). Treatment is conservative, but if doubt exists about the diagnosis, antibiotics should be given.

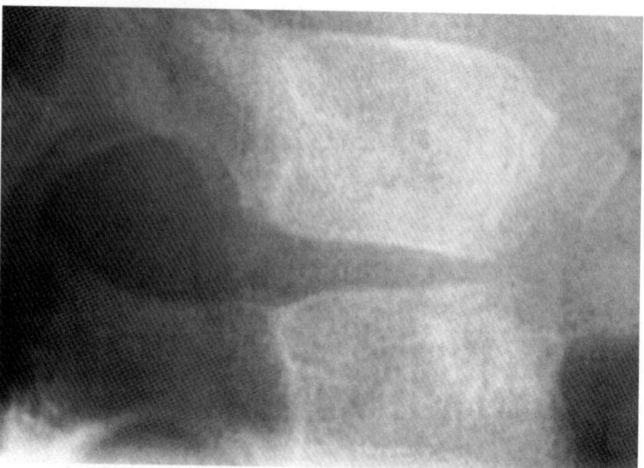

Figure 16.8 Discitis: the radiograph shows narrowing of the disc space without vertebral body end plate destruction

KEY LEARNING POINTS

- Most bone tumours present with a mass on careful clinical examination.
- A bone tumour should never be considered benign without seeking an expert opinion.
- Persistent, non-specific bone pain, which occurs at night is consistent with a bone tumour.
- Acute lymphoblastic leukaemia may present with an identical clinical picture to JIA, a normal full blood count or subtle features such as a low normal platelet count, which is atypical in JIA.
- The incidence of rheumatic fever in children is increasing in industrialized countries and should be considered in a child with a painful, migratory polyarthritis.
- Septic arthritis may be particularly difficult to diagnose, especially in the neonate, but should be excluded in all children with a monoarthritis.
- Tuberculosis is increasing in incidence and can cause a septic arthritis with an indolent progress, or a reactive arthritis, and should be considered in patients at risk.
- In the miserable younger child with arthritis or bone pain consider neuroblastoma.

AUTOIMMUNE DISORDERS

Inflammatory bowel disease

CASE STUDY

A 13-year-old boy had developed arthritis at the age of 8 years. His disease was never very well controlled despite methotrexate, and he had persistent episodes of ankle swelling which were painful. However, even when he was relatively well without active synovitis he was a pale and lacked energy, with an Hb 10.5 g/dL, albumin 33 g/L and an ESR of 22 mm/h. At 13 years, he had several episodes of diarrhoea. This became more persistent, and was associated with mucus production. Diagnosis: The arthritis of inflammatory bowel disease, and subsequent appearance of previously occult inflammatory bowel disease.

Children with inflammatory bowel disease may develop an associated arthritis. The inflammatory bowel disease may present with little or no bowel features, but be identified through failure to thrive, anaemia or hypoalbuminaemia out of proportion to the arthritis.

There are two characteristic patterns of joint involvement. The commonest is a peripheral large joint arthritis (ankles and knees predominantly). This arthritis responds to good control of the bowel disease and exacerbations occur with flares of bowel inflammation. Sulfasalazine is useful in controlling both bowel inflammation and arthritis. The second pattern, which is less common in children, but may develop later in life, involves a progressive, central spinal ankylosis, which is progressive irrespective of bowel involvement.

Sarcoidosis

Sarcoid is a rare cause of arthritis in childhood. A florid synovitis, characteristically without much pain or restriction of movement of the joints, occurs and the synovitis may be transient. It is associated with uveitis and an erythematous skin rash, which may present in the neonate, and erythema nodosum. The other systemic manifestations such as hilar lymphadenopathy and lung involvement are less common in childhood.

Connective tissue disorders

Juvenile dermatomyositis

CASE STUDY

An 11-year-old girl presented with acute appendicitis, which was treated and she was well, but she was noted to have persistently raised aspartate aminotransferase (AST) and alanine aminotransferase (ALT) levels, and an ESR of 45 mm/h. Over the course of a year she developed difficulty climbing stairs, and brushing her hair because of pain and weakness. She developed an erythematous rash on her cheeks, knuckles and knees over the summer, and had calcium nodules on her elbows. Her creatine kinase (CK) and lactose dehydrogenase (LDH) were not raised. Diagnosis: Juvenile dermatomyositis.

Juvenile dermatomyositis (JDM) is an important differential diagnosis in the child presenting with weakness. The commonest idiopathic inflammatory myopathy in children is dermatomyositis. Rarely, muscle weakness without rash can occur as polymyositis (5 per cent). There are two peaks of disease: the first occurring in the toddler and young school-age child, and the second in the teenage years. The onset of JDM is acute in 50 per cent of cases with rapid onset of weakness and rash, although the rash may appear first followed by progressive muscle weakness. The painful proximal myopathy is characterized by difficulties in walking, cycling, climbing steps and dressing, especially combing the hair. In younger children loss of gross motor milestones may occur. Gottron sign is seen in the hands as a red discoloration of the skin which often scars over the metacarpophalangeal, proximal interphalangeal and distal interphalangeal joints, and extensor surfaces of the knees, ankles and elbows (Figure 16.9). Malar erythema and purple telangiectasia develops over the eyelids (called a heliotrope rash). A consistent sign in JDM is nailfold capillary dilatation and infarction, visible to the naked eye in more than 95 per cent of cases.

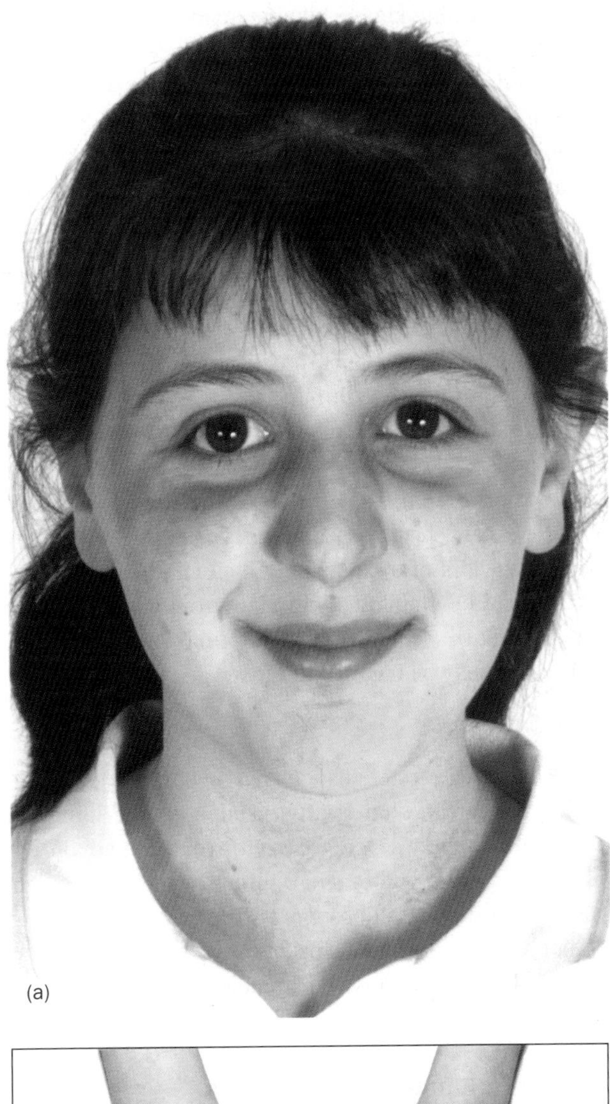

(a)

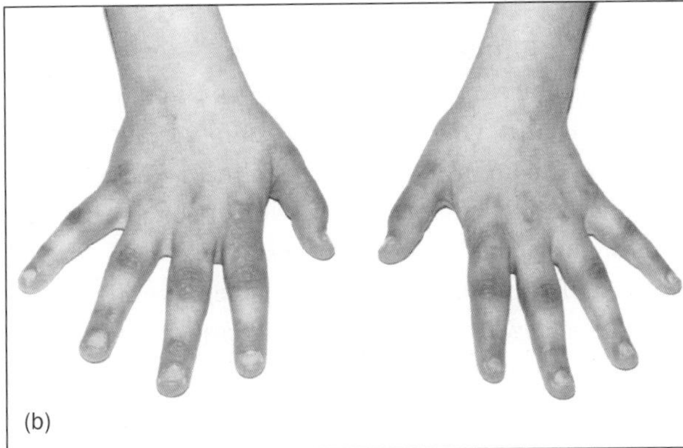

(b)

Figure 16.9 (a) The facial rash of juvenile dermatomyositis, including a purple (heliotrope) rash over the eyelids, malar erythema and erythema on the neck in a photosensitive distribution. (b) Gottron papules over the metacarpophalangeal and distal and proximal interphalangeal joints. The erythema around the nailfolds is associated with dilated nailfold capillaries

AETIOLOGY

Juvenile dermatomyositis is caused by a vasculitis which leads to loss of arterioles and capillaries and subsequent decrease in capillary to muscle fibre ratio. The aetiology remains unclear but both genetic and infectious factors have been implicated. Antinuclear antibodies are present in 80 per cent of cases. Untreated the disease can extend to involve both striated and smooth muscle, so that apart from skeletal involvement, gastrointestinal and cardiac involvement may occur. The rash is typically accompanied by the deposition of calcium in the skin, especially over bony prominences, subcutaneous tissues and fascial planes. The incidence of calcinosis is falling with more aggressive treatment. The rash is photosensitive and exposure to strong sunshine may not only aggravate the rash but also precipitate a flare-up of the myositis.

DIAGNOSIS

Diagnosis is based on the typical skin features, clinical evidence of inflammatory muscle disease and supported by evidence of muscle involvement such as elevated muscle enzymes (creatine kinase, alanine aminotransferase (ALT) and aldolase in 75 per cent of cases). Muscle biopsy shows perivascular lymphocytic infiltrate with muscle atrophy but for straightforward cases has been superseded by MRI of muscle which also allows serial monitoring of muscle inflammation. Clinical assessment of changing weakness is more useful than muscle enzymes, which do not accurately reflect disease activity and are poor for monitoring disease progress. Traditional manual muscle testing is too crude to identify significant weakness in many children. The history of functional problems (dressing, walking upstairs, etc.) and in performing tasks such as rising from a chair, climbing on an examination couch and sit-ups, may reveal weakness, and children may use tricks to compensate for weakness (as in the Gowers sign). Profound weakness can occur very quickly, including respiratory failure and loss of swallowing. Children with severe disease should be monitored with daily respiratory function tests and assessment of swallowing function. A period of ventilation may be required in the most severe cases.

TREATMENT

For mild disease steroids tapered over a 6–12-month period may treat what is often a monophasic illness in childhood. In more severe cases intravenous methylprednisolone is used, with a small group of the most severe cases requiring immunosuppressive treatment ranging from methotrexate and ciclosporin to intravenous immunoglobulin and cyclophosphamide depending on the severity of disease.

Systemic lupus erythematosus

Systemic lupus erythematosus is an autoimmune multisystem disorder which is often diagnosed late in those children with an insidious onset of illness. Features such as fatigue and lethargy, fever, weight loss, arthralgia, mouth ulcers and diffuse alopecia are typical of SLE, albeit non-specific. The differential diagnosis may be difficult and wide (infection, malignancy), and clinical features may overlap with other childhood connective tissue diseases such as dermatomyositis. Children can present with illnesses such as idiopathic thrombocytopenic purpura, and be well for many years before the full picture of SLE emerges. They can present acutely and very unwell with severe nephritis or neurolupus. The diagnosis of SLE requires interpretation of clinical features (Figure 16.10) and investigations (Table 16.5).

The estimated incidence of lupus is 0.8 per 100 000 children, rising to 12.3 per 100 000 in teenage girls. It is commonest in African-Caribbeans, followed by East Asians, Asians from the Indian subcontinent and the white population.

NEONATAL SYSTEMIC LUPUS ERYTHEMATOSUS

Neonatal SLE is caused by the transplacental passage of maternal anti-Ro IgG autoantibodies during pregnancy. The mother may be asymptomatic. The baby presents with congenital heart block which usually requires cardiac pacing after birth. Less frequently, the baby is born with a widespread rash involving mainly the face and trunk, consisting of several small, sharply delineated areas of vasculitic rash (see Figure 16.10). These can be photosensitive, but usually resolve before the first birthday.

TREATMENT OF SYSTEMIC LUPUS ERYTHEMATOSUS

The mainstays of drug therapy are steroids and immunosuppressants. Oral prednisolone helps to gain disease control. In severe cases with vasculitis, cerebral or severe renal involvement intravenous methylprednisolone and cyclophosphamide are required. Steroids are reduced to a minimum once disease control is achieved. The addition of azathioprine has a sparing effect on the dose of prednisolone, and methotrexate is increasingly used. Hydroxychloroquine is useful in controlling skin manifestations and gives some protection against cardiovascular disease. Non-steroidal anti-inflammatory drugs may be helpful for arthritis. Sunlight may worsen the skin manifestations and precipitate a flare of systemic manifestations. Anti-UVA and B sunblock should be used all year round.

OUTCOME OF SYSTEMIC LUPUS ERYTHEMATOSUS

The disease is characterized by relapses and remissions. Multidisciplinary management including involvement of multiple specialities (renal, rheumatology, dermatology, neurology), and careful handover to adult care is critical to successful management of these children. Outcome has improved with better therapy for renal and cerebral involvement, but these remain important causes of increased morbidity and mortality. As survival has improved, management to reduce the late, adult sequelae of secondary premature cardiovascular disease and osteoporosis are important.

Mixed connective tissue disease/ overlap syndromes

Patients may exhibit features of different connective tissue diseases concurrently, particularly SLE, dermatomyositis, systemic sclerosis and less often rheumatoid arthritis. The common features at presentation are arthritis, Raynaud phenomenon and thickened oedematous skin of the fingers and face and the presence of an extractable nuclear antigen against ribonuclear protein (RNP). Children may

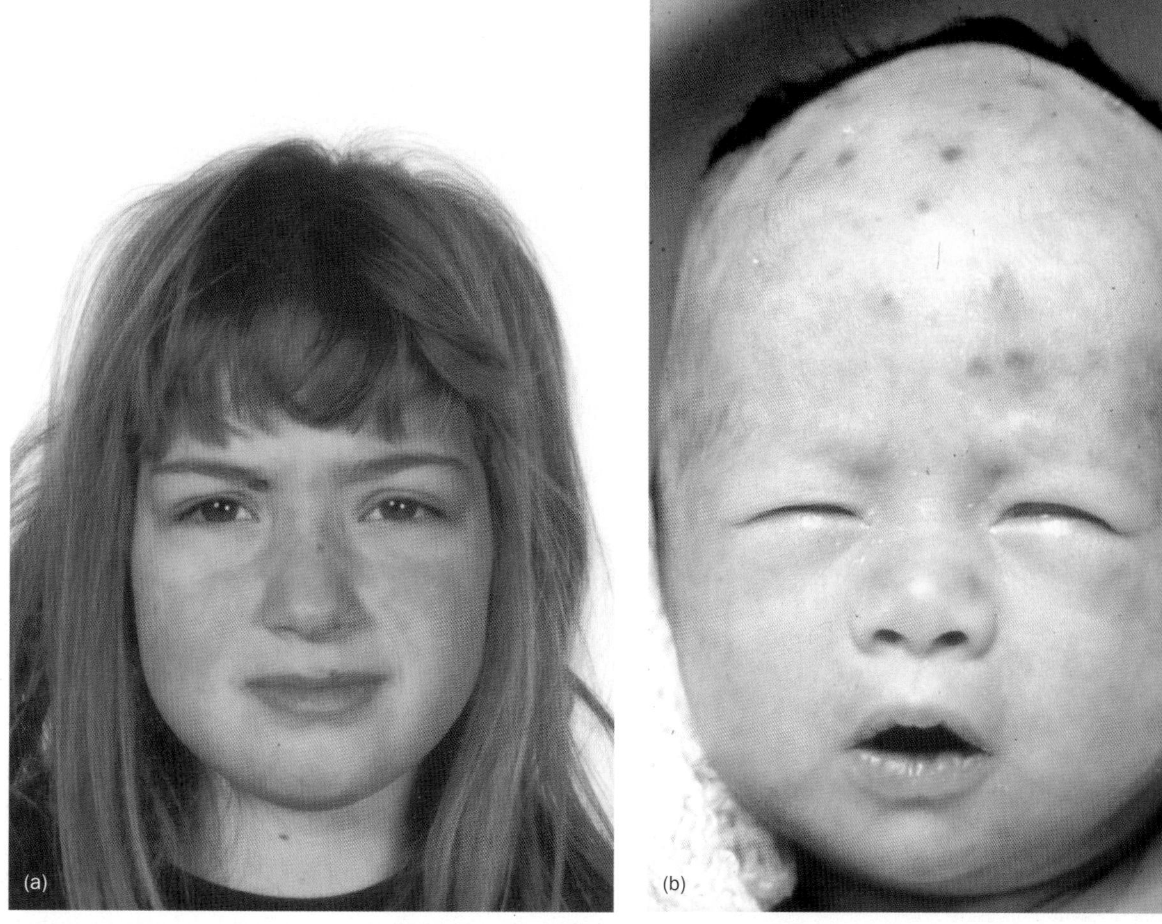

Figure 16.10 (a) The butterfly rash of systemic lupus erythematosus (SLE) showing sparing of the nares, and folliculitis. Note also the cushingoid appearance of this girl. (b) Neonatal systemic lupus erythematosus showing rash

Table 16.5 Clinical features of systemic lupus erythematosus (SLE): common or important features

System	Characteristics
Mucocutaneous	Numerous rashes occur; butterfly rash (malar rash) in 50 per cent of children, discoid lesions which scar, including a scarring alopecia, photosensitive rash, tender vasculitic lesions typically on the tips of fingers and toes, oral ulceration (often painless and palatal), diffuse alopecia, dilated nailfold capillaries, Raynaud phenomenon, livido reticularis
Musculoskeletal	Non-erosive arthritis and tenosynovitis; myositis
Neurological	Peripheral neuropathies, cerebrovascular accidents, psychosis, seizures, encephalopathy
Haematological	Typically a persistent lymphopenia; neutropenia, anaemia of chronic disease, autoimmune haemolytic anaemia, thrombocytopenia
Immunological	The production of autoantibodies is typical; antinuclear antibody, dsDNA and anti-Smith particularly associated; polyclonal increase in immunoglobulins, particularly IgG
Renal	SLE causes all types of glomerulonephritis; nephrotic syndrome
Serositis	Pleurisy and pericarditis typically without large effusions
Other	Hepatosplenomegaly, fever, lymphadenopathy; profound tiredness very common and underrecognized; weight loss, anorexia; erythrocyte sedimentation rate raised with normal C-reactive protein

later evolve into SLE, systemic sclerosis or rheumatoid arthritis. Treatment depends on the clinical manifestations but most patients need steroids and methotrexate for adequate disease control.

Systemic sclerosis/scleroderma

This is similar to the adult disease, but is rare in childhood, although no good epidemiological data exist. Of unknown cause, it is characterized by multisystem

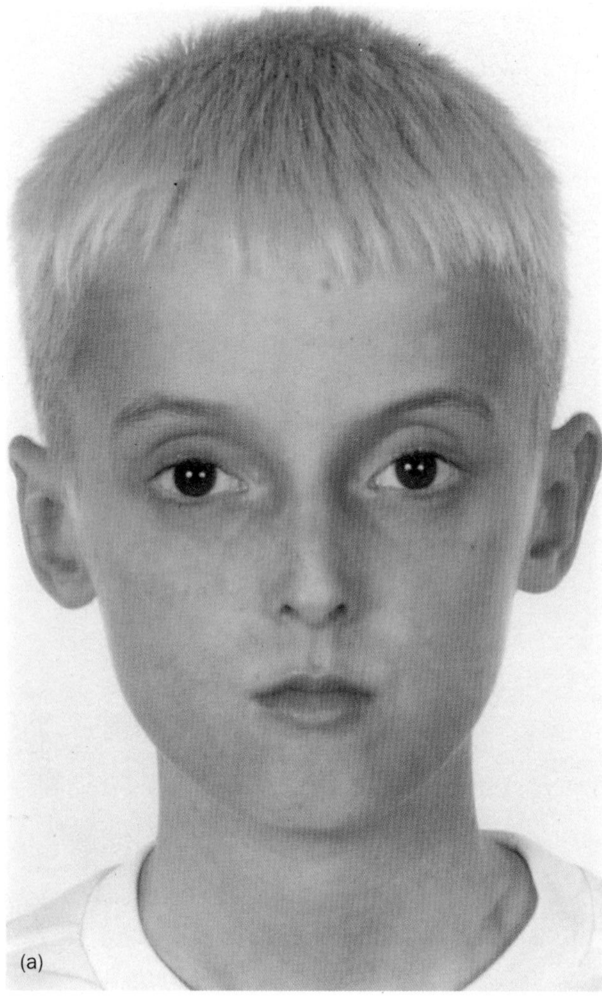

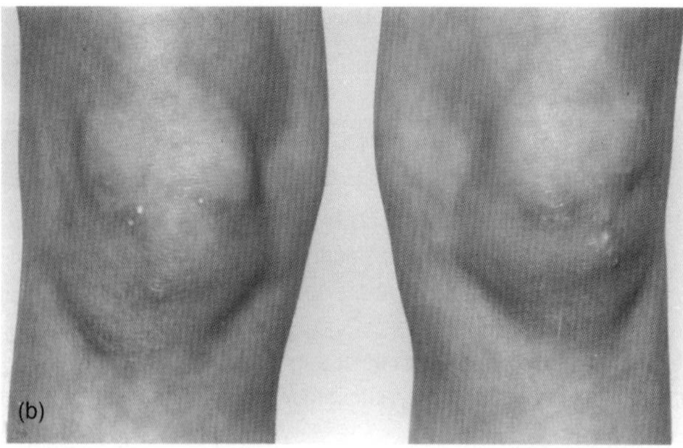

Figure 16.11 Systemic sclerosis. Note the typical features with telangectasia, tight skin, loss of lip volume, poor mouth opening and beaked nose

involvement, which may be difficult to control, and is associated with a poor outcome. Raynaud phenomenon may be an early and common feature. Skin tightening is progressive often after a period of oedema, particularly in the fingers. The skin feels waxy, tight and hard, and it is most noticeable on the face and hands, which may develop contractures (Figure 16.11). Telangectasia and calcinosis occur, especially over extensor surfaces. Sicca syndrome (dry mouth and eyes) is often present. Arthritis does occur, but loss of fingertip pulp and infarction of bone are commoner features. Involvement of the gastrointestinal tract most commonly affects the oesophagus, with reduced motility, reflux and dysphagia. Pulmonary, cardiac and renal involvement is associated with a poor prognosis. Meticulous management, infection control, skin care, monitoring of renal and pulmonary function and judicious use of immunosuppression is the mainstay of management.

Localized sclerodermas

These are important in childhood, and are commoner in children than adults. Although classifications divide these into morphea and linear scleroderma, both may coexist in the same patient (Figure 16.12), and the management principles are the same. Morphea affects a local area of skin, most commonly on the trunk. It develops gradually, often starting with a purplish colour, becoming pale and thickened, and keeping a purple edge. The skin is tight and waxy to touch. Most morphea lesions eventually become inactive and scarred in appearance. These lesions may affect breast development or other soft tissue structures. Linear scleroderma also produces a gradually progressive lesion which is shiny, often ivory coloured or sometimes pigmented. In addition to a poor cosmetic result, these lesions can affect the underlying muscle, fat and bone and may affect local growth, including skull growth; where they cross a joint, it results in contractures. There is no evidence base for treatment. Steroids and immunosuppressives are used, but the natural history of these lesions is to stop progressing after a variable amount of time.

Vasculitis

Henoch–Schönlein purpura

Henoch–Schönlein purpura (HSP) is the commonest childhood vasculitis, with an incidence between 13.5 and 24.0 per 100 000 children under 14 years old, falling with increasing age. It is a multisystem disorder affecting the skin, joints (in 60–84 per cent) particularly ankles and knees, gastrointestinal tract with pain and gastrointestinal bleeding, and kidneys. The aetiology is unknown although preceding infection, particularly upper respiratory tract infection is found in most children, and there is a seasonal variation in incidence supporting an infectious aetiology. No single organism has been found to be associated with HSP.

For most children, HSP is diagnosed by the appearance of the rash (Figure 16.13), and is a self-limiting

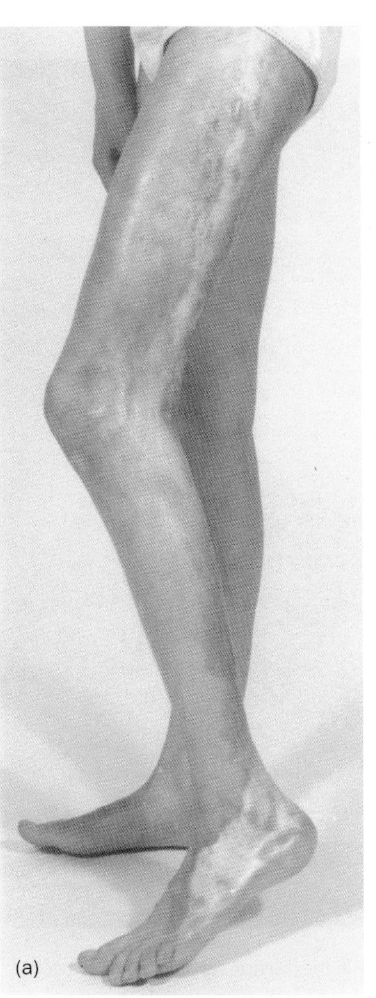

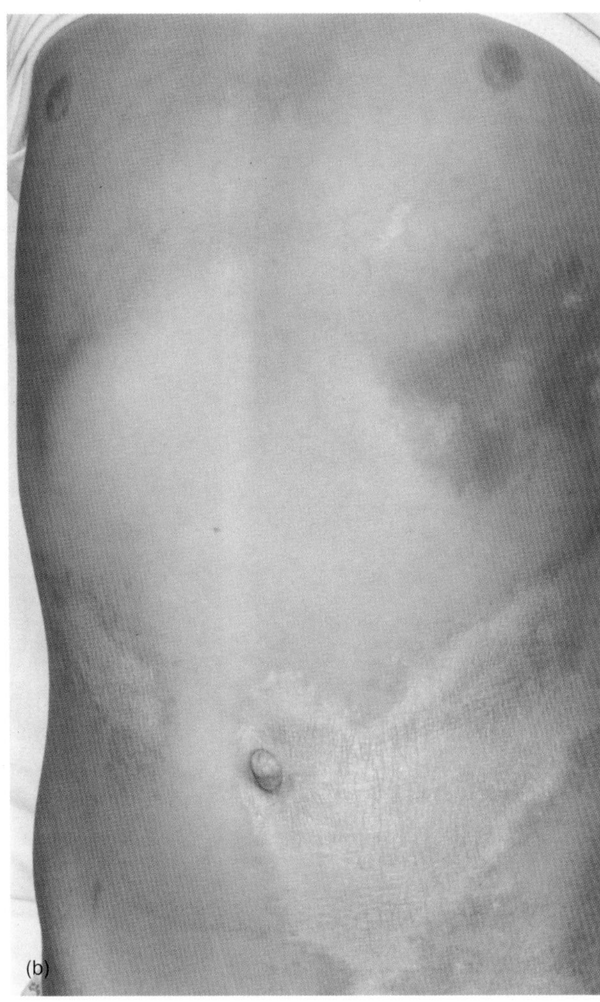

Figure 16.12 Localized scleroderma, left panel showing linear scleroderma, right panel showing morphea and linear scleroderma

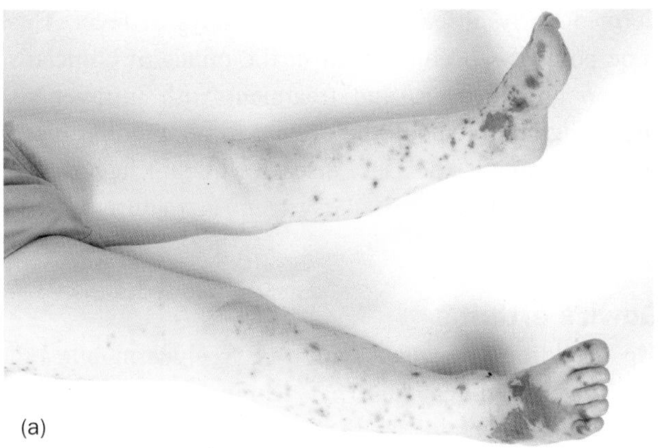

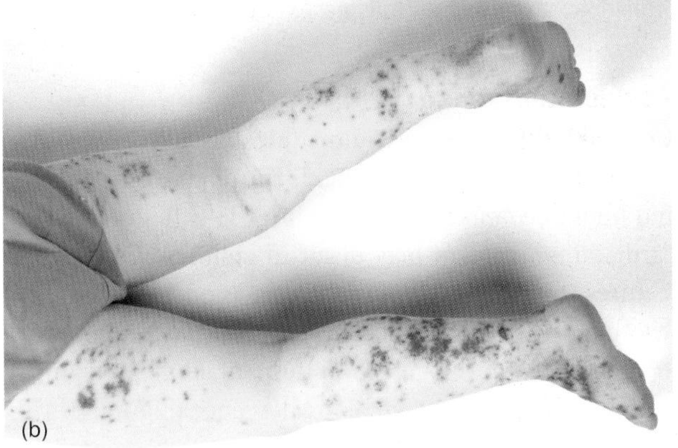

Figure 16.13 The palpable purpuric rash of Henoch–Schönlein purpura in the classic distribution around the lateral malleoli, the ventral aspects of the feet, the buttocks and the extensor aspects of the legs. The rash may start with urticaria.

illness complicated by arthritis and abdominal pain. However, a significant number develop nephritis with an estimated 1 per cent developing endstage renal failure. Five to 15 per cent of children requiring dialysis have Henoch–Schönlein purpura. There is some suggestion that steroids may change the long-term outcome, and prednisolone is effective for joint and abdominal pain. In the UK, most children are managed conservatively with

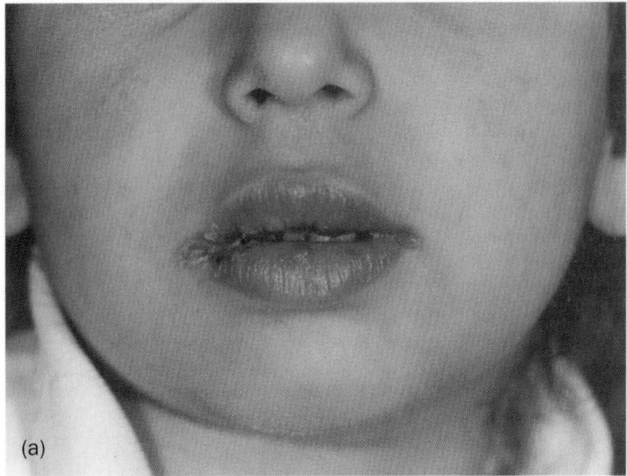

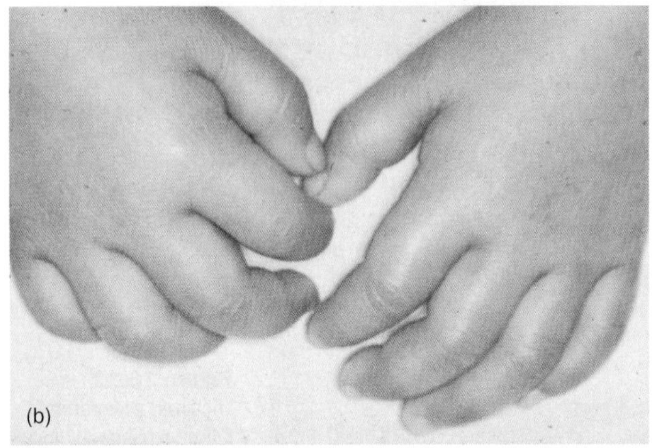

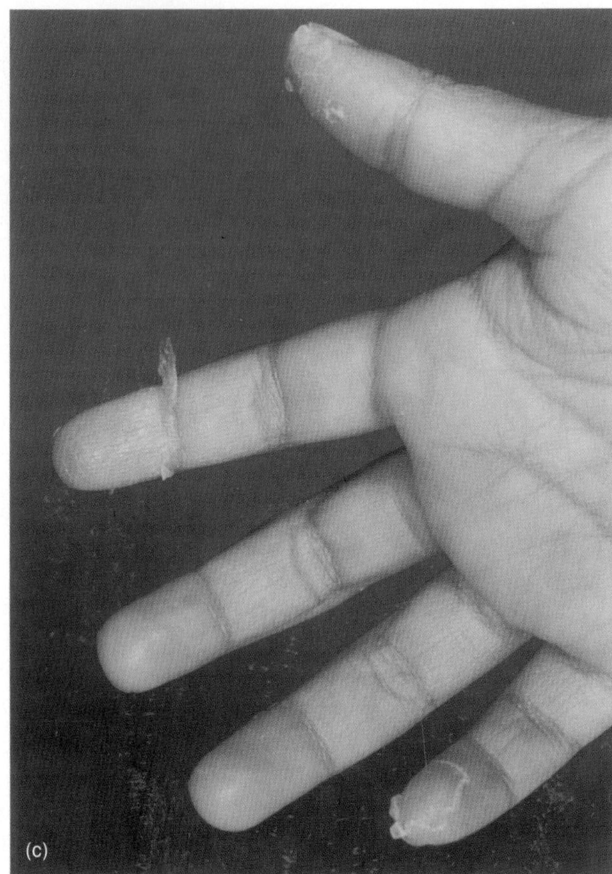

Figure 16.14 Clinical features of Kawasaki disease. (a) Mucositis. (b) The fingers are oedematous early in the disease, (c) progressing to peeling

NSAIDs for pain, and expectant management. Crescentric glomerulonephritis is treated with cyclophosphamide, high-dose steroids and plasma exchange.

Kawasaki disease

Kawasaki disease is an idiopathic vasculitis typically occurring in the pre-school child. The diagnosis is clinical and mimics common childhood infections (Figure 16.14). Cardiac involvement may occur in children with partial features, especially the very young (under 18 months) who have a worse prognosis (Table 16.6). It is important to recognize the changing pattern of clinical features from presentation through convalescence (Figure 16.15). The aetiology is unclear, but infection is suggested by current epidemiological and immunological evidence. No single organism has been identified. The incidence is estimated at 2/100 000 children in the UK, but is doubled in children under 5 years, much higher in Japan and migrants of far eastern origin. The incidence of cardiac artery aneurysms has fallen from 20 per cent to under 5 per cent with the early use of intravenous immunoglobulin. This is associated with a fall in early mortality from myocardial infarction from 1 per cent to <0.2 per cent. The original trials of intravenous immunoglobulin defined 'early' disease as before 10 days of fever. This time point has become fixed in the minds of clinicians for no good reason, and treatment with intravenous immunoglobulin should be offered to all children diagnosed as having Kawasaki disease who still have fever. These children are also at risk from premature atherosclerosis later in adult life.

Down's arthritis

Most children with Down syndrome are hypermobile and may get associated pain. Less commonly, Down syndrome can be complicated by an inflammatory arthritis, further adding to the burden of disability in these children. The arthritis is destructive and responds poorly to steroids and immunosuppression.

KEY LEARNING POINTS

- Muscle weakness in dermatomyositis may be subtle. The history, and examination of

Table 16.6 Clinical features of Kawasaki disease

Feature	Characteristic
Fever (100 per cent)	High (40°C) remittent fever unresponsive to antibiotics but does respond to antipyretics and intravenous immunoglobulin
Conjunctivitis (85 per cent)	Bilateral, non-purulent
Lymphadenopathy (70 per cent)	Cervical lymph node at least 1.5 cm in diameter, non-purulent
Rash (80 per cent)	Polymorphous rash particularly on the trunk and perineum; perineal desquamation occurs later
Oral (90 per cent)	Erythema of oropharynx, strawberry tongue, fissured lips
Extremities (70 per cent)	Oedema of palms and soles early (and often unrecognized), may be red/brawny; later desquamation (often diagnosed at this stage)
Cardiac involvement	Early: myositis (arrhythmias or congestive cardiac failure)/pericarditis; aneurysms develop later so echocardiography should be performed after six weeks; myocardial infarction can occur as a late complication of aneurysms
Misery/irritability (100 per cent)	Probably secondary to an aseptic meningitis
Arthritis (common)	

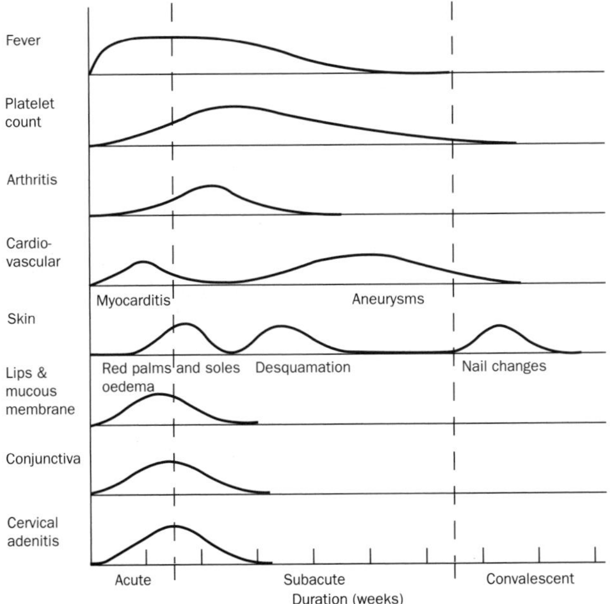

Figure 16.15 Time course of Kawasaki disease

tasks such as rising from a chair and Gowers sign are more valuable than traditional scales of muscle power.

- Systemic lupus erythematosus (SLE) may have an insidious onset in children with non-specific features such as lethargy, fever, mouth ulcers and diffuse alopecia as the prominent features.
- The liver transaminases (AST and ALT) may be confused with muscle isoenzymes. Levels of muscle enzymes do not correlate with clinical assessment of weakness, and may be normal long before the child is well.

- Arthritis may be the presenting feature of a number of systemic diseases in children. In particular inflammatory bowel disease may present with little or no bowel features, but be identified through failure to thrive, anaemia or hypoalbuminaemia out of proportion to the arthritis.
- Kawasaki disease should be considered in the younger child with misery and painful joints.

MECHANICAL

Slipped capital femoral epiphysis (SCFE)

CASE STUDY

A 10-year-old girl presented having been under the care of her family doctor for several months with pain in her knee. She denied trauma. The pain was poorly localized and associated with a limp. Examination showed that she walked with an externally rotated foot and a limp. She had no abnormal physical findings around the knee, in particular there was no tenderness or effusion. Flexion of the hip was painful and restricted. Anteroposterior and frog lateral views of her hip show a slipped capital femoral epiphysis.

This is an uncommon condition, which occurs in children in early adolescence. Girls are affected at an earlier age than boys. The aetiology is poorly understood, but is thought to be related to the rapid period of skeletal growth and to the susceptibility of the proximal femoral physis to shear forces. It is also associated with hypothyroidism, radiotherapy, chronic renal failure and growth hormone treatment. The presentation is usually insidious, but may occasionally be acute with severe pain and inability to bear weight. Hip pain is frequently referred to the knee because of the shared nerve supply to the hip joint and to the skin on the medial side of the knee. Adolescents with knee pain and no physical signs in the knee should be assumed to have a SCFE until proved otherwise. Treatment is surgical with percutaneous *in situ* pinning. Twenty per cent of cases will either present with bilateral SCFE or develop a contralateral slip.

Legg–Calvé–Perthes disease

Perthes disease, as it is commonly known, is a poorly understood condition, which, in European populations, commonly affects children between the ages of 4 and 8 years. The cause is unclear, but the effects are due to necrosis of part of the femoral capital epiphysis. The dead bone is gradually replaced by living bone, but during this process, which may last several years, the femoral head is at risk of deforming. A deformed head increases the risk of developing secondary osteoarthritis. The prognosis relates to the age of the child at presentation, the sex of the child, the pattern of head involvement and the ultimate congruency of the hip joint. Young boys tend to do better than older girls. Treatment is variable, but may involve simply observation, cast treatment or surgery.

Anterior knee pain

Anterior knee pain is very common in children. Most children describe pain on the front of the knee, which is worse going up and down stairs and after sitting with the knee bent for prolonged periods of time. Difficulty straightening the knee after sitting is common. Physical findings are usually few although there may be retropatellar tenderness or crepitus and the pain may be reproduced by patellofemoral compression. The exact cause of the pain is unclear and there are many theories. Pain does not correlate with thinning or fibrillation of articular cartilage seen at arthroscopy, so the term chondromalacia is best avoided. The natural history of the condition is for the pain to persist in most children, but it becomes less of a problem to the child as they get older. This is in contrast to Osgood–Schlatter disease (tibial tuberosity pain and swelling), which always resolves around the time of skeletal maturity. The management of anterior knee pain involves explanation of the course of the condition, activity modification and physiotherapy.

Accidental injury

In children, fractures are very common and accidents remain the commonest cause of death, despite injury prevention programmes. Multiple injuries in children are uncommon. The commonest injuries are as a result of simple falls and affect the wrist and forearm. There is a seasonal variation in the incidence of fractures with more occurring in the summer time (and on sunnier days) than in the winter. Fractures in children behave differently to those in adults in a number of ways. Children's capacity for remodelling is greater because of growth but there is also a potential for growth disturbance when fractures involve the physis. Healing is quicker, without the complications of immobilization seen in adults, allowing conservative management rather than operative fixation. An acutely painful joint with a history of minor trauma in a young child should raise the possibility of other diagnoses such as JIA, non-accidental injury, or septic arthritis.

In the adolescent serious trauma causing a haemarthrosis, fracture or ligamentous injury is associated with immediate onset of swelling, clearly associated with the trauma. A gradual onset of joint swelling over a longer time course should raise the possibility of other diagnoses such as JIA.

Non-accidental injury

Non-accidental injury is an important differential diagnosis for children presenting with musculoskeletal pain, refusal to weight bear, joint effusions, or skin lesions which mimic vasculitis. The child with poorly explained trauma, haemarthrosis, and unexplained bruises, limb pain or pseudoparalysis should be investigated for non-accidental injury. Radiological survey may show multiple fractures, including the typical, but subtle metaphyseal fractures (see Figure 16.3) or marked periosteal reaction resulting from the pulling and twisting actions associated with non-accidental injury. Self-abuse in an older child can cause joint swelling as in the example of a teenager repeatedly hitting his knee with a hammer. Sexual abuse may present with gonococcal arthritis.

Minor abnormalities of gait and posture

Clinical confidence in diagnosing simple abnormalities of gait and posture allows the management of these problems with good explanation to the family, and simple orthoses where necessary.

Hypermobility

Benign generalized hypermobility is a common normal finding in children. Children who are hypermobile are often good at sport such as ballet and gym. Hypermobility is commoner in girls, and people of African–Caribbean origin. It often runs in families (Figure 16.16). Hypermobility can present in infancy and should be considered in those children presenting with delayed walking and hypotonia of their lower limbs in the absence of neurological or other abnormalities. Hypermobility presents to doctors when it is associated with pain. It can be diagnosed using the Carter–Wilkinson criteria (Table 16.7), and asking the children to demonstrate their own contortionist tricks. The pain is typically worse during or after exercise and may be associated with transient swelling of the joints. Often orthoses for flat feet can improve posture at the ankle, knee, hip and lumbar spine and reduce pain. Children should be encouraged to be active as maintaining normal muscle bulk also helps maintain a normal posture, and reduces pain. Nocturnal idiopathic pain is commoner in these children. The evidence that these children are predisposed to osteoarthritis or long term postural abnormalities is poor.

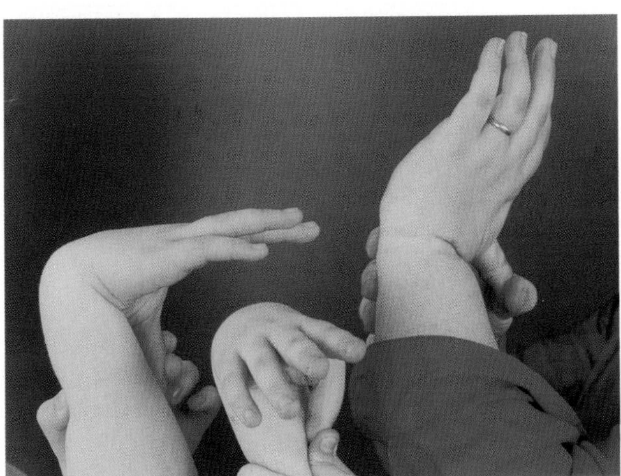

Figure 16.16 Benign familial hypermobility

Table 16.7 Beighton's modification of the Carter-Wilkinson criteria for hypermobility

Criterion	Score
Palms flat on the floor with knees extended	1
Opposition of thumb to flexor aspect of forearm	2
Hyperextension of fingers parallel to extensor aspect of forearm	2
Hyperextension of elbows by more than 10°	2
Hyperextension of knees by more than 10°	2
Score (1 mark for each, including right and left, hypermobile if >6)	**9**

Pes planus

Flat feet is a common parental concern. Young children all have flat feet, and some ankle valgus (see Figure 16.1). In most children flat feet improve over time and remain pain free. Some children do get pain in their feet, however these are the minority. There is controversy about the relation of physiological flat feet to knee, ankle and back pain. Simple well-fitting orthoses can correct postural abnormalities, and remove the pain in some children. There is, however, no evidence that shoes or orthoses permanently alter the shape of the foot over time.

Rare associations with hypermobility

Hypermobility is a feature of very rare connective tissue diseases such as Ehlers–Danlos and Marfan syndromes. Ehlers–Danlos is a group of inherited disorders of connective tissue that are characterized as a group by true dislocations of large joints (not just patellar dislocation common in children, particularly teenage girls, or partial subluxation of shoulder or knees which is found in benign hypermobility) and papery atrophic scars and easy bruising following minor skin trauma. Vascular abnormalities occur in rare types of Ehlers–Danlos and may lead to vessel rupture or gastrointestinal bleeding. Marfan syndrome is characterized by an arm span greater than the height, a high arched palate, lens subluxation, arachnodactyly and aortic root dilation, aneurysm formation and mitral valve prolapse. Individuals are often tall.

Stickler syndrome is an uncommon autosomal dominant condition, associated with micrognathia and a cleft or high-arched palate at birth. Severe myopia (>−10 dioptres) develops during childhood and is associated with a high-risk of retinal detachment and blindness. Early degenerative changes in joint surfaces occur, leading to a destructive painful arthropathy. Management is mostly supportive.

Stress fractures and shin splints

Stress fractures occur with repetitive activity in weight-bearing areas of the growing skeleton. They may be insidious in onset, exacerbated by exercise and often occur in the foot (metatarsal shaft, navicular, calcaneum). Radiographs may be normal before callus has developed. Shin splints is a syndrome characterized by pain on the anterior aspect of the lower shin and typically numbness in the fourth toe, brought on by activity and relieved by rest. They result from overuse of the posterior tibial muscle, and treatment is symptomatic and must be accompanied by activity modification.

Nocturnal idiopathic pain (night pains)

Night pains and growing pains are diagnostic labels that are frequently badly applied to children with unexplained pain. Growing pains is a poor term which should be avoided as these pains occur during the period of slowest growth in childhood and are unrelated to growth. Night pains occur in children aged 3–10 years. The child typically awakes during the night crying with leg pain. The parents soothe the child, usually finding that massage helps, sometimes using simple analgesia. The child then falls back to sleep over a short period of time and the next day is well without any swelling or limp. In some children, nocturnal pain may have a clear association with exercise the day before. The pains characteristically are felt bilaterally in the calves, shins and thighs. Unilateral pain raises the possibility of a local more serious cause such as malignancy or osteomyelitis. Any child with a limp, tenderness, swelling or persistent pain continuing into the day should be investigated for an alternative explanation. Management of night pains is with explanation, reassurance and simple analgesia.

KEY LEARNING POINTS

- Insidious onset of pain in adolescents with knee pain but with a normal knee on examination should be assumed to have SCFE until proved otherwise.
- Children between 4 and 8 years of age with hip pain, or pain referred to the knee, should be investigated for Perthes disease.
- The history of trauma – appropriate force or not – and the temporal relation between the trauma and development of joint signs are critical in the differential diagnosis of accidental trauma from non-accidental injury, septic arthritis, JIA or osteomyelitis.
- Distinguishing minor problems such as anterior knee pain, Osgood–Schlatter disease and benign hypermobility from more sinister pathology requires confidence, skill and practice in clinical examination.
- Non-accidental injury may present with joint effusions and is a medical emergency with a significant morbidity and mortality (2 per cent). Subtle, metaphyseal fractures, often without callus formation, should be sought on radiological skeletal survey, or bone scan where the fractures appear as hot spots.

METABOLIC AND GENETIC

Rickets covers several distinct diseases of ossification (Table 16.8 and Figure 16.17).

Scurvy

CASE STUDY

A 9-year-old boy presented with weakness, loss of ability to walk upstairs unaided, and pain in his legs and back. He then developed a fever, and was admitted to hospital with a rapidly falling haemoglobin reaching 5.6 g/dL over the course of a week. He had a perifollicular petechial rash on the legs, peripheral oedema, and bleeding gums. He had a spontaneous haemorrhage behind his right knee despite sitting in a flexed position in the hospital bed. His bone marrow showed ineffective haematopoiesis. Diagnosis: Scurvy. This boy had no fruit or vegetables in his diet. The sudden fall in haemoglobin with an intercurrent infection is typical.

Lack of vitamin C (ascorbic acid) prevents the development of normal collagen, resulting in intradermal and subperiosteal haemorrhage. Subperiosteal haemorrhage is painful, and haemarthroses may occur. Radiographs may demonstrate subperiosteal new bone formation.

Gout

Gout is exceedingly rare in childhood, except where hyperuricaemia is caused by other underlying disease such as renal failure, malignancy or glycogen storage disease. Lesch–Nyhan syndrome is a sex-linked disorder of uric acid metabolism with predominantly central nervous system effects, and gouty arthritis does not occur until late adolescence or adulthood.

Haematological disorders

Sickle cell anaemia

During a sickle cell crisis, acute arthritis and bone pain can be incapacitating. Secondary osteonecrosis can occur. Septic arthritis in these patients may be caused by otherwise atypical organisms, such as *Salmonella* spp.

Haemophilia

With improved management and factor VIII available joint destruction from repeated intra-articular haemorrhage is

Table 16.8 The causes of rickets

Type	Cause/biochemistry	Clinical features
Vitamin D deficiency [1]	Lack of light ± lack of dietary vitamin D	Pain in joints and tenderness over the bones, bowing of the long bones, and splaying of the rib cage, proximal muscle weakness
Calcium deficiency [2]	Reduced calcium absorption (e.g. coeliac disease/scleroderma/inflammatory bowel disease)	
Hypophosphataemic (vitamin-D-resistant) [3]	Impaired parathormone-dependent proximal renal tubular reabsorption of phosphate	Infancy: short stature, bowing of the legs, ectopic calcification, low serum phosphate with normal calcium; sex-linked recessive or autosomal dominant, occasionally sporadic
Vitamin-D-dependent		
Type 1 [4]	Defect in renal 1-hydroxylase	Autosomal recessive; develop rickets before the age of 2 years
Type 2 [5]	End organ unresponsiveness to 1, 25-dihydroxyvitamin D_3	Rare, but features of rickets in early infancy and before 1 year; also alopecia and absence of eye lashes
Hypophosphatasia [6]	Decreased serum alkaline phosphatase from impaired parathormone-dependent proximal tubular resorption of phosphate	Rare autosomal recessive presenting with severe rickets and fractures. Band keratopathy, proptosis, papilloedema, early loss of teeth, chondrocalcinosis and pseudogout
Numbers in square boxes relate to those in Figure 16.17.		

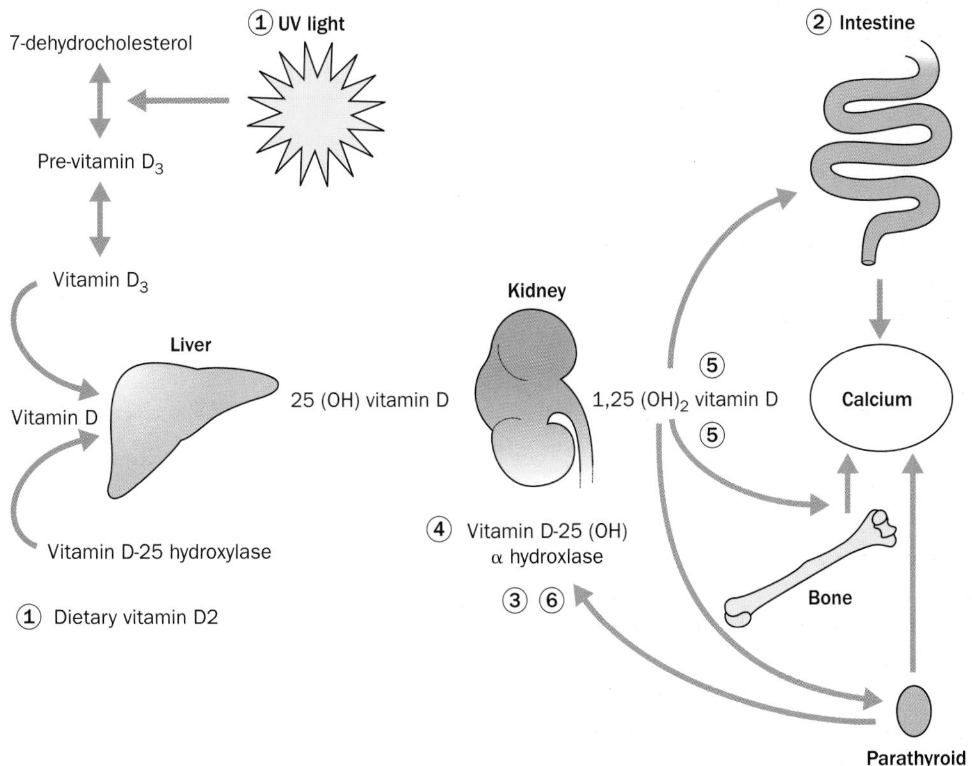

Figure 16.17 The metabolism in rickets

becoming less common in haemophilia. Soft tissue haemorrhage can also occur. Management of an acute bleed consists of rest, splinting the joint and factor VIII replacement.

Cystic fibrosis

A small number of children with cystic fibrosis develop episodic arthritis, most probably reactive in origin, others develop a progressive erosive arthritis. Hypertrophic pulmonary osteoarthropathy also occurs.

Skeletal dysplasias

Skeletal dysplasia encompasses a huge group of ill understood and defined conditions, of which achondroplasia is the commonest. These conditions can broadly be divided into abnormalities of the epiphyses, diaphyses or metaphyses. There is a profound impact on growth, and disproportionate growth occurs. The management is supportive for these often severely disabled children, many of whom have poor mobility, function and pain and extraskeletal features. Genetic support is also required.

NEONATAL

Congenital limb abnormalities

It is important to have a working knowledge of some of the commoner congenital abnormalities seen in neonates. It is essential that families receive accurate, consistent and appropriate information about their baby's condition following delivery. The source may be a local paediatrician, geneticist or paediatric orthopaedic surgeon. There are many support groups available for these families. Ultrasound allows prenatal diagnosis of many congenital limb anomalies, enabling discussion of the findings with an orthopaedic surgeon during pregnancy. Many congenital talipes equinovarus (CTEV) deformities seen on ultrasound are postural and will not require treatment.

Congenital limb malformations

Table 16.9 summarizes the classification of upper limb congenital malformations, which can also be applied to lower limb congenital abnormalities. Limb anomalies can be associated with systemic conditions. The most widely known is the link between radial deficiencies (radial club hand) with the VACTERL spectrum (*v*ertebral anomalies, *a*nal anomalies, cardiac, *t*racheoesophageal, *r*adial aplasia, renal and *l*imb anomalies) thrombocytopenia and Fanconi anaemia. Congenital longitudinal deficiencies of the lower limb are less likely to be associated with visceral involvement.

The proportionate difference in the leg lengths at birth remains constant throughout growth so that a 20 per cent discrepancy at birth will result in a 20 per cent discrepancy at skeletal maturity. The treatment options are the use of either a prosthesis or limb lengthening depending on factors, such as the size of the limb length difference and the condition of the foot. In general, severe discrepancies (Figure 16.18) or a foot that has less than three rays are best treated with a prosthesis rather than limb reconstruction.

Congenital foot deformities

The aim of management of all foot deformities is to achieve a painless, supple and plantigrade foot that will

Table 16.9 Congenital limb malformations of the upper limb

Proposed aetiology	Example	Management
Failure of formation		
Transverse terminal deficiencies	Congenital amputations	Supportive, occupational therapy, occasionally prosthetics
Longitudinal deficiencies	Radial club hand	Surgical involving centralization of the wrist and tendon transfers
	Cleft hand	Possible surgery
Failure of differentiation		
Syndactyly	Simple syndactyly	Surgical correction
Duplication		
Polydactyly	Accessory digits	Surgical
Overgrowth		
Macrodactyly		Conservative or amputation
Undergrowth	Thumb hypoplasia	Possible surgery
Congenital constriction band	Band indentation	Possible surgical release
	Congenital amputations	As above
Generalized skeletal abnormalities	Madelung deformity	

enable normal shoes to be worn. Many parents fear that their child's foot deformity, no matter how minor, will affect their ability to walk. It is well recognized that children with severe deformities such as untreated CTEV will walk despite problems with callosities and footwear. There is no evidence to suggest that minor toe anomalies (such as overlapping toes) delay or significantly affect walking.

Congenital talipes equinovarus

The prevalence of CTEV is 2 per 1000 live births. The aetiology is unknown and most are sporadic isolated anomalies. The condition can be associated with neuromuscular disorders such as neural tube defects or in conditions such as arthrogryposis. There is a familial tendency and it is associated with hip dysplasia. The diagnosis is clinical (Figure 16.19). The ankle is in equinus and the heel in varus, the midfoot adducted and the forefoot appears supinated. Whereas postural deformities appear similar to true CTEV, *all* components of a postural deformity can be fully corrected and may spontaneously improve with time. Treatment of CTEV is initially conservative with serial casting or strapping. Surgery in one form or another will be required in the majority of children, but this can range from either a simple Achilles' tenotomy under local anaesthetic to a more comprehensive release.

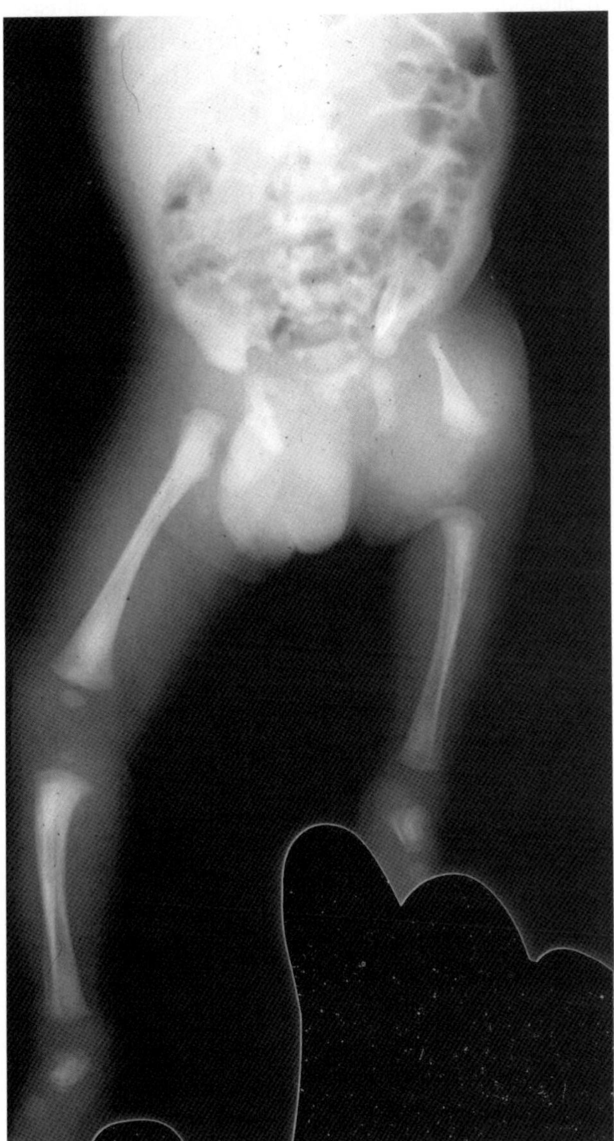

Figure 16.18 Congenital femoral deficiency. A radiograph of the lower limbs of a child with severe congenital short femur (proximal focal femoral deficiency). Note the abnormal hip joint on the affected side and the foot lying at the level of the contralateral knee. There would be a very high risk of complications during limb lengthening in this child. The child was managed with a prosthetic limb

Congenital convex pes valgus

Congenital convex pes valgus (congenital vertical talus) is much less common than CTEV. The clinical picture is quite different (Figure 16.20). The foot has been likened to a Persian slipper. The ankle is in equinus and the forefoot abducted and dorsiflexed. This deformity is usually associated with an underlying cause, such as neuromuscular condition or a chromosomal abnormality. Treatment is surgical.

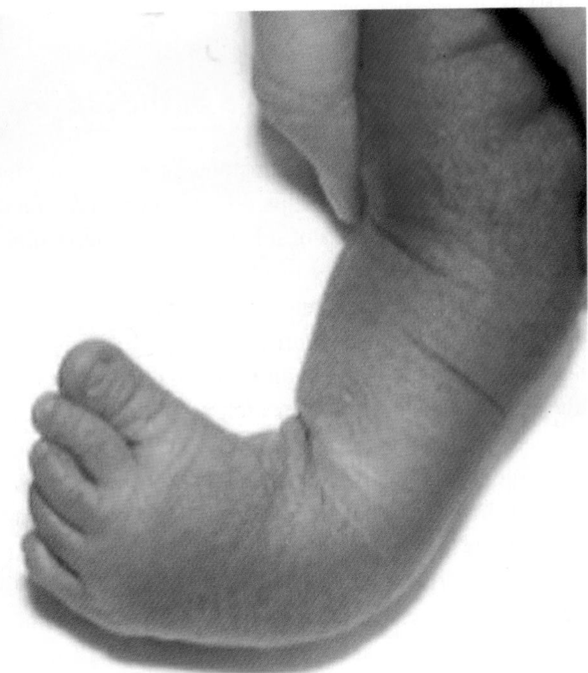

Figure 16.19 Typical congenital talipes equinovarus (CTEV). Photograph of atypical CTEV in which the hindfoot is fixed in equinus and varus. There is also forefoot adduction and cavus

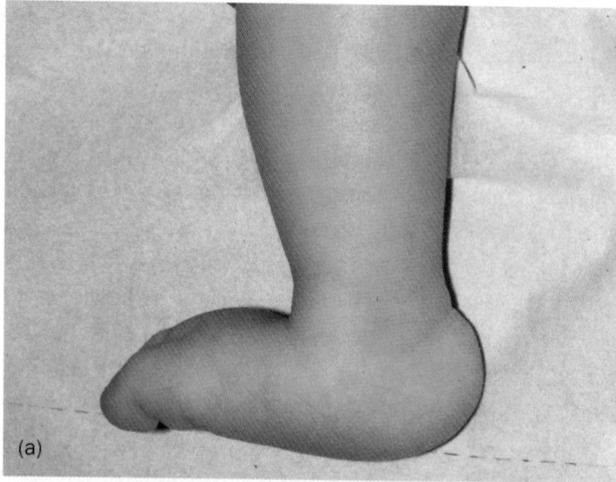

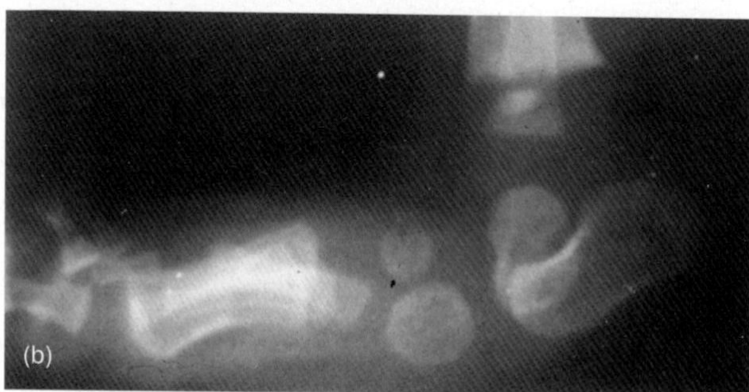

Figure 16.20 Congenital convex pes planus. This shows the clinical and radiographic appearances of CCPV (congenital vertical talus). Note the rocker bottom appearance of the sole of the foot. The radiograph shows that the calcaneus and talus are in equinus and the forefoot is dorsiflexed. The navicular (unossified) will be sitting on the dorsum of the talar neck

Developmental dysplasia of the hip

Some hips are dislocated or unstable at birth and some are dysplastic. Dysplastic hips do not have an adequate acetabulum and are at risk of subluxation. This recognition has prompted the change in the name of the condition from congenital dislocation of the hip to developmental dysplasia (or displacement) of the hip (DDH). It is important to differentiate between an unstable hip and a 'clicky' hip. The vast majority of clicks felt around the hip in the neonate are ligamentous in origin and are not associated with true instability. Instability means that there is movement of the femoral head in or out of the socket. Currently all neonates are screened for DDH by clinical examination before discharge from hospital. Dysplastic hips may be stable, which explains the increasing use of ultrasound as an adjunct to clinical examination. There is an intense debate on the most effective method for screening for DDH, ranging from ultrasound screening of all neonates to targeting only those at high risk. The aim of screening is to attempt to reduce the incidence of osteoarthritis of the hip secondary to dysplasia. Dysplasia and subluxation concentrate the forces across the hip joint over a smaller surface area, predisposing to osteoarthritis of the hip. Surgery aims to improve these mechanical disadvantages but residual dysplasia is common.

The prevalence of neonatal hip instability is thought to be 2 per cent at birth, however the majority stabilize within the first few weeks of life. The prevalence drops to 1.5 per 1000 at 2 months of age. DDH is commoner in girls. The risk is higher in children with a breech presentation after 35 weeks' gestation, in those with a foot deformity or congenital muscular torticollis, in those with a family history of DDH in a first degree relative and in those with oligohydramnios. Fixed prenatal hip dislocations are seen in neuromuscular conditions, but the majority of cases of DDH are not associated with other skeletal or visceral anomalies. Ligamentous laxity and position *in utero* are thought to be important aetiological factors.

Examination of the hip is part of the routine postnatal check. It is very difficult to elicit the signs of hip instability in a child who is not relaxed. The examination comprises two parts, Barlow test and Ortolani test. Both are performed with the child supine on a firm surface. The hips and knees are flexed to 90° and any difference in the length of the femurs noted. The examining hand is positioned with the thumb over the lesser trochanter and the middle finger over the greater trochanter (Figure 16.21). It is easier to examine one hip at a time and it may be useful to stabilize the pelvis with the other hand. The hip is abducted slightly and the thumb of the examining hand used to push the lesser trochanter posteriorly. This is known as the Barlow test and will identify a hip which is located, but can be dislocated posteriorly out of the socket. The Ortolani test involves gently abducting the hip. The middle finger is used as a 'watching finger'. If the hip is dislocated it will usually reduce on hip abduction. The middle finger will detect the movement anteriorly over the posterior rim of the socket. Neither of these tests is accompanied by an audible click – the word used by Ortolani to describe the sensation of movement experienced during his test has been translated into English as 'clunk'. This is misleading and accounts for the misconception that all 'clicky' hips are unstable – they are not.

Ultrasound is the most effective modality for identifying abnormal hips in the neonatal period and during the first three to four months of life. Radiographs are more useful thereafter (Figure 16.22). Traditionally all unstable hips were treated with an abduction orthosis from birth, but the natural history of the untreated condition is for the majority of unstable hips to become stable in a short period of time. Some clinicians therefore believe that it is acceptable to monitor unstable hips closely with clinical examination and ultrasound before implementing

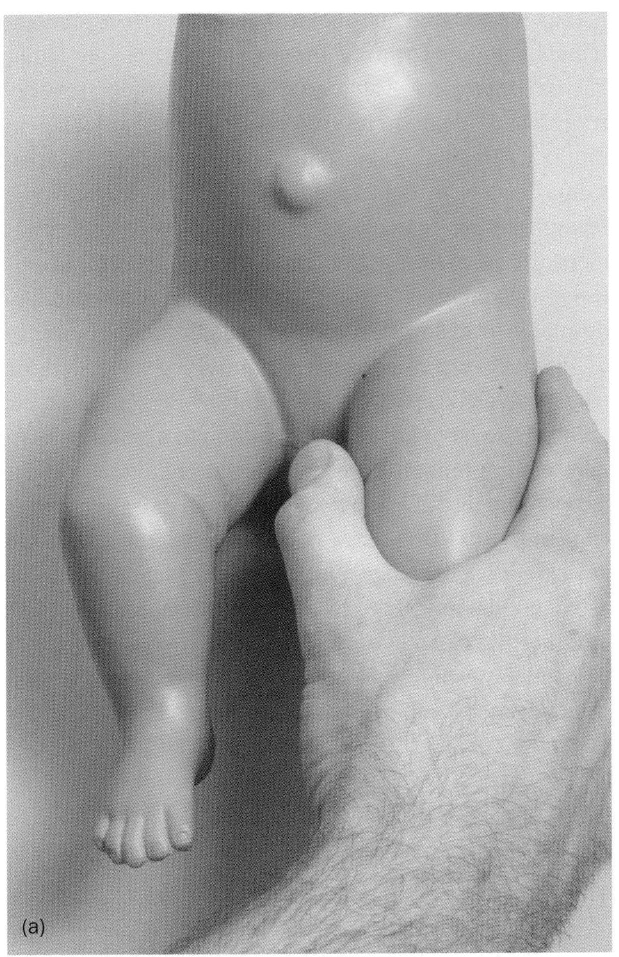

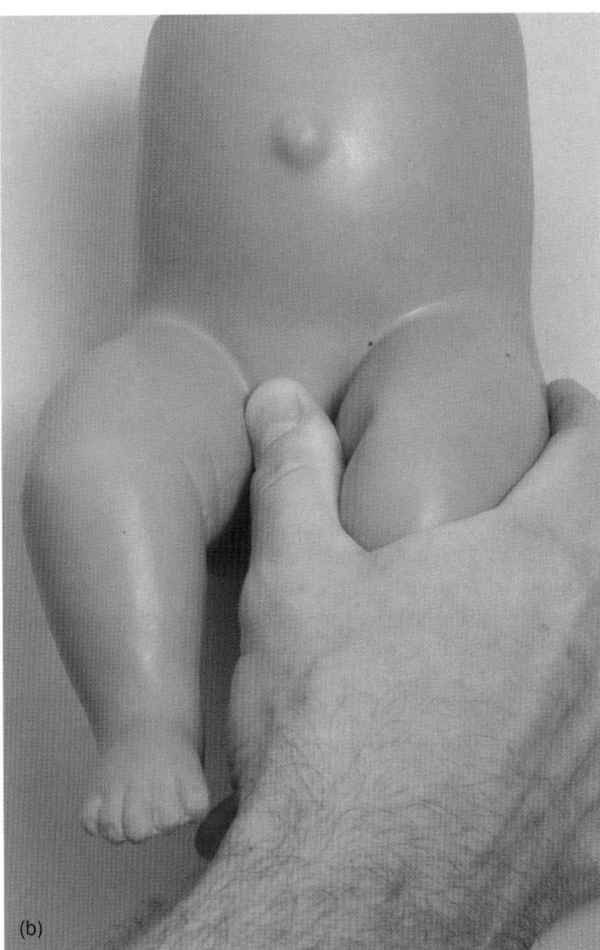

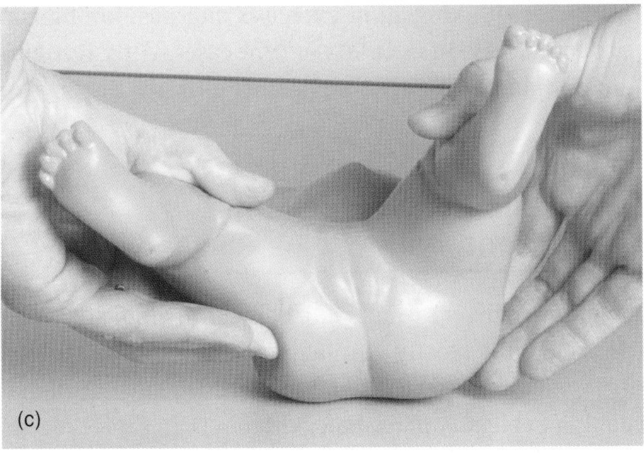

Figure 16.21 Examination for developmental dysplasia of the hip (DDH). The figure shows the examination for DDH on a training mannequin (Baby Hippy®). (a) The baby should be relaxed and examined on a firm surface. The hip and knee are flexed by the examiner. The index or middle finger is placed on the greater trochanter of the femur and the thumb over the lesser trochanter on the medial side of the thigh. (b) Barlow's manoeuvre involves pushing the femoral head posteriorly and feeling whether or not the femoral head moves posteriorly out of the socket. Ortolani's test is performed to demonstrate the reduction of a dislocated hip that occurs during hip abduction. The index or middle finger will feel the femoral head relocate with abduction (c)

treatment. Approximately 12 weeks of treatment with either the Pavlik harness or von Rosen splint is usually successful.

In the child over 3 months it is difficult to demonstrate hip instability. The most reliable signs of hip dysplasia or dislocation after this age are of restriction in the range of abduction at the hip and of shortening of the limb (Figure 16.23). Measuring leg lengths with a tape measure is very inaccurate and impractical in small children. Children presenting after walking will usually have a short leg gait. Walking at a normal age should not discourage investigation of DDH. Delay in walking because of DDH is only a matter of days, rather than months. Treatment of DDH is usually with simple abduction splints until the age of around 6 months of age when their use becomes impractical. Thereafter plasters are more appropriate. After the age of 1 year, open reduction is more likely to be required, with either femoral or pelvic surgery in addition.

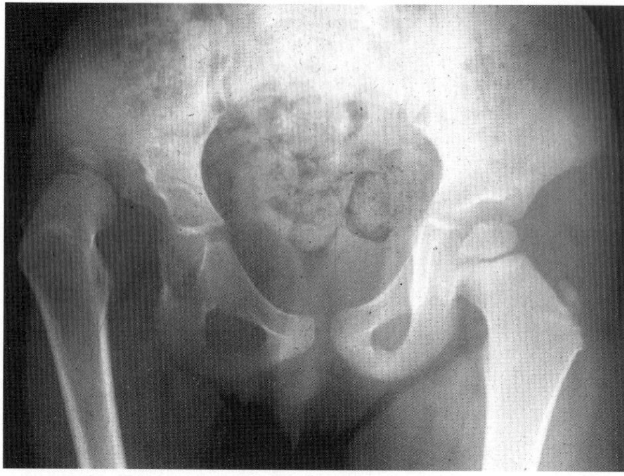

Figure 16.22 Imaging of developmental dysplasia of the hip (DDH) in a 3-year-old child. The radiograph shows the right femoral head lying out of the socket displaced posteriorly and superiorly

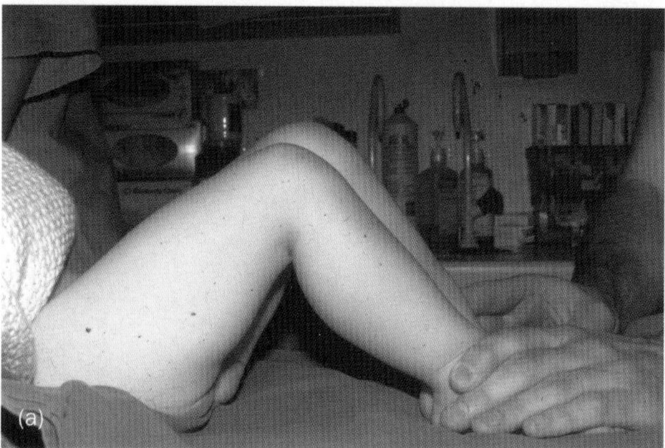

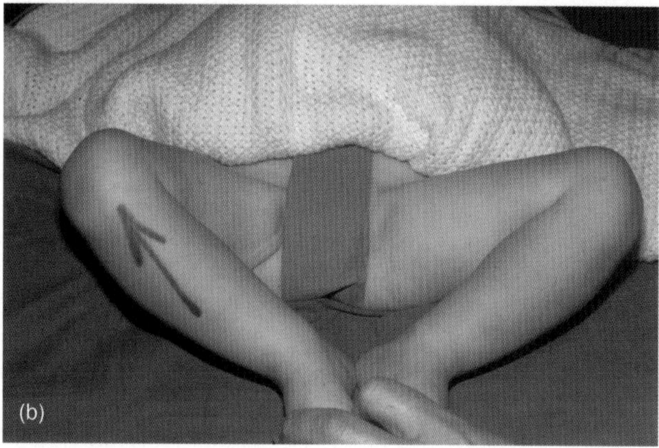

Figure 16.23 Developmental dysplasia of the hip in an older child. The clinical photographs show the leg length discrepancy (a) and restriction of abduction (b) seen in a child with a dislocated right hip. Examination of the limbs in this way with the child supine, the pelvis level and the hips and knees flexed, is a useful way to demonstrate a leg length discrepancy in a young child

Brachial plexus palsy

Erb palsy is the common term used for brachial plexus palsy (BPP), although strictly speaking this refers to a particular lesion affecting the upper part of the brachial plexus (C5/6). Brachial plexus palsy can affect predominately the upper trunks, the lower trunks or the whole plexus (Klumpke). The nerve lesions vary in severity from root avulsion to lesions 'in continuity' such as neurapraxia. Brachial plexus palsy is associated with macrosomia, maternal diabetes and difficult delivery. Prompt recognition of this condition is important so that treatment can be started early. This will help to prevent soft tissue contractures around the shoulder and secondary dysplasia or dislocation of the shoulder joint. The range of full recovery is between 50 and 95 per cent. Those who recover biceps function before 2–3 months of life are likely to have full function, although a small number may require tendon transfers later in childhood. Asymmetrical upper limb movements should raise the suspicion of a BPP. Other causes of pseudoparalysis should be carefully excluded, in particular septic arthritis, osteomyelitis anywhere in the upper limb, and fractures of either the clavicle or humerus. Early orthopaedic and physiotherapy referrals are required. Nerve conduction studies may be indicated at a later stage.

Torticollis

Congenital muscular torticollis is associated with a palpable 'tumour' in around half of the infants. It is important to reassure the family that this is not a neoplastic condition. The cause is poorly understood, but conservative treatment with stretching exercises and positioning can produce success in over 90 per cent cases. Early recognition and an experienced physiotherapist are the keys to success.

Metabolic bone disease in the preterm baby

Premature delivery results in a baby born at an age when the skeleton is mostly cartilaginous. Continuing skeletal ossification after birth depends on an adequate nutritional supply of calcium, phosphate, vitamin D and trace metals amongst other requirements. Nutritional intake is usually poor because of the problems associated with prematurity. Total parenteral nutrition (TPN) fluids do not contain enough calcium and phosphate to meet the high requirements of the rapidly growing preterm baby. Special preterm formula feeds and supplementation of breast milk and TPN fluids with extra calcium, phosphate and trace metals helps in reducing this problem. Impaired ability by the immature liver and kidney to hydroxylate vitamin D contributes to poor ossification and may be overcome by increasing the daily dose of vitamin D supplements to 800–1000 IU/day. Trace metals, especially copper, are needed for ossification. Copper reserves in the fetal liver are deposited between 28 and 32 weeks' gestation. Babies born before 28 weeks' gestation are likely to become copper deficient unless copper supplements are given in TPN and orally when tolerated. This helps prevent the osteopenia, fractures and radiological 'rickets-like' changes associated with copper deficiency. Dexamethasone and diuretic therapy in the treatment of chronic lung disease causes increased calcium loss from bone contributing to the osteopenia. Weekly measurements of calcium, phosphate, alkaline phosphatase and copper levels should be part of the routine monitoring of the extremely preterm baby.

KEY LEARNING POINTS

- Children with isolated deformities such as CTEV or a leg length discrepancy will walk. Minor abnormalities do not delay or significantly affect walking.
- The proportionate difference in limb lengths at birth remains constant throughout growth.
- Congenital convex pes valgus is usually associated with an underlying cause such as a neuromuscular or genetic condition.
- Most clicks felt around the hip in the neonate are ligamentous and not associated with true instability.
- Practise and experience in hip examination in the neonate is essential to recognize true DDH.
- To identify DDH ultrasound is the preferred imaging up to the age of 3–4 months, thereafter radiographs.
- Prompt recognition of Erb palsy is important to improve prognosis.

PSYCHOLOGICAL

Non-organic musculoskeletal pains

In children, pain without an organic cause is a common problem. It should not be dismissed. Particular skill is required to make the diagnosis confidently without perpetuating a never-ending search for an organic cause. The diagnosis should be conveyed to the family without the loss of face on the child's behalf. A management plan with appropriate expectations of the outcome should be prepared. In many of these children the search for a diagnosis goes on for a long time, and they have huge disability and miss out on schooling and social development. Doctors hide behind a plethora of names, but fail to give these children a way to get better 'with grace'. The first step is to recognize the distinct clinical features of these syndromes.

Localized idiopathic pain syndrome

This is also known as reflex sympathetic dystrophy, reflex neurovascular dystrophy, algodystrophy, complex regional pain syndrome types I and II, Sudeck atrophy, shoulder-hand syndrome, traumatic angiospasm, algoneurodystrophy, causalgia, etc. There is typically a history of remembered or supposed trauma. Typically, the pain is not severe at the time of the incident, but becomes so with time (hours/days). Colour and temperature changes occur. The affected limb becomes purple and cool to the touch. The limb may become oedematous. The pain increases until the patient develops allodynia (pain due to a stimulus that does not normally cause pain, e.g. gently stroking the limb, the draft from the door, inability to tolerate the bedclothes at night). There may be non-organic features such as inability to cut fingernails because the nails hurt. The patients describe the pain as excruciating. The child becomes unable to dress and cannot attend school. Painkillers have no effect and immobilization by plaster casts or splints exacerbate the problem. The affected limb is held immobile and nursed. The patient may be hypervigilant, describing in laborious detail the variation of the pain in the limb often with complex drawings (with no anatomical basis), or detailed descriptions/diaries.

Pain amplification syndromes

Again, several names have been applied to these conditions, and the name may reflect the predominant symptom, e.g. musculoskeletal pain and fibromyalgia, tired all the time, myalgic encephalomyelitis. Typically these children have disturbed sleep, fibromyalgia trigger sites, and features of pain with characteristic features as in the local pain syndromes. These children often have other related conditions such as irritable bowel, tension headaches either concurrently or in the past history. There are often features of anxiety and depression. Occasionally there may be a previous history of severe illness, such as a now treated malignancy. Pain syndromes often occur in conjunction with chronic disease such as diabetes or arthritis. There may be an important perpetuating psychological event, such as physical or sexual abuse, or unhappiness about areas such as parental tensions, or the death of a favourite pet, but a psychological event is not invariable.

Management of pain syndromes

Make the diagnosis, and stop investigating. Ongoing investigations suggest a degree of uncertainty in the doctor's mind. The patient should be confident that the doctor believes and understands the extent of the pain. Dismissing the symptoms as psychological or of no serious organic cause perpetuates the problem. Explanation as to how pain can exist without an organic cause is important. A graded exercise programme and graded reintroduction to school are all critical. A skilled physiotherapist is invaluable in providing a programme supporting recovery. A psychologist's input is valuable, offering techniques such as cognitive behavioural therapy, advice on sleep hygiene and relaxation techniques. The team should offer a programme of care allowing the child to control the pain, regain their mobility, self-confidence and dignity.

KEY LEARNING POINTS

- Making a confident, non-judgemental diagnosis without perpetuating the search for an organic cause is key.
- It is vital to learn the features of these conditions so that the diagnosis is made by recognition of the features, rather than reached by exclusion of multiple possible diagnoses. If there is an important differential diagnosis to be excluded all investigations should be completed before embarking on a management plan.
- These conditions are better managed by physiotherapists and psychologists rather than by doctors with a medical model of illness. A supported graded programme of recovery should be offered.

COMMON SCENARIOS

The approach to the child with a limp

Acute onset of limp has a significant organic cause until proved otherwise (Figure 16.24). A proper history and full examination are mandatory. In a child with a limp

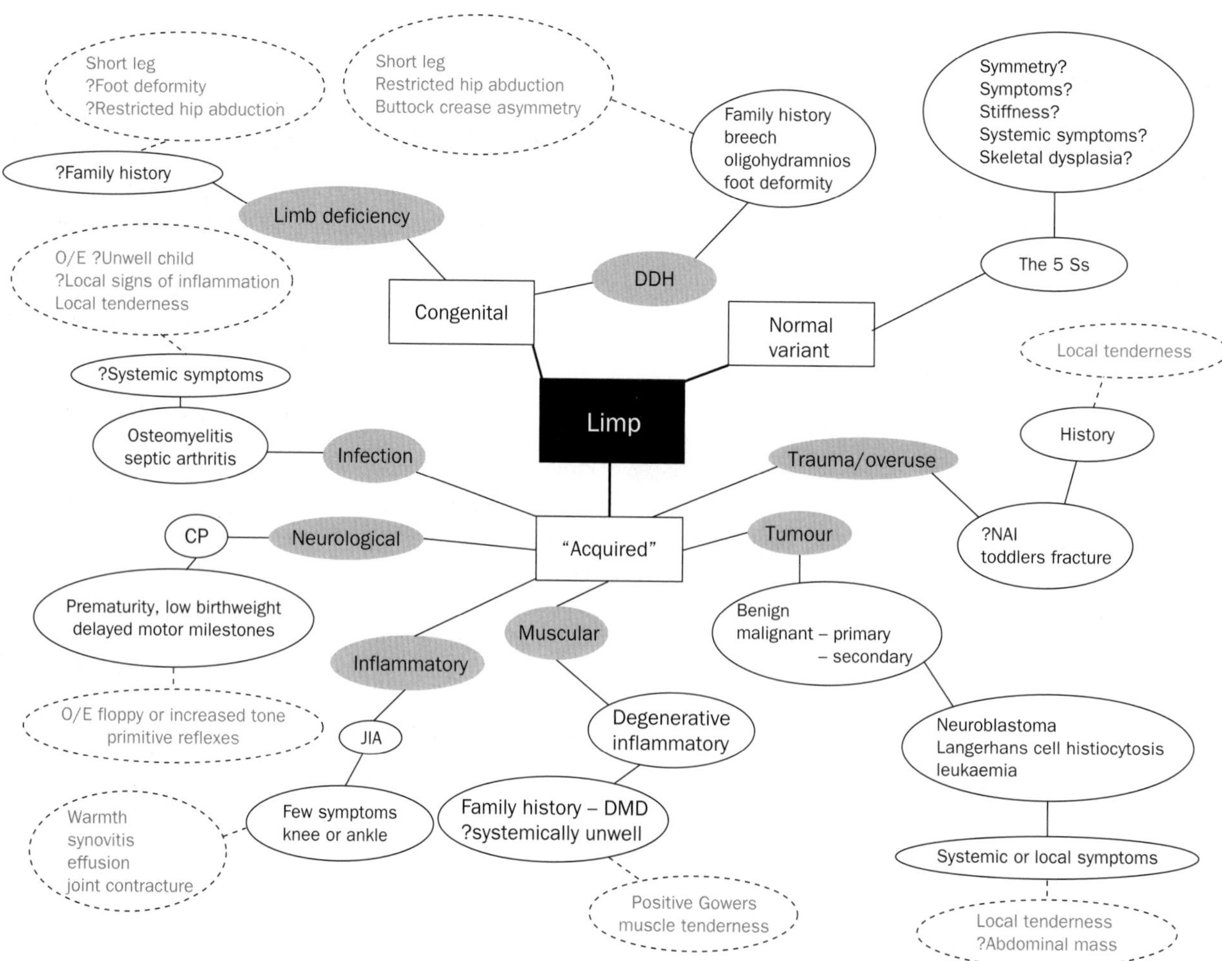

Figure 16.24 Differential diagnosis of a child with a limp

exclusion of pathology in the foot (ingrowing toenail, dactylitis and trauma, enthesitis), ankle, knee, and hip as well as the long bones is essential for tenderness and swelling. The spine should be examined for normal posture, movement and for areas of tenderness. Intra-abdominal, pelvic and retroperitoneal pathology should also be considered. Warning signs that should alert the physician to the likelihood of important underlying pathology are:

- a young child
- night pain associated with a daytime limp
- limitation of movement of joints or abnormalities of movement such as Trendelenburg gait
- systemic features.

Investigations which may be helpful include:

- Radiographs
- Bone scintigraphy
- MRI
- Full blood count and ESR.

Approach to back pain in children and adolescents

There is a high prevalence of non-specific back pain in children in different studies suggesting the presence of a demonstrable cause in between 50 and 85 per cent of cases. In adolescents most back pain is due to poor posture and prolonged sitting in one position such as slumped in front of the television or video game console. However, more serious causes of backache should always be excluded.

A proper history and full examination are mandatory in the assessment of a child with back pain. There are seven important warning signs that should alert the doctor to the likelihood of important underlying pathology. These are:

- a child under 4 years of age
- back pain causing functional disability and persisting at night
- pain causing the child to miss out on sports/enjoyed activities
- pain lasting longer than 4 weeks
- postural shift of the trunk due to splinting of the back to decrease the pain
- limitation of motion due to pain
- neurological abnormalities.

Useful investigations in a child with back pain include:

- Full blood count
- ESR
- Blood culture
- HLA-B27
- Plain radiograph of spine
- MRI of spine
- Radioisotope scan.

KEY LEARNING POINTS

- Back pain and/or a limp in a *young* child have an organic cause until proved otherwise.
- Examination skills, which are maintained by regular practise, are critical in recognizing musculoskeletal pathology and normality in the child.
- Remember the life-threatening differential diagnoses of malignancy and non-accidental injury in the differential diagnosis of the child with a musculoskeletal presentation.

FURTHER READING

Benson MKD, Fixsen JA, Macnicol MF (2001) *Children's Orthopaedics and Fractures*, 2nd edn. Edinburgh: Churchill Livingtone.

Cassidy J, Petty R (1995) *Textbook of Pediatric Rheumatology*, 3rd edn. Philadelphia: WB Saunders.

Isenberg DA, Miller JJ (1999) *Adolescent Rheumatology*. London: Martin Dunitz Ltd.

Maddison P, Isenberg DA, Woo P, Glass DN (1998) *Oxford Textbook of Rheumatology*. 2nd edn. Oxford: Oxford University Press.

Lightman S, Towler HMA (1998) *Fundamentals of Clinical Ophthalmology: Uveitis*. London: BMJ Books.

Southwood TR, Malleson P (1993) *Arthritis in Children and Adolescents*. London: Bailliére Tindall.

Chapter 17

Paediatric ophthalmology

William Newman

The visual system is a highly complex structure, all parts of which are susceptible to disorder or disease. The cornea and lens focus the visual scene on the retina. The image is clearest in the centre (the fovea) and is less clear towards the periphery. There are many millions of photoreceptors. The cones serve day and colour vision and are most tightly packed in the centre but are present throughout the retina. The rods become sensitive under darkened conditions and serve night vision that is less clear and has no colour. The image data are passed via bipolar cells to the ganglion cell fibres that pass down the optic nerves to synapse in the lateral geniculate bodies. There are approximately 1.2 million fibres in each optic nerve. The optic nerves fibres from the nasal retina (serving temporal visual field) cross at the optic chiasm, and the optic tracts thereafter contain the information from one hemifield (the left optic tract and beyond subserves the right hemifield and the right side the left hemifield). The tracts pass to the lateral geniculate body and from there to the visual cortex in the posterior occipital lobes. The upper fibres passing over the top of the lateral ventricles serve the lower visual fields. The lower fibres, which loop into the temporal lobes around the lateral horns of the lateral ventricles, serve the upper visual fields.

Basic image analysis takes place in the occipital lobes. The temporal lobes serve the function of recognition, route finding and visual memory. The pathway between the occipital lobes and the temporal lobes is known as the ventral stream. The posterior parietal lobes analyse the visual scene and accord attention to objects of interest. They plot the coordinates of the object of interest, passing the data to the motor cortices to facilitate accurate movement of the body through three-dimensional visual space. The pathway between the occipital lobes and the parietal lobes is known as the dorsal stream.

EMBRYOLOGY OF THE EYE AND ASSOCIATED DISORDERS

A clear idea of the development of the eye and visual pathway helps in the understanding of congenital and associated systemic disorders.

Embryological development

The development of the eye begins at day 22 *in utero* with the optic sulci appearing as pits in the inner aspect of the neural plate. The sulci invaginate to form the hollow optic vesicles. The cavity of the optic vesicle, which goes on to form the subretinal space, is continuous with the future third ventricle via the lumen in the optic stalk. At this critical point, the optic vesicle transforms by invagination to become a goblet-shaped optic cup. The thickened retinal disc and the lens placode also invaginate by day 29. By day 36, the lens vesicle separates from the surface ectoderm, and lens epithelial cells enclose the lens cavity, which is surrounded by a basal lamina that later forms the lens capsule. At day 39, a wave of mesenchyme passes over the rim of the optic cup giving rise to the corneal endothelium, corneal stroma, the iris stroma and iridocorneal angle.

The invagination process leaves a temporary longitudinal fissure extending from the optic fissure into the optic stalk. It is through this that the hyaloid artery, a branch of the ophthalmic artery, gains access to the retrolenticular space. By about day 44 the growing edges of the fissure meet and start to fuse in the mid optic stalk progressing proximally and distally. The completed distal margins will form the aperture of the pupil. The proximal end of the fusion represents the entry point of the hyaloid vessels, which become the central retinal vasculature. By this point, the embryo is 30 mm in length and the developing eye is about 2 mm in diameter.

Retinal development comprises synapse formation by 4–5 months, photoreceptor outer segment by month 5 and retinal vasculature development between 16 weeks and birth. From this brief description of the ocular development, it can be seen that an insult at a particular time can result in specific defects, some of which are described below.

Congenital malformations

Anophthalmia

Anophthalmia (absent eye) results from failure of optic vesicle formation.

Microphthalmia

In microphthalmia (macroscopically small eye), there is formation of the optic vesicle but subsequent development is incomplete.

Coloboma

Coloboma is a notch, break or fissure in an ophthalmic structure and is due to a defect of closure of the embryonic fissure of the eye in the fifth week of intrauterine development. This lies inferonasally and is usually where the defect lies. The lesion varies from a small defect in the posterior retina causing a chorioretinal defect (which may not affect vision) to one that includes all the tissues along the fissure. The latter results in a chorioretinal defect and may also involve the optic nerve posteriorly and the lens and iris structures anteriorly. Commonly the iris is underdeveloped inferiorly giving rise to a slit-like pupil. If the chorioretinal defect affects the macular or there is significant involvement of the optic nerve then there may be consequent visual impairment and associated nystagmus. Colobomas may be associated with many chromosomal and developmental abnormalities. It is important to examine the parents as it is also found as an autosomal dominant trait.

The CHARGE syndrome is a multiorgan disorder comprising: *c*oloboma, *h*eart disease, *a*tresia choanae, *g*enital hypoplasia and *e*ar malformation.

Morning glory syndrome

Morning glory syndrome is an axial defect of the distal optic stalk as it meets with the optic vesicle and is a large excavation defect of the optic disc. Importantly, it is associated with basal encephalocele and midline and facial abnormalities.

Lens

The lens is particularly vulnerable to intrauterine insults such as rubella that cause cataract and a salt and pepper retinopathy. Abnormalities of lens development may give rise to small or round lenses, colobomatous defects and anterior or posterior bulges (lenticonus) of the lens or cataract.

Persistent hyperplastic primary vitreous

Besides defects of fusion of developing intraocular structures there may be disorders of regression. Persistent hyperplastic primary vitreous (PHPV) results from persistent embryonic fibrovascular tissue. This draws the ciliary processes inwards so they become visible. It is usually associated with cataract. The presence of the retrolental mass gives rise to a white pupil (leukocoria) and is a differential diagnosis of retinoblastoma. Ultrasound examination, however, shows the pathology to be anterior to the retina.

Aniridia

This condition comprises a macroscopically absent iris and is usually bilateral. It may occur sporadically or be inherited in an autosomal dominant fashion for which a defect has been found in the PAX6 gene on chromosome 11. This gene is responsible for various inductive interactions during development of the ocular structures. As a result, there may be associated abnormalities of the lens, including cataract, dislocation of the lens and abnormal optic discs and foveae. Patients often have nystagmus, photophobia and poor vision and go on to develop glaucoma in 50–75 per cent of cases. As the children get older, they may suffer a corneal epithelial keratopathy, which can prove difficult to treat.

The deletion on chromosome 11 in sporadic aniridia is larger than that of familial aniridia and may encompass the Wilms tumour locus, resulting in the association of nephroblastoma (Wilms tumour) in up to a third of cases of sporadic aniridia. These children need to undergo DNA analysis to seek the deletion of the Wilms tumour locus.

Congenital glaucoma

Congenital glaucoma is due to disorganization of the drainage angle during development and includes the persistence of a membrane (Barkan membrane) over the inner surface of the drainage angle. This is treated by dividing the membrane surgically (goniotomy or trabeculotomy).

Congenital nasolacrimal duct obstruction

Canalization of the solid columns of cells near the lacrimal sac takes place at about 3 months *in utero*. However, a membrane may persist at the lower end of the lacrimal sac at birth giving rise to epiphora. Most cases clear spontaneously during the first 12 months of life. Probing of the nasolacrimal duct is carried out in those cases which persist.

Table 17.1 Genetic disorders involving ocular defects

Autosomal dominant	Autosomal recessive	X-linked	Other
Corneal dystrophies	Corneal dystrophy (macular)	Norrie disease	Leber's hereditary optic neuropathy (mitochondrial inheritance)
Marfan syndrome	Homocystinuria	Incontinentia pigmenti	Myopathies (Kearns-Sayre syndrome) (mitochondrial inheritance)
Ehlers-Danlos syndrome	Sulphite oxidase deficiency	Juvenile retinoschisis	Retinoblastoma (13q14) (RB1 tumour suppressor gene)
Aniridia	Hyperlysinaemia	Retinitis pigmentosa	
Congenital cataract	Familial ectopia lentis	Albinism	
Myotonic dystrophy	Anterior lenticonus	Choroideraemia	
Colobomata	Congenital cataract		
Myelinated nerve fibres	Oculocutaneous albinism		
Stickler syndrome	Goldmann-Favre disease		
Tritanope colour blind	Retinitis pigmentosa		
Retinitis pigmentosa	Stargardt disease		
Best viteliform dystrophy	Fundus flavimaculatus		
	Gyrate atrophy		
	Neimann-Pick disease		
	Metachromatic leucodystrophy		
	Tay-Sachs disease		
	Mucopolysaccharidoses		

GENETICS

It is important to realize that many ocular defects have a genetic basis (Table 17.1). Many of the inborn errors of metabolism present with ocular signs and symptoms – some examples are given below.

Inborn errors of metabolism

Optic atrophy associated with progressive loss of vision:

- Batten disease
- Canavan disease
- Cockayne syndrome
- Tay–Sachs disease
- Leber hereditary optic neuropathy

Corneal opacity causing progressive reduction in the clarity of vision:

- Fabry disease
- Mucopolysaccharidoses

Lens subluxation (displacement) predisposing to dislocation:

- Homocystinuria
- Marfan syndrome
- Sulphite oxidase deficiency

Glaucoma:

- Mucopolysaccharidoses

Pigmentary retinopathy:

- Abetalipoproteinaemia
- Batten disease
- Hurler syndrome

Cherry red spot at the macula due to intracellular deposit of GM2 ganglioside:

- Tay–Sachs disease

Ptosis:

- Kearns–Sayre syndrome

Cataract:

- Galactosaemia
- Galactokinase deficiency
- Hypocalcaemia
- Cockayne syndrome
- Lowe syndrome

Abnormal eye movements:

- Niemann–Pick disease type C
- Gaucher disease
- Canavan disease

DEVELOPMENT OF THE EYE AND VISUAL SYSTEM

For a clear image to be focused on the retina, the ocular medium must be transparent with no obstruction to the visual axis and the retina must be fully formed. The focusing power of the cornea and intraocular lens needs to be closely calibrated to the length of the eyeball for the image to be brought into focus on the retina. If the refractive power of either the cornea or the lens is too high or the length of the eye is too short then the image is projected 'behind' the retina and the eye is long sighted or hypermetropic. Most infants and young children are mildly long sighted (+2 D with a standard deviation of 2 D) but they compensate for this by accommodation, which increases the focusing power of the lens inside the eye. To correct hypermetropia convex (or positive) lenses (which magnify the eye) are worn. When the cornea/lens combination is too powerful or the length of the eye too long, the image falls in front of the retina and the eye is myopic or short sighted. The concave (negative) lenses worn to correct myopia make the eye look smaller.

KEY LEARNING POINTS

Summary of normal visual development:

- 0–2 weeks: acuity 6/400–6/60; behaviour – limited visual attention, inaccurate fixation, immature pursuit eye movements.
- 2–6 weeks: acuity 6/180–6/45; behaviour – attentive to faces, pursuit and oculokinetic eye movements developing.
- 6–12 weeks: acuity 6/130–6/24; behaviour – good central fixation and ocular alignment, accurate smooth pursuit.
- 6 months and over: acuity 6/90–6/9; behaviour – reaches for toys, accurate saccades and pursuit, stereopsis developing.

CLINICAL EXAMINATION

The history

- Clinical features seen by the parents, i.e. what was the first thing the parents thought was wrong and has there been any change in these features since they were first noticed?
  - Visual behaviour
  - Abnormal wobbly eye movements
  - Squint (ensure that the parents understand what you mean, i.e. a 'turn' in the eye)
  - Dislike of the light/dark
  - Watery eye
    - Does anything improve or make the abnormality worse?
- What do the parents think the child can see?
- How is the child progressing in comparison with his or her peers?
- General health
- Medication
- Any family history of eye problems or other problems?
- Antenatal and birth history
- Are the parents related?

Appearance

The assessment of visual function begins with the child entering the room and should be initially directed towards observation looking for:

- dysmorphic features
- appearance of eye lids, telecanthus, epicanthal folds or ptosis, and the alignment of the eyes
- epiphora
- photophobia.

The child's initial visual behaviour

This of course varies with the age of the patients – from observing the babe in arms looking at the carer's face to a toddler playing with toys or a teenager looking at objects around the room.

Red reflex

The red reflex can be elicited by using an ophthalmoscope with the lens set at zero and at a distance of a few feet in a dim room.

Testing for ocular alignment (squint)

Corneal reflex

Shine the torch light from about a metre and observe the central corneal reflexes, which are normally just nasal to the centre of the cornea (Figure 17.1). In the squinting eye, the reflex will either be more temporal as in a convergent squint or more nasal as in a divergent one.

Cover test

This is an extension of testing corneal reflexes. With the child looking at the light the eye that is thought to be

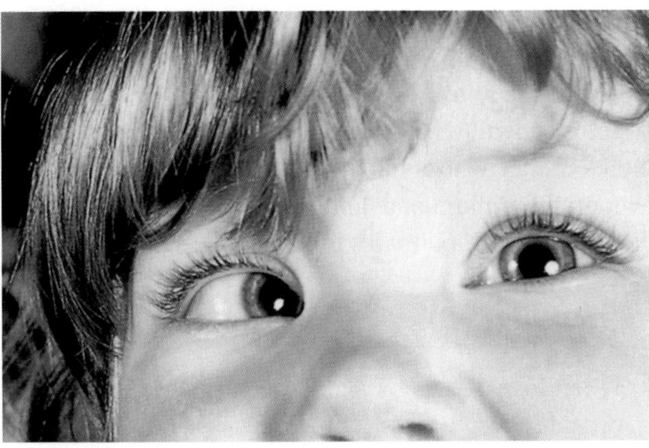

Figure 17.1 Corneal light reflections in squint (from Cockburn F, Carachi R, Goel, NK, Young DG (eds) *Children's Medicine and Surgery*. London: Arnold)

fixing on the target (and looking straight) is covered while you look at the eye you think is squinting. You are looking to see if there is any movement of that eye to take up fixation. If the eye moves outwards there is a convergent squint; if it moves inwards there is a divergent squint. If it does not move, there is probably no squint or the eye does not see. As the child gets older and more cooperative, the light is replaced by the use of fixation targets both at distance and near.

KEY LEARNING POINT

The combination of clear, bright and equal red reflexes with central corneal reflexes and no eye movement during the cover test suggests that there is no significant refractive error, no squint and no opacity within the optics of the eye. This information can be obtained quickly with the use of a direct ophthalmoscope.

Visual acuity

The visual acuity is a measure of the resolution of the visual system measured at maximum contrast (black on white). It is a robust measure of the smallest high contrast target that can be seen. Different methods are used at different ages.

Preferential looking (0–2 years)

This method is used in preverbal children and relies on the observation that infants will preferentially look at a patterned object rather than a blank stimulus. Large grey cards that have a patterned stimulus on one side and blank on the other with a central peep hole are usually used.

The principle is to present the cards to the children starting with larger targets sequentially getting smaller. The cards are presented at differing orientations, the examiner watching to see where the child looks. If the child looks (moves the eyes to take up fixation) in the correct direction for three out of four presentations the next smallest size is used.

Picture matching and naming (2–4 years)

An example of this is the Kay picture test, a flip book of 25 isolated line pictures. There are versions for 3 m or 6 m testing and a matching chart, so if the child cannot or will not verbalize the name of the target they can point to it on the matching chart.

Snellen and LogMAR acuities

The standard visual acuity chart is the Snellen chart. The size of the letters becomes progressively smaller further down the chart, and each line is labelled with a number. The lowest line that can be seen is the visual acuity expressed as a fraction. The denominator (lower number) corresponds to the number associated with the lowest line read on the chart (and is the distance at which the letter subtends five minutes of arc at the eye). The numerator (upper number) denotes the distance between the patient and the chart (usually 6 m). The fractions are usually expressed in metres (e.g. 6/18) or in feet (e.g. 20/60).

The spacing between the letters varies with each line and the decrease in the size of the letters from line to line is not uniform. These problems are addressed by the use of LogMAR acuity charts or cards; however, the recording of acuity is different in that it is the *log* of the *min*imum *a*ngle of *r*esolution.

Colour vision

The most commonly used test of colour vision is the Ishihara colour test. The Ishihara colour plates were designed to detect congenital red-green colour blindness, which occurs in about 6 per cent of white males.

Visual fields

Assessment of the visual field is possible without the use of complex equipment, and although limited to the detection of gross field defects it may be carried out in young children.

In infants, the examiner sits in front of them and a second examiner introduces a bright object from behind into the infant's visual field. The point at which the infant initiates a saccade or head movement to look at the object is the point at which the edge of the visual field is. Similarly, this can be done with a small white ball on the end of a black stick in older children. As cooperation improves, finger matching techniques can be used progressing to direct confrontation techniques using a small ball on a stick target and asking the child to indicate when the ball is seen.

Binocular testing is effective if the visual field defect is homonymous but not otherwise. By about the age of 6 years many children will be able to perform formal Goldmann perimetry.

Pupillary examination

In the first few months of life, the infant tends to have small pupils that are minimally responsive to light. It is not unusual to have a small degree of difference in pupillary diameter (anisocoria). Abnormalities of pupillary reaction are difficult to interpret in infants as accurate assessment requires accurate fixation because of the relation between convergence and miosis. Thus although testing for a light reaction and near reaction may be easily done, testing for a relative afferent pupillary response is much more difficult.

Swinging flashlight test

The patient looks at a distant target. A bright light is shone from below at one pupil and then briskly moved to the other pupil. On moving the light from the first pupil both pupils start to dilate, which is reversed when the fellow pupil is illuminated. Unilateral or asymmetrical optic nerve pathology results in both pupils dilating instead of constricting when the affected side is illuminated.

There is no anisocoria when there is a relative afferent pupillary defect (RAPD), and no RAPD in the presence of anisocoria unless there is additional pathology of the afferent visual pathway.

Ophthalmoscopy

Ophthalmoscopy presents a particular challenge, as proximity to the child is required, along with shining a bright light, which the child almost invariably will look at directly, and they will have a small pupil. It is considerably easier if the pupil is dilated (cyclopentolate 0.5 per cent and phenylephrine 2.5 per cent).

You need to be proficient at examining an adult with the direct ophthalmoscope before starting on a child. The approach varies depending on age, but creating some sort of game usually helps: 'Let's see what you had for breakfast.'

Start with the ophthalmoscope lens set at zero and the illumination set at about 50 per cent; some children will tolerate the red-free light (the green filter) better. Children commonly look directly at the light giving you a view of the fovea. To view the optic disc an interesting target is shown to the other eye of the child from behind the examiner who approaches the eye to be examined temporally to illuminate and visualize the optic disc and then follow the landmarks of the retinal vessels.

KEY LEARNING POINTS

When investigating visual problems always consider:

- detailed history
- visual acuity/behaviour
- colour vision
- pupil responses
- visual fields
- eye movements
- examination of the eye.

INVESTIGATIONS

Electrophysiology

Electrophysiological testing of the retina and afferent visual pathway can be helpful in making a diagnosis and in objectively estimating visual acuity. The adoption of the correct testing protocol necessitates knowledge of the suspected pathology.

The visual evoked potential

The visual evoked potential (VEP) is a measure of neuronal activity extending from the ganglion cells in the retina through the optic nerve chiasm to the primary visual cortex. The main uses in children are to check the integrity of the visual pathway and to give an objective estimate of visual acuity. This has the advantage of requiring little cooperation from the child, and neonates can be tested in this way. This is a useful test in the apparently blind baby who is not fixing and following when a VEP shows a good response which matures with time, indicating that one can be cautiously optimistic that the diagnosis will be delayed visual maturation.

The electroretinogram

The electroretinogram (ERG) tests the aggregate electrical response of the retina to a stimulus. It is a useful test in the investigation of visual loss in the presence of a normal looking retina. Most retinal dystrophies show abnormality of both rod and cone responses. However, some show specific defects such as in achromatopsia (rod monochromatism), where the cone response is absent, or congenital stationary night blindness, in which the rod response is abnormal.

In visual loss for which there is no anatomically demonstrable cause on clinical examination, electroretinography detects retinal pathology and the VEP detects visual pathway pathology. If both are normal, disturbances of the higher visual pathways or functional visual impairment are suspected.

KEY LEARNING POINTS

- The VEP is essentially a test of the visual pathway and is particularly affected by intrinsic disease of the optic nerve.
- The ERG is a test of retinal function.

Ultrasound

Ultrasound examination of the eye is non-invasive and is particularly helpful in a number of situations.

- When there is no view of fundus, due to opacity in the visual pathway, to exclude any posterior segment abnormality such as retinal detachment or intraocular tumour.
- To study the structure, blood flow and echogenicity of an intraocular mass (e.g. the echo patterns of calcification are indicative of retinoblastoma).
- In the setting of a suspected swollen optic disc, examination of the nerve head can be carried out to exclude buried optic nerve head drusen.
- To measure optic nerve sheath diameter in suspected intracranial hypertension, when the nerve sheath is dilated.
- In proptosis or suspected orbital mass, the delineation of the mass (if it is in the anterior orbit or just behind the globe), its position, structure and any internal blood flow can be ascertained.

Neuroradiology

The decision about which is the most appropriate imaging should be taken in conjunction with the radiologist.

Indications for computed tomography (CT) and magnetic resonance imaging (MRI)

CT scanning

- Proptosis
- Orbital cellulitis (bone involvement, subperiosteal abscesses)
- Optic nerve tumour (calcification in meningiomata)
- Orbital tumours
- Orbital bone pathology/fractures

MRI

- Pituitary/parasellar tumours
- Midline abnormalities in optic nerve hypoplasia
- Cerebral visual impairment

KEY LEARNING POINTS

- Ultrasound is a very useful and non-invasive investigation when an opacity precludes a view of the retina.
- When requesting MRI and CT, make sure the radiologist is aware what you are looking for – if possible discuss your requirements first.

SCREENING FOR DISEASE

Postnatal check

The purpose of postnatal screening is to look for any obvious morphological abnormalities of the eyes and surrounding tissues and to check for the presence of a red reflex in each eye. If there is any significant abnormality, in particular, an abnormal red reflex, the neonate should be referred urgently as the abnormal red reflex may indicate opacity in the eye such as retinoblastoma or cataract.

Universal visual screening

The most appropriate time for universal screening of vision and the detection of squint and amblyopia is between 4 and 5 years of age. The purpose is to check vision and detect, investigate and treat any squint or amblyopia.

The tests should include the minimum of:

- observation of appearance, including head postures
- test uniocular vision
- perform a cover test
- test ocular movements.

Table 17.2 Opthalmological disorders required specific screening

Disorder	Problem	Criteria for screening
Retinopathy of prematurity	Untreated – retinal detachment	Birth weight of less than 1500 g or 31 or less weeks' gestational age
Retinoblastoma	Inherited nature of bilateral (and to a much lesser extent) unilateral retinoblastoma	Screening under anaesthetic at 3-monthly intervals until the results of chromosomal analysis are available, and continued if the child has the RB1 gene until the age of about 5 years
Juvenile idiopathic arthritis	Visual loss from cataract, glaucoma, band keratopathy and maculopathy in asymptomatic iritis	Risk is assessed on the basis of the number of joints, time of onset and the result of the antinuclear antibody test (see Table 17.2)
Diabetes mellitus	Asymptomatic retinopathy	Starting at puberty, annual dilated funduscopy
von Hippel-Landau disease siblings	This is an genetic condition, the gene being located on chromosome 3. Early diagnosis reduces morbidity and mortality from haemangioblastomas and renal cell carcinoma	The Cambridge protocol includes annual dilated funduscopy from the age of 5 years

Table 17.3 Targeted screening for children with juvenile idiopathic arthritis (JIA)

Risk group	Criteria	Review periods
High risk	Early-onset pauciarticular disease – Antinuclear antibody (ANA) positive	3-monthly review for one year
		6-monthly review for five years Annual review thereafter
Medium risk	Pauciarticular disease – ANA negative Polyarticular disease – ANA positive	6-monthly review for five years Annual review thereafter
Low risk	Systemic JIA, B27-associated JIA, disease starting after the age of 11 years	Annual review

Targeted screening

Children at a high risk of ophthalmic disease or visual disability either because of a genetic predisposition, such as congenital nystagmus, cataract or retinitis pigmentosa, or a morphological abnormality, such as craniofacial disorders (hydrocephalus) or neurological disorders (neurodegenerative diseases) should be assessed. Some disorders require specific screening (Table 17.2).

KEY LEARNING POINT

Uveitis is common in juvenile idiopathic arthritis and may be asymptomatic; therefore children should be screened (Table 17.3).

PARTICULAR PROBLEMS

The problems in this section relate to the consideration of differential diagnoses of a specific sign or symptom rather than a particular disease.

The apparently blind infant

CASE STUDY

A 4-month-old baby boy has been referred because the health visitor has noticed that the infant does not appear to fix or follow, although his parents think he does look, for instance, look around when they enter a room. There is no relevant past medical or family history. On examination there are random eye movements, he does not consistently fix and follow a bright light. The pupils are sluggish to respond to a light. Examination of the optic discs reveals that they are very small, hypoplastic, exhibiting the double ring sign.

The diagnosis is likely to be optic nerve hypoplasia. The infant should have electrodiagnostic testing (VEP), an MRI to look for associated midline abnormalities (septum pellucidum, ectopic posterior pituitary) and should be referred for a neuroendocrine assessment for associated pituitary/hypothalamic defects. This child is likely to have severe visual impairment and a sensitive but realistic approach needs to be taken with the parents.

Babies do not all fix and follow at birth, but by about 6 weeks they have at least started to do so. Concern is usually registered by the parents or health visitor that the baby is not fixing and following, attentive to faces, or making visually appropriate behaviour. There are several differential diagnoses, as bilateral deficit of the optics of the eye, the eyes themselves, the neurological visual pathway or the motor pathways to the extraocular muscles may give rise to the appearance of visual inattention. It is important to distinguish those who have severe visual impairment from those who, while they exhibit blind behaviour, in fact have a remedial or treatable cause such as bilateral cataract and those with delayed visual maturation or saccadic initiation failure who will develop visual behaviour subsequently.

In the absence of specific clues to suggest a genetic or perinatal cause, one should systematically examine the eyes.

- Abnormal eye movements
  - Head thrusts – saccadic initiation failure
  - Nystagmus – primary or secondary to ocular disease
    - pendular – albinism/aniridia/achromatopsia/optic nerve hypoplasia
    - searching – optic nerve hypoplasia/Leber congenital amaurosis
- Morphologically abnormal eyes
  - Small eye (microphthalmos)
  - Corneal opacity
  - Abnormal iris
    - Iris transilluminates – albinism
    - Absent – aniridia
- White pupil
  - Cataract
  - PHPV
  - Retinopathy of prematurity
  - Retinoblastoma
- Pupillary responses
  - Bilateral sluggish response – prechiasmal disease (optic nerve or retinal disease)
  - Relative afferent pupillary defect – asymmetric retinal or optic nerve disease
- Cycloplegic retinoscopy
  - High refractive error, myopic or hypermetropic
- Vitreous opacity
  - PHPV
  - Retinopathy of prematurity
  - Retinoblastoma
  - Haemorrhage
- Optic disc
  - Large defect in disc
  - Coloboma
  - Small with double ring sign – optic nerve hypoplasia
- Macula
  - Very light pigmentation – albinism
  - Large defect – coloboma
  - Retinal folds – congenital/retinopathy of prematurity (Figures 17.2 and 17.3)
  - Mass/tumour – retinoblastoma
- No abnormality of the eye
  - Delayed visual maturation
  - Saccadic initiation failure
  - Leber congenital amaurosis
  - Retinal cone/rod dystrophy
  - Cerebral abnormalities – developmental and acquired such as perinatal anoxia/haemorrhage/meningitis/hydrocephalus

In the absence of an abnormality of the eyes (including cycloplegic refraction) or neurology, the investigation should proceed to electrophysiological studies (Table 17.4)

The visually impaired child

CASE STUDY

A 12-year-old girl attending the local special school has a principal diagnosis of spastic cerebral palsy. Because of her problems with mobility and speech she is considered to be intellectually slow. She had never been seen by an optician or by an ophthalmologist. She attended with her five siblings, because there was a suspicion of autosomal dominant hereditary optic neuropathy in her father and one of her brothers. Indeed, not only did she have signs of optic neuropathy, but she also had significant astigmatism and refractive error. She was prescribed appropriate spectacles and low vision aids and registered partially sighted.

> **KEY LEARNING POINT**
>
> Children with other handicaps can be difficult to assess but this should be done as such children have a higher incidence of strabismus, refractive errors and other significant ocular problems.

Effects of visual impairment on development

Severe visual impairment has a profound effect on general development. Lack of sight means that the child is not rewarded by the parents' smiles or body language and equally the parents do not have the reward of the child's smile, as the child cannot mimic what is not seen. The process of seeing, touching and understanding is disrupted. Head control is poor at birth, and while there is motivation and feedback that the child wishes to raise the head to see, this mechanism is lacking in visually impaired children. The result is delayed motor development. The lack of visual feedback impedes language development. These problems become more profound when there are associated neurological abnormalities and, in particular, if there is associated deafness.

- Circadian rhythms are often abnormal in those who are completely blind. This can be very disruptive as

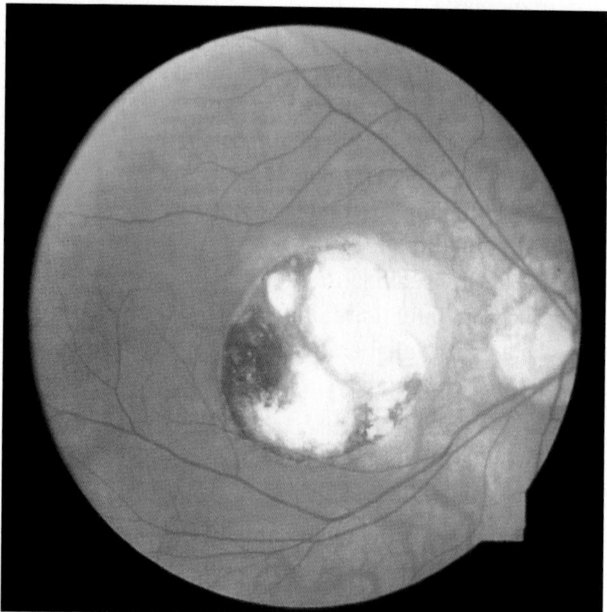

Figure 17.2 Retinopathy of prematurity in a preterm baby (from Cockburn F, Carachi R, Goel, NK, Young DG (eds) (1996) *Children's Medicine and Surgery*. London: Arnold)

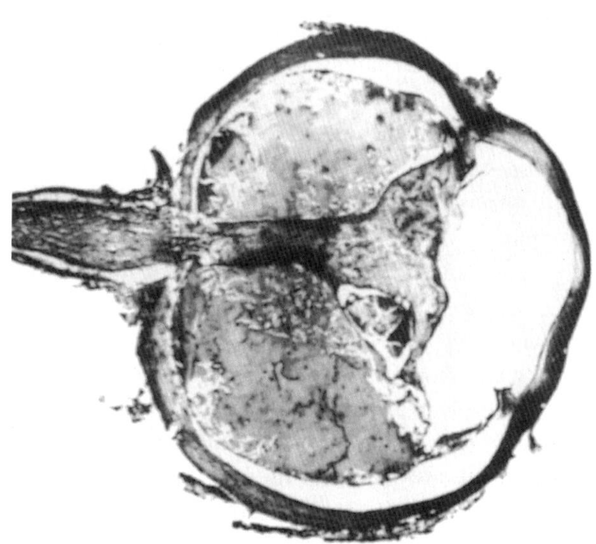

Figure 17.3 Complete retinal detachment in fully established retrolental fibroplasia (from Cockburn F, Carachi R, Goel, NK, Young DG (eds) (1996) *Children's Medicine and Surgery*. London: Arnold)

Table 17.4 Electrophysiological studies in the apparently blind infant

Disorder	Electroretinography	Flash visual evoked potential	Pattern visual evoked potential	Imaging
Delayed visual maturation	Normal	Normal	Normal	Normal
Saccadic initiation failure (includes oculomotor apraxia, cogans oculomotor apraxia)	Normal	Normal	Normal	Normal
Leber congenital amaurosis	Abnormal/absent	Abnormal	Absent	Normal
Achromatopsia	Abnormal, absent flicker response	Abnormal	Abnormal	Normal/not indicated
Congenital stationary night blindness	Abnormal, reduced scotopic B wave	Abnormal	Abnormal	Normal/not indicated
Optic nerve hypoplasia	Normal	Abnormal	Abnormal	Check for midline abnormalities
Cerebral visual impairment	Normal	Abnormal	Abnormal	Abnormal

sleep patterns are not normal. Treatment with melatonin may have a role.

- Poverty of facial expression. Explain to parents – bonding and later social interaction (analogy of a monotonic voice).
- No visual memory and difficulty mapping surroundings/permanence/perspective.
- Disturbing habits such as eye poking, looking into bright (warm) lights, rocking.

KEY LEARNING POINTS

- The diagnosis of visual impairment is devastating for both the child and the parents.
- Make sure both the parents and the child understand what you have told them.
- Support this with appropriate documentation, and appropriate local support from the general practitioner, Royal National Institute of the Blind, local sensory service and the community paediatric vision team.
- Children should be referred for a full developmental assessment.

The needs of visually impaired children

ASSESSMENT

Visual acuity is a measure of the threshold of the limit of vision. In visually impaired children, however, this measure may be somewhat artificial and a measure of their functional ability is required.

Vision is required for communication, access to information and mobility. The assessment should address the following list starting with the question: How well do the parents think their child can see? The response often generates a wealth of useful information and allows you to fill in the gaps with questions directed towards:

- Depending on age, the size and types of toys, books, size of print the child uses. This gives an idea of functional vision.
- The distance at which the child can recognize people and interpret facial expression.
- Can the child see better for near which is usually the case as the objects are visually enlarged by proximity (which can be the case when the macula is damaged)?
- Specific problems related to light or dark (suggestive of a retinal dystrophy or pigmentary disorder such as albinism) that need to be identified.
- Any problems with navigation around either a floor or a room. Bumping into things that may be on one side or another is suggestive of a visual field defect.
  - There is no point in presenting material of any size or using a low vision aid in the area of the visual field deficit, it still will not be seen.
- Spatial awareness, problems with stairs, steps or kerbs or flat floor interfaces, which are due to disorders or central processing or inferior visual field defects.
- Problems picking out faces in a crowd or objects from a toy box, facial recognition, or problems with moving objects. These all suggest a cognitive visual processing problem.

Further assessment with refraction funduscopy, assessment of ocular motility, electrophysiology and neurodevelopmental assessment are all helpful towards building up a picture of the child's abilities and assessment of educational needs.

Environment

MOBILITY

A safe environment is required with clear paths and no obstructions. Where stairs are encountered, for instance at school, these may require banisters and assistants and that the child learns the routine routes between classes. Depending on the level of visual impairment, stairs may be brightly coloured or doors for specific rooms or drawers may be of specific colours, patterns or marks. It is often helpful to have door frames and changes in the direction of corridors marked with high contrast to the background to facilitate navigation. This gives greater independence and builds self-confidence.

PRESENTATION OF INFORMATION

Clear, enlarged, high-contrast information is presented under good illumination with little glare. Visual acuity is a measure of the smallest print that can be read. This is not the same as the size that is comfortable to read, which is several point sizes larger. It is this latter size that should be determined for the purposes of schooling.

Although this concept may be obvious with print, it is often forgotten when presenting pictures. There is more information in terms of colours and the details of the picture may be smaller than can be seen, e.g. a clock face may be large but the numbers may be too small to be seen.

LIGHTING

This needs to be assessed on an individual basis and depends on the underlying disorder. It is wise to avoid lighting from the front, which may increase glare, and look for task-orientated lighting that is uniform. Increased illumination may help with optic nerve disorders but probably may need to be reduced for retinal disorders with cone dysfunction.

Low vision aids

Low vision aids (LVAs) magnify the size of the object being viewed at the expense of reducing the visual field (e.g. magnifying a word at the expense of being to see the whole line). Each child requires individual assessment by an appropriately trained individual, often an optometrist. There should be a clear understanding of the objective of the LVA, how large the object needs to be magnified for easy viewing and at what distance the objects are, e.g. reading a textbook or reading the 'blackboard'. Children often do not want to use a LVA as they do not want to be different from others.

The four main types of visual aids

Simple magnifiers: magnifier; bar magnifier

- Usually handheld or on a stand which is placed close to the object being viewed, usually print
- Helpful for reading but not for writing (cannot get under the magnifier)
- Portable, relatively easy to use and cheap

Telescopes

- May be handheld or more commonly incorporated into spectacles (like surgical operating loupes)
- Can be modified for distance or near, no problem with writing, but mobility with them on is difficult
- Portable, not as easy to use, more expensive
- They can feel uncomfortable because of the weight and draw attention to the child.

Close circuit television (CCTV)

- Fixed, variable magnification, which may be adjusted for distance, more usually near
- Excellent for reading, can manipulate background, contrast and brightness
- Expensive, not portable

Computer

- Teaching material and books produced in electronic format
- Able to change type size, foreground/background colour, automated presentation for more fluent reading
- Moderately expensive, can be portable, but often limited to material specifically produced for the system

Education

There is no universal recommendation based on any particular ocular disease or acuity level, as the visual disability is very variable within a population with the same disorder and acuity. Education provision should be based on assessment as outlined above as part of a multidisciplinary approach from all the professionals involved. To this end one of the most important aspects is communication between the team, the parents and the child. With appropriate support, many visually impaired children progress well at mainstream schools whereas others benefit from attending schools for the visually impaired.

KEY LEARNING POINTS

- Registration as visually impaired: this can only be done by a consultant ophthalmologist.
- Registration is based on the best corrected visual acuity with both eyes open.
- Partial sight registration is considered if the visual acuity is less than 6/18.
- Blind registration is considered if the visual acuity is 3/60 or worse.
- One is not considered significantly visually impaired if there is sight in one eye.

Failing vision in a school-age child

CASE STUDY

Two children present: a 5-year-old who fails the school eye test and an 11-year-old who has been having problems seeing the classroom blackboard. The local optometrist finds a variable response to a formal sight test with a vision of about 6/24 in both that he is unable to improve. He arranges to see them again to perform a cycloplegic refraction. This reveals that they both have significant refractive errors, and when appropriate glasses were prescribed, both children's vision improved significantly.

Younger children often fail the school eye test because they are long sighted (hyperopic). Children who are short sighted are often identified when they start high school and require good distant acuity.

In children of school age who are failing due to visual problems it is important to obtain a clear history from the child and parents, including a full family history, and try to determine if the visual loss is acquired or congenital and if only recently noticed.

KEY LEARNING POINT

In unilateral visual loss, it is more usual to notice a squint, or the failure of an eye test at school, and it would be unusual to present with failing 'vision'. This usually occurs only in disorders that affect the visual pathway bilaterally. The children often overcome such difficulties and only complain of problems or start being noticed to have problems at school when the second eye becomes significantly involved.

Examination

- Visual acuity
  - Distance/near/colour (each eye separately and both eyes together)
- Pupil responses
- Visual fields
- Ocular movement
  - Nystagmus
- Proptosis
- Refraction
  - High myopia/hypermetropia/astigmatism

In the presence of a normal examination then the differential diagnosis is between

- Retinal dystrophy
- Cerebral visual impairment
- Functional visual loss

Further investigations may be required such as:

- VEP
- ERG
- MRI

The red eye

CASE STUDY

An 18-month-old infant presented with a red right eye with a watery discharge. There was a history of a previous mild chemical injury (kitchen cleaner) to the same eye a month previously, from which, according to the hospital, he had recovered completely. He had been started on chloramphenicol, but this had been changed to gentamicin due to failure to improve. The infant now will not open his eye.

Two weeks of antibiotics would usually resolve most bacterial conjunctivitis, and in any case most bacterial and viral causes of conjunctivitis are self-limiting and would have started to improve. Bacterial causes are usually bilateral viral may remain unilateral – thus the antibiotics are not really helping. Trying to swab the conjunctiva would not be helpful while on the antibiotics, and would probably be difficult to do. Indeed both chloramphenicol and gentamicin can cause allergy and can be toxic to the ocular surface. One should stop all topical therapy for 48 hours and review.

CASE STUDY (continued)

After 48 hours of stopping all topical therapy, there was no improvement and the eye was examined under anaesthetic. This revealed a dendritic ulcer and a swab confirmed herpes simplex virus-type infection. The symptoms resolved after 10 days of topical aciclovir eye ointment.

Equally the examination could have revealed:

- Uveitis
- Foreign body under the eye lid
- Retinoblastoma.

KEY LEARNING POINT

If conjunctivitis does not settle after seven days of antibiotics do not just change to a more toxic preparation – consider an alternative diagnosis. Stop all topical therapy for at least 24 hours before taking a swab.

Conjunctiva

Disorders affecting the conjunctiva

Infection

- Ophthalmia neonatorum
- Bacterial
- Chlamydial
- Viral

Inflammation

- Blepharoconjunctivitis
- Trauma
- Foreign body

- Chemical
- Nasolacrimal duct obstruction
- Allergic eye disease
- Molluscum contagiosum

Acute oedema

- Acute urticarial response

Ophthalmia neonatorum

True ophthalmia neonatorum is unusual, that is neonatal conjunctivitis with redness, oedema and discharge at birth acquired from the maternal genital tract. The principal organisms to consider are *Neisseria gonorrhoeae*, *Chlamydia* and herpes simplex virus. The most serious is *Neisseria* as the organism can produce proteases that may penetrate intact corneal epithelial cells and cause corneal ulceration in the absence of trauma in an otherwise healthy eye. Chlamydial infection is commoner and is important to identify as the baby may go on to develop associated pneumonia.

DIAGNOSIS

It is not possible to distinguish the organism from the appearance of the conjunctivae and swabs in the appropriate medium should be taken for culture and sensitivity and for polymerase chain reaction (PCR) techniques for chlamydia and herpes. In babies with positive results, arrangements should be made for screening the parents.

KEY LEARNING POINT

Ophthalmia neonatorum from herpesvirus, *Neisseria* or *Chlamydia* is usually acquired from a pre-existing maternal genital infection. Parents should be advised to attend for screening and treatment for themselves.

Bilateral purulent conjunctivitis

In older children most infections are either bacterial in origin (*Haemophilus* and *Pneumococcus* are the commonest) or viral, which are self-limiting. A culture is required for severe cases and topical treatment may be administered such as chloramphenicol. Gentamicin and the fluoroquinolones are less commonly used.

Unilateral conjunctivitis

This is commonly due to a viral infection such as adenovirus (8, 11, 19). It is easily transmitted and may spread through nursery and school communities. Children should avoid contact for about 14 days. Most episodes are self-limiting and require no treatment. In severe infections, vision may be reduced because of infiltrates in the cornea and problems because of the formation of membranes particularly on the tarsal conjunctiva.

Herpes simplex

Primary herpes simplex can affect one eye with an associated skin eruption on the eyelids and preauricular and submandibular lymphadenopathy. Recurrent infection tends to affect the cornea. Treatment if required is with topical antiviral agents (e.g. aciclovir), particularly if there is involvement of the cornea with a dendritic ulcer.

Allergic eye disease

ACUTE ALLERGY

This is due to a type I hypersensitivity reaction, often occurring in children and young adults when they encounter an antigen to which they have become sensitized. This group often also exhibits signs and symptoms of atopy. The symptoms vary from a sudden onset of unilateral marked conjunctival chemosis associated with itching, a watering eye and eyelid oedema, which comes on acutely and then starts to resolve over the next four hours, resolving by the next day.

SEASONAL ALLERGIC CONJUNCTIVITIS

Hay fever presents with mild-to-moderate itching and some redness and watering of the eyes associated with high pollen counts. Pre-emptive treatment with topical mast cell stabilizing agents, such as sodium cromoglicate, used regularly whether symptomatic or not during the known problem period may reduce the symptoms. In the more severe and chronic form, often known as **vernal or atopic keratoconjunctivitis**, children may develop chronic redness with thickening of the eyelid tissues and the formation of large conjunctival papillae and chronic stringy mucous discharge from the tarsal conjunctiva. This causes severe itching, and the lid changes cause a partial ptosis. This may progress to involve the cornea, usually its superior half (i.e. the part in close proximity to the upper eye lid) causing a keratitis and sometimes severe ulceration.

STEVENS–JOHNSON SYNDROME (ERYTHEMA MULTIFORME MAJOR)

This acute necrotizing vasculitis associated with immune complex deposition occurs in otherwise healthy children following exposure to a trigger factor, which may be a drug such as the sulphonamides or infections like herpes simplex, but often no precipitating factor is identified.

The rash lesions are described as 'target lesions' as they are bullous areas into which a central haemorrhage has occurred. They appear in crops. The mucous membranes of the mouth and the conjunctiva are affected. This results in ulceration, secondary infection, and later severe scarring and foreshortening of the conjunctiva resulting in a mechanical in-turning of the lashes and lid margin with secondary exposure and damage to the cornea. Treatment in the acute event is multidisciplinary (in conjunction with paediatricians, dermatologists and ophthalmologists) with ocular lubricants, systemic steroids, prevention of secondary infection and possibly the use of large bandage contact lenses to protect the cornea.

Abnormalities of the red reflex

CASE STUDY

A 4-year-old girl was brought in by her mum because she had noticed that the child had a white pupil on the right. Mum mentioned that three months earlier she had noticed that she had a white pupil in a photograph but had not thought it important. On examination, the right pupil was obviously white, middilated and unresponsive. There was a right relative afferent pupil defect. The child was fractious and uncooperative with examination of the eye. However, she did cooperate with an ocular ultrasound that revealed the vitreous cavity was filled with a mass that was highly reflective and solid. This is consistent with a diagnosis of retinoblastoma.

A white pupil is never normal, and implies significant pathology with obstruction of the visual axis and reflection of the light by abnormal tissues. It is always associated with reduction in vision in the affected eye. The red reflex can be elicited by using an ophthalmoscope with the lens set at zero and at a distance of a few feet in a dim room. With the illumination at about 50 per cent, direct the illumination towards the child so both eyes are within the cone of the illumination from the ophthalmoscope. One should then see a red reflex bilaterally through the ophthalmoscope.

The white pupil, called leukocoria, is usually obvious to the examiner, or becomes obvious when testing for the red reflex. The cause is an obstruction to the visual axis, which when light is reflected from it causes a white/ dull reflection, or a defect in the normal retina revealing the underlying white sclera causing the same. It is important to exclude retinoblastoma or any other treatable condition.

If there is no view of the fundus due to opacity, an ultrasound should be carried out to reveal the nature and location of the opacity. Ultrasound is very good at delineating the anatomy of the eye, particularly in terms of PHPV behind the lens, retinal detachment, areas of high reflectivity within a mass suggesting calcification and thus the diagnosis of retinoblastoma. Where there are multiple abnormalities such as cataract and retinal/cerebral dysfunction it is useful to obtain an ERG and VEPs to ensure there is realistic possibility of visual improvement before embarking on surgery.

Sequence of examination:

- Red reflex
- Pupil responses
- Dilated funduscopy with examination of lens, vitreous and retina
- Ultrasound
- CT scan

Possible abnormalities:

- Lens
  - Cataract (Figure 17.4)
  - PHPV
  - Vitreoretinal abnormality
  - Retinal detachment
    - Retinopathy of prematurity
    - Coats disease
  - Retinal haemorrhage
  - Endophthalmitis
- Retinal mass
  - Retinoblastoma
  - Toxocariasis
- Retina
  - Myelinated nerve fibres
- Chorioretinal abnormality
  - Coloboma
  - Toxoplasmosis (Figure 17.5).

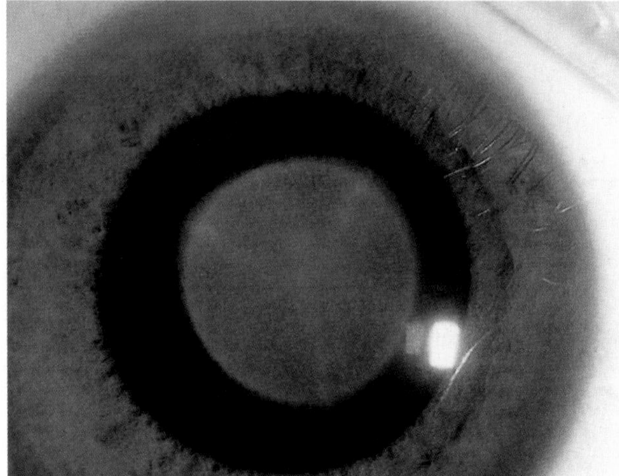

Figure 17.4 Congenital cataract (from Cockburn F, Carachi R, Goel, NK, Young DG (eds) (1996) *Children's Medicine and Surgery*. London: Arnold)

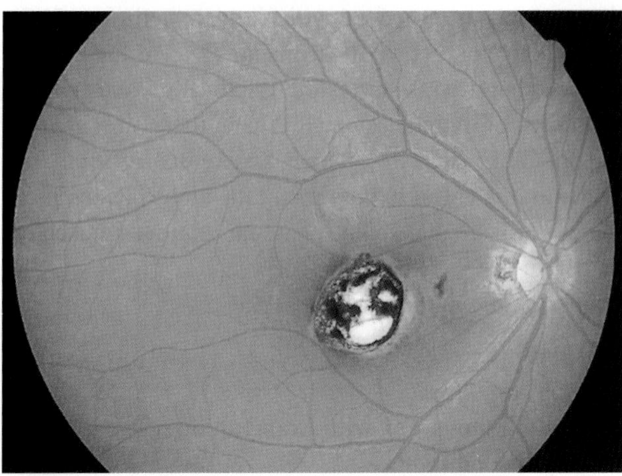

Figure 17.5 Choroidoretinitis caused by *Toxoplasma* (from Cockburn F, Carachi R, Goel, NK, Young DG (eds) (1996) *Children's Medicine and Surgery*. London: Arnold)

KEY LEARNING POINTS

Features of the red reflex

Normal red reflex
- No nystagmus (nystagmus is easily seen in this manner).
- An equal red reflex and corneal reflex suggests that the eyes are aligned.

A uniformly present but dull reflex
- Bilateral cataracts.
- High refractive error in both eyes.

Normal red reflex in one eye and dull reflex in the other
- The eye with the dull reflex is not fixing and has a squint.
- The eye with the dull reflex has a high refractive error.
- Unilateral cataract in the eye with the dull reflex.

Absent red reflex
- Anterior segment opacity such as corneal scar or hyphaema.
- Cataract; PHPV.
- Vitreous opacity from haemorrhage or retinoblastoma (Figure 17.6).
- Reduced reflex due to retinal detachment or retinopathy of prematurity.

White reflex (leukocoria)
- Anterior eye: cataract; PHPV.
- Mass in the vitreous: retinoblastoma; toxocariasis.
- Coloboma: exudative vitreoretinopathy; retinal detachment (retinopathy of prematurity).

The appearance of the red reflex forms the basis on which photoscreening is undertaken.

The swollen optic disc

CASE STUDY

A 14-year-old girl while in Canada developed a febrile illness associated with a headache, lethargy and weakness. She was admitted with weakness and swollen optic discs. It was considered that she might have had a demyelinating episode and consideration was given to treating her with intravenous methylprednisolone. However, she had a distance acuity of 6/5 each eye, N5 for near with both eyes, she managed to read all the Ishihara colour plates and visual field testing revealed an enlarged blind spot. Careful review of the history revealed that when she got up quickly or bent over she had a visual disturbance (obscuration). Examination revealed brisk pupil responses and bilateral disc swelling with no obvious spontaneous venous pulsation. MRI showed no evidence of demyelination and lumbar puncture confirmed a raised opening pressure. Her symptoms settled without treatment over the next 10 days. Her optic discs and visual fields returned to normal over three weeks.

In optic neuritis the vision is nearly always reduced in particular colour vision, and there is a central scotoma, in comparison with raised intracranial pressure where acuity is not affected, colour testing is normal and there is an enlarged blind spot on visual field testing.

Papilloedema

The term papilloedema is reserved for bilateral pathological swelling of the optic discs due to raised intracranial pressure. There is oedematous swelling of the discs with local capillary dilation and obscuration of some of the vessels by the axonal oedema, and splinter haemorrhages at the disc margins. The normal spontaneous venous pulsations are absent. In children, the commonest cause is hydrocephalus, an intracranial mass or idiopathic intracranial hypertension (IHH, formerly known as benign

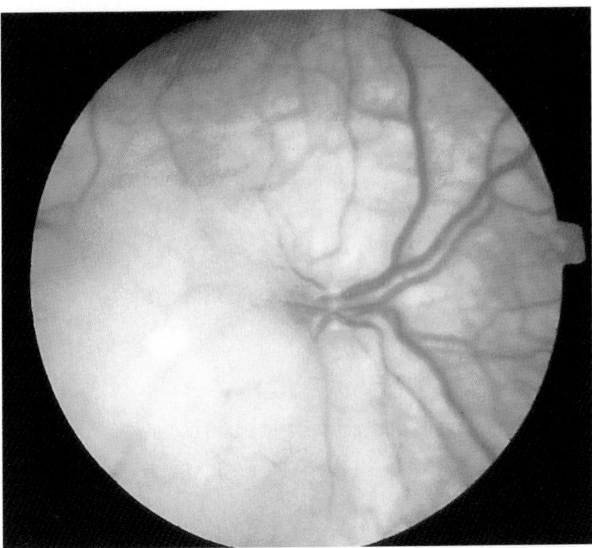

Figure 17.6 Retinoblastoma (from Cockburn F, Carachi R, Goel NK, Young DG (eds) (1996) *Children's Medicine and Surgery*. London: Arnold)

intracranial hypertension (BIH)). In older children, visual disturbances in the form of transient visual loss when bending down or coughing (called obscurations) may be noted. On visual field testing the blind spot is enlarged and there is peripheral visual field constriction; central vision is not affected until late. The abducent nerves (VI cranial nerves) may be damaged as a result of raised intracranial pressure resulting in a convergent squint.

Chronic disc oedema may result in secondary optic atrophy and visual loss.

Optic neuritis and retrobulbar neuritis

This may be post-infectious and presents with a rapid decline in visual acuity, which may be down to perception of light unilaterally or bilaterally over a period of a few days. There is usually an associated relative afferent pupil defect and in optic neuritis disc swelling is usually found. Visual evoked potentials show reduced amplitudes and delayed latencies. Visual recovery is the norm but takes a few weeks and it is not unusual to find secondary optic atrophy developing. In the majority of children no underlying systemic abnormality is found and recurrence is unusual.

Apparent optic disc swelling

The optic disc may look swollen because of anatomical variation, that is the disc is small and crowded and is elevated and lacks the normal physiological cup, but there is no oedema or vascular change or visual deficit. Intrinsic abnormalities of the disc such as optic disc drusen may give a similar appearance and with time the glistening drusen become visible. There is no treatment for drusen, which may cause progressive visual field defects in adulthood. Diagnosis is by ultrasound of the optic nerve head, demonstrating highly reflective bodies within the optic nerve head at low gain.

KEY LEARNING POINTS

Papilloedema
- Oedema of the disc with vascular changes and disc haemorrhages.
- Good vision with enlarged blind spot and peripheral visual field constriction.
- Progressive in the absence of treatment with enlarging blind spot and reducing peripheral field, and finally central field loss with reduction in visual acuity.

Optic neuritis
- Oedema of the disc with vascular changes.
- Poor vision with central visual field loss.
- Vision usually improves within six weeks, although optic atrophy may develop.

Apparent optic disc swelling
- Elevated small disc, absent cup, no vascular changes.
- Good vision, usually no visual field loss.
- No change on serial observation.

Optic disc drusen
- Small disc with absent cup and abnormal vascular trifurcations.
- Good vision and initially no field loss.
- The drusen are often not visible but can be found with ultrasound.
- Over many years the drusen become visible.
- There may be associated progressive visual field defects.

Proptosis

CASE STUDY

A 14-year-old girl presented with intermittent horizontal double vision, and pain behind the eye. Her parents had thought the right eye to be protruding more than the left. On examination her eyelids

Table 17.5 Preseptal versus orbital cellulitis

Sign	Preseptal cellulitis	Orbital cellulitis
Systemically unwell	Sometimes	Yes
Lid erythema and swelling	Yes	Yes
Reduced visual acuity	No	If optic nerve involved
Reduced colour vision	No	If optic nerve involved
Eye proptosed	No	Yes
Conjunctival oedema	No	Yes
Reduced eye movements and tense orbit	No	Yes
RAPD	No	If optic nerve involved
Investigations	If systemically unwell – blood cultures	CT scan of orbits and sinuses and blood cultures
Admit	Yes, if systemically unwell; if older and well can be treated as an outpatient	Yes
Treatment	Broad-spectrum antibiotics cephalosporin) Rehydration	Parenteral broad-spectrum antibiotics (e.g. flucloxacillin and third-generation cephalosporin) Rehydration
Surgery	No	Yes – if clinical signs suggest actual or incipient optic nerve involvement and imaging demonstrates sinus involvement and subperiosteal collections emergency drainage is performed usually by a paediatric otolaryngologist

CT, computed tomography; RAPD, relative afferent pupillary defect.

were erythematous, the conjunctiva red and infected, particularly medially and laterally, she was able to open her eyes, and on measurement the right eye was proptosed by 2 mm. She had horizontal double vision when she moved her eyes away from the centre and seemed to have restriction of eye movements in all directions of gaze. Her visual acuity was equal in both eyes as was her colour vision. There was no evidence of a relative afferent pupil defect. The diagnosis was considered an inflammatory process within the orbit. The differential diagnosis included orbital cellulitis, myositis, dysthroid eye disease or an orbital tumour. She was admitted and started on systemic antibiotics. A CT scan of the orbits was requested. This was reported as being consistent with orbital cellulitis, showing a small subperiosteal abscess as a result of sinus disease from the adjacent ethmoids. Her visual function was monitored daily by the ophthalmologists (visual acuity, colour vision, pupil responses), and there was no evidence of optic nerve compression. The clinical signs and symptoms resolved over the next seven days.

Proptosis: differential diagnosis

Proptosis is the protrusion of the eye from the orbit to an abnormal degree and is most obvious when unilateral. There are many causes of this appearance, which include a large diameter eye in unilateral high myopia or congenital glaucoma, both of which cause apparent rather than real proptosis. True proptosis is due to a space-occupying lesion within the orbit, which may be a dermoid cyst, orbital infection, orbital haemorrhage or orbital tumours, or swelling due to changes with the orbital muscles and fat as in thyroid eye disease.

SPONTANEOUS ORBITAL HAEMORRHAGE (ORBITAL VENOUS ANOMALIES/ORBITAL VARICES/ORBITAL LYMPHANGIOMA)

Sudden-onset proptosis or variable proptosis with the Valsalva manoeuvres can be a result of vascular anomalies within the orbit. Investigation by ultrasound and CT scan demonstrates the presence of vascular abnormality or blood-filled cysts within the orbit. Treatment in the absence of a progressive compressive optic neuropathy is conservative with serial ultrasound and observation, with management of any associated amblyopia. The haematinic cysts may take 6–12 months to resolve.

OPTIC NERVE GLIOMA

There is an association with neurofibromatosis type 1. These tumours present with gradual-onset proptosis with associated strabismus and visual decline. Histologically they are low-grade pilocytic astrocytomas and are an intrinsic tumour of the optic nerve or chiasm. On CT scan they show a characteristic enlargement of the nerve with kinking. Treatment is conservative as there is often spontaneous remission.

OPTIC NERVE SHEATH MENINGIOMA

Is a local tumour of the optic nerve sheath. Patients usually present with a decline in acuity due to compression of the optic nerve. CT scan shows an encased optic nerve of normal diameter with flecks of calcification within the tumour sheath.

RHABDOMYOSARCOMA

This presents with rapidly progressive proptosis, or sometimes as orbital cellulitis unresponsive to conventional treatment. They present around the age of 6 years. Imaging shows a well delineated uniform density irregular mass, which may extend intracranially. A biopsy confirms the diagnosis and the primary treatment is chemotherapy.

PERIOCULAR CELLULITIS

The commonest cause of cellulitis is spread of infection from the adjacent sinuses. Preseptal cellulitis is anterior to the orbital septum and orbital cellulitis extends into the orbit (Table 17.5). The former is commoner. In both, there is often a preceding upper respiratory tract infection. The child is febrile and systemically unwell (more so with orbital involvement). Both have well demarcated erythema and swelling of the eyelids. However, in orbital cellulitis there is infection and inflammation within the orbit. This gives rise to conjunctival chemosis, proptosis of the eye and reduced and painful movement of the eye. There may be displacement of the globe from an associated subperiosteal abscess.

The management of orbital cellulitis should be multidisciplinary with a clear lead team (usually the paediatric team or paediatric otolaryngologists), with early and regular review by the paediatric ophthalmologist. Prompt recognition and treatment of orbital cellulitis is important as the complications not only include optic neuropathy but cavernous sinus thrombosis and intracranial abscess.

FURTHER READING AND USEFUL WEBSITE

Taylor D, Hoyt C (1996) *Practical Paediatric Ophthalmology*. London: Blackwell Science.

Taylor D (ed) (1997) *Paediatric Ophthalmology*, 2nd edn. London: Blackwell Science. www.emedicine.com

Chapter 18

Dermatology

Rosemary Lever and A David Burden

The skin is one of the largest organs in the body. Its primary function is to provide physical protection by acting as a barrier between the internal systems of the body and the environment. It also has important sensory, immunological, endocrine and thermoregulatory functions.

CLINICAL FEATURES AND INVESTIGATIONS

Descriptive dermatology

The first step in making a diagnosis of dermatological disease is careful examination of the skin in a good light to establish a morphological diagnosis such as 'dermatitis'. From this starting point, further information concerning the onset and progression of the eruption, along with other factors in the patient's history, will enable a more precise or even an aetiological diagnosis (e.g. 'allergic contact dermatitis'). However, without a clear description of the cutaneous changes, the chance of making a reliable diagnosis is small. When examining the skin, three aspects of the physical signs should be systematically analysed:

- distribution of the rash
- morphology of the primary lesion
- configuration of the lesions.

The **distribution** of the rash can best be seen from the end of the bed with the child suitably undressed. The areas of the body affected should be noted, in particular the following.

- Does the rash affect the body symmetrically?
- Is its location primarily central (affecting trunk and head) or peripheral (affecting mainly the limbs)?
- Does it mainly affect flexural areas or extensor surfaces?
- Does the distribution reflect points of exposure to ultraviolet radiation (face, hands and forearms) or a contact allergen?
- Is the distribution typical of a common skin disease, e.g. seborrhoeic dermatitis, psoriasis, atopic dermatitis, acne, etc.?

Next, the **morphology** of a primary lesion should be assessed. This involves close inspection and may require a magnifying lens. In general, a lesion of recent onset should be examined before it has been modified, for instance by scratching. Many rashes are monomorphic (all primary lesions are similar) but sometimes a rash may have several different primary lesions, e.g. a maculopapular rash. The common primary lesions are defined in Table 18.1 and for each, the colour, contour, size and shape (Table 18.2) should be recorded. The surface should be carefully examined for scaling (defective desquamation) or crusting (dried serum). It is useful to try to localize the lesion anatomically into the epidermis, dermis or subcutaneous tissue by inspecting the overall architecture, the surface (scaling or crusting implying an epidermal component), the colour (remember the epidermis does not have a vascular supply) and by palpation for depth.

For red lesions, it is important to determine whether the lesion blanches on pressure (implying intravascular blood) or fails to blanche (suggesting extravascular erythrocytes) as seen in purpura. This may easily be achieved with pressure from a glass slide – a technique called diascopy that also allows the colour and nature of any dermal abnormality to be examined. **Dermatoscopy** (epiluminescence microscopy) is an extension of this technique in which mineral oil is first applied to the lesion, which is then examined with a handheld 10 times magnifying lens with a contact plate. The oil reduces scattering of light at the stratum corneum, allowing the epidermis to appear translucent and assisting in the examination of pigmented structures in the epidermis such as moles.

Another useful way of illuminating the skin is with the **Wood light**. This is a long wavelength (320–400 nm) ultraviolet light from which most visible wavelengths have been filtered. It accentuates epidermal pigmentation enabling vitiligo and the ash leaf macules of tuberous

Table 18.1 Common primary skin lesions

	Definition	Example
Macules and patches	Circumscribed flat areas of altered colour (macule <1 cm, patch >1 cm)	Vitiligo
Papules and nodules	Circumscribed palpable solid elevations (papule <1 cm, nodule >1 cm)	Viral wart
Plaque	An elevated, flat-topped area of skin >2 cm diameter	Psoriasis
Blisters (vesicles and bullae)	Visible collections of clear fluid in the skin (vesicle <5 mm, bulla >5 mm)	Herpes simplex
Pustule	A blister containing pus	Acne
Wheal	A transient area of dermal oedema often surrounded by erythema	Urticaria
Ulcer	Full thickness loss of epidermis with damage to dermis; heals with scarring	Aplasia cutis
Erosion	Loss of epidermis, which heals without scarring	Following rupture of a blister in epidermolysis bullosa simplex

Table 18.2 Shapes of primary lesions

Shape	Definition	Example
Discoid	A filled circle	Discoid eczema
Annular	An empty circle or ring	Tinea corporis
Arcuate	An incomplete circle	Urticaria
Targetoid	Multiple concentric rings	Erythema multiforme
Polycyclic	Rings fusing together	Neonatal lupus erythematosus
Reticulate	A fine net-like pattern	Cutis marmorata
Linear	A straight line	Epidermal naevus

sclerosis to be more easily seen. Also, some infective agents fluoresce, for example *Microsporum* spp. of tinea capitis that appears yellow-green.

Finally, the **configuration** of the lesions should be examined. Primary lesions may overlap each other to become confluent or may be discrete. They may be arranged at random or may be grouped. Grouped lesions may form patterns such as rings (as in granuloma annulare) or lines (e.g. psoriasis with the Koebner phenomenon). One important pattern in paediatric dermatology is the development of linear lesions as a developmental abnormality along the Blaschko lines (Figure 18.1). These are thought to represent lines of embryological neuroectodermal migration and do not correspond to known vascular or dermatomal patterns. Diseases that follow this pattern often represent genetic mosaicism either due to somatic mutation (e.g. linear epidermal naevus) or lyonization in X-linked traits (e.g. incontinentia pigmenti).

Investigations in dermatology

Bacterial swabs

The area of skin with the greatest degree of exudate should be chosen and recorded. A moistened swab should be briskly rubbed over the affected area and placed in bacterial transport medium for bacterial culture.

Viral infection

The Tzanck smear is occasionally used as a simple rapid test to identify the cytopathic changes produced in keratinocytes by viruses. An erosion or blister base is gently scraped with a scalpel blade, the material transferred to a glass slide, and stained as for a blood film for microscopic examination. To identify the virus, material can be obtained for polymerase chain reaction (PCR), electron microscopy or viral culture. These techniques are mainly used for identification of herpes viruses. Fluid can be aspirated from vesicles and transported immediately to the laboratory for electron microscopy. Swabs for culture are sent to the laboratory in viral transport medium.

Fungal scrapes

The fungi that cause tinea infections involve the stratum corneum, which can be sampled by skin scraping. The edge of a lesion where scaling is most apparent is gently scraped with a scalpel blade, allowing the fragments of scale to fall onto a dark piece of paper. This is then folded and posted to a mycology laboratory for microscopic examination and fungal culture. For suspected fungal nail infections, clippings of the nail plate and subungual debris are collected and in tinea capitis, plucked hair and scalp scrapings are sent.

Immunological testing

Different allergic mechanisms produce very different morphological patterns in the skin (Table 18.3). Therefore, the first step in the diagnosis of skin allergy is to carefully examine the clinical features. Investigation of allergic reactions types 1–3 relies largely upon sending appropriate

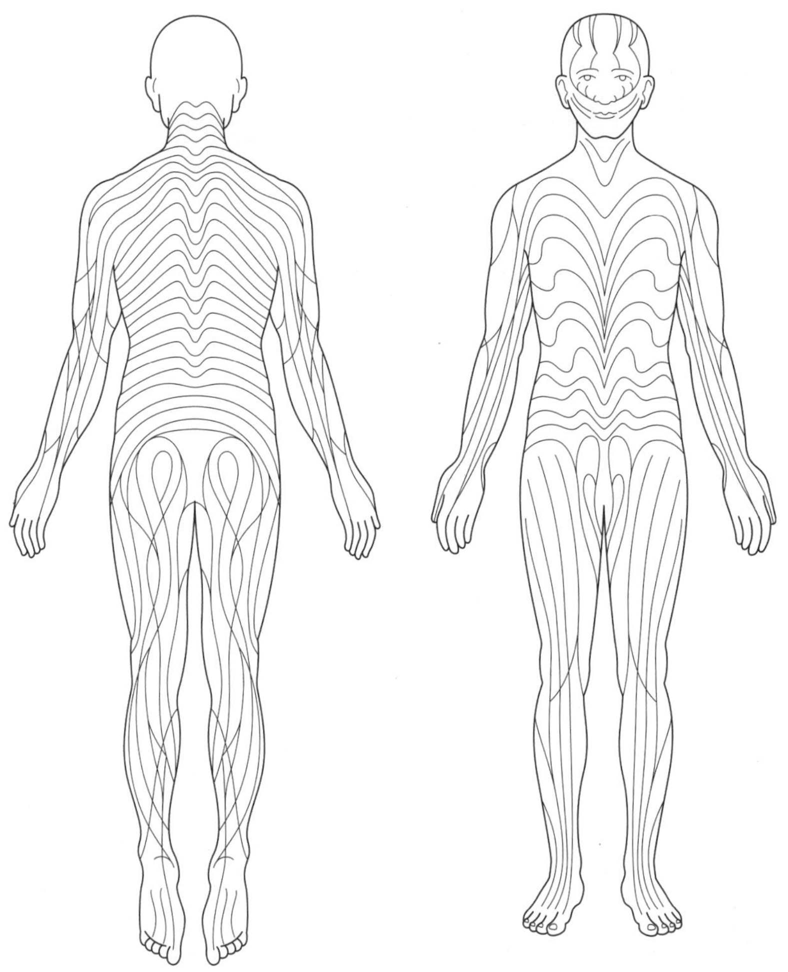

Figure 18.1 Blaschko lines – these are thought to represent lines of embryological neuro-ectodermal migration

Table 18.3 Allergic reactions in the skin (Gell and Coombs classification)

Type	Mechanism	Example	Relevant investigation
I	Immediate IgE-mediated reaction	Acute urticaria	Prick test Serum antibody (e.g. RAST)
II	Antibody directed against cell-bound antigen	Autoimmune blistering disease	Detection of circulating or fixed antibody by immunofluorescence or ELISA
III	Circulating immune complex (Arthus reaction)	Cutaneous vasculitis	Measure circulating immune complexes
IV	T-cell-mediated delayed hypersensitivity reaction	Allergic contact dermatitis	Patch testing

ELISA, enzyme-linked immunosorbent assay; RAST, radio allergosorbent testing.

blood samples to the laboratory to detect specific antibody. The investigation of contact dermatitis on the other hand is a clinical procedure (patch testing). Discs containing the relevant suitably diluted antigens are placed on the upper back for 48 hours. They are removed and the first reading made. A final reading is made after a further 48 hours. A positive response consists of a patch of localized dermatitis under a particular disc, present at the first and second readings but not present in normal controls. This test is more difficult to carry out in children than in adults because the patches can become dislodged by physical activity or water. Also, a younger child's back is relatively small, which restricts the number of antigens that can be applied at one time.

Skin biopsy

The skin has a limited number of microscopic reaction patterns, many of which are quite subtle. If you do not provide the pathologist with a relevant differential diagnosis, you are unlikely to obtain an accurate report. The commonest means of obtaining skin for pathological examination are incisional biopsy and punch biopsy. These generally require an injectable local anaesthetic and may be made less painful by the prior application of a topical anaesthetic cream. The commonest incisional biopsy is elliptical and consists of two-thirds lesional skin and one-third adjacent normal skin. This allows the pathologist to examine the edge of the lesion, which is often helpful. When taking the biopsy, remember which anatomical layer you are expecting the pathology to be in and ensure the biopsy is of a suitable depth. For instance, in erythema nodosum the pathology is in the subcutaneous fat and can easily be missed if the biopsy is not deep enough. When taking a biopsy from a widespread rash, it is very important to select the most informative lesion to biopsy. This is generally the most recent undamaged lesion.

Punch biopsy is a more rapid technique and therefore well suited to younger children. Smaller specimens are obtained and non-lesional skin cannot generally be included. Sterile disposable punch biopsies are available which have circular cutting blades in a range of diameters, commonly 3 mm and 4 mm. Specimens are generally sent to the laboratory in formalin but occasionally fresh material may be required, for example for immunofluorescence studies or microbiological culture.

Principles of treatment

Topical therapy

In choosing a suitable topical preparation, the vehicle that contains the active ingredient is more important than with oral medication. For acute exudative conditions, soaks, creams or lotions are more suitable. For chronic, dry, scaly dermatoses, greasy ointments are more effective and, as they do not contain preservatives, they are less likely to produce an allergic contact dermatitis. However, ointments can be less cosmetically acceptable for regular use as they leave a shiny residue on skin and can mark clothing, paper, etc. For older children, and to maintain compliance, it may be acceptable to restrict the use of an ointment to a night-time application, using a cream during the day.

It is difficult to specify a dose when prescribing topical therapy. There is a tendency for doctors to prescribe and patients to apply too small an amount of the preparation. Moisturizers should generally be prescribed in large quantities of up to 500 g per week. The **fingertip unit** (the amount of cream squeezed from a tube from the tip of an adult's index finger to the first joint) has been suggested as a guide to the amount of topical corticosteroid needed for various body sites at different ages (Table 18.4). As one fingertip unit weighs about 0.5 g, you can easily calculate how much cream to prescribe per week. For instance, the back of the trunk of a 6 year old child requires 5 fingertip units per application and twice daily application requires a prescription of 35 g per week.

Table 18.4 Dose of cream in fingertip units for different body sites at various ages

Body site	3–6 months	1–2 years	3–5 years	6–10 years
Face and neck	1	1.5	1.5	2
Arms and hands	1	1.5	2	2.5
Legs and feet	1.5	2	3	4.5
Front of trunk	1	2	3	3.5
Back of trunk	1.5	3	3.5	5

It should be remembered that topical therapy might be absorbed systemically. This is especially the case in young children as their body surface area is relatively great and in neonates as the barrier function of their skin is immature. Particular care should be paid to prescription of salicylic acid (metabolic acidosis, salicylism), silver sulfadiazine (kernicterus), urea (uraemia), iodine (hypothyroidism), neomycin (neural deafness) and topical anaesthetics (methaemoglobinaemia).

Cryotherapy

Cryotherapy uses freezing to produce controlled cell death and is useful in treating viral warts and molluscum contagiosum. Liquid nitrogen is the most widely used agent and may be applied directly using a cotton bud or sprayed onto the lesion. The duration of the freeze and the number of cycles of freezing and thawing should be recorded and will depend on the nature of lesion being treated. Common complications include pain, blistering and pigmentary disturbance.

Phototherapy

Phototherapy using ultraviolet wavelength 280–320 nm (ultraviolet B) or 320–400 nm combined with a photosensitizing psoralen (PUVA) is useful in treating several widespread inflammatory dermatoses, such as psoriasis or atopic dermatitis. However, its use in children is restricted to severe disease unresponsive to other modalities, because of concerns about carcinogenicity, which may be greater in this age group.

Laser therapy

Oxyhaemoglobin, deoxyhaemoglobin and melanin are the principal pigments in the skin and can be targeted by laser light of a wavelength that coincides with the peak of their absorption curve. Using the principle of selective photothermolysis, the cells containing pigment can be destroyed with relatively little damage to surrounding structures. The most frequently used lasers in clinical practice are the pulsed dye laser, Q-switched ruby laser, potassium-titanyl-phosphate (KTP), and Q-switched neodymium:yttrium aluminum garnet (Nd:YAG) lasers, which differ in their wavelength and pulse duration.

Laser therapy is being investigated for many clinical indications but in the paediatric age group they are most frequently used for the portwine stain type of vascular malformation, ulcerated haemangiomas and spider telangiectases. Lasers are also being developed for some benign pigmented lesions such as lentigenes. Complications of laser therapy include pigmentary and textural change in the treated skin. Of particular concern in children is pain control, as most lasers will produce a pricking sensation in the skin. Local anaesthesia is generally preferred but general anaesthesia may be given when treating large areas repeatedly in young children.

ANATOMY, EMBRYOGENESIS AND FUNCTION

The skin is a complex organ composed of many types of cell that form the epidermis, dermis and subcutaneous fat, all of which are tightly bound to each other. The epidermis is a keratinizing stratified squamous epithelium primarily composed of keratinocytes and consisting of four recognizable layers: the basal layer, the spinous layer, the granular cell layer and the stratum corneum. In the spinous layer, keratinocytes produce the intermediate filament protein keratin that provides a cytoskeleton and at the cell surface inserts into adhesion structures called desmosomes. In the outermost layers of the epidermis, keratinocytes undergo cornification to produce the stratum corneum. During this process:

- the cell nucleus is lost by apoptosis
- keratin filaments in the cytoplasm are cross-linked under the influence of filaggrin
- proteins in the plasma membrane such as involucrin are cross-linked under the action of a specific epidermal transglutaminase to form a rigid cell envelope
- lipids stored in lamella bodies in the cell cytoplasm are extruded into the intercellular space where they form water-impermeable lipid sheets surrounding the cornified envelope.

The other two major cell types in the epidermis are melanocytes and Langerhans cells. Melanocytes are derived from neuroectoderm and migrate to the basal layer of the epidermis between 8 and 12 weeks of embryogenesis. The major biological function of melanocytes is to produce the pigment melanin. Melanin is transported in melanosomes via the dendritic processes of the melanocyte to neighbouring keratinocytes where it forms a cap over the cell nucleus that protects DNA from the mutagenic effects of ultraviolet radiation. Langerhans cells are professional antigen presenting cells of bone marrow origin. They are located primarily in the spinous layer where their dendritic processes form a net to trap antigens, following which Langerhans cells migrate from the epidermis via dermal lymphatics to regional lymph nodes where they present the antigen to naive lymphocytes as the afferent limb of the primary immune response.

The epidermis lies on a complex basement membrane to which it is connected by adhesion structures within the basal keratinocyte called hemidesmosomes, which contain adhesion molecules such as plectin, type XVII collagen and $\alpha_6\beta_4$ integrin. The basement membrane consists of a more superficial lamina lucida that is rich in laminin 5, and a deeper electron dense lamina densa consisting of type IV collagen and laminin 1. The lamina densa is attached to the underlying dermis by type VII collagen that inserts into anchoring plaques in the superficial dermis.

The dermis provides much of the tensile strength of the skin. The main cell type is the fibroblast, which synthesizes collagen and elastin fibres and ground substance rich in glycosaminoglycans (mucopolysaccharides). The dermis contains a microvascular network and a rich sensory nerve supply. There are resident macrophages, mast cells and dermal dendritic cells in addition to transient cells such as trafficking T lymphocytes involved in immunosurveillance.

The subcutaneous fat is important as an energy store and in thermal insulation. The adipocytes are divided into lobules by fibrous septae, which carry the blood supply.

Adnexal structures

Eccrine sweat glands are epidermal structures that extend into the dermis. They play a major role in thermoregulation. Hair follicles and nails also develop from the epidermis but the terminal differentiation of the keratinocytes produces a distinct set of hard keratins that form the hair shaft and nail plate. Hair differs from epidermis and other adnexal structures in that cell proliferation and growth occur cyclically, with distinct phases of fibre growth (anagen), arrest (catagen) and quiescence (telogen) when the fibre has reached its definitive length. The final length of hairs is determined mainly by the duration of the anagen phase.

Sebaceous glands and apocrine glands are derivatives of the hair follicle and release their secretions onto the skin surface through the opening of the hair follicle.

Embryogenesis

Skin is derived from two germ layers. Ectoderm and neuroectoderm give rise to the epidermis, and mesoderm gives rise to the dermis. By 28 days estimated gestational age, the epidermis consists of a basal cell layer and periderm. By month 2 melanocytes can first be detected between basal cells and periderm. The epidermis starts to become stratified during the second trimester. Hair follicles start to develop at about 80 days' gestation and continue in a cephalocaudal direction during the fourth month. Nail development can first be detected at about 8 weeks' gestation, keratinization of the nail plate starts at about 11 weeks and the nail plate reaches the tip of the fingers by about 32 weeks. Sebaceous, eccrine and apocrine glands develop during the third to fifth months.

NEONATAL DERMATOLOGY

At term, the skin is generally well developed structurally although there may be slightly reduced thermal sweating. In the preterm neonate, the skin is immature both structurally and functionally. In babies born before 34 weeks' gestation, the barrier function is impaired, causing increased evaporative loss of water and making the baby prone to hypernatraemic dehydration and also energy loss through heat of evaporation. Within two to three weeks of birth, an adequate barrier function has developed regardless of gestational age. The skin of the premature baby is also prone to mechanical injury such as shearing due to an immature dermo–epidermal junction and dermis. Skin care of the neonate is extremely important and involves good hygiene (for instance handwashing by staff and parents), minimal use of adhesive tapes, the frequent application of a bland emollient such as liquid paraffin, and an assumption that whatever is placed on the skin can be absorbed.

Transient neonatal rashes

See Table 18.5 for an overview of transient neonatal rashes.

> **CASE STUDY**
>
> A 2-day-old healthy baby boy born at term develops red patches 1–2 cm in diameter and a few small pustules on the posterior trunk.

Erythema toxicum neonatorum

Erythema toxicum neonatorum (ETN) (Figures 18.2 and 18.3) is a self-limiting eruption of unknown cause that affects up to a half of healthy mature neonates.

Table 18.5 Transient neonatal rashes

	Age at onset	Prevalence (%)	Morphology	Distribution	Associated features	Outcome
Erythema toxicum neonatorum	1-7 days	30-50	Small red patches and pustules	Mainly trunk and face	Term babies	Resolves in one week
Transient neonatal pustular melanosis	Birth	1-5	Small pustules followed by hyperpigmentation	Forehead, ears, neck, back	Black skin	Resolves in two to three months
Neonatal acne	1-3 weeks	1	Red papules and pustules; no comedones	Cheeks, forehead, scalp		Resolves in first month
Miliaria crystallina	0-1 week	Uncommon	Non-inflammatory vesicles	Forehead	Overheating	Resolves in a few days
Miliaria rubra	1-4 weeks	~1	Red papules, vesicles and pustules	Neck and trunk	Overheating	Resolves in a few days
Neonatal lupus erythematosus	Birth to a few weeks	Rare	Red scaly patches; annular lesions	Mainly face, around eyes	Maternal Ro antibody; congenital heart block	Resolves by 6 months
Subcutaneous fat necrosis of newborn	0-4 weeks	Rare	Firm subcutaneous nodules and plaques	Back of trunk, buttocks, cheeks	Hypercalcaemia	Resolves by 6 months

Red macules and wheals, with or without small pustules rich in eosinophils, develop on the trunk and face between days 1 and 3 and usually resolve within the first week without treatment. It is generally easy to diagnose without investigation but other causes of pustule formation should be considered, for instance neonatal acne, miliaria crystallina, neonatal candidia-sis, superficial staphylococcal infection and incontinentia pigmenti. A variant of ETN seen in dark-skinned races is described as **transient neonatal pustular melanosis**. At birth, tiny pustules may be present which rapidly rupture to leave a ring of scale and subsequently hyperpigmented macules that may last for several months.

Neonatal acne

Neonatal acne is a pustular eruption of the face and scalp in the first month of life. It lacks comedones, which are normally the hallmark of acne. It is questionable whether it is in fact a form of acne and more recently, the term neonatal cephalic pustulosis has been introduced along with a theory that it is caused by *Malassezia* yeasts. It should be distinguished from infantile acne, which occurs after the first month of life and has the features of adolescent acne, including comedone formation.

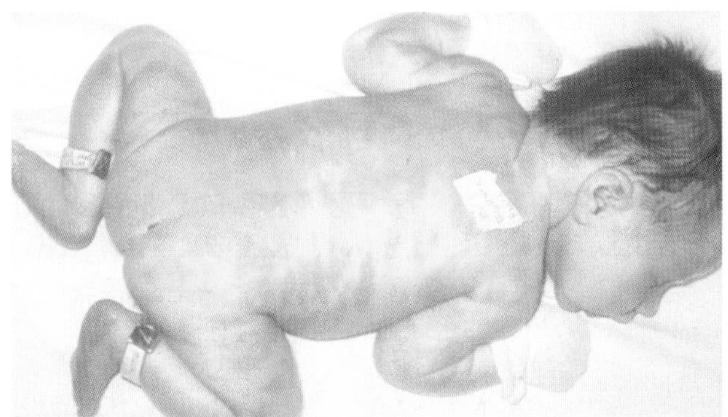

Figure 18.2 Erythema toxicum neonatorum showing widespread erythema and pustules

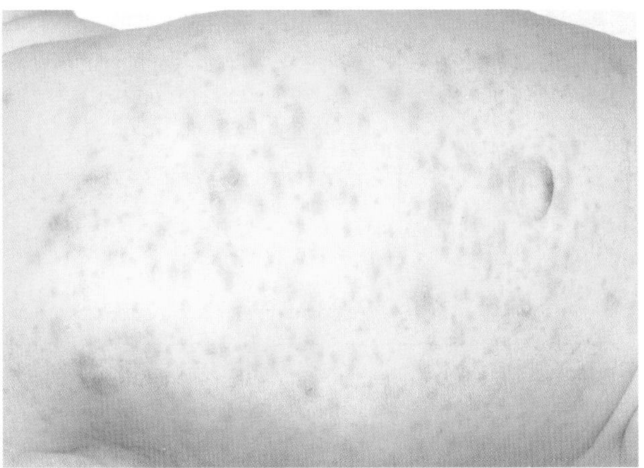

Figure 18.3 A close up view of erythema toxicum neonatorum

Miliaria

This describes the effects of occlusion of the eccrine sweat duct at various levels, usually associated with overheating. If blocked at the level of the stratum corneum tiny superficial non-inflammatory vesicles develop, particularly on the forehead, and are called **miliaria crystallina.** The vesicles rapidly rupture and desquamate over about one week. **Miliaria rubra** (sometimes called 'prickly heat') is due to occlusion of the duct within the spinous layer of the epidermis. It presents as red papules with superimposed vesicles and pustules, commonly on the neck.

Two rarer self-limiting eruptions should be remembered because of important systemic associations. **Subcutaneous fat necrosis of the newborn** affects babies in the first few weeks of life and is characterized by firm, circumscribed flesh-coloured to blue subcutaneous nodules or plaques with a predilection for the trunk, buttocks, thighs and cheeks. It is commoner in babies born by caesarean section with fetal distress and resolves spontaneously over a few months. Hypercalcaemia occurs in about 25 per cent of cases and may be delayed by up to two months.

Neonatal lupus erythematosus

This occurs due to transplacental transmission of maternal anti-Ro or anti-La antibodies (Figure 18.4). About a half of affected infants have skin lesions and 10 per cent of these also have congenital heart block. Skin lesions may be present at birth or develop over the first few weeks of

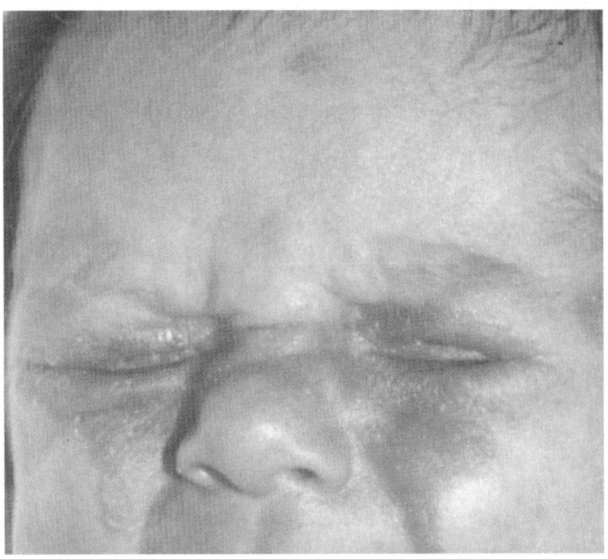

Figure 18.4 Neonatal lupus erythematosus with typical symmetrical peri-ocular involvement

life, sometimes triggered by ultraviolet light. The morphology is of red scaly patches, sometimes annular, that appear especially on the periorbital and malar regions of the face (see Chapter 16, Figure 16.10) The lesions may respond to a moderate potency topical corticosteroid and all affected infants should be advised about sun avoidance. The eruption fades over a few months, sometimes leaving atrophy and telangiectases.

Vascular anomalies

> **CASE STUDY**
>
> A 4-month-old infant presents with an enlarging red nodule on the left cheek. She has had this since 6 weeks of age.

Vascular anomalies are classified into **vascular tumours** and **vascular malformations**, which are then subclassified according to the vascular structure involved. This biological classification is useful prognostically and in planning treatment.

Infantile haemangiomas

'Strawberry naevi' (Figure 18.5) are the only common vascular tumours in infancy and affect up to 10 per cent of the population by the age of 1 year. They are five times more common in girls than boys and are also commoner in premature neonates. They may be present at birth as an area of telangiectases or bruising but more often they are first noticed at 4–8 weeks as either a superficial bright red plaque or a deeper nodule. The head is most frequently affected although any site may be involved. The natural history is very distinctive with a phase of rapid growth over the first 9–12 months of life followed by a gradual involution over five to 10 years. Occasional haemangiomas are fully formed at birth and in this situation they frequently involute rapidly. With rare exceptions, and in contrast with vascular malformations, haemangiomas are not associated with other syndromes. Complications and associations of infantile haemangiomas are listed in Table 18.6. The Kasabach–Merritt phenomenon (a bleeding diathesis due to platelet sequestration within the lesion) is now recognized to complicate kaposiform haemangioendothelioma (KHE) and sometimes tufted angiomas, rather than common infantile haemangiomas. Kaposiform haemangioendothelioma is rare, affects both sexes equally and usually presents as a congenital vascular nodule without the growth and involuting pattern of infantile haemangiomas.

Uncomplicated infantile haemangiomas do not usually require active intervention but should be carefully monitored, sometimes with serial photography, and the family often require emotional support as they await the

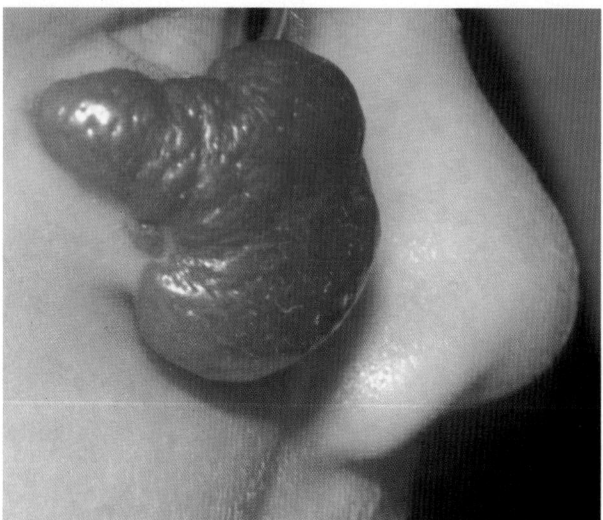

Figure 18.5 Early proliferating infantile haemangioma; in this site vision is threatened and systemic treatment may be necessary

Table 18.6 Associations and complications of infantile haemangiomas

Complication/association	Features
Ulceration, bleeding and infection	Most often on lip, perineum and rapidly enlarging lesions
Impairment of function	Particularly peri-ocular causing amblyopia but also ear and nostril
Residual disease	Fibrofatty lump, superficial telangiectases
Benign neonatal haemangiomatosis	Multiple, widespread, small, superficial haemangiomas
Diffuse neonatal haemangiomatosis	As above but with symptomatic involvement of other organs especially the liver
Laryngeal haemangioma	Associated with haemangiomas of 'beard' area of face
PHACE syndrome	Posterior fossa brain malformation, haemangioma, aortic coarctation, cardiac defects, eye abnormalities

PHACE, *p*osterior fossa malformations, large cervical *h*aemangioma, *a*rterial anomalies of the head and neck, *c*oarctation of the aorta and cardiac defects, *e*ye anomalies and sternal cleft.

involution of the lesion. Larger, disfiguring and complicated haemangiomas may require treatment. In the growth phase, intralesional corticosteroid injections or systemic corticosteroids (3–5 mg/kg per day) are often effective. Otherwise, surgical excision or reduction may be necessary. Laser therapy is not generally useful, except sometimes in healing ulcerated haemangiomas or in treating residual telangiectases.

Vascular malformations

In contrast with infantile haemangioma, **vascular malformations** affect both sexes equally, are generally fully formed at birth and do not involute. Despite this they are sometimes loosely and confusingly referred to as haemangiomas in the literature. They are subclassified according to the vessel involved into capillary (portwine stain), venous, arteriovenous, lymphatic and combinations of the above. **Portwine stains** (Figure 18.6) present as pink-red patches with a predilection for the face and which do not generally cross the midline. When the distribution of the ophthalmic division of the trigeminal nerve is affected, about 10 per cent have involvement of the eye, underlying leptomeninges and brain (Sturge–Weber syndrome). Other syndromic associations are listed in Table 18.7. Portwine stains tend to become darker and nodular with age. They can often be improved during childhood by laser therapy depending on their site, colour and extent.

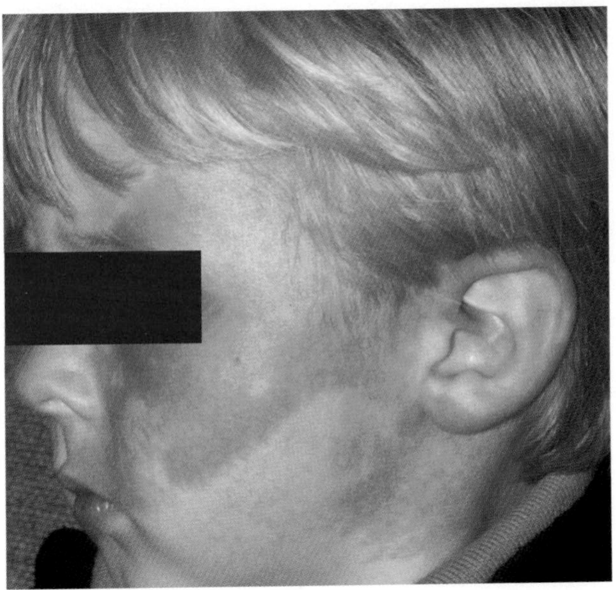

Figure 18.6 Port wine stain in the distribution of the trigeminal nerve: ocular involvement should be considered

VENOUS MALFORMATIONS

Venous malformations present as a blue subcutaneous or mucosal nodule that is compressible and may enlarge with coughing or straining. They may appear similar to deep infantile haemangiomas but the natural history (present at birth and enlarges at the same rate as the child) helps to distinguish them. If treatment is necessary on functional or cosmetic grounds, they may respond to carefully planned intralesional injection of sclerosant and/or surgical excision.

LYMPHATIC MALFORMATIONS

Lymphatic malformations are either macrocystic (previously referred to as cystic hygromas) or microcystic (lymphangioma circumscriptum). Macrocystic lymphatic malformations are present at birth as a subcutaneous cystic swelling often involving the neck and axilla. Microcystic lymphatic malformations usually develop later during childhood and present as grouped vesicles containing clear or blood-stained fluid.

ARTERIOVENOUS MALFORMATIONS

These are locally aggressive and very difficult to treat adequately. They can simulate portwine stains but can be distinguished by their high flow rate, which causes local

Table 18.7 Selected syndromes associated with vascular malformations

	Malformation	Extracutaneous features
Sturge-Weber syndrome	Portwine stain in distribution of ophthalmic division of trigeminal nerve	Eye abnormalities (glaucoma, buphthalmos); leptomeningeal and brain involvement; epilepsy
Klippel-Trelaunay syndrome	Low-flow capillary-venous-lymphatic malformation of a limb	Limb overgrowth; varicose veins of same limb
Parkes-Weber syndrome	High-flow capillary-arterio-venous malformation of a limb	Limb overgrowth; sometimes high-output cardiac failure
Proteus syndrome	Large portwine stains, lymphatic malformations or low-flow capillary-venous-lymphatic malformation	Multiple including asymmetrical bone overgrowth; macrodactyly; cerebriform hyperplasia of soles; epidermal naevi; lipomas; café-au-lait macules

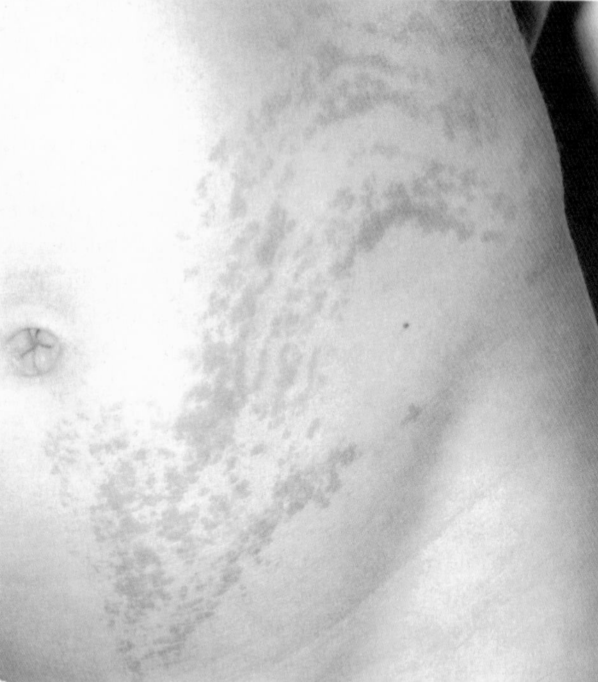

Figure 18.7 Linear verrucous epidermal naevus following the lines of Blaschko

warmth and sometimes a bruit. The high flow rate can be confirmed using Doppler ultrasound – the only other high flow vascular anomalies are some deep infantile haemangiomas.

Epidermal naevi

Linear verrucous epidermal naevi (Figure 18.7)

These are keratinocyte naevi present in about 1:1000 children. They are usually present at birth as small or large areas of light brown papules that become papillomatous over years. They are frequently linear in configuration and follow the lines of Blaschko. An inflammatory variant with psoriasiform features is recognized (*i*nflammatory *l*inear *v*errucous *e*pidermal *n*aevi – ILVEN). They are usually an isolated finding but very occasionally may be associated with developmental abnormalities of central nervous system, skeleton and eye ('epidermal naevus syndrome' or Schimmelpenning syndrome). Other epidermal naevus syndromes are Proteus syndrome and CHILD syndrome (congenital *h*emidysplasia with *i*chthyosiform naevus and *l*imb *d*efects)

Organoid naevi (sebaceous naevus)

These are variants of epidermal naevi derived from adnexal structures, particularly sebaceous and apocrine glands (Figure 18.8). They produce yellow plaques, oval or linear in shape, which mainly affect the head. When the scalp is involved they often present as a patch of alopecia. After puberty these lesions are recognized to occasionally develop neoplastic growths such as syringocystadenoma papilliferum, trichoblastoma and basal cell carcinoma. For this reason some authorities recommend routine removal in childhood. However, the risk of developing an aggressive neoplasm is very small and often it is acceptable to keep these lesions under observation.

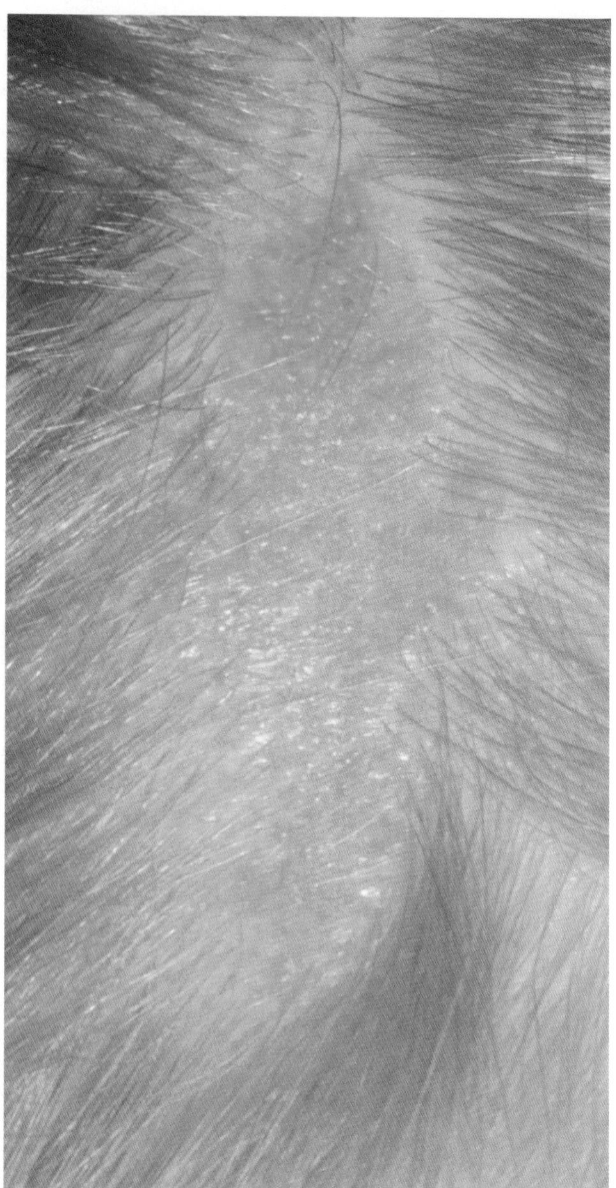

Figure 18.8 Organoid (sebaceous) naevus in the scalp. This shows the characteristic orange-yellow colour and associated alopecia

Dermal naevi

Congenital smooth muscle hamartoma

This is not uncommon (1:2500) and represents a naevus of the arrector pili muscle. It presents usually on the trunk as a tan-coloured dermal plaque with overlying hypertrichosis. Occasionally the muscle can be seen to ripple if gently stroked. They are of no significance and seem to fade with time.

Connective tissue naevi

Connective tissue naevi are single or multiple, skin-coloured dermal plaques or nodules due to the deposition of collagen or elastin. They are not generally present at birth but appear during the first few years. Elastic tissue naevi are sometimes associated with osteopoikilosis (Buschke–Ollendorf syndrome) and collagenomas are sometimes associated with tuberous sclerosis, when they are called shagreen patches.

Dermal melanocytoses

Due to an optical effect, the normal brown colour of melanin appears blue if situated deep within the dermis. The dermal melanocytoses are thought to represent arrested embryonic migration of melanocytes from the neural crest to the epidermis. This is most commonly seen in **mongolian spots**, which consist of large grey-blue patches affecting principally the lower back. These are present in 80 per cent of dark-skinned races and tend to fade with time. **Blue naevi** are common in all races and present in early childhood, or less frequently at birth, as small papules of a dark blue/black colour often on the dorsa of the hands and feet or the buttock area.

Melanocyte naevi

Congenital-type melanocytic naevi consist of nests of melanocytes in the epidermis and dermis visible at birth or within the first few years of life. They are classified by size into small (less than 1.5 cm diameter), intermediate (1.5 cm to 20 cm diameter) and large (greater than 20 cm diameter). **Small and intermediate congenital melanocytic naevi** occur in 1 per cent and 0.1 per cent of the population, respectively, and present as round or oval brown macules or plaques. They often but not invariably produce coarse hair and with time the surface may become rougher or even papillomatous. Pigmentation can be variable through the lesion and the centre is often darker or contains darker foci. Speckled lentiginous naevus is a variant consisting of a circumscribed light-tan coloured macule studded with small, darkly pigmented macules. In contrast to large congenital melanocytic naevi, it is not clear that small and intermediate lesions have an increased malignant potential. If the risk is elevated, it is only marginally so, and therefore the management of these lesions is largely determined by cosmetic considerations. **Large congenital melanocytic naevi** (LCMN) (Figure 18.9) occur in approximately 0.01 per cent of neonates and usually

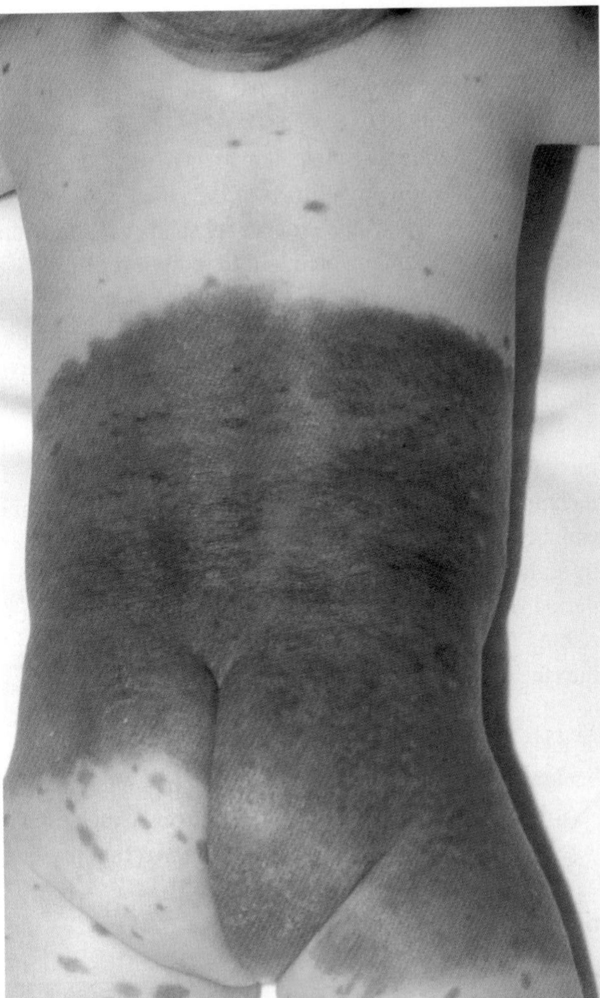

Figure 18.9 Giant congenital melanocytic naevus with associated numerous smaller congenital melanocytic naevi. These children have an increased lifetime risk of melanoma

affect the trunk, particularly the lower back and buttocks. They are often associated with smaller congenital naevi that are more widely distributed. In addition to the substantial disfigurement that they may produce, two major complications should be remembered. Melanoma, which is often aggressive, develops in 5 per cent to 10 per cent of individuals with LCMN, usually before puberty. This should always be suspected when darker areas develop within LCMN or if they develop papules, nodules or ulceration. A few children with LCMN develop neurocutaneous melanosis in which the leptomeninges may be infiltrated with melanocytes. This is more commonly associated with LCMN in the lumbosacral area or affecting the head and neck. Neurocutaneous melanosis can vary from clinically silent disease detected by magnetic resonance imaging (MRI) scanning, to symptomatic disease usually associated with obstructive hydrocephalus. In those with symptomatic disease the prognosis is poor. Up to 50 per cent develop leptomeningeal melanoma.

Acquired melanocytic naevi (moles) develop in virtually all older children and become particularly numerous during the teenage years. By the end of childhood the average individual will have 20–50 benign acquired naevi, the number varying due to genetic factors and early sun exposure. In contrast to the congenital type of melanocytic naevi, acquired naevi are smaller (up to 5 mm diameter), evenly pigmented and less often hair bearing. Up to 5 per cent of the population develop the atypical mole syndrome – large numbers of moles that have irregular shape and pigmentation. Both the atypical mole syndrome and a large number of clinically typical acquired naevi are risk factors for the later development of melanoma, particularly if there is a family history of melanoma. Melanomas are very rare before puberty and can be distinguished from melanocytic naevi by their irregular shape or colour and relentless growth over a period of weeks and months. As in adult melanoma, the risk of metastasis is dependent on the depth of growth into the dermis and early diagnosis is paramount. This can be difficult in children because of the very low prevalence of melanomas in this age group compared with acquired benign naevi, which also have a growth phase in children.

Spitz naevus (known in the past as 'juvenile melanoma') is a clinically distinctive melanocytic naevus that presents usually in the first decade of life as a red or red-brown, round or oval, dome-shaped papule or nodule usually on the face or upper limb. They are clinically benign but careful clinical–pathological correlation is necessary as the histological appearance can closely simulate a melanoma.

Napkin rashes

The napkin area is commonly affected by inflammatory dermatoses as shown in Table 18.8.

CASE STUDY

A 6-month-old infant presents with a napkin rash, which has been troublesome for the past six to eight weeks.

Irritant napkin dermatitis

This is a common condition that affects the napkin area and classically spares the skin folds. Outside the napkin area, the rest of the skin is normal. It is thought to be due to the irritant effects of faeces and urine. It is commoner after a bout of diarrhoea and may complicate the use of broad-spectrum antibiotics. It is now much less frequent

Table 18.8 Napkin dermatitis

Condition	Clinical features	Associated clinical features	Investigations	Treatment	Prognosis
Irritant (napkin) dermatitis	Napkin area only; spares skin folds	None	None	Steroids/anti-yeast + ichthyol preparations	Good
Seborrhoeic dermatitis	Bright red well demarcated; scaly	Scalp: scaly; flexural	Bacteriology	Steroid/anti-yeast; 1% ichthyol/zinc ointment	Clears <9/12
Atopic eczema	Napkin area usually spared	Facial eczema; extensor limbs; trunk	Usually unnecessary	Steroid/anti-yeast; 1% ichthyol/zinc ointment	Variable
Candidiasis	Yellowish erythematous + scale	Satellite lesions	Bacteriology	Topical imidazoles; nystatin	Good
Psoriasis	Well-demarcated; erythema	Check scalp; extensors of knees and elbow	None	Topical steroids ± weak tars	Tends to persist
Bullous impetigo	Discrete erythematous lesions; superficial scaling	May affect other sites	Bacteriology	Antibiotics	Excellent
Dermatitis enteropathica	Persistent napkin 'dermatitis'	Lesions: corners of mouth, nose and eyes; irritability, failure to thrive; hair changes; photophobia	Serum zinc	Zinc supplements for life	Good with treatment
Langerhans cell histiocytosis	Persistent napkin 'dermatitis'	Scalp involvement; brownish skin lesions; systemic involvement; diabetes insipidus	Biopsy and electron microscopy Staging	Variable Chemotherapy	Variable

in the Western world because of the considerable improvement in disposable nappies. Most cases respond well to a moderately potent topical steroid. Combined steroid/anticandidal formulations are preferable to prevent secondary colonization with *Candida*. Simple barriers creams or 1 per cent ichthyol in zinc ointment are also useful. For the very acute weeping napkin dermatitis wet dressings, such as 1 per cent ichthyol in calamine lotion, are the treatment of choice.

Seborrhoeic dermatitis

Seborrhoeic dermatitis is characterized by a confluent shiny intense erythema affecting the whole napkin area including the skin folds. Despite this striking erythema, which may also affect the scalp and flexures, these babies are placid and content. In contrast to atopic eczema or scabies, they do not appear to be itchy. There is often heavy scaling of the scalp that may also affect the eyebrows.

This condition is now uncommon in hospital practice in the UK, although this may simply reflect a change in the referral pattern rather than a true change in the incidence of the condition.

The prognosis is generally good with most cases clearing by the age of 9 months, with the exception of a subgroup that overlaps with atopic eczema. These infants have the classic clinical features of seborrhoeic dermatitis but are either itchy or have a positive family history of atopy. The prognosis in these infants should be more guarded.

Atopic eczema

In the vast majority of infants with atopic eczema the napkin area is spared. However, this site may be involved in children with widespread involvement. These children usually have the typical distribution seen in infants with involvement of the face and dribble area, the extensor aspects of the limbs and the trunk. In contrast to seborrhoeic dermatitis this is an intensely itchy, distressing condition.

Candidiasis

In infants with candidiasis, the lesions are often yellowish and slightly scaly plaques. Satellite lesions are a helpful diagnostic sign and oral candidiasis may also coexist. A swab should be sent for microscopic examination and culture. The condition responds well to topical anticandidal preparations.

Psoriasis

This is rare in infancy. However, it can occur at any age and infants may present with involvement of the napkin area. The affected area is a salmon-pink colour that is very well demarcated. It lacks the typical psoriatic scale seen in other sites. Moderately potent steroid/anticandidal preparations can be used alone or in combination with clean tar-based ointments. Psoriasis responds much less well to treatment than the eczematous conditions.

Bullous impetigo

This commonly affects the napkin area and may complicate infection of the umbilical cord in neonates. Bullous impetigo is usually staphylococcal in origin (*Staphylococcus aureus*, phage type 2). Clinically the lesions are discrete erythematous denuded areas with cigarette-paper-like scaling. Intact bullae are rarely seen because of the high level of the split in the epidermis. A bacteriological swab should be taken to confirm the diagnosis, to identify the organism and provide antibiotic sensitivities. If the affected area is very localized topical antibiotics may be effective, but systemic antibiotics are needed for more extensive involvement. Flucloxacillin is the antibiotic of choice for staphylococcal infection unless the child is sensitive to penicillin.

The napkin area may also be affected in other **generalized conditions** such as scabies, herpes simplex, chronic bullous disease of childhood and HIV infection.

Diagnoses not to miss

Most children with a napkin rash have one of the above common conditions. However, it is important not to miss two important conditions that may present with an atypical unusually persistent rash in the napkin area. **Acrodermatitis enteropathica** (Figure 18.10) is a very rare condition but should be considered when an infant presents with a persistent nappy rash that is unresponsive to topical treatment with moderately potent topical

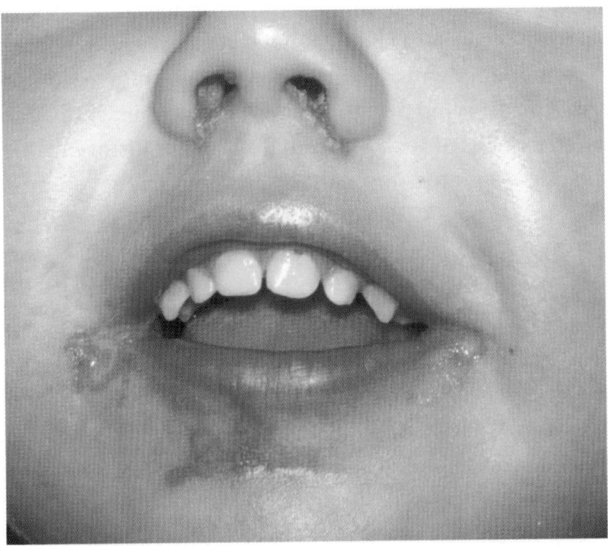

Figure 18.10 Acrodermatitis enteropathica showing the characteristic peri-orificial distribution. This child presented with a persistent nappy rash

steroids. Other helpful diagnostic signs are eroded moist areas affecting the corners of the mouth, nose and eyes. The classic triad is dermatitis, diarrhoea and alopecia. The hair is fine and sparse. Nail involvement may occur and the child may fail to thrive and be irritable. The condition is due to zinc deficiency and should be confirmed by a serum zinc level. Zinc deficiency may be acquired and secondary to nutritional problems. This form is transient. In the inherited autosomal recessive form there is a lifelong inability to absorb sufficient zinc from the gastrointestinal tract. Zinc supplements lead to a rapid improvement in all the clinical features. Lifelong zinc supplementation is needed for the inherited form.

Cutaneous involvement occurs in 40 per cent of patients with **Langerhans cell histiocytosis** (LCH) and commonly affects the napkin area, scalp and back. The lesions are brownish papules, which may be purpuric. In the napkin area the lesions are more marked in the inguinal folds and these may become eroded. Some children present initially with scaly involvement of the scalp that may be misdiagnosed as seborrhoeic dermatitis. Others present later with diabetes insipidus and these may have a history of problems with the scalp. The disease may be confined to the skin and be a self-limiting condition. Bone cysts are common and multisystem involvement may occur (page 613). Cutaneous lesions may respond to treatment with topical steroids or to topical nitrogen mustard. Children with multisystem disease may require chemotherapy.

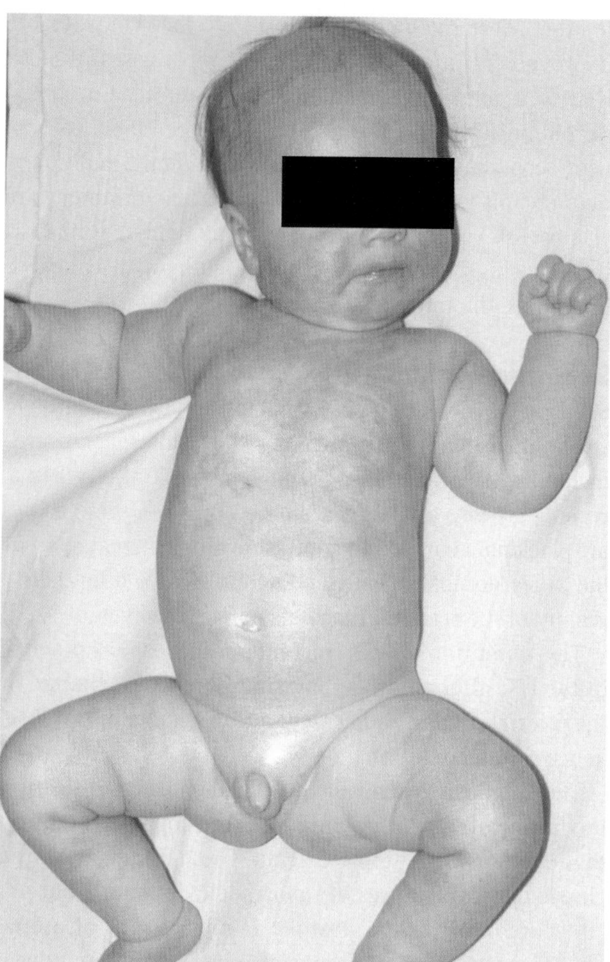

Figure 18.11 Atopic eczema in an infant with widespread involvement but relative sparing of the napkin area

ATOPIC ECZEMA

Atopic eczema (Figure 18.11) is the commonest cause of referral of a child to a paediatric dermatology clinic. The prevalence of the condition varies worldwide but affects up to 20 per cent of children in the Western world. It most commonly presents in early infancy and 95 per cent of cases present under the age of 5 years. Atopic eczema is often associated with a personal or family history of the allergic respiratory diseases (asthma and hay fever).

Clinical features

The predominant symptom at all ages is itch and children tend to be irritable and sleep poorly. During infancy, atopic eczema classically affects the face, dribble area and the extensor aspects of the limbs. In the severer forms the trunk may also be extensively involved although the napkin area itself is usually spared. Flexural involvement is the characteristic distribution in the older child and adolescent. Persistent hand eczema is often a continuing problem at all ages.

Genetics and aetiology

Family studies have demonstrated that the phenotype of atopic eczema is highly heritable and genetic loci have been identified on chromosomes 1, 3, 17 and 20. Patients with atopy show an exaggerated response to common environmental antigens, though the cause for this is still not clearly understood. In most patients the total IgE and specific IgEs to one or more of the inhalant and other allergens are raised. However, atopic eczema is primarily a T-cell-mediated condition with an imbalance of the Th1 and Th2 helper cells. There is often a peripheral eosinophilia and eosinophils form part of the infiltrate in early lesions.

Management

First-line treatment

Children with atopic eczema do not tolerate wool next to their skin well. Cotton underwear is often helpful. Some children also have an irritant reaction to the washing powders used. It is generally best to use a non-biological, non-fragranced powder. Immunization should be encouraged.

TOPICAL TREATMENT

Moisturizers

All children with atopic eczema should use liberal amounts of moisturizers both regularly and frequently. During infancy, a greasy moisturizer such as 50 per cent liquid paraffin in white soft paraffin or Vaseline® is preferable. As the children get older, personal preference becomes more important and a lighter cream such as aqueous cream or one of the proprietary brands is often more acceptable in this age group. It is important that adequate amounts of moisturizers are prescribed. A teenager or adult will require up to 500 g/week. Many families also find a bath oil useful – unfragranced preparations are preferable.

Topical steroids

Most children will require regular treatment with topical steroids. A weak steroid such as 1 per cent hydrocortisone ointment for facial use and a moderately potent steroid such as clobetasol butyrate for the trunk and limbs are acceptable for maintenance treatment. Some families find the intermittent use of a potent steroid (class 2) such as mometasone more effective and more convenient. However, for maintenance treatment, steroids of this potency should not be used more than once a week or five times a month. It is often helpful to apply a tar preparation such as 1 per cent ichthyol in zinc ointment or tar impregnated bandages over the topical steroids.

Topical tacrolimus

Topical tacrolimus can be an effective therapeutic option in moderately severe eczema that has failed to respond to topical steroids. It is also useful in the peri-ocular area, a site where topical steroids are relatively contraindicated. Its usefulness is sometimes limited by the common side effect of a burning sensation on application. Topical tacrolimus seems to be a safe alternative to topical steroids in the short and medium term, but its long-term safety has yet to be established. Sun protection should be used if it is used on sun-exposed sites.

BANDAGING

Bandaging is a very important part of the management of atopic eczema, particularly in the younger child with severe disease. These can be applied dry or wet as in the wet wrap technique of bandaging.

An oral sedative **anti-histamine** may be useful at night for those children who sleep poorly because of itch.

MANAGEMENT PLAN

Families need a plan for maintenance treatment (as outlined above). In addition, a rescue plan is necessary for flares. In general, an increase in topical steroid potency is necessary. Thus if 1 per cent hydrocortisone (class 4 – weak) is used for maintenance treatment an increase to a moderately potent steroid (class 3) such as clobetasol butyrate may be adequate. However if a class 3 steroid is used as maintenance, a class 2 steroid will be needed for five to seven days.

Many flares are secondary to bacterial infection and will require treatment with a systemic antibiotic. Flucloxacillin is the treatment of choice unless the child is sensitive to penicillin.

Second-line treatment: allergen avoidance

FOOD

During infancy, adverse reactions to food may be an important factor in the aetiology of eczema in those referred to secondary care. It is worth asking if there is a history suggestive of food allergy. Some infants (aged <2 years) may merit further investigation: a white cell differential count to check for an eosinophilia and an IgE screen to common ingested and inhaled allergens (radio-allergosorbent testing (RAST) or skin prick tests). A positive specific IgE is not in itself diagnostic of food allergy. Although the specific IgE level (or wheal size in skin prick test) can give a reasonable guide for some of the allergens (eggs, peanuts and fish) they are less helpful for others (milk and wheat). Reactions to milk and wheat may also be delayed and be associated with gastrointestinal symptoms suggesting that these allergies may be mediated by a different pathway. False-negative specific IgEs are uncommon but do occur. False-positive results are much more common, particularly in the older child. Test results therefore should be interpreted with caution.

The real test of food allergy in atopic eczema is whether the eczema improves when the food is withdrawn and flares on its reintroduction. The two commonest allergens are eggs and milk. If in doubt, it is reasonable to withdraw the food(s) for six weeks as a trial. However, the diet should only be continued if definite clinical benefit results. If the diagnosis remains in doubt, formal food challenges may be necessary.

All children on a restricted diet should be supervised by a paediatric dietitian. This is important to make sure that the allergen is completely avoided and that the diet is nutritionally adequate. Growth and weight should be monitored in all children on restricted diets.

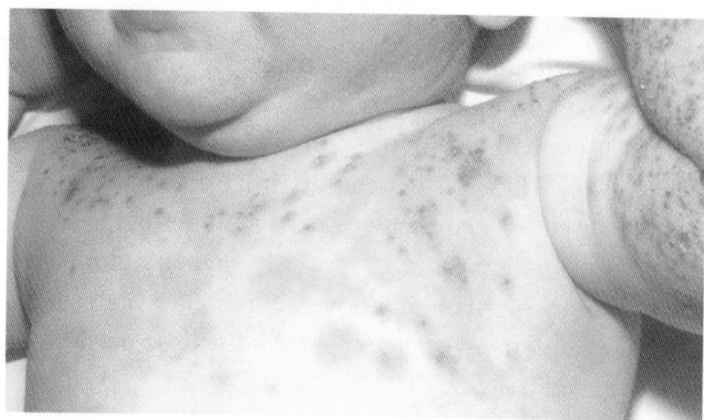

Figure 18.12 Eczema herpeticum showing typical monomorphic discrete erosions in a child with atopic eczema

INHALANT SENSITIVITY

In the older child or adult, sensitivity to the inhalant allergens often predominates. House dust mite and grass are the two allergens that are most difficult to avoid. Animal dander is another potent allergen and the family of atopic children should be advised not to have domestic pets.

COMPLICATIONS

Secondary bacterial infection

This is the commonest complication, usually caused by *S. aureus* although streptococci can also be responsible. Clinically infected eczema needs a course of an appropriate antibiotic. However, even in the absence of clinical infection, *S. aureus* can be isolated from the majority of swabs from older children and adults. This colonization contributes to the inflammatory process in atopic eczema but satisfactory treatment to reduce it is still awaited.

Herpes simplex virus

It is also important to recognize infection with herpes simplex (Figure 18.12). Children with atopic eczema do not handle this virus normally and the lesions may be much more widespread (Kaposi varicelliform eruption or eczema herpeticum). It classically presents as small discrete erosions. Swabs should be taken for virological examination and treatment started empirically with aciclovir while awaiting the results.

Allergic contact dermatitis

The development of contact allergy is a problem for some patients with persistent disease. The commonest allergens involved are nickel and fragrances. However, medicament sensitivity is being increasingly recognized.

Third-line treatment

Some children have severe eczema and fail to respond to topical treatment alone. Phototherapy has been given, using UVB and PUVA, and high-dose UVA_1 phototherapy could be considered. Systemic steroids, ciclosporin and azathioprine have all been used in the treatment of severe, unresponsive atopic eczema.

BLISTERING DISORDERS

Blisters (vesicles and bullae) are an important clinical sign of a heterogeneous group of conditions encompassing:

- infective conditions such as impetigo and staphylococcal scalded skin syndrome, herpes simplex and hand, foot and mouth disease
- genodermatoses (epidermolysis bullosa, bullous ichthyosiform erythroderma and incontinentia pigmenti)
- immunobullous diseases (chronic bullous disease of childhood), dermatitis herpetiformis, pemphigus and pemphigoid)
- a miscellaneous localized group (acute dermatitis, pompholyx, insect bites, phytophotodermatitis).

The history and age of onset are both important factors in the differential diagnosis of the blistering disorders.

Blistering in the neonatal period

Causes of blistering in the neonate

Genetic

- Epidermolysis bullosa
- Bullous ichthyosiform erythroderma
- Incontinentia pigmenti
- Porphyria

Autoimmune

- Pemphigoid of pregnancy
- Bullous pemphigoid
- Pemphigus
- Chronic bullous disease of childhood

Infection

- Congenital herpes simplex
- Congenital syphilis
- Bullous impetigo
- Staphylococcal scalded skin syndrome

Miscellaneous

- Sucking blisters
- Urticaria pigmentosa
- Infantile acropustulosis
- Acrodermatitis enteropathica

Table 18.9 Acquired blistering

Condition	Frequency	Clinical features	Investigations	Treatment
Herpes simplex	Common; may be recurrent	Primary stomatitis: recurrent/ vesicles Atypical in atopic eczema: small discrete erosions	Swab for virological electron microscopy	Aciclovir: topical/oral/ systemic
Impetigo	Common; heals without scarring	Erosions with superficial scale	Bacteriological swab	Oral/topical antibiotics
Pompholyx	Relatively common	Blisters: palms and soles	Bacteriology	Potassium permanganate soaks Potent topical steroids
Erythema multiforme	Common	Target lesions and mucosal involvement Blistering less common	Look for precipitating cause	Treatment of underlying condition
Chronic bullous disease	Rare	Perineal and facial lesions: erythematous plaques with marginal subepidermal bullae (string of pearls sign)	Bx and immuno-fluorescence Linear IgA deposition	Sulfapyridine/dapsone Spontaneous remission after 3+ years
Dermatitis herpetiformis	Uncommon	Tense subepidermal blisters: knees and elbows	Bx and immuno-fluorescence IgA granular pattern	Dapsone; gluten free diet
Phytophoto dermatitis	Uncommon	Linear blistering H/O exposure to sunlight and plants, e.g. giant hogweed	Clinical, history and examination	Avoidance of plants
Pemphigus and pemphigoid	Very rare	Blistering/erosions	Immunofluorescence	Potent topical steroids

Bacterial infections are the commonest cause of blistering in this age group and may give rise to bullous impetigo or more rarely to staphylococcal scalded skin syndrome. **Congenital herpes simplex virus infection** is rare but should be considered in a sick neonate with a vesicular eruption. The genodermatoses are considered separately below.

Blistering in infants and children

See Table 18.9 for acquired blistering disorders. Bacterial and viral infections remain the commonest cause. An **acute dermatitis** can also cause a vesicular eruption as may be seen in an acute allergic dermatitis. **Pompholyx** affects the palms or soles, although this is uncommon in children. **Insect bites** sometimes give rise to quite marked localized blistering. **Erythema multiforme** is a relatively common condition although the bullous form is only rarely seen. The **immuno-bullous** disorders are all very rare in children and the two commonest are IgA mediated.

Chronic bullous disease of childhood

This predominantly affects young children. It is characterized by small tense blisters around the edge of lesions – the so-called string of pearls sign. The lesions are distributed predominantly in the perineal region and on the limbs. Immunofluorescence is diagnostic and shows linear deposition of IgA at the basement membrane. The condition usually goes into spontaneous remission within a few years.

Dermatitis herpetiformis

Dermatitis herpetiformis only rarely affects children. It is an intensely itchy condition, so much so that intact blisters are rarely seen. The lesions are distributed predominantly on the extensor aspects of the limbs. The diagnosis is confirmed by histology of a fresh lesion and immunofluorescence shows a granular pattern of IgA along the basement membrane. There may be an associated gluten enteropathy and patients should be on a gluten-free diet. Dapsone is usually effective in this condition.

Some of the **porphyrias** may present with blistering on exposed sites. It is usually easy to recognize a **phytophotodermatitis** because of the linear blistering on exposed sights. The blistering reaction is caused by the combination of exposure to sunlight together with a photosensitizer in plants such as giant hogweed.

GENODERMATOSES

Epidermolysis bullosa

This is a group of genetically determined skin diseases that produce mechanically induced blistering of the skin varying in severity from minor to life-threatening disease (Figure 18.13). Based on the level of the skin at which blistering can be seen by electron microscopy, epidermolysis bullosa has traditionally been classified into:

- Epidermolysis bullosa simplex: mutations in keratins (K5 and K14) cause an intraepidermal split within the basal keratinocytes
- Junctional epidermolysis bullosa: mutations in laminin 5 causes a cleavage within the lamina lucida
- Dystrophic epidermolysis bullosa: mutations in type VII collagen cause a cleavage below the lamina densa in the basement membrane zone split in the lamina lucida.

Over the past decade the molecular genetic basis of many of these diseases has been unravelled. The basic clinical and genetic features of the commoner subtypes of epidermolysis bullosa are shown in Table 18.10. Epidermolysis bullosa presents with skin fragility, blistering and subsequent erosions. Blisters and erosions may be present at birth but their extent does not reliably predict the subsequent severity of the disease. Although epidermolysis bullosa simplex is usually a relatively benign type, the Dowling Meara form can present in the neonatal period with fairly extensive blistering. In contrast, some have seemingly mild and relatively limited disease at birth that becomes progressively much more extensive and severe. It is therefore important to establish a precise diagnosis by ultrastructural or genetic studies before discussing the prognosis. In general the more severe types are autosomal recessive.

The milder autosomal dominant forms usually present later in childhood with blistering at sites of trauma. In the milder forms of epidermolysis bullosa simplex, blistering is often restricted to the palms and soles. Similarly in the dominant dystrophic form blistering may be restricted to the knees, elbows and feet and hands and milia formation may be seen. After repeated blistering in the recessive dystrophic forms of the disease, scarring

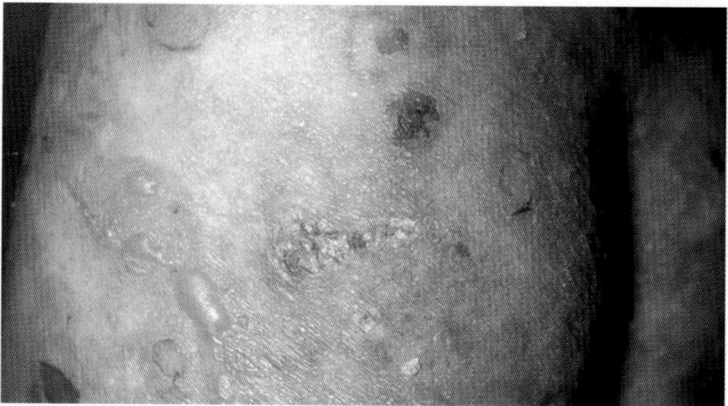

Figure 18.13 Severe epidermolysis bullosa showing subepidermal blisters and subsequent erosions on the buttocks

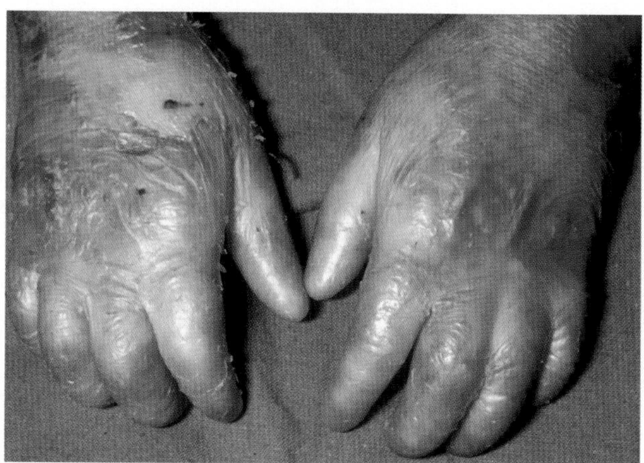

Figure 18.14 Recessive dystrophic epidermolysis bullosa with erosions, scarring, fusion of the fingers and loss of fingernails

and joint contractures can develop and ultimately squamous cell carcinoma of the skin (Figure 18.14).

Junctional epidermolysis bullosa is subdivided into the lethal (Herlitz) type and the non-lethal type. Extreme skin fragility is present at birth and mucosal involvement may also be present, giving rise to a hoarse cry and stridor. In the lethal form death may occur in early infancy, usually from infection. In contrast, those in the non-lethal group may survive into adult life. Nail abnormalities may also be associated. In the more severe varieties of epidermolysis bullosa, involvement of the larynx, eye, respiratory tree, gastrointestinal tract and genitourinary tract may cause problems and chronic anaemia may develop.

At present there is no curative treatment but supportive care is critically important and often a multidisciplinary team approach is useful. Parents and carers should be instructed in gentle handling of the skin and the use of appropriate dressing techniques. Attention should also be focused on growth, nutrition, anaemia, dental hygiene, constipation and the early detection of squamous cell carcinoma of the skin. Genetic counselling requires accurate subclassification of the disease and the identification of the specific mutation.

For other congenital blistering disorders see Table 18.11.

Table 18.10 Congenital blistering disorders: epidermolysis bullosa (EB)

Type	Level of split	Subtype	Mode of inheritance	Morphology	Gene
EB simplex	Intraepidermal	Weber-Cockayne	AD	Blisters restricted to palms and soles; hyperhidrosis; worse in summer; heals without scarring	Keratin 5 or 14
		Dowling-Meara	AD	May be severe in infancy ± involvement oral mucosa Annular configuration of blisters in major flexures Blistering of palms and soles with hyperkeratosis	Keratin 5 or 14
		Koebner	AD	Generalized blistering	Keratin 5 or 14
		EB-MD	AR	Similar to junctional EB clinically Muscular dystrophy	Plectin
Junctional EB	Lamina lucida	Herlitz (lethal)	AR	Severe skin fragility; generalized blisters and non-healing crusted erosions especially around mouth, pharynx, nails Mucosal involvement: hoarseness and stridor Nail and teeth dystrophies Persistent failure to thrive; often lethal	Laminin 5
		Non-Herlitz (non-lethal)	AR	Similar to Herlitz but gradually less severe; growth failure less prominent; alopecia; oral and ocular erosions	Laminin 5 or collagen 17
		EB-PA	AR	Similar to Herlitz Pyloric atresia	$\alpha_6\beta_4$ integrin
Dystrophic EB	Sublamina densa	Recessive	AR	Severe skin fragility; blisters and erosions particularly of hands, feet and limbs; heal with milia and severe scarring and contracture Oesophageal blisters and strictures Hair: scarring alopecia Fusion of fingers	Collagen 7
		Dominant	AD	Mild phenotype Blistering at sites of trauma: knees, hands and feet Heals with milia, mild atrophic scarring; nail dystrophies	Collagen 7

AD, autosomal dominant; AR, autosomal recessive.

Table 18.11 Other congenital blistering disorders

Condition	Inheritance	Clinical features	Investigations	Mutation
Bullous ichthyosiform erythroderma	FH +ve AD >50 per cent Sporadic	Infancy: erythroderma, blistering Childhood: hyperkeratosis Palmoplantar hyperkeratosis Skin infections common	Biopsy: epidermolytic hyperkeratosis	Keratin gene mutations (K1 and K10)
Incontinentia pigmenti	Sex-linked dominant Lethal in males	Three stages: Crops of small tense vesicles Warty Hyper/hypopigmentation Associated: eye and neurological abnormalities	Biopsy early Eosinophils in vesicles	NEMO gene
Porphyrias	Uncommon	Photosensitivity Blisters on exposed sites	Porphyrin screen	

Ichthyoses

These are a group of conditions characterized by generalized, dry, scaly skin resulting from a genetically determined abnormality in cornification. This may present in the neonatal period as scaling erythroderma or as the development of a collodion baby, in which the skin is encased in shiny adherent film. Ichthyoses are generally treated with greasy emollients and in the more severe forms, topical or systemic retinoids may improve the condition of the skin. Genetic counselling requires an accurate diagnosis of the type of ichthyosis and a knowledge of the mode of inheritance. In a few instances this may now be assisted by molecular genetic studies.

Ichthyosis vulgaris (autosomal dominant ichthyosis vulgaris)

This is the commonest ichthyosis, affecting about 1:250 of the population and can be very mild. It is not usually present in the neonate but typically first appears at age of about 6 months as light-coloured fine scales on the trunk and extensor limbs. It typically spares the face, limb flexures and palms. The gene mutation is not known.

X-linked recessive ichthyosis

This affects 1 in 2000 boys. Compared with autosomal dominant ichthyosis vulgaris, the scales are larger, darker and more adherent. The trunk and limbs are affected and although the face is spared, the sides of the neck are typically involved. In this condition there is deficiency of steroid sulphatase, which is usually due to deletion of the gene on Xp22.3, rather than a point mutation. Steroid sulphatase is also expressed in the placenta and about a third of affected children are born after a prolonged or complicated labour. About 10 per cent of affected boys have a contiguous gene defect resulting in cryptorchidism. The diagnosis of X-linked recessive ichthyosis can be confirmed by assays of steroid sulphatase activity in blood or by molecular genetic techniques.

Autosomal recessive ichthyoses

These are a group of clinically and genetically heterogeneous severe ichthyoses. They normally present with a collodion membrane at birth and the ichthyosis is often associated with marked erythema. The face is frequently affected and ectropion and eclabion may develop. Two clinically recognizable forms are described: lamellar ichthyosis in which large, dark plate-like scales develop with little erythema and non-bullous ichthyosiform erythroderma in which the scaling is finer and erythema more intense. The molecular basis for some causes of lamellar ichthyosis has been shown to be mutations in keratinocyte transglutaminase I.

Bullous ichthyosiform erythroderma (epidermolytic hyperkeratosis)

This is an autosomal dominant trait that often presents in the neonate with blistering and erythroderma. During the first few years of life the blistering and erythema diminish and hyperkeratosis develops in a linear manner particularly in the limb flexures. This disease is due to a mutation in keratin 1 or 10. Ichthyosis may also form part of a more generalized syndrome as shown in Table 18.12.

Neurofibromatosis

Neurofibromatosis (NF)1 (Figure 18.15) affects about 1:5000 of the population and is an autosomal dominant

Table 18.12 Syndromes associated with ichthyosis

Disorder	Inheritance	Mutation	Clinical features
Sjögren-Larsson	AR	Fatty aldehyde dehydrogenase	Hyperkeratosis; mental retardation; spastic paraplegia
Trichothiodystrophy	AR	DNA helicase in some	Variable ichthyosis; hair shaft abnormality; mental retardation; short stature; photosensitivity
Netherton syndrome	AR	SPINK 5	Ichthyosiform erythroderma; hair shaft abnormality; atopy; failure to thrive
Conradi-Hünermann	X-linked dominant	Emopamil binding protein	Psoriasis-like erythema and scaling along Blaschko lines; short stature; chondrodysplasia punctata
Neutral lipid storage disease	AR	Recycling of triacylglycerol to diacylglycerol	Ichthyosiform erythroderma; multisystem lipid accumulation with liver; neurological and ocular involvement

AR, autosomal recessive.

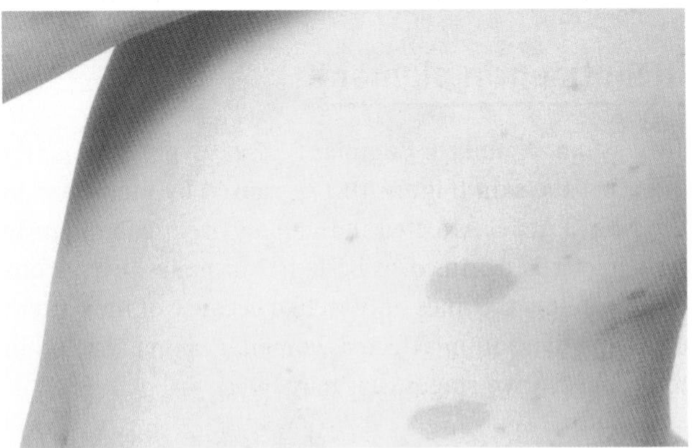

Figure 18.15 Café-au-lait macules: an early sign of neurofibromatosis

trait with high penetrance and high rate of new mutation. The NF1 gene encodes a GAP protein named neurofibromin. Mutation analysis is difficult in clinical practice because of the large size of gene and the lack of mutation hot spots. Diagnosis therefore still relies on clinical features as described by a 1998 National Institutes of Health (NIH) consensus conference (see below) and requires two criteria to be met in an individual. Café-au-lait macules (CALMs) are frequently the first and most obvious manifestation of NF1. They may be present at birth and consist of light brown macules and patches with well-defined edges affecting any area of skin except palms and soles. Café-au-lait macules are not specific to NF1; they also occur in NF2 and McCune–Albright syndrome. Ten per cent of the normal population also has one or two CALMs (particularly dark-skinned races). Children with six or more CALMs should be monitored during childhood for the development of other features of NF1. Other relatively early features of NF1 are Lisch nodules and axillary freckling. Lisch nodules are asymptomatic pigmented iris hamartomas that usually appear between 5 and 10 years of age. They are elevated and can be distinguished from common melanocytic naevi, which are flat. Freckles in the axilla, inguinal region and side of the neck may appear between 3 and 15 years of age and look like small CALMs (1–3 mm in diameter).

NIH consensus diagnostic criteria for neurofibromatosis 1

- Six or more café-au-lait macules: ⩾5 mm diameter in a child, ⩾15 mm diameter in an adult
- Two or more neurofibromas or one plexiform neurofibroma
- Freckling in the axillary or inguinal region
- Two or more iris hamartomas (Lisch nodules)
- Optic glioma
- Distinctive osseous lesions (e.g. sphenoid wing hyperplasia or thinning of long bone cortex)
- First-degree relative with NFI

Neurofibromas often do not develop until after the age of 10 years. The commonest neurofibromas arise from dermal nerve endings, most frequently on the trunk, and vary in number in an unpredictable manner from several to thousands. The overlying skin is usually pink, the lesions are very soft and when pressed they tend to invaginate – the so-called 'button-holing' sign. Less frequently, neurofibromas arise from major nerve trunks and may cause neurological symptoms, in contrast with dermal neurofibromas. When plexiform neurofibromas develop they are usually of early onset (1–2 years of age). They can occur anywhere on the body as a large subcutaneous swelling with ill-defined margins.

There are no specific treatments for NF1 that prevent the various manifestations of the disease. An annual examination in a multidisciplinary clinic is recommended, particularly to assess complications of NF1 and to provide genetic counselling.

Complications of neurofibromatosis 1

Neurological
- Intellectual handicap
- Epilepsy
- Central nervous system tumour
- Optic glioma
- Spinal neurofibroma
- Peripheral nerve sarcoma

Orthopaedic
- Scoliosis
- Pseudoarthritis of tibia and fibula

Ophthalmological
- Congenital glaucoma

Other
- Renal artery stenosis and hypertension
- Phaeochromocytoma

Tuberous sclerosis complex

Tuberous sclerosis complex (TSC) 1 and TSC2 (Figure 18.16) are autosomal dominant disorders caused by mutations in the genes for hamartin and tuberin, respectively. Diagnosis is criterion based, the major criteria being cutaneous, neurological, renal and cardiac. The cutaneous features include hypomelanotic macules, connective tissue naevi (forehead plaques and shagreen patches), and angiofibromas (adenoma sebaceum). Hypomelanotic macules (ash leaf macules) are generally present a birth. They can be any shape and are usually multiple. They are commonest on the trunk and limbs and can be more easily identified with a Wood lamp. It is not uncommon to see a single hypomelanotic macule in a normal child. Shagreen patches usually develop during adolescence as a dermal plaque, usually in the lumbar region. Forehead plaques have a similar appearance but may develop earlier during childhood. Angiofibromas typically develop from the age of 2 years as red papules and nodules symmetrically affecting the nasolabial folds, cheeks and chin. Periungual fibromas generally develop from adolescence into adulthood. They more frequently affect the toes than fingers and appear as a papule arising from the proximal nail fold and produce a linear depression in the nail plate.

Incontinentia pigmenti

This is an X-linked dominant disease predominantly affecting the skin (Figure 18.17), caused by mutations in the NEMO gene. Affected individuals are predominantly girls and it is assumed to be lethal in males. Cutaneous lesions follow the lines of Blaschko because of the pattern of X-inactivation in affected women. Lesions develop in four consecutive stages that may overlap:

- Stage 1 – lasts for up to six months of age. Vesicles and pustules develop
- Stage 2 – linear verrucous plaques
- Stage 3 – linear and whorled hyperpigmentation, not necessarily in the same areas of skin affected by stages 1 and 2
- Stage 4 – occurs in adults and is characterized by hypopigmented atrophic lines, which can be very subtle.

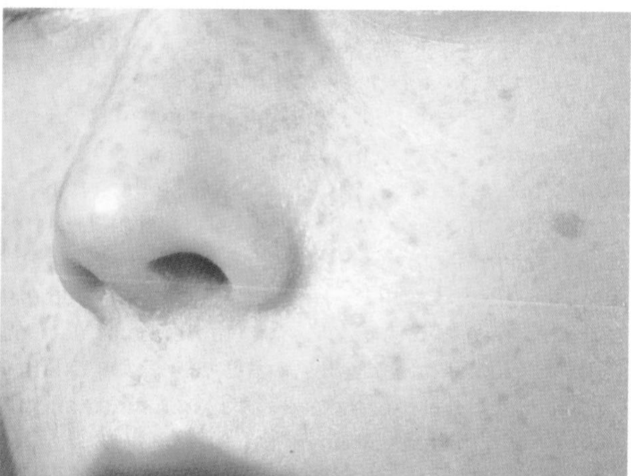

Figure 18.16 Angiofibromas (adenoma sebaceum), a major diagnostic criterion of tuberous sclerosis

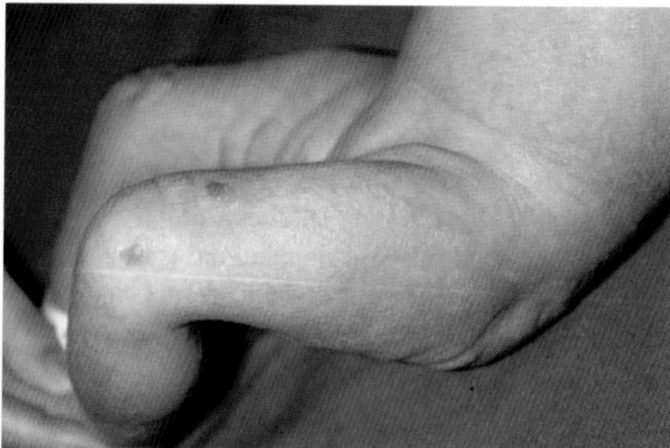

Figure 18.17 Vesiculation of the thigh in a girl as an early manifestation of incontinentia pigmenti

Other less common manifestations of the disease include a nail dystrophy, scarring alopecia, hypodontia and unilateral aplasia of the breast. Mental retardation and seizures develop in about 10 per cent.

Albinism

Albinism refers to a group of diseases characterized by inherited disorders of melanin production. In most cases the pattern of inheritance is autosomal recessive. Clinically there is congenital, partial or complete absence of pigment from skin and hair, and involvement of the iris and retina associated with photophobia, decreased visual acuity and nystagmus. Although traditionally classified into tyrosinase positive and negative based on the activity of a key enzyme in melanin biosynthesis, recent molecular genetic studies have identified at least 10 subtypes. In most subtypes the risk of cutaneous malignancy is greatly increased and regular surveillance should be undertaken. Affected individuals need to be advised on reducing their exposure to ultraviolet radiation by appropriate sun-avoidance behaviour, clothing and sun blocks.

Piebaldism

This is an autosomal dominant condition due to mutations in *c*-kit, which encodes a melanocyte receptor tyrosine kinase. Loss of function mutations result in failure of melanocyte migration to the skin, which presents at birth as symmetrically distributed, well-defined patches of depigmentation. This can simulate vitiligo but differs in being non-progressive and congenital.

Ectodermal dysplasia

This is a diverse group of over 150 rare disorders of development of two or more ectodermal structures (hair, teeth, nails, sweat glands, other ectodermal structures). They are classified by phenotype according to the pattern of involvement of ectodermal structures and in most the molecular mechanisms are not known. Two well-defined syndromes are presented to illustrate the group. **X-linked hypohidrotic ectodermal dysplasia** (Christ-Siemens-Touraine syndrome) mainly affects hair, teeth and sweat glands. Affected boys often present in infancy with hyperthermia due to inability to thermoregulate due to an absence of eccrine sweat glands. They have distinctive facial features with frontal bossing, saddle nose and sparse, lightly pigmented hair. Dentition is delayed and erupted teeth are often small and peg-shaped.

AEC Syndrome (ankyloblepharon – ectodermal dysplasia – cleft palate, or Hay Wells syndrome) is a very rare autosomal dominant condition. Ankyloblepharon describes partial thickness filiform fusion of the eyelid margins. The remainder of the skin is red and scaly, scalp hair is sparse and wiry, the nails are often thickened and hypodontia is common. Cleft palate, with or without cleft lip, is present in about 75 per cent of cases.

Xeroderma pigmentosum

Xeroderma pigmentosum is a rare autosomal recessive disease caused by defects in DNA repair mechanisms. There is genetic locus heterogeneity, and eight subtypes or complementation groups of varying severity are recognized. The skin appears normal at birth but is photosensitive and within the first few years of life, irregular freckling and dryness develop, initially affecting the photo-exposed areas of the face and hands. This subsequently becomes more generalized and the anterior compartment of the eyes are frequently sun damaged. Skin cancers of all types (basal cell carcinoma, squamous cell carcinoma and melanoma) start to develop before the age of 10 years. A progressive neurological deterioration affects some complementation groups. Diagnosis can be confirmed by studying the effects of ultraviolet radiation on cultured fibroblasts. Management of affected individuals depends on rigorous photoprotection and early surgical excision of skin cancers.

INFECTIONS

See Table 18.13 for an overview of paediatric dermatological infections.

CASE STUDY

A neonate presents with a five-day history of the development of discrete discoid lesions in the napkin area. These are somewhat crusted with a superficial scale. Initially, only one or two lesions were present but more are developing each day.

Impetigo

Impetigo is characterized clinically by honey-gold crusts. It is usually a straightforward clinical diagnosis. Most children with impetigo are diagnosed and treated in the community. Thus children presenting to secondary care

Table 18.13 Infections

	Frequency	Distribution	Clinical features	Organism	Treatment	Prognosis/complications
Bacterial						
Impetigo	Very common	Face/any site	Golden crusts	*Staphylococcus aureus*; *Streptococcus* group A	Systemic/topical antibiotics	Excellent
Bullous impetigo	Common	Any site	Superficial erosions and scale	*S. aureus* usually	Systemic/topical antibiotics	Excellent
Staphylococcal scalded skin syndrome	Uncommon	Face and flexures	Toxic/febrile/superficial erosions and cigarette paper scale	*S. aureus* phage type 3/toxin		Usually good
Erysipelas	Uncommon in childhood	Any/face/perianal	Toxic/febrile; bright red erythema	*Streptococcus* group A	Penicillin V	Excellent
Viral						
Herpes simplex: primary	Common	Oral	Gingival stomatitis	Herpes simplex type 1	Oral aciclovir	Good
Herpes simplex: secondary	Common	Perioral	'Cold sores'	Herpes simplex type 1	Antiseptics/topical/ oral aciclovir	Good; erythema multiforme
Herpes simplex recurrent	Fairly common	Face/fingers	Recurrent localized vesicles	Herpes simplex type 1	Topical or oral aciclovir	Good; erythema Multiforme
Herpes simplex secondary to atopic eczema	Common	Any	Toxic/punched out erosions	Herpes simplex type 1	Oral aciclovir	Usually good
Molluscum	Common	Any	Dome-shaped shiny umbilicated papules	Pox virus	Nil/mild trauma/ cryotherapy	Good; develop natural immunity – 12–18 months
Warts	Common	Hands/face/ plantar/genital	Skin-coloured papules/ filiform/plantar	Papillomavirus	Nil/topical keratolytics/cryotherapy	Good
Yeast						
Candida	Common	Young children Oral; napkin area	White mucosal plaques; erythematous scaly lesions + satellite lesions	*Candida albicans*	Nystatin/topical anticandidal	Excellent
Chronic candida paronychia	Uncommon	Young children Periungual	Erythema and bolstering of nail folds	*Candida albicans*	Antiseptics/topical imidazoles	Protracted course
Mucocutaneous candidiasis	Rare	Young children Mouth/nails	Oral/nail dystrophies	*Candida* + Immuno-deficiency	Systemic/anticandidal	
Fungal	Common	Any age; Feet; body; hair; nails	Interdigital maceration; erythematous plaques with peripheral scale; patchy alopecia; nail dystrophy	*Tinea rubrum* + others Scrape/plucked hair/ nail clippings	Topical or systemic antifungals	Usually good

are usually treatment failures or have an atypical clinical picture. This may be due to inadequately treated infections. A bacteriological swab should be taken to identify the infecting organism and to establish antibiotic sensitivity. This is becoming increasingly important in the face of rising antibiotic resistance, particularly in penicillin-sensitive patients. *S. aureus* is usually the causative organism, but *Streptococcus pyogenes* may be involved alone or in combination with *S. aureus*.

Bullous impetigo

The lesions (Figure 18.18) are usually localized but may be fairly extensive, as in the above case study. Intact bullae are not commonly seen, as they tend to rupture because of the high level of the epidermal split. Superficial erosions with peeling of the skin are characteristic. Bacteria can be isolated from the lesions.

Treatment

A topical antibiotic may be adequate for very localized disease. To minimize the development of antibiotic resistance, a five-day course of treatment should be completed and then the tube discarded. In general, antibiotics that are not available for systemic use are to be preferred for topical use.

For more extensive disease, or for children who are systemically unwell, a course of an oral antibiotic such as flucloxacillin is the antibiotic of choice for staphylococcal infections and penicillin for streptococcal infections. Children with combined infections should receive both antibiotics.

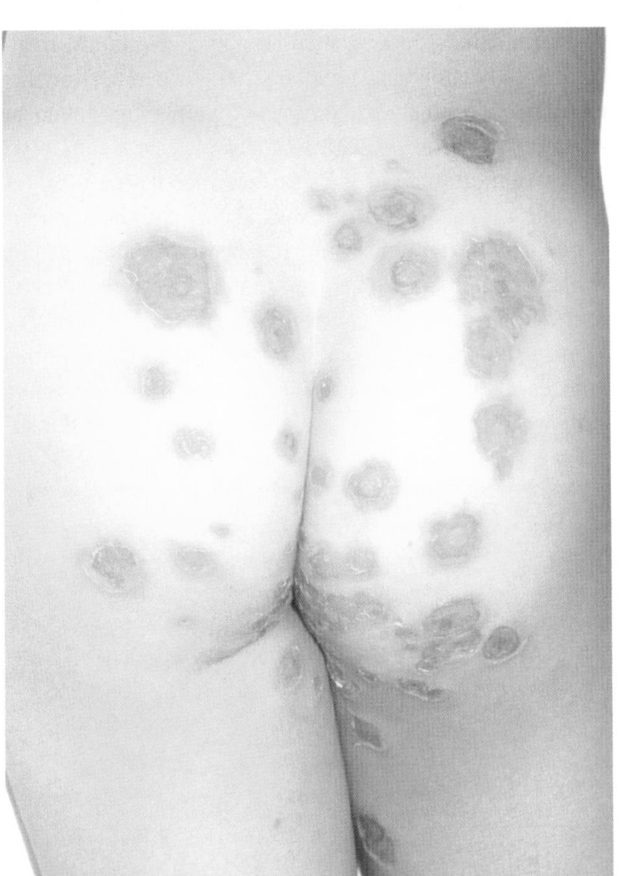

Figure 18.18 Bullous impetigo with characteristic erosions on a typical site

Staphylococcal scalded skin syndrome

Staphylococcal scalded skin syndrome (Figure 18.19) is an uncommon condition that predominantly affects young children. The primary focus of infection may be in the nasopharynx, conjunctivae or the umbilicus in neonates or may remain unidentified. Bacteria, usually *S. aureus* (phage type 2), release epidermolytic toxins into the general circulation and cause the characteristic clinical picture. Children are febrile and systemically unwell. Erythema develops which is often most marked in the flexures. Subsequently superficial erosions develop with the typical cigarette-paper-like desquamation of the skin. The clinical appearances are usually diagnostic but if the diagnosis is in doubt a skin biopsy will confirm the high level split in the epidermis that differentiates this from the deeper level of the split found in toxic epidermal necrolysis (TEN). Bacteria are not isolated from the denuded areas but may be isolated from the primary focus if this has been identified.

Treatment

Systemic antibiotics are indicated to treat the primary focus of infection and thus halt further production of the toxins. Adequate analgesia is often necessary for the first 48–72 hours, as the child can be quite uncomfortable. Skin care is needed to protect the denuded area using non-adherent

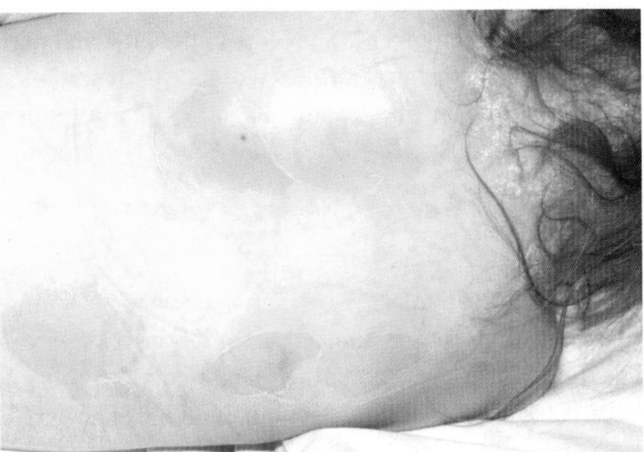

Figure 18.19 Staphylococcal scalded skin syndrome: superficial erosions with cigarette paper-like desquamation

dressings. Water and electrolyte balance needs monitoring because of the loss of skin barrier. With treatment, the condition usually resolves fairly rapidly, although there is a small mortality. The skin lesions heal without scarring.

Erysipelas

This is a superficial streptococcal infection of the skin which is uncommon in young children, although it is seen more frequently in adults. The portal of entry is not always visible and streptococci may not be isolated from the skin surface. It is usually a clinical diagnosis and is recognized by the characteristic well-demarcated erythema. Patients are usually systemically unwell and febrile. The condition responds rapidly to treatment with penicillin. The oral route is usually adequate but the intravenous administration may be needed if the child is very toxic.

Herpes simplex

Primary herpes simplex may present acutely with a gingivostomatitis (see Chapter 6).

Recurrent herpes simplex virus (HSV) infection

The commonest form of secondary infection is the 'cold sore', which may be a recurrent problem. Cold sores are so common that many sufferers do not seek medical advice. Prodromal symptoms of tingling or pain may precede the vesicular eruption. Herpes simplex may be provoked by fever caused by an intercurrent infection and may also be provoked by sunlight. The severity of the condition shows a wide variation. Other sites may be affected, and the herpetic whitlow is a well-recognized entity affecting a finger.

Diagnosis

In all cases of recurrent herpes simplex it is important to make a definitive diagnosis. Children are usually free of lesions when seen in a routine outpatient clinic and need to be seen acutely at the onset of symptoms so that swabs or vesicular fluid can be taken from early lesions. Once the diagnosis has been made the early use of aciclovir may abort subsequent attacks.

Complications

Secondary infection is the commonest complication that needs treating. Herpes simplex infection of the eye can cause dendritic ulcers and other ocular complications. If HSV is suspected an urgent ophthalmological review is essential.

Herpes simplex is also a well-recognized cause of **erythema multiforme** (EM). Typically the cold sore antedates EM by 10 days or so. However, the interval can be very much shorter and in some patients HSV and EM may almost coincide or the preceding HSV infection may even pass unrecognized.

Molluscum

See Figure 18.20. This typically affects young children. Successive crops of lesions develop until the child develops their own natural immunity, usually in 12–18 months. Molluscum may be complicated by infection and/or secondary eczema. Parents are often keen for active treatment. This can include mildly traumatizing the lesions and different techniques are available. An antiseptic paint should then be applied to prevent secondary infection. Other options include cryotherapy but this is a painful procedure for small children. A number of topical agents such as cantharidin and potassium hydroxide are being investigated and these may prove useful alternatives.

Warts

Warts are very common. They are caused by the human papillomavirus (HPV), a small DNA virus. Many subtypes have been identified. Most warts resolve spontaneously given time, but some persist and may need topical treatment with keratolytics or podophyllin (for plantar warts) or cryotherapy with liquid nitrogen. Cryotherapy should be repeated every three weeks until clearance or for up to six cycles. **Genital warts** are a cause for concern because of the possible association with sexual abuse. Although genital warts are a sexually transmitted disease in adults, genital warts in children may be acquired innocently by vertical transmission from the mother *in utero* or during delivery. Warts can also be spread by direct contact with other affected family members or indirectly from swimming baths or towels. The virus can also lie latent in the skin.

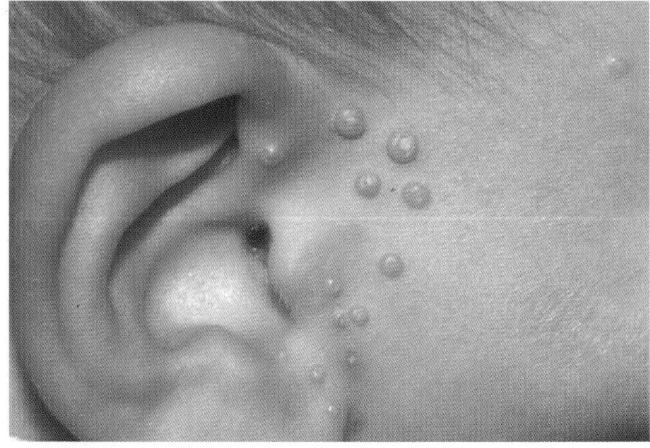

Figure 18.20 Molluscum contagiosum: grouped umbilicated papules

Extensive genital warts in young children may require surgical removal under a general anaesthetic. However, the treated areas can be quite sore postoperatively so a period of observation to allow natural resolution is usually sensible in the first instance. Topical agents such as imiquimod may also be worth a trial.

Yeast infections

Candidiasis

Yeast infections with *Candida* are common in infants, giving rise to the typical white plaques with oral involvement (thrush) and to localized erythematous slightly scaly plaques in the napkin area (napkin candidiasis). *Candida* can be isolated from a swab, or by skin scrapings and/or a strip of adhesive tape from the napkin area. **Mucocutaneous candidiasis** is a rare condition occurring in children with an underlying T-cell abnormality. Clinically it is characterized by severe and persistent oral candidiasis despite adequate treatment and by severe disfiguring nail dystrophies.

Chronic paronychia

This is not uncommon in young children who suck their fingers. Clinically persistent erythema and bolstering of the nail folds is associated with a nail dystrophy. Combination treatment with a topical antiseptic such as povidone and a topical azole is often only partially successful. Topical corticosteroids may be helpful in some individuals.

Mucocutaneous candidiasis

Mucocutaneous candidiasis is a rare condition occurring in children with an underlying T cell abnormality. Clinically it is characterized by severe and persistent oral candisiasis despite adequate treatment and by severe disfiguring nail dystrophies.

Fungal infections

Some fungi only affect humans (the so-called anthrophilic infections) whereas others predominantly affect animals and humans are only infected by chance. **Tinea pedis** is common and is usually caused by *Trichophyton rubrum* but may be caused by *T. interdigitale* and *Epidermophyton* spp. The condition usually responds well to treatment. **Tinea corporis** is less common. Affected children are usually in contact with an infected animal such as a cat (*Microsporum canis*) or guinea pig. **Tinea capitis** (Figure 18.21) usually presents with localized alopecia and the affected areas may fluoresce under a Wood lamp. Plucked hairs are needed for mycological examination as some fungi only affect the hair bulb. Infection with cattle ringworm presents more acutely with kerion (Figure 18.22). The differential diagnosis is of an acute scalp abscess. However, the association of the typical clinical features with a history of exposure should suggest the diagnosis. Because of the brisk inflammatory response fungi are not always identified. It is an important condition to diagnose correctly as permanent alopecia can result if the condition is unrecognized. **Fungal nail infections** (tinea unguium) more commonly affect the toenails than the fingernails. Topical treatment is usually ineffective and systemic treatment is needed if the lesions are symptomatic or the family is keen for active treatment.

Topical agents such as the imidazoles or terbinafine are usually effective in tinea pedis and in tinea corporis if the plaque size is fairly limited. Extensive skin involvement and infection of the hair and nails usually requires systemic treatment for four to six weeks. Griseofulvin is usually effective for infections of the skin and hair but is much less successful in nail infections. For toenail infections an 18-month course of treatment with griseofulvin

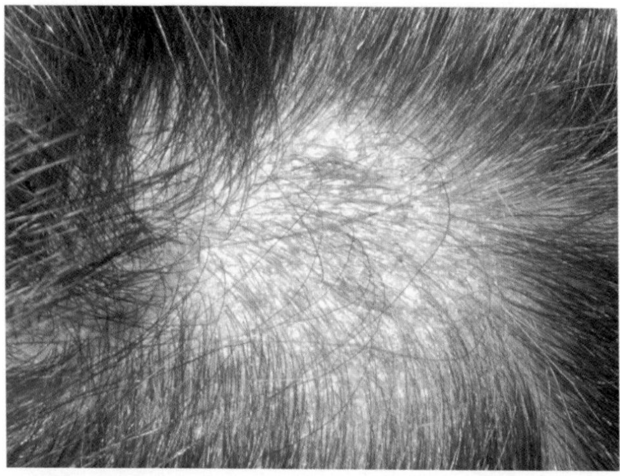

Figure 18.21 Tinea capitis showing a patch of scaling with associated hair loss

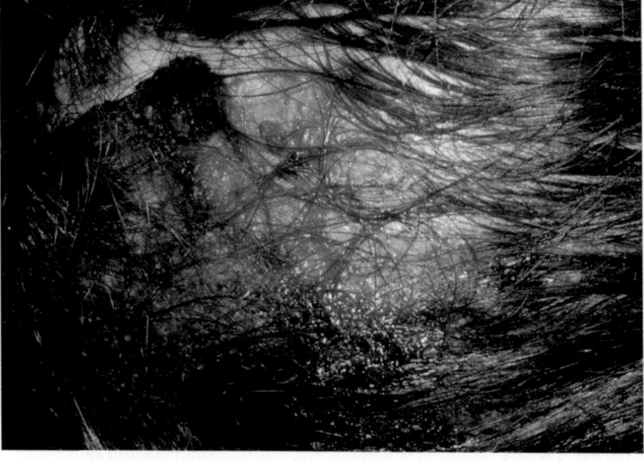

Figure 18.22 Kerion, an inflammatory mass that is often mistaken for a pyogenic abscess. Often caused by cattle ringworm

is usually necessary, in contrast to terbinafine where a three-month course is usually adequate. Currently terbinafine is only licensed for adults although it has been used effectively in children.

INFILTRATIONS

CASE STUDY

A 1-year-old infant presents with several yellow brown patches and plaques on the trunk. His mother reports that they sometimes blister.

Cutaneous mastocytosis

Urticaria pigmentosa (Figure 18.23) typically presents in the first 2 years of life with multiple yellow-brown macules, papules and plaques, mainly on the trunk and proximal limbs. Less often, only one or two lesions are present and are called mastocytomas. If the lesions are gently rubbed, histamine is released from the mast cells, producing a wheal-and-flare reaction or blister (Darier sign). No treatments are particularly effective in clearing the lesions but when the onset is in childhood they tend to clear spontaneously. It is important that the child is advised to avoid histamine-releasing agents such as opiate analgesics and aspirin. The least common of the childhood cutaneous mastocytosis is diffuse cutaneous mastocytosis, which is characterized by widespread infiltration by mast cells. It usually presents as blistering in infancy and subsequent leathery thickening of the skin, sometimes with a yellow discoloration.

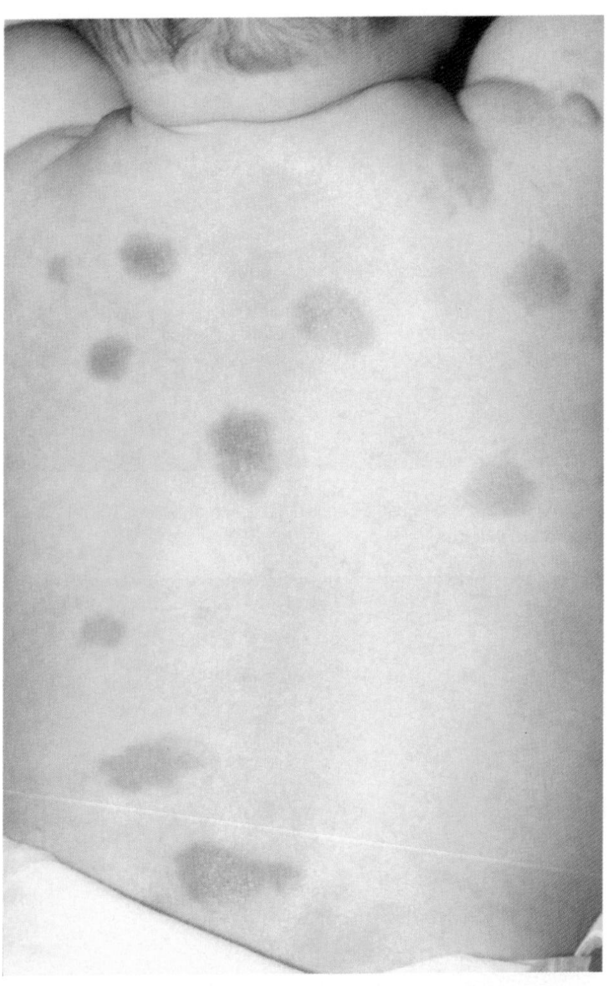

Figure 18.23 Multiple mastocytomas as a manifestation of urticaria pigmentosa. These lesions urticate if rubbed

Cutaneous histiocytosis

Langerhans cell histiocytosis (LCH, class I histiocytosis)

Langerhans cell histiocytosis is often first diagnosed in the skin, which is affected in 40 per cent of cases. Occasionally the skin is the only organ affected and the disease can spontaneously regress. The lesions are small papules frequently containing purpura and which tend to become confluent. There is often secondary erosion and crusting. The lesions preferentially affect the scalp, flexures and napkin area. It is frequently misdiagnosed as seborrhoeic dermatitis, from which it can be distinguished by the presence of purpura and erosions.

Non-Langerhans cell histiocytosis (class II histiocytosis)

Juvenile xanthogranuloma is a benign accumulation of lipid-laden macrophages within the dermis. It typically presents as a dome-shaped red nodule 2 mm to 20 mm in diameter that gradually turns yellow-brown. One or several lesions may be present and they generally resolve spontaneously over the first few years of life. **Benign cephalic histiocytosis** is a rare entity that presents as small yellow-brown papules, usually on the forehead and cheeks. These resolve over a few years leaving small atrophic scars.

Other cutaneous nodules are summarized in Table 18.14.

HAIR ABNORMALITIES

Hair abnormalities may be congenital or acquired (Figure 18.24 and Table 18.15).

Table 18.14 Infiltrations

	Peak age at onset	Morphology	Distribution	Associations	Outcome
Histiocytosis					
Langerhans cell histiocytosis	1–4 years	Confluent papules containing purpura with secondary crusting and erosions	Scalp; flexural areas; trunk	Systemic involvement	Variable
Juvenile xanthogranuloma	0–1 year	Red or yellow dome-shaped papule	Head; neck; upper trunk	Eye involvement; neurofibromatosis 1; leukaemia	Regression over three to six years
Benign cephalic histiocytosis	0–3 years	Small yellow-brown papules	Head	None	Regression with scarring
Mastocytosis					
Mastocytoma	0–1 year	One to five yellow-brown dermal nodules which urticate when rubbed	Limbs	None	Gradual involution
Urticaria pigmentosa	0–1 year	Five or more brown dermal nodules which urticate when rubbed	Trunk	Occasional systemic involvement	50 per cent resolve by adolescence
Diffuse cutaneous mastocytosis	0–1 year	Subepidermal blister and skin thickening	Generalized	Frequent systemic involvement	Blisters stop after a few years

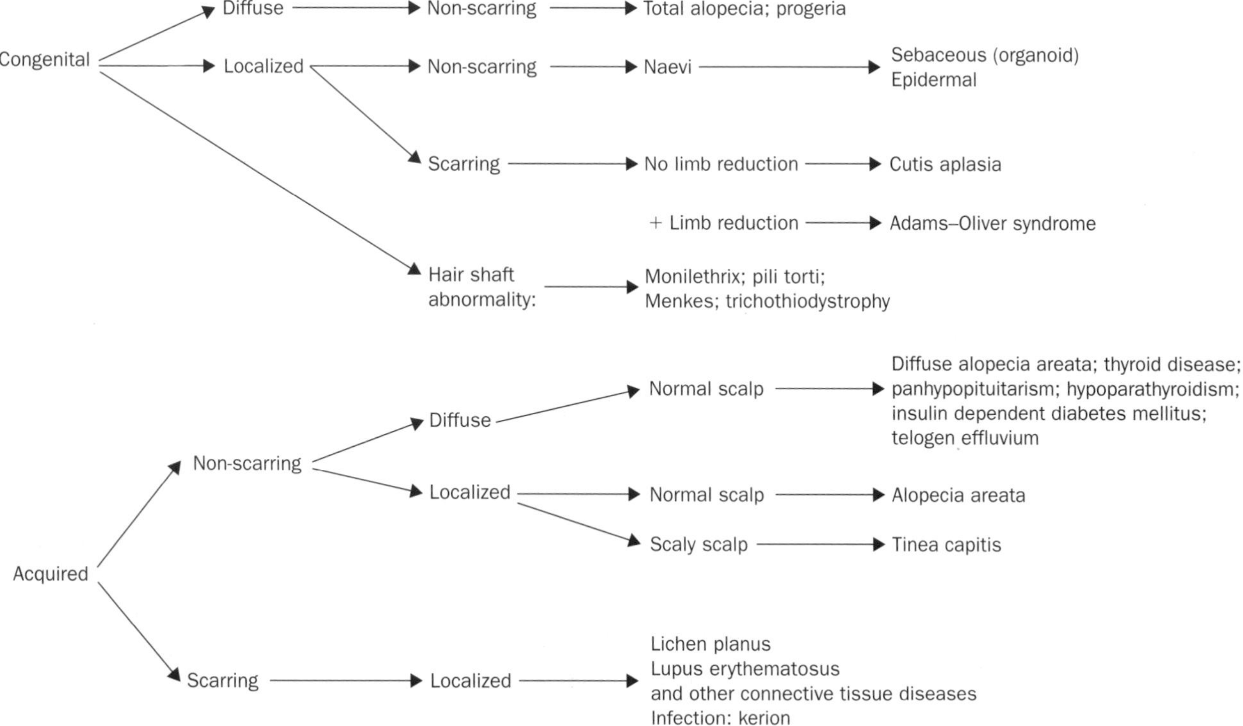

Figure 18.24 Hair loss

Table 18.15 Hair loss: investigations and treatment

Types	Clinical features	Key investigations	Management/outcome
Acquired: localized non-scarring			
Alopecia areata	Well-circumscribed normal scalp; exclamation mark hairs; localized/ diffuse/totalis/universalis ± loss eyelashes/eyebrows; nail pitting	None necessary	Topical steroid scalp applications/ irritants; outlook usually good; may recur
Diffuse hair loss; diffuse alopecia areata	Diffuse; normal scalp	Ferritin; full blood count; Thyroid function tests	Correct underlying cause; diffuse alopecia areata outlook usually good
Tinea capitis	Scaly scalp; localized	Plucked hair for mycology	Oral antifungals
Trichotillomania	Broken short hairs; localized	None	Psychological support
Androgenic alopecia	Frontal thinning and at vertex; male pattern baldness; uncommon in children	None	Treatment unsatisfactory
Congenital			
Cutis aplasia Absence of skin	Scalp commonest site (80 per cent) Localized; single or multiple; variable size; varied morphology; superficial erosions to deep ulceration	None	May heal with scarring Larger lesions may need plastic surgery Trauma from scalp electrodes
Adams–Oliver syndrome	Solitary or multiple scalp defects; limb reduction; congenital heart disease	Clinical diagnosis	Scalp lesions may need corrective surgery
Sebaceous naevus	Yellowish-orange lesion	Biopsy if diagnosis in doubt	Increased risk of malignant change in adult life; consider excision

Alopecia areata

CASE STUDY

An 8-year-old boy presents with a three-month history of the development of bald patches in his hair. There is considerable concern within the family.

Alopecia areata (Figure 18.25) presents with well-circumscribed patches of hair loss. The underlying scalp is normal and exclamation mark hairs may be seen (Figure 18.26). The condition is usually localized but total loss of scalp hair (alopecia totalis) may occur and, in the most severe form, loss of all body hair (alopecia universalis). The loss of eyelashes and eyebrows may also be seen. Pitting of the fingernails may be an associated clinical feature. The family history for alopecia areata may be positive (5–25 per cent). Regrowth is usually spontaneous with white hairs initially. Topical treatment is largely unsatisfactory. A trial of a topical steroid scalp application or an irritant may be worthwhile.

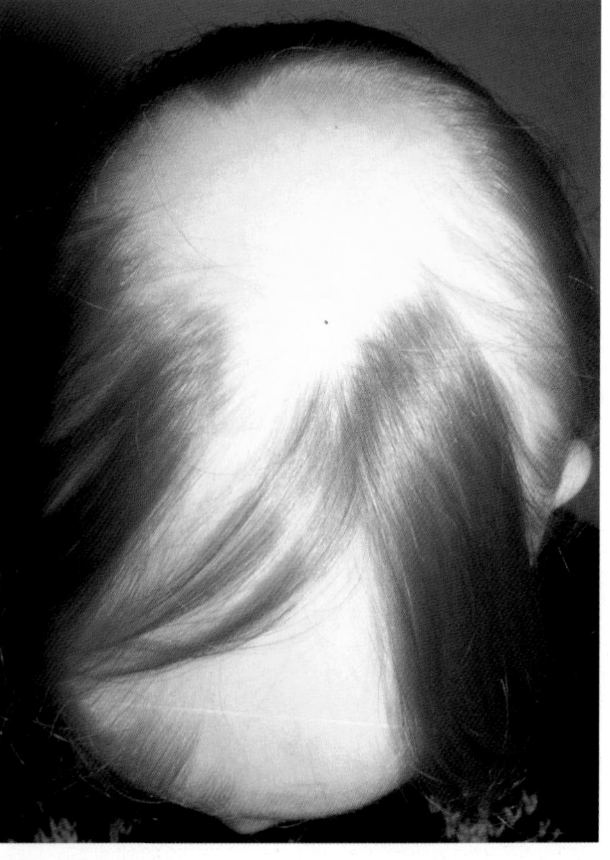

Figure 18.25 Extensive alopecia areata: well defined areas of complete hair loss

The prognosis for complete regrowth is usually good although permanent hair loss may occur. The condition can also recur. Adverse prognostic features include a personal history of atopy and hair loss affecting the hair margin in the occipital region (ophiasis). The longer the duration of the alopecia the worse the outlook for regrowth.

Aetiology

Alopecia areata is usually grouped with the autoimmune diseases. Usually no clear initiating factor can be identified although in some children stress or intercurrent illness may be causally related.

Diffuse hair loss

> **CASE STUDY**
>
> A 9-year-old girl presents with a four-month history of thinning of the hair.

This may be due to a **diffuse form of alopecia areata** and behaves in a similar way to the localized form above. **Diffuse hair loss** may also follow any serious illness. Other causes include sideropenia and thyroid disease. Both hyperthyroidism and hypothyroidism are rare causes of hair loss. In hypothyroidism the texture of the hair is also coarser. It is worth checking ferritin level in addition to a full blood count in these children and, for completeness, thyroid function tests to make sure there is no remediable cause.

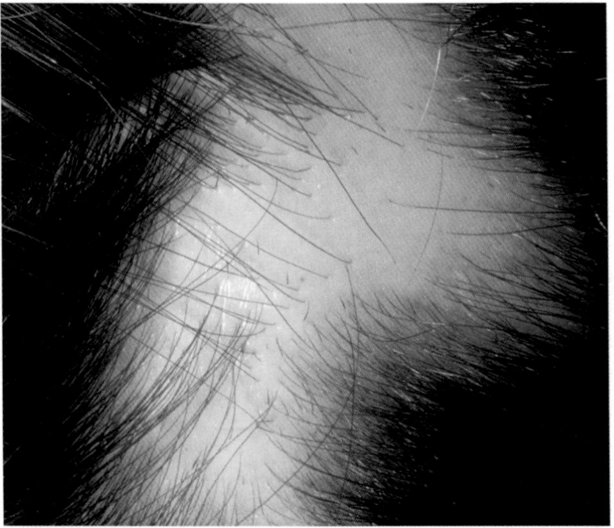

Figure 18.26 Close up of a patch of alopecia areata showing exclamation mark hairs. In contrast to tinea, there is no scaling of the scalp

CONGENITAL ABSENCE OF SKIN (CUTIS APLASIA)

This is the absence of skin at birth. The majority (80 per cent) of lesions affect the scalp. There is usually only a single lesion but multiple may occur. The morphology of the lesions varies from superficial erosions to deeper ulcerations and these may heal with scarring. If there is a large area of scarring alopecia plastic surgery may be necessary for cosmetic reasons when the child is older. Cutis aplasia may be associated with limb reductions as in the Adams–Oliver syndrome.

GENERALIZED RED RASHES OF CHILDHOOD

Infants and young children

> **CASE STUDY**
>
> A 5-month-old infant is referred with a two-month history of a generalized skin rash with marked facial involvement. He is irritable and is sleeping very poorly. His mother is exhausted.

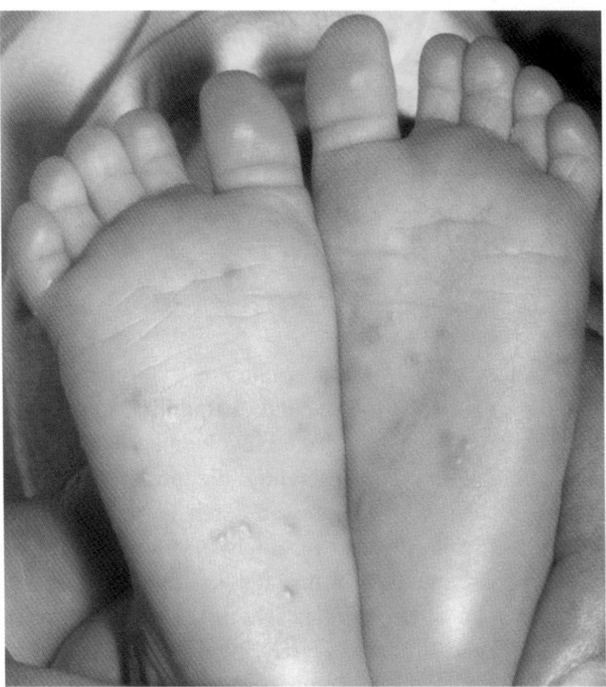

Figure 18.27 Scabies in an infant: in an itchy child, examine the soles as lesions on this site are very suggestive of scabies

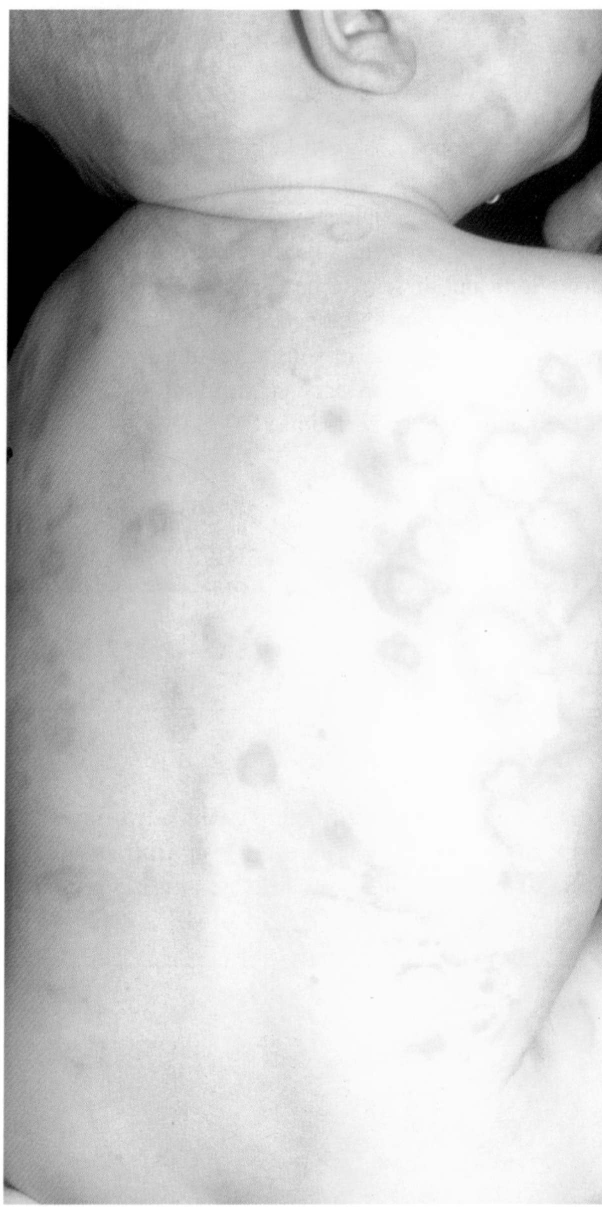

Figure 18.28 Urticaria: itchy evanescent (less than 24 hours) wheals

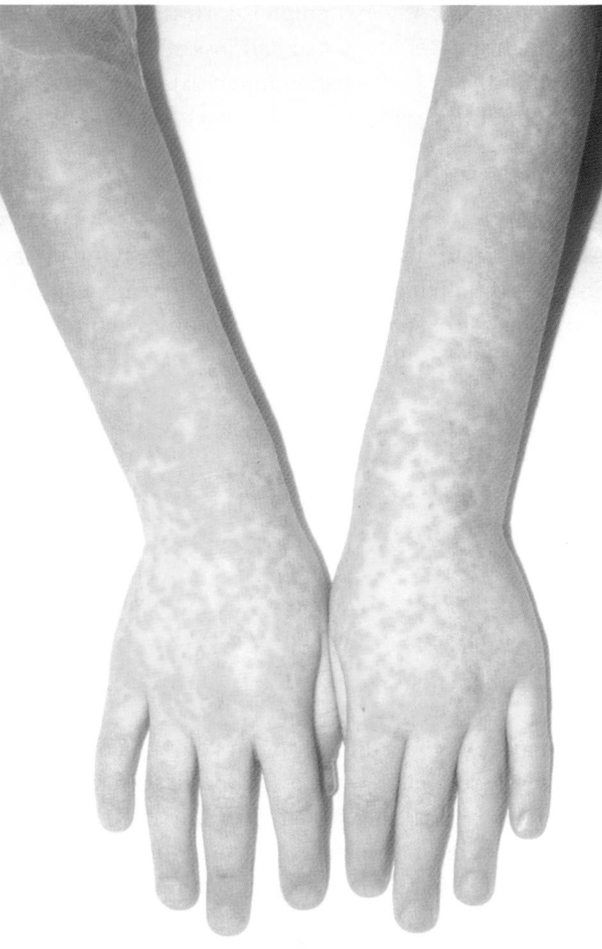

Figure 18.29 Toxic erythema - a blanching erythematous rash in a child often associated with a viral infection. In contrast to urticaria, lesions are more persistent

In this age group **atopic eczema** is the most likely diagnosis. The history of itch, irritability and sleep disturbance is typical and facial involvement is common in young children. The differential diagnosis would also include scabies, which causes an extensive non-specific dermatitis. **Scabies** is also very itchy. Typically the soles of the feet are involved in this age group (Figure 18.27), in contrast to atopic eczema where the soles are only rarely affected. The face is rarely involved. A recent history of a similar itchy eruption affecting other family members is almost diagnostic. **Seborrhoeic dermatitis** is uncommon and would be unlikely in an infant who is very itchy, although this diagnosis should be considered in placid infants. Typically the scalp, flexures and napkin area are involved and scaling is often a prominent feature.

The transitory nature of wheals (<24 hours) should make it easy to recognize **urticaria** (Figure 18.28). In some young children, urticaria is associated with intercurrent viral infections, although frequently no cause can be identified. A number of viral infections can also cause a diffuse blanching red rash (**toxic erythema** (Figure 18.29) which can affect children of all ages).

Older children and teenagers

Generalized red rashes may be eczematous, dermal as in urticaria or scaly and/or psoriasiform (Tables 18.16 and 18.17).

Table 18.16 Red rashes of childhood

Condition	Frequency/onset	Itchy	Morphology and distribution	Associations	Investigations/treatment	Outcome
Atopic eczema	Common: up to 15 per cent of children Onset <2 years: 90 per cent	Very	Infants: face and extensors limbs Older children: Flexural	Asthma and hay fever	Moisturizers and topical steroids; bandaging; antihistamines	Overall good May persist to adult life
Seborrhoeic dermatitis	Now uncommon	No	Scalp, flexures/scaly and napkin area	Overlap with atopic eczema	Topical steroids + anticandidal creams/ ointments	Clears <9/12
Allergic contact dermatitis	Uncommon in children Incidence increases with increasing age	Yes	Varies with allergen	–	Patch testing; allergen avoidance; topical steroids	Variable
Scabies	Common all ages	Very	Diffuse. Infants: soles Older children: interdigital webs and wrists	Other family members affected	Permethrin preparations	Excellent
Non-specific dermatitis	Common	Yes	Generalized – secondary scabies Localised – secondary molluscum	Scabies; molluscum	Treat underlying condition	Good
Urticaria	Common	Yes	Individual lesions short-lived <24 hours	Majority – nil	3/12 oral antihistamines; (non-sedative) can be persistent	Variable
Toxic erythema	Common	Variable	Maculopapular	Viral infections; adverse drug reactions	Treat underlying condition	Usually good
Erythema multiforme	Uncommon	Variable	Acral target lesions $\pm$ mucosal involvement	Herpes simplex; adverse drug reaction	Treat underlying condition	Usually good
Psoriasis	Uncommon in first decade	Variable	Scalp and extensors Guttate form: children	Positive family history; arthritis	Topical preparations including: tar, dithranol, calcipoitriol	Variable May persist
Pityriasis rosea	Uncommon in children	Sometimes	Herald patch Bathing trunks distribution Collarette of scale	None	Usually unnecessary	Excellent Spontaneous resolution
Tinea corporis	Uncommon	Rarely	Erythematous plaques Peripheral scale	Scrapings for mycology	Topical/systemic antifungals	Excellent

Table 18.17 Facial rash

	Frequency	Clinical features	Associations	Investigations	Management	Comments
Atopic eczema	Common	Infants – cheeks and chin	Asthma, hay fever	If indicated	Moisturizers	May persist
Acne: infantile	Rare	Pustules: cysts; comedones	None	None	Topical benzylperoxide ± erythromycin	
Acne vulgaris	Common	Pustules: cysts; comedones	None	None as a routine	Erythromycin or tetracyclines >12 years	May scar
Acne: steroid-induced	Uncommon	Monomorphic pustules	Long-term systemic steroids, e.g. for transplants		Erythromycin; tetracyclines >12 years	More resistant to treatment
Perioral dermatitis	Uncommon	Perioral pustules	Potent topical steroids	–	Erythromycin; tetracyclines >12 years	
Tuberous sclerosis	Uncommon	Adenoma sebaceum (fibroangiomas); ungual fibromas; shagreen patch; hypomelanotic macules	Epilepsy; retinal; cardiac; renal		Genetic counselling	See Chapter 3
Psoriasis	Uncommon in first decade	Scalp; extensor limbs	Arthritis	–	Topical steroids face and scalp; scalp – keratolytics	
Acute urticaria	Common	Wheals (last <24 hours)	None/viral infections/drug rashes; rarely identified	Rarely helpful	Oral antihistamines	Good
Chronic urticaria	Common	>6/52 Wheals		Rarely helpful	3/12 Oral antihistamines	May persist
Congenital hereditary angiodema	Rare	Painless facial swellings and other sites	Abdominal pain; connective tissue diseases	C1 inhibitor level and functional assay	Tranexamic acid/cyproterone acetate; C1 inhibitor (emergency use)	Persistent
Dermatomyositis	Uncommon	Violaceous rash eyelids and fingers; extensor limbs	Muscle weakness	CK; C/T screen; MRI muscles	See Chapter 16	
Systemic lupus erythematosus	Uncommon	Erythematous plaques in photosensitive distribution	Joint, renal; haematological Photosensitivity	C/T screen	Sun blocks; topical steroids; hydroxychloroquine	See Chapter 16
Hydroa vacciniforme	Rare	Photosensitive; vesicles heals with scarring	Ocular involvement	Photo testing	Photoprotection: sun blocks; appropriate clothes	
Porphyrias: erythrocyte protoporphyria	Rare	Acute photosensitive (sunburn); Superficial scarring	Cholestatic hepatitis	Porphyrin screen; LFTs; phototesting	Photoprotection as hydroa β-carotene	Defective ferrochelatase

CK, creatine kinase; C/T, connective tissue; LFTs, liver function tests; MRI, magnetic resonance imaging.

Eczematous rashes

> **CASE STUDY**
>
> A 9-year-old boy presents with a six-week history of a very itchy eczematous rash. He has never had any skin problems before but his younger brother has also been itchy recently.

The commonest diagnosis in this age group is still atopic eczema although the differential diagnosis is wider as the child gets older. It is not uncommon for atopic eczema to clear in childhood and to recur again later. However it is unusual for eczema to present for the first time at this age. In this age group the rash of atopic ezcema typically affects the flexures.

Non-specific dermatitis may also occur in association with other **infections** such as molluscum contagiosum and head lice. If the dermatitis is localized to the occipital area, remember also to examine the scalp for lice and/or nits. Treatment is that of the underlying condition, but it is important to avoid topical steroids in areas affected by molluscum; 1 per cent ichthyol in zinc ointment is a useful substitute.

Scabies is common in this age group and the history is usually relatively short as in this boy (unless the child also has pre-existing eczema). Other family members or friends are also frequently affected. The dermatitis is non-specific so it is important to examine carefully the sites of predilection for the presence of burrows, which are usually localized to the finger webs and wrists. The soles are not involved in this age group, but in older boys involvement of the genital area is a helpful diagnostic sign.

Dermal rashes

URTICARIA

This is common at all ages and may be associated with dermographism. Once the transitory nature of the lesions is recognized the diagnosis is usually straightforward. Urticaria is divided arbitrarily into acute and chronic forms, based on a history of less than or more than six weeks, respectively. A cause is more commonly identified in acute urticaria, which may be associated with viral infections, adverse drug reactions or with food allergy. However, even in acute urticaria a cause is often not identified. In chronic urticaria a cause is more rarely identified and investigations are seldom helpful. The condition usually responds well to a non-sedative antihistamine, which should be given on a regular daily basis for three months. This condition is frequently misdiagnosed by paediatricians as erythema multiforme (Figure 18.30). However the distribution, morphology and transitory nature of the lesions should differentiate the two conditions.

ERYTHEMA MULTIFORME

In erythema multiforme the history is relatively short and the diagnosis is made by recognizing the typical target lesions that are distributed peripherally on the limbs. These lesions persist for several days or longer and are morphologically distinct from urticarial wheals. Mucosal involvement is also common in erythema multiforme and may affect the mouth, eyes and perineal regions (Figure 18.31). Erythema multiforme is a reactive process, which is most commonly secondary to herpes simplex but may be precipitated by many other causes including mycoplasma, bacterial and viral infections. There is a spectrum of severity in erythema multiforme. The skin alone may be involved or may be associated with mucosal involvement, which can be severe. Some patients with severe mucosal involvement require inpatient treatment if they cannot take enough oral fluids.

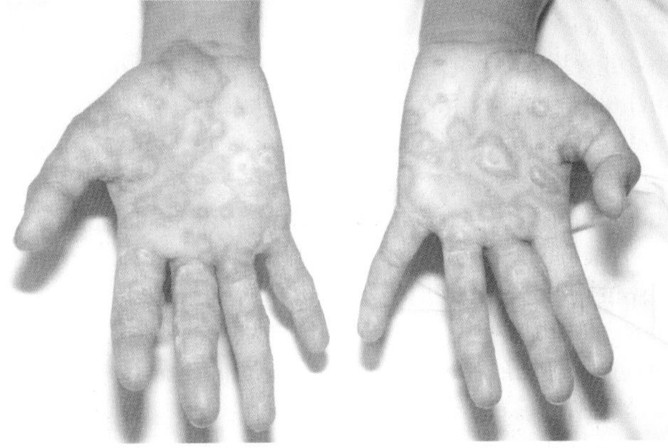

Figure 18.30 Erythema multiforme: classical target lesions, some with bullae, which usually affect the extremities

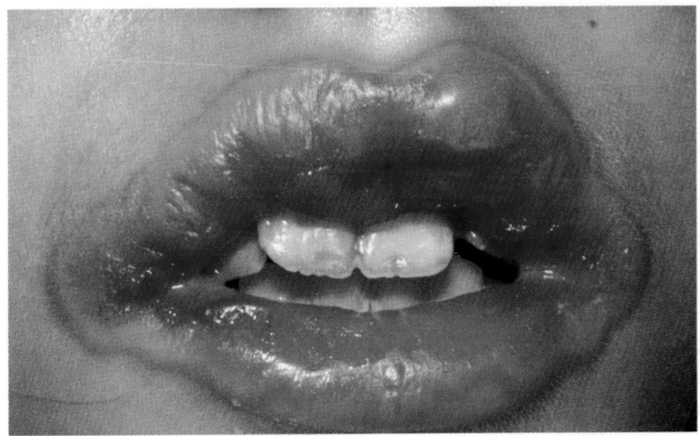

Figure 18.31 Erythema multiforme: mucosal involvement is common although not often this severe

Toxic epidermal necrolysis

This is a severe and potentially fatal condition. Although there may be an overlap between Stevens–Johnson syndrome and TEN, it is pathogenically distinct. It may be precipitated by a number of causes including graft-versus-host disease but is most commonly caused by an adverse drug reaction. These patients may need to be admitted to an intensive care unit. Good skin care is essential using non-adherent dressing. Careful attention to fluid balance and heat loss is needed. Intravenous γ-globulins, steroids and ciclosporin have been used in this condition.

Psoriasiform and scaly rashes

PSORIASIS

Psoriasis is uncommon in the first decade of life but the incidence then rises and reaches a peak in the third decade. There are two distinct clinical patterns seen in childhood: the typical large plaque-type, which is the commonest form in adults, and guttate (rain drop) psoriasis, which is commoner in children (Figure 18.32). If psoriasis is suspected clinically, ask specifically for a family history of the condition and examine the sites of predilection – scalp, extensor surfaces and nails. Typically well-demarcated erythematous scaly plaques affect the extensor aspects of the knees and elbows. Scalp involvement is common and nail dystrophies may occur including nail pitting, onycholysis (separation of the nail plate from the nail bed) and subungual hyperkeratosis. Itch may occur in psoriasis, although is less commanding than that of eczema. **Guttate psoriasis** typically follows a streptococcal sore throat infection. The lesions are small plaques like the adult form in miniature. Guttate psoriasis must be distinguished from pityriasis rosea (see below). Other forms include **generalized pustular psoriasis**, which is rare. This is characterized by sheets of sterile monomorphic pustules. The child is often febrile and is systemically unwell. This condition carries a mortality and immunosuppressant agents (steroids, ciclosporin) or retinoids may be required. Topically only bland preparations such as 1 per cent ichthyol in calamine lotion should be used. These children need good nursing care, adequate analgesia and attention to the fluid and electrolyte balance.

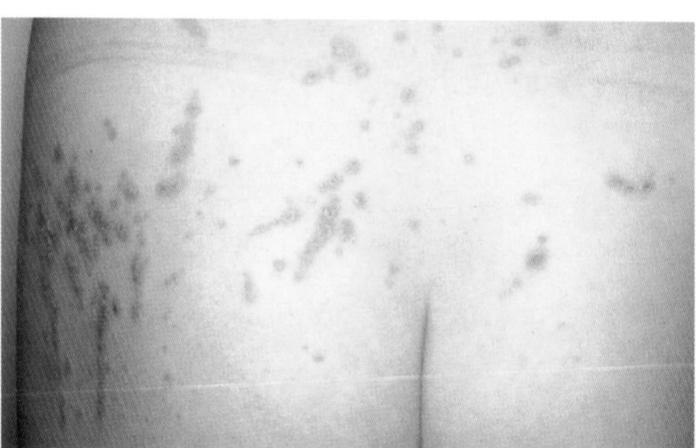

Figure 18.32 Guttate psoriasis: well-defined, red, scaly papules. Scratching in this itchy boy is producing the Koebner phenomenon

PITYRIASIS ROSEA

This may be mistaken for psoriasis. Typically, a single large erythematous plaque is the first sign of the condition – a herald patch. Subsequently the eruption becomes more widespread and has a classic distribution, the so-called Victorian bathing trunks distribution, which affects the trunk and proximal parts of the limbs. The individual lesions are oval, pinkish yellow with peripheral scale. No cause has yet been identified although it is thought to be of viral origin. The condition usually resolves spontaneously in six to eight weeks and any one individual only has one attack in their lifetime. Treatment is often unnecessary but topical steroids can be used if the condition is very itchy for symptomatic relief.

Tinea corporis

Tinea corporis is not very common in children. It is usually acquired by direct contact with infected animals such as cats or other domestic pets such as guinea pigs. It is presents as a slowly expanding erythematous plaque with a peripheral scale.

FACIAL DERMATOSES

The face is affected in many conditions and may provide helpful diagnostic clues in a number of systemic disease, in particular the connective tissue diseases and the photosensitive disorders. The facial dermatoses can be conveniently be subdivided into

- Eczematous lesions
- Pustular lesions
- Facial lumps
- Part of a generalized condition.

Eczematous lesions

CASE STUDY

A 12-year-old girl presents with a three-month history of an itchy facial rash. She is very upset about it and is now refusing to go to school. She had atopic eczema as a baby but this cleared several years ago. She is otherwise well. On taking a careful more detailed history, two important facts emerge. Firstly, this girl had her ears pierced several years ago and she is aware that cheap earrings irritate her ears. She also seems to have a problem with some perfumes.

In young children with **atopic eczema**, the face is often one of the most severely affected areas, classically affecting the cheeks, chin and dribble area. The lesions may be crusted and eroded if secondarily infected. Facial involvement is also common in older children and adolescents with atopic eczema, often affecting the eyelids and periorbital areas.

Seborrhoeic dermatitis

Striking facial involvement may be seen, but the condition is scaly rather than crusted and is not very itchy. There is often accentuation over the eyebrows and marked 'cradle cap'.

Allergic contact dermatitis

Allergic contact dermatitis is relatively uncommon in children, although the incidence rises with increasing age. As in the above case study, the history is usually of fairly short duration and is of an itchy eruption that is localized initially to the site of contact, e.g. the ears or neck of teenage girls with nickel allergy, but can become more widespread with time. Allergic contact dermatitis can also develop as a complication of atopic eczema. This possibility should be considered when there is an unexplained deterioration in the eczema in a child who was previously well controlled. Fragrances are the most frequent allergen but nickel, lanolin and other constituents of topical medicaments such as cetylstearyl alcohol and topical steroids are also all well recognized. Patch testing should be considered in such patients.

Pustular lesions

Infantile acne

Infantile acne is a rare condition but an important one to recognize if permanent scarring is to be avoided. It should be distinguished from neonatal acne, from which it is quite distinct. Infantile acne is a self-limiting condition, and is thought to be an effect of circulating maternal androgens. It is commoner in boys. Two distinct patterns are seen: one with the typical inflammatory pustules and comedones seen in 'teenage acne'. The other is predominantly cystic and comedones are often not seen. The treatment of choice is erythromycin taken orally. A few children may also require a course of the vitamin A derivative isotretinoin, as for teenage acne.

Acne vulgaris

This is a very common condition, with its maximum incidence in the teenage years. The diagnosis is usually straightforward. The rash is polymorphic with lesions including comedones (blackheads and whiteheads), papules and pustules. It classically involves the central greasy triangle of the face and may also affect the trunk, particularly the upper back.

Milder cases may respond to a number of topical agents including benzyl peroxide. Moderate or more severe forms will also require extended courses of systemic antibiotics (minimum course – three months). Oral tetracyclines are the drugs of choice but cannot be used in children under 12 years because of the discoloration they cause to the secondary dentition. In this age group erythromycin is a useful substitute. The aim of treating acne is to control the condition while it is still active to try to prevent permanent scarring.

Nodules and cysts may both develop in severe cases and there may also be extensive involvement of the trunk. Such patients will often require a course of isotretinoin. This drug is a hospital-only prescription and has a number of side effects, including dryness of the lips, muscle pains, hyperlipidaemia and abnormal liver function tests. It is important to remember that the retinoids are teratogenic in females. Women of childbearing age should normally be on an oral contraceptive. This decision is less easy in younger girls but the issue should be raised and fully discussed with the family.

Steroid-induced acne

This is a rarer condition seen in patients on long-term oral steroids. The eruption is more monomorphic and comedones are much less apparent. The condition is also much more difficult to treat unless the steroids can be discontinued.

Perioral dermatitis

Perioral dermatitis is a rare condition in young children. It is often secondary to the use of topical steroids on the face. It tends to be self-perpetuating as attempts to withdraw the topical steroids can cause the condition to flare. Systemic treatment with a three-month course of erythromycin or tetracycline (in those >12 years) is usually effective. During this time the topical steroids should be stopped.

Facial lumps

The facial lesions of **tuberous sclerosis** may sometimes be misdiagnosed as acne. This can be avoided if the morphology of the lesions is carefully examined. The facial lesions of tuberous sclerosis are monomorphic papules – the so-called adenoma sebaceum. Histologically these are fibroangiomas. Clinically the differential diagnosis would include benign adnexal tumours but the distribution and morphology of the lesions should suggest the diagnosis.

Generalized conditions

Facial lesions may be part of generalized conditions such as **psoriasis** or **urticaria** and which occasionally may only affect the face. Psoriasis typically affects the hairline with a yellow, erythematous scaly eruption. It can be difficult to make the diagnosis if the condition only affects this site.

Urticaria is very common and facial lesions are usually just part of a more generalized eruption. Urticaria may be associated with angioedema, and more rarely angioedema may occur alone. **Congenital hereditary angioedema** is rare but is an important condition to recognize. It is due to a deficiency of C1-esterase inhibitor; 85 per cent of cases have a quantitative deficiency, in the remaining 15 per cent the level is normal but there is a functional abnormality. The condition often presents with painless facial swelling after dental treatment. Similar localized swellings can occur on other sites after trauma but the history of trauma is often minimal or absent. Stress is another provoking factor. Abdominal pain is a well-recognized clinical feature of the condition. Tranexamic acid can be given for prophylaxis, for example, before dental treatment. This drug is also useful in shortening the duration of the episodes of swelling or abdominal pain. Cyproterone acetate is an alternative. C1-inhibitor concentrate is also available for the treatment of an acute episode if associated with laryngeal obstruction.

Connective tissue diseases

Involvement of the face can provide useful clinical clues to the diagnosis of a number of the connective tissue diseases. The connective tissue disorders are multisystem diseases and are also covered in Chapter 16.

Dermatomyositis

This classically causes a violaceous discoloration of the eyelids and periorbital area. The colour and distribution of the skin lesions are both important diagnostic clues (see Figure 16.9a, page 499). Look specifically for the reddish-purple streaking along the dorsal aspects of the fingers with Gottron papules (see Figure 16.9b). Capillary loops are often seen around the nail folds. More extensive skin involvement may be present, involving particularly the extensor aspects of the limbs but the back may also be involved. The cutaneous features are usually associated with a myositis, although either may occur independently and one may precede the other. Most children with muscle involvement need systemic treatment as suggested in Chapter 16.

Systemic lupus erythematosus

This classically presents with an erythematous butterfly facial rash (Figure 18.33) in a photosensitive distribution, which spares the orbits and shaded areas under the nose and chin (see Figure 16.10a, page 501). Patients may also have the Raynaud phenomenon. Many patients will require systemic treatment for renal, joint or central nervous system involvement. However, treatment with potent topical steroids may useful for cutaneous disease either alone or in association with systemic treatment. Hydroxychloroquine is often useful as the first of the second-line agents, particularly in those patients with predominantly cutaneous involvement.

It is also very important that all these patients receive sensible sun advice (see below) as sunlight can be a trigger for lupus erythematosus.

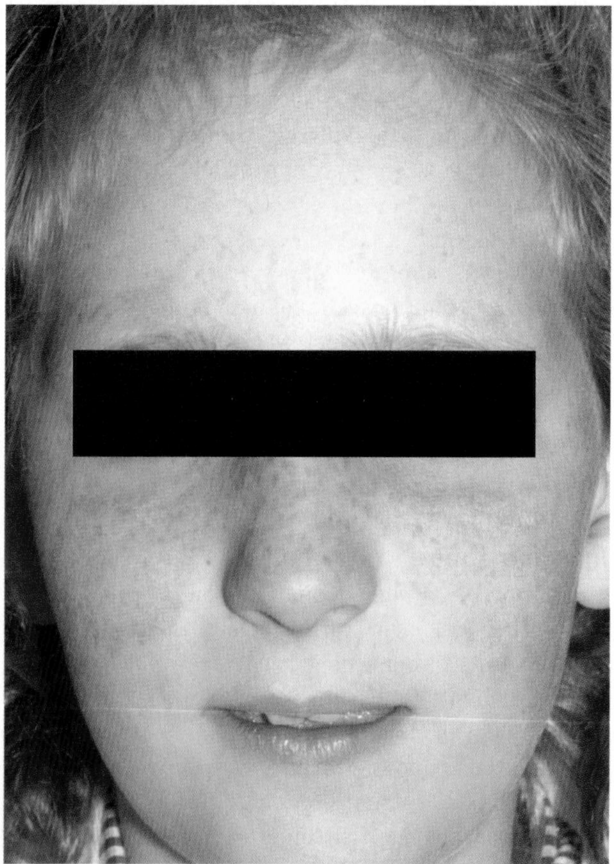

Figure 18.33 Lupus erythematosus

Photodermatoses

The photodermatoses are a heterogeneous group of disorders, all of which are characterized by abnormal photosensitivity. **Polymorphic light eruption** (prickly heat) is the commonest condition. It is commoner in the second and third decades but can also affect children. Patients present with itchy erythematous papules and plaques in exposed sites 24–48 hours after sun exposure. The condition is usually worse in spring or early summer and the skin may become less sensitive over the summer months. **Hydroa vacciniforme** is a rare condition that usually presents during early childhood. It is important to recognize so that the family receives appropriate advice. Children usually present acutely within hours of sun exposure with a vesicular eruption that often becomes crusted. Typically lesions affect the face, but the backs of the hands may also be affected. Lesions heal with pockmark scarring. Clinically, the lesions may look herpetic and as herpes simplex may also be provoked by sunlight the diagnosis may be delayed. Helpful diagnostic features of hydroa include symmetry of the lesions, scarring and photosensitive distribution. For completeness, children should be investigated to exclude the other photosensitive diseases. The condition may improve during adolescence.

Other idiopathic **photodermatoses** include actinic prurigo, juvenile spring eruption, solar urticaria. All are rare and merit referral for photo-testing in a specialized unit. It is important also to remember **xeroderma pigmentosa** (see Genodermatoses, page 556) and the cutaneous porphyrias

Porphyrias

The porphyrias are a group of disorders caused by defects in haem synthesis. All are rare but investigations for porphyria should be considered in children presenting with a history suggestive of photosensitivity. Blood, urine and faeces for porphyrin analysis should be sent in light-protected containers. The conditions are subdivided into the hepatic porphyrias and those involving erythrocytes.

Erythrocyte protoporphyria is one of the commonest of these rare diseases and is due to a deficiency of the enzyme ferrochelatase, which leads to an accumulation of protoporphyrins. It may present in early childhood but can be difficult to diagnose. The family may give a history of unexplained screaming in a child after sun exposure. However, the link with sun exposure may not be appreciated initially as the reaction may be delayed from a few minutes to an hour. In addition, the reaction may also occur through windows, as the activating wavelengths are the 400 nm range, which can pass through window glass. Initially this causes a burning sensation followed a few hours later by the development of skin lesions on exposed sites.

The diagnosis should be suspected clinically from the history and by the presence of fine scarring in light exposed sites on examination. The diagnosis is confirmed by measuring porphyrins in the blood. There may be associated liver disease, which is usually mild but liver function tests should be done.

MANAGEMENT

In common with other photodermatoses, patients should receive sensible sun avoidance advice:

- Avoid bright sunlight, particularly the mid-day sun.
- Wear appropriate clothing and a sun hat.
- Use high sun protection factor sun creams. Sun creams that also contain a physical block in the form of titanium are preferable as they cover a wider range of the UV spectrum.

If the child is very light sensitive – in the UVA or visible range – additional measures such as screening window glass may be necessary.

SUMMARY

Paediatric dermatology is a big subject. This chapter has only covered the commoner skin problems and briefly mentioned some of the more important ones. More detailed information of these and other skin conditions can be found in reference textbooks of paediatric dermatology.

FURTHER READING

Eichenfield LF, Frieden IJ, Esterly NB (2001) *Textbook of Neonatal Dermatology*. Philadelphia: WB Saunders.

Freedberg IM, Eisen AZ, Wolff K, *et al.* (1999) *Dermatology in General Medicine*, 5th edn. New York: McGraw-Hill.

Harper J, Orange A, Prose N (2000) *Textbook of Pediatric Dermatology*. Oxford: Blackwell Science.

White GM, Cox NH (2000) *Diseases of the Skin. A Color Atlas and Text*. Edinburgh: Mosby.

Chapter 19

Haematology and oncology

Brenda ES Gibson

HAEMATOLOGY

DEVELOPMENT OF HAEMATOPOIESIS

Haematopoiesis begins in the yolk sac at around 3 weeks' gestation, enters the hepatic and the bone marrow phases at 6 weeks' and 20 weeks' gestation respectively and is established in the bone marrow by birth.

Embryonic haemoglobin (Hb) gene expression starts at 3 weeks' gestation and the chains produced combine with alpha (α-chains) and gamma chains (γ-chains) produced in the hepatic phase to form embryonic haemoglobins (Hb Gower, Hb Portland). Fetal haemoglobin, Hb F ($\alpha_2\gamma_2$) is dominant after the 8th week. Beta (β-chain) gene expression starts as early as 10 weeks' gestation but does not begin to replace gamma gene expression until 7 months' gestation, when the switch from fetal to adult haemoglobin occurs. Fetal red cells express virtually no delta genes (Table 19.1). At birth the neonate has around 80 per cent Hb F, 20 per cent Hb A and trace amounts of Hb Bart's, whereas adult red cells contain less than 1 per cent Hb F, 2–3 per cent Hb A2 and the remainder is Hb A. The switch from Hb F to Hb A synthesis is precisely timed and genetically predetermined by the post-conception age. Fetal red cells are large and progressively decrease in size as gestation advances but even at birth are larger than adult red cells.

Normal neonatal haematopoiesis

- The neonate's mean corpuscular volume (MCV) is increased at birth, but falls gradually over the first 6 months of life to that of the older child.
- The neonate's blood film has macrocytes, stomatocytes, echinocytes, schizocytes, Howell–Jolly bodies and occasional spherocytes as normal findings.

Table 19.1 Globin chain development

Stage of development	Haemoglobin (Hb)	Globin chain constitution
Embryonic	Hb Gower I	$\zeta_2\,\epsilon_2$
	Hb Gower II	$\alpha_2\,\epsilon_2$
	Hb Portland	$\zeta_2\,\gamma_2$
Fetal	Hb F	$\alpha_2\,\gamma_2$
	Hb Bart's	γ_4
Adult	Hb A2	$\alpha_2\,\delta_2$
	Hb A	$\alpha_2\,\beta_2$

- The platelet count in term and preterm babies is greater than 150×10^9/L.
- The reticulocyte count is higher in babies, particularly preterm babies, than in adults in the first days and weeks of life and then falls to adult values.
- Marked neutrophilia is present during the first hours of life and then declines (Table 19.2). Lymphocytes are predominant after the first 3–5 days of life and remain so for the first 4 years. An absolute lymphocyte count of less than 2.0×10^9/L should alert the clinician to the possibility of immunodeficiency.
- Low intrauterine oxygen tension stimulates erythropoietin production and this high erythropoietin level is responsible for the newborn's high haemoglobin level at birth. Following birth, the increase in oxygen tension causes erythropoietin suppression and a physiological fall in haemoglobin production (physiological anaemia). The haemoglobin nadir occurs at 9 weeks of age (to around 10 g/dL in healthy infants). The postnatal fall in haemoglobin is earlier and the nadir lower in preterm babies. This reduction in haemoglobin is partially compensated for by an increase in Hb A, which gives up oxygen readily, unlike Hb F, which is a high affinity haemoglobin. The fall in haemoglobin in turn

Table 19.2 Variation in haematological parameters during the first year of life (mean values)

	Haemoglobin (g/dL)	Mean corpuscular volume (fL)	WCC ($\times 10^9$/L)	Neutrophils ($\times 10^9$/L)	Lymphocytes ($\times 10^9$/L)
Term	16.5	108	18.1	11.0	5.5
2 months	11.5	96	10.8	3.8	6.0
3-6 months	11.5	91	11.9	3.8	7.3
1 year	12.0	78	11.4	3.5	7.0

results in increased erythropoietin production and a subsequent rise in haemoglobin.

- Postnatally, in healthy infants Hb A2 does not rise to adult values until 5–6 months of age.
- The normal blood volume in infancy is 85 mL/kg.

THE COAGULATION CASCADE

Blood must circulate as fluid, but when a vessel wall is breached it has to be repaired quickly to prevent blood loss. A very large number of proteins are involved in the initiation and propagation of clot formation, and a similarly large number are involved in inhibiting the process. Thrombin generation involves two pathways: extrinsic and intrinsic (Figure 19.1), but the extrinsic is the pathway thought to be primarily responsible for initiating haemostasis. The complex reactions involved take place on membrane surfaces, which provide negatively charged phospholipid.

The extrinsic pathway is initiated when tissue factor (TF) binds the enzyme activated factor (F)VII (FVIIa). This complex can activate either FX or FIX. Activated FIX (FIXa) complexes with FVIIIa to activate FX. Factor Xa, formed either by the TF/FVIIa complex or by the FVIIIa/FIXa complex, interacts with FVa to convert prothrombin to thrombin. Thrombin then cleaves fibrinogen to insoluble fibrin. Thrombin can also regulate clotting by binding with thrombomodulin to activate protein C to activated protein C (APC). Activated protein C complexes with protein S and this complex inactivates FVa and FVIIIa. These two co-factors are critical for prothrombin and FX activation and their proteolytic inactivation blocks further thrombin generation.

The intrinsic pathway is thought less important than the extrinsic pathway for initiating haemostasis. This pathway is initiated when FXII binds to a foreign surface such as collagen and is proteolysed by prekallikrein (PK). On the surface, FXIIa interacts with high molecular weight kininogen (HMWK) and the complex activates FXI. FXIa then activates FIX to FIXa, which, once activated, binds to FVIIIa to generate FXa, which in turn binds to FVa and converts prothrombin to thrombin.

The prothrombin time (PT) measures the extrinsic pathway (FI, II, V, VII, X) and the activated partial thromboplastin time (APTT) measures the intrinsic pathway (FI, II, V, VIII, IX, X, XI, XII, PK, HMWK). The thrombin clotting time (TCT) measures the conversion of fibrinogen to fibrin. It is prolonged when fibrinogen is low from consumption, from hypo/dysfibrinogenaemia or in the presence of inhibitors such as heparin and fibrin degradation products (FDPs)/D-dimers. Protamine sulphate neutralizes heparin and shortens the TCT in its presence. The Reptilase® time is prolonged in the presence of hypofibrinogenaemia but is not affected by the presence of heparin.

Normal neonatal haemostasis

- The haemostatic system is profoundly influenced by age and is immature at birth. This is reflected in reduced levels of both procoagulants and inhibitors of haemostasis. Both are more marked in the preterm than in the term baby. Reference ranges, which reflect both gestational and postnatal age, are necessary for diagnostic purposes.
- Coagulation proteins do not cross the placental barrier but are synthesized by the fetus from 10 weeks' gestation onwards. FVIII, FV and fibrinogen are within the normal adult range in the term and preterm baby at birth, whereas the von Willebrand factor (vWF) is above the adult range. The fact that FVIII levels are normal at birth allows the accurate diagnosis of haemophilia A at birth, regardless of severity. Increased levels of vWF at birth mean that testing for the commoner types of vWD (quantitative defects) should be delayed until around 6 months of age.
- The vitamin K-dependent factors (II, VII, IX, X) are around 50 per cent of adult values at birth and

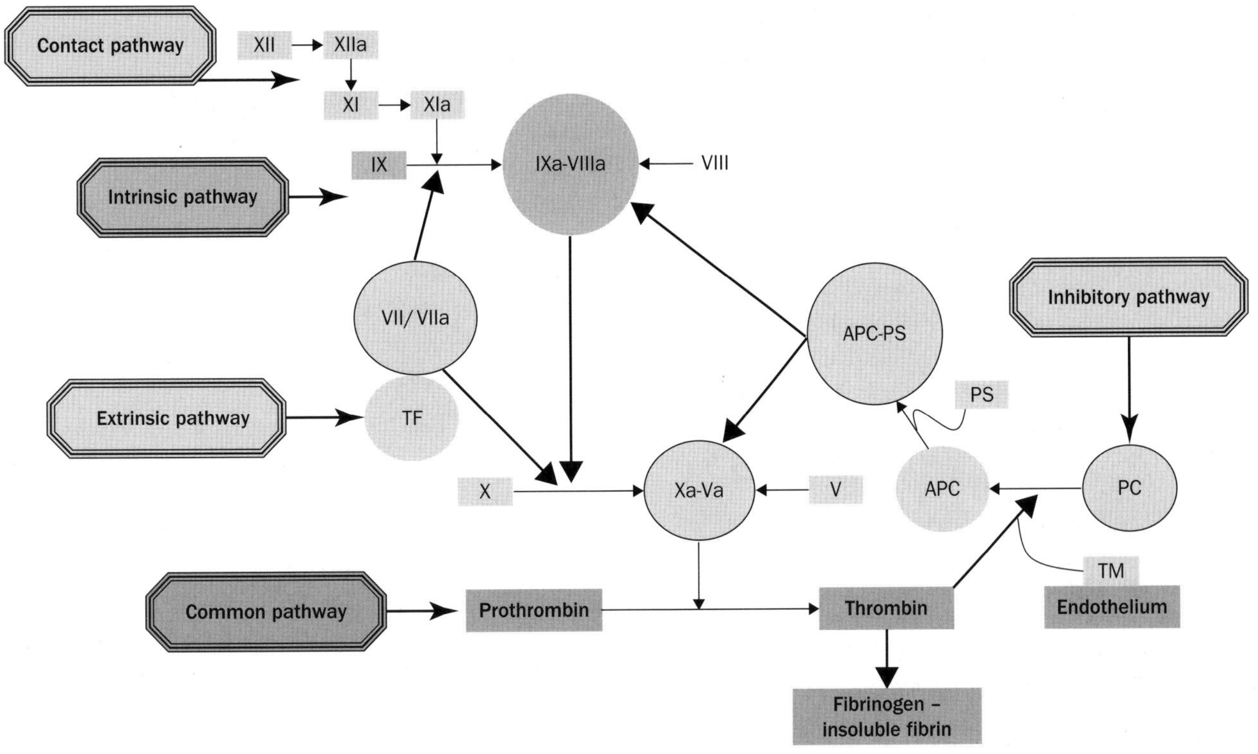

Figure 19.1 Pathways of the coagulation cascade. APC, activated PC; PC, protein C; PS, protein S; TF, tissue factor; TM, thrombomodulin

further reduced in the premature neonate. The contact factors (XI, XII, PK and HMWK) are reduced to 30–50 per cent of normal at term, whereas FXIII is 70 per cent of normal.

- Of the commonly used screening tests, the PT is only minimally prolonged in the healthy term baby and shortens within the first month of life, whereas the APTT may be more prolonged, because of the reduced levels of contact factors which have a disproportionate effect on the APTT compared with reduced levels of FVIII or IX. It shortens to the normal adult range by 2–6 months of age. The TCT is usually normal.
- The inhibitors of coagulation, antithrombin, heparin co-factor II, protein C and protein S (both vitamin K-dependent proteins) are around 50 per cent of normal at birth and α-2-macroglobulin is increased.
- The net effect of these changes is that neonatal plasma has a reduced capacity to generate thrombin to around 50 per cent of that of adult plasma. Thrombin inhibition is slower in neonatal plasma but the overall capacity is similar to that of adults.
- Plasminogen levels are about 50 per cent of adult values in the term baby and further reduced in the preterm baby, resulting in a reduced rate of plasmin generation in neonatal plasma compared with adult plasma.
- The bleeding time, which is the best *in vivo* test of platelet–vessel-wall interaction, is shorter in the first week of life than in adulthood and this probably reflects increased levels of vWF antigen and activity, together with the increased red cell size and haematocrit of the infant. This has no clinical implications.

KEY LEARNING POINT

Age-related reference ranges are necessary for diagnostic purposes.

DIFFERENTIAL DIAGNOSIS OF ANAEMIA

Anaemia is defined as a haemoglobin level that is more than two standard deviations below the age-appropriate mean. A reduced haemoglobin level can result from one of two pathophysiological mechanisms:

- defective production of red cells
- excessive destruction/loss of red cells due to:
  - haemolysis
  - haemorrhage.

The reticulocyte count, which is increased in the presence of increased red cell production, but not in defects of red cell production, distinguishes the two mechanisms. A reticulocytosis is seen in haemolysis, blood loss, the response to haematinic treatment and during the recovery phase of red cell aplasia.

Red cell morphology is useful in the differential diagnosis of anaemia. Defects of haemoglobin production (cytoplasmic maturation) tend to give rise to microcytic red cells, whereas defects of DNA synthesis (nuclear maturation) are usually associated with the production of macrocytic red cells. Marrow failure syndromes give rise to normocytic or macrocytic red cells.

- Microcytic, hypochromic red cells: iron deficiency, thalassaemia trait, sideroblastic anaemia, lead poisoning.
- Normochromic, normocytic red cells: acute blood loss, anaemia of chronic disease (can be microcytic), haemolysis.
- Macrocytic red cells: megaloblastic anaemia (B_{12} and folate deficiency), liver disease, myelodysplasia, hypothyroidism, aplastic anaemia, reticulocytosis, normal in the neonate.

KEY LEARNING POINTS

- Anaemia can result from reduced production or increased destruction/loss of red cells.
- The distinction between these two mechanisms is made on the basis of the reticulocyte count, which is increased in the presence of increased red cell production but not in defects of red cell production.
- Red cell morphology is important in the diagnosis of anaemia. Defects of haemoglobin production give rise to microcytic red cells, defects of DNA synthesis give rise to macrocytic red cells and marrow failure syndromes give rise to normocytic or macrocytic red cells.

Classification of red cell production disorders

Defects of haemoglobin production
- Iron deficiency
- Anaemia of chronic disorders
- Sideroblastic anaemia
- Lead poisoning

Defects in erythroid cell maturation
1 Nuclear maturation defects
   - Cobalamin (vitamin B_{12}) deficiency
   - Folate deficiency
   - Hereditary abnormalities of cobalamin or folate metabolism
   - Other metabolic defects associated with megaloblastic anaemia (Lesch–Nyhan syndrome; orotic aciduria; thiamine-responsive megaloblastic anaemia)
2 Congenital dyserythropoietic anaemias

Defects in marrow 'environment' or erythroid stem cells
1 Marrow failure
   - Aplastic anaemia
   - Marrow infiltration
   - Pure red cell aplasia: Diamond–Blackfan syndrome; parvovirus; transient erythroblastopenia of childhood; drugs
2 Inadequate erythropoietin production
   - Chronic renal disease
   - 'Anaemia of chronic disorders'
   - Anaemia of prematurity

Adapted from Lilleyman JS and Hann IM (eds) (1992) *Paediatric Haematology*, 1st edn. Edinburgh: Churchill Livingstone.

Iron deficiency

Iron deficiency is the commonest cause of anaemia at all ages but is particularly prevalent in infants and young children, whose rapid growth demands a large iron supply that can outstrip the available iron in the diet. Non-haemopoietic manifestations of iron deficiency may also be important in the developing child.

The majority of body iron is in the form of haemoglobin with about 10 per cent in iron-containing proteins in non-haem tissues (e.g. myoglobin and cytochromes) and further 10–15 per cent stored intracellularly as ferritin or its degradation product, haemosiderin. Iron taken up by intestinal mucosal cells and iron recirculated from haem by macrophages is transported in plasma bound to transferrin. Transferrin is synthesized primarily in the liver, at a rate inversely related to iron stores and therefore is increased in iron deficiency and reduced in iron overload.

The serum iron, transferrin level (measured as total iron binding capacity: TIBC) and particularly the percentage saturation of the plasma transferrin indicate the amount of iron available to the tissues. Total iron binding capacity is normally about 33 per cent saturated, and when it falls below 16 per cent in adults and lower in children there is insufficient iron available to support erythropoiesis. Small amounts of intracellular ferritin are secreted into the plasma and therefore serum ferritin is an indirect measure of intracellular iron and body iron stores. Ferritin is an acute phase protein and is increased by inflammatory disease and plasma ferritin may be normal even in the absence of iron stores.

Causes of iron deficiency

EFFECT OF GROWTH

The haemoglobin and stored iron accumulated during fetal development is relatively independent of maternal iron stores. Iron stores are rarely depleted in the term baby before 6 months of age, but this can occur earlier in the preterm baby who has a faster growth rate and less stored iron. Iron deficiency is therefore most likely to occur between 6 months and 2–3 years of life. A further period of rapid growth during adolescence and menstrual loss in girls increase the risk of iron deficiency in this age group.

EFFECT OF DIET

Breast milk and cows' milk are low in iron, although the iron in breast milk is more available. Formula milk is fortified with iron. Iron insufficiency in the infant can be reduced by:

- continuing breastfeeding until 6 months (or by use of an iron-supplemented formula)
- avoiding cows' milk
- weaning to iron-containing/fortified foods by the age of 6 months.

Low birth weight, exclusively breast-fed infants need at least 2–4 mg/kg iron per day, starting no later than 2 months of age. Infants between 6 months and 3 years require 1 mg/kg iron per day. Preterm infants receiving erythropoietin require at least 6 mg/kg iron per day. The recommended daily intake of iron for children 4–10 years of age is 10 mg and for adolescents 18 mg.

Occult gastrointestinal blood loss can be associated with unprocessed cows' milk feeding in early infancy. Iron deficiency is commoner among Asian children who are more likely to be vegetarian. Convenience foods are often low in iron. Red meat, eggs and green vegetables are sources of iron.

BLOOD LOSS

- Perinatal: fetal–maternal haemorrhage, twin–twin transfusion, placenta previa or abruption
- Gastrointestinal: fresh cows' milk intolerance, parasites (hookworm), non-steroidal analgesics, Meckel diverticulum (painless intermittent blood loss), haemorrhagic telangiectasia, peptic ulcer, inflammatory bowel disease
- Malabsorption
  - Coeliac disease

Clinical features

ANAEMIA

- Pallor of the mucous membranes, palms and nail beds
- Tiredness and listlessness
- Systolic flow murmur

NON-HAEMATOLOGICAL

- Skin and gut: koilonychia, glossitis, oesophageal web
- Muscles: diminished work/exercise performance, independent of anaemia
- Nervous system: diminished attention span and reduced cognitive performance – even children with depleted iron stores but no anaemia may be at risk
- Pica
- Immunity: diminished cell-mediated immunity and impaired neutrophil activity

Diagnosis

Laboratory testing can help identifying the various stages of iron deficiency from depletion of iron stores to frank anaemia. The diagnosis of mild anaemia may be difficult. Erythrocyte protoporphyrin (EPP) is a measure of iron supply to the red cell and is raised in iron deficiency. There are age-related differences in the tests used to assess iron status (Table 19.3).

DIFFERENTIAL DIAGNOSIS OF LOW HAEMOGLOBIN AND LOW MCV

There are causes of a low haemoglobin and a low MCV other than iron-deficiency anaemia, where iron replacement is unnecessary and can accentuate iron overload.

- β-Thalassaemia trait
  - The MCV is usually disproportionately low compared with the mild anaemia, whereas the MCV and haemoglobin levels generally correlate in iron-deficiency anaemia.
  - The red cell count is usually raised in β-thalassaemia but reduced in iron-deficiency anaemia.
  - Ferritin should be normal in thalassaemia but reduced in iron-deficiency anaemia.
  - Hb electrophoresis or high-performance liquid chromatography (HPLC) confirms the diagnosis of β-thalassaemia. In β-thalassaemia trait the Hb F and Hb A2 are both elevated, but when iron deficiency and β-thalassaemia trait coexist, the Hb A2 may not be raised in the presence of iron

Table 19.3 Results of laboratory tests of iron status

Iron status	Test	Result at different ages	
		0.5–17 years	>17 years
Iron sufficient	• Ferritin (μg/L)	>12	>13
	• Transferrin saturation (%)	>10	>16
	• EPP (μmol/molhaem)	<100	<80
Iron depleted non-anaemic	• Ferritin (μg/L)	<12	<13
	• Transferrin saturation (%)	>10	>16
	• EPP (μmol/molhaem)	<100	<80
Iron deficiency anaemia	• Ferritin (μg/L)	<12	<13
	• Transferrin saturation (%)	<10	<16
	• EPP (μmol/molhaem)	>100	>80
	• Hb	↓	↓
	• Red cell morphology	Hypochromic: microcytic	Hypochromic: microcytic

Hb, haemoglobin; EPP, erythrocyte protoporphyrin.

Adapted from Lilleyman JS, Hann IM, Blanchette V (Eds) (1999) *Paediatric Haematology*, 2nd edn, Edinburgh: Churchill Livingstone.

depletion. Haemoglobin electrophoresis or HPLC should be repeated when the child is iron replete.

- α-Thalassaemia trait
  - There may be only a mild reduction in Hb and MCV; Hb electrophoresis, HPLC, DNA studies are required to confirm the diagnosis.
- Anaemia of chronic disorders
- Lead poisoning

TREATMENT

Replacement should be with oral iron using any of the ferrous salts and should continue for three to six months. Parenteral iron should be avoided except in exceptional circumstances.

Anaemia of chronic disorders

Anaemia is common in acute or chronic inflammatory or infective disease. The anaemia is initially normochromic normocytic but may progress to a microcytic hypochromic anaemia. It results from a reduction in available iron (due to trapping in macrophages of iron released from red cells for reuse) rather than a true deficiency. The inflammatory process blunts the normal erythropoietin response to anaemia. The serum ferritin level is high and may remain so in the presence of coincidental iron deficiency. A bone marrow aspirate stained for macrophage iron stores may be the most certain means of determining whether coincidental iron deficiency is present or not.

Sideroblastic anaemia

Sideroblastic anaemia is characterized by a population of hypochromic, microcytic red cells in the peripheral blood, punctate basophilia and ring sideroblasts in the bone marrow. Ringed sideroblasts are erythroblasts with large iron granules (iron-laden mitochondria) forming a partial or complete ring around the nucleus. A failure to utilize iron for synthesis of haem within the mitochondria leads to a microcytic anaemia and iron accumulation. The serum ferritin and serum iron levels are high with a reduced TIBC and near-complete saturation. Sideroblastic anaemia can be inherited or acquired. Inherited forms of sideroblastic anaemia usually follow an X-linked pattern and may be due to a deficiency of aminolevulinic acid synthase (ALA) synthase and be pyridoxine responsive. Acquired sideroblastic anaemia can be associated with myelodysplasia, drugs or lead poisoning.

Lead poisoning

Chronic lead ingestion is commonest among infants and small children. Lead absorption is increased by dietary deficiency of iron. Anaemia is a late manifestation of lead poisoning and only seen in severe cases and/or in the presence of coexistent iron deficiency. The anaemia is normochromic or slightly hypochromic with mild reticulocytosis secondary to mild haemolysis; itself secondary to mitochondrial damage. Basophilic stippling is characteristic. The bone marrow may show increased sideroblasts, sometimes with ring sideroblasts. Children with symptomatic lead poisoning require treatment with chelation therapy with dimercaprol and calcium EDTA.

Thalassaemia syndromes

The thalassaemic syndromes are disorders of haemoglobin synthesis that result in reduced synthesis of one or more of the globin chains of haemoglobin. A microcytic hypochromic anaemia results.

Developmental changes in haemoglobin synthesis

Human haemoglobins have a tetrameric structure consisting of two globin chains from the alpha cluster (ch16) and two globin chains from the beta cluster (ch11). During development there is a switch in production of α-like globin chains from ζ to α, while production of β-chains switches first from embryonic ε to fetal γ and then, at around 32 weeks' gestation, from fetal γ to adult β-chains. At birth, about 70–90 per cent of circulating Hb is Hb F. A slight excess of γ over α-chain production results in trace amounts of γ tetramers (Hb Bart's) even in normal babies. After birth, the percentage proportion of Hb F falls to around 5–20 per cent at 4 months, and to below 2 per cent at 1 year.

Classification of the thalassaemias

These are classified according to the particular globin chain involved, i.e. α, β, δβ, and γδβ types. Where no α or β-chains are produced the thalassaemias are described as α^0 or β^0, to distinguish them from α+ and β+ thalassaemias, where there is some synthesis but at a reduced rate. Reduction in chain synthesis produces a microcytic hypochromic anaemia and a relative excess of one of the other globin chains. In α-thalassaemia, excess γ-chains (in fetal life) and then β-chains (in adult life) form Hb Bart's (γ4) and Hb H (β4), respectively.

Prevalence of thalassaemia

The thalassaemias are widely distributed through the Mediterranean, the Middle East, India, southeast Asia and Africa. The distribution parallels that of falciparum malaria for which the trait appears to confer a selective advantage.

α-Thalassaemia

The normal alpha genotype is αα/αα. The severity of α-thalassaemia syndromes correlates to the number of remaining functioning α-globin genes. The molecular defects are very varied and are generally due to gene deletions (Table 19.4). The deletion of one of the duplicated α-globin genes gives rise to α+-thalassaemia (or α-thalassaemia 2), whereas loss of both α-globin genes gives rise to α^0-thalassaemia (or α-thalassaemia 1). The clinically important types of α-thalassaemia are the Hb Bart's hydrops fetalis syndrome (−/−) and Hb H (−α/−) disease.

HB BART'S HYDROPS FETALIS SYNDROME

Infants with Hb Bart's hydrops fetalis syndrome are usually of southeast Asian, Greek or Cypriot origin and are stillborn or die within hours of birth. They are pale with massive hepatosplenomegaly and generalized oedema. Almost all of their haemoglobin is Hb Bart's which is a very high oxygen affinity haemoglobin and therefore non-functional. Hb A and Hb F are absent. Hb Portland (20 per cent) allows survival to term. The parents are obligate carriers of α^0-thalassaemia.

Table 19.4 α-Thalassaemias

Gene deletion	Laboratory findings
−α/αα	**Silent carrier/α-thalassaemia trait** MCV:MCH normal or mildly reduced Red cells normochromic or mildly hypochromic Hb Bart's 1–2 per cent at birth Hb electrophoresis/HPLC normal Diagnosis requires α-globin gene mapping
−α/−α − −/αα	**α-Thalassaemia trait** MCV:MCH reduced Mild hypochromic microcytic anaemia Hb Bart's 2–10 per cent at birth Occasional Hb H inclusions in − −/αα Hb electrophoresis/HPLC normal Diagnosis requires α-globin gene mapping

Hb, haemoglobin; HPLC, high-performance liquid chromatography.

HB H DISEASE

Children with Hb H have a single functioning α gene, a variable anaemia (range 7–10 g/dL) and splenomegaly. Haemoglobin H inclusion bodies (β-tetramers) are insoluble, shorten the red cell lifespan and result in a chronic haemolytic anaemia. Children usually survive into adult life, but the anaemia may become more marked with progressive splenomegaly and be improved by splenectomy. Patients require folic acid supplements. Transfusion dependence and severe iron overload are unusual. The blood film shows hypochromic, microcytic red cells, polychromasia and moderate reticulocytosis. Haemoglobin H inclusion bodies are present and electrophoresis or HPLC show 5–40 per cent Hb H (or Hb Bart's in the neonate) and Hb A. One parent will be a heterozygote for α^0-thalassaemia and the other for α+-thalassaemia.

α-THALASSAEMIA CARRIER STATE

This is a difficult state to diagnose after the neonatal period. Loss of two α-globin genes usually gives rise to reduced red cell indices, an increased red cell count and hypochromic, microcytic red cells. Hb Bart's (2–10 per cent) is present at birth and, later, very occasional Hb H inclusions may be present in − −/αα thalassaemia. A single chain deletion is particularly difficult to diagnose because red cell indices may overlap with the normal range. Haemoglobin Bart's is present in small amounts at birth. α-Globin gene mapping is indicated only if accurate diagnosis for antenatal counselling is necessary.

β-Thalassaemia

See the section on Core problems (page 605).

Vitamin B_{12} and folate deficiency

Causes of vitamin B_{12} deficiency

DIETARY CAUSES

Vitamin B_{12} combines with intrinsic factor produced in the stomach by parietal cells and is carried to the terminal ileum where it is absorbed. It is provided by foods of animal origin, fish, meat, eggs and milk. Adults have stores of approximately 3 mg (enough for at least 3–4 years) and a neonate has stores of 50 μg. Uncomplicated dietary deficiency will cause megaloblastic anaemia only in exceptional circumstances in childhood, e.g. vegan for many years; baby born with very low stores due to maternal vitamin B_{12} deficiency and then breastfed vitamin B_{12}-deficient milk.

MALABSORPTION

- Juvenile pernicious anaemia (gastric atrophy, achlorhydria, antibodies to intrinsic factor)
- Congenital vitamin B_{12} malabsorption – Imerslund–Grasbeck syndrome (abnormality of the ileal receptor for the cobalamin–intrinsic factor complex)
- Congenital deficiency of intrinsic factor (no antibodies to intrinsic factor)
- Transcobalamin II deficiency (absence of the main transport protein)
- Inborn errors of cobalamin metabolism
- Post gastrectomy
- Crohn disease
- Ileal resection
- Intestinal blind loop syndrome
- Fish tapeworm

Causes of folate deficiency

DIETARY CAUSES

Folate is absorbed unchanged in the duodenum and jejunum. It is provided by most foods including meat and vegetables. In the adult, stores last 3–4 months and the daily requirement is 200 μg, but is much higher in the infant on a weight basis at 20–50 μg. Pure dietary deficiency is uncommon except in severe malnutrition, but it can occur in children on special diets.

INCREASED REQUIREMENTS

- Haemolytic anaemia
- Dyserythropoietic anaemia

MALABSORPTION

- Coeliac disease

DRUGS

- Anticonvulsants – phenytoin
- Antimetabolites – methotrexate

Clinical and haematological features of vitamin B_{12} and folate deficiency

- Anaemia
- Glossitis
- Mild jaundice (due to ineffective erythropoiesis)
- Low platelet count
- Low white cell count (WCC)
- Neurological sequelae (not in folate deficiency)

Investigation of vitamin B_{12} and folate deficiency

- The anaemia is megaloblastic and the neutrophil and platelet counts may also be low in severe deficiency.
- Blood film red cells are increased in size and may be round or oval macrocytes (macro-ovalocytes); hypersegmented neutrophils may be present.
- Red cell indices: the MCV is elevated.
- Bone marrow shows marked erythroid hyperplasia; erythroblasts are larger than normal (megaloblasts) with lacy, finely stippled nuclei. There is nuclear/cytoplasmic asynchrony due to relative immaturity of the nucleus compared to cytoplasm. Other marrow cells show megaloblastic change, e.g. giant metamyelocytes. Erythropoiesis is ineffective.
- Haematinic assays – low levels of:
  - Vitamin B_{12}
  - Red cell folate
  - Serum folate
- A clinical and haematological response to the deficient factor confirms the diagnosis.
- Schilling test: Vitamin B_{12} is first given IM to saturate the storage sites. This is followed by oral radiolabelled hydroxycobalamin. Because the storage sites are saturated by the previously given IM vitamin B_{12}, a percentage of the oral vitamin B_{12} is excreted in the urine. The urine is then collected for 24 hrs and the amount of excreted radiolabelled vitamin B_{12} quantified. A reduction in the expected amount of radiolabelled vitamin B_{12} excreted suggests reduced absorption. The radiolabelled vitamin B_{12} is next given along with intrinsic factor, which is required for its absorption. Improved excretion suggests a problem with reduction or absence of intrinsic factor production. If there is no increase in vitamin B_{12} excretion when given with intrinsic factor this suggests that the problem is at the level of the terminal ileum.

Treatment

Treat the underlying cause and give folate or vitamin B_{12} supplements. In vitamin B_{12} deficiency due to malabsorption or the absence of intrinsic factor, vitamin B_{12} should be given intramuscularly.

Aplastic anaemia

Aplastic anaemia may be constitutional or acquired. There is peripheral pancytopenia with anaemia, neutropenia, thrombocytopenia and reticulocytopenia. Bone marrow examination shows a marked reduction or absence of normal haematopoietic precursors, which are replaced by hypocellular fatty tissue. In addition to a bone marrow aspirate, a trephine biopsy should be carried out to exclude sampling errors and confirm marrow hypoplasia.

Constitutional causes

- Fanconi anaemia
- Dyskeratosis congenita
- Schwachman syndrome

Acquired causes

- Idiopathic
- Post infection: especially hepatitis
- Drugs
- Radiation
- Chemicals: benzene, insecticides
- Paroxysmal nocturnal haemoglobinuria
- Pre-leukaemia

Fanconi anaemia

This disorder is recessively inherited. Pancytopenia usually develops in childhood, most frequently in the first decade, and thrombocytopenia frequently develops first. There is a predisposition (about 10 per cent) to leukaemia, usually myelomonoblastic. This is usually preceded by the appearance of an abnormal clone characterized by monosomy 7. Other malignancies include hepatoma, carcinomas and lymphoma.

Patients show a number of congenital defects including dysmorphia, short stature, microcephaly, cardiac defects, learning difficulties, abnormal skin pigmentation, skeletal (hypoplasia of the thumb and forearm) and renal deformities.

Laboratory findings include macrocytic anaemia, neutropenia and thrombocytopenia. The Hb F level is raised and a bone marrow/trephine biopsy confirms the reduced cellularity. The diagnosis of Fanconi anaemia is confirmed by abnormal chromosomal fragility demonstrated by excessive chromatic breaks following exposure to mitomycin C.

Treatment includes supportive care, androgen therapy and bone marrow transplantation; only the last is curative. Androgen therapy is associated with an increased incidence of hepatic tumours and patients receiving androgen therapy should be serially evaluated for this complication.

Dyskeratosis congenita

This rare disorder is characterized by skin pigmentation, leucokeratosis of the mucous membranes and nail dystrophy. Presentation is usually in the first decade. Bone marrow failure develops in some but not all patients in the second or third decade and carcinomas may appear in the leucokeratotic lesions. The haematological changes are those of a progressive macrocytic anaemia and pancytopenia.

Shwachman syndrome

This disorder is characterized by short stature, exocrine pancreatic insufficiency and neutropenia, which can progress to pancytopenia. A number of patients acquire a clonal disorder characterized by monosomy 7 and progress to acute myeloid leukaemia.

The differential diagnosis of cytopenia and growth retardation includes Fanconi anaemia, Shwachman syndrome, Diamond–Blackfan anaemia and dyskeratosis congenita.

Idiopathic aplastic anaemia

The onset of symptoms is usually acute but can be more chronic. The symptoms are those of pancytopenia – pallor, tiredness, infection, bruising and petechiae secondary to anaemia, neutropenia and thrombocytopenia. Aplastic anaemia is classified by its severity, which in turn dictates treatment.

Treatment of aplastic anaemia

Criteria for severe aplastic anaemia

Blood

- Neutrophil count less than 0.5×10^9/L
- Platelet count less than 20×10^9/L
- Reticulocyte count less than 20×10^9/L

Marrow

- Severe hypocellularity (<25 per cent cellularity)
- Moderate hypocellularity (25–50 per cent) with less than 30 per cent of the residual cells being haematopoietic

Severe aplastic anaemia is defined by any two peripheral blood criteria and either marrow criteria.

Very severe aplastic anaemia is defined by a neutrophil count of less than 0.2×10^9/L.

The pathogenesis is complex but the fact that the marrow hypoplasia can be reversed by immunosuppression suggests that the hypoplasia is in part immune mediated.

Severe idiopathic aplastic anaemia in childhood with aggressive treatment has a survival in the region of 80 per cent. Treatment is aimed at supporting patients through the aplastic phase until recovery of the marrow occurs and at restoring normal marrow activity.

Supportive care includes platelet transfusions, which should be kept to a minimum to prevent sensitization, and aggressive treatment of infections (bacterial and fungal) related to neutropenia with broad-spectrum antibiotics and antifungals in the absence of a response.

The treatment of choice for children with severe aplastic anaemia and a histo-compatible sibling donor is bone marrow transplantation. Those without a donor should receive immunosuppression with antilymphocyte globulin followed by ciclosporin. Unrelated bone marrow transplantation is associated with a high procedure-related mortality and should be reserved for those children without a histo-compatible sibling donor and who fail immunosuppression.

Diamond–Blackfan syndrome

This disorder presents in early infancy, usually in the first year of life. It is characterized by a severe macrocytic or normochromic anaemia, reticulocytopenia and a paucity of red cell precursors in the bone marrow. White cell and platelet precursors are normal. Most cases are sporadic but familial cases occur. Approximately 25 per cent of affected children have at least one congenital abnormality (10 per cent with abnormalities of the thumb). Short stature is common and characteristic facial features are described of a snub nose, wide-set eyes and a thick upper lip. The red cells show features of fetal erythropoiesis, macrocytosis and a raised Hb F. A small number of children develop neutropenia or thrombocytopenia.

About two-thirds of patients respond to steroids and can be maintained on very small doses. A few patients have spontaneous remission and become steroid independent. About one third either do not respond or become refractory to steroids having once responded. These patients may become transfusion dependent and require chelation to treat iron overload. Bone marrow transplantation has been used in a small number of cases.

Transient erythroblastopenia of childhood

Transient erythroblastopenia of childhood is characterized by severe anaemia and reticulocytopenia in a previously healthy child. A history of a viral illness a few weeks earlier is common. Most cases occur after the first year of life with a peak incidence at 2 years of age. The red cells are normochromic normocytic, MCV is not elevated and the Hb F level is not raised, all of which helps differentiate this disorder from Diamond–Blackfan syndrome. The marrow shows a paucity of red cell precursors. The anaemia recovers spontaneously and steroids are not indicated. Red cell transfusion should be avoided if possible.

Anaemia of prematurity

Although the haemoglobin level falls after birth (physiological anaemia), it falls faster and further in the premature baby. Suboptimal erythropoietin production is thought to be responsible.

Haemolytic disorders

Haemolysis is the increased breakdown of red cells, resulting in shortening of the normal red cell lifespan. The red cell lifespan in children is 120 days, 60–80 days in neonates and even shorter in premature babies. Anaemia develops if the increase in marrow activity and the consequent reticulocytosis cannot compensate for the increased rate of red cell destruction. The diagnosis requires evidence of both increased red cell destruction and increased marrow activity.

Diagnosis

- Reticulocyte count: This may be reported as an absolute count (normal range 25–75 × 10^9/L) or as a percentage of the total number of erythrocytes present (normal range 0.5–1.5 per cent). The degree of reticulocytosis usually reflects the degree of compensatory marrow response.
- Unconjugated bilirubin: About 1 per cent of red cells are broken down daily and the haemoglobin degraded to bilirubin. An increase in the unconjugated bilirubin suggests an increase in degraded haemoglobin.
- Blood film: Reticulocytes appear on a blood film as polychromatic cells and are increased in haemolysis. Other specific red cell abnormalities suggestive of haemolysis include spherocytes, red cell fragments or bite cells; the last are associated with an unstable

haemoglobin or glucose 6-phosphate dehydrogenase (G6PD) deficiency.

- Haptoglobins: These are produced in the liver and bind free haemoglobin to form a complex that is cleared rapidly. The level of free haptoglobin falls when production is outmatched by clearance of the haptoglobin/haemoglobin complex. This usually occurs when the rate of red cell destruction is approximately twice the normal. Haptoglobins are extremely low or even absent in the first month of life.
- Plasma and urine-free haemoglobin: Free haemoglobin does not appear until all available haptoglobin has been depleted; haemoglobinuria then results. Haemoglobin is absorbed by the renal tubular epithelium and this is excreted into the urine as haemosiderin when epithelial cells are shed.

The detection of urinary haemosiderin suggests ongoing, previous or intermittent chronic haemolysis, because haemosiderin will be detected for weeks after the last haemolytic episode.

In haemolytic anaemias, a stable haemoglobin level can only be maintained by an increase in bone marrow erythropoietic activity. Parvovirus infects the colony-forming units-erythrocyte (CFU-E) and prevents their maturation. Suppression of bone marrow activity due to parvovirus in a patient with chronic haemolysis (e.g., hereditary spherocytosis), may cause a sudden fall in haemoglobin due to an aplastic crisis.

Classification of haemolytic disorders

Inherited haemolytic disorders

Defects in the structure of the red cell membrane

- Hereditary spherocytosis
- Hereditary elliptocytosis
- Hereditary stomatocytosis

Defects of erythrocyte metabolism

- G6PD deficiency
- Pyruvate kinase deficiency
- Other enzyme disorders

Qualitative haemoglobin disorders

- Stable variants – sickle cell disease
- Unstable variants

Quantitative haemoglobin disorders

- Impaired globin chain synthesis
- Thalassaemias

Acquired haemolytic disorders

Immune

- Autoimmune
- Alloimmune haemolytic disease of the newborn
- Maternal autoimmune haemolytic anaemia

Non-immune

- Infection
- Mechanical – microangiopathic haemolytic anaemia
- Drug-induced
- Paroxysmal nocturnal haemoglobinuria

Adapted from Lilleyman JS and Hann IM (eds) (1992) *Paediatric Haematology*, 1st edn. Edinburgh: Churchill Livingstone.

Disorders of the red cell membrane

Red cell membrane defects include hereditary spherocytosis, hereditary elliptocytosis, hereditary pyropoikilocytosis, hereditary acanthocytosis and hereditary stomatocytosis. These disorders have characteristic morphological features.

Disorders of red cell metabolism

The mature red cell is dependent on the anaerobic metabolism of glucose for its energy requirements. There are a number of pathways of red cell metabolism involving red cell enzymes, and enzyme abnormalities are a rare cause of haemolytic anaemia. The commonest enzyme deficiency to produce acute haemolysis is G6PD deficiency and pyruvate kinase deficiency is the commonest enzyme deficiency to cause chronic haemolysis.

The red blood cell enzyme profile in neonates is different from that in older children with some enzymes increased and others decreased.

Diagnosis/associations

- Morphology: There are no specific red cell morphological abnormalities associated with the majority of enzymopathies. In G6PD deficiency, during haemolytic crisis 'bite cells' may be seen and echinocytes in pyruvate kinase deficiency.
- Inheritance G6PD is X-linked but the majority of enzymopathies are autosomal recessive.
- Clinical associations: Favism (haemolysis after ingestion of fava beans) or the precipitation of haemolysis by oxidant drugs suggests G6PD deficiency. Nervous and muscular symptoms are associated with some enzymopathies. Cyanosis

may be due to methaemoglobinaemia, secondary to methaemoglobin reductase deficiency or one of the M-type haemoglobinopathies.

Glucose 6-phosphate dehydrogenase deficiency

Glucose 6-phosphate dehydrogenase is the first enzyme in the hexose monophosphate shunt and catalyses the conversion of glucose 6-phosphate to 6-phosphogluconate. There are more than 300 variants. Glucose 6-phosphate dehydrogenase B is the normal enzyme found in white and most black people. Glucose 6-phosphate dehydrogenase A is the commonest variant associated with haemolysis and is found in 10–15 per cent of African–Americans. Glucose 6-phosphate dehydrogenase Mediterranean is the commonest variant in white people of Mediterranean origin and G6PD Canton is the commonest in Asia. Glucose 6-phosphate dehydrogenase deficiency may protect against malaria. It is X-linked and haemolysis is mainly confined to males. Most variants of G6PD deficiency cause acute haemolytic episodes and not chronic haemolysis. These episodes are precipitated by oxidant drugs, infections and fava beans in G6PD Mediterranean and G6PD Canton but not G6PD A. Haemolysis in the neonatal period is common. During acute episodes 'bite cells' are seen on the peripheral smear and specific supra vital stains may show Heinz bodies. Glucose 6-phosphate dehydrogenase levels are measured by a specific enzyme assay. The level may be falsely high during haemolytic crisis because reticulocytes have a higher enzyme concentration. Patients should be educated about which drugs to avoid and should be supported through acute episodes.

Pyruvate kinase deficiency

This is inherited in an autosomal recessive manner. Although rare, it is the commonest red cell enzyme deficiency in north Europeans. The disease has a variable clinical course but usually the anaemia is moderate to severe. About one-third present in the neonatal period (anaemia and jaundice). The anaemia may improve as the child gets older. The occasional echinocyte may be seen on the peripheral smear. Diagnosis requires measurement of red cell pyruvate kinase enzyme activity. There is poor correlation between the degree of haemolysis and the enzyme activity level. Splenectomy may help severely affected individuals.

Qualitative haemoglobin disorder

Haemoglobin variants may be stable or unstable. Unstable haemoglobins denature either spontaneously or in response to oxidant stress. The clinical picture is variable and the abnormality may involve the α or β chains. Stable haemoglobin variants include Hb S, Hb C, Hb E and Hb SC.

Alloimmune haemolytic disease of the newborn (HDN)

Alloimmune HDN is due to placental transfer of maternal antibody. The commonest red cell antibodies involved remain anti-D followed by anti-c. Haemolysis is maximal at birth and decreases as the level of maternal antibody in the baby's circulation falls. The severity of haemolysis varies but can be sufficiently severe to require intrauterine transfusion or exchange transfusion and may lead to intrauterine death.

The Kleihauer test is an acid solution test carried out on maternal blood. Haemoglobin F in fetal cells is acid resistant so that fetal cells remain pink while maternal cells become colourless. The percentage of fetal red blood cells in the maternal blood and the amount of fetomaternal haemorrhage can be calculated and determines the dose of anti-D required to prevent sensitization of a Rhesus (Rh)-negative mother.

ABO haemolytic disease in the newborn

ABO HDN is due to IgG anti-A and anti-B crossing the placenta and causing haemolysis in an ABO incompatible fetus. It is usually only a problem in mothers with blood group O and occurs in 20 per cent of at-risk pregnancies (3 per cent of all births). It is rare for babies to have clinical problems and the blood films are often the most striking abnormality. ABO incompatibility is associated with marked spherocytosis. The A and B antigens are not well developed in babies and this probably explains some of the mildness of the clinical course. The mother's blood group is usually O and the baby group A. The mother will have significant IgG anti-A and anti-B titres.

Haemolysis due to ABO and Rh incompatibility in the neonate can be easily differentiated. The direct antiglobulin test (DAT) is strongly positive in Rh incompatibility but negative or weakly positive in ABO incompatibility. Spherocytes are not seen in haemolysis secondary to Rh incompatibility but the reticulocytosis may be marked. The haemolysis associated with Rh incompatibility is much more severe than that of ABO incompatibility. ABO incompatibility can affect the first pregnancy whereas in Rh incompatibility the first pregnancy sensitizes the mother and stimulates her to produce anti-D. Each subsequent pregnancy is more severely affected.

However, in Rhesus incompatibility the firstborn child can be affected if the mother has been sensitized by a previous event.

Microangiopathic haemolytic anaemia

The blood film shows red cell fragmentation. The commonest cause in children is haemolytic uraemic syndrome (renal failure, red cell fragmentation and thrombocytopenia), but it is also seen in children with burns and with haemolysis secondary to some types of heart valve prosthesis.

Paroxysmal nocturnal haemoglobinuria

This disorder is very uncommon in childhood and the characteristic features are those of acquired chronic intravascular haemolysis with haemosiderinuria, pancytopenia and thrombocytopenia. The diagnosis is made by the acidified serum lysis test (Ham test) or by FACS analysis for expression of the GPI-anchored proteins. It is a clonal disorder, which can be associated with marrow hypoplasia and a predisposition to venous thrombosis.

Infection

Bacterial sepsis can be associated with microangiopathic haemolytic anaemia complicating disseminated intravascular coagulopathy. Viral infections can cause autoimmune haemolytic anaemia (AIHA). Malaria (*Plasmodium falciparum*) is an important cause of haemolysis.

SCREENING FOR SICKLE CELL DISEASE AND β-THALASSAEMIA SYNDROMES

Haemoglobin electrophoresis or HPLC is the most important diagnostic test for haemoglobinopathies. In haemoglobin electrophoresis, a control and patient sample are electrophoresed on a gel and the width of the band corresponds to the percentage of the haemoglobin type that contributes to the total haemoglobin in the sample being tested.

High performance liquid chromatography is a process in which a mixture of molecules (normal and variant haemoglobins) with a net positive charge is separated into its components by their absorption on to a negatively charged chromatography column followed by their elution. Haemoglobins eluted from the column are represented graphically and automatically quantified by spectroscopy. Test results should be compared with normal haemoglobin values for different ages (Table 19.5). In sickle cell disorders the MCV is normal. Patients who have a high percentage of Hb S and low MCV probably have an Hb S/thalassaemia variant or iron deficiency.

Table 19.5 Screening for sickle cell disorders and β-thalassaemia syndromes

Healthy infant	Hb A 20% Hb F 80%
Healthy child	Hb A 97% Hb F 0.5% Hb A2 2.5%
Hb SS	Most of the haemoglobin present is Hb S Hb F is raised Hb A is absent - no β-chain production Parents - both have sickle cell trait - Hb AS Reduced MCV suggests co-inheritance of α-thalassaemia trait or iron deficiency
Hb AS	Hb A 60% Hb S 30–40%
Hb SC	Hb S 45–50% Hb C 45–50% Parents - one has Hb AS and one has Hb AC
Hb S/β^0 thalassaemia	Major haemoglobin present is Hb S Hb F is raised Hb A is absent - some β-chain production MCV reduced Differentiated from Hb SS with α-thalassaemia trait by parental studies Parents - one has Hb AS and one has β^0-thalassaemia trait
Hb S/β^+ thalassaemia	Major haemoglobin present is Hb S Hb F is raised Hb A is absent - no β-chain production MCV reduced Parents - one has Hb AS and one has β^+-thalassaemia trait
Thalassaemia major	Hb F 75–90% Hb A2 5–8% Hb A is absent Values apply to untransfused patient
Thalassaemia minor/trait	Hb A 90–95% Hb A2 3.5–7% Hb F 1–3%

Note: Stated haemoglobin values are approximate examples.

Hereditary persistence of fetal haemoglobin

Hereditary persistence of fetal haemoglobin is not associated with any clinical problems.

DISORDERS OF COAGULATION

Disorders of coagulation may be inherited or acquired. Inherited disorders are likely to present in infancy or childhood and are discussed later in Core problems (page 608).

Acquired disorders of coagulation

Disseminated intravascular coagulation – older child

- Infection, e.g. meningococcal, disseminated varicella
- Giant haemangioma (Kasabach–Merritt syndrome)
- Purpura fulminans
- Acute anaphylaxis
- Burns
- Heatstroke
- Hypothermia
- Head injury/trauma
- Haemolytic transfusion reaction
- Haemorrhagic shock
- Acute promyelocytic leukaemia
- Metastatic solid tumours

Disseminated intravascular coagulation – neonate

- Hypoxia/acidosis
- Infection
- Dead twin fetus
- Abruptio placenta
- Necrotizing enterocolitis
- HDN

Vitamin K deficiency

Hepatocellular disease

Congenital heart disease

Renal disease

Disseminated intravascular coagulation is the commonest acquired coagulopathy. It can be secondary to infection, hypovolaemia, hypoxia, malignancy, trauma, burns, Kasabach–Merritt syndrome, transfusion reactions and acute anaphylaxis. It can be acute and severe or chronic and low grade. In children, one of the most fulminant of DICs follows meningococcal septicaemia. In DIC, the coagulation system is triggered, with excess formation of fibrin resulting in disseminated microthrombi, coincident coagulation factor and platelet consumption and secondary fibrin(ogen)lysis. Laboratory findings consist of thrombocytopenia, anaemia with red cell fragmentation on the blood film, prolonged PT, APTT and TCT, low fibrinogen and elevated FDPs or D-dimers. Red

Table 19.6 Coagulation parameters in common required coagulation disorders

Test	Vitamin K deficiency	Liver disease	Disseminated intravascular coagulation
Platelet count	N	N*	L
PT	P	P	P
APPT	P	P	P
TCT	N	N	P
FDPs/D-Dimers	N	N or R	R
Low factor assays	II, VII, IX, X	II, V, VII, IX, X	I, II, V, VIII, IX, X

* Thrombocytopenia may be present in liver disease due to hypersplenism, and platelet dysfunction is not uncommon. Cardiac and renal disorders can also be associated with haemostatic abnormalities.

L, low; N, normal; P, prolonged; R, raised.

cell changes generally only occur if the condition has been present for a number of days.

Microthrombi formation can lead to the syndrome of purpura fulminans, which is characterized by peripheral gangrene involving the fingers, toes, nose and earlobes. This can follow meningococcal, pneumococcal and streptococcal infections and, rarely, varicella. A similar picture is seen in children with homozygous deficiency of protein C.

Treating the underlying cause and correcting hypovolaemia and hypoxia are as important as correcting the clotting abnormalities with replacement therapy. Vitamin K deficiency and liver disease are other important causes of acquired coagulopathy. It should be possible to differentiate liver disease from vitamin K deficiency (Table 19.6). In the latter only the vitamin K-dependent factors (II, VII, IX and X) are low, whereas in liver disease all factors produced by the liver fall.

Replacement therapy

Vitamin K deficiency should be corrected with vitamin K alone except in the presence of active bleeding when coagulation products containing the vitamin K dependent factors are indicated. Vitamin K should always be included in the treatment of a coagulopathy associated with liver disease. Replacement therapy in DIC may include platelet concentrates, fresh frozen plasma (FFP), which contains all clotting factors and cryoprecipitate as a concentrated source of fibrinogen. Virus-inactivated FFP and cryoprecipitate are now available. In the presence of peripheral gangrene, protein C concentrate may be beneficial.

PRINCIPLES UNDERLYING TRANSFUSION OF BLOOD PRODUCTS

The British Clinical Standards in Haematology (BCSH) has recently published a transfusion guideline for neonates and older children. Advances in neonatal intensive care, extracorporeal membrane oxygenation (ECMO), cardiac bypass surgery, bone marrow and solid organ transplantation, and the management of haemoglobinopathies and malignancy means that any child requiring transfusion will be among the most intensively transfused of all hospital patients. Furthermore, children and, in particular, neonates, often need highly individualized products. Safety in blood transfusion has attracted a great deal of resource and in no age group is it more important than children, because of the probable intensity of their transfusion requirements and their potential life expectancy.

While most attention and resource is focused on guaranteeing the microbiological safety of blood, transfusion-related infection is now a small risk compared to the risk of an error in administration. All hospitals in the United Kingdom are required to report all blood transfusion-related errors to the Serious Hazards Of Transfusion committee (SHOT). The annual reports of this committee repeatedly show that the greatest number of errors are due to the administration of the wrong blood or blood product to the wrong patent. Every hospital should have a transfusion committee responsible for producing local guidelines for the safe administration of blood and blood products and for educating those involved.

- Blood and blood products should only be prescribed if truly clinically indicated.
- Alternatives to blood products should always be considered.
- Recombinant products should be used where available.
- Virus-inactivated products should be used in the absence of recombinant products if the blood component can be virus inactivated. Two virus inactivated FFP products are available – solvent detergent (SD) FFP and methylene-blue-treated (MB) FFP.
- Red cells and platelets are not virus inactivated and are sourced from donors in the UK.

Every unit of blood collected in the UK is now screened for the following:

- antihuman immunodeficiency virus (anti-HIV) 1 and 2 antibodies
- antihepatitis C virus (anti-HCV) antibody
- HCV by nucleic acid test (NAT)
- antihuman T-lymphotrophic virus (anti-HTLV) antibodies
- syphilis.

Selected units are also screened for anticytomegalovirus (anti-CMV) antibody. The risk of transmitting infection from blood or non-virus-inactivated blood components is (figures from the Scottish National Blood Transfusion Service):

- HIV – 1 in 4 000 000
- HCV – <1 in 1 000 000
- HBV – 1 in 200 000
- HTLV – 1 in 5 000 000
- Bacteria – 1 in 2000–10 000

The risk of transfusion-transmitted variant Creutzfeldt–Jakob disease (vCJD) at present is unknown. However, the following measures have been introduced in the UK to reduce/remove the risk:

- Since 1999, all cellular blood components have been leucocyte-depleted at source.
- The Department of Health recommends that all children born after January 1996 and therefore not exposed to bovine spongiform encephalitis (BSE) in the food chain should receive either SD FFP or MB FFP sourced from outwith the UK, where BSE and vCJD are not endemic. Although this may increase the risk of other transfusion-transmissible diseases that are more prevalent in those areas, these can be eliminated by virus inactivation procedures that do not inactivate prions but do reduce the overall risk.

Recommendations

- Components for transfusion *in utero* and to infants under 1 year of age must be prepared from blood donated by donors who have given at least one previous donation within the past two years which was negative for all microbiological markers.

- CMV-seronegative blood should be transfused to:
  - infants in their first year of life, but this recommendation is under review. Those at greatest risk are fetuses and infants weighing less than 1.5 kg.
  - recipients of haematopoietic stem cells transplants
  - patients with cellular immunodeficiency.

Leucocyte-depleted blood significantly reduces the risk of CMV transmission, and in an emergency where CMV-seronegative blood is not available, transfusion of leucocyte-depleted blood is an acceptable alternative.

- Red cells and platelets should be irradiated for:
  - intrauterine transfusion (IUT)
  - exchange transfusion
  - top-up transfusion after IUT of red cells or platelets
  - when the donation is from a first- or second-degree relative or an HLA-selected donor.
- Platelet and plasma compatibility:
  - Platelets should be ABO and RhD identical or compatible with the recipient (see Table 19.8).
  - FFP should be ABO compatible with the recipient (see Table 19.8).
  - Platelets contain enough red cell stroma to stimulate Rh immunization. Therefore RhD-negative girls who receive RhD-positive platelets should receive anti-D immunoglobulin.
- Transfusion testing for neonates and infants within the first four postnatal months:
  - Small volume transfusions can be given repeatedly over the first 4 months of life without further serological testing, provided that there are no atypical maternal red cell antibodies in the maternal/infant serum, and the infant's DAT is negative when first tested.
  - If either the antibody screen or the DAT (or both) are positive, serological investigation or full compatibility testing will be necessary.
- Age of blood:
  - Red cells for exchange transfusion or large volume transfusion should be 5 days old or less.
  - Red cells for small volume transfusion (10–20 mL/kg) can be used up to 35 days old or less if in SAG-M (saline adenine glucose-mannitol) or similar additive solution or 28 days old or less if in CPD (citric phosphate dextrose).
- SAG-M or similar additive solution:
  - Red cells for exchange transfusion or similar large volume transfusion to infants less than 6 months of age should be collected into CPD and not SAG-M, because of concerns about the toxicity of the additive solutions. There is no evidence that SAG-M causes detriment in infants over the age of 6 months.

Table 19.7 Component volumes to be transfused to children and neonates

Component	Volume
Red cell concentrates	
Exchange transfusion	
For a term baby	80–160 mL/kg
For a preterm baby	100–200 mL/kg
Top-up transfusion	Desired Hb (g/dL) – actual Hb × weight (kg) × 3 (usually 10–20 mL/kg)
Platelet concentrates	
Children weighing <15 kg	10–20 mL/kg
Children weighing >15 kg	Single apheresis unit/ standard pool
Fresh frozen plasma	10–20 mL/kg
Cryoprecipitate	5–10 mL/kg

Hb, Haemoglobin.

Table 19.8 Choice of ABO group for blood products for administration to children

Patient's ABO group	ABO group of blood products to be transfused		
	Red cells	Platelets	FFP*
O			
First choice	O	O	O
Second choice	–	A	A or B or AB
A			
First choice	A	A	A or AB
Second choice	O		–
B			
First choice	B	B	B or AB
Second choice	O		–
AB			
First choice	AB	AB	AB
Second choice	A, B	A	A
Third choice	O†		

* Group O FFP should only be given to Group O patients.
† Group O components which test negatively for 'high titre' anti-A and anti-B should be selected.
FFP, fresh frozen plasma.

Indications for prophylactic platelet transfusion in children with thrombocytopenia as a result of reduced production

Platelet count $<10 \times 10^9$/L

Platelet count $<20 \times 10^9$/L and one or more of the following:

- severe mucositis
- DIC
- anticoagulant therapy
- platelets likely to fall $<10 \times 10^9$/L before next evaluation
- risk of bleeding due to local tumour infiltration

Platelet count 20–40 $\times 10^9$/L and one or more of the following:

- DIC in association with induction therapy for leukaemia
- extreme hyperleucocytosis
- prior to lumbar puncture or central venous line insertion.

PREVENTION OF INFECTION IN THE ASPLENIC CHILD: IMMUNIZATION PROPHYLAXIS

Life-threatening infection is a major long-term risk after splenectomy. Splenic macrophages have an important role in filtering and phagocytosing the bacteria in the circulation. Most serious infections are due to encapsulated bacteria such as *Streptococcus pneumoniae*, *Haemophilus influenzae* type B, and *Neisseria meningitides* (meningococcus). Patients at risk include:

- those who have undergone surgical removal
- those with congenital asplenia
- those with functional hyposplenism secondary to Hb SS, Hb SC, thalassaemia major, lymphoproliferative diseases, coeliac disease, inflammatory bowel disease, dermatitis herpetiformis, and post bone marrow transplantation (splenic irradiation).

Asplenic children under 5 years have an infection rate of over 10 per cent, much higher than in adults (<1 per cent). The risk of dying of serious infection is lifelong, although most infections occur in the first two years after splenectomy with up to one-third by five years after splenectomy.

Recommendations

All children with an absent or dysfunctional spleen should receive appropriate immunization and advice on lifelong antibiotic prophylaxis.

PNEUMOCOCCAL IMMUNIZATION

Polyvalent pneumococcal vaccine should be given at least two weeks before splenectomy to optimize antibody response. All other at-risk children should be immunized at the first opportunity, but immunization should be delayed at least six months after immunosuppressive chemotherapy or radiotherapy. Children under the age of 2 years have a reduced ability to mount an antibody response to polysaccharide antigens and are at risk of vaccine failure. They should receive a conjugate vaccine, which may provide a more reliable serological response. Reimmunization is currently recommended every five years.

H. INFLUENZAE TYPE B IMMUNIZATION

H. influenzae type B vaccine should be given prior to splenectomy and to hyposplenic previously non-immunized children. There is no recommendation to revaccinate.

MENINGOCOCCAL C CONJUGATE VACCINE

In the UK, meningococcal infection is most commonly due to group B strain (60 per cent) followed by group C (40 per cent). Meningococcal C conjugate vaccine is part of routine childhood immunization. It should be given prior to splenectomy and to hyposplenic previously non-immunized children. There is no recommendation to revaccinate. Those travelling abroad should receive protection against group A infections with meningococcal plain polysaccharide A and C vaccine.

INFLUENZA VACCINATION

This is recommended yearly.

ANTIBIOTIC PROPHYLAXIS

Prophylactic oral phenoxymethyl penicillin is first choice and for those allergic to penicillin erythromycin should be used. Prophylaxis should be lifelong although compliance is a problem. Patients developing infection despite prophylaxis should be admitted immediately to hospital and receive systemic antibiotics. Vaccine failure occurs and despite vaccination and prophylactic antibiotics, breakthrough infections can occur.

OTHER RECOMMENDATIONS

Patients should carry a card with information about their lack of spleen. They may wish to wear a MedicAlert®

disc. They should be educated on the potential risk of travel, particularly with regard to malaria and about the risks of animal and tick bites.

ONCOLOGY

GENETIC AND ENVIRONMENTAL FACTORS PREDISPOSING TO CHILDHOOD MALIGNANCY

Most childhood malignancies probably require a combination of inherited susceptibility and candidate exposure. There is evidence in childhood leukaemia for genetic factors – identical twins are at increased risk and those with Down syndrome or DNA fragility, e.g. Fanconi anaemia. In lymphoid malignancies, the second event is probably a delayed and abnormal response at an age when lymphoid tissue is developing rapidly. The Epstein–Barr virus (EBV) is thought to play a role in Burkitt lymphoma, Hodgkin disease and other forms of non-Hodgkin lymphoma (NHL). Radiation and radiotherapy are implicated, but there is no evidence for electromagnetic fields or environmental background radiation. Alkylating agents are associated with an increased risk of secondary leukaemia.

LEUKAEMIA

Acute leukaemia accounts for approximately one-third of all childhood cancers in the UK with about 80 per cent of cases being due to acute lymphoblastic leukaemia (ALL) and the remainder due to acute myeloid leukaemia (AML). Chronic myeloid leukaemia and myelodysplasia are rare.

Acute lymphoblastic leukaemia (ALL)

The peak incidence is between 2 and 6 years (median 4 years) with a male:female ratio of 1.2:1. The presenting symptoms are due to:

1 Marrow infiltration with blasts and subsequent failure of normal haematopoiesis:
   a anaemia – pallor, tiredness, headache, dizziness
   b thrombocytopenia – bruising, bleeding, retinal haemorrhage
   c neutropenia – pyrexia, infection.
2 Organ infiltration:
   a lymphadenopathy and hepatosplenomegaly
   b bone pain/limp – due to involvement of the periosteum and bone
   c anterior mediastinal mass – correlates closely with T-cell disease
   d skin infiltrates – seen in infants
   e central nervous system (CNS) disease – occurs in approximately 1–2 per cent at presentation, may be asymptomatic or present with headache and vomiting or cranial nerve palsies
   f testicular involvement – at presentation is rare
   g weight loss and anorexia.

Investigations

- Full blood count (FBC) and blood film:
  - Anaemia and thrombocytopenia of variable degrees
  - Neutropenia is generally present
  - WCC may be normal, increased or decreased
  - Lymphoblasts are generally seen on the blood film but patients can have ALL with no circulating blasts – termed 'aleukaemic leukaemia'.
- Bone marrow:
  - Morphology – blasts are classified by their morphological appearances into L1 (80–85 per cent), L2 (10–15 per cent) and L3 (2–3 per cent) based on cell size, nuclear/cytoplasmic ratio, nuclear irregularity and number of nucleoli.
  - Cytochemistry – special stains which distinguish between ALL and AML have largely been replaced by immunophenotyping. Periodic acid Schiff (PAS) shows block positivity in c-ALL and acid phosphatase polar positivity in T-cell ALL.
  - Immunophenotype – monoclonal antibodies differentiate cells of lymphoid or myeloid lineage and within lymphoid lineage subtype to pre-pre-B or common ALL (Ia+, CD10+, CD19+, tdt$\pm$), B-cell ALL, null ALL and T-cell ALL. Seventy per cent of children with ALL have common ALL.
  - Cytogenetics – refers to the number and structural changes in the chromosomes in the leukaemic clone in the bone marrow: high hyperdiploid ($>$50), hyperdiploid (47–50), normal (46), hypodiploid ($<$45) and structural abnormalities called non-random translocations.
- Lumbar puncture:
  - Cell count and cytospin to examine for leukaemic blasts.
- Biochemistry:
  - Urea and electrolytes, liver function tests, urate, immunoglobulins.
- Viral serology:
  - Baseline chickenpox and measles titres.
- Radiology:
  - Chest X-ray to detect mediastinal mass or pleural effusion (important prior to general anaesthesia for bone marrow), abdominal ultrasound to assess

organomegaly (children with bulky disease and large involved kidneys are at risk of tumour lysis syndrome).

Prognostic factors

Prognostic factors may be influenced by the treatment given.

- WCC and age are important prognostic indicators and are used to stratify treatment. Children with a WCC greater than $>50 \times 10^9$/L and those more than 10 years of age have a less favourable outcome than those who are younger with a lower WCC. Infants less than 1 year of age have a particularly poor outlook.
- Gender: girls have a more favourable prognosis than boys.
- Immunophenotype: common ALL or B-lineage disease does better than T-cell ALL. Mature B-cell ALL is more characteristic of a Burkitt type lymphoma than a leukaemia and is treated as such.
- Cytogenetics: hyperdiploidy and t(12,21) are favourable; near haplodiploid, t(9,22) and t(4,11) are poor prognostic indicators. AML 1 amplification also appears to be associated with a poor outlook.

Management

- Supportive care: children should receive adequate intravenous hydration and allopurinol before starting treatment. They may require red cell and platelet support to correct anaemia and thrombocytopenia and antibiotics for febrile neutropenia.

CHEMOTHERAPY

The outlook for standard-risk ALL is now at least 70–80 per cent and this is achieved with combination intensive chemotherapy. The rate of cell kill is a very important prognostic indicator (the faster the disease clears the better the outcome) and is used to modify treatment. Treatment of ALL is arbitrarily divided into:

- Induction therapy: This refers to the initial weeks of treatment, which aims to eradicate disease from the bone marrow and allow it to repopulate with normal cells. Children are stratified by their age ($<10>$ years) and by WCC ($<50 \times 10^9$/L) to the intensity of their induction therapy. The combination of dexamethasone (superior to reprednisolone because of better control of CNS disease), vincristine and asparaginase ±daunorubicin, depending on the child's age and WCC, results in remission in at least 95 per cent of children.
- Intensification/consolidation: The intensity is tailored to the prognostic group. Combination chemotherapy is used to prevent drug resistance developing.
- CNS-directed treatment: CNS-directed therapy is important in reducing the risk of CNS relapse, although dexamethasone and intensive chemotherapy contribute. Intrathecal methotrexate, high-dose systemic methotrexate and cranial radiation have been employed. Cranial radiation is now reserved for the treatment of CNS leukaemia because of its associated neuropsychological impairment and learning difficulties. Intrathecal methotrexate is currently used in the UK.
- Maintenance/continuing chemotherapy: This involves daily 6-mercaptopurine, weekly methotrexate and four weekly vincristine and dexamethasone. Presently in the UK, boys receive treatment for three years and girls for two years.
- Co-trimoxazole (Septrin®) is given throughout as prophylaxis against *Pneumocystis carinii* pneumonia (PCP).

Acute myeloid leukaemia (AML)

The presenting symptoms are similar to those of ALL, with lethargy, pallor, purpura, fever and infection. FAB M4–M5 subtypes are characterized by extramedullary disease, including skin and gum infiltration, lymphadenopathy and CNS involvement. Other rare presenting features are myeloblastic chloromas, which are solid masses of myeloblasts which can develop around the orbits, spinal cord or cranium. M3 is associated with haemorrhage secondary to DIC, which may be made worse with induction therapy.

A transient myeloproliferative disorder is seen in some neonates with Down syndrome and the blast cells characterized as megakaryoblasts. Although it resolves spontaneously, some of these children subsequently develop AML.

Investigations

This is similar to those for ALL. Important differences include:

- Blood film:
  - The blasts are larger than those of ALL and in certain subtypes can contain inclusions referred to as Auer rods. These are seen only in AML.
- Bone marrow:
  - Morphology – blasts are subclassified by their morphological appearance and cytochemistry into a number of FAB (French American British classification) subtypes (M0–M7) distinguished

by degree of differentiation and cell type (myeloblasts, promyeloblasts, myelomonoblasts, monoblasts, erythroblasts, megakaryoblasts).
- Cytochemistry – Sudan Black and myeloperoxidase positively stain myeloblasts and non-specific esterase monoblasts.
- Immunophenotype – CD33 and CD13 are the most important myeloid markers recognizing myeloid and monocytic lineages.
- Cytogenetics – these are the most important prognostic indicators in AML:
  - favourable cytogenetics: t(15,17), t(8,21) and inv(16)
  - unfavourable cytogenetics: −5, −7, del(5q), ab(3q), complex karyotype.
- It is recognized that cytogenetic abnormalities characterize subtypes of AML (e.g. t(8,21) present in some patients with M2) and that the genetic change determines the biology of the leukaemia and the clinical outcome. In response to this the World Health Organization (WHO) has produced a new classification for AML incorporating morphologic, immunophenotypic, genetic and clinical features. This aims firstly to define leukaemias that are biologically homogeneous and secondly to be of clinical relevance. The WHO classification has four major categories:
  - acute myeloid leukaemia with recurrent genetic abnormalities
  - acute myeloid leukaemia with multi-lineage dysplasia
  - acute leukaemia, therapy related
  - acute leukaemia, not otherwise categorized.

Treatment

Treatment is stratified by cytogenetic group and response to initial treatment. About 90 per cent of children with AML achieve remission with one or two courses of intensive combination chemotherapy. Generally a total of four blocks of treatment is given.

Allogeneic bone marrow transplantation is reserved for those who respond slowly to chemotherapy or have unfavourable cytogenetics. The disease-free survival is now in the region of 60 per cent, but there is significant mortality associated with treatment due mainly to infection.

NEPHROBLASTOMA

Nephroblastoma originates in the developing renal tissue, the metanephric blastoma and may be associated with congenital anomalies such as aniridia, hemihypertrophy, genitourinary tract abnormalities and Beckwith–Wiedemann syndrome.

Children present with an abdominal mass, although a minority have haematuria and fewer hypertension at diagnosis. Biopsy or nephrectomy are required for a tissue diagonsis. Imaging by ultrasound, computed tomography (CT) scanning or magnetic resonance imaging (MRI), surgical findings (capsule status, lymph node involvement, intra-abdominal spread) and the histology stage of the disease. The stage of disease at diagnosis determines which treatment modalities are used and may include surgery, chemotherapy and radiotherapy.

NEUROBLASTOMA

Neuroblastoma is the commonest extracranial solid tumour of childhood and originates from the sympathetic nervous system. The tumour may occur in the abdomen, thorax or head and neck region, when children may present with Horner syndrome. Spinal cord compression may occur when the tumour grows through intravertebral foramina. In infants, liver and skin involvement may be seen. Opsomyoclonus (myoclonic jerking and random eye movements, 'dancing eyes') or cerebellar ataxia are present in a small number of cases and may be associated with a favourable outcome, although these specific symptoms may persist. Increased levels of urinary catecholamines homovanillic acid (HVA) and 4-hydroxy-3-methoxymandelic acid (HMMA) support the diagnosis. Ultrasound, CT and MRI scanning are used to assess the extent of the primary tumour and the presence of metastases. Metastatic bone disease is detected by bone marrow examination, bone scan and metaiodobenzylguanidine (MIBG) scanning; MIBG labelled with iodine-131 can also be used to demonstrate primary, residual and recurrent tumour masses.

Age and stage at diagnosis determine outcome, which is also influenced by the biological factors of N-myc amplification and DNA ploidy. Combination treatment with chemotherapy, surgery, radiotherapy and high-dose chemotherapy with stem cell rescue are used. Infants with stage IVS disease who do not have life-threatening complications may have resolution of their disease without any therapy. Stage IV neuroblastoma outside infancy has a grim outlook.

HODGKIN DISEASE (HD)

In Hodgkin disease, the malignant cells are multinucleated Reed–Sternberg and mononuclear Hodgkin disease cells. It is a disease of older childhood and the commonest presentation is with painless cervical lymphadenopathy with or without a mediastinal mass.

Stage I – disease confined to a single node or group of nodes.

Stage II – disease involves two or more groups of nodes on the same side of the diaphragm.

Stage III – disease involves nodes above and below the diaphragm.

Stage IV – disseminated involvement of one or more organs or tissues (e.g. lung, liver, bone marrow) with or without associated lymph node enlargement.

The presence of 'B' symptoms (fever, night sweats and loss of >10 per cent of body weight) confers a less favourable prognosis. Histologically, Hodgkin disease is classified into nodular sclerosis, lymphocyte depleted, lymphocyte dominant and mixed cellularity. Disease stage is determined by CT or MRI scanning. Chemotherapy is the mainstay of treatment.

NON-HODGKIN LYMPHOMA (NHL)

Non-Hodgkin lymphomas represent a heterogeneous group of lymphoid malignancies, which in childhood are high grade, and of immature B- or T-lineage. Non-Hodgkin lymphoma constitutes about 5 per cent of all childhood malignancies.

Stage I
- a single nodal or extranodal area with the exclusion of mediastinum and abdomen.

Stage II
- a single tumour (extranodal area) with regional node involvement
- two or more nodal areas on the same side of the diaphragm
- two single (extranodal) tumours with or without regional node involvement on the same side of the diaphragm
- a primary gastrointestinal tumour, with or without involvement of associated mesenteric nodes only, grossly completely resected.

Stage III
- two single tumours (extranodal) on opposite sides of the diaphragm
- two or more nodal areas above and below the diaphragm
- all primary intrathoracic tumours
- all extensive primary intra-abdominal disease
- all paraspinal and epidural tumours.

Stage IV
- any of the above with initial CNS and/or bone marrow involvement.

B-cell disease commonly presents with an abdominal mass and T-cell disease with a mediastinal mass with or without a pleural effusion. There may be compression of vital organs such as the urinary tract in abdominal disease and airway and/or superior vena caval obstruction with thoracic disease. Disease extent is determined by CT/MRI scanning, lumbar puncture and bone marrow aspiration. The diagnosis may be made from examination of pleural fluid, bone marrow or biopsy of an involved lymph node or lesion.

Treatment is with chemotherapy. The initial course of therapy may be complicated by tumour lysis if the tumour is bulky and these patients should receive high-dose fluids and a xanthine oxidase inhibitor such as rasburicase or allopurinol prior to chemotherapy to prevent this complication.

RHABDOMYOSARCOMA

Rhabdomyosarcoma is the commonest soft-tissue sarcoma in children, and it is thought to arise from primitive mesenchymal cells committed to developing into striated muscle. It may be associated with congenital anomalies of the genitourinary tract and with neurofibromatosis. Rhabdomyosarcoma may arise anywhere in the body, notably the orbit, parameningeal area, genitourinary tract and extremities. A fifth of patients have metastatic disease at presentation. Full staging is performed by CT or MRI scanning, bone scan and bilateral bone marrow aspirates and trephine. Multimodality treatment involving surgery, chemotherapy and radiotherapy is required. The outcome is dependent on stage and histology.

BRAIN TUMOURS

Brain tumours are the commonest malignant solid tumours in childhood; half arise in the posterior fossa and include medulloblastomas, cerebellar and brain stem tumours. The clinical presentation of brain tumours varies and the non-specific symptoms may lead to a delay in diagnosis. Features of raised intracranial pressure include headaches, vomiting and, in infants, a rapidly increasing head circumference. Specific neurological abnormalities related to the tumour site may also be present. Dependent on the site, histology and clinical condition of the patient, combinations of surgery, radiotherapy and chemotherapy are used. Radiotherapy is avoided in infants because of concerns of treatment-related neurotoxicity. In survivors, there may be significant cognitive, neuroendocrine and physical disability. These patients must be managed by a multidisciplinary team with input from neurologists, endocrinologists and psychologists as well as oncologists.

STEM CELL TRANSPLANT

Bone marrow, peripheral blood and cord cells are all sources of stem cells for bone marrow transplantation. Stem cell transplantation may be characterized as autologous (recipient's own stem cells), syngeneic (twins' stem cells) or allogeneic (stem cells from sibling, non-sibling related or unrelated donor).

Indicators for stem cell transplantation

- High risk ALL and AML in first complete remission (CR)
- Relapsed ALL or AML
- Chronic and accelerated phase CML
- Myelodysplasia
- Stage IV solid tumours
- Relapsed HD and NHL
- Thalassaemia major/sickle cell disease
- Immunodeficiency/inborn errors of metabolism
- Aplastic anaemia

Allogeneic stem cell transplantation is generally employed in leukaemia and primary bone marrow disorders whereas high dose chemotherapy with autologous stem cell rescue is used in solid tumours. Intensive chemotherapy with or without total body irradiation is given as conditioning prior to the return of stem cells to eradicate any residual disease or haematopoietic tissue. Children less than 3 years of age and those with benign disease do not receive irradiation but chemotherapy alone. The stem cells, which are infused, are pluripotent and over the next three to four weeks will repopulate the host bone marrow and produce red cells, white cells and platelets.

A number of complications are associated with allogeneic stem cell transplantation:

- Graft rejection.
- Infection: Bacterial, fungal and viral. Bacterial and fungal infections dominate during the early period of neutropenia, and viral infections later. Cytomegalovirus is a particular risk after stem cell transplantation, and children who have intensive immunosuppression are also at risk of adenovirus, parainfluenza and respiratory syncytial virus (RSV).
- Graft-versus-host disease (GVHD): In this condition the donor lymphocytes (graft) react against recipient (host) cells. Graft-versus-host disease is divided into acute (first 100 days post bone marrow) or chronic (after 100 days). Acute GVHD can affect any organ, but is classically thought of as affecting the skin (rash), gut (diarrhoea) and liver (hepatitis), whereas chronic GVHD resembles a connective tissue disorder.
- Veno-occlusive disease of the liver (VOD): This is due to damage to the hepatic vessels caused by drugs and radiation during conditioning and is commoner in patients with pre-existing liver disease.
- Haemorrhagic cystitis: Cyclophosphamide can cause cystitis and haemorrhage in the bladder wall.

Children undergoing stem cell transplantation are at high risk of infection and should receive antimicrobial prophylaxis against fungus, *Pneumocystis carinii* pneumonia (PCP), CMV (if indicated by serological status of donor and recipient) and varicella zoster. Immunoglobulin replacement is given to those who are severely immunocompromised and at increased risk of viral infection. Ciclosporin or tacrolimus is given to prevent GVHD. All blood products should be CMV negative and irradiated to prevent transfusion-associated GVHD.

The mortality associated with autologous stem cell rescue is <5 per cent, and with sibling allogeneic stem cell transplantation 5–10 per cent, whereas that of unrelated stem cell transplantation is higher at around 20 per cent. Despite the risk of allogeneic stem cell transplantation, the greatest risk post transplant for patients with malignant disease remains relapse of the underlying disease.

SIDE EFFECTS OF CHEMOTHERAPY AND RADIOTHERAPY

These can be divided into early and late side effects.

Early side effects

- Chemotherapy-induced marrow suppression – thrombocytopenia and neutropenia.
- Haemorrhage – rare when platelet count $>10 \times 10^9$/L, except in the presence of sepsis.

- Infection – bacterial and fungal infections occur during periods of neutropenia. Viral infections (chickenpox, shingles, herpes simplex and measles) are a risk with continuing immunosuppression. Bacterial infections in neutropenia may be with Gram-positive or Gram-negative organisms. Children with febrile neutropenia should receive broad-spectrum antibiotic cover with an aminoglycoside and a β-lactam. Children with indwelling intravenous catheters who remain pyrexial despite broad-spectrum antibiotics should receive treatment to cover possible line-related coagulase negative staphylococcal infection. Antifungal therapy should be considered for persistent fever. Prior to starting antibiotics appropriate cultures should be taken (blood cultures, urine, throat swab, stool) and a chest radiograph if indicated.
  Co-trimoxazole is given throughout treatment for ALL to prevent PCP.
- Nausea and vomiting – controlled by antiemetics.
- Mucositis and poor nutrition.
- Alopecia.
- Tumour lysis syndrome – leukaemia/cancer cells lyse with chemotherapy. Intracellular electrolytes are released with resultant hyperuricaemia, hyperkalaemia, hyperphosphataemia and hypocalcaemia. Renal obstruction can occur secondary to urate and calcium phosphate precipitation in the kidneys. Patients at risk of tumour lysis are those with a high WCC and/or bulky organomegaly. They should receive intravenous hyperhydration and xanthine oxidase inhibitors, rasburicase or allopurinol before starting chemotherapy. Alkalinization of the urine with intravenous sodium bicarbonate is no longer thought appropriate. Electrolytes and urine output should be carefully monitored.
- Hepatotoxicity – most chemotherapeutic agents can cause hepatic dysfunction. Veno-occlusive disease/ portal hypertension is a recognized complication of thiopurines.
- Coagulation abnormalities – coagulation abnormalities can be associated with sepsis. Asparaginase interferes with protein metabolism and produces low levels of functional fibrinogen and antithrombin. This more often results in thrombosis than bleeding.
- Neurotoxicity – vincristine can lead to peripheral neuropathy and a syndrome of inappropriate antidiuretic hormone excretion (SIADH) with hyponatraemia and seizure activity.
- Steroid-related problems – steroids can produce weight gain, fluid retention, hypertension, glucose intolerance, mood changes and a cushingoid appearance.
- Haemorrhagic cystitis – this can occur with cyclophosphamide and may be aggravated by viral infection.

Late side effects

- Endocrine problems – radiotherapy can damage the pituitary or gonads resulting in growth retardation, delayed puberty, hypothyroidism (radiation damage to the thyroid) and hypopituitarism. Spinal irradiation can cause impairment of spinal growth.
- Sterility/infertility – this occurs with both radiation to the gonads and certain chemotherapeutic agents.
- Cataracts – this can occur following irradiation to the lens.
- Cardiotoxicity – anthracyclines (daunorubicin, doxorubicin, epirubicin, idarubicin) are associated with a reduction in the fractional shortening and ejection fraction. The dose limit is stated to be 450 mg/m^2, but much lower doses can cause cardiotoxicity especially in young children.
- Cognitive dysfunction – all CNS-directed (cranial irradiation, high dose intravenous methotrexate and intrathecal chemotherapy) treatment is probably associated with cognitive impairment. Cranial irradiation is the most damaging and produces the greatest degree of learning difficulties. Young children are particularly vulnerable and cranial irradiation is avoided below the age of 3 years.
- Avascular necrosis – this can follow steroid therapy and radiation. Teenagers are particularly at risk and girls are affected more than boys.
- Second tumours.

CORE PROBLEMS

THROMBOCYTOPENIC PURPURA

CASE STUDY: Idiopathic thrombocytopenic purpura

A 2-year-old boy presented with a 24-hour history of widespread petechiae and purpura. He had had a trickle of blood from one nostril the previous day. He had no previous history of easy bruising. He had

had an upper respiratory tract infection two weeks earlier. He was on no medication and previously healthy. Examination revealed widespread petechiae and purpura. He had a small patch of eczema behind one knee. There were no other abnormalities and, in particular, he had no lymphadenopathy or hepatosplenomegaly. His Hb was 11.5 g/dL, WCC 8.7×10^9/L, neutrophil count 3.4×10^9/L and platelet count 2×10^9/L. The blood film was normal except for the absence of platelets. Biochemistry was normal.

The likeliest diagnosis is idiopathic thrombocytopenic purpura (ITP). Idiopathic thrombocytopenic purpura is a diagnosis of exclusion. In boys, it is important to consider congenital thrombocytopenias. Wiskott–Aldrich syndrome is characterized by the triad of eczema, thrombocytopenia and immunodeficiency. In this boy there was no suggestion that thrombocytopenia had been present from birth or that he had been abnormally susceptible to infection. He was on no drugs to implicate drug therapy. Meningococcal septicaemia is a differential diagnosis of a widespread petechial rash but unlikely in a well child. The absence of lymphadenopathy and organomegaly and any abnormality on the blood film other than thrombocytopenia make an infiltrative process in the bone marrow very unlikely.

Haemolytic uraemic syndrome is in the differential diagnosis of profound thrombocytopenia but excluded by the lack of red cell fragmentation and normal biochemistry. Furthermore, a patient with this disorder rarely manifests the same degree of purpura as those with ITP. Non-accidental injury, which can present with excessive bruising, is excluded by the abnormal platelet count.

Thrombocytopenia is defined as a platelet count of less than 150×10^9/L and can result from failure of production, which can be congenital or acquired (Table 19.9), or increased destruction, which may be immune or non-immune mediated (Table 19.10).

Table 19.9 Childhood thrombocytopenia due to reduced platelet production

Congenital	
Reduced or absent megakaryocytes	**Normal numbers of megakaryocytes**
Thrombocytopenia with absent radii syndrome Fanconi anaemia Other megakaryocytic thrombocytopenia	Wiskott–Aldrich syndrome (eczema, thrombocytopenia, immune deficiency) May–Hegglin syndrome (giant platelets and neutrophil inclusions) Bernard–Soulier syndrome (mild thrombocytopenia and giant platelets) Epstein syndrome (nerve deafness and nephritis) Grey platelet syndrome Montreal syndrome Mediterranean thrombocytopenia Other hereditary thrombocytopenias Metabolic disorders Inherited megaloblastic anaemia
Acquired	
Aplastic anaemia/myelosuppression Idiopathic Drug-induced Toxin-induced Radiation-induced Hepatitis-associated Marrow replacement Leukaemia Metastic malignancy Megaloblastic anaemias	

Idiopathic thrombocytopenic purpura

The term idiopathic thrombocytopenic purpura refers to immune-mediated thrombocytopenia unassociated with any underlying disease and has a probable incidence of 4 per 100 000 children per year. It is classified as acute (80–90 per cent) or chronic (10–20 per cent); the latter defined as ITP lasting for more than six months. The two types are probably two distinct entities characterized by differences in age, sex and mode of presentation. Recurrent or relapsing ITP is also described and is considered a subtype of chronic ITP.

Acute ITP usually presents with a sudden onset of bruising and petechiae in an otherwise well child. Minor epistaxis and subconjunctival haemorrhage are relatively common and mucocutaneous bleeding and haematuria are less often present. The peak age is 2–4 years with a male:female ratio of 1:1. A history of a preceding upper respiratory tract infection is common.

In contrast, chronic ITP often has a more insidious onset with easy bruising noted for a number of weeks/months before presentation. The male:female ratio is 1:2 and girls older than 10 years of age are particularly at risk.

Table 19.10 Childhood thrombocytopenia due to shortened platelet survival

Immune mediated	Non-immune mediated
Idiopathic thrombocytopenic purpura (ITP) Neonatal (maternal) ITP Neonatal alloimmune thrombocytopenia Infection Autoimmune disorders (SLE, Evan Syndrome) Drug-induced (heparin, sodium valproate, phenytoin, carbamazepine) Malignant disease Post-transfusion purpura	Disseminated intravascular coagulation Haemolytic uraemic syndrome Thrombotic thrombocytopenic purpura Kasabach-Merritt syndrome - giant haemangioma Cyanotic congenital heart disease Liver disease Perinatal aspiration syndromes Neonatal undefined Phototherapy Intravascular prosthesis Drug-induced

History

Idiopathic thrombocytopenic purpura is a diagnosis of exclusion of other causes of thrombocytopenia (see Tables 19.9 and 19.10). These include leukaemia, aplastic anaemia, familial thrombocytopenia, drug-related thrombocytopenia, connective tissue disorders and specific infections. From the history and examination it is important to exclude a family history of bruising, recent weight loss, joint pain or swelling, rashes, fevers, lymphadenopathy and hepatosplenomegaly. The presence of any of these findings should raise doubt of the diagnosis of ITP.

Full blood count

The platelet count will be low and often is $<10 \times 10^9$/L, whereas the WCC and haemoglobin should be normal, unless there has been active bleeding which is rare. There should be no abnormality on the blood film other than the absence of platelets.

Other investigations

The bone marrow findings in ITP are not diagnostic and megakaryocytes may be normal or increased in number in keeping with peripheral destruction. A bone marrow is indicated only in the presence of an atypical presentation, abnormal findings on physical examination or abnormalities other than absent platelets on the blood film. It may also be indicated to exclude other pathology, if the course of the ITP is not typical, when the platelet count does not recover within a few months or so, or if steroids are to be considered as treatment, because these may partially treat an unsuspected case of leukaemia and jeopardize the chance for long-term survival. Even if steroids are to be given it may not be necessary to carry out a bone marrow, if there is no other indication.

IgG autoantibodies to platelet-specific antigens should not be routinely performed. They are of little value diagnostically and do not distinguish between acute or chronic ITP. They are, however, much more often found in chronic ITP than acute ITP. Investigations should be minimal. It is worth screening for CMV in infants less than 1 year of age with apparent ITP and for autoantibodies in teenage girls, who are at risk of chronic ITP associated with an underlying immune disorder.

Prognosis and management

- About 80–90 per cent of children with ITP will have a spontaneous remission within six months, and in 50 per cent this will have occurred within two to three months.
- Despite very low platelet counts of even less than 10×10^9/L, major haemorrhage is rare and the only symptoms are usually bruising. Life-threatening intracranial haemorrhage is a very rare event with a recently reported incidence of 1:500, but the risk is probably cumulative over time. Where it arises it is usually associated with trauma or a vascular anomaly.
- The patient should be treated and not the platelet count. Haemorrhagic symptoms justify treatment, bruising alone does not. Therefore, children with mucous membrane bleeding or problematic epistaxis may require treatment, whereas those who only have bruising do not, irrespective of their platelet count.
- Treatment approaches include observation, steroids or intravenous immunoglobulin. Limited trials suggest that intravenous immunoglobulin is associated with a faster recovery of the platelet count than steroid therapy and both are associated with a faster recovery than no therapy. There is no difference in long-term outcome between these three approaches.
- Intravenous immunoglobulin acts by blocking FC receptors in the spleen but is expensive and, although it appears to be microbiologically safe, is a blood product.
- Steroids suppress antibody formation and carry the risk of general immunosuppression, weight gain, hyperglycaemia and hypertension. At present in the UK, most children who receive treatment do so with corticosteroids. These should be given for a period of

two weeks and then withdrawn, irrespective of the platelet count, to avoid side effects. Intravenous immunoglobulin is best reserved to raise the platelet count in chronic ITP when it is necessary to overcome haemorrhagic problems or to allow dental extractions or surgical procedures.

- Splenectomy should be reserved for children with problematic chronic ITP or those who have had an intracranial haemorrhage. About 70 per cent of children respond. Children who undergo splenectomy should have pneumococcus and *H. influenzae* type B (HIB) vaccine prior to and penicillin prophylaxis after splenectomy.
- Therapy for children with chronic ITP who fail to respond to splenectomy, or those in whom splenectomy is inappropriate, include anti-D immunoglobulin (to Rhesus D positive patients only) or immune suppression.
- Platelet transfusions are only used in the face of active bleeding, particularly intracranial bleeding when large doses are necessary, because transfused platelets will be rapidly destroyed by circulating autoantibody.
- In the presence of active intracranial bleeding in ITP, craniotomy may be indicated and an emergency splenectomy may be carried out at the same time, with the procedures covered by large platelet transfusions, intravenous immunoglobulin and high doses of methylprednisolone. With this approach, mortality is historically less than 50 per cent.

Neonatal thrombocytopenia

- Neonatal alloimmune thrombocytopenia: In this disorder there is feto-maternal incompatibility of platelet-specific antigens, most commonly platelet-specific antigen HPA-1 (PL^{A1}). The mother is HPA-1 (PL^{A1})-negative and anti-HPA-1 (PL^{A1}) antibodies pass to the fetus. The maternal platelet count is normal, but the otherwise well infant is profoundly thrombocytopenic. Diagnosis is confirmed by the presence of IgG alloantibody in the maternal serum, which reacts with the father's (and infant's) platelets. The infant remains thrombocytopenic for one to three weeks. Intracranial haemorrhage, ante- and postnatally, occurs in about 10 per cent of severely affected babies. First born infants are affected and subsequent siblings are equally or more severely affected.
- Neonatal ITP: These infants are born to mothers with active or previous ITP. There is no correlation between the platelet count of the mother and infant, and only about 50 per cent of babies born to mothers with active or previous ITP are affected. The platelet count is rarely less than 50×10^9/L or clinically significant.
- Infection (including TORCH infections – toxoplasmosis, rubella, CMV, herpes simplex, syphilis)
- Birth asphyxia
- Sepsis/DIC
- Congenital abnormalities such as Wiskott–Aldrich syndrome, TAR syndrome
- Kasabach–Merritt syndrome
- Maternal drugs
- Congenital tumours, e.g. leukaemia/neuroblastoma
- Undefined thrombocytopenia.

Thrombocytopenia is common in sick term and preterm babies. An incidence of 22 per cent was reported in one large study of unselected consecutive neonates admitted to a regional intensive care unit. The underlying cause is thought to be a shortened platelet survival, secondary to a number of factors, but primarily infection.

Thrombocytopenia outwith the neonatal period

- Immune thrombocytopenia associated with infection: Infections include infectious mononucleosis, HIV, CMV, rubella, varicella, toxoplasmosis, malaria, mumps, measles and measles vaccine.
- Drug-induced immune thrombocytopenia: Important drugs causing thrombocytopenia include heparin, sodium valproate, carbamazepine, phenytoin and co-trimoxazole.
- DIC: See section on acquired disorders of coagulation (page 588).
- Autoimmune disorders:
  - Systemic lupus erythematosus (SLE) – associated with a lupus anticoagulant
  - Evan syndrome – immune-mediated thrombocytopenia and autoimmune haemolytic anaemia
  - Immune thrombocytopenia associated with lymphoma – most commonly seen with Hodgkin disease, more rarely with NHL.

Haemolytic uraemic syndrome

Haemolytic uraemic syndrome (HUS) is characterized by the triad of microangiopathic anaemia, thrombocytopenia and renal failure. The platelet count may be moderately or markedly reduced due to shortened platelet survival, but coagulation screening tests are usually normal or only slightly abnormal, suggesting that the thrombocytopenia is not part of a consumptive coagulopathy. There may be a prodromal illness of abdominal pain and bloody diarrhoea. The epidemic form of HUS is often associated with enteropathogenic *Escherichia coli*, but *Shigella* and echovirus can also be causative organisms.

The cause of the thrombocytopenia is unknown, but it may be that the toxin damages vascular endothelium releasing high molecular multimers of vWF antigen, which cause platelet aggregation. HUS may be epidemic or sporadic. The epidemic variety probably follows an infective insult and the sporadic type may be a more heterogeneous group with a number of aetiologies.

Thrombotic thrombocytopenic purpura (TTP), whilst similar to HUS, with the same classic triad of haemolytic anaemia, thrombocytopenia and renal failure, is a more serious multiorgan disorder with fever, neurological disturbances and a guarded outcome.

Congenital heart disease

Children with cyanotic congenital heart disease and secondary polycythaemia may have thrombocytopenia. The severity of the thrombocytopenia may be related to the degree of polycythaemia.

Liver disease

Thrombocytopenia in liver disease is due in part to congestive splenomegaly and partly to shortened platelet survival secondary to consumption.

Thrombocytopenia and absent radii (TAR)

This disorder is characterized by profound thrombocytopenia associated with skeletal abnormalities, including hypoplastic or absent radii. The physical deformities are nearly always symmetrical. It is recessively inherited. The severity of the thrombocytopenia is greatest in the first year of life and thereafter the platelet count improves. The platelets are of normal size. The marrow shows reduced megakaryocytes with those present being small and dysplastic. Myeloid hyperplasia is common. Associated disorders include early failure to thrive and gastrointestinal bleeding due to cows' milk allergy, cardiac defects, dysplasia of the jaw and clavicles and congenital dislocated hips.

Fanconi anaemia

Thrombocytopenia is usually the first haematological abnormality to appear in this disorder. It rarely presents in the neonatal period and most commonly develops around the age of 6–7 years.

Wiskott–Aldrich syndrome

This disorder is characterized by a triad of eczema, thrombocytopenia and immunodeficiency. It has an X-linked inheritance. The immune deficiency involves both cellular and humoral immunity with absent or reduced isoagglutinins, progressive lymphopenia and failure to produce antibodies to some antigens after an appropriate challenge. The severity of the thrombocytopenia is variable, and may be marked. The degree of bruising is more severe than would be expected from the platelet count, suggesting that these boys have both thromboctopenia and a platelet function defect. The platelets are small with a mean platelet volume of about half that of normal platelets. Platelet function studies are abnormal and suggest a storage pool defect. The presence of platelet specific IgG suggests an immune mediated component to the thrombocytopenia in addition to a failure of production and a frequently observed good response to splenectomy supports this. Therefore despite the risks of splenectomy in an immunocompromised child, splenectomy may be justified. Bone marrow transplantation is the only curative treatment for this disorder.

Platelet function abnormalities

Glanzmann thrombasthenia

The inheritance is autosomal recessive. Platelet aggregation studies show complete failure to respond to ADP, collagen, thrombin and ristocetin. The glycoprotein IIb/IIIa complex on the membrane of the platelets is absent/reduced or abnormal resulting in failure of platelets to bind to fibrinogen. Both the platelet count and morphology are normal, but the bleeding time is markedly prolonged.

Bernard–Soulier syndrome

The inheritance is autosomal recessive. The disorder is characterized by moderate thrombocytopenia with giant morphologically abnormal platelets. The bleeding time is markedly prolonged. Platelet aggregation is normal with ADP and collagen, but absent to ristocetin. The GPIb/IX/V glycoprotein receptor complex on the platelet which carries the receptor for vWF and GPV is absent/reduced or abnormal. The platelet vWF subendothelial interaction is an essential step for the initial adhesion of platelets to damaged blood vessels. Plasma vWF is normal.

SPHEROCYTOSIS

CASE STUDY

A 4-year-old girl presented with a three-day history of intermittent fever, vomiting, lethargy and increasing jaundice. She attended nursery school and several of her playmates had what was thought to be viral gastroenteritis. She had had neonatal jaundice and required phototherapy. There was no family history of blood disorders elicited but a family member had undergone a splenectomy. At presentation she was pale and icteric. She had no significant lymphadenopathy or hepatomegaly, but had 6-cm splenomegaly. Her height was on the 10th centile and her weight on the 3rd centile. Examination was otherwise normal with the exception of a cardiac flow murmur. Her Hb was 4.6 g/dL, WCC 2.7×10^9/L, neutrophil count 1.5×10^9/L, platelet count 51×10^9/L and reticulocyte count 50×10^9/L. Numerous spherocytes were noted on her peripheral smear. Her total bilirubin was elevated at 151 μg/L with an unconjugated bilirubin of 141 μg/L. Alanine aminotransferase (ALT) and aspartate aminotransferase (AST) were normal and direct Coombs' test was negative. She was IgM positive for Parvo B19.

The differential diagnosis is that of a haemolytic anaemia (anaemia and hyperbilirubinaemia) characterized by spherocytosis. The commonest causes in this age group are hereditary spherocytosis and autoimmune haemolytic anaemia. Supporting a diagnosis of hereditary spherocytosis is her impressive splenomegaly (suggesting this had in part been longstanding), neonatal jaundice, a family history of splenectomy and negative direct Coombs' test. Her reticulocytopenia, borderline neutropenia and moderate thrombocytopenia are secondary to an aplastic crisis associated with parvovirus infection. Patients with chronic haemolysis are at particular risk. Her pancytopenia improved with folic acid supplements.

Hereditary spherocytosis

Hereditary spherocytosis has a frequency of 1 in 5000 people of north European extraction, but appears to be less common in other ethnic groups. Seventy-five per cent of cases are inherited in an autosomal dominant fashion; in the remainder, the inheritance may be autosomal recessive, a new mutation or autosomal dominant with reduced penetrance.

Spectrum deficiency has been described in the majority of patients with HS and the degree probably correlates with the severity of the haemolysis. The deficiency of the spectrum protein leads to increased membrane fragility and the red cells are removed by the spleen.

Clinical features

The severity of haemolysis varies from very mild to very severe, although the majority have mild to moderate haemolysis characterized by anaemia, jaundice (unconjugated) and splenomegaly. Anaemia is the commonest presentation but children may be asymptomatic. Many adults and older children have compensated haemolysis with little or no anaemia. The reticulocyte count is almost always raised. A sudden exacerbation of a previously mild or moderate anaemia may occur following a viral illness usually due to an increased rate of haemolysis or transient marrow aplasia. Pigmented gall stones are rare but can occur in children.

Neonatal hereditary spherocytosis

In 30–50 per cent of children with hereditary spherocytosis there is a history of significant neonatal jaundice. This is usually evident within the first 48 hours of life and phototherapy and, occasionally, exchange transfusion may be necessary. The diagnosis is difficult because the film appearances may not be typical and spherocytes are routinely seen on neonatal blood films. There is no evidence that those who are symptomatic as neonates have more severe haemolysis later in life.

Diagnosis and management

Spherocytes are usually easily identified on the blood film. The osmotic fragility test is commonly performed and whereas it is usually increased a normal osmotic fragility test does not exclude the diagnosis. It may be normal in the presence of an increased reticulocyte count. It also does not differentiate between the causes of spherocytosis and is positive in all cases of haemolytic anaemia where spherocytosis is present. The cryohaemolysis test and the eosin 5-maleimide (EMA)-binding test have a higher predictive value. In the neonatal period, the non-incubated osmotic fragility test is unreliable. Fetal red cells are more osmotically resistant than adult cells and as a result although the incubated test may be abnormal, the non-incubated test may be normal. Family history or studies may help in differentiating hereditary spherocytosis from other causes of spherocytosis in the neonate. Very occasionally, atypical cases may require measurement of erythrocyte membrane proteins to clarify the nature of the membrane disorder.

Treatment usually consists of folic acid supplementation, but these may not be required in very mild cases. Splenectomy is not usually necessary during childhood and adolescence for mildly affected individuals, but moderately and severely affected individuals will benefit from splenectomy. Because of the risks of post-splenectomy infection, splenectomy should be postponed until late childhood unless the disease interferes with normal growth and development. Following splenectomy the red cell abnormalities persist but haemolytic and aplastic crises cease. The risk of gall stone development decreases. The risk of pneumococcal infection can probably be reduced by the administration of prophylactic penicillin and pneumococcal and HIB vaccine should be given prior to splenectomy. All should be appropriately counselled about the infection risk.

Causes of spherocytosis

- Hereditary spherocytosis
- ABO incompatibility in the neonate
- Autoimmune haemolytic anaemia
- Bacterial sepsis
- Hereditary pyropoikilocytosis
- Burns

Autoimmune haemolytic anaemia

In childhood, AIHA is generally acute and self-limiting. There is usually a history of preceding viral illness. In older children, autoimmune haemolysis may be the presenting symptom of a multisystem autoimmune disease. Autoimmune haemolytic anaemia can be warm or cold.

Warm autoimmune haemolytic anaemia

- Idiopathic
- SLE
- Rheumatoid arthritis
- Hodgkin disease
- Evan syndrome
- Drugs

In warm AIHA IgG antibodies and/or complement bind to red cells at a temperature greater than 37°C. Warm AIHA is mainly idiopathic (60 per cent), or associated with thrombocytopenia in Evan syndrome (20 per cent). The remaining 40 per cent are associated with autoimmune/immune dysregulation disorders, e.g. SLE, rheumatoid arthritis, HD and drugs. Intravenous penicillin is the most commonly implicated drug. Warm-type AIHA can be severe and life threatening.

Treatment initially consists of steroids but for those who do not respond immunosuppression has been used, including ciclosporin, cyclophosphamide and high-dose intravenous immunoglobulin. Splenectomy may be indicated. Blood transfusion may be necessary. The DAT will be positive and all blood crossmatched will be incompatible. The least incompatible blood should be transfused, if clinically indicated.

Cold autoimmune haemolytic anaemia

Cold antibody AIHA produces IgM autoantibodies that bind to the red cells at temperatures less than 37°C. This usually follows infections with mycoplasma and infectious mononucleosis. The disorder is acute and self-limiting and haemolysis tends to be milder than in warm AIHA because the thermal range of the antibody may be clinically insignificant. Treatment is usually unnecessary. Blood, if necessary, should be warmed before transfusions. Steroids are not helpful.

Paroxysmal cold haemoglobinuria

- Non-specific viruses
- Measles vaccine
- Varicella

A biphasic antibody with anti-P specificity may be present. This antibody, Donath–Landsteiner, is IgG, fixes to red cells in the cold and generates complement-mediated lysis when the temperature rises to 37°C, resulting in paroxysmal cold haemoglobinuria. Children generally present after a non-specific viral infection. Paroxysmal cold haemoglobinuria is usually a benign and self-limiting condition requiring only supportive therapy. The diagnosis is confirmed by the Donath–Landsteiner lysis test.

Investigations

- Blood count – isolated low haemoglobin
- Reticulocytosis
- Blood film – may show anisocytosis, polychromasia, and spherocytosis in warm AIHA and cold agglutinins in cold AIHA (these cause a falsely elevated MCV and disappear on warming the blood sample to 37°C)
- Direct antiglobulin test is positive with IgG and/or C3-coating in warm AIHA. In cold AIHA the red cells may be coated with complement.
- Positive Donath–Landsteiner lysis test in paroxysmal cold haemoglobinuria.

β-THALASSAEMIA

β-Thalassaemia is a more serious disorder than α-thalassaemia. Individuals with β-thalassaemia develop normally *in utero* but become anaemic during the first few months of life and thereafter may require lifelong blood transfusion.

The molecular defects are varied but more often arise from point mutations than deletions. The clinical severity of β-thalassaemia ranges through thalassaemia minor (usually symptomless), thalassaemia intermedia (anaemia and splenomegaly but not transfusion dependent) to thalassaemia major (transfusion dependent) and depends on the number of β-thalassaemia genes inherited and whether gene expression is reduced or absent.

β-Thalassaemia major

Thalassaemia major arises from homozygous β-thalassaemia or the inheritance of compound heterozygous β-thalassaemia and presents in the first year of life with failure to thrive, poor feeding, recurrent respiratory infections, pallor and massive hepatosplenomegaly. Infants with thalassaemia intermedia have a milder disorder and may present later in the second year of life.

- Severe anaemia with markedly hypochromic red cells, anisocytosis, basophilic stippling and nucleated red cells on the peripheral film.
- The MCV is reduced but less so than in β-thalassaemia trait.
- The bone marrow shows massive erythroid hyperplasia.
- An unconjugated hyperbilirubinaemia reflects the shortened red cell survival and ineffective erythropoiesis.
- In β^0-thalassaemia, the only haemoglobin that can be produced is Hb F, but a variable amount of Hb A is produced with β^+-thalassaemia genes. These should be measured by electrophoresis or HPLC.

MANAGEMENT OF THALASSAEMIA MAJOR

- In the absence of transfusion death may occur within the first year or two of life.
- With inadequate transfusion, ineffective erythropoiesis leads to massive marrow expansion driven by erythropoietin, resulting in gross deformities of the skeleton with lacey trabecular pattern on radiographs and thickening and overgrowth of the zygomata of the skull. Progressive splenomegaly and hypersplenism contribute to the severity of the anaemia. Intercurrent infection, leg ulcers and a hypermetabolic state with weight loss, fever and secondary gout occur. The erythroid expansion leads to increased gastrointestinal iron absorption with resultant iron overload even in the absence of regular blood transfusion.
- With adequate transfusion, early growth and development is usually normal. The aim of transfusion is to maintain a haemoglobin level that inhibits ineffective erythropoiesis, marrow expansion and bone deformity and allows normal growth. By suppressing ineffective erythropoiesis it also reduces the likelihood of splenomegaly and hypersplenism and suppresses excess iron absorption from the gut. The haemoglobin should be maintained between 10 and 14 g/dL with a pretransfusion haemoglobin of 10–11 g/dL. Patients should have their red cells genotyped to reduce the risk of sensitization with repeated transfusions.
- Transfusion requirements should be carefully documented and monitored. If transfusion requirements rise disproportionately to the increase in size of the child, hypersplenism should be suspected and splenectomy may be beneficial. It should be delayed until after the fifth year of life wherever possible because of the risk of post-splenectomy infection.
- Iron chelation: This should be started to prevent iron overload before the third birthday and hopefully when the infant is dry at night. Desferrioxamine is the only chelating agent in clinical use and is given by subcutaneous infusion overnight. Iron is excreted in the stools and urine. Ferritin should be used to monitor iron load. A small dose of vitamin C given concurrently increases the urinary iron excretion. Compliance can be poor, particularly in the teenage years.
- Toxicity includes retinal damage, sensorineural deafness and growth retardation, all being more common in patients with low body iron stores receiving high doses of desferrioxamine.
- Iron overload can lead to cardiac, liver and endocrine complications, which are reduced by chelation. Testosterone or oestrogen supplements may be required for secondary hypogonadism, which is usually related to hypothalamic-hypopituitary dysfunction. Growth hormone may also be required. Insulin will be necessary for those who develop diabetes as a result of pancreatic iron overload. A multidisciplinary approach is therefore important.
- Patients should receive folic acid supplements to prevent folate deficiency, secondary to the increased demands of increased erythropoiesis.
- Bone marrow transplantation is the only curable option but at present reserved for those with fully compatible HLA sibling donors.

β-Thalassaemia minor

Heterozygotes for β-thalassaemia are typically asymptomatic. The haemoglobin is slightly reduced (9–12 g/dL) and the red cell count is high. The red cell indices are markedly reduced (MCV 60–70 fL and MCH 18–22 fL). The Hb A2 is increased (4–7 per cent), as is the Hb F. The Hb A2 may not be elevated in iron depletion.

δβ-Thalassaemia and hereditary persistence of fetal haemoglobin

The δβ-thalassaemias are characterized by the absence of δ and β-globin chain production and increased levels of Hb F. Because of the compensatory γ-globin production homozygotes have a milder disease than those with thalassaemia major.

Thalassaemia intermedia

Patients with thalassaemia intermedia are symptomatic but have a milder clinical course than those with thalassaemia major and are not transfusion dependent. The molecular basis is varied and includes the co-inheritance of a gene that enhances Hb F (gamma chain) production or the co-inheritance of α-thalassaemia in a patient with β^+-thalassaemia; both situations improve the balance between α and β-chain production. It is important to identify these individuals at presentation because they will not require transfusion or chelation.

SICKLE CELL DISEASE

Sickle cell disease is caused by a single base mutation, which results in the substitution of valine for glutamic acid at the sixth codon of the β-globulin chain. When deoxygenated, sickle haemoglobin polymerizes and the red cell becomes sickle shaped. The subsequent red cell membrane damage leads to haemolysis and the rigid sickle cells block the blood flow in the microcirculation.

The degree of sickling correlates with the concentration of Hb S. The condition does not usually present before 6 months of age, and the disease severity may be modified by high levels of Hb F. The important sickling syndromes are homozygous sickle cell disease (Hb SS) and the double heterozygous states Hb SC disease (Hb SC) and sickle β-thalassaemia (Hb S β-thal). In Africa, about a third of all births are carriers for the sickle cell trait and are Hb AS(Hb A + Hb S) heterozygotes.

Diagnosis

The blood film features are those of sickle cells, hypochromasia, microcytosis, target cells, polychromasia and numerous crenated red cells. Most infants are functionally asplenic by 1 year of age because of repeated splenic infarction and features of hyposplenism may be noted on the peripheral smear. High-performance liquid chromatography or haemoglobin electrophoresis demonstrates more than 80 per cent Hb S. Investigation of double heterozygous states is essential, both for treating the patient and for antenatal diagnosis, which can be made on chorionic villous biopsy in the first trimester of pregnancy. The sickle test detects around 20 per cent Hb S and therefore does not distinguish carriers from those with the disease.

Clinical features and complications

Anaemia

The degree of anaemia is variable and tends to remain stable in any individual patient. The anaemia is due to chronic haemolysis and the unconjugated bilirubin is increased. Children with Hb SC have a higher haemoglobin level than those with Hb SS. A fall in haemoglobin may follow marrow suppression after viral infections, particularly parvovirus.

Infection

The increased risk of infection is multifactorial but includes hyposplenism and, defective optimization. Causative organisms include *Pneumococcus*, *H. influenzae* and *Salmonella*. The risk of pneumococcal infection is particularly high and is greatest in the first 2 years of life. Prophylactic penicillin results in an 80 per cent reduction in the infection rate in infancy between 3 and 36 months of age, and, therefore, penicillin prophylaxis should be started in any child with sickle cell disease by the age of 4 months. Immunization prophylaxis should be as recommended in the section on Prevention of infection in the asplenic child (see page 593).

Acute painful crises

These result from vascular occlusive episodes and may be provoked by infection, dehydration and cold. Pain most frequently occurs in the bone, muscles and abdomen, but may occur anywhere. In the hand/foot syndrome, dactylitis due to infarction of the metacarpals and metatarsals results in painful swelling of the hands and feet.

Treatment of painful crisis is supportive and includes fluid replacement, pain relief and appropriate antibiotics. There is an increased risk of osteomyelitis.

Splenic sequestration

This is a life-threatening condition due to the rapid sequestration of red cells in a rapidly enlarging spleen. It is characterized by the sudden onset of pallor, breathlessness, abdominal pain and splenic enlargement. Urgent blood transfusion may be indicated. Splenic sequestration crises often recur and it is an indication for elective splenectomy after recovery.

Stroke

Cerebrovascular occlusion can lead to hemiplegia and cranial nerve palsies. The risk of recurrence is high and it is an indication for hypertransfusion. Many patients with sickle cell disease have subtle neurological damage, even in the absence of major radiological evidence.

Other complications

- Acute chest syndrome – characterized by lung consolidation, often bilateral, on the chest X-ray and may be due to a combination of infection and infarction. The symptoms are those of fever, increasing dyspnoea, tachycardia and chest pain. Patients may deteriorate rapidly and this complication is life threatening. Monitoring should include the measurement of oxygen saturations out of oxygen supplementation to detect increasing respiratory compromise. Top-up or exchange transfusion may be necessary.
- Pigmented gall stones
- Priapism
- Renal papillary necrosis with haematuria leading to loss of concentrating ability by tubules
- Leg ulcers
- Pulmonary hypertension
- Aseptic necrosis of the femoral head
- Delay of growth and puberty
- Congestive cardiac failure
- Blindness due to retinal infarction and detachment

Treatment

- Acute painful crisis – analgesia, fluids and antibiotics.
- Blood transfusion should only be given when absolutely clinically indicated. This avoids iron overload and sensitization. Regular transfusion can suppress erythropoiesis and keep the Hb S concentration less than 30 per cent, a level that prevents complications, but is only indicated for severe complications such as stroke. Exchange transfusion may be indicated in stroke or acute chest syndrome and, following these crises, affected children should have regular transfusion to prevent recurrence.
- Supportive care – asplenic prophylaxis, folic supplements.
- Genetic counselling.
- At present the role of BMT is limited.
- Some patients benefit clinically from hydroxyurea, which raises the Hb F level.

Sickle cell trait

Sickle cell trait is not usually associated with symptoms, except for renal abnormalities of microscopic haematuria and a concentrating defect. However, when exposed to extreme hypoxic conditions, sickling infarcts may occur, particularly in the spleen, and the trait may carry a slight increased risk of thrombotic events.

HAEMOPHILIA

CASE STUDY

An 11-month-old infant presented with a large haematoma on his forehead, which he had bumped on the side of his cot. He was noted to have raised bruises on his shins, which had appeared since he started crawling. There was no family history of a bleeding disorder. A coagulation screen showed him to have a PT of 12.6 s, APTT >120 s, FVIII:C <1 IU/dL, vWF:Ag 80 IU/dL, vWF activity 90 IU/dL and platelet count 250×10^9/L.

The FVIII:C of <1 IU/dL confirms the diagnosis of severe haemophilia A. Severely affected boys typically present outwith the neonatal period when they begin crawling and bumping into objects, or attempting to stand and fall. At least 30 per cent of cases of severe haemophilia A have no family history and arise from a spontaneous mutation. An infant with excessive bruising is sometimes wrongly diagnosed as being the victim of non-accidental injury.

Haemophilia A and B and von Willebrand disease are the commonest inherited bleeding disorders. von Willebrand factor is a carrier protein for FVIII:C in plasma, protecting it from degradation. Thus patients with severe vWD, who lack vWF, have very low levels of FVIII:C.

Haemophilia A and B

Deficiency

Haemophilia A and B are due to deficiencies of the procoagulants FVIII:C and FIX:C respectively (true deficiency or non-functional protein).

Incidence

Severe haemophilia A and severe haemophilia B occurs in 1:10 000 and 1:50 000 males, respectively.

Inheritance

This is X-linked recessive. About 30 per cent are due to new mutations. Extreme lionization of the normal X chromosome in female carriers may result in FVIII:C activity less than 50 IU/dL and in clinical bleeding problems when haemostatically challenged. Diverse genetic defects give rise to the same clinical disorder.

Clinical symptoms

Haemophilia A and B result in clinically indistinguishable bleeding disorders of variable severity. The severity is classified according to the FVIII:C or FIX:C activity in the plasma and is consistent within families: severe <1 IU/dL, moderate 1–5 IU/dL and mild >5 IU/dL. This classification provides a good indicator of the likely frequency and severity of bleeding episodes. Fifty per cent of boys are severely affected. Bleeding may occur at any site, but typically boys with severe haemophilia present with apparently spontaneous recurrent haemarthrosis, deep muscle bleeds, easy bruising, subcutaneous haematomas and mouth bleeds from a traumatically torn frenulum. Intracranial haemorrhage following minor trauma is a small but constant risk. Moderately affected boys may have haemarthrosis or soft tissue haematomas after mild trauma, although not spontaneously, whereas mildly affected boys only bleed after significant trauma or after dental extraction or surgery.

Diagnosis

Activated partial thromboplastin time is prolonged due to low levels of FVIII:C or FIX:C. FVIII:C or FIX:C levels are low, confirming the diagnosis and classifying the severity. In haemophilia A the vWF:Ag and ristocetin co-factor activity (measurement of vWF activity) are normal because the vWF molecule is unaffected. In both haemophilia A and B the bleeding time and PT are normal. Additional investigations include the exclusion of a FVIII:C inhibitor and identification of the molecular defect for family studies and antenatal diagnosis.

Von Willebrand disease

Deficiency

von Willebrand disease is a disorder of the vWF, which is responsible for the adherence of platelets to damaged endothelium. It is caused by either a quantitative or a qualitative deficiency of the vWF in which the structure and function of the molecule are abnormal. vWF circulates in the plasma as a series of polymers of variable molecular weight. The size of the vWF multimers is important because the largest have the greatest affinity for the vWF receptors on platelets.

Incidence

It is a common disorder in its many heterogeneous forms and may be as common as 1:100.

Inheritance

It is an autosomal disorder, usually inherited in a dominant manner, and thus affects both sexes equally. Autosomal recessive forms and double heterozygosity exists. The gene is situated on chromosome 12, but homologous sequences have been localized to chromosome 22. A variety of genetic defects have been identified.

Clinical symptoms

Bleeding is mild in most cases and restricted to mucocutaneous bleeding, easy bruising, epistaxis, menorrhagia and post-surgical and post-traumatic bleeding. Homozygous or double heterozygous vWD results in severe bleeding clinically similar to, but milder than, haemophilia A with symptoms which may include haemarthrosis and muscle haematomas in addition to the mucous membrane bleeding of vWD. This is because components of the FVIII–vWF complex, including FVIII:C, vWF:Ag and ristocetin co-factor activity, are all markedly reduced. FVIII:C levels may be as low as 2 IU/dL.

Diagnosis

von Willebrand disease is classified by the multimeric structure of vWF in plasma and platelets. The bleeding time is prolonged because of abnormal platelet adhesion. The APTT is prolonged relative to the reduction in FVIII:C, which is variably reduced. The vWF:Ag and ristocetin co-factor activities (vWF activity) are reduced. The multimeric pattern is variably abnormal. The PT is normal.

Management of inherited bleeding disorders

- Children with inherited bleeding disorders should be referred to a regional paediatric haemophilia centre where the family will have access to a haemophilia sister for support, appropriate physiotherapy and dental care.
- All patients likely to receive regular blood products should be vaccinated against hepatitis A and B.
- Alternatives to blood products should be used if appropriate and, when not, recombinant products should be given to children to obviate the risk of viral transmission. Desmopressin acetate (DDAVP®) may raise the FVIII:C level two to four times its basal level and into the haemostatic range in mild haemophilia A.

- Most patients with severe haemophilia A will require FVIII concentrate and this should be recombinant. FVIII 1 U/kg will raise the FVIII:C level by 2 IU/dL and has a half-life of 8–12 hours. For mild haemorrhage a level of 30 IU/dL is required, for established haemarthrosis a level of around 50 IU/dL and for surgery 80–100 IU/dL.
- Haemophilia B replacement is with FIX concentrate. FIX concentrate 1 U/kg raises the FIX:C level by approximately 1 IU/dL and the half-life is approximately 24 hours. Minimum level of FIX:C of 20 IU/dL is necessary for early bleeding episodes, 40 IU/dL for more advanced muscle or joint bleeding and an initial level of 60 IU/dL for surgery.
- Treatment of mild vWD is with desmopressin if this has been shown to raise the vWF and FVIII:C into a haemostatic range. If not, treatment is with vWF concentrates or FVIII concentrates, which contain adequate amounts of vWF. By definition, these will not be FVIII recombinant products and should be viricidally treated.
- Boys with severe haemophilia A and B generally receive prophylactic treatment thrice and twice weekly, respectively. This will greatly reduce the frequency of bleeds and hopefully will translate into reduced arthropathy.
- About 10 per cent of boys with haemophilia A develop antibodies to FVIII:C when FVIII replacement fails to stop bleeding. Recombinant FVII is now used to bypass the inhibitor. A smaller percentage (6 per cent) of boys with haemophilia B develop inhibitors.
- The problems seen in haemophilia are changing as the treatment advances. Recombinant products will hopefully stop the transmission of viral infection and the resultant liver disease. Prophylaxis will reduce damage to joints with less painful chronic arthropathy and the need for joint replacement later in life. Home treatment allows a more normal life with less dependency on the haemophilia centre. However, the immune modulation associated with recombinant product may lead to an increase in inhibitor formation.

CERVICAL LYMPH NODE ENLARGEMENT

CASE STUDY

An 11-year-old girl presented with a two-month history of a painless right-sided neck swelling. She had no history of infection but had received a course of antibiotics and had not shown any improvement. She had had no contact with tuberculosis. She was otherwise asymptomatic and, in particular, had not lost any weight and had had no fever or night sweats. On examination she had bilateral supraclavicular lymphadenopathy, more marked on the right side. She had no axillary or inguinal lymphadenopathy and no organomegaly. A chest radiograph showed hilar lymphadenopathy and the supraclavicular lymphadenopathy was confirmed by a CT scan, which also showed paratracheal and subcarinal lymphadenopathy. There was no airway compression. Her spleen was mildly enlarged. On pathological examination the lymph node biopsied was that of Hodgkin disease.

The differential diagnosis of lymphadenopathy is:

- Reactive nodes secondary to infection
- Granulomatous conditions
- Malignant infiltration

Reactive nodes secondary to infection

Lymphadenopathy is extremely common in children and mostly represents the response to local or generalized infections as a result of antigenic stimulation. The majority of children experience some form of cervical lymph node enlargement at some time between 2 and 12 years of age. Children have a larger lymphoid mass than adults as well as a brisker response following exposure to new antigens.

The commonest cause of lymphadenopathy is infection within the drainage area of the lymphoid chain involved, which, for throat, ear, nose and scalp, is the cervical lymph nodes. It is important to differentiate lymphadenopathy secondary to infection from that of an infiltrative process.

A history of infection should be sought. This may be generalized in viral infection or localized in bacterial infection. Non-pathological occipital and post-auricular nodes mostly occur in younger children, whereas older children tend to have cervical and submandibular lymphadenopathy. Enlarged nodes in the supraclavicular region are rarely, if ever, reactive, and therefore lymphadenopathy in this area is highly significant.

Erythema, tenderness or fluctuation suggests acute inflammation with possible abscess formation. The size of the lymph node is less helpful in determining its pathology than site and texture. Malignant nodes are often discrete and hard, whereas reactive nodes are soft and rubbery. Identification of the specific organism may be difficult. A blood count and film may show a neutrophilia associated with bacterial infection or the presence of atypical lymphocytes in viral infections, particularly infectious mononucleosis. Viral titres may be helpful, as may local cultures.

Granulomatous conditions

A history of contact with tuberculosis, household cats and the presence or absence of systemic symptoms should be sought. Tuberculosis nodes may be matted.

Malignant infiltration

Enlargement of mediastinal nodes in the presence of cervical lymphadenopathy raises the likelihood of a malignant process, although hilar and mediastinal lymphadenopathy may be due to respiratory tract infection. The commonest malignancies causing lymphadenopathy are Hodgkin disease, NHL and leukaemia, although neuroblastoma, rhabdomyosarcoma and thyroid cancer can also cause cervical lymphadenopathy.

Biopsy is required in the following situations:

- abscess formation
- a significant increase in size, failure to respond and no resolution following treatment with antibiotic therapy
- supraclavicular nodes
- hard or matted nodes and nodes fixed to surrounding structures
- development of new symptoms, e.g. weight loss, pyrexia, night sweats.

HEPATOSPLENOMEGALY

CASE STUDY

A 3-year-old girl presents with a two-week history of lethargy, irritability, anorexia and fever. She has moderate cervical and axillary lymphadenopathy and marked hepatosplenomegaly. Her blood count shows her to be pancytopenic with haemoglobin 6 gm/dL, WCC 2.1×10^9/L, neutrophil count 0.4×10^9/L and platelet count 20×10^9/L. Blasts are not identified on the peripheral smear. She has a transaminitis and a coagulopathy with prolongation of PT and APTT, hypofibrinogenaemia and raised D-dimers. Triglycerides are elevated. A bone marrow aspirate shows marked hypocellularity with prominent haemophagocytosis. She is the youngest of four children who are all healthy.

Haemophagocytic lymphohistiocystosis is the likeliest diagnosis. This may be familial or sporadic and may be associated with infection. The syndrome is characterized by marked fever, pancytopenia, hepatosplenomegaly, profound hypofibrinogenaemia and high triglycerides. The CNS is commonly involved at presentation with irritability and vomiting. If related to infection, CMV, EBV, herpes simplex, varicella zoster and adenovirus may be implicated.

The clinical course is variable. When secondary to infection, the symptoms may resolve spontaneously if supported through the pancytopenia and coagulopathy. Non-infective causes require immunosuppression with chemotherapy, and the prognosis is more guarded. Bone marrow transplantation may be curative.

Causes of hepatosplenomegaly:

- Infection – CMV, EBV, toxoplasmosis, malaria, visceral leishmaniasis
- Histiocytic disorders – Langerhans' cell histiocytosis, haemophagocytic lymphohistiocystosis
- Storage disease
- Leukaemia/lymphoma – ALL, AML, Hodgkin disease, NHL, juvenile myelomonocytic leukaemia, myelodysplasia
- Portal hypertension

MASSES DETECTED CLINICALLY AND RADIOLOGICALLY

- Masses may be benign or malignant.
- Mediastinal masses may present with:
  - airway obstruction – stridor, dyspnoea, desaturation
  - superior vena cava obstruction – swelling and venous congestion of head and neck.
- Abdominal masses may present with inferior vena cava obstruction – oedema of the legs.
- Pelvic masses may present with obstruction of renal tract.
- Paraspinal masses may present with paraplegia.

Benign masses

These may be abscesses, lymphadenopathy secondary to infection, cysts and loaded colon (constipation).

Malignant masses

- Mediastinal
  - Hodgkin disease
  - NHL
  - ALL
  - Neuroblastoma
  - Teratoma
- Abdominal
  - Wilms tumour
  - Neuroblastoma
  - Hepatoblastoma
  - NHL
- Pelvic
  - Rhabdomyosarcoma
  - Teratoma

FURTHER READING

Lilleyman JS, Hann IM, Blanchett VS (eds) (1999) Paediatric haematology, 2nd edn. Edinburgh: Churchill Livingstone.

Pinkerton CR, Plowman N, Pieters R (2004) Paediatric oncology. London: Hodder Arnold.

Chapter 20

Surgical topics

Robert Carachi

NECK LUMPS

Anatomy and pathology of neck swellings

Swellings in the neck are common, with over 200 lymph nodes present. These nodes are the natural safeguard against infection once it has entered into the body through the oral or nasal cavities. Enlarged lymph nodes are the commonest lumps to be found in the neck of a child. Following a sore throat or acute tonsillitis the jugulodigastric lymph nodes in the neck enlarge. Lymphadenitis may be aborted by the body's natural defences or by antibiotics; however, if this does not happen then it may progress to an abscess. The glands usually affected are commonly found in the anterior triangle of the submandibular region and these may become matted together to form a firm tender mass. Discoloration of the skin and fluctuation are not early features, as the glands lie deep to the deep cervical fascia. Abscess formation is usually caused by penicillin-resistant *Staphylococcus aureus*. Surgical drainage is the treatment of choice.

In the differential diagnosis of swellings in the neck, consider the swellings arising from the midline and those arising from a more lateral position.

Midline swellings:
- Lymph node
- Dermoid
- Thyroglossal cyst

Lateral swellings:
- Lymph node
- Branchial cyst
- Cystic hygroma

Midline swellings

CASE STUDY

A 9-year-old boy had a swelling and discharging sinus in the submental region for six months. This started as a lump and was treated by the general practitioner with several courses of antibiotics. Examination of the mouth revealed a lower incisor dental abscess as the cause with regional lymphadenitis. A radiograph confirmed this and after appropriate dental treatment it cleared up.

Submental lymph nodes usually result from a dental root abscess that drains into the submental nodes. Occasionally these discharge pus and a persistent fistula may result with chronic infection.

Dermoid cysts can be found anywhere in the midline of the body and the neck is not an unusual place to find them. These sometimes arise from the suprasternal notch; they are firm to feel and do not usually get infected. These can be confused clinically with thyroglossal cysts.

Thyroglossal cysts are midline swellings (Figure 20.1) arising from the remnants of the thyroid gland and can be found along a tract from the foramen caecum at the base of the tongue to the isthmus of the thyroid. These cysts vary in size and characteristically move up and down with protrusion of the tongue. The cyst lining is often squamous but may contain mucus-secreting cells and respiratory epithelium. They are subject to recurrent infection and may present as a painful swelling, which may be fluctuant suggesting the presence of a thyroglossal abscess. Surgical removal involves excision of the middle portion of the hyoid bone and removal of the complete tract from

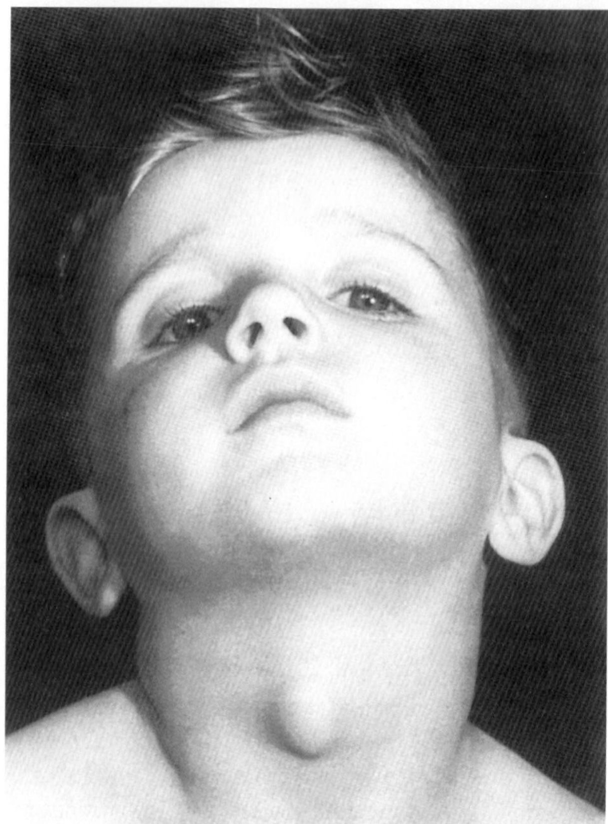

Figure 20.1 A boy with at thyroglossal cyst (from Cockburn F, Carachi R, Goel, NK, Young DG (eds) (1996) *Children's Medicine and Surgery*. London: Arnold)

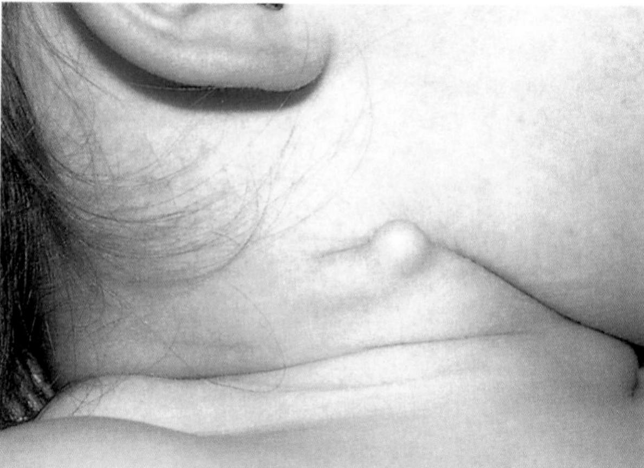

Figure 20.2 A branchial cyst (from Cockburn F, Carachi R, Goel, NK, Young DG (eds) (1996) *Children's Medicine and Surgery*. London: Arnold)

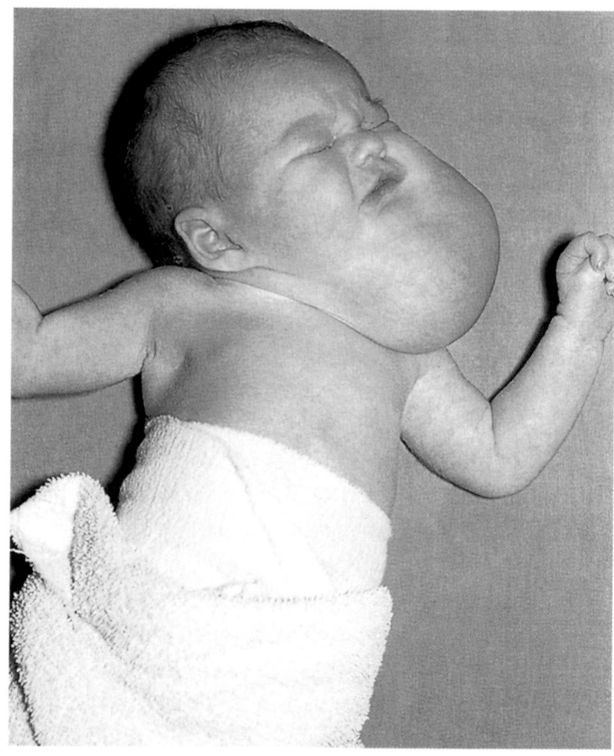

Figure 20.3 A baby with cystic hygroma (from Cockburn F, Carachi R, Goel, NK, Young DG (eds) (1996) *Children's Medicine and Surgery*. London: Arnold)

which the thyroglossal cyst arises. This procedure should be delayed for several weeks if an abscess is present.

Lateral swellings

More recently, the recurrence of tuberculosis in the UK, and atypical mycobacteria especially, should be considered when there are large matted lymph nodes. Other rare causes of lateral swellings in the neck include lymphoma (Hodgkin and non-Hodgkin lymphoma) and metastases from tumours elsewhere.

Branchial cyst remnants (Figure 20.2) are epithelial remnants derived from the branchial arches and may give rise to cysts, sinuses and fistulae. Infection may result in localized cellulitis and abscess formation. Portions of the first and second branchial arches may persist and give rise to several anomalies. Persistence of a first arch occurs when the lower end opens below the border of the mandible and the upper end in the external auditory canal. Careful inspection of the auditory canal is essential – otherwise these will be missed. Persistence of the second arch is commoner and opens in the tonsillar fossa and the skin over the anterior border of the lower one third of the sternomastoid. The tract passes between the internal and external carotid arteries and the glossopharyngeal nerve. These branchial cysts may be seen in infancy or become apparent in childhood. They may present as a painless swelling or indeed may, if a fistula is present, have a continuous discharge of fluid, which is often opalescent.

Cystic hygroma (Figure 20.3) is caused by a disorganized lymphatic system and is predominantly found in the neck. The natural history is of variable growth and regression; the growth occasionally is arrested by infection. These are usually multilocular cysts although unilocular ones do exist and quite commonly they infiltrate the surrounding tissues including the neck muscles and the base of the tongue. The clinical picture is that of a soft fluctuant lobulated mass in the neck which transilluminates. Ultrasound and computed tomography (CT) scans are useful to define the extent of these lesions prior to treatment. Injection of sclerosing substances (e.g. OK432) may be used to destroy cysts. In most cases the treatment is by surgical excision.

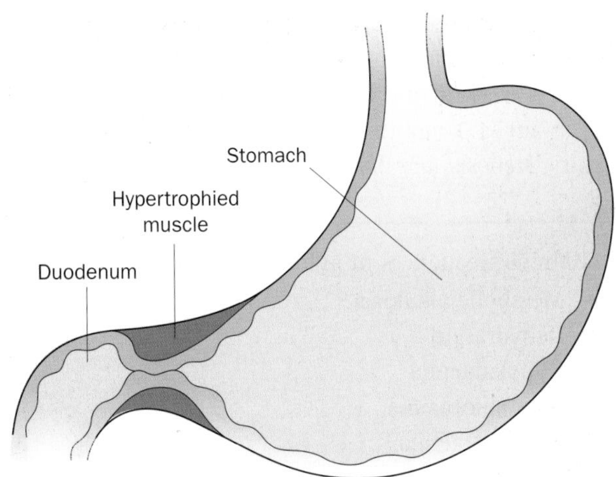

Figure 20.4 Pyloric stenosis in infants (from Cockburn F, Carachi R, Goel, NK, Young DG (eds) (1996) *Children's Medicine and Surgery*. London: Arnold)

KEY LEARNING POINTS

- Always inspect the mouth in the presence of a neck lump.
- Lymph nodes are the commonest cause of neck lumps.

VOMITING

Vomiting in some infants becomes more troublesome than the mouth full of regurgitation, which is commonplace. Vomiting may be due to gastro-oesophageal reflux that occurs more frequently and more easily in infants; they have a transverse oval abdominal cavity compared with adults who have a vertical oval abdominal cavity, which may alter the angulation between the oesophagus and stomach. If the infant is gaining weight satisfactorily, there is no need for major concern. When vomiting is persistent, treatment with thickened feeds and additional therapy with alginate preparations (Gaviscon®) may help.

Children with a hiatus hernia and gastro-oesophageal reflux merit surgery if they fail to thrive or have recurrent respiratory tract problems due to the aspiration of feeds.

Infantile hypertrophic pyloric stenosis

Hypertrophy of the smooth circular muscle of the pylorus results in a mass (tumour) that obstructs passage of feeds from the stomach to the duodenum (Figure 20.4). The pyloric lumen is narrow and deformed by the mucosa being compressed inwards.

CASE STUDY

A 5-week-old baby boy had a five-day history of vomiting which occurred about 30 minutes after every feed. The vomit became projectile and was never bile stained. He was irritable and had dry nappies for the past 12 hours. Examination revealed a dehydrated infant who had lost weight and was just above his birth weight of 3.5 kg. He had a test feed which showed visible left-to-right peristalsis and a mass like an 'olive' could be palpated in the midline. Biochemistry tests showed a metabolic alkalosis. A diagnosis of pyloric stenosis was made.

CLINICAL FEATURES

The symptoms in pyloric stenosis are those of a high obstruction with loss of fluids, electrolytes and calories. Males are more often affected and the sex ratio is 4:1. The cardinal signs are projectile vomiting, visible peristalsis and a palpable pyloric tumour. The infant becomes oliguric and constipated and shows evidence of dehydration with wrinkling of the skin and emaciation if not diagnosed early. Vomiting starts after the first week with regurgitation of feeds followed by vomiting that becomes more forceful and frequent. The vomitus may contain blood from a secondary gastritis. The common age of presentation is 3–9 weeks, but some present after the first week of life and others may not present until the infant is 3 months old. Rarely, 1:100 patients with pyloric stenosis may have bile in the vomit.

Main consequences of pyloric stenosis
- Metabolic alkalosis
- Dehydration
- Hypokalaemia
- Hypochloraemia
- Hyponatraemia
- Gastritis
- Anaemia
- Jaundice
- Prerenal uraemia

The technique of examination is important for eliciting the signs. Seated comfortably on the left of the patient, the clinician inspects the abdomen of the baby while the baby sucks either the breast or a teat. In good light, it is possible to see the distended stomach through the abdominal wall with visible peristalsis passing from left to right across the epigastrium. Palpating a pyloric tumour is difficult. The clinician rests the fingers of the left hand gently on the abdomen and the fingertips feel slowly up under the liver edge from the central to right upper abdomen. Palpation should be carried out while the infant is having a test feed, and, with patience, a rounded tumour about the size of an olive can be felt. If the tumour cannot be palpated and there is doubt about the diagnosis, then an ultrasound by an experienced ultrasonographer can confirm its presence.

Electrolyte imbalance develops where there has been delay in diagnosis. Adequate intravenous replacement of fluids and electrolytes is essential prior to operation. The infant is treated by pyloromyotomy. Postoperatively, feeds are gradually reintroduced over 48 hours and infants usually make a speedy recovery.

Bile-stained vomiting

MALROTATION

Bile-stained vomiting is often due to a surgical cause. In extrinsic duodenal obstruction, bands are associated with incomplete rotation of the mid-gut. These peritoneal bands extend from the caecum and terminal ileum towards the right hypochondrium, under the surface of liver, gall bladder or posterior parietal wall. Obstruction usually occurs a few days after birth when the increased motility of the gut causes these bands to drag across the duodenum. Incomplete rotation commonly referred to as malrotation is present and this is sometimes complicated by volvulus (twisting) of the mid-gut loop. The twisting of the mid-gut (Figure 20.5) frequently causes venous and subsequently arterial obstruction at the root of the mesentery and so the viability of the whole of the mid-gut can become impaired. Prompt diagnosis is essential to prevent ischaemia and infarction of the bowel. The baby frequently feeds normally for the first few days and then develops bile-stained vomiting, but after the volvulus occurs, there may be passage of blood per rectum. For reasons that remain unclear, there is a 4:1 male to female incidence of this disorder.

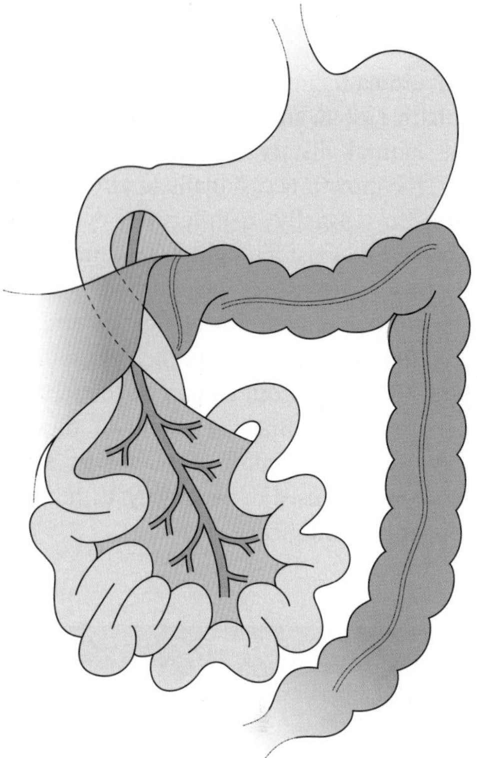

Figure 20.5 Malrotation and volvulus (from Cockburn F, Carachi R, Goel, NK, Young DG (eds) (1996) *Children's Medicine and Surgery*. London: Arnold)

On examination of the infant, often no clear clinical signs can be detected. If peritonism has developed, the viability of the bowel has already become impaired. Straight radiograph of abdomen does not give the clear-cut picture seen in intrinsic duodenal obstruction. There may be a fluid level only in the stomach. The duodenum is never dilated to the degree that is it is with intrinsic obstruction. An important sign, which is sometimes not appreciated, is lack of normal distribution of gas throughout the bowel. Contrast studies of the upper gastrointestinal tract will demonstrate the failure of the duodenum in crossing the midline. Treatment of extrinsic duodenal obstruction requires immediate laparotomy. Ladd's procedure, i.e. dividing the peritoneal bands, broadening the root of the mesentery and returning the bowel to the abdominal cavity, is the operation of choice. Postoperatively there is commonly a delay of 72 hours before gut motility recovers. The long-term outlook is good but 10 per cent of children may, in succeeding years, develop an adhesion obstruction, which may require laparotomy.

KEY LEARNING POINTS

- Bile-stained vomiting is often due to a surgical cause
- Malrotation and volvulus are the most serious causes to consider.

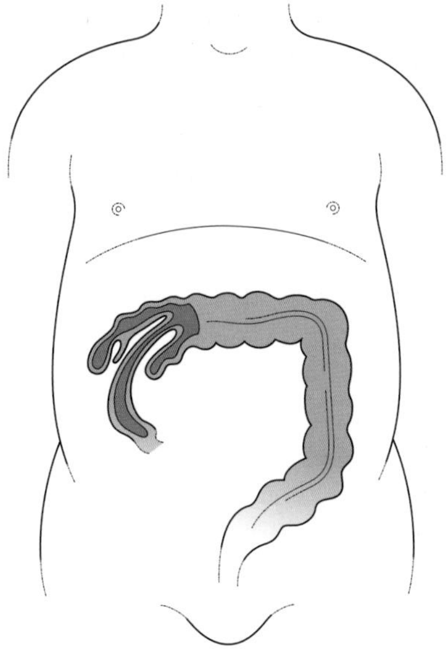

Figure 20.6 Ileocolic intussusception (from Cockburn F, Carachi R, Goel, NK, Young DG (eds) (1996) *Children's Medicine and Surgery*. London: Arnold)

ABDOMINAL PAIN

Intussusception

Intussusception is a telescoping of one portion of the bowel into the adjacent segment (Figure 20.6). Most cases of intussusception (over 60 per cent) occur during the first year of life but the condition is rarely seen under the age of one month. The peak incidence is between the fourth and ninth months, and boys are more frequently affected than girls (3:2). In infants, there is rarely any demonstrable cause and a change from milk to a more solid diet may alter peristalsis in such as way as to initiate an intussusception. Infective causes have been sought but no pathogen has been found to cause intussusception. Enlarged mesenteric glands are almost always found at operation and although the glands may be secondary to the intussusception, they may also be associated with a preceding lymphoid hyperplasia from infection. Only rarely is a definite mechanical factor found to be responsible for initiating the investigation. In older children, Meckel's diverticulum or a polyp may be at the apex and lead point of an intussusception, but definite anomalies such as Meckel's diverticulum are found in only 2 per cent of patients. Other underlying causes include angiomas, lymphoma and intestinal haematoma. In the UK, the peak incidence occurs in the winter months. There is no relation between intussusception and seasonal diarrhoea, but upper respiratory infections commonly precede the onset of intussusception. Ileoileal and colocolic are uncommon in childhood and 90 per cent are ileocolic or ileocaecal. Where the mesentery of the caecum and ascending colon has failed to obliterate, the caecum is mobile and the apex of the intussusception may reach the sigmoid or even the rectum where it may be felt by digital rectal examination. As the ileum advances through the ileocaecal valve, its mesentery soon becomes constricted. Consequently, the venous return is obstructed resulting in oedema and congestion. The obstruction of blood supply may be followed by gangrene of the intussuscipiens. Obstruction of the lumen of the bowel is a consequence of intussusception but symptoms and signs usually result in the infant or child presenting before intestinal obstruction is clearly established.

Clinical features

The patient is usually a healthy vigorous baby boy of 3 months or older who was previously well. Onset is dramatic, as the child, without warning, screams, drawing up his knees as though in abdominal pain and becomes pale. The attack ceases as suddenly as it began and in a few minutes the child seems at peace and may even pass a stool and fall asleep. The mother is reassured by the apparently quick recovery and may postpone seeking medical advice. After a short lapse of time, varying from minutes to several hours, another similar attack of colic occurs. This continues to recur at shorter and shorter intervals. A feature in these children is the pallor during spasms, probably due to a vasovagal reaction. Vomiting is frequent in these episodes. Pain is not always a constant feature. The other common sign is the passage of mucus and blood per rectum (redcurrant jelly stools). If the diagnosis is delayed, signs of intestinal obstruction supervene.

Abdominal examination often reveals a sausage-shaped mass to the right of the umbilicus or in the right hypochondrium. There is no peritonism but tenderness or guarding directly over the mass may make its delineation difficult. Rectal examination demonstrates no faeces in the lumen, but blood and/or mucus is often present on the examining finger. The most important factor causing delay in diagnosis is the association of the idea of intestinal obstruction with intussusception. The triad of colic, vomiting and abdominal distension are late signs.

In the older child, the picture is less dramatic. Severe colic is not an outstanding feature and blood may not be passed per rectum for hours or even days after onset. The child usually experiences periodic attacks of colic and shows little interest in food. Between attacks the abdomen is soft and no mass may be felt.

Diagnosis

The diagnosis can be made on the history alone. Plain radiographs of the abdomen may reveal a soft tissue mass with signs of intestinal obstruction such as dilated loops and fluid levels. Ultrasound examination of the abdomen is often helpful in making the diagnosis. An air enema or a barium enema will confirm the diagnosis and in 60 to 70 per cent of patients reduction of the intussusception may be successful. This procedure is both diagnostic and therapeutic. During this procedure backflow of barium or air into the small bowel is essential to ensure there is complete reduction of the intussusception.

The differential diagnosis includes volvulus, which may present a similar picture, but there is seldom remission of pain. Palpation of the abdomen reveals an ill-defined swelling usually in the central area. Ultrasound (Figure 20.7) and radiographs will differentiate these. Gastroenteritis is perhaps the commonest cause of difficulty in diagnosis. However, the onset in gastroenteritis is less dramatic and the colic rarely severe. The rectum in this case contains loose faeces or foul-smelling watery stools. Temperature is usually elevated and vomiting

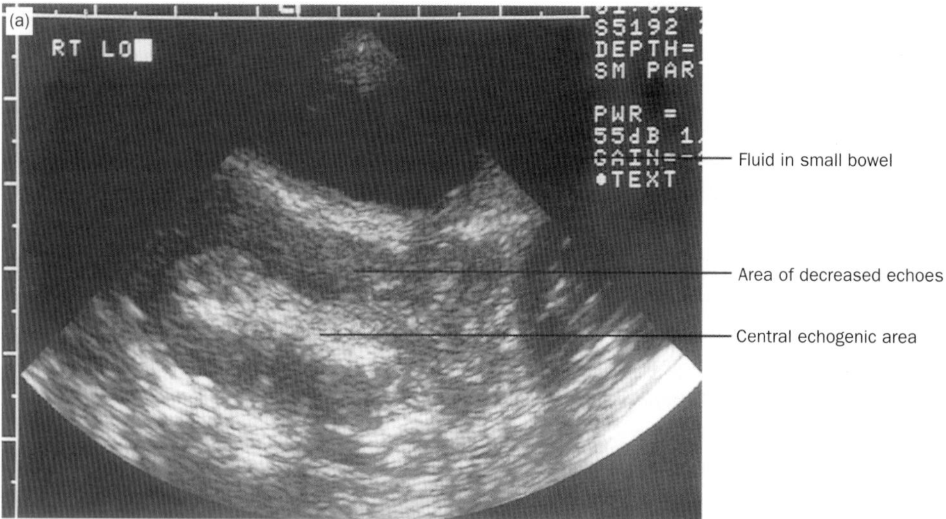

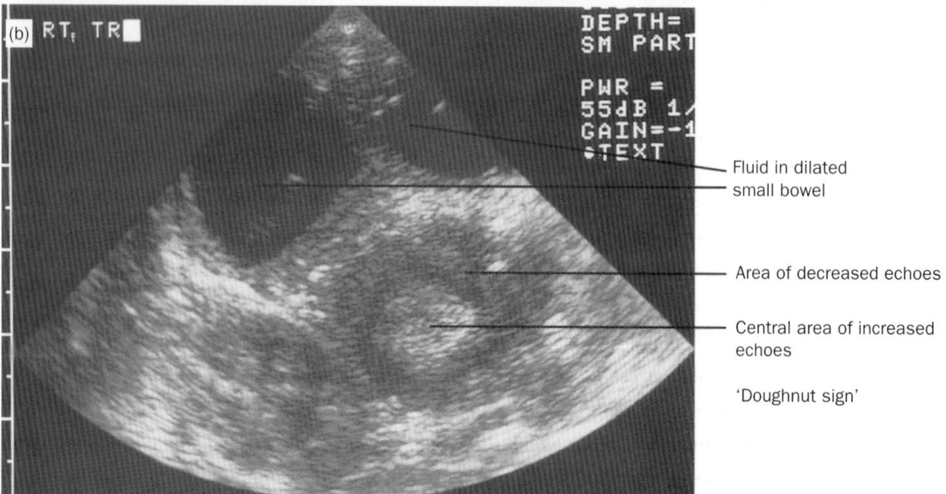

Figure 20.7 Ultrasound scan of intussusception. (a) Longitudinal scan. (b) Transverse scan (from Cockburn F, Carachi R, Goel, NK, Young DG (eds) (1996) *Children's Medicine and Surgery*. London: Arnold)

may be a prominent feature. Palpation of the abdomen of a child with gastroenteritis reveals no tumour but a generalized tenderness may be present. On auscultation, there is increase in bowel sounds. In older children (aged 3 years or more), Henoch–Schönlein purpura may cause difficulty in the differential diagnosis. Blood in the rectum may be accompanied by loose motions and there is evidence of haemorrhagic effusions elsewhere. A child with Henoch-Schönlein purpura may develop haemorrhage in the wall of the bowel and show signs of intussusception and indeed intestinal obstruction.

Management

The management of a child in whom intussusception is suspected should commence with intravenous infusion of dextrose–saline solution and monitoring of peripheral and core temperatures while results of blood investigations are awaited. If there are signs of shock then plasma should be given initially to expand the intravascular volume. The blood haematocrit, urea and electrolytes should be checked and high-dependency nursing care given. Many of the children who are entering into the phase of shock no longer exhibit signs of irritability and restlessness but lie still and uncomplaining between spasms. The clinical condition of these children is vulnerable to rapid deterioration. Peripheral and core temperatures should be measured and a 3°C or a greater gap indicates a requirement for more fluid replacement.

If the child has signs of peritonism, no attempts should be made at reduction and once resuscitation has been fully achieved, which includes administration of intravenous antibiotics (e.g. metronidazole and either a cephalosporin or aminoglycoside), the child should be taken to theatre. Operative reduction can be achieved in most instances. In some cases where there is delay in diagnosis and the viability of the bowel is impaired or where reduction cannot be achieved, resection of the affected bowel and end-to-end anastomosis is performed. Once there is a return of peristalsis, then enteral feeds can be started and intravenous infusion reduced. The child who does not require surgery needs to be in hospital for a couple of days to ensure the intussusception has not recurred.

Recurrent intussusception occurs in 2 per cent of patients. The interval between the intussusceptions varies from 24 hours to several years. Peutz–Jeghers syndrome, which is characterized by the presence of small intestinal polyps associated with pigmentation of the buccal mucosa, may be a cause of recurrent intussusception.

KEY LEARNING POINTS

- Intussusception is an important cause of abdominal pain in an infant.
- The diagnosis must be considered early to avoid morbidity and mortality.

Acute appendicitis

Anatomy and pathology of the appendix

There is marked variation in the anatomy of the appendix. The appendix is attached to the posterior medial quadrant of the caecum. In childhood, the appendix lies in a retrocaecal position in 70 per cent of patients. Obstructive appendicitis is common in childhood, the obstruction being caused by a kink, a faecolith, or the scar of a previous attack of inflammation. When inflammation occurs, there is accumulation of purulent exudate within the lumen and a closed loop obstruction is established. Blood supply to the organ is diminished by distension or by thrombosis of the vessels and gangrene occurs early in children. Free fluid drains into the peritoneal cavity as a result of irritation, and, within a few hours, this fluid is invaded by bacteria from the perforated appendix or from organisms translocating the inflamed but still intact appendix. Peritoneal infection may remain localized by adhesions between loops of intestine, caecal wall and parietal peritoneum. There is danger in administering a purgative in these children because it increases intestinal and appendicular peristalsis, and perforation and dissemination of infection are more likely to occur.

CASE STUDY

A 9-year-old boy had a 48-hour history of central colicky abdominal pain associated with anorexia nausea and vomiting of food stuff. The pain became more constant and settled in his lower abdomen and is associated with fever and persistent vomiting. Examination revealed a fit boy who was distressed, had low-grade pyrexia and localized tenderness and guarding in the right iliac fossa. A full blood count showed white blood cell count (WBC) 18 000/mm^3, raised C-reactive protein (CRP; 30 mg/L) and slightly elevated urea. A plain radiograph of the abdomen revealed a faecolith in the right iliac fossa and some fluid levels. A diagnosis of acute appendicitis was made.

Clinical features

Appendicitis may present as:

- Uncomplicated acute appendicitis
- Appendicitis with local peritonitis
- An appendix abscess or diffuse peritonitis

The onset of symptoms is vague and initially may be of a general nature. Only a third of younger patients are seen in hospital within 24 hours of onset of abdominal symptoms, and in a high percentage of these young patients the appendix has ruptured before admission. The diagnosis is made late in many cases. Reasons for delay in diagnosis include failure to suspect appendicitis in a child under 4 years of age and the poor localization of pain by the younger child. Although often not severe, the pain appears to come intermittently and irritability, vomiting and diarrhoea may result in the mistaken diagnosis of gastroenteritis. Psoas spasm from irritation of the muscle by the inflamed appendix may cause flexion of the hip resulting in a limp, thus distracting attention from the abdomen and directing it to the hip joint. Vomiting occurs in most patients. The child is usually pyrexial but the temperature is only moderately elevated to between 37°C and 38.5°C. Temperatures higher than this usually suggest upper respiratory tract infections or occasionally diffuse peritonitis from appendicitis. A history of constipation is uncommon and many patients have a history of diarrhoea.

The clinical features in the older child are similar to those in the adult. Abdominal pain is usually followed by nausea and vomiting. The pain begins centrally and later shifts to the right iliac fossa. If the appendix is retrocaecal, abdominal pain and tenderness may be slight. If the child has a pelvic appendix then tenderness may again be slight, or absent, or elicited only on rectal examination. Anorexia is a common accompanying sign.

Clinical examination

The child with acute appendicitis is usually anorexic, listless and does not wish to be disturbed. There is often a characteristic foetid odour and the tongue is furred. The child is usually irritable, crying and uncooperative. Low-grade pyrexia is usual but the temperature seldom exceeds 38.5°C. Inspection alone may be significantly informative while attempting to gain the child's confidence. The most important physical sign on abdominal examination is the area of maximum tenderness located in the right iliac fossa and the presence of rebound tenderness. If this is not defined, then a gentle digital rectal examination should be made and tenderness may be elicited or a mass felt in the pelvis in patients with a pelvic appendix.

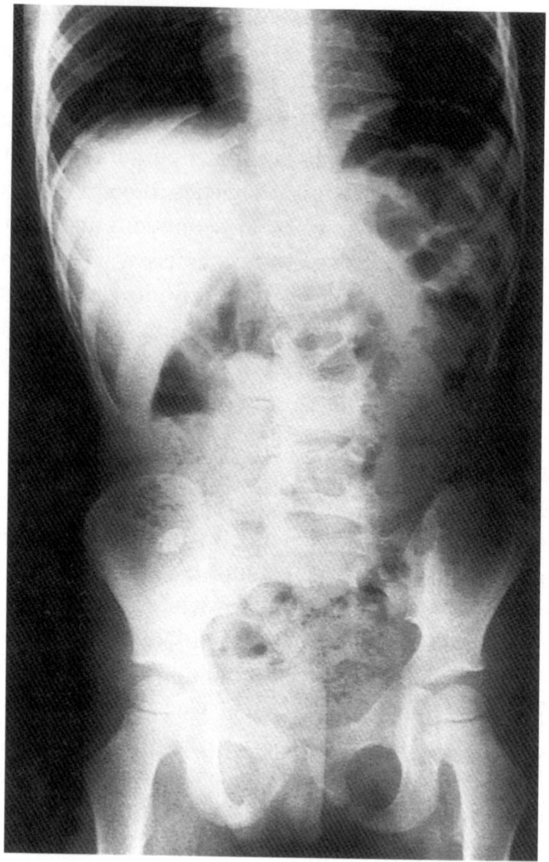

Figure 20.8 Radiograph of abdomen in acute appendicitis. Faecolith, scoliosis with psoas spasm, dilated loop of bowel with fluid level and loss of fat line cell are seen (from Cockburn F, Carachi R, Goel, NK, Young DG (eds) (1996) *Children's Medicine and Surgery*. London: Arnold)

Urine should be checked for presence of bacteria or white cells and also to exclude glycosuria or significant proteinuria. Leucocytosis is usually present in children with acute appendicitis but a normal white cell count does not exclude the diagnosis. The child with diffuse peritonitis may have a low white cell count. Plain radiograph of the abdomen often shows useful signs of acute appendicitis (Figure 20.8).

Differential diagnosis

The differential diagnosis of acute appendicitis includes numerous other disorders, the commonest of which is upper respiratory tract infection. Presence of a common cold, sinusitis, acute tonsillitis, pharyngitis may all be associated with acute non-specific mesenteric lymphadenitis. This is the commonest condition to be differentiated from acute appendicitis. The presence of enlarged glands elsewhere in the body accompanied with an upper respiratory tract infection may suggest this condition. Fever may be absent, but temperatures can be very high. Abdominal tenderness is not as acute as that in appendicitis. It is usually more generalized and not localized to the right iliac fossa, and there is no rebound tenderness. The presence of a cough, increased respiratory rate and runny nose may suggest a respiratory infection. Examination of the chest is mandatory to pick up any signs of consolidation as right lower lobe pneumonia may result in referred pain occurring in the right lower quadrant of the abdomen. Constipation can cause abdominal pain, nausea and vomiting, with tenderness over the distended caecum. It can be easily mistaken for acute appendicitis. Faecal masses may be felt per abdomen or on digital rectal examination. Usually following a suppository, satisfactory evacuation of the colon and rectum will bring rapid relief to patients whose symptoms are caused by constipation.

Pyelonephritis and infection of the kidney and renal pelvis can usually be differentiated by a higher temperature, pus cells in the urine, and tenderness over one or the other kidney in the renal angle.

ABDOMINAL TRAUMA

Abdominal trauma, accidental or non-accidental, may cause injury to the abdominal viscera. A plain radiograph of the abdomen should be done and serum amylase tested to exclude the presence of traumatic or idiopathic pancreatitis and pneumoperitoneum.

GASTROENTERITIS

In gastroenteritis and dysentery there may be severe cramping and abdominal pain. The pain and tenderness may be more marked over the distended caecum. Other members of the family may have similar symptoms or diarrhoea. Rectal examination can help differentiate between a pelvic appendicitis and appendicitis with pelvic peritonitis from gastroenteritis.

INFECTIVE HEPATITIS

Infective hepatitis may occur in epidemic form but in an isolated case may simulate appendicitis. The temperature is usually elevated and the child complains of a headache with nausea, vomiting, abdominal pain and tenderness. On examination, the liver is enlarged and tender. The child may or may not be jaundiced depending on whether he is seen in the prodromal phase of the disease. Examination of the urine usually reveals the presence of bile salts, but urobilinogen may be present.

INTESTINAL OBSTRUCTION

Intestinal obstruction may be due to incarceration of a hernia, secondary to anomalies, e.g. a volvulus around a vitello-intestinal remnant, or adhesions following previous abdominal operations. Vomiting, abdominal colic, abdominal distension and constipation are the usual signs. After a thorough clinical examination, plain radiographs of the abdomen in the erect and supine positions should be taken to differentiate intestinal obstruction from appendicitis.

PRIMARY PERITONITIS

Primary peritonitis is an uncommon diagnosis and almost always affects females. There is a diffuse infection of the visceral and parietal peritoneum usually due to a pneumococcus. With the peritonitis there is exudation of fluid to the peritoneal cavity. Mesenteric lymph nodes are swollen. Diffuse abdominal pain, vomiting, dehydration and high fever are the main features and diarrhoea may be present initially but is usually followed by constipation. Rectal examination usually is suggestive of a pelvic appendicitis as there is diffuse tenderness and heat present. The white blood cell count is usually grossly elevated between 20 000 and 50 000/mm^3. The diagnosis is usually made at laparotomy when peritonitis is found but the appendix is normal.

RENAL CAUSES

Severe abdominal pain and vomiting may occur during passage of a renal calculus. Hydronephrosis due to blockage of the pelviureteric junction by stricture, stone or aberrant vessel may present with abdominal pain and nausea. The pain and tenderness are maximal in the flank. Red or white cells may be found in the urine. Haemolytic uraemic syndrome may present with acute abdominal pain and may be confused with acute appendicitis. The presence of fragmented red blood cells on a blood film and also the presence of oliguria are suggestive of this disease.

CROHN DISEASE

Crohn disease is an unusual diagnosis in childhood, but the incidence is increasing in Western countries. It can present with all the symptoms of acute appendicitis and at operation the terminal ileum is found to be acutely inflamed and thickened. A biopsy confirms the diagnosis and barium meal and follow-through very often indicates the presence of other affected areas of the gut.

TORSION

Torsion of the right cord or testis may be confused with acute appendicitis, but this is less likely with torsion of the left testis. Routine examination should always include the inguinal regions and the scrotum.

INFLAMMATION OF THE MECKEL DIVERTICULUM

Inflammation of the Meckel diverticulum and intussusception in older children may simulate acute appendicitis. Other medical conditions that should be considered are those of diabetes mellitus, cyclical vomiting and Addison disease. The onset of menstruation may simulate appendicitis and many girls have recurring attacks of lower abdominal pain, sometimes for a year before menstruation actually begins. Pain associated with torsion of an ovary or an ovarian cyst may also present with signs similar to those of acute appendicitis.

THREADWORMS

It is not uncommon for both adults and children to harbour threadworms (pinworms) without noticeable symptoms. Many symptoms and signs have been ascribed to the presence of threadworms including weight loss, poor appetite, nausea, vomiting and chronic abdominal pain.

CARCINOID TUMOUR

Carcinoid tumour in the appendix is rare in childhood but the tumour may obstruct the lumen of the appendix and lead to obstructive appendicitis. It is far more common to find this as an incidental finding on histopathological examination of the removed appendix. In cases where it is present in the tip of the appendix, no further follow-up is necessary. In older children, if a carcinoid exists in the caecal region there is a chance of invasive disease with subsequent evidence of the carcinoid syndrome. Treatment should include a right hemicolectomy and careful follow-up with an MIBG scan and measurement of 5-hydroxyindoleacetic acid (5-HIAA).

Treatment

The treatment of the child with acute appendicitis is early operation. In the toxic child with peritonitis, time may be profitably spent in combating toxaemia and dehydration. It is important to resuscitate the patient and start intravenous antibiotics before surgery is undertaken. In such cases, metronidazole (Flagyl®), ceftazidime or cefotaxime should be given intravenously. The administration of intravenous antibiotics given as three doses pre-, per- and postoperatively with peritoneal lavage in children with peritonitis has considerably reduced the incidence of postoperative complications. Early appendectomy is indicated in the child with an appendix abscess. This hastens the recovery period and allows much earlier discharge from hospital.

The best access to the appendix with minimal disturbance to the peritoneal cavity is through a grid-iron or lance incision following which appendectomy is performed. There is an increasing trend to carry out appendectomy by minimal invasive surgical techniques rather than 'open' operation.

KEY LEARNING POINTS

- Acute appendicitis is the commonest pathology in children with an acute abdomen.
- Delay in diagnosis causes high morbidity.
- Localized tenderness in the right iliac fossa is the most important diagnostic sign.
- Ultrasound in expert hands is useful.

THE GROIN AND GENITALIA

Embryology and anatomy

Stage one

The testes arise high in the posterior abdominal wall at the level of the renal bud. They migrate down into the deep inguinal ring controlled by a hormone, the mullerian inhibitory factor (MIF). The gubernaculum then guides the testes to their eventual location in the superficial inguinal ring at seven months of gestational age.

Stage two

This stage is dependent on fetal testosterone released from the fetal testes and on an intact genitofemoral nerve, which mediates substances (MIF) which cause contraction of the gubernaculum to guide the testes into the scrotum. In 95 per cent of term babies this occurs in the ninth month period of gestation.

Groin swelling

Inguinal hernia is one of the commonest surgical problems in childhood; it is invariably of the indirect type. Boys are affected 10 times more commonly than girls and the incidence in both sexes under 12 years of age is 10 per 1000 live births. The right testis descends at a later date than the left, and, accordingly, the processus vaginalis is closed off later on the right side. This probably accounts for the greater frequency of right-sided inguinal hernia (right-sided 60 per cent versus left-sided 20 per cent). The indirect inguinal hernia passes down the tract of the processus vaginalis to the inguinal canal to appear near the skin surface at the external inguinal ring. The hernia usually contains the pampiniform plexus of veins, the vas deferens and its artery and the cremasteric coverings. Thirty per cent of premature babies develop an inguinal hernia.

Clinical features

A hernia may be discovered at or shortly after birth and a very large scrotal hernia may appear during the first week of life. Most commonly hernias are first noticed during the second or third month and recognition occurs following a period of coughing or crying. The contents of a hernia (small intestine) reduce spontaneously when the infant ceases to cry or strain, also it can be reduced by simple taxis. At times there may be a good history of recurrent swelling but no inguinal swelling can be found during the examination. The clinical findings may be only those of a thickened spermatic cord on the site of the hernia. A hernia may be incarcerated (trapped), causing intestinal obstruction; rarely this may proceed to gangrene of the bowel. When this happens there is evidence of cellulitis of the scrotum and the groin region and any attempts to try to reduce the hernia should be strongly resisted. The infant needs emergency surgery. The testis likewise on that side may suffer ischaemia as a result of the obstruction; this is a common complication in the first six months of life and rarer in older children.

In a girl, an inguinal hernia is a rare event and presents as a lump in the groin. The infant is usually well with no complaint, this hernia may contain a prolapsed ovary and pain may be caused by attempts to reduce it into the peritoneal cavity. During surgical exploration it is important to ensure that the hernia does contain an ovary and not a testis because in a number of cases these children have an underlying testicular feminization syndrome. If there is uncertainty, a biopsy to confirm the nature of the gonad should be carried out because testicular tissue has to be removed since there is a high incidence of malignancy in later life.

Trauma

Trauma to the testis presents with a haematoma of the scrotum that makes it impossible to examine. Ultrasound can demonstrate a viable or an ischaemic testis, in which case surgical intervention is indicated. A painful scrotum can also occur during other systemic illnesses such as Henoch-Schönlein purpura and also hypoproteinaemic oedema secondary to acute nephritis.

Tumour

Occasionally a testicular tumour may be mistaken for a hernia although this is usually painless and presents as an enlarged testicle in a child. The commonest tumours are orchioblastoma and other germ cell tumours.

Hydrocele

A patent processus vaginalis (PPV) allows fluid to enter into the scrotum from the peritoneal cavity. Hydrocele (Figure 20.9) of the tunica vaginalis usually presents as a blue hue, which appears in the inguinal scrotal region. It is often possible to get above a hydrocele whereas it is impossible to reduce it because the neck of the hydrocele is very narrow and tortuous. Most hydroceles disappear spontaneously by the age of 3 years (80 per cent). The remainder require ligation and division of the PPV together with drainage of the hydrocele. Transillumination of a hydrocele, although helpful, is not diagnostic since children's tissues contain a high percentage of fluid and transilluminate easily. A testicular tumour in a child has been mistakenly diagnosed as a hydrocele because it transilluminated.

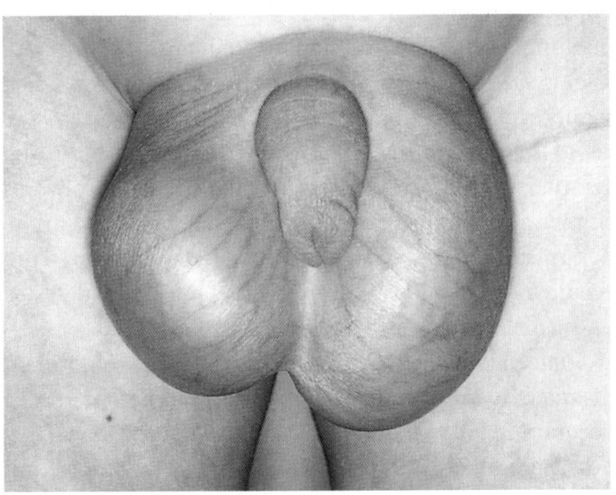

Figure 20.9 Bilateral hydroceles in a child (from Cockburn F, Carachi R, Goel, NK, Young DG (eds) (1996) *Children's Medicine and Surgery*. London: Arnold)

Genitalia

The 'absent' testis – cryptorchidism

The testes normally descend into the scrotum by seven months' gestation. They lie at the deep inguinal ring and by the ninth month they descend into the scrotum. At birth 95 per cent of term babies should have palpable testes in the scrotum. In premature babies this figure is 75 per cent. Failure of descent of the testes along the line of descent is termed undescended testes or cryptorchidism. Testes develop best when in the scrotum, the lower body temperature allows for proper development of the testes. There is an increased risk of sterility and possibly malignancy in boys who have intra-abdominal testes. There is, however, a lack of evidence to suggest conclusively that an undescended testis inevitably proceeds to develop either complete sterility and/or malignancy.

The retractile testis is a normal physiological variation. Testes are retractile in small children due to the strong 'cremasteric reflex'. Under warm conditions testes can be coaxed to come down into the scrotum and remain there. The cause of defective descent of the testis is unknown although there is an increased incidence of malformation of the testes and epididymis in this group. The scrotum is often atrophic. Cryptorchidism is commonly right sided and is bilateral in fewer than 25 per cent. There is evidence that the testes should be in the scrotum by the second or third year of life to prevent further atrophy that would occur if they remained in the peritoneal cavity. Ultrasound and laparoscopy are required for diagnosis of bilateral undescended testes and impalpable testes.

Some patients with cryptorchidism have chromosomal disorders, which need to be investigated. Ectopic testes account for 10 per cent of undescended testes. They descend normally in the inguinal canal and then are pulled into unusual locations, e.g. the perineum. Orchidopexy is easy to perform because the testicular vessels are on a long leash.

Torsion of the testis or its appendages

Torsion (Figure 20.10) involves twisting of the spermatic cord and the vessels resulting in venous congestion and infarction of the testis. The testis is painful and swollen and the cremasteric reflex retracts the enlarged tender swollen testis out of the scrotum into the groin. Pain may be referred to the abdomen and torsion may be missed if the genitalia are not examined. Doppler ultrasound examination is useful and urgent surgical intervention is indicated. Neonatal torsion of the testis is rarely salvageable but should be operated on to remove the dead testis and orchidopexy should be carried out on the contralateral testis to prevent a similar occurrence on the other side.

Epididymo-orchitis

Infection of the testis or epididymis is uncommon before puberty and orchitis associated with mumps is rare before the age of 12 years. Orchitis may appear during the course of systemic bacterial infection. Swelling and oedema after torsion or trauma may closely simulate orchitis but with such trauma the onset is sudden. Epididymo-orchitis is more likely to occur in boys with abnormal communication between the vas and ureter. Doppler ultrasound of the epididymis shows increased flow in epididymo-orchitis, whereas in torsion of the testis there is no flow.

Idiopathic scrotal oedema

Idiopathic scrotal oedema is a condition not uncommon and usually unilateral. The aetiology is obscure but may be caused by an allergic phenomenon. The scrotum on the affected side is red, swollen, indurated and the redness extends into the groin and into the perineal region. The testis can usually be palpated and is not tender. This condition usually subsides spontaneously within two to three days (Figure 20.11).

Varicocele

Varicocele is usually described as a scrotum feeling like a bag of worms, this is due to abnormal communications within the pampiniform plexus of veins of the testis. This diagnosis can only be made when the child is standing up because on lying down these veins empty and cannot be palpated. It is unusual for this condition to be mistaken for torsion of the testis. Very rarely, this may be a physical sign of an obstructive lesion in the left kidney because of the testicular veins draining into the left renal vein.

Painful foreskin

ANATOMY AND PATHOLOGY

During the years when an infant is incontinent and in nappies, the glans is protected by the prepuce. Despite

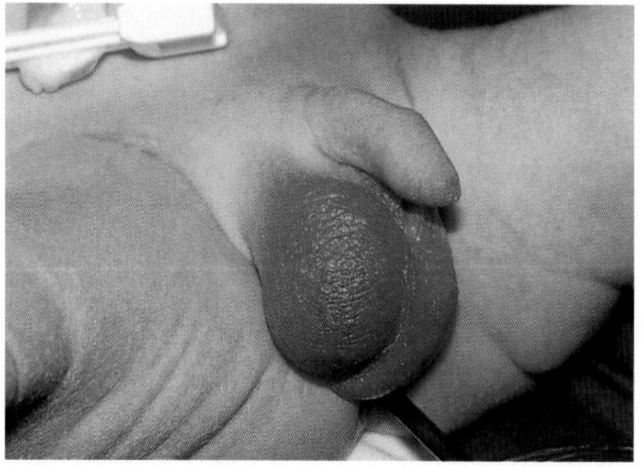

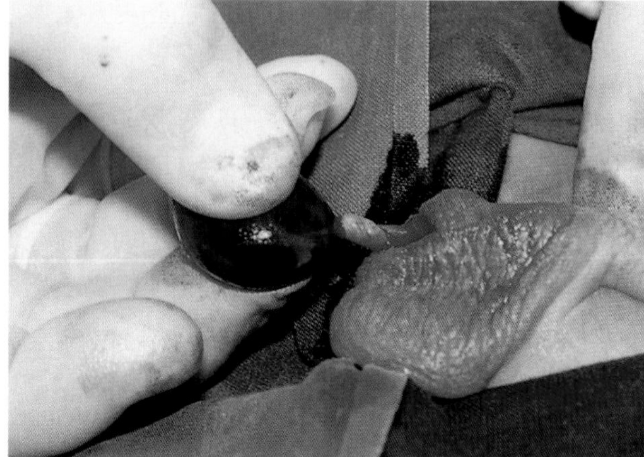

Figure 20.10 Torsion with necrotic testis in a neonate (from Cockburn F, Carachi R, Goel, NK, Young DG (eds) (1996) *Children's Medicine and Surgery*. London: Arnold)

this protection, it is easily traumatized. At birth, fewer than 5 per cent of foreskins are retractable and it is only gradually over the next decade that the foreskin becomes freely retractable. In a little more than 50 per cent the external meatus of the urethra or the glans can be displayed but the infant has adequate space to pass urine. This situation can be regarded with equanimity in the pre-school child unless the smegma which forms and collects around the coronal sulcus becomes infected, causing balanitis with sometimes retention of urine. Treatment with baths, analgesics and antibiotics usually quickly settles the child. When a second attack of balanitis occurs it is more likely that recurrent infection may ensue and, after treatment of the infection, the foreskin is retracted and the retained smegma is cleared out under anaesthesia. Circumcision may also be performed to prevent recurrence of this condition.

BALANOPOSTHITIS

Balanoposthitis is inflammation of the glans under the surface of the prepuce and may be due to retained smegma, poor hygiene or may be associated with an ammoniacal dermatitis. There is redness, pain and swelling and creamy purulent discharge from beneath the prepuce. The condition usually subsides with baths and antibacterial treatment, for example, co-amoxiclav (Augmentin®). Circumcision may be performed as already mentioned after the inflammation has subsided. Foreskin adhesions to the glans are not uncommon and prevent full retraction of the foreskin. Normally most are gone by school age but persistence causes retention of smegma in the coronal sulcus and can cause irritation.

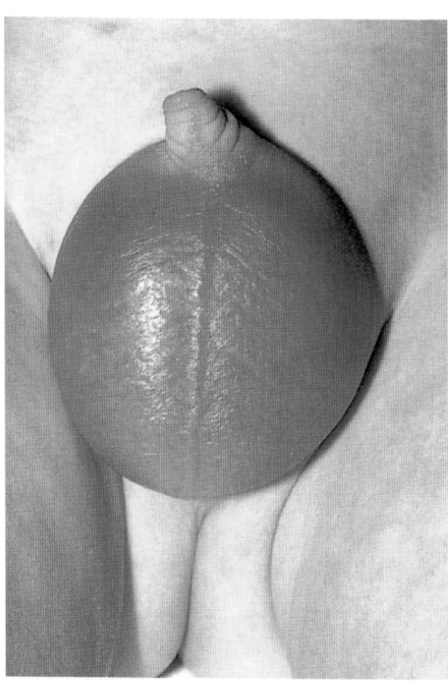

Figure 20.11 Idiopathic scrotal oedema (from Cockburn F, Carachi R, Goel, NK, Young DG (eds) (1996) *Children's Medicine and Surgery*. London: Arnold)

PHIMOSIS

In phimosis (Figure 20.12), there is a tight prepuce that does not allow retraction of the foreskin and in severe cases may obstruct urinary flow. Forceful retraction of foreskin in early life may cause fissuring of the meatus

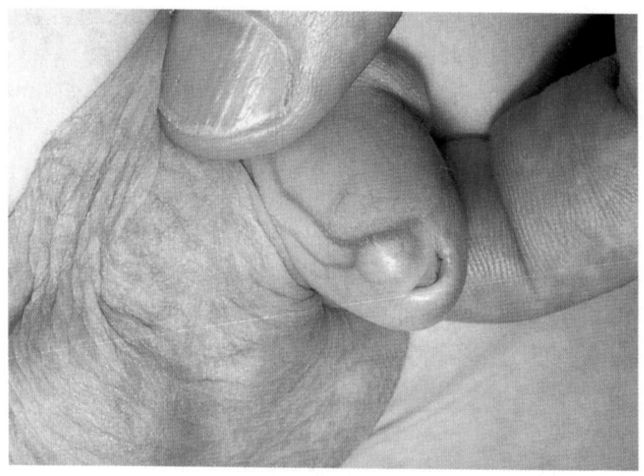

Figure 20.12 Phimosis. The tight prepuce does not allow retraction of the foreskin (from Cockburn F, Carachi R, Goel, NK, Young DG (eds) (1996) *Children's Medicine and Surgery*. London: Arnold)

Table 20.1 Key surgical issues in children

Key symptoms	Key diagnosis	Other related conditions
Neck lump	Cervical lymphadenitis	Dermoid cyst Thyroglossal cyst Branchial cyst Cystic hygroma
Vomiting	Infantile hypertrophic pyloric stenosis	Gastro-oesophageal reflux
Abdominal pain	Acute appendicitis	Mesenteric adenitis Intussusception Volvulus
Groin swelling	Inguinal hernia	Hydrocele
Painful scrotum	Torsion of the testis and appendages	Epididymo-orchitis Idiopathic scrotal oedema Varicocele Trauma, tumour
Absent testis	Cryptorchidism	Inguinal node
Painful foreskin	Balanoposthitis	Phimosis Labial adhesions

of the foreskin with scarring and progression to phimosis. True phimosis is rare in early childhood and usually occurs in the 5–10-years age group. Phimosis is associated with balanitis xerotica obliterans. If a tight prepuce is retracted this may cause constriction, i.e. paraphimosis, resulting in oedema of the glans and the mucous membrane. A general anaesthetic may have to be administered and a small dorsal slit made. The definitive treatment is circumcision.

LABIAL ADHESIONS

At birth the labia rarely may appear to be fused and the infant may not pass urine. In early infancy this is a relatively common and probably acquired condition and the infant's genitalia are otherwise normal. Adhesions are rarely dense and separation can usually be accomplished with finger pressure on a swab held laterally on the labia. Oozing of blood is negligible in this condition. Application of Vaseline® with each change of nappy for 72 hours will usually prevent any readhesion. Separation of the labia can be achieved later on in childhood by using Emla® cream as a local anaesthetic or a general anaesthetic may be needed before separation of the labia.

Table 20.1 gives an overview of the key surgical conditions in paediatrics.

KEY LEARNING POINTS

- Torsion of the testes is the most serious condition to consider in the 'acute scrotum'.
- Undescended testes need orchidopexy before the age of 2 years.
- True phimosis is rare. Avoid retraction of the foreskin early in life.

FURTHER READING

Atwell JD (1998) *Paediatric Surgery*. London: Arnold.

Puri P (2003) *Newborn Surgery*. London: Arnold.

Chapter 21

Tropical paediatric medicine

Brian Coulter

CHILD HEALTH IN LOW-RESOURCE COUNTRIES

Mortality

In developing countries infant mortality (deaths under 1 year per 1000 live births) has fallen from 124 to 59 between 1960 and 1998 (UNICEF, 2000). Neonatal mortality (deaths in first week) accounts for 40–70 per cent of all deaths under 1 year. Mortality among the under-5s (deaths under 5 years per 1000 live births) fell from 193 to 86 between 1960 and 1998 but still remains over 100 in 40 countries (Dabis *et al.*, 2002). However, many of the gains in mortality have been offset by increased mortality from acquired immune deficiency syndrome (AIDS) especially in sub-Saharan Africa. Causes of mortality in children are outlined in Table 21.1.

Methods to reduce neonatal deaths centre on improving women's health and nutrition, birth spacing, access to a trained/skilled birth attendant and, for complicated pregnancies, a well-organized and equipped health centre or hospital. Antenatal care should include treatment of sexually transmitted diseases (STDs) and other infections, tetanus immunization, iron supplements, antimalarials (if appropriate) and human immunodeficiency virus (HIV) testing (if counselling and laboratory facilities are available). At birth, the trained attendant should have the skills for basic resuscitation, clean cord care and routine neonatal care. They should be taught to recognize conditions such as asphyxia, respiratory distress, infections and jaundice, and they should know how to manage low birth weight babies. Early and exclusive breastfeeding should be emphasized.

Methods to reduce infant and childhood deaths include health education of parents to recognize early signs of illnesses, e.g. dehydration, respiratory distress and level of consciousness, and seek aid promptly. Improvement in primary healthcare (including availability of drugs), referral systems and transport are essential components.

Table 21.1 Major causes of infant and child mortality in developing countries*

Neonates	1–59 months	5–12 years
Birth asphyxia/trauma	Pneumonia	Septicaemia
Low birth weight	Septicaemia	Malignancies
Septicaemia	HIV infection	HIV infection
Neonatal tetanus	Meningitis/ encephalitis	
Congenital syphilis	Malaria†	
Congenital abnormalities	Anaemia†	
	Dehydration	
	Malnutrition	
	Measles	

*Prevalence of HIV infection, malaria, anaemia and malnutrition will vary geographically, and measles with immunization levels. Other causes include trauma, snake bite, intestinal obstruction due to *Ascaris lumbricoides*, rheumatic heart disease and renal disorders.

†In tropical countries malaria and anaemia are major causes of mortality.

HIV, human immunodeficiency virus.

The Integrated Management of Child Illness (IMCI) promoted by the World Health Organization (WHO) and UNICEF is a strategy for identification and management of childhood illness from 1 week to 5 years at primary care level. It is being incorporated into healthcare systems for many countries. Its ability to improve child health has yet to be evaluated.

Public health problems

Major underlying causes of morbidity and mortality in children are poverty, illiteracy, lack of clean water and sanitation, poor hygiene and overcrowding with exposure to frequent viral, bacterial or parasite infections (especially malaria).

Immunization

The standard immunization schedule in the Expanded Programme for Immunization (EPI) is outlined in the box below. In addition, in some countries immunization is given for hepatitis B virus (HBV), yellow fever (sub-Saharan Africa) and meningococcal A and C (meningitis belt of Africa); HBV is given at birth, 6 and 14 weeks and yellow fever at 9 months. Some countries give or are considering conjugated *Haemophilus influenzae* type B (HIB) vaccine; HIB and MMR are usually available at private clinics.

Standard immunization schedule

Birth – BCG, OPV0
6 weeks – DPT1, OPV1
10 weeks – DPT2, OPV2
14 weeks – DPT3, OPV3
9 months – Measles

For babies born to HIV-infected mothers, the EPI immunization schedule is administered as usual, including bacille Calmette Guérin (BCG) vaccine at birth. Two doses of measles vaccine are given at 6 and 9 months. If BCG is missed at birth and the child is suspected of having symptomatic HIV infection, BCG is not given. Yellow fever vaccine is also contraindicated for symptomatic HIV-infected children.

A major problem with immunization is poor infrastructure for administration, breaks in the 'cold change' and lack of knowledge about its benefits especially among the poor, illiterate section of the population. Administration is also difficult with nomadic groups.

Diagnostic facilities

Diagnostic facilities in government hospitals are often limited, and where undertaken by poorly paid and unsupervised technicians may be inaccurate. Basic investigations usually include stool microscopy, urinalysis (microscopy, blood, protein and glucose), CSF (Gram stain, protein and glucose), haemoglobin and total white blood cell (WBC) count, and smear for malaria and other parasites. Chest radiographs are often available on payment only and frequently are of poor quality. Bacterial cultures are seldom available. Basic chemical pathology may be available, but results are often delayed. Thus, one of the main constraints in training doctors in some developing countries is the inability to investigate patients properly and develop their diagnostic skills.

Management issues

Poor, underresourced and under-staffed health centres and hospitals may be under-used and conversely the better health facilities may be grossly overcrowded. Major constraints are 'user fees' where parents have to pay for attendance/admission, investigations and treatment. This frequently excludes the poorest members of society whose only option is to resort to traditional medicine. Across-the-counter availability of drugs is usual which is responsible for high levels of antibiotic resistance. Many drugs produced by disreputable firms are ineffective, and are commonly found in markets and pharmacies in developing countries.

Tuberculosis and HIV infection

Tuberculosis and HIV infection in children are commonly interlinked. Frequently, babies are born into families where the mother is HIV-infected and there is also open tuberculosis among the family members. In addition, the clinical features of tuberculosis may be very difficult to distinguish from HIV infection, especially in children with lymphocytic interstitial pneumonitis (LIP) or other HIV-related pulmonary disorders.

Tuberculosis

Contact tracing is rarely practised in developing countries thus, children with symptomatic tuberculosis are just the 'tip of the iceberg' of tuberculous infection in the community.

Mycobacterial culture is seldom available and a smear of gastric aspirates has low sensitivity (2 per cent), thus confirmation of tuberculosis is rarely achieved. In addition, the tuberculin test is frequently non-reactive in children with malnutrition, advanced disease and HIV infection. In hospitals where culture facilities are available, induced sputum or nasopharyngeal aspiration may be more convenient than gastric aspiration. Culture positivity for *Mycobacterium tuberculosis* is seldom more than 30–40 per cent by any of these methods. As the vast majority of children (>80 per cent) who have had neonatal BCG are tuberculin-negative by 2 years or so, the tuberculin test may be undertaken and read as normal (positive reaction >10 mm). Frequently, the diagnosis of tuberculosis, especially pulmonary, is made by a response to tuberculous chemotherapy in children who have failed to respond to a course of standard antibiotics, referred to as 'therapeutic trial'. Once detected and treated, mortality in childhood tuberculosis is low unless there is HIV infection.

HIV infection in sub-Saharan Africa

Approximately 95 per cent of childhood HIV infections are in developing countries, the majority of which are in sub-Saharan Africa. In east, central and southern Africa, 20–30 per cent of women attending government antenatal clinics in cities are infected with HIV. Currently rates as high as 45 per cent are reported from southern Africa, e.g. Zimbabwe, Botswana, Lesotho and Swaziland. Conversely, over the past 10 years or so, rates have fallen from 28 to 10–12 per cent in Kampala, Uganda, associated with, among other things, improved health education.

Mother-to-child vertical transmission (MTCT) rates are calculated approximately as follows: 5 per cent in the last two months of pregnancy; 10 per cent during delivery; 5 per cent in the first two months, postnatally and up to 5 per cent during the period of continued breastfeeding (De Cock *et al.*, 2000). Thus, MTCT rates in breastfeeding societies are approximately 25–30 per cent with breastfeeding accounting for one-third to one-half of MTCT.

The majority of HIV-infected women are unaware of their HIV status, and many of the few who know conceal this information from their partners and families for fear of divorce and family disruption. Due to high death rates of parents from AIDS, approximately 10–15 per cent of children in areas of high HIV endemicity are orphans. Fortunately, most are able to be absorbed into the extended family.

In developing countries, there is often rapid progression to AIDS in HIV-infected children. As co-trimoxazole prophylaxis is rarely given, *Pneumocystis carinii* pneumonia is an important cause of death in the first six months of life. Common illnesses include diarrhoea, pneumonia, severe skin disorders, chronic discharging ears, malnutrition, tuberculosis and, in east/central Africa, Kaposi sarcoma. Mortality for cohorts of HIV-infected Ugandan children was 34 per cent at 12 months, 50 per cent at 21 months, and 75 per cent at 5 years (Marum *et al.*, 1997).

Features that differentiate HIV infection from malnutrition

Marasmus (commoner than kwashiorkor)
- Failure to respond to nutritional rehabilitation

Lymphadenopathy
- Early infancy
- Generalized
- Large nodes

Dermatitis
- Papules, nodules
- Ulcers
- Widespread and severe

Candidiasis
- extensive and severe

Parotid enlargement

Discharging ears

Finger clubbing

Prevention of MTCT

Neither routine antenatal HIV testing nor antiretrovirals (ARVs) are generally available for most women in Sub-Saharan Africa. Thus, perinatal HIV transmission is not controlled and mothers do not benefit from counselling regarding breastfeeding. Short-course ARV therapy at low cost may result in substantial reductions in perinatal MTCT as long as the mother does not breastfeed. Nevirapine given as a single dose during labour and a single dose to the neonate within 72 hours may reduce MTCT by 47 per cent at a cost of US$4. In the PETRA trial, zidovudine + lamivudine given from 36 weeks' gestation and postnatally for seven days to mother and baby resulted in an MTCT rate of 5.7 per cent at six weeks compared with 15.3 per cent for placebo (Dabis and Ekpini, 2002). However, in breastfeeding mothers MTCT rates at 18 months were 15 per cent and 22 per cent, respectively.

Certain centres in sub-Saharan Africa supported by international funds are now offering universal HIV screening of women, nevirapine during the perinatal period, counselling regarding infant feeding and sometimes polymerase chain reaction (PCR) testing of the infant at 6 weeks. Mothers who opt to give artificial feeds (by cup and spoon) are offered free milk for six months. Those who decide to breastfeed are advised to give breast milk exclusively for three to six months. Also, trials of ARVs in mothers and infants during the breastfeeding period are in progress. However, many mothers despite being offered free artificial milk opt to breastfeed because of the stigma associated with artificial feeding.

Where the above facilities are unavailable, WHO/UNICEF's advice for mothers who do not know their HIV status and where there is no safe alternative, is to exclusively breastfeed for four to six months then wean on to an artificial milk formula, e.g. fresh cows' milk (diluted by one third with added sugar) given by cup and spoon.

DISEASES CAUSED BY PARASITES

Definitions

Parasites require an animal (or plant) host ± a vector for survival and completion of their life cycle. Some parasites are confined to tropical countries because their vector thrives in a warm environment, e.g. mosquitoes; warm water, snails for schistosomiasis, or require warm, moist soil for survival, e.g. hookworm.

Helminths are parasitic worms and include nematodes (roundworms) and platyhelminths (flatworms) which are divided into trematodes (flukes) and cestodes (tapeworms). Soil-transmitted helminths are also referred to as geohelminths. Protozoa are unicellular organisms, e.g. malarial parasite, leishmaniae, trypanosomes and amoebae.

Transmission

Diseases caused by soil-transmitted helminths are particularly related to poor hygiene. Two common causes are:

- indiscriminate defaecation (or using human faeces for manure) on open soil, beside rivers or pools, etc.
- contamination of food and water by faeces, infected fingers or flies.

Infection by geohelminths begins when young children crawl on contaminated soil and put things in their mouths. Other methods of transmission include close contact with animals and their faeces, particularly dogs, e.g. in toxocariasis, hydatid disease; by larvae burrowing through the skin, e.g. in disease caused by hookworms, schistosomiasis; or where the parasite is injected into the blood by a bite of a mosquito or fly, e.g. malaria, filariasis, trypanosomiasis or leishmaniasis.

Approach to diagnosis

History

Knowledge of the geographical distribution of major parasites is helpful (Coulter, 2002). The following history should be obtained: where the child was born, countries where the child has lived or visited and duration, especially of the last visit. Other important information includes malaria prophylaxis, exposure to mosquitoes, swimming in lakes and rivers (schistosomiasis), eating raw plants or fish (food-borne flukes), exposure to animals (e.g. pups – toxocariasis) and recent illnesses, skin lesions or bites and their treatment.

Investigations

The following is a guide to specimens required for parasitological diagnosis.

- Blood smear
  - Thick films – malarial parasites, trypanosomes, microfilaria (filariasis) and *Borrelia* (*B. duttoni*, bacteria that cause relapsing fever)
  - Thin film – for identifying species
- Serology
  - In toxocariasis, amoebiasis, hydatid disease, leishmaniasis, trypanosomiasis (African and South American), schistosomiasis, cysticercosis, malaria and filariasis
  - Serology is less helpful for people who have lived in an endemic area (and may have had past infection) as opposed to non-immune people who recently visited an endemic country
- Stool
  - In amoebiasis (warm, fresh stool to detect trophozoites), for geohelminths, *Schistostoma mansoni* (may require concentration test), *Strongyloides stercoralis* (for larvae not eggs, also stool culture), tapeworm eggs or gravid segments
  - Adhesive tape (Sellotape) slide for *Enterobius vermicularis* (pin worm)
- Urine
  - For *S. haematobium* (mid-day, urine should be sedimented and filtered)
- Bone marrow
  - In visceral leishmaniasis
- Aspiration/biopsy
  - Rectal biopsy – for *S. mansoni*
  - Lymph node aspiration – in Gambian trypanosomiasis
  - Skin snip – in onchocerciasis
  - Smear, aspiration or biopsy – in cutaneous leishmaniasis

Particular problems

In this section specific drug treatment will be mentioned only briefly. More detailed management can be found in *Medicines for Children* (Royal College of Paediatrics and Child Health, 2003), the *British National Formulary* (*BNF*) and standard textbooks.

Malaria

Malaria is caused by *Plasmodium falciparum*, *P. vivax*, *P. malariae* and *P. ovale*.

- *P. falciparum* causes cerebral malaria and may be fatal in non-immune individuals.

- *P. vivax* and *P. ovale* may cause recurrent attacks of malaria.
- *P. malariae* is associated with the nephrotic syndrome in some parts of the world.
- *P. falciparum* is found in many tropical countries but particularly sub-Saharan Africa.
- *P. vivax* is common in the Indian subcontinent.

Of about 2000 cases of imported malaria occurring in the UK per annum, 15 per cent are in children. About half the cases are caused by *P. falciparum*, a third by *P. vivax* and the remainder by *P. ovale* and *P. malariae*. This brief account of malaria will be mainly confined to *P. falciparum*.

LIFE CYCLE

The female *Anopheles* mosquito (bites from dusk to dawn) injects saliva containing sporozoites into the blood stream. The sporozoites enter the liver cells and pre-erythrocytic schizonts are formed within hepatic sinusoids. Merozoites are produced and invade the red blood cells (RBCs). Rupture of RBCs results in anaemia and stimulation of cytokine production, e.g. tumour necrosis factor (TNF), causing symptoms of malaria. Some merozoites develop into gametocytes. The mosquito ingests the gametocytes. Sexual cycle occurs and sporozoites are produced. *P. vivax* and *P. ovale* may remain in the liver in a dormant phase (hypnozoite), which is responsible for recurrent attacks of malaria.

CLINICAL FEATURES

The incubation period is approximately two to four weeks. Symptoms include high-grade fever alternating with cold sweats, rigors, headache, vomiting, myalgia and arthralgia. There is usually hepatosplenomegaly.

COMPLICATIONS

In hyper or holoendemic areas, cerebral malaria is common in young children (under 5s) before they develop sufficient immunity. In hypoendemic areas and in non-immune visitors, cerebral malaria may occur in any age group. Typical features are altered consciousness, convulsions, coma, metabolic acidosis, hypoglycaemia and sometimes decorticate or decerebrate posturing. There may be pulmonary oedema, jaundice (in older children and adults), oliguria and, sometimes, haemoglobinuria. Mortality may be 15–30 per cent and about 10 per cent may have neurological sequelae, which in some children may improve or resolve. In endemic areas, pregnant women (especially primigravidae) are prone to severe anaemia and involvement of the placenta results in intrauterine growth retardation – malaria is an important cause of low birth weight in tropical countries.

Children with immunity to *P. falciparum* may present with uncomplicated malaria – fever and a positive blood slide, or a positive blood slide may be detected by coincidence in children with other conditions, e.g. pneumonia or gastroenteritis.

DIAGNOSIS AND INVESTIGATIONS

A thick blood smear is needed for diagnosis and a thin blood smear to detect the species. The level of parasitaemia relates to severity. Blood glucose should be checked. If meningitis is suspected, lumbar puncture should be undertaken unless the Glasgow Coma Score is <8 or raised intracranial pressure is suspected, when antibiotics should be given and a delayed lumbar puncture undertaken, if indicated.

MANAGEMENT

For *P. falciparum*, standard treatment is quinine for seven days. If resistance to quinine is suspected a single dose of pyrimethamine with sulfadoxine (Fansidar®) should be given on day 7 of quinine treatment. If Fansidar resistance is considered, give doxycycline for seven days in children over 12 years. For children under 12 years, clindamycin is an alternative. If the patient has altered consciousness, is seriously ill or unable to take quinine orally, they should be given it intravenously 20 mg/kg over four hours then 10 mg/kg every 8–12 hours until the child can take orally.

Severe cases require careful monitoring to detect and treat dehydration/shock, anaemia, metabolic acidosis, hypoglycaemia, seizures, pulmonary oedema and oliguria. For mild and uncomplicated cases Fansidar (single dose) or mefloquine (single or divided doses) may be given. For children coming from areas of multidrug resistance, e.g. south-east Asia or the Amazon basin, specialist advice should be sought.

For *P. vivax*, *P. ovale* and *P. malariae* malaria, chloroquine is the drug of choice. To eradicate *P. vivax* and *P. ovale* from the liver, primaquine 250 µg/kg per day is given for 14 days. Check glucose 6-phosphate dehydrogenase (G6PD) activity first as primaquine may cause haemolysis in these cases.

PREVENTION

In endemic areas if children can be persuaded to sleep under insecticide-impregnated (e.g. pyrethroids) bed nets, morbidity (especially anaemia) and mortality is reduced by 25 per cent or more. For non-immune subjects visiting endemic areas, see *BNF* or *Medicines for Children* for preventive measures and prophylaxis.

Leishmaniasis

Leishmaniasis is caused by *Leishmania*, a protozoan whose reservoir is in animals, e.g. rodents and dogs, and in some areas (e.g. India) in humans. The vector is the female sandfly. Clinical types of the disease are:

- Cutaneous (CL): *L. tropica*, *L. major*, *L. mexicana* and *L. amazonensis* in Central and South America
- Mucocutaneous (MCL): *L. braziliensis* in South America
- Visceral (VL): *L. donovani* (India), *L. infantum* (Mediterranean) or *L. chagasi* (South America)

Details of geographical distribution can be found in standard textbooks. This information is important regarding type of disease and drug sensitivity.

LIFE CYCLE

When the sandfly bites an infected animal (or human) it swallows amastigotes. The amastigote develops into a promastigote (has flagellum), which is injected into man by the sandfly. It penetrates local tissue macrophages, loses its flagellum and becomes an amastigote. This may remain in skin (CL) (local macrophages) or invade the mucosa (MCL) or be taken up by circulating macrophages and transported to the reticuloendothelial system (VL) depending on the type of *Leishmania*.

CUTANEOUS LEISHMANIASIS (ALEPPO BUTTON, DELHI BOIL)

Single or multiple nodules appear on exposed areas, especially the face or extremities and usually ulcerate. Most heal spontaneously within months to a year or so.

Management

Multiple, large or disfiguring lesions, especially on the face, require treatment. Local application of ointment containing 15 per cent aminosidine and 12 per cent methylbenzethonium chloride or oral fluconazole may be tried. If unsuccessful, parenteral (or local) sodium stibogluconate should be given for three weeks.

MUCOCUTANEOUS LEISHMANIASIS (ESPUNDIA)

Metastatic lesions occur on nasal or oropharyngeal mucosa and may progress to destruction of local tissue.

Management

Stibogluconate is given parenterally for six to eight weeks.

VISCERAL LEISHMANIASIS (KALA-AZAR)

Epidemics occur in northeast India and in southern Sudan where mortality is very high amongst displaced people. Where VL and HIV infection coexist as in the Mediterranean littoral, VL is difficult to eradicate. Incubation period may be up to two to four months or longer. VL presents with fever, anaemia and splenomegaly (Figure 21.1). Oedema occurs in longstanding cases associated with hypoalbuminaemia. There is pancytopenia.

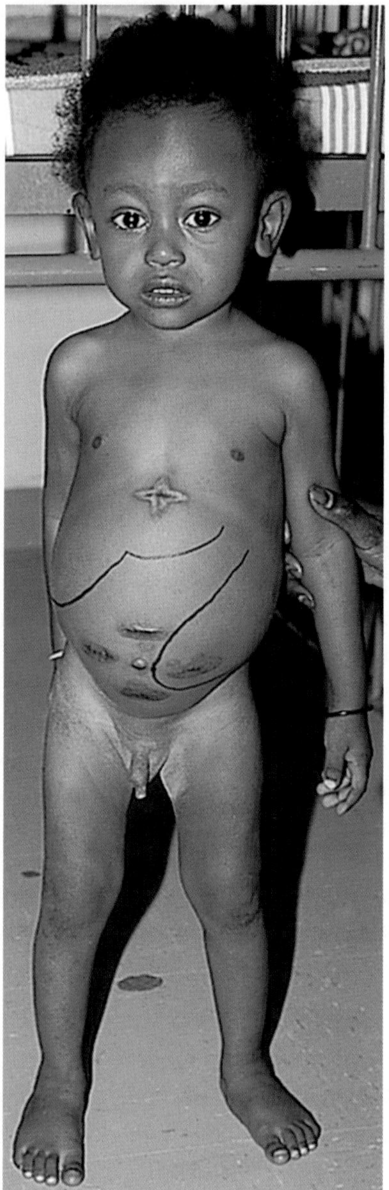

Figure 21.1 An 18-month-old Libyan child with visceral leishmaniasis. Clinical features were fever, anaemia, hepatosplenomegaly and pancytopenia

Diagnosis

The diagnosis is confirmed by detecting amastigotes on microscopy of aspirates of bone marrow or spleen (PCR and culture is available). Serology may be useful in patients from non-endemic areas. Antigen tests in urine are available.

Management

- Liposomal amphotericin (expensive) 3 mg/kg, total dose of 30 mg/kg, given over 10 days or 3 mg/kg on days 1–5, 14 and 21.
- Pentavalent antimonials (Sb^V), i.e. sodium stibogluconate (Pentostam®) or meglumine

antimoniate (Glucantime) 20 mg Sb^V/kg intravenously (IV) or intramuscularly (IM) (painful) daily for four weeks (six weeks in cases from resistant areas). Electrocardiogram changes, elevated hepatic transaminases and amylase levels are common.
- Aminosidine 16–20 mg/kg IV or IM daily for three to four weeks.
- Trials of miltefosine in children are in progress.

Other drugs include standard amphotericin B and pentamidine, both of which are toxic. Unless child is very sick, symptomatic improvement occurs within a few days. Prolonged follow-up (at least a year) is required because of risk of relapse.

African trypanosomiasis

There are two forms of African trypanosomiasis. Gambian trypanosomiasis is caused by *Trypanosoma brucei gambiense*, has a human reservoir, progresses slowly and occurs in west and central Africa. Rhodesian trypanosomiasis is caused by *T.b. rhodesiense*, has a wild animal reservoir, is a more rapid subacute disease and occurs in east and southern Africa. The vector is the tsetse fly.

There are two stages: the haemolymphatic (stage 1) and the meningo-encephalitic (stage 2), which is the 'sleeping sickness' phase. Death may occur in stage 1 in Rhodesian trypanosomiasis and is invariable in stage 2 trypanosomiasis if not adequately treated.

DIAGNOSIS

Trypanosomes may be detected in (i) thick blood films, but a more sensitive technique may be required (quantitative buffy coat); (ii) in aspirates from enlarged lymph nodes (commonly on the back of the neck) in Gambian disease; and (iii) in cerebrospinal fluid (CSF). In stage 2, raised lymphocyte count and protein are found in the CSF. Serological tests are available, e.g. card agglutination test (CAT) which detects anti-trypanosomal IgM.

MANAGEMENT

Drugs for treatment of trypanosomiasis are toxic and require experience in their use. Pentamidine isethionate is used for stage 1 Gambian disease and suramin for Rhodesian disease. For stage 2, suramin and melarsoprol are given. Resistance to melarsoprol occurs and eflornithine is an alternative for stage 2 Gambian disease.

American trypanosomiasis

American trypanosomiasis occurs in Latin and Central America and is caused by *T. cruzi*, which is deposited on the skin of the host from infected faeces of triatomae bugs. Reservoirs are small animals and humans; the disease is also transmitted through blood transfusion.

CLINICAL FEATURES

Infection occurs when the infected faeces of the bug are scratched through a wound or bite in the skin or enter through the conjunctiva. The resulting conjunctivitis is called Romaña sign. The **acute phase** is seen in young children and includes fever, lymphadenopathy, hepatosplenomegaly, generalized oedema and myocarditis. The **chronic phase** occurs in adults and is a chronic debilitating disease associated with cardiomyopathy, megaoesophagus and megacolon.

DIAGNOSIS

Trypanosomes are usually detected in the blood during the acute phase. Serological tests are useful.

MANAGEMENT

The acute phase is treated with nifurtimox or benznidazole. Drug treatment of the chronic phase is less effective and the main aspects of care are the management of cardiomyopathy (e.g. pacemakers) and the gastrointestinal disorders.

Amoebiasis

Amoebiasis is an invasive disease caused by *Entamoeba histolytica*. Infection results from sewage contamination of water supplies, food handlers and person-to-person transmission.

LIFE CYCLE

Cysts are ingested and trophozoites (amoebae) escape from cysts, dividing into more trophozoites. The trophozoites invade the mucosa of colon resulting in ulcer formation. Some trophozoites form cysts, and cysts are excreted in faeces.

CLINICAL FEATURES

Entamoeba histolytica is considered to have two forms: *E. dispar* and *E. histolytica*. *E. dispar* is associated with mild or asymptomatic disease and passage of cysts in stool. The invasive form of disease is caused by *E. histolytica*. Clinical features include colitis with bloody diarrhoea, liver abscess, less commonly extension to the lung (usually right) and pericardium, and rarely the brain.

DIAGNOSIS

Trophozoites with haemophagocytosis or cysts are detected in fresh warm stools of patients with colitis. Diagnosis may also be made by lower endoscopy. In hepatic abscess, amoebae may not be detected in stool and confirmation is by serology.

MANAGEMENT

Asymptomatic intestinal carriage is treated with diloxanide furoate, 20 mg/kg per day in three divided doses for 10 days. For colitis or liver abscess, metronidazole 30–50 mg/kg in three divided doses is given for five to

10 days. Tinidazole (50–60 mg/kg for three to five days) is an alternative. Diloxanide furoate is also given as a luminal amoebicide for 10 days. Aspiration of the liver abscess may be required if rupture is suspected or if there is failure to respond to treatment by three to five days.

Gut nematodes

Intestinal helminths or geohelminths may infect over 80 per cent of children in some communities, however, probably only those with the heaviest burdens 5–10 per cent will have symptomatic disease. Many children have multiple intestinal helminths. In industrialized countries, most intestinal helminths will have been contracted abroad apart from *Enterobius vermicularis* (pin or thread worm), *Toxocara canis* (toxocariasis), *Trichinella spiralis* (trichinosis) and some tapeworms.

Diagnosis is by detection of eggs in the stool for *Ascaris lumbricoides*, *Trichuris trichiura* and hookworm, and larvae in stool for *Strongyloides stercoralis*. Eosinophilia is common especially early on in infection.

CASE STUDY: Geohelminths

A 6-year-old boy from a rural background presented with a three-day history of bilious vomiting, abdominal distension and constipation. Plain erect radiograph of abdomen demonstrated fluid levels. Full blood count showed a low-grade eosinophilia. At laparotomy a large number of adult *A. lumbricoides* worms were found to be causing obstruction of the small intestine. Post-operatively stool microscopy demonstrated eggs of *A. lumbricoides*, *Hymenolepis nana* and *Entamoeba coli* cysts. The presence of *H. nana* and *E. coli* in addition to *A. lumbricoides*, supported frequent exposure to highly contaminated soil.

ASCARIS LUMBRICOIDES

This is a very common worm of worldwide distribution.

Life cycle

After ingestion of eggs, larvae hatch and penetrate the small bowel, moving to the liver in the portal system. They enter the general circulation, then the lungs, trachea and oesophagus. Adult worms develop in small intestine and eggs are produced by the female worm and passed in faeces. Adult worms live for about a year or so.

Complications

In heavy infections, there may be malabsorption, which is more likely to be symptomatic in children already malnourished. Obstruction of gut, biliary or pancreatic ducts is a life-threatening complication. A hypersensitivity reaction to larvae of *A. lumbricoides* (also in hookworm and *T. canis* infection) when passing through the lungs may cause a 'Löffler syndrome' with cough, dyspnoea and wheeze.

Management

Mebendazole 100 mg twice daily for three days or albendazole 400 mg in a single dose. Repeat in two to three weeks if necessary.

TRICHURIS TRICHIURA (WHIPWORM)

In heavy infection, this is an important cause of disease in developing countries.

Life cycle

After ingestion of eggs, larvae hatch and worms attach to the mucosa of caecum. In heavy infections, they may extend to rectum. The eggs are passed in faeces.

Clinical features

These include bloody diarrhoea, rectal prolapse, growth failure, clubbing of fingers and hypoalbuminaemia (rarely oedema).

Management

Mebendazole 100 mg twice daily for three days or albendazole 400 mg for three days. Repeat in two to three weeks if necessary.

ENTEROBIUS VERMICULARIS (PIN OR THREAD WORM)

This is a very common infection worldwide, many of which are asymptomatic. Usually detected by parents when the worm appears in the stool or around the anus.

Life cycle

After ingestion of eggs, worms develop in the caecum, appendix and upper colon. Gravid females migrate from the colon to the anus (usually at night) and deposit eggs, which stick to the perianal skin (these remain viable for up to three weeks). When the infected child scratches their anus, eggs are ingested from infected fingers or clothing (autoinfection). Other sources of infection include bath water and inhalation of contaminated house dust. Worms die within six to eight weeks, thus without autoinfection the disease usually resolves spontaneously. However, 'retroinfection' may occur where larvae migrate from the anus back into the colon to continue the cycle. Pin worms may be vectors for *Dientamoeba fragilis*, which may be a cause of colitis.

Clinical features

Symptoms include anal pruritus with local excoriation, vulval pruritus, dysuria and discharge if the worm migrates to the vulva, and sleeplessness. Rarely in girls, worms may migrate to the internal genital tract and cause pelvic inflammatory disease (Tandon *et al.*, 2002). Pin worms may be detected in neonates and young infants.

Diagnosis

Diagnosis is by applying adhesive tape to the anus in the morning before washing and applying it to a microscopic slide. Repeating the procedure on three to five consecutive days increases the sensitivity.

Management

Mebendazole 100 mg or albendazole 400 mg as a single dose, repeat in two weeks time. Usually, all the children in a household are treated. In intractable cases, mebendazole 100 mg may be given weekly for up to three months and to other family members if indicated.

Hygiene measures include keeping nails short, washing hands and scrubbing nails before meals and after defaecation. Pants and, if necessary, gloves should be worn at night. The perianal areas should be washed before bedtime and in the morning. Night and underclothes should be washed daily.

Mebendazole should be avoided during the first trimester of pregnancy and in infants under 1 year. For infants under 1 year, hygiene measures may suffice until they can be treated with mebendazole after 1 year or piperazine 65 mg/kg per day may be given for seven days.

HOOKWORM

Hookworm is an important cause of anaemia in older children and adults. It is caused by *Ancylostoma duodenale* and *Necator americanus*. *A. duodenale* is commoner in subtropical and temperate areas whereas *N. americanus* is widespread in the tropics.

Life cycle

The larvae enter the skin, especially the feet ('ground itch', dermatitis) and migrate to the lungs, trachea, oesophagus and attach to the jejunum. Worms develop and eggs are passed in stool. The larvae hatch in soil. *A. duodenale* may cause infection through ingestion of larvae but they do not migrate. Worms may live for a year or longer. Each worm may suck up to 0.5 mL of blood per day, amounting to 100–150 mL/day.

Clinical features

Iron-deficient anaemia is the main complication but heavy infections in children already malnourished may result in hypoalbuminaemia, micronutrient deficiency, oedema and heart failure.

Management

Mebendazole 100 mg twice daily for three days or albendazole 400 mg daily for three days and iron supplements.

MASS CAMPAIGNS

Mass campaigns of regular treatment of school children for geohelminths with albendazole and, if indicated, combined with praziquantel for schistosomiasis are effective. Of course they miss children who do not go to school and who may be more vulnerable to infection by parasites. There is evidence that mass treatment of children may improve rates of growth and in some studies improved cognitive function has been demonstrated (Coulter, 2002).

CUTANEOUS LARVA MIGRANS (CREEPING ERUPTION)

This is commonly caused by the dog hookworm *Ancylostoma caninum*. The larvae penetrate the epidermis (but not the dermis), fail to develop and wander 'aimlessly' in the epidermis. They are usually found in the feet but may be found on the buttocks of infants from sitting on the ground. Parents reporting movement of the worms in the skin aids diagnosis.

Management

Local application of thiabendazole: 0.5 g tablet is ground-up with 5 g petroleum jelly and applied every 12 hours under an occlusive dressing. For multiple infections, albendazole 10 mg/kg may be given in divided doses for five days.

VISCERAL LARVA MIGRANS (VLM)

This is caused by *Toxocara canis*, an ascaris-like worm in dogs, which is unable to complete its cycle in humans. It is distributed worldwide.

Life cycle

Adult bitches or hosts such as mice or rats ingest eggs. The larvae migrate particularly to mammary glands and pups are infected through transplacental or transmammary routes. The worms develop in the intestines of pups and eggs are passed in stool. In a child who has ingested the eggs (of pup or adult dogs), larvae migrate from the intestine and lodge in tissues such as retina or brain, as they are unable to complete their cycle. As larvae do not develop into worms in human intestine, children are not infectious – pups are highly infectious.

Clinical features

- In the VLM stage, there may be fever, hepatomegaly, wheezing and marked eosinophilia. It is unusual to detect eye lesions during this stage.
- Larvae trapped in retina cause a local granuloma and visual impairment. The lesion may be mistaken for retinoblastoma (with resultant enucleation of the eye), the phakoma of tuberous sclerosis or granulomata associated with cysticercosis.

Diagnosis

A marked eosinophilia is characteristic in VLM but the count may be within normal limits in retinal lesions. Serology is the main diagnostic tool but is less sensitive in ocular lesions than in VLM.

Management

Visceral larva migrans is self-limiting, but in severe cases, drug therapy may alleviate symptoms. Albendazole, 10 mg/kg for seven days is probably the drug of choice. Diethylcarbamazine given for seven to 10 days in increasing doses is an alternative. Systemic or local steroids are used for ocular lesions. Laser therapy or surgery may also be indicated.

STRONGYLOIDES STERCORALIS

Strongyloidiasis is uncommon in children and prevalence increases with age. Light infections are often asymptomatic but may lead to 'larva currens' (see below).

Life cycle

Larvae penetrate the skin and migrate to the small intestine (route not certain). The female worm develops and burrows into the crypts of Lieberkühn glands. Eggs hatch in glands and rhabditiform larvae burrow through intestinal mucosa and are excreted in stool. Larvae in soil either develop into an infective larval stage or free-living adult worms which then mate and reproduce infective (filariform) larvae. Autoinfection possibly occurs when infective larval stage develops in and then invades intestine (instead of being excreted), or by re-entry through the perianal area. Hyperinfection is an exaggeration of the above process when larvae penetrate the intestine with massive autoinfection. Immunosuppressed patients, particularly those on corticosteroids are at particular risk.

Clinical features

Autoinvasion of anal skin by larvae may cause 'larva currens'. Heavy intestinal infections may result in malabsorption. Eosinophilia is common. Because of autoinfection, infection may persist for decades.

Management

Treatment is with albendazole 400 mg daily for three days. Ivermectin is an alternative. Hyperinfection is difficult to eradicate and requires prolonged treatment (up to two weeks).

CESTODES (TAPEWORMS)

Tapeworms have definite and intermediate hosts. Humans are the definite host for *Hymenolepis nana, Taenia saginata* (beef tapeworm) and *T. solium* (pork tapeworm) and cattle and pigs are intermediate hosts for *T. saginata* and *T. solium*, respectively. *H. nana* (dwarf tapeworm) is a common tapeworm found in stools of children and is usually asymptomatic. Heavy infections may be associated with diarrhoea and abdominal pain. If required, treatment is as for *T. saginata.*

Distribution of *T. saginata* infection is worldwide. *T. solium* is common in Central and South America, Asia and East Africa.

Life cycle

When a person eats undercooked beef/pork containing onchospheres of *T. saginata* or *T. solium* encysted in muscle (cysticerci), onchospheres excyst in intestine and develop into adult worms. Gravid proglottides (segments) of the female containing fertilized eggs are passed in stool and eaten by cows/pigs. The eggs release onchospheres, which pass through intestinal wall, lodge in muscle and develop into cysticerci.

Cysticercosis occurs when eggs of *T. solium* (either from the person or from another infected person) are ingested. Larvae released from eggs migrate and encyst in tissues such as subcutaneous tissue, muscle, central nervous system (neurocysticercosis), eye or myocardium.

Clinical features

Infection by *T. saginata* and *T. solium* is usually asymptomatic (except when cysticercosis occurs). Heavy infections may be associated with abdominal pain and diarrhoea.

Management

Treatment is with praziquantel 10 mg/kg in single dose before breakfast. Niclosamide is an alternative. Following treatment, faeces are highly infectious.

NEUROCYSTICERCOSIS

Neurocysticercosis may manifest with epilepsy, raised intracranial pressure or meningoencephalitis. The cysts may be detected on computed tomography (CT) scan of the brain. Serology may be helpful.

Management

Treatment of neurocysticercosis requires experience. Spontaneous resolution occurs and thus efficacy of antiparasitic drugs is difficult to assess. Albendazole, 15–20 mg/kg is given in two divided doses for seven to 14 days and repeated, if necessary. Dexamethasone, 0.6 mg/kg is given for one week and tailed off over two to three days. Standard anticonvulsants are given for epilepsy.

HYDATID DISEASE

CASE STUDY

A 10-year-old girl from a nomadic family presented with a tender swelling in the right hypochondrium. She also had mild dyspnoea. Cautery marks were present over the abdominal mass. There was slight tenderness and dullness on percussion of the left posterior chest wall. Chest radiograph showed a round cystic mass in the left lower zone. Abdominal ultrasound also demonstrated a cystic mass in the left lobe of the liver. Serology for *Echinococcus granulosa* was positive. The cautery had been performed by a traditional medicine practitioner nine months earlier as a treatment for the abdominal swelling.

Hydatid disease is caused by *E. granulosa*. Dogs are the definitive hosts and animals such as sheep, cattle, goats and camels are intermediate hosts. Hydatid disease is common in sheep-farming areas and where there is intimate contact between dogs and people.

Life cycle

When a dog eats hydatid cyst in carcass of a sheep, the worm develops in the intestine. The eggs are passed in stool and ingested by sheep (or human). Larvae develop into hydatid cysts in liver, lung or less commonly peritoneal cavity, brain or bone.

Clinical features

Many cysts are asymptomatic. Symptoms are due to pressure effects of cysts (Figure 21.2). Leakage or rupture of a cyst may cause an anaphylactic reaction.

Diagnosis

Ultrasound is effective in detecting cysts especially if daughter cysts are seen inside the cyst wall. Serological examination is a sensitive test. It must be undertaken in any situation where operative treatment is considered for lesions that could be hydatid cysts because of the risk of anaphylaxis.

Management

Asymptomatic cysts require no treatment. Accessible large cysts are excised or they may be aspirated under ultrasound guidance. A scolicidal agent, e.g. cetrimide, is injected into the cyst to sterilize it before removal.

Albendazole is used pre- and postoperatively and for inaccessible and multiple cysts. Four-week cycles of

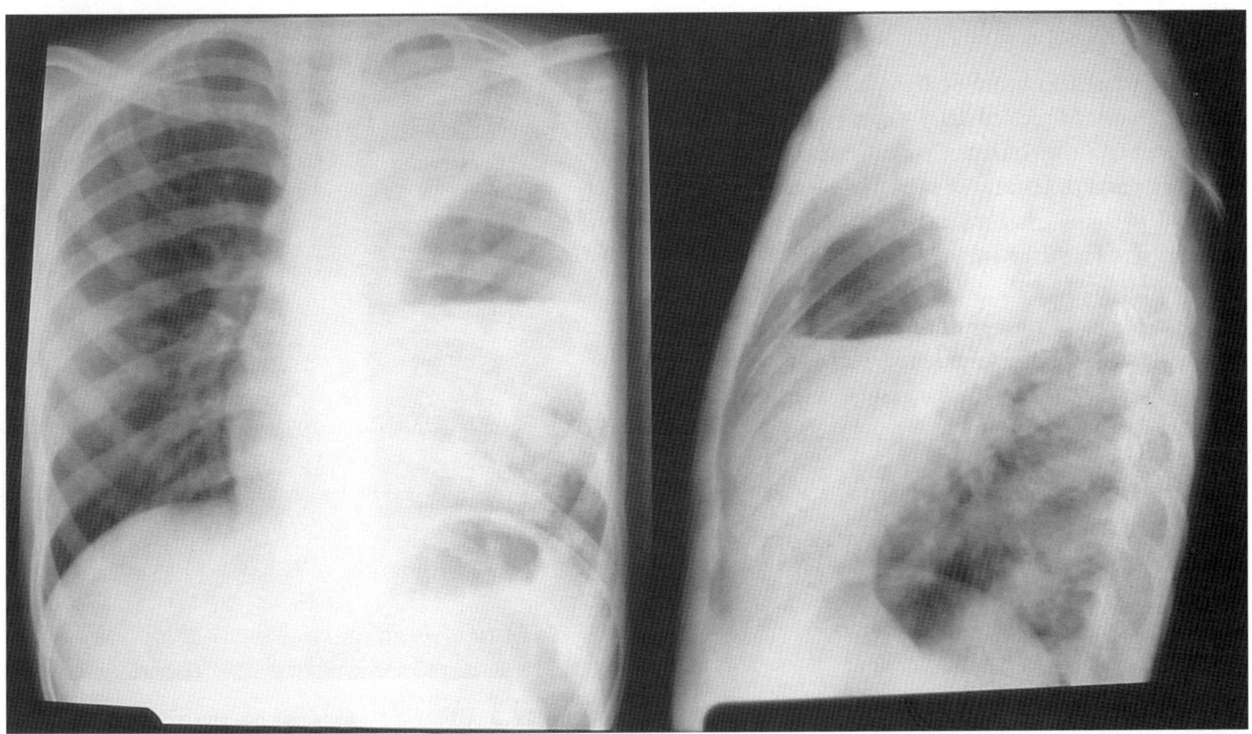

Figure 21.2 Chest radiographs showing hydatid cyst of left lung

15–20 mg/kg per day in two divided doses are given followed by two weeks free between cycles.

Schistosomiasis

CASE STUDY

A 15-year-old Egyptian boy presented with haematuria which had been present for over a year. It was most prominent at the end of micturition (terminal haematuria). Blood pressure was 140/90 mmHg. Urine microscopy showed numerous RBCs and *Schistosoma haematobium* ova. Abdominal ultrasound demonstrated bilateral dilated ureters from the level of the vesicoureteric junction with distension of renal pelvices. There was a rim of calcification in the bladder wall.

Schistosomiasis occurs in areas where there is a combination of warm, fresh water containing specific snails and indiscriminate urinary or faecal excretion of *Schistosoma* eggs by humans. Three species of *Schistosoma* cause the majority of schistosomial infections (Table 21.2).

In *S. haematobium* infection, a chronic granulomatous process in the bladder and lower ureter results in obstructive uropathy. There may be complete or partial resolution with treatment (praziquantel) as long as the person does not contract further infections.

LIFE CYCLE

Eggs are passed in urine or stool into fresh water containing snails. Miracidia hatch from eggs, penetrate the snails and replicate into cercariae. Cercariae are released into water and penetrate the skin. The cercariae lose their tail and become schistosomulae, which are transported to lungs and reach the left side of the heart. They are distributed throughout the body. Schistosomulae that reach the liver develop into mature worms and adult males and females copulate. Copulating pairs migrate to egg-laying sites (*S. haematobium* – vesical veins; *S. mansoni*, *S. japonicum* – superior and inferior mesenteric veins). The eggs of *S. haematobium* and *S. mansoni/S. japonicum* pass either into tissue and cause immune reactions and fibrosis or escape into the lumen of the urinary or intestinal tract, respectively, and are excreted.

Table 21.2 Schistosomiasis

Schistosoma spp.	Organs involved	Geographic area
S. haematobium	Urinary tract	**Africa**, Middle East
S. mansoni	Intestines, liver	**Africa**, Middle East, **South America**
S. japonicum	Intestines, liver	**China, Indonesia, Philippines**

CLINICAL FEATURES AND COMPLICATIONS

S. haematobium

The main symptom is terminal haematuria. Complications include obstructive uropathy, calcification of the bladder and lower parts of ureter and bladder calculi.

S. mansoni *(and* S. japonicum*)*

Clinical features of *S. japonicum* infection are generally similar to infection with *S. mansoni*. The main symptom is bloody diarrhoea, which results in anaemia. A protein-losing enteropathy may also occur. Complications include hepatic fibrosis, portal hypertension and granulomatous polyps in the large intestine. Nephrotic syndrome may be associated with *S. mansoni* (Figure 21.3).

Schistosoma granulomas may cause spinal cord lesions and rarely involve the brain; pulmonary hypertension is also a complication. Chronic *Salmonella* infection may occur in both *S. haematobium* and *S. mansoni* infections.

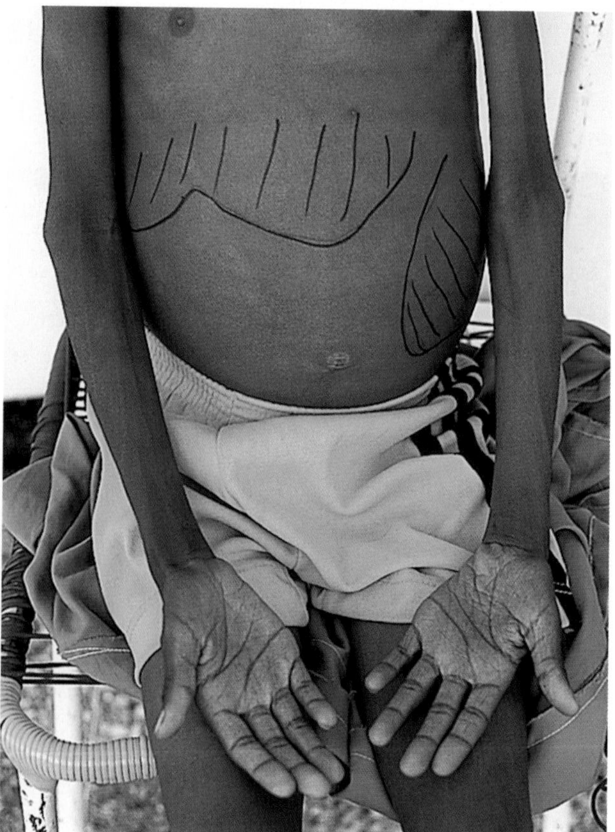

Figure 21.3 A 14-year-old Sudanese boy who presented with haematemesis due to *S. mansoni* and portal hypertension. Note predominant enlargement of left lobe of the liver

DIAGNOSIS

S. haematobium

A mid-day urine specimen (if possible) should be sediment or filtered before undertaking microscopy for eggs. For prevalence surveys, dip sticks of urine for blood and protein are useful.

S. mansoni

Stool smear is taken for eggs. If this is negative, a concentration method should be used.

Serological examination is useful for diagnosis in non-immune travellers to endemic areas.

MANAGEMENT AND FOLLOW-UP

Praziquantel is effective against all forms of schistosomiasis, 40 mg/kg is given in two divided doses four to six hours apart. For heavy *S. mansoni* infections and for *S. japonicum* 60 mg/kg is given. Repeat urine or stool examination at 2 and 4–6 months. The viability of eggs should be determined. A further dose of praziquantel may be required.

NUTRITION IN DEVELOPING COUNTRIES

Over 50 per cent of child deaths among the under 5s are associated with malnutrition. The interaction between infection and nutrition is a key factor. Infection is associated with a number of problems including anorexia, malabsorption due to gastroenteritis, suppression of protein synthesis and enhanced catabolism, and suppression of the immune system. Nutritional deficiency causes atrophy of organs, e.g. gut mucosa, heart and the reticuloendothelial system. Impaired function of the immune system results in severe and prolonged infections.

Breastfeeding

The WHO estimates that 1.5 million deaths a year could be prevented by effective breastfeeding (WHO, 1993). In most traditional societies, mothers breastfeed for at least 12 months and commonly for 18–24 months or longer. However, in many societies breastfeeding is *not exclusive*. Colostrum is often discarded and babies may not be put on the breast for 24–48 hours. Prelacteal feeds include water, formulae and a wide range of herbal and other concoctions. After establishing breastfeeding, supplements may be given as early as 1 month of age. Mothers who are unable to or choose not to breastfeed may be stigmatized (see section on HIV infection).

Breast milk provides substantial protection against infection, particularly during the period of exclusive breastfeeding (4–6 months), but in poor societies, especially for uneducated mothers, this protection may continue to a certain degree as long as the mother breastfeeds; and, in addition, it continues to provide important nutrients, particularly animal protein and energy (Figure 21.4). However, prolonged breastfeeding without introduction of adequate complementary (weaning) foods will result in inadequate weight gain and when the mother stops breastfeeding frank malnutrition may ensue.

The advantages, problems and suggestions for improvement in breastfeeding practices are outlined in Table 21.3. The WHO/UNICEF has an international code of marketing of breast milk substitutes that has been adopted by most governments of developing countries (but not all industrialized countries).

Staples and weaning diets

At 4 months, mothers should begin the introduction of additional foods and the infant should be well established on a weaning diet by 6 months. A major problem is the inadequacy of complementary foods in the poorer and less educated families. They are often single staple,

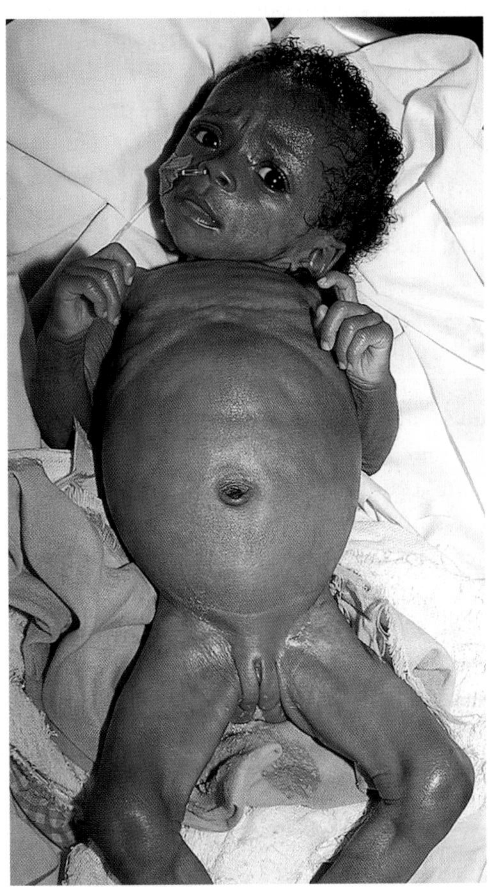

Figure 21.4 A 6-week-old neonate in Sierra Leone. The mother bottle fed the infant from birth. She has persistent diarrhoea with gross abdominal distension and is marasmic

Table 21.3 Breastfeeding in developing countries

Advantages	Problems	Improvement
Reduced infection especially diarrhoea* Enhanced child survival and nutrition Contraception (lactational amenorrhoea 6–9 months)	Colostrum discarded Not exclusive breastfed† HIV infection (see page 631) Commercial promotion of artificial milk Poor support from health care staff Working mothers Specific: Poor milk flow Engorgement Breast abscess	Antenatal preparation Suckling within a half-hour of birth If supplements required, should be given by cup and spoon (not bottle) Training of healthcare staff to support breastfeeding and in management of specific problems Working mothers: Maternity leave Creches at work

* Particularly if infant is exclusively breastfed.

† Exclusive breastfeeding: no supplements in first 4–6 months. Even in hot climates no fluid other than breast milk is required.

HIV, human immunodeficiency virus.

thin and watery gruels which are bulky with low energy density and high phytate levels and are often contaminated. High phytate levels reduce bioavailability of nutrients such as zinc, iron and calcium.

A **staple** is the common food used in a community, e.g. wheat, sorghum, maize, millet, rice, potatoes, cassava or plantain (bananas). Its **biological value** is limited by being low in essential amino acids, e.g. lysine for cereal grains and in addition, tryptophan in maize. This can be rectified by giving legumes, e.g. groundnuts, beans, chickpeas and lentils which contain these amino acids. If families can afford it, animal protein, which contains all the essential amino acids, will provide a rich source of protein, e.g. milk, eggs and fish. In general, weaning diets in developing countries are low in energy and have borderline levels of protein except when the staples comprise potatoes, yams, cassava and plantains, which contain very low protein levels. Energy is increased by the addition of oil and sugar. Dark green leaves of plants provide additional iron and vitamin A. Cultural practices such as fermentation of foods reduces bacterial load and germination makes food more digestible.

Cultural attitudes and taboos

In traditional societies, there are a wide variety of cultural attitudes and taboos regarding breastfeeding and diets for children, many of which have an adverse effect on infant nutrition. Discarding colostrum and too early introduction of supplementary fluids or foods have already been mentioned above. A mother may wean her infant from the breast if she considers her milk to be 'bad' or poisoned. The latter may occur if she has extramarital sexual desires or intercourse. In sub-Saharan Africa, sexual intercourse while breastfeeding is taboo in many societies. Children may not be fed or fluids may be restricted when they have diarrhoea. 'Rich foods' may be regarded as harmful when a child is sick. Eggs may be taboo for children.

Particular problems

Vitamin A deficiency

Vitamin A is important for the integrity of the epithelium, e.g. the eye, gastrointestinal, respiratory and renal tracts and for normal mucociliary function. Deficiency results in secretion of keratin instead of mucus, resulting in epithelial cells becoming hard and dry and prone to infection. Vitamin A is also important for normal function of the immune system. Retinol (preformed vitamin A) is found only in animals, especially in the liver. Important sources are fish liver oils, liver, dairy produce and eggs. The provitamin β-carotene is the main source of vitamin A in developing countries. Foods with a high β-carotene level include red palm oil, carrots, dark green leaves and generally most vegetables with yellow-red colour, e.g. mangoes and tomatoes. Only about a third of the β-carotene content of diet is absorbed and many children in poor societies are deficient in vitamin A stores. Ninety

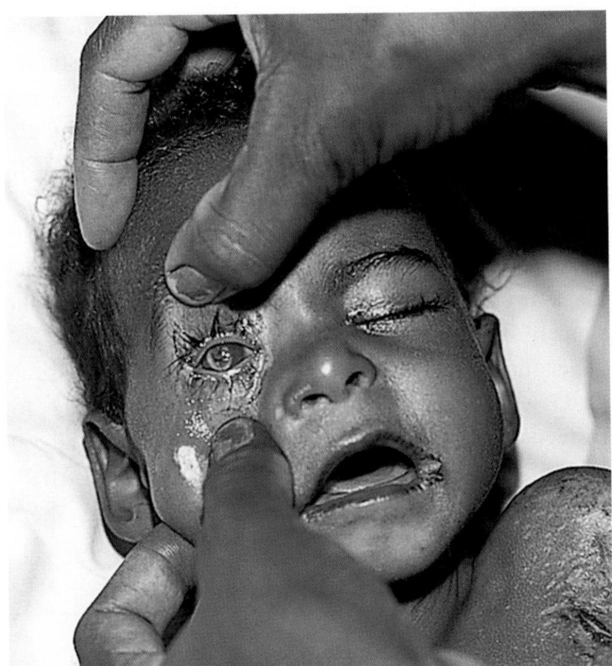

Figure 21.5 An 18-month-old Sudanese infant with keratomalacia of the right eye associated with vitamin A deficiency, severe malnutrition and recent measles

per cent of vitamin A is stored in the liver (as retinyl palmitate). At birth, fetal stores are relatively low but are quickly enhanced by colostrum and mother's milk if her diet has adequate vitamin A content.

Deficiency of vitamin A may result from dietary insufficiency, impaired absorption, increased demand (e.g. measles), reduced distribution (e.g. low retinol binding transport proteins) and impaired uptake and metabolism due to other micronutrient deficiencies (e.g. zinc).

XEROPHTHALMIA

Xerophthalmia is the most important cause of blindness in children in low-resource countries. The spectrum of xerophthalmia varies according to the level of deficiency of vitamin A and the presence of precipitating factors such as measles, herpes simplex or other local or systemic infections. Vitamin A is essential for production of rhodopsin (visual purple), a photosensitive pigment of the rods of the retina, which is responsible for appreciation of vision in dim light. Clinical features include night blindness, conjunctival xerosis (Greek *xeros*, dry; *ophthalmos*, eye), Bitot spots, corneal xerosis and the most severe form – corneal ulceration and keratomalacia (due to colliquative necrosis) (Figure 21.5). Bitot spots are foamy lesions usually found on the temporal bulbar conjunctiva and may persist despite treatment. Children presenting with keratomalacia often have additional problems including malnutrition, measles, diarrhoea or respiratory disorders and mortality is high.

GENERAL MORBIDITY AND MORTALITY

Randomized controlled trials of regular four monthly supplements of vitamin A to children 6 months to 5 years of age in Nepal, India and sub-Saharan Africa have demonstrated reduced mortality by up to 30 per cent (Fawzi *et al.*, 1993). Diarrhoea-associated mortality (but not pneumonia mortality) is reduced. Morbidity in HIV-infected children is also decreased, especially that due to diarrhoea. Vitamin A given during severe measles reduces both morbidity and mortality (D'Souza and D'Souza, 2002). The mechanism of benefit from regular supplementation with vitamin A in deficient children may be due to upregulation of the immune system.

PREVENTION

All children with malnutrition or measles are given high dose(s) of vitamin A. Lactating mothers are given high dose of vitamin A within six weeks of delivery and children are given regular vitamin A supplements (combined with vitamin E) from 6 months to 5 years, four to six monthly. Fortification of food, e.g. sugar or salt, is practised in some countries.

Beriberi

Beriberi is caused by thiamine (B_1) deficiency. Thiamine acts as a co-enzyme (thiamine pyrophosphate) in carbohydrate metabolism providing energy for cell metabolism. Deficiency results in incomplete carbohydrate metabolism with accumulation of pyruvic and lactic acids. Brain, nervous tissue and heart muscle utilize large amounts of glucose and they are particularly vulnerable to thiamine deficiency. Clinical syndromes include dry beriberi (polyneuropathy), wet beriberi (high output cardiac failure with peripheral dilation), a mixture of the two and Wernicke encephalopathy due to involvement of the brain. Aphonia (weak cry) is associated with involvement of the recurrent laryngeal nerve.

Beriberi is associated with consumption of a diet which mainly comprises polished rice. It also occurs in alcoholics. Thiamine is contained in the husk (pericarp) and the embryo of whole cereals, both of which are removed during milling and polishing of rice. Parboiling prior to milling retains some of the thiamine content. An additional factor in the aetiology of beriberi is the presence of antithiamin substances in foods such as raw freshwater fish, shellfish, fish paste, betel nut and fermented tea leaves (Butterworth, 2001). Infantile beriberi is still a problem in East Asia, particularly northeastern Thailand where milled 'sticky rice' is popular. Also, brown rice takes longer to cook and has a cultural stigma in being associated with 'poor' people. Beriberi occurs in any part of the world and in any age group where polished rice and food containing thiaminases are the main diet.

INFANTILE BERIBERI

Infantile beriberi occurs in breastfed infants whose mothers are deficient in thiamine. The child presents with severe cardiac failure and often has a weak cry (aphonia). There is a dramatic response to parenteral thiamine (50 mg daily for three days). Mothers should be treated as well.

PREVENTION

This involves health education regarding a varied diet and improved milling methods of rice. In high risk areas refugees are particularly vulnerable.

Pellagra

> **CASE STUDY: Secondary pellagra**
>
> An 8-year-old white boy presented to Accident and Emergency with pigmentation of face, neck, hands and forearms. His mother did not think he had been exposed to excessive sunshine. However, he had recently been commenced on isoniazid because of contact with his grandfather who had tuberculosis.
>
> The rash typical of pellagra, which is seen, especially in Africa, in people whose diet comprises mainly maize flour. However, it is also seen in individuals on isoniazid, which may lead to deficiency of vitamin B_6 (pyridoxine), which is required for synthesis of nicotinamide from tryptophan.

Pellagra is caused by a combination of niacin (nicotinic acid) and tryptophan deficiency. The active form of niacin is nicotinamide which is a component of the respiratory co-enzymes NAD (nicotinamide adenosine dinucleotide) and NADP concerned with tissue oxidation. Deficiency results in widespread metabolic disturbance, particularly in processes that depend on glucose for energy. Prominent among the organs affected are the skin (photosensitivity), gastrointestinal tract (mucosal atrophy) and the central nervous system (demyelination of brain and spinal cord) accounting for the triad of 'dermatitis, diarrhoea and dementia'.

Niacin is widely distributed in plant and animal foods, particularly in meat, wholemeal cereals and pulses. However, in many cereals, especially maize, most of the niacin is in a bound unabsorbable form. It can be synthesized in the body from the essential amino acid tryptophan, but tryptophan is first required for formation of proteins and only excess is available for synthesis of niacin. Pyridoxine, and also thiamine and riboflavin, are necessary co-enzymes for conversion of tryptophan to nicotinamide.

Pellagra used to be a widespread disease in areas where maize and, to a lesser extent, sorghum are staples. The practice of soaking maize in lime water, which increases the bioavailability of niacin, abolished the disease in Mexico and Central America. Sporadic cases continue to be reported, especially among refugees.

Diagnosis is based on the sharply demarcated skin lesions on areas exposed to sunlight – hands, feet and neck (Casal necklace). Glossitis, gastrointestinal symptoms and signs of other nutritional deficiencies are common.

Secondary pellagra may be seen in children on isoniazid, which antagonizes pyridoxine (co-enzyme for conversion of tryptophan to nicotinamide), and also in alcoholics, 'slim disease' associated with AIDS in Africa, malabsorption syndromes and Hartnup disease.

Scurvy

> **CASE STUDY**
>
> A 5-year-old Indian girl presented with painful limbs, easy bruising and gingival bleeding. Her diet mainly comprised chapatti, sugar and tea. She refused vegetables and fruit. When venepuncture was undertaken, multiple petechiae appeared on her arm distal to the tourniquet (positive Hess test). Her haemoglobin was 5.5 / 100 mL and the film showed a hypochromic microcytic picture. However, the WBC and platelet count were normal and no blast cells were detected. Bone radiograph demonstrated dense lines at the ends of the metaphyses along the provisional zones of calcification (white line of Frankel) with generalized demineralization and a thin cortex. Low blood levels of vitamin C and excessive retention after an IV infusion of vitamin C confirmed the diagnosis of scurvy.

Scurvy is due to deficiency of ascorbic acid (vitamin C) due to severe dietary lack of citrus fruits and fresh vegetables. The name ascorbic acid is derived from the term 'without scorb or scurvy'. Ascorbic acid activates enzymes responsible for hydroxylation of protocollagen proline and lysine to collagen hydroxyproline and hydroxylysine. In scurvy, fibroblasts in the skin, bone and blood vessels produce defective collagen and there is failure of deposition of intercellular ground substance in bone. Symptoms relate to capillary fragility in skin, mucosal membranes and the periosteum of bone. Ascorbic acid is a co-factor for a large number of enzymes. It is required in tyrosine metabolism, conversion of folic to folinic acid, absorption of iron from intestines and release of steroids from the adrenal gland. Ascorbic acid cannot be produced in the body and evidence of scurvy may occur within a few months of experimental dietary deficiency – in the past it has devastated armies, sailors and populations affected by war.

Scurvy has been recognized since ancient times. In 1747, James Lind, a surgeon in the Royal Navy, undertook a successful clinical trial of citrus fruits in the treatment of a severe outbreak of scurvy in sailors on a cruise in the English Channel (Dunn, 1997). However, it was not until 1795 that routine issue of lemon juice was introduced and scurvy was virtually abolished in the navy. Scurvy is still reported from refugee camps in famine areas where, nowadays, perifollicular haemorrhage in older children and adults is a commoner manifestation than frank scurvy. However, though rare, scurvy is still seen in industrialized countries and occurs when a child is on a diet severely deficient in fruits, vegetables and commercial foods fortified with ascorbic acid (Riepe *et al.*, 2001). In the past, infantile scurvy was common in poor families whose children were fed with limited diets such as evaporated milk formula or cows' milk in which ascorbic acid was destroyed by boiling. Breast fed infants may develop scurvy if their mother's diet is deficient in ascorbic acid.

Clinical features of scurvy include irritability, anaemia, gingival haemorrhages (absent in the edentulous infant or elderly), and tenderness and swelling over the legs associated with peritoneal haemorrhage. The 'beads' of scorbutic rosary are sharper than the swellings of rickety rosary. The infant lies in a 'frog position' and resents handling. Differential diagnosis includes leukaemia, juvenile arthritis and osteomyelitis. Radiological features include demineralization, giving a ground-glass appearance of bone, which is enclosed by a well demarcated, pencil-point, thin cortex in the metaphysis and epiphyses; widening and increased density of the provisional zone of calcification, the white line of Frankel, is typical. A spur, the result of fracture and healing of the ends of the provisional zone of calcification is also characteristic.

Low fasting levels of ascorbic acid in serum or better, the white cell platelet layer (buffy coat), are supportive of scurvy. Diagnosis is confirmed by estimation of urine ascorbic acid following a parenteral test dose when over 80 per cent should normally be excreted.

Zinc deficiency

Trace metals, such as zinc, copper, iron and selenium, tend to be low among poor children on diets with low bioavailability of micronutrients, also due to recurrent infections which cause both increased loss and increased demand. Micronutrients are low in malnourished children, but estimation is complicated by factors such as low transport proteins.

Zinc is a very important micronutrient, essential for protein and nucleic acid synthesis, cell development and division. The immune system, skin and gastrointestinal tract are tissues with the highest rates of protein synthesis and are the most likely to be affected by zinc deficiency. Zinc deficiency, as seen in acrodermatitis enteropathica, is associated with reduced intestinal water and sodium absorption. Loss of zinc from the body is mainly via the intestine due to epithelial cell desquamation, and, in hot climates, appreciable losses may occur through sweat. Diarrhoea leads to severe zinc depletion and levels are low in malnutrition.

Breast milk has high bioavailability. Zinc is found in a wide variety of foods including animal protein, whole grains and legumes. However, absorption is variable and is affected by phytates, fibre and a number of inorganic elements including iron and calcium. Thus, in developing countries, where animal protein is limited by costs (and culture), the majority of children have to depend on zinc from plant foods which have reduced bioavailability.

Recent research has indicated a potent role for zinc in the management of acute diarrhoea in developing countries (Fontaine, 2001). Supplements with zinc 10–20 mg/day for 14 days are effective in reducing the severity of acute diarrhoea and also the duration, thus the risk of persistent diarrhoea. There are proposals to provide zinc in oral rehydration solutions for routine use in children with diarrhoea. However, vomiting is a problem and the exact formulation requires further research. Zinc is also important in the management of persistent diarrhoea (Roy *et al.*, 1998) and in the resuscitation and rehabilitation phases of severe malnutrition (see below).

Severe malnutrition in developing countries

Growth

In developing countries, approximately 38 per cent of under 5s are stunted, 31 per cent are underweight and 9 per cent are wasted (Onis and Blossner, 1997). Rates may vary geographically and are particularly affected by famine, war, forced migration and depression in the economy.

Definitions

The WHO definitions of severe malnutrition are outlined below. In sub-Saharan Africa, where most cases of kwashiorkor (oedematous malnutrition) are seen, the Wellcome classification is commonly used (Table 21.4).

WHO classification of severe malnutrition (WHO, 1999)

Weight for height
- Standard deviation (or Z) score: ≤3
- Percentage of median National Child Health Statistics (NCHS)/WHO reference: <70 per cent

Oedema: Irrespective of weight or height

Aetiology

The aetiology of malnutrition is multifactorial and includes socioeconomic factors, absence or failure of breastfeeding, inadequate weaning diet and infection (Table 21.5). Malnutrition commonly increases during the 'hungry' or rainy season. This is when families are planting the new crops, at a time when the previous year's harvest is exhausted and prices in the market have risen. It frequently dates from the time when the infant or child is taken off the breast or suffers a severe infection, e.g. measles. If breastfeeding is stopped in the first 6 months or so of life, particularly if the infant is bottle fed, malnutrition, usually marasmus, is common and mortality is high (Figure 21.4). If a child is having adequate breast milk but is failing to thrive consider an infection e.g. tuberculosis or HIV infection.

Kwashiorkor is commoner where staples have a low protein : energy ratio, e.g. root crops – cassava, yams and bananas (e.g. Matoke in Uganda), or a maize diet (poor bioavailability of protein). Foods that are low in protein are also often low in important micronutrients such as zinc and copper.

Why one child develops oedematous malnutrition (kwashiorkor) and another only wasting (marasmus) when both are apparently exposed to similar nutritional inadequacy and infection is not known (Coulter, 1999). Both will have had dietary deficiency of energy or have a degree of wasting. Dietary deficiency of essential amino acids and genetic variability, whereby the child has increased demand for protein or inability to adapt to its deficiency may be a factor in kwashiorkor, but this has not been proved.

Increased free radical activity has been demonstrated, particularly in kwashiorkor (Golden, 1998). This may be partly due to deficiency of micronutrients, e.g. zinc, copper and selenium, which are essential for formation of antioxidant metalloenzymes such as superoxide dismutase. Other antioxidants include vitamins such as β-carotene, E, C and riboflavin. Thus, when a child with nutritional deficiency and inadequate levels of antioxidants is exposed to stress such as infection or toxins, severe disturbance of metabolism may occur. In tropical countries, aflatoxins are commonly detected in foods, e.g. groundnuts, where the warmth and humidity promote the growth of the fungus *Aspergillus flavus*. Children with

Table 21.4 Wellcome classification

Weight per cent of standard*	Oedema	
	Present	Absent
60–80	Kwashiorkor	Underweight
<60	Marasmic-kwashiorkor	Marasmus

* Median of National Child Health Statistics (NCHS) (Wellcome Trust Working Party, 1970).

Table 21.5 Factors associated with malnutrition

Socioeconomic factors	Nutritional factors	Infection
Lack of education	Food insecurity:	Immunosuppression
Poverty	General	HIV infection
Poor hygiene and sanitation	Seasonal	Persistent diarrhoea
Low birth weight	Cultural practices and taboos	Acute lower respiratory tract infections
Intrafamilial:	Maldistribution of food within the family	Measles
Divorce, separation	Inadequate weaning diets	
Working mothers	Vitamin A, zinc and other micronutrient deficiencies	
Unemployment		
Sending a child away to be looked after by a relative		
Inadequate medical and nutritional support		

HIV, human immunodeficiency virus.

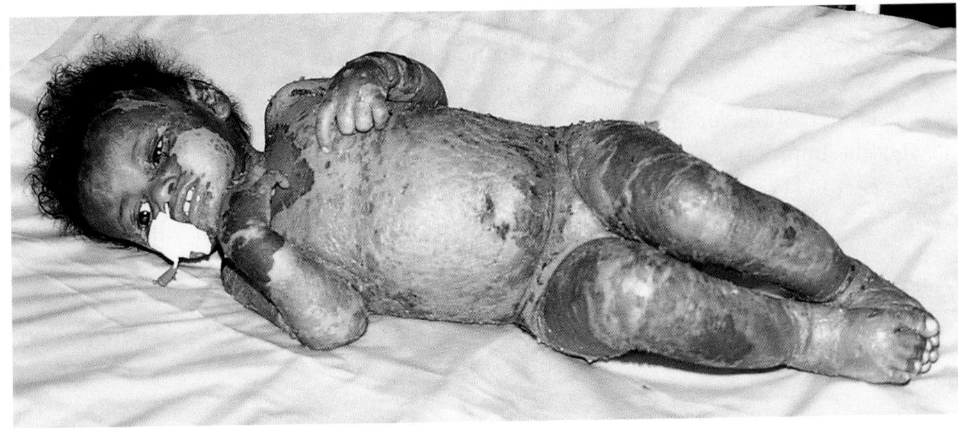

Figure 21.6 An 18-month-old Sudanese infant who developed kwashiorkor following measles six weeks previously. There is generalized oedema and flaky paint skin changes. The liver was enlarged to 6 cm below the costal margin

kwashiorkor are less able to metabolize aflatoxins than marasmic or normal children and in some cases aflatoxins might be an additional factor in the aetiology of kwashiorkor by promoting free radical generation and/or causing liver dysfunction (Coulter, 1999).

Clinical features

The main clinical findings in marasmic children are wasting of subcutaneous tissue. Hair changes are seen in longstanding cases. Features of kwashiorkor include hair changes – dyspigmentation (loss of pigment) and easy (painless) pluckability of hair – and flaky paint peeling and desquamation of hyperpigmented skin exposing hypopigmented areas underneath (Figure 21.6). Other physical signs include angular stomatitis, cheilosis (dry, cracked lips) and xerophthalmia due to vitamin A deficiency. The liver may or may not be enlarged but on histological examination is fatty. This is due to failure of transport proteins to remove fat from the liver. In kwashiorkor, the main chemical pathology finding is low serum albumin levels.

Management

The management of severe malnutrition is outlined in WHO guidelines (WHO, 1999). Essential details are as follows:

- Phase I: Dehydration is treated with an oral, low sodium solution supplemented with a mineral mix containing potassium, magnesium, zinc and copper. This is followed by a low protein/low energy milk (F75) supplemented with the mineral mix (see above). Mortality is high during the resuscitation phase and care regarding hyponatraemia, hypoglycaemia and overhydration is important.
- Phase II: Phase I is followed by the rehabilitation (phase II) when a high protein/energy formula (F100) is given to promote catch-up growth. High-dose vitamin A is given with multivitamins and folic acid. Iron supplements are delayed, i.e. for two weeks until the child shows a response to treatment. Antibiotics, e.g. ampicillin and gentamicin, are given routinely to all children with severe malnutrition. Children are discharged when they reach 80–90 per cent expected weight for height by which time the mother should have received nutritional education. Follow-up is undertaken as an outpatient at a nutritional rehabilitation unit.

Mortality ranges from 5 to 50 per cent with a median of 20–30 per cent. This depends on a number of factors including the level of illness and malnutrition on admission and the standard of care the child receives.

Prevention

Prevention of malnutrition is complex. Essential factors include health education, family planning, promotion of breastfeeding, education regarding weaning diets, treatment of infections, detection of weight faltering and, most important, education of women.

REFERENCES

Butterworth RF (2001) Maternal thiamine deficiency: still a problem in some world communities. *Am J Clin Nutr* **74**: 712–13.

Coulter JBS (1999) Malnutrition related disease. *Curr Paediatr* **9**:27–33.

Coulter JBS (2002) Global importance of parasitic disease. *Curr Paediatr* **12**:523–33.

D'Souza RM, D'Souza R (2002) Vitamin A for preventing secondary infection in children with measles – a systematic review. *J Trop Pediatr* **48**:72–7.

Dabis F, Ekpini ER (2002) HIV-1/AIDS and maternal and child health in Africa. *Lancet* **359**:2097–104.

Dabis F, Orne-Aliemann J, Perez F, *et al.* (2002) Working Group on Women and Child Health. Improving child health: the role of research. *BMJ* **324**:1444–7.

De Cock KM, Fowler MG, Mercier E, *et al.* (2000) Prevention of mother-to-child HIV transmission in resource-poor countries: translating research into policy and practice. *JAMA* **283**:1175–82.

Dunn PM (1997) James Lind (1716–94) of Edinburgh and the treatment of scurvy. *Arch Dis Child* **76**:F64–F65.

Fawzi WW, Chalmers TC, Herrera MG, Mosteller F (1993) Vitamin A supplementation and child mortality: a meta-analysis. *JAMA* **269**:898–903.

Fontaine O (2001) Effect of zinc supplementation on clinical course of acute diarrhoea. *J Health Popul Nutr* **19**:339–46.

Golden MHN (1998) Oedematous malnutrition. *Br Med Bull* **54**:433–44.

Marum LH, Tindyebwa D, Gibb D (1997) Care of children with HIV infection and AIDS in Africa. *AIDS* **11**(suppl B):S125–S134.

Onis M de, Blossner M (1997) WHO Global database on child growth and malnutrition. WHO/NUT/97.4. Geneva: Programme of Nutrition, World Health Organization.

Riepe FG, Eichmann D, Oppermann HC, Schmitt HJ, Tunnessen WW (2001) Picture of the month: infantile scurvy. *Arch Pediatr Adolesc Med* **155**:607–8.

Roy SK, Tomkins AM, Mahalanabis D, *et al.* (1998) Impact of zinc supplementation on persistent diarrhoea in malnourished Bangladeshi children. *Acta Pediatr* **87**:1235–9.

Tandon T, Pollard AJ, Money DM, Scheifele DW (2002) Pelvic inflammatory disease associated with *Enterobius vermicularis*. *Arch Dis Child* **86**:439–40.

UNICEF (2000) *The State of the World's Children 2000*. New York: UNICEF.

Wellcome Trust Working Party (1970) Classification of infantile malnutrition. *Lancet* **ii**:302–3.

World Health Organization (1993) *Infant and Child Nutrition*. Geneva: WHO.

World Health Organization (1999) *Management of Severe Malnutrition: a Manual for Physicians and Other Senior Health Workers*. Geneva: WHO.

FURTHER READING

Cook GC, Zumla A (eds) (2002) *Manson's Tropical Diseases*. London: Harcourt Publishers Ltd.

Peters W, Pasval G (eds) (2002) *Tropical Medicine and Parasitology*, 5th edn. London: Mosby.

Waterlow JC (ed) (1992) *Protein-Energy Malnutrition*. London: Edward Arnold.

Appendix A

Biochemistry

Peter Galloway

A GUIDE TO CLINICAL CHEMISTRY VALUES

The values given are a guide to the normal range but local laboratories may vary from these because of differing methodologies and nomenclature. If in any doubt, check with the laboratory, asking specifically if they know whether the reference range covers the age of interest. When interpreting an analyte, the pathophysiological processes need to be considered; in particular inflammation and acute phase response, such that analytes increase (e.g. copper, α-1-antitrypsin) or decrease (e.g. iron, zinc).

Those where large differences occur when compared to adult reference ranges are in italic.

Blood

Acid–base [H^+]	38–45 nmol/L	*pH* 7.35–7.42
Neonates especially premature		*pH 7.2–7.5*
pCO_2	4.5–6.0 kPa	(32–45 mmHg)
pO_2	11–14 kPa	(78–105 mmHg)
Bicarbonate [HCO_3^-]	22–27 mmol/L	
Preterm/<1 month	*17–25 mmol/L*	
Base excess	−4 — +3 mmol/L	

Plasma: electrolytes and minerals

Sodium		135–145 mmol/L
Potassium	Newborns	4.3–7.0 mmol/L
	Older children	3.5–5.0 mmol/L
Chloride		95–105 mmol/L
Calcium	Preterm	1.5–2.5 mmol/L
	First year	2.25–2.75 mmol/L
	Children	2.25–2.70 mmol/L
Phosphate (lower in breast fed)	Preterm	1.4–3.0 mmol/L
	First year	1.2–2.5 mmol/L
	Children	0.9–1.8 mmol/L
Magnesium	Children	0.7–1.0 mmol/L
Copper	Birth to 4 weeks	5.0–12.0 μmol/L
	17–24 weeks	5.0–17.0 μmol/L
	25–52 weeks	8.0–21.0 μmol/L
	>1 year	12.0–24.0 μmol/L
Zinc		9.0–18.0 μmol/L
Iron	<3 years	5.0–30.0 μmol/L
	>3 years	15.0–45.0 μmol/L
Ceruloplasmin	Newborn	0.05–0.26 g/L
	Children	0.25–0.45 g/L
Ferritin	Infant	20–200 ng/mL
	Children	*10–100 ng/mL*

Plasma: other analytes

Acetoacetate (incl. acetone)		<0.3 mmol/L
AFP <6 months *(Very high levels especially if premature – rapid fall over a week expected)*		
	>6 months	<10 U/mL
Alkaline phosphatase	Newborn	<800 U/L
	Children	100–500 U/L
Alanine aminotransferase (ALT)	Infants	10–60 U/L
	Children	10–40 U/L
Ammonia	Preterm	<200 μmol/L
	Newborn	50–80 μmol/L
	Infants and children	10–35 μmol/L
Amylase		<200 U/L

Ascorbic acid		15–90 μmol/L
Aspartate aminotransferase (AST)	<4 weeks >4 weeks	40–120 U/L 10–50 U/L
Bilirubin total (preterm greater)	Cord blood Term day 1 Term days 2–5 >1 month	<50 μmol/L <100 μmol/L <200 μmol/L <20 μmol/L
Cholesterol	Cord blood Newborn Infants and children	1.0–3.0 mmol/L 2.0–4.8 mmol/L 2.8–5.7 mmol/L
Cortisol	Neonates use Synacthen test Diurnal variation after 10 weeks post-term	
Creatine kinase (CK)	Newborn Infants Children	<600 U/L <300 U/L <200 U/L
Creatinine	Newborn	90–120 μmol/L
	(Reflects maternal level and declines over first month)	
	Infants and children	20–80 μmol/L
Creatinine clearance	0–3 months 12–24 months Older children	30–70 mL/min/1.73 m^2 50–100 mL/min/1.73 m^2 90–120 mL/min/1.73 m^2
C-reactive protein (CRP)		<7 mg/L
Folic acid		***10–30 nmol/L***
Follicle-stimulating hormone (FSH)		<3 U/L
Gammaglutamyl-transferase (γGT)	Newborn 1–6 months >6 months	<200 U/L <120 U/L <40 U/L
Glucose	Newborn (<48 h) Infants and children	2.2–5.0 mmol/L 3.0–5.0 mmol/L
Glycosated haemoglobin		4.1–6.1% (DCCT aligned)
17 OH Progesterone	>4 days	<13 nmol/L >60 confirms CAH
Insulin	Fasting *(Always measure glucose)*	<13 mU/L

Lactate (blood)	Newborn Infants and children	<3.0 mmol/L 1.0–1.8 mmol/L
Lactate dehydrogenase (LDH)	<1 month 1–12 months 1–6 years 6–9 years >9 years	550–2100 U/L 400–1200 U/L 470–920 U/L 420–750 U/L 300–500 U/L
Lipids – Triglycerides	Fasting	0.3–1.5 mmol/L
Luteinizing hormone (LH)		<1.9 U/L
Osmolality		275–295 mmol/kg
Protein – Total	Newborn Infants Children	45–70 g/L 50–70 g/L 60–80 g/L
– Albumin	Newborn Infants and Children	25–35 g/L 35–50 g/L

– Immunoglobulins (g/L)

	IgG	IgA	IgM
Newborn	2.8–6.8	0–0.5	0–0.7
Infants	3.0–10.0	0.2–1.3	0.3–1.5
Children >3 years	5.0–15.0	0.4–2.5	0.4–1.8

Pyruvate (blood)		50–80 μmol/L
	(Ratio lactate/pyruvate > 20 abnormal)	
Free Thyroxine (T_4)	<1 month >1 month	6–30 pmol/L 9–26 pmol/L
Thyroid-stimulating hormone (TSH)	1–30 days 1 month–5 years >5 years	0.5–16 mU/L 0.5–8 mU/L 0.4–6 mU/L
Tri-iodothyronine (T_3)	Newborn Infants and children	0.5–6.0 nmol/L 0.9–2.8 nmol/L
Urea	*(Neonates often 1.0–5.0 mmol/L)*	2.5–6.0 mmol/L
Uric acid	<9 years	0.11–0.3 mmol/L

Vitamin A	Preterm	0.09–1.7 μmol/L
	<1 year	0.5–1.5 μmol/L
	1 year–6 years	0.7–1.7 μmol/L
	>6 years	0.9–2.5 μmol/L
25 Hydroxy vitamin D		>15 nmol/L 25–100 nmol/L
Vitamin E (α-tocopherol)	<2 months	2–8 μmol/L
	1–6 months	5–14 μmol/L
	2 years	13–24 μmol/L

Urine

The kidney develops rapidly over the first year of life. Its handling of many filtered compounds is substantially different, for example:

Urine calcium	Birth–6 months	<2.4 mmol/mmol Creatinine
	6–12 months	0.09–2.2 mmol/mmol Creatinine
	1–3 years	0.06–1.4 mmol/mmol Creatinine
	3–5 years	0.05–1.1 mmol/mmol Creatinine
	7 years to adult	0.04–0.07 mmol/mmol Creatinine
Urine phosphate	7–12 months	1.2–19 mmol/mmol Creatinine
	1–3 years	1.2–12 mmol/mmol Creatinine
	3–6 years	1.2–8 mmol/mmol Creatinine
	Adult	0.8–2.7 mmol/mmol Creatinine

CSF

Protein	<1 month	0.26–1.2 g/L
	1–3 months	0.1–0.8 g/L
	>3 months	0.1–0.5 g/L

Appendix B

Haematology

Brenda Gibson

Table B1 Red Blood cell values at various stages: mean and lower limit of normal (−2 SD)

Age	Haemoglobin (g/dL)		Haematocrit (%)		Red cell count ($\times 10^{12}$/L)		MCV (fL)		MCH (pg)		MCHC (g/dL)	
	Mean	−2 SD	Mean	−2 SD	Mean	−2 SD	Mean	−2 SD	Mean	−2 SD	Mean	−2 SD
Birth	16.5	13.5	51	42	4.7	3.9	108	98	34	31	33	30
1 month	14.0	10.0	43	31	4.2	3.0	104	85	34	28	33	29
1 year	12.0	10.5	36	33	4.5	3.7	78	70	27	23	33	30
8 years	13.5	11.5	40	35	4.6	4.0	86	77	29	25	34	31

Table B2 Normal leucocyte counts

Age	Total leucocytes ($\times 10^9$/L)		Neutrophils ($\times 10^9$/L)			Lymphocytes ($\times 10^9$/L)			Monocytes ($\times 10^9$/L)		Eosinophils ($\times 10^9$/L)	
	Mean	(range)	Mean	(range)	%	Mean	(range)	%	Mean	%	Mean	%
Birth	18.1	(9.0-30.0)	11.0	(6.0-26.0)	61	5.5	(2.0-11.0)	31	1.1	6	0.4	2
1 month	10.8	(5.0-19.5)	3.8	(1.0-9.0)	35	6.0	(2.5-16.5)	56	0.7	7	0.3	3
1 year	11.4	(6.0-17.5)	3.5	(1.5-8.5)	31	7.0	(4.0-10.5)	61	0.6	5	0.3	3
8 years	8.3	(4.5-13.5)	4.4	(1.5-8.0)	53	3.3	(1.5-6.8)	39	0.4	4	0.2	2

Reproduced with permission from Dallman PR (1977) in: Rudolph A (ed.) Pediatrics, 16th edn. New York: Appleton-Century-Coofts, p. 1111.

Table B3 Haematology reference ranges

Test	Range
Ferritin	12-70 μg/L
Serum folate	3-7 μg/L
Red cell folate*	97-668 μg/L
Vitamin B_{12}	170-960 μg/L
Prothrombin time*	9.5-12.5 s
Activated partial thromboplastin time*	20-29.5 s
Thrombin time*	13-16 s
Fibrinogen:functional	1.5-4 g/L
D-dimer*	<0.3 mg/L
Reptilase time*	16-21 s
Bleeding time (template)	2-9.25 min
Platelet count	150-400 $\times 10^9$/L
Haemoglobin F (adult value by 6-12 months)	<2%
Haemoglobin A_2 (adult value by 4 months)	1.5-3.2%
Erythrocyte sedimentation rate	1-5 mm/h

* Assay and reagent specific.

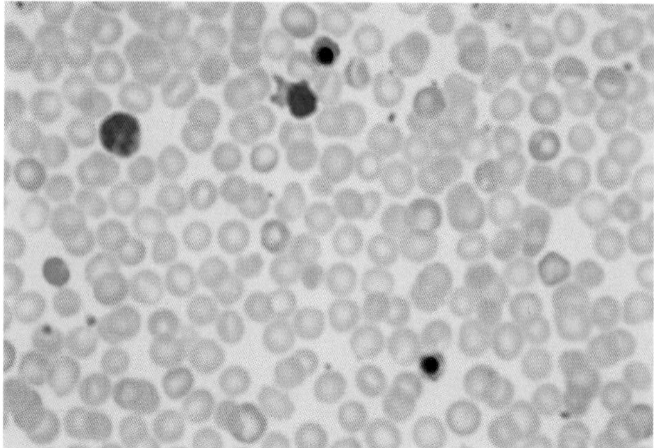

Figure B1 Blood film of a healthy preterm baby showing polychromasia and nucleated red cells.

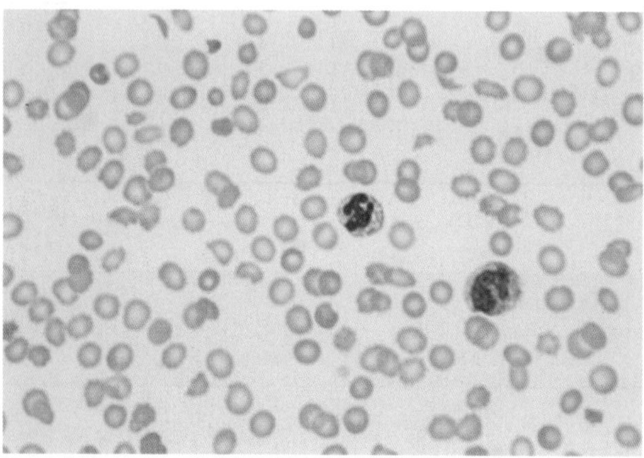

Figure B2 Blood film of septic preterm infant showing spherocytes red cell fragments and irregularly concentrated red cells.

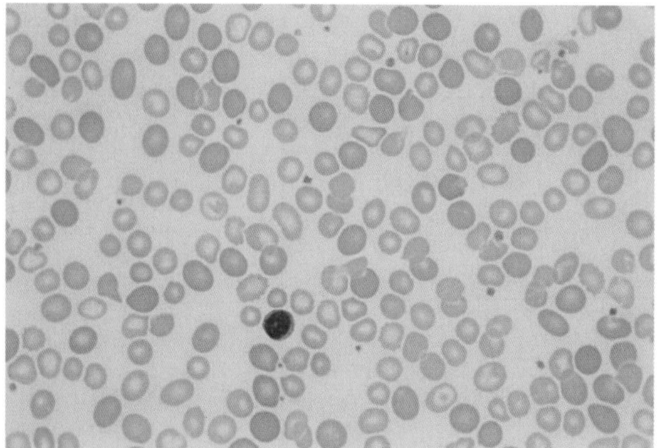

Figure B3 Blood film of patient with iron deficiency anaemia on iron replacement. Diamorphic blood film with dual populations of hypochromic, microcytic red cells and normochromic, normocytic red cells.

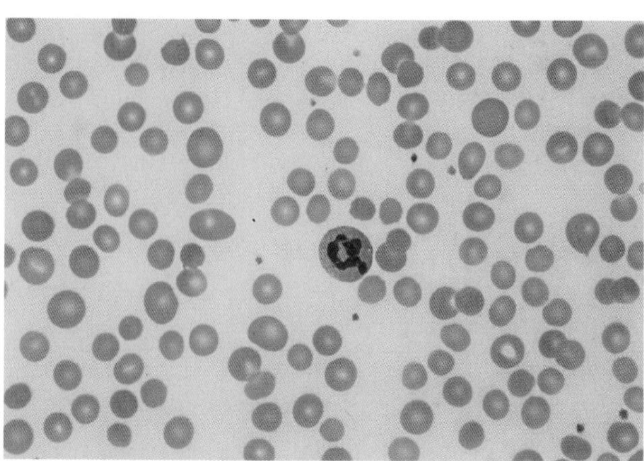

Figure B4 Blood film of patient with folate deficiency showing oval macrocytes with a hypersegmented neutrophil.

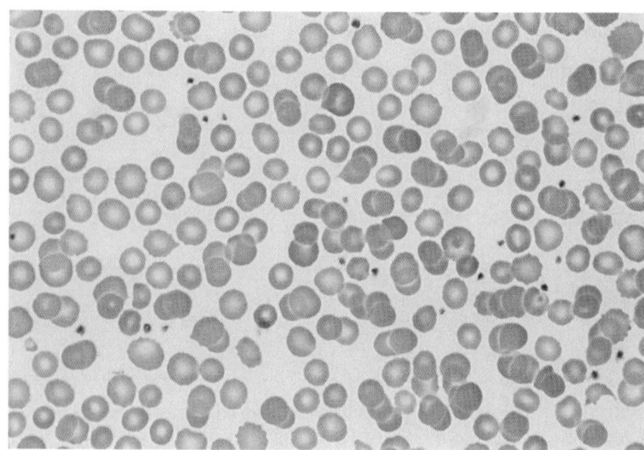

Figure B5 Blood film of patient with a high reticulocyte count showing marked polychromasia.

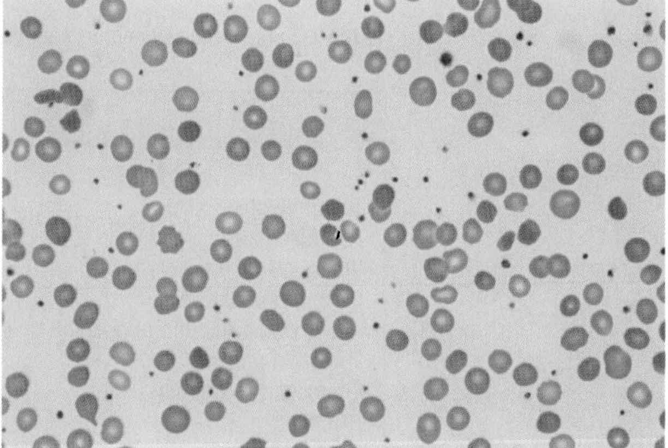

Figure B6 Blood film of patient with hereditary spherocytosis showing numerous spherocytes and polychromasia.

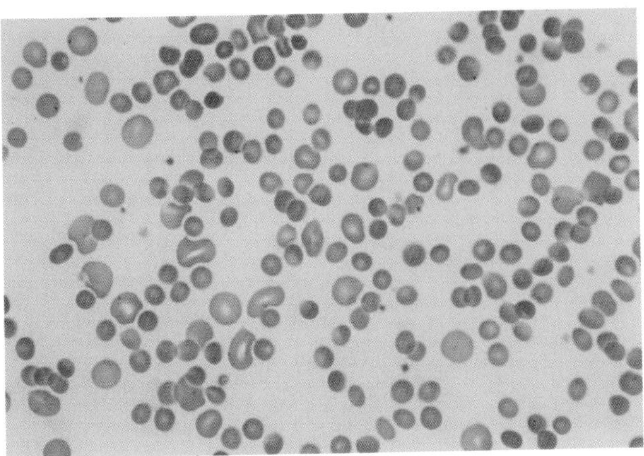

Figure B7 Blood film of patient with autoimmune haemolytic anaemia showing polychromasia and spherocytes.

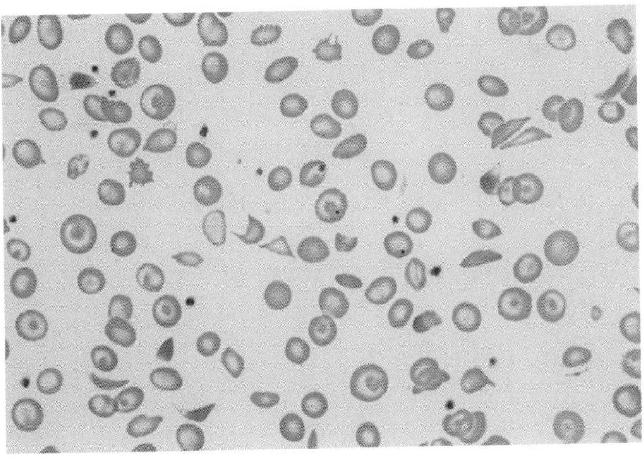

Figure B8 Blood film of patient with sickle cell anaemia showing sickle cells, target cells and Howell-Jolly bodies.

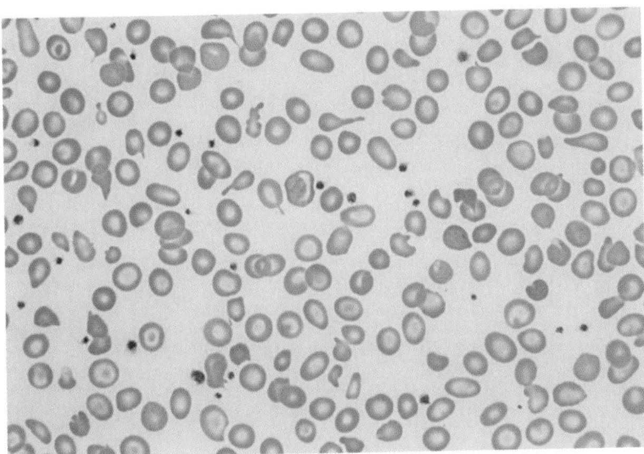

Figure B9 Blood film of patient with thalassaemia showing anisocytosis, hypochromasia, poikilocytosis and target cells.

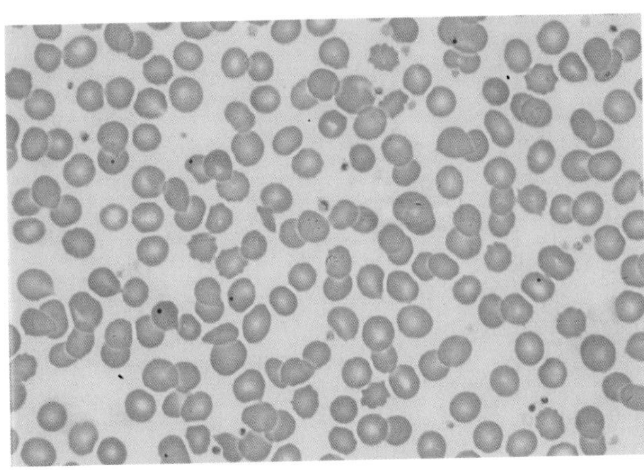

Figure B10 Post splenectomy blood film showing Howell-Jolly bodies.

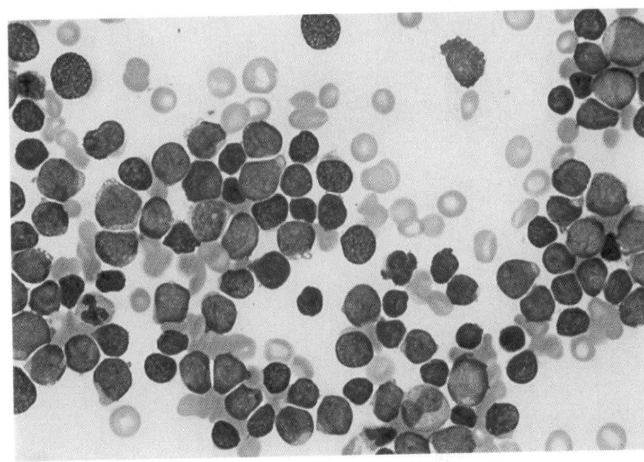

Figure B11 Bone marrow of patient with acute lymphoblastic leukaemia showing normal haematopoietic tissue replaced by lymphoblasts.

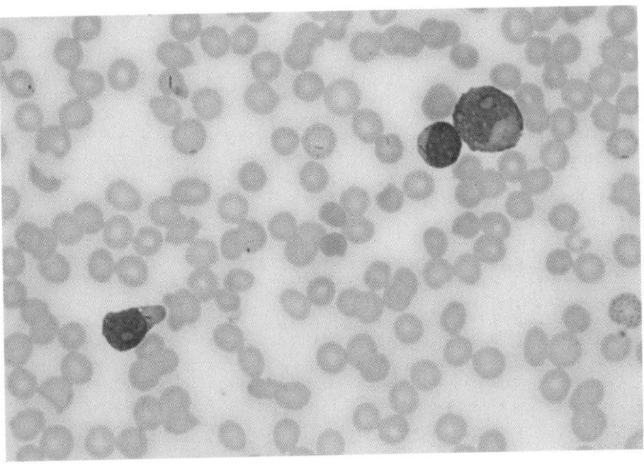

Figure B12 Blood film of a patient with acute myeloid leukaemia showing a myeloblastic with an Auer rod.

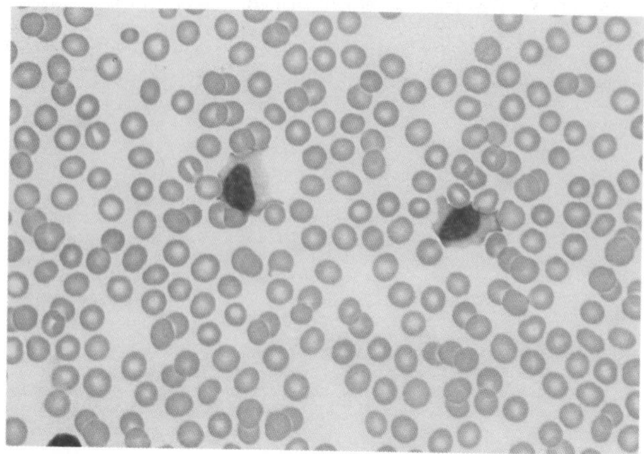

Figure B13 Blood film of patient with glandular fever showing atypical mononuclear cells.

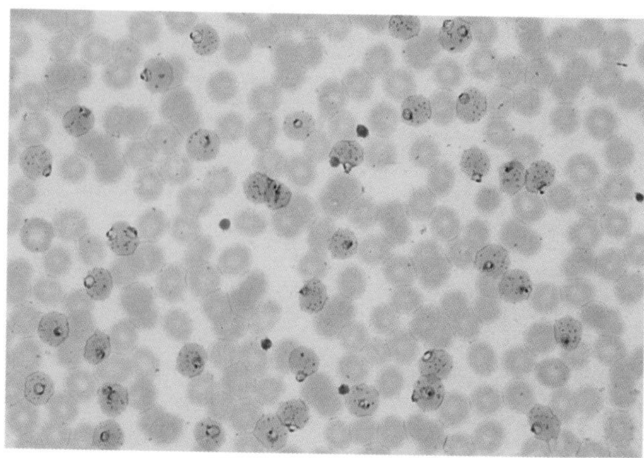

Figure B15 Blood film of patient with malaria plasmodium falciparum showing trophozoites.

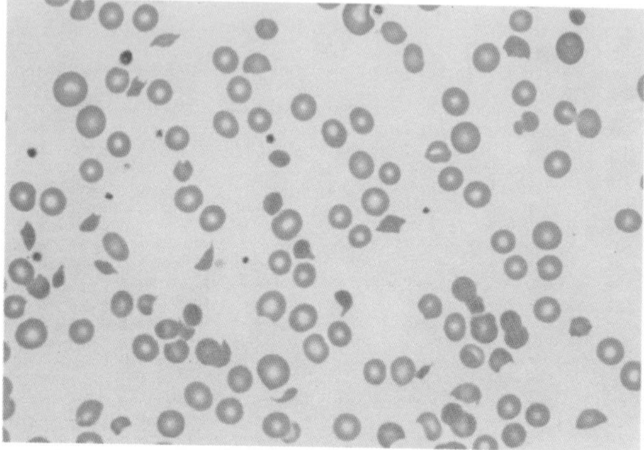

Figure B14 Blood film of patient with haemolytic uraemic syndrome showing polychromasia, microspherocytes and red cell fragments.

Appendix C

Age and gender specific blood pressure centile data

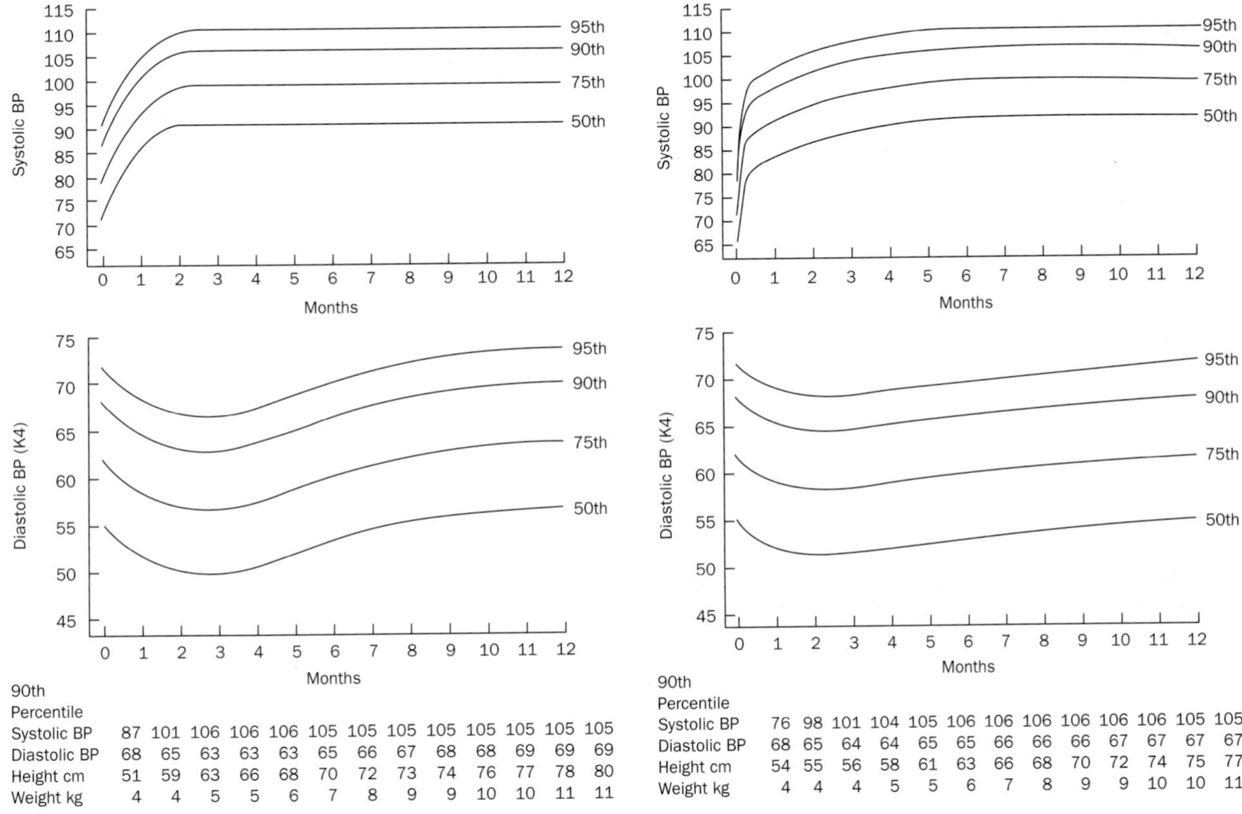

90th Percentile													
Systolic BP	87	101	106	106	106	105	105	105	105	105	105	105	105
Diastolic BP	68	65	63	63	63	65	66	67	68	68	69	69	69
Height cm	51	59	63	66	68	70	72	73	74	76	77	78	80
Weight kg	4	4	5	5	6	7	8	9	9	10	10	11	11

Figure C1 Age-specific percentiles of BP measurements in boys – birth to 12 months of age; Korotkoff phase IV (K4) used for diastolic BP. Reproduced with permission from Task Force on Blood Pressure Control in Children (1987) Report on the second task force on blood pressure control in children. *Pediatrics* 79, 1–25

90th Percentile													
Systolic BP	76	98	101	104	105	106	106	106	106	106	106	105	105
Diastolic BP	68	65	64	64	65	65	66	66	66	67	67	67	67
Height cm	54	55	56	58	61	63	66	68	70	72	74	75	77
Weight kg	4	4	4	5	5	6	7	8	9	9	10	10	11

Figure C2 Age-specific percentiles of BP measurements in girls – birth to 12 months of age; Korotkoff phase IV (K4) used for diastolic BP. Reproduced with permission from Task force on Blood Pressure Control in Children (1987) Report on the second task force on blood pressure control in children. *Pediatrics* 79, 1–25

Table C1 Blood pressure levels for boys by age and height percentile

Age, y	BP percentile	SBP, mmHg							DBP, mmHg						
		Percentile of height							Percentile of height						
		5th	10th	25th	50th	75th	90th	95th	5th	10th	25th	50th	75th	90th	95th
1	50th	80	81	83	85	87	88	89	34	35	36	37	38	39	39
	90th	94	95	97	99	100	102	103	49	50	51	52	53	53	54
	95th	98	99	101	103	104	106	106	54	54	55	56	57	58	58
	99th	105	106	108	110	112	113	114	61	62	63	64	65	66	66
2	50th	84	85	87	88	90	92	92	39	40	41	42	43	44	44
	90th	97	99	100	102	104	105	106	54	55	56	57	58	58	59
	95th	101	102	104	106	108	109	110	59	59	60	61	62	63	63
	99th	109	110	111	113	115	117	117	66	67	68	69	70	71	71
3	50th	86	87	89	91	93	94	95	44	44	45	46	47	48	48
	90th	100	101	103	105	107	108	109	59	59	60	61	62	63	63
	95th	104	105	107	109	110	112	113	63	63	64	65	66	67	67
	99th	111	112	114	116	118	119	120	71	71	72	73	74	75	75
4	50th	88	89	91	93	95	96	97	47	48	49	50	51	51	52
	90th	102	103	105	107	109	110	111	62	63	64	65	66	66	67
	95th	106	107	109	111	112	114	115	66	67	68	69	70	71	71
	99th	113	114	116	118	120	121	122	74	75	76	77	78	78	79
5	50th	90	91	93	95	96	98	98	50	51	52	53	54	55	55
	90th	104	105	106	108	110	111	112	65	66	67	68	69	69	70
	95th	108	109	110	112	114	115	116	69	70	71	72	73	74	74
	99th	115	116	118	120	121	123	123	77	78	79	80	81	81	82
6	50th	91	92	94	96	98	99	100	53	53	54	55	56	57	57
	90th	105	106	108	110	111	113	113	68	68	69	70	71	72	72
	95th	109	110	112	114	115	117	117	72	72	73	74	75	76	76
	99th	116	117	119	121	123	124	125	80	80	81	82	83	84	84
7	50th	92	94	95	97	99	100	101	55	55	56	57	58	59	59
	90th	106	107	109	111	113	114	115	70	70	71	72	73	74	74
	95th	110	111	113	115	117	118	119	74	74	75	76	77	78	78
	99th	117	118	120	122	124	125	126	82	82	83	84	85	86	86
8	50th	94	95	97	99	100	102	102	56	57	58	59	60	60	61
	90th	107	109	110	112	114	115	116	71	72	72	73	74	75	76
	95th	111	112	114	116	118	119	120	75	76	77	78	79	79	80
	99th	119	120	122	123	125	127	127	83	84	85	86	87	87	88
9	50th	95	96	98	100	102	103	104	57	58	59	60	61	61	62
	90th	109	110	112	114	115	117	118	72	73	74	75	76	76	77
	95th	113	114	116	118	119	121	121	76	77	78	79	80	81	81
	99th	120	121	123	125	127	128	129	84	85	86	87	88	88	89
10	50th	97	98	100	102	103	105	106	58	59	60	61	61	62	63
	90th	111	112	114	115	117	119	119	73	73	74	75	76	77	78
	95th	115	116	117	119	121	122	123	77	78	79	80	81	81	82
	99th	122	123	125	127	128	130	130	85	86	86	88	88	89	90
11	50th	99	100	102	104	105	107	107	59	59	60	61	62	63	63
	90th	113	114	115	117	119	120	121	74	74	75	76	77	78	78

(Continued)

Table C1 *(Continued)*

Age, y	BP percentile	SBP, mm Hg							DBP, mmHg						
		Percentile of height							Percentile of height						
		5th	10th	25th	50th	75th	90th	95th	5th	10th	25th	50th	75th	90th	95th
	95th	117	118	119	121	123	124	125	78	78	79	80	81	82	82
	99th	124	125	127	129	130	132	132	86	86	87	88	89	90	90
12	50th	101	102	104	106	108	109	110	59	60	61	62	63	63	64
	90th	115	116	118	120	121	123	123	74	75	75	76	77	78	79
	95th	119	120	122	123	125	127	127	78	79	80	81	82	82	83
	99th	126	127	129	131	133	134	135	86	87	88	89	90	90	91
13	50th	104	105	106	108	110	111	112	60	60	61	62	63	64	64
	90th	117	118	120	122	124	125	126	75	75	76	77	78	79	79
	95th	121	122	124	126	128	129	130	79	79	80	81	82	83	83
	99th	128	130	131	133	135	136	137	87	87	88	89	90	91	91
14	50th	106	107	109	111	113	114	115	60	61	62	63	64	65	65
	90th	120	121	123	125	126	128	128	75	76	77	78	79	79	80
	95th	124	125	127	128	130	132	132	80	80	81	82	83	84	84
	99th	131	132	134	136	138	139	140	87	88	89	90	91	92	92
15	50th	109	110	112	113	115	117	117	61	62	63	64	65	66	66
	90th	122	124	125	127	129	130	131	76	77	78	79	80	80	81
	95th	126	127	129	131	133	134	135	81	81	82	83	84	85	85
	99th	134	135	136	138	140	142	142	88	89	90	91	92	93	93
16	50th	111	112	114	116	118	119	120	63	63	64	65	66	67	67
	90th	125	126	128	130	131	133	134	78	78	79	80	81	82	82
	95th	129	130	132	134	135	137	137	82	83	83	84	85	86	87
	99th	136	137	139	141	143	144	145	90	90	91	92	93	94	94
17	50th	114	115	116	118	120	121	122	65	66	66	67	68	69	70
	90th	127	128	130	132	134	135	136	80	80	81	82	83	84	84
	95th	131	132	134	136	138	139	140	84	85	86	87	87	88	89
	99th	139	140	141	143	145	146	147	92	93	93	94	95	96	97

The 90th percentile is 1.28 SD, the 95th percentile is 1.645 SD, and the 99th percentile is 2.326 SD over the mean. Reproduced with permission from the National High Blood Pressure Education Program Working Group on High Blood Pressure in Children and Adolescents (2004). The fourth report on the diagnosis, evaluation and treatment of high blood pressure in children and adolescents *Pediatrics* 114, 555–576.

Table C2 BP levels for girls by age and height percentile

Age, y	BP percentile	SBP, mmHg							DBP, mmHg						
		Percentile of height							Percentile of height						
		5th	10th	25th	50th	75th	90th	95th	5th	10th	25th	50th	75th	90th	95th
1	50th	83	84	85	86	88	89	90	38	39	39	40	41	41	42
	90th	97	97	98	100	101	102	103	52	53	53	54	55	55	56
	95th	100	101	102	104	105	106	107	56	57	57	58	59	59	60
	99th	108	108	109	111	112	113	114	64	64	65	65	66	67	67
2	50th	85	85	87	88	89	91	91	43	44	44	45	46	46	47
	90th	98	99	100	101	103	104	105	57	58	58	59	60	61	61
	95th	102	103	104	105	107	108	109	61	62	62	63	64	65	65
	99th	109	110	111	112	114	115	116	69	69	70	70	71	72	72
3	50th	86	87	88	89	91	92	93	47	48	48	49	50	50	51
	90th	100	100	102	103	104	106	106	61	62	62	63	64	64	65
	95th	104	104	105	107	108	109	110	65	66	66	67	68	68	69
	99th	111	111	113	114	115	116	117	73	73	74	74	75	76	76
4	50th	88	88	90	91	92	94	94	50	50	51	52	52	53	54
	90th	101	102	103	104	106	107	108	64	64	65	66	67	67	68
	95th	105	106	107	108	110	111	112	68	68	69	70	71	71	72
	99th	112	113	114	115	117	118	119	76	76	76	77	78	79	79
5	50th	89	90	91	93	94	95	96	52	53	53	54	55	55	56
	90th	103	103	105	106	107	109	109	66	67	67	68	69	69	70
	95th	107	107	108	110	111	112	113	70	71	71	72	73	73	74
	99th	114	114	116	117	118	120	120	78	78	79	79	80	81	81
6	50th	91	92	93	94	96	97	98	54	54	55	56	56	57	58
	90th	104	105	106	108	109	110	111	68	68	69	70	70	71	72
	95th	108	109	110	111	113	114	115	72	72	73	74	74	75	76
	99th	115	116	117	119	120	121	122	80	80	80	81	82	83	83
7	50th	93	93	95	96	97	99	99	55	56	56	57	58	58	59
	90th	106	107	108	109	111	112	113	69	70	70	71	72	72	73
	95th	110	111	112	113	115	116	116	73	74	74	75	76	76	77
	99th	117	118	119	120	122	123	124	81	81	82	82	83	84	84
8	50th	95	95	96	98	99	100	101	57	57	57	58	59	60	60
	90th	108	109	110	111	113	114	114	71	71	71	72	73	74	74
	95th	112	112	114	115	116	118	118	75	75	75	76	77	78	78
	99th	119	120	121	122	123	125	125	82	82	83	83	84	85	86
9	50th	96	97	98	100	101	102	103	58	58	58	59	60	61	61
	90th	110	110	112	113	114	116	116	72	72	72	73	74	75	75
	95th	114	114	115	117	118	119	120	76	76	76	77	78	79	79
	99th	121	121	123	124	125	127	127	83	83	84	84	85	86	87
10	50th	98	99	100	102	103	104	105	59	59	59	60	61	62	62
	90th	112	112	114	115	116	118	118	73	73	73	74	75	76	76
	95th	116	116	117	119	120	121	122	77	77	77	78	79	80	80
	99th	123	123	125	126	127	129	129	84	84	85	86	86	87	88
11	50th	100	101	102	103	105	106	107	60	60	60	61	62	63	63
	90th	114	114	116	117	118	119	120	74	74	74	75	76	77	77

(Continued)

Table C2 *(Continued)*

Age, y	BP percentile	SBP, mmHg							DBP, mmHg						
		Percentile of height							Percentile of height						
		5th	10th	25th	50th	75th	90th	95th	5th	10th	25th	50th	75th	90th	95th
	95th	118	118	119	121	122	123	124	78	78	78	79	80	81	81
	99th	125	125	126	128	129	130	131	85	85	86	87	87	88	89
12	50th	102	103	104	105	107	108	109	61	61	61	62	63	64	64
	90th	116	116	117	119	120	121	122	75	75	75	76	77	78	78
	95th	119	120	121	123	124	125	126	79	79	79	80	81	82	82
	99th	127	127	128	130	131	132	133	86	86	87	88	88	89	90
13	50th	104	105	106	107	109	110	110	62	62	62	63	64	65	65
	90th	117	118	119	121	122	123	124	76	76	76	77	78	79	79
	95th	121	122	123	124	126	127	128	80	80	80	81	82	83	83
	99th	128	129	130	132	133	134	135	87	87	88	89	89	90	91
14	50th	106	106	107	109	110	111	112	63	63	63	64	65	66	66
	90th	119	120	121	122	124	125	125	77	77	77	78	79	80	80
	95th	123	123	125	126	127	129	129	81	81	81	82	83	84	84
	99th	130	131	132	133	135	136	136	88	88	89	90	90	91	92
15	50th	107	108	109	110	111	113	113	64	64	64	65	66	67	67
	90th	120	121	122	123	125	126	127	78	78	78	79	80	81	81
	95th	124	125	126	127	129	130	131	82	82	82	83	84	85	85
	99th	131	132	133	134	136	137	138	89	89	90	91	91	92	93
16	50th	108	108	110	111	112	114	114	64	64	65	66	66	67	68
	90th	121	122	123	124	126	127	128	78	78	79	80	81	81	82
	95th	125	126	127	128	130	131	132	82	82	83	84	85	85	86
	99th	132	133	134	135	137	138	139	90	90	90	91	92	93	93
17	50th	108	109	110	111	113	114	115	64	65	65	66	67	67	68
	90th	122	122	123	125	126	127	128	78	79	79	80	81	81	82
	95th	125	126	127	129	130	131	132	82	83	83	84	85	85	86
	99th	133	133	134	136	137	138	139	90	90	91	91	92	93	93

The 90th percentile is 1.28 SD, the 95th percentile is 1.645 SD, and the 99th percentile is 2.326 SD over the mean. Reproduced with permission from the National High Blood Pressure Education Program Working Group on High Blood Pressure in Children and Adolescents (2004). The fourth report on the diagnosis, evaluation and treatment of high blood pressure in children and adolescents *Pediatrics* 114, 555–576.

Appendix D

Surface area nomograms in infants and children

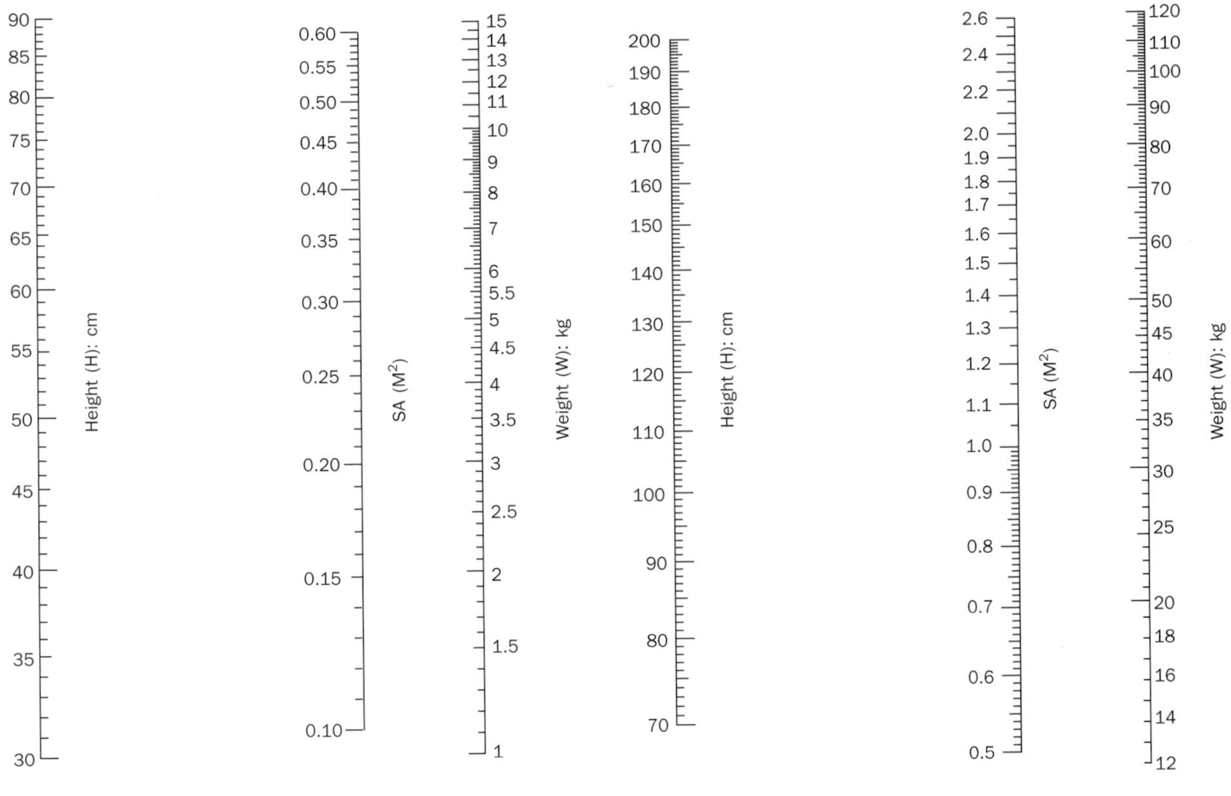

$$SA = W^{0.5378} \times H^{0.3964} \times 0.024265$$

Figure D1 Nomogram representing the relationship between height, weight and body surface area in infants. Reproduced with permission from Haycock G *et al.* (1978) Geometric method for measuring body surface area: a height-weight formula validated in infants, children and adults. *J Pediatrics* 93, 62–66

$$SA = W^{0.5378} \times H^{0.3964} \times 0.024265$$

Figure D2 Nomogram representing the relationship between height, weight and body surface area in children and adults. Reproduced with permission from Haycock G *et al.* (1978) Geometric method for measuring body surface area: a height-weight formula validated in infants, children and adults. *J Pediatrics* 93, 62–66

Index

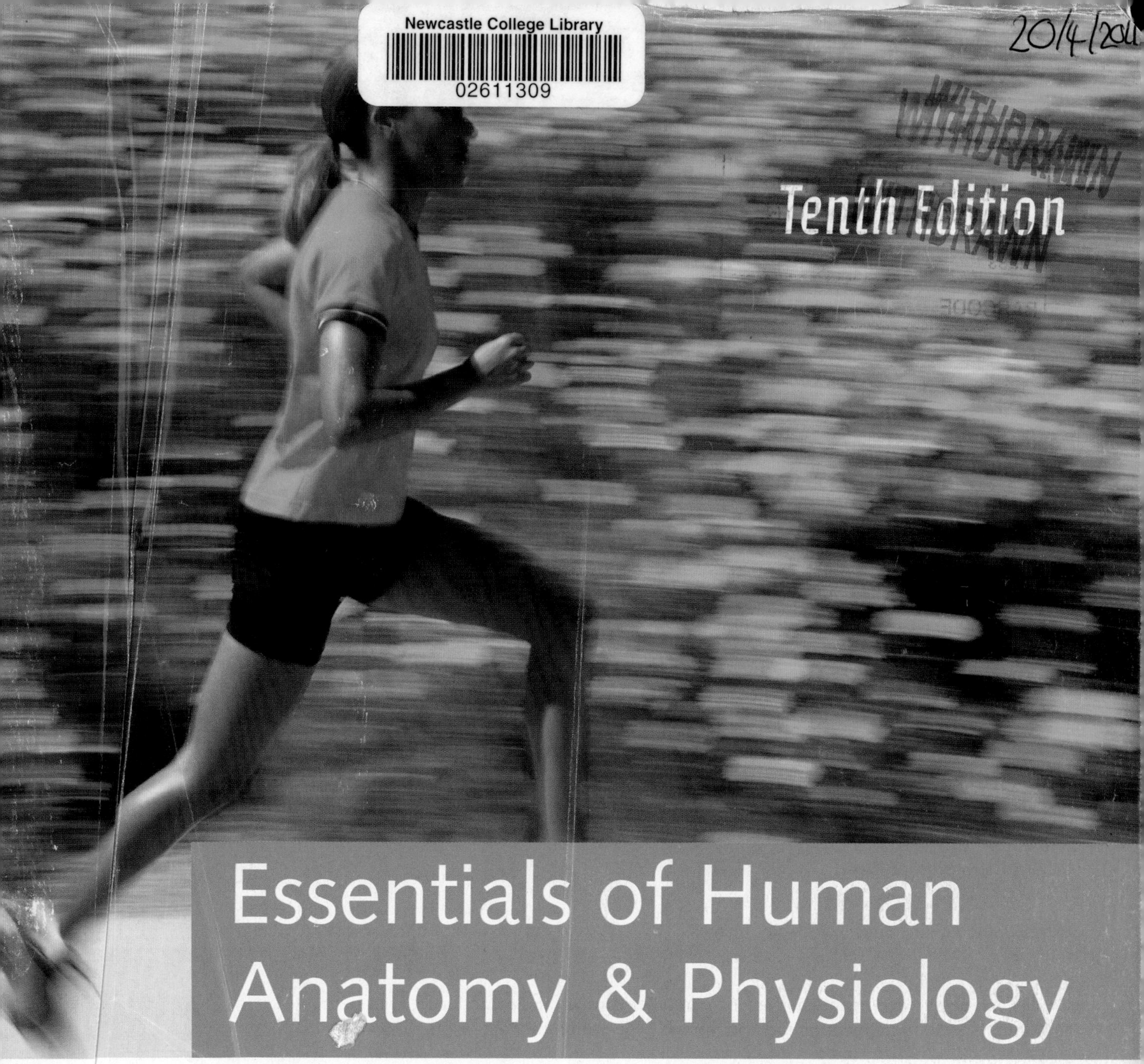

Tenth Edition

Essentials of Human Anatomy & Physiology

Elaine N. Marieb, R.N., Ph.D.,
Holyoke Community College

Benjamin Cummings
Boston Columbus Indianapolis New York San Francisco Upper Saddle River
Amsterdam Cape Town Dubai London Madrid Milan Munich Paris Montréal Toronto
Delhi Mexico City São Paulo Sydney Hong Kong Seoul Singapore Taipei Tokyo

Executive Editor: *Deirdre Espinoza*
Associate Project Editor: *Shannon Cutt*
Director of Development: *Barbara Yien*
Editorial Assistant: *Ashley Williams*
Art Development Manager: *Laura Southworth*
Development Editor: *Anne A. Reid*
Managing Editor: *Deborah Cogan*
Production Manager: *Michele Mangelli*
Production Supervisor: *David Novak*
Copyeditor: *Anita Wagner*
Proofreader: *Martha Ghent*
Compositor: *Nesbitt Graphics, Inc.*
Art Coordinator: *Linda Jupiter*
Interior Design: *tani hasegawa*
Cover Designer: *Jodi Notowitz*
Illustrators: *Imagineering STA Media Services Inc.*
Photo Researcher: *Kristin Piljay*
Senior Manufacturing Buyer: *Stacey Weinberger*
Marketing Manager: *Derek Perrigo*
Director, Media Development: *Lauren Fogel*
Media Producer: *Erik Fortier*

Cover Photo Credit: Chris Cole/Getty Images.

Credits and acknowledgments borrowed from other sources and reproduced, with permission, in this textbook appear on the appropriate page within the text or on p. 595.

Benjamin Cummings
is an imprint of

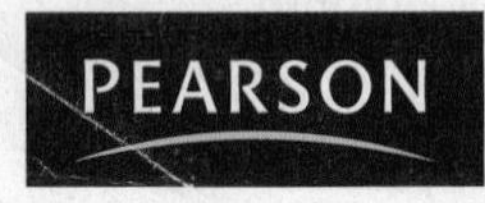

ISBN: 0-321-73552-8
ISBN: 978-0-321-73552-2

1 2 3 4 5 6 7 8 9 10—WBC—14 13 12 11 10